KU-034-800

Willard and Spackman's Occupational Therapy

CONTRIBUTING AUTHORS

M. Carolyn Baum, B.S., O.T.R.
Clinical Director, Occupational Therapy Services, Washington University School of Medicine, St. Louis, Missouri

Mary Margaret Daub, Ed.M., O.T.R.
Assistant Professor, College of Allied Health Professions, Temple University, Philadelphia, Pennsylvania

Elizabeth B. Devereaux, M.S.W., O.T.R.
Assistant Professor, Department of Psychiatry, Marshall University School of Medicine, Huntington, West Virginia

Elnora M. Gilfoyle, B.A., O.T.R., F.A.O.T.A.
Private Practice, Boulder, Colorado

Doris Gordon, M.S., O.T.R.
Chairperson, Department of Occupational Therapy, Elizabethtown College, Elizabethtown, Pennsylvania

Ann P. Grady, B.A., O.T.R., F.A.O.T.A.
Director, Occupational Therapy, The Children's Hospital, Denver, Colorado

Celestine Hamant, M.S., O.T.R.
Associate Professor and Director of Occupational Therapy Services and Affiliate Program, Indiana University Medical Center, Indianapolis, Indiana

Carole Ann Hays, M.A., O.T.R., F.A.O.T.A.
Director, Division of Practice, The American Occupational Therapy Association, Inc., Rockville, Maryland

L. Irene Hollis, B.S., O.T.R., F.A.O.T.A.
Director of Occupational Therapy, Hand Rehabilitation Center, The University of North Carolina, Chapel Hill, North Carolina

Helen L. Hopkins, M.A., O.T.R., F.A.O.T.A.
Associate Professor of Occupational Therapy, College of Allied Health Professions, Temple University, Philadelphia, Pennsylvania

Margaret Howison, B.S., O.T.R.
Director of Occupational Therapy, Elizabethtown Hospital for Children and Youth, and Instructor, Elizabethtown College, Elizabethtown, Pennsylvania

A. Joy Huss, M.S., O.T.R., R.P.T., F.A.O.T.A.
Associate Professor of Occupational Therapy, University of Minnesota, Minneapolis, Minnesota

Linda Ann Johnson, B.A., O.T.R.
Head Occupational Therapist, Robison Jewish Home, Portland, Oregon

Nancy Allen Kauffman, B.S., O.T.R.
Teacher, Perceptual-Motor Skills, Cornman Diagnostic Center, Philadelphia School System, Philadelphia, Pennsylvania

Dorothy L. Kester, O.T.R.
Chief, Vocational Services, Delaware Curative Workshop, Wilmington, Delaware

Ruth Ellen Levine, Ed.M., O.T.R.
Assistant Professor of Occupational Therapy, College of Allied Health Professions, Temple University, Philadelphia, Pennsylvania

Maude H. Malick, B.S., O.T.R.
Director of Occupational Therapy and Out of Center Services, Harmarville Rehabilitation Center, Pittsburgh, Pennsylvania

Joyce Perella, B.S., O.T.R.
Instructor in Occupational Therapy, Elizabethtown College, Elizabethtown, Pennsylvania

Marianne Rozycka, B.S., O.T.R.
Assistant Director, Department of Occupational Therapy, Moss Rehabilitation Center, Philadelphia, Pennsylvania

Reba M. Sebelist, M.S., O.T.R.
Instructor in Occupational Therapy, Elizabethtown College, Elizabethtown, Pennsylvania

Bonnie Sherry, B.S.
Rehabilitation Home Economist, Harmarville Rehabilitation Center, Pittsburgh, Pennsylvania

Mary A. Silberzahn, M.A., O.T.R.
Private Practice, Sensory Integrative Specialist, and Faculty Member of the Center For The Study of Sensory Integrative Dysfunction, Los Angeles, California

Helen D. Smith, M.O.T., O.T.R.
Associate Professor of Occupational Therapy, Tufts University—Boston School of Occupational Therapy, Boston, Massachusetts

Elinor Anne Spencer, B.A., O.T.R.
Chief Occupational Therapist, Eastern Maine Medical Center, Bangor, Maine

Elizabeth Gordon Tiffany, M.Ed., O.T.R., F.A.O.T.A.
Assistant Professor of Occupational Therapy, College of Allied Health Professions, Temple University, Philadelphia, Pennsylvania

Gail Tower, M.S., L.P.T.
Assistant Professor of Physical Therapy, College of Allied Health Professions, Temple University, Philadelphia, Pennsylvania

Ann Starnes Wade, M.S., O.T.R.
Clinical Instructor of Occupational Therapy, Occupational Therapy Division, School of Allied Medical Professions, The Ohio State University, Columbus, Ohio

Elizabeth June Yerxa, Ed.D., O.T.R., F.A.O.T.A.
Chairperson, Department of Occupational Therapy, University of Southern California, Downey, California

Willard and Spackman's Occupational Therapy/Fifth Edition

Edited by

Helen L. Hopkins, M.A., O.T.R., F.A.O.T.A.

Associate Professor of Occupational Therapy
College of Allied Health Professions
Temple University
Philadelphia, Pennsylvania

Helen D. Smith, M.O.T., O.T.R.

Associate Professor of Occupational Therapy
Tufts University—Boston School of Occupational Therapy
Boston, Massachusetts

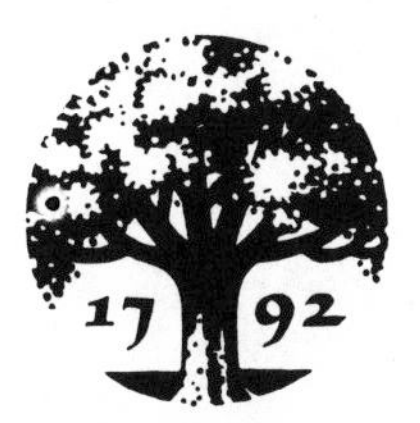

J. B. LIPPINCOTT COMPANY
PHILADELPHIA
NEW YORK SAN JOSE TORONTO

Distributed in Great Britain by
Blackwell Scientific Publications
London Oxford Edinburgh

Printed in the United States of America

2 4 6 8 9 7 5 3

Library of Congress Cataloging in Publication Data

Willard, Helen S., ed.
Willard and Spackman's Occupational therapy.

Includes bibliographies and index.
1. Occupational therapy. I. Spackman, Clare S. II. Hopkins, Helen L. III. Smith, Helen D. IV. Title. V. Title: Occupational therapy.
RM736.W48 1978 615'.8515 78-4607
ISBN 0-397-54216-X

To our families, friends, coworkers, and students
with appreciation for their support and understanding
and
to all past, present, and future occupational therapists.

Give a man a fish, and you feed him for a day. Teach a man to fish, and you feed him for a lifetime. Chinese Proverb

CONTENTS

FOREWORD

When thirty-two years ago we agreed to edit what was then called *Principles of Occupational Therapy* it never occurred to us that in 1976 we should at last be passing on the editorship of *Occupational Therapy*. It is with pleasure that we give this task to two of our coworkers and friends—Helen L. Hopkins and Helen D. Smith—who have accepted the responsibility of editing the fifth edition while we become editors emeriti.

Forty-two authors have contributed to the first four editions. To them go our warmest thanks and appreciation. The third and fourth editions have been translated into Japanese and the fourth into Spanish.

During this time our field has changed and grown immeasurably. The present edition reflects recent changes and will add much to the knowledge and understanding of occupational therapy today.

Clare S. Spackman
Helen S. Willard

PREFACE

As editors of this fifth edition of *Willard and Spackman's Occupational Therapy* we determined that this would be the appropriate time to change the format. Therefore the subject matter has been rearranged in an attempt to make it a unified whole rather than a compilation of contributions.

The book has been divided into ten parts: (1) history, (2) theory and philosophy, (3) approaches for intervention, (4) evaluation process and procedures, (5) treatment process and procedures, (6) general areas of practice, (7) special areas of practice, (8) organization and administration, (9) consultancy and research, and (10) projections for the profession.

Part 1 gives an historical perspective on the profession, discussing its genesis and development from ancient origins to the present time. Part 2 deals with the current basis for theory and philosophy in occupational therapy. Current occupational therapy practice appears to be based in three broad areas—human growth and development, scientific and medical knowledge, and the activity process—and each is described.

Part 3 discusses the occupational therapy process as one using problem solving procedures. Three approaches currently used in occupational therapy practice are identified as developmental, rehabilitation/habilitation, and occupational behavior. The developmental approach includes a number of subapproaches, including neuromuscular reflex, neurodevelopmental, neurophysiological, proprioceptive neuromuscular facilitation, neurobehavioral or sensory integrative, behavioral, and psychoanalytical. An overview of each of the approaches is given. Each approach allows for varying frames of reference to be used as the rationale for treatment planning and treatment implementation, depending upon the type of patients or clients and the philosophy, preferences, biases, and expertise of the therapist as well as the goals and interests of the patients or clients. Four elements are identified as the organizing principles that give occupational therapy its essence, that is, the patient or client, the therapist and therapeutic relationship, the activity, and the context or setting for treatment. The six phases of the occupational therapy process described include initial evaluation, development of treatment objectives, treatment planning, treatment implementation, on-going evaluation, and termination of treatment.

Part 4 describes the evaluation process and specific occupational therapy evaluation procedures that are used in practice. Part 5 describes the treatment process and specific treatment procedures utilized in practice. These procedures include therapeutic application of activity, activities of daily living, homemaking, orthotics, and prevocational training. A section on human sexuality has been added.

Part 6 identifies six general areas in which occupational therapists practice. These include psychiatry and mental health, functional restoration, minimal brain dysfunction, pediatrics, general medicine and surgery, and gerontology. Part 7 deals with eight special areas of current occupational therapy practice, including those covered in previous editions (problems with special senses, i.e., blind and deaf, cerebral palsy, and amputations). Several other areas are included in this edition: mental retardation, burns, hand rehabilitation, educational settings, and community home health care in both urban and rural settings.

Part 8 deals with the management of occupational therapy services. Report writing, personnel management, legal liability, and accountability issues of concern to the profession are included. Part 9 describes the new roles of consultant and researcher open to the occupational therapy professional. Part 10 discusses the profession today and makes projections for the future. Appendices and a Glossary complete and define the outlook of the book.

Our attempt to provide comprehensive coverage of the profession is evident in our choice of twenty-eight authors. Twenty six are practicing occupational therapists, one is a practicing physical therapist, and one is a rehabilitation home economist. Authors work in nine universities and numerous clinics and community settings in fourteen states. Contributions from some authors are presented as complete chapters, while some contributions are included as sections of larger chapters in order to provide continuity of subject matter.

We thank the authors for their excellent contributions and assistance in providing a comprehensive overview of the profession. We also thank our secretaries, Lorraine Witkowski, Deborah Smith, and Norma Springer, for their assistance. Special thanks are due our friends Theresa McCoy for typing and editorial assistance and Jennifer Tiffany for copy-editing and design suggestions. Special appreciation is expressed to Elizabeth Tiffany for suggestions, collaboration, and support in the planning, development, and execution of an enormous task; and to Eleanor D. Mora of J. B. Lippincott Co. for her excellent editorial assistance.

Part One History

1

An Historical Perspective on Occupational Therapy

Helen L. Hopkins

The term "occupation" has long been recognized as a requirement for survival and, to varying degrees, as a source of pleasure. The term "occupational therapy" may seem to indicate use of "work" as treatment but those pioneers who fashioned the profession believed that the health of individuals was influenced by "the use of muscles and mind together in games, exercise and handicraft" as well as in work.[1] This, then, is the basis for the use of work, exercise, and play as modalities of treatment in occupational therapy.

In order to obtain a perspective of the profession of occupational therapy it is necessary to trace the history of the use of "occupation" from its ancient origins until the present time. The origin and development of the profession will be traced through the description of the foci of those persons within the field upon whose efforts and ideas occupational therapy practice has been based.

ANCIENT ORIGINS OF OCCUPATION FOR TREATMENT

Evidence can be found that the healing qualities of work, exercise, and play were recognized and utilized thousands of years ago. The interrelationship of these three aspects of occupational therapy was also recognized early in the history of civilization.

Exercise (Physical Training)

There is evidence that as early as 2600 B.C. the Chinese taught that disease was caused by organic inactivity and thus used physical training for the promotion of health. They came to utilize a series of medical gymnastics called Cong Fu, which they felt could not only prolong life but would ensure immortality of the soul.[2]

The ancient Persians realized the beneficial effects of physical training and about 1000 B.C. utilized it to fit their youth for military duty. They used a systematic course of physical training which began at age 6 and continued through adult years. This resulted in the production of an army of physically fit, able-bodied fighters.

Among the ancient Greeks, physical training was developed to a high degree. Socrates (400 B.C.) and Plato (347 B.C.) understood the relationship between physical status and mental health and Aristotle

(340 B.C.) felt that the "education of the body must precede that of the intellect."[3] The Athenians used physical training for its cultural and social aspects while the Spartans used it to build military manpower.

Hippocrates, the father of medicine (359 B.C.), and Galen, his successor (200 A.D.), recommended that their patients exercise in the gymnasiums as a means of recovering from illness. The Roman Asclepiades (100 B.C.) advocated massage, therapeutic baths, and exercises for improving diseased conditions. Scientific medicine is indebted to the interest of the early Greeks and Romans in physical training.[4]

Recreation (Play)

Play, games, and pastimes were a part of the life of all primitive people as is evidenced by the toys, drawings, and sculptures found in excavations of ancient Egypt, Babylonia, and China as well as in the cultural remains of the Aztecs and Incas of the western hemisphere. The ancient Egyptians' inscriptions on stone depict the game of draughts, stately dances, the playing of the harp and lute, and children playing with balls, dolls, and jumping jacks.

The Egyptians in 2000 B.C. and the Greeks in 420 B.C. described diversion and recreation as a means of treating the sick.[5] One hundred years before Christ, Asclepiades, the Roman, recommended activity treatment for patients with mental diseases. This included diversions and entertainment, but only the diversional value was recognized.

In the fifth century A.D. Caelius Aurelius of Sicca (Africa) recommended a careful regime for convalescents that included walks, reading, theater performances, and throwing the discus. Traveling, especially sea voyages, was described as useful for treatment.

During the Dark Ages play was frowned upon by the Church and was regarded as evil, but its mental and physical influence were again recognized during the Renaissance period.

Work

Records from 3400 B.C. indicate that in Egypt even men of leisure were involved in outdoor work and did not spend their days in idleness. The typical nobleman is pictured as being fond of nature and of working in his garden planting trees, "laying out arbors, excavating a pool, lining it with masonry, and filling it with fish."

The writings of the ancient Hebrews make reference to the beneficial effects of work on the body and mind. The ancient Greeks also recognized the value of work. Socrates said, "A man should inure himself to voluntary labor, and not give up to indulgence and pleasure, as they beget no good constitution of body nor knowledge of mind."

In 17 A.D. Livy, the historian, wrote "Toil and pleasure in their nature opposites are linked together in a kind of necessary connection." The value of alternating work and play was stressed by Phaedra, a writer of the first century who said "The mind ought sometimes to be diverted that it may return the better to thinking." Thus, the interrelatedness of work, exercise and play were recognized 2,000 years ago.[2]

THERAPY AND MEDICINE IN THE EIGHTEENTH AND NINETEENTH CENTURIES

Occupational therapy is intimately related to humane treatment. It was not until the last quarter of the eighteenth century, when people on both sides of the Atlantic began to regard others as equals, and fought for this equality, that the practical application of occupational therapy was begun.[6] It was in the midst of the French Revolution (1786) that *Philippe Pinel* introduced work treatment in the Bicêtre Asylum for the Insane near Paris. In his book published in 1801, he describes his methods as "prescribed physical exercises and manual occupations." He said these should be employed in all mental hospitals because "rigorous executed manual labor is the best method of securing good morale and discipline. The return of convalescent patients to their previous interests, to the practice of their profession, to industriousness and perseverance have always been for me the best omen of final recovery."[7] This is the first reference in the literature to medically prescribed use of work for remediation.

On the other side of the Atlantic, where colonists were striving for equality and independence, the first hospital in the colonies, the Pennsylvania Hospital, was established in Philadelphia in 1752. Benjamin Franklin had been involved in drafting the petition for establishing this hospital and it was probably at his suggestion that inmates who were able were provided with the light manual labor of spinning and carding wool and flax. In 1798 *Benjamin Rush, M.D.*, one of the signers of the Declaration of Independence, advocated work as a remedial measure for patients in this hospital.[8] In an address to the Board of the Pennsylvania Hospital in 1810 Rush advised that "certain kinds of labor, exercise, and amusements be contrived for them, which should act at the same time, upon their bodies and minds. The advantages of labor have been evidenced in foreign hospitals as well as our own, in a greater number of recoveries taking place."[9]

In Germany, *Johann Christian Reil*, recommended the use of work for treatment of the insane and also suggested the use of exercise and a special hospital gymnasium along with patient participation in dramatic productions and fine arts. Reil's writings give evidence of what was probably the first use of psychodrama in the treatment of the insane.[10]

In the early 1800s *Samuel Tuke*, an English Quaker established Retreat Asylum for the Insane at York, England. He used work or occupation therapy as Pinel did but placed special emphasis on humane treatment or treating of patients as rational beings who have capability of self-restraint. He called it "moral treatment." Neither chains nor corporal punishment were used and all patients wore clothes and were induced "to adopt orderly habits" and "participate in exercise and labour."[11]

In 1840 *F. Leuret* wrote a book *On the Moral Treatment of Insanity*. He said all psychiatrists recommend diversions and work to prevent the effects of idleness and boredom. He stressed the improvement of habits and the development of a consciousness of society. He utilized exercise, drama, music, and reading along with manual labor.[12] Moral treatment was virtually synonymous with the principles and practice of occupational therapy; this was probably the first book entirely devoted to occupation therapy.

Many Americans visited Europe following the Revolutionary War and observed the treatment of the insane at European hospitals. *Thomas Scattergood*, a Quaker minister who visited Retreat, brought back to America the principles of "occupation and nonrestraint." These principles were used at Friends Asylum for the Insane in Philadelphia, a hospital which he had helped to establish. The hospital was opened in May 1817 and continues to serve the mentally ill today. *Thomas Eddy* was another visitor to Retreat. A New York merchant and a member of the Society of Friends, he was so impressed with the improved care of the insane that he submitted suggestions for the "moral management" of the insane to the Governors of the Lunatic Asylum of the New York Hospital. As a result of his suggestions, in 1821 the Bloomingdale Asylum was opened in New York City and began moral management including occupation therapy. This hospital continues today as the Westchester Division of the New York Hospital. In 1818 McLean Asylum opened near Boston under the supervision of *Rufus Wyman, M.D.* He established, and was probably the first physician in this country to supervise, a program of occupation therapy.[13]

Around 1843, an innovation, regular classroom instruction, was introduced as a part of the care of the mentally ill in hospitals in both Europe and the United States. In 1844 *Amariah Brigham*, superintendent of the Utica State Hospital in New York stated that "employment to be of benefit to the patient should not consider the question of gainful occupation, but should divert the patient from his morbid fancies, engage his attention, stimulate his interest, and lead him to resume natural and healthy methods of thought and occupation."[14] The idea that only the therapeutic value to the patient should be considered in selecting the activity was a new and important advance toward the more scientific use of occupation as therapy.

The period of maximum use of occupation therapy in the United States occurred during the lifetime of *Thomas Story Kirkbride, M.D.* He became superintendent of the Pennsylvania Hospital in 1840 and began a program of mental care that stressed occupation therapy. He said the value cannot be measured in dollars and cents but must be judged in regard to the restoration of comfort to the inmates of the hospital. Crafts, amusements, and hospital occupations were used therapeutically. Kirkbride helped to organize the Association of Asylum Medical Superintendents, which later became the American Psychiatric Association. Through this association, Kirkbride influenced its members regarding the value of occupation therapy.[15]

During the eighteenth and nineteenth centuries

work or occupation therapy was utilized primarily in the care of the mentally ill patients. The only mention in the literature of occupation therapy for the physically disabled was in a book published in 1780 in which a physician in the French Cavalry, *Clement-Joseph Tissot*, gave detailed instructions for the use of crafts and recreational activities for disabilities of muscles and joints following disease or injury.[16]

The effective development of work or occupation therapy continued in the United States through 1860. Then it declined suddenly and its emphasis on the therapeutic value of work was lost for more than a quarter of a century. There seem to be several causes for this period of disuse. Physicians became too busy with increasing responsibilities to take sufficient personal interest in work or occupation therapy. There was a lack of public interest and insight and an underestimation of the therapeutic value of occupation as well as "the real returns as compared to the incidental returns or possible economic proceeds from the treatment."[17] The economic pressures felt in all hospitals during and after the Civil War were also a cause for the decline of occupation therapy.

GENESIS OF OCCUPATIONAL THERAPY PROFESSION IN THE UNITED STATES

Forerunner of the Profession—Adolf Meyer's Philosophy

Toward the end of the nineteenth century, work as a therapeutic agent was again utilized in the treatment of the mentally ill in the United States. In a paper presented in December 1892, Adolf Meyer, a psychiatrist, reported that "the proper use of time in some helpful and gratifying activity appeared to be a fundamental issue in the treatment of the neuropsychiatric patient."[18] In 1895 Meyer's wife, Mary Potter Brooks Meyer, a social worker, introduced systematic type of activity into the wards of a state institution in Worcester, Massachusetts. She was also the first social worker to provide a systematic program to help patients, their families, and the physician.

Meyer's philosophy of treatment and of occupational therapy had a marked impact on the philosophy and history of the profession. His philosophy as stated in the first volume of the first official organ of the profession, published in 1922, was

> Our conception of man is that of an organism that maintains and balances itself in the world of reality and actuality by being in active life and active use, i.e. using and living and acting its time in harmony with its own nature and the nature about it. It is the use that we make of ourselves that gives the ultimate stamp to our every organ.[19]

Meyer described rhythms of life that must be kept in balance even under difficulty. These were work and play, rest and sleep. He said balance was attained by actual doing and practice, with a program of wholesome living as the basis for wholesome thinking, feeling, and interest. He felt that personality was fundamentally determined by performance.[18]

Meyer described mental illness as "a problem of living" and not merely as a disease of structure and function or of a toxic nature. He said because there was habit deterioration, systematic use of time and interest became both an obligation and a necessity. His statement from the yearbook of the Chicago School of Civics and Philanthropy (1908–1911) is the first reference in the literature that indicates that conflicts occur through poor adaptation and that occupation may influence and enhance human adaptiveness:

> During the last decade, we have come to realize more than ever that while some mental disorders are due to toxic conditions, others are rather due to conflicts through poor adaptation. In these conditions a training in normal activities and a culturation of fruitful interests are the sanest and only efficient point of attack.[20]

Thus Meyer felt that the treatment of the mentally ill must be a blending of work and pleasure that included both recreation and productive activity. He said "the pleasure in achievement, a real pleasure in the use of one's hands and muscles and a happy appreciation of time" should be used as incentives in the management of patients and should replace the use of repressive rules. The goal for patients was to create an "orderly rhythm and sense of a day simply and naturally spent."[18]

Meyer said the philosophy of the occupational therapy worker should be "an awakening to the full meaning of time as the biggest wonder and asset of our lives and the valuation of opportunity and performance as the greatest measure of time." Patients must have the realization of reality and a full sense of actuality. This was to be accomplished by providing opportunities rather than prescriptions, opportunities "to do, to plan and to create."[18]

Interpersonal relationships were also an important part of Meyer's philosophy of occupational therapy for he felt that personal contact with instructors and helpers brought out an interchange of experiences and resources. Instructors had to be resourceful and respect the native capacities and interests of their patients.[18]

Adolf Meyer had thus provided the profession of occupational therapy with a philosophy upon which it could build.

Founders of the Profession

Susan E. Tracy

Susan E. Tracy probably can be called the first occupational therapist for, in 1905, during her training as a nurse, she noticed the benefits of occupation in relieving nervous tension and making bedrest more tolerable for patients. In working with orthopedic bedfast patients she felt occupation was important because "happiness and contentment will certainly prove conducive to rest, and absolute rest is the foremost condition of recovery." She saw occupation as an important adjunct to drug treatment and also felt that instruction in self-help was important. Tracy believed that wholesome interests could be substituted for morbid ones and could carry over into the patient's life after discharge from the hospital. She also saw interpersonal relationships between the teacher or nurse and the patient as an important factor in the success of occupation treatment.[21]

Tracy began her work with the mentally ill when she became director of the Training School for Nurses at the Adams Nervine Asylum in Boston. It was here that in 1906 she developed the first systematic training course in occupation to prepare instructors for teaching patient activities. Up until this time it was felt that craftsmen were probably the best teachers of patients in craft activities. Since limitations were imposed on patients because of illness or disease, it was determined that persons with medical training would be better qualified because they would recognize signs of fatigue or eyestrain and know the limitations caused by various diseases or injury. Thus the nurse seemed to be the most qualified person to teach occupation to patients. Tracy felt "Kindergartners" (teachers of small children) could also qualify but would have to become nurses first. She also cautioned that the variety in activity choices must be great in order to meet individual patient requirements.

In 1910 the first book on occupations, *Studies in Invalid Occupations, A Manual for Nurse and Attendants,* was published. This was a compilation of Tracy's lectures with an illustrated guide for the use of activities with patients. The book was primarily a craft book, giving methods of teaching and explaining the rationale for use of specific activities for many patient diagnoses in different types of settings (bed, ward, workshop, home). In this book Tracy describes her concept of occupation by using a quote from John Dewey:

> By occupation is not meant any kind of "busy work" or exercise that may be given to a child to keep him out of mischief or idleness when seated at his desk. By occupation I mean a mode of activity on the part of the child which reproduces or runs parallel to some form of work carried on in the social life . . . The fundamental point of the psychology of an occupation is that it maintains a balance between the intellectual and the practical phases of experience.[22]

Tracy felt that occupations chosen can help retain connections with the social life, provide tangible relations between the individual and other people and their needs, and thus "self-respect is preserved and ambition fostered."[21]

Tracy encouraged the use of occupation for treatment by conducting numerous training courses. In 1911, she conducted the first course in occupation at a general hospital, Massachusetts General Hospital Training School for Nurses. In 1914, as director of the Experiment Station for the Study of Invalid Occupations in Jamaica Plains, Massachusetts, she provided instruction for three classes of students:

"(1) To invalids, whether inside or out of institutions, (2) To pupil nurses, in order to enlarge their practical equipment and (3) To Graduate Nurses who have felt the need of the work and may become teachers."[23] The course description from a flier on the course is as follows:

> Each patient is considered in light of his threefold personality—body, mind and spirit.
>
> The Aim is likewise threefold:
> 1. The patient's physical improvement
> 2. His educational advancement
> 3. His financial betterment
>
> The Method is based upon a threefold principle:
> 1. The realization of resources
> 2. The ability to initiate activities
> 3. The participation in such activities of both sick and well subjects.[23]

Through her training courses Tracy did much to disseminate knowledge in regard to use of occupation for treatment of both physically and mentally ill patients.

Herbert J. Hall

In 1904 Herbert J. Hall began to prescribe occupation for his patients as medicine to regulate life and direct interest. He called this the "work cure."[24]

In 1906 Harvard University became interested in work as a form of treatment and gave Hall a grant of one thousand dollars "to assist in the study of the treatment of neurasthenia by progressive and graded manual occupation." Hall established a workshop in Marblehead, Massachusetts, where he used, as treatment, the crafts of handweaving, woodcarving, metalwork, and pottery "because of their universal appeal and the normalizing effect of suitable manual work." He said, "Suitable occupation of hand and mind is a very potent factor in the maintenance of the physical, mental and moral health in the individual and the community."[25]

Hall felt that nurses and social service workers should be trained in the use of work as treatment. Therefore he began a training program for young women at Devereaux Mansion in Marblehead, Massachusetts, around 1908. In 1915 Hall published *The Work of Our Hands—A Study of Occupations for Invalids*.[26] He divided invalid occupation into "diversional" occupation for those patients in advanced stages of incurable diseases and "remedial" occupation for those patients for whom there was therapeutic and economic value in remedial work.

Eleanor Clark Slagle

In 1908 a training course in occupations for hospital attendants was given at the Chicago School of Civics and Philanthropy, which was directed by Graham Taylor. Jane Addams, the director of Hull House, along with Julia Lanthrop and Taylor, influenced the development of a number of courses to meet the needs of the community. Lanthrop developed the course for hospital attendants with the purpose of substituting "the educational for the custodial idea in the daily care of the mentally unsound." "Attendants learned games, arts, crafts, and hobbies which they could use to reach their patients." The philosophy of the program was that the work of the attendant was educational and the "methods were those used by the best teachers of little children—teaching the use of muscles and mind together in games, exercises and handicraft."[27] These concepts were reinforced by Adolf Meyer who worked with Addams and Lanthrop and supported their work for the improvement of the care of the mentally ill in state hospitals in Illinois.

Up until this point in the development of occupational therapy, the persons most qualified to be occupation workers had fallen into three categories of social workers, nurses, and kindergarten or crafts teachers. There were those who believed that nurses had the most desirable background because they had medical training and thus had higher qualifications for working with the sick and disabled. Lanthrop, however, believed that "occupational treatment was to have a large future in hospital treatment and that this service should be carried on by persons specifically educated for it."[28] This controversy continued for many years as courses designed for nurses or teachers were developed throughout the United States.

Eleanor Clark Slagle, a social work student in the Chicago School of Civics and Philanthropy, became concerned about the detrimental effects of idleness on the patients at Kankakee State Hospital. Consequently she enrolled in Miss Lanthrop's first course in Curative Occupations and Recreations for attendants and nurses in Institutions for the Insane given at the Chicago School of Civics and Philanthropy. Following her completion of the course in July 1911, she conducted a similar course at the State Hospital in Newberry, Michigan. She then went to Phipps Psychiatric Clinic in Johns Hopkins Hospital in Baltimore under Meyer where she was the director of the Occupational Therapy Department for two years and conducted classes for nurses in "handiwork for dispensary patients."[29] In 1915 Slagle organized the first professional school for occupational therapists, the Henry B. Favill School of Occupations, in Chicago. She served as the director of this school from 1918 to 1922. At this school, Slagle used her background in social work. Special instruction was given in invalid occupations along with experience in working with mentally ill patients in order to develop the "Habit Training" method of treatment, based on the use of occupation. She based this method on the concept that "for the most part, our lives are made up of habit reactions" and "occupation usually remedially serves to overcome some habits, to modify others and to construct new ones to the end that habit reactions will be favorable to the restoration and maintenance of health."[30] Remedial occupation implied training in conduct, in habit training and in the art of doing things in a socially acceptable manner. This method stressed the interdependence of mental and physical components; the need to build on the habit of attention; the need to analyze occupations; and the need to grade activity from simple to complex, to go from the known to the unknown, and to provide tasks that are of increasing interest and require increasing degrees of concentration. Included in the program were craft activities, preindustrial and vocational work as well as games, folk dancing, gymnastics, and playground activities. This type of rehabilitation program attempted to create a balanced program of work, rest, and play for mentally ill patients.

Slagle, in the development of her habit training program, built on the philosophy of Meyer and provided a model of treatment that was utilized in occupational therapy for mentally ill patients until the early 1950s.

William Rush Dunton, Jr.—Father of the Profession

William Rush Dunton, Jr.'s endeavors on behalf of occupational therapy, as a practitioner, as a theoretician, as a philosopher, and as an officer of the national group, assured him the title of "father of occupational therapy." He was involved in the use of occupational therapy as treatment of mental patients as early as 1895. When he was staff psychiatrist at Sheppard and Enoch Pratt Asylum in Baltimore in 1895, a metalworking shop was fitted for treatment of patients. Later other crafts were added and, in 1908, a teacher in arts and crafts was engaged to instruct patients.[31] As Dunton observed his patients as they were engaged in occupations, he noted how important it was to have someone trained to direct their activities and he became aware of the care required to place a patient in the right activity. Thus, in 1911, after studying Tracy's book on invalid occupations, he undertook the responsibility of conducting a series of classes on occupations and recreation for nurses at Sheppard and Enoch Pratt Asylum. In 1912 he was placed in charge of the occupations and recreation program at the hospital and his classes for nurses became an ongoing process.[32]

In 1915 the first complete textbook on occupational therapy, *Occupational Therapy—A Manual for Nurses*,[33] written by Dunton, was published. This book outlined the basic tenets or cardinal rules in applying occupation therapy. He said occupation's primary purpose was "to divert the patient's attention from unpleasant subjects, to keep the patient's train of thought in more healthy channels, to control attention, to secure rest, to train in mental processes by educating hands, eyes, muscles, etc., serve as a safety valve, to provide a new vocation."[33] The greatest part of this book dealt with simple activities which the nurse could use or adapt to treatment of patients.

George Edward Barton

Up until this time, the use of activity for therapy had been called by many titles such as moral treatment, work treatment, work therapy, occupation treatment, occupational reeducation, and ergotherapy. It was not until December 1914, at a meeting in Boston of hospital workers and the Massachusetts State Board of Insanity, that the term "occupational therapy" was introduced by a layman, *George Edward Barton*. Barton, an architect, became an advocate of this treatment after his own illness, during which he experienced the beneficial effects of directed occupation. He consequently organized an institution called Consolation House in Clifton Springs, New York, where, by means of occupations, people could be retrained or adjusted to gainful living. Barton described the purposes of occupational therapy as "to divert the patient's mind, to exercise some particular set of muscles or a limb, or perhaps merely to relieve the tedium of convalescence." He felt that "these activities may have little if any practical value beyond the immediate purpose they serve. . . . the idea is to give that sort [of activity] which will be preliminary to and dovetailed with the real vocational education which is to begin as soon as the patient is able to go farther along." He felt that the fundamental principle upon which occupational therapy rested was "not making of an object but the making of a man." He defined occupational therapy as the "science of instructing and encouraging the sick in such labors as will involve those energies and activities producing a beneficial therapeutic effect."[34]

FOUNDING OF THE NATIONAL SOCIETY FOR THE PROMOTION OF OCCUPATIONAL THERAPY

Shortly before the United States entered World War I, a number of persons who were actively interested in providing occupation for patients decided that an association of workers to exchange views would be advantageous. Thus, in March 1917 at a meeting held at Consolation House, the National Society for the Promotion of Occupational Therapy was formed, incorporated and chartered under the laws of the District of Columbia. The objects of the association as noted in the constitution were "the advancement of occupation as a therapeutic measure, the study of the effects of occupation upon the human being, and the dissemination of scientific knowledge of this subject."[35] The title of the organization gives some indication of its character, for its membership included medical doctors, social workers, teachers, nurses, and artists whose main interests were in other areas. They did, however, recognize an inadequacy in the care of the sick and disabled which they felt might be filled by the technique called occupational therapy. The charter members of this society were George E. Barton, Eleanor Clark Slagle, William Rush Dunton, Jr., Susan C. Johnson (occupational therapist at Montefiore Hospital in New York), Isabel G. Newton (Barton's secretary), and Thomas B. Kidner (vocational secretary of the Military Hospital Commission of Canada). Susan B. Tracy was unable to attend the meeting but was elected as an active member and incorporator of the society. A total of 14 active, 7 associate, and 26 sustaining members were elected to the society of which Barton became the first president.

The first annual meeting of the society was held in September 1917 in New York City.[36] The presentations at this conference were centered on the theme "The Reconstruction of the Mentally and Physically Disabled." Dunton spoke and proposed a system of vocational education whereby the convalescent, while still in the hospital, could be evaluated and taught useful occupations which would be meaningful and useful on discharge.[37] His plan included a plan for community action and canvassing of local businesses to determine if they would hire handicapped but trained persons.

Dunton was elected president of the society at this meeting, a post which he held for two years. While he was president it became apparent that there was a need for local organizations for exchange of ideas and concepts. Dunton began organizing a cohesive group in the state of Maryland. Soon other states followed this lead and a pattern of local organizations becoming affiliated with the national organization was established. This basic pattern remains today.[32]

This marked the beginning of the professional organization of occupational therapy in the United States. In 1920, the name was changed to its present title, the American Occupational Therapy Association.

In 1918, at the second annual meeting of the National Society for the Promotion of Occupational Therapy, Dunton delivered nine cardinal rules to guide practice. These were expanded to fifteen principles by a committee of therapists. Out of these fifteen principles came the first universal definition of occupational therapy: "A method of treatment by means of instruction and employment in productive occupation." The objectives were "To arouse interest, courage and confidence; to exercise the mind and body in healthy activities; to overcome functional disability; and to re-establish a capacity for industrial and social usefulness."[38]

In a second book, *Reconstruction Therapy*, published in 1919, Dunton further delineated the basic tenet upon which the profession of occupational therapy is based in the Credo for occupational therapists:

> That occupation is as necessary to life as food and drink.
> That every human being should have both physical and mental occupation.
> That all should have occupations which they enjoy, or hobbies. These are the more necessary when the vocation is dull or distasteful. Every individual should have at least two hobbies, one outdoor and one indoor. A greater number will create wider interests, a broader intelligence.
> That sick minds, sick bodies, sick souls may be healed through occupation.[39]

The Maryland Psychiatric Quarterly, edited by Dunton, from its inception in 1911, published articles relating to occupations and amusement. This journal became the official organ of the National Society for the Promotion of Occupational Therapy when it was founded in 1917. In 1922, the *Archives of Occupational Therapy* was first published and became the official organ of the American Occupational Therapy Association. In 1925, the title of this journal was changed to *Occupational Therapy and Rehabilitation*. This was the official organ of the association until 1947 when the American Occupational Therapy Association assumed the total responsibility for publication of its own organ and entitled it *American Journal of Occupational Therapy*.

EXPANSION DURING WORLD WAR I

Shortly after the entrance of the United States into World War I, the nation was faced with wounded men in need of rehabilitation. Slagle approached the armed forces and pleaded the cause of therapy as a means of treating the wounded. After initial opposition, Surgeon General Gorgas of the Army authorized the appointment of Reconstruction Aides to serve in Army hospitals.[40] The National Committee for Mental Hygiene initially recruited six aides to serve in European-based hospitals of the American Expeditionary Forces. The success of this small group was such that in September 1917 General John J. Pershing cabled to Washington from Paris requesting 200 young women to serve in Army hospitals overseas.[41] Thus, directives from the Medical Department of the Army, dated January 1918 (Class 1) and March 1918 (Class 2), established training programs for two groups of reconstruction aides (Class 1, physiotherapy, and Class 2, occupational therapy).

The physiotherapy aides were to be trained "to give massage and exercise and other remedial treatment to the returned soldiers," while the occupational therapy aides were to be trained "to furnish forms of occupation to convalescents in long illnesses and to give to patients the therapeutic benefit of activity." Rigid criteria were established for applicants including at least a high school education with experience in some profession such as social work or library science. Applicants had to be at least 25 years old, be citizens of the United States or one of its allies, and have theoretical knowledge and practical experience in various crafts. Initial intensive courses were given at the Henry B. Favill School in Chicago under Slagle and at the Teachers College of Columbia University in New York and the Boston School of Occupational Therapy (the Franklin Union) in Boston. The courses ranged from 6 to 12 weeks in length and included lectures on psychology of the handicapped, fatigue and the work cure, personal hygiene, anatomy, kinesiology, ethics, and hospital administration. Classes in the use and application of crafts included woodwork, weaving, cordwork, beadwork, basketry, and ceramics. Field work and practice in local hospitals were also a vital part of the training program.[42,43]

As requests for reconstruction aides increased, other emergency war courses were established throughout the country. Between April 1918 and July 1921, 25 schools had graduated 1685 reconstruction aides, of whom 460 served overseas.[44] Reconstruction aides were civilian employees who worked with patients in orthopedic and surgical wards as well as working with those suffering from nervous or mental disorders.

Occupational therapy for the treatment of physical dysfunction gained impetus during this period and the scientific approach to the treatment of physical disabilities was begun.

Bird T. Baldwin

In the *Army Manual on Occupational Therapy*, Bird T. Baldwin gives this explanation of occupational therapy:

> Occupational therapy is based on the principle that the best type of remedial exercise is that which requires a series of specific voluntary movements involved in the ordinary trades and occupations, physical training, play or the daily routine activities of life. Our curative shops are now being organized and graduated on the principle which will enable us ultimately to isolate, classify, repeat and to a limited degree, standardize and control the type of movements involved in the particular occupational and recreational operations. The patient's attention is repeatedly called to the particular remedial movements involved; at the same time the movements have the advantage of being initiated by the patient and of forming an integral and necessary part of the larger and more complex series of coordinated movements. The purposive nature of the movements and the end products of the work offer a direct incentive for sustained effort; the periodic measurement of the increase in range and strength of movement makes it possible for the patient to watch his recovery from day to day. . . . The records also enable the examiner to determine which mode of treatment leads to the greatest and most consistent gains in a particular case. . . .[45]

It was during this period that devices were developed to measure range of motion and strength; thus more scientific recording was made possible. The kinesiological analysis of activities begun during the war allowed activities to be chosen based on specific physical limitation. Adapted pieces of equipment were devised. They provided specific motions for increasing range of motion and strength, and their use was then applied for the remediation of selected disabilities.

By the end of World War I thousands of soldiers in the United States had received some form of occupational therapy and the profession was beginning to gain public support.

Baldwin made a valuable contribution through the development of evaluation and treatment procedures for restoration of physical function and dissemination of these by publication in the Army Manual.

POST WORLD WAR I TO WORLD WAR II

Many of the schools for training reconstruction aides closed permanently following World War I. The demand for trained occupational therapists in civilian hospitals caused the reopening of the Boston School of Occupational Therapy in the fall of 1919, followed shortly by the opening of the Philadelphia School of Occupational Therapy and the St. Louis School of Occupational Therapy. These schools continue to function today. The Boston School is now located in Tufts University, the Philadelphia School is located in the University of Pennsylvania, and the St. Louis School is located in Washington University.

The American Occupational Therapy Association established "Minimum Standards for Courses of Training in Occupational Therapy"[46] in 1923. At this time several war emergency schools were disbanded because of their inability to meet requirements. The minimum standards included a prerequisite of a high school education and a 12-month course of not less than 8 months of theoretical work and 3 months in practice. The establishment of standards did much to raise the status of the profession. However, the schools of occupational therapy trained therapists as teachers of crafts, or occupations, which would help individuals move from acute illness to vocational training. Many therapists gained knowledge of anatomy, kinesiology, and medical conditions through postgraduate courses and developed principles of specific treatment to restore physical function on an empirical basis.[47]

The caliber of publications in the official journal of the Association, however, did not reflect a scientific basis for the profession. Articles generally were undocumented, unscientific, and inconclusive and fell into three categories: (1) description of occupational therapy as it was practiced at various hospitals, (2) helpful hints on crafts, and (3) the relationship of occupational therapy to other medical services.[47] Ethel Bowman, Associate Professor of Psychology at Goucher College, described the problem of the profession in 1922 as follows:

> Literally there is no psychology of occupational therapy today. Although there is abundant material for such, it is, at present, unorganized. In speaking of the psychology of a subject, we may mean that the known facts of scientific psychology have been given practical application, or that the peculiarly psychological aspects of the subject have been singled out and subjected to specific study by the methods which psychology has found applicable in its problems of pure science. In neither of these meanings have we a psychology of occupational therapy.[48]

In spite of the lack of scientific approach, occupational therapy was being utilized in both civilian and military hospitals throughout the United States. After their experiences during the war, physicians recognized the value of occupational therapy and established units in many general and children's hospitals. Treatment was based on the principles advocated by Dunton in 1915. These principles advocated that treatment be prescribed and administered under constant medical supervision and correlated with other treatment of the patient; treatment should be directed to individual needs; treatment should arouse interest, courage, and confidence; treatment should exercise mind and body in healthy activity; treatment should overcome disability and reestablish capacity for industrial and social usefulness; occupation should be regulated and graded as a patient's strength and capabilities increased; employment in groups is advisable to provide opportunity for social adaptation; and the only reliable measure of the treatment is the effect on the patient.[49]

In 1923 the Federal Industrial Rehabilitation Act made it a requirement that every general hospital dealing with industrial accidents or illness provide occupational therapy as an integral part of its treatment. There was a demand for graduates of accredited schools, in spite of budget cuts in hospitals during the Depression, demonstrating an increasing recognition of the necessity for constructive occupation in the maintenance of mental and physical health.[50,51]

By 1928 there were six schools of occupational therapy. In addition to the Boston, Philadelphia, and St. Louis Schools of Occupational Therapy, Milwaukee Downer College, the University of Minnesota, and the University of Toronto in Canada had accredited programs. Each of these met the minimum standard of nine months didactic and three months clinical preparation. Each gave a diploma in occupational therapy with the University of Minnesota giving a bachelor's degree as well. The Minnesota program was discontinued in 1931 because of low enrollment and the resignation of the director.[52]

In 1927 Everett Elwood recommended that the American Occupational Therapy Association safeguard the profession and maintain high standards by requiring all practitioners to be licensed and by utilizing a national examination to qualify graduates of the accredited schools.[53]

In 1931 a National Registry of all qualified occupational therapists was established "for the protection of hospitals and institutions from unqualified persons posing as occupational therapists." When the association issued its first registry in 1932, 318 therapists were listed, all qualified by a rigid set of standards.[40] Registration required that therapists have one year of active practice under an experienced therapist and be recommended by that therapist.

In March 1931 the American Occupational Therapy Association requested that the American Medical Association undertake inspection and approval of the occupational therapy schools. Because the American Medical Association had experience in medical education and had investigated medical schools and teaching hospitals, the Council on Medical Education and Hospitals agreed to undertake the survey. The inspection began in November 1933. Following the inspection, meetings were held with representatives from the American Occupational Therapy Association, the Council on Physical Medicine, and the Council on Medical Education and Hospitals. The result of these meetings was the drafting of the "Essentials of an Acceptable School of Occupational Therapy." The "Essentials" were adopted by the Council on Medical Education and Hospitals in February 1935 and were ratified the following June by the House of Delegates of the American Medical Association at its Annual Meeting.[54]

The thirteen schools of occupational therapy in operation were classified in 1938 and only five schools met the essentials and were approved. They were the Boston, Philadelphia, and St. Louis Schools of Occupational Therapy and Milwaukee Downer College and the University of Toronto in Canada. Kalamazoo State Hospital School of Occupational Therapy received tentative approval. The "Essentials" increased the length of the program to 25-calendar months plus an additional 9 months of hospital practice training. The requirements expanded the theoretical basis of the profession by adding emphasis in biological and social sciences and clinical medicine. Clinical practice was expanded to include experience in mental, tuberculosis, children's, and orthopedic hospitals. Although degree courses were available at Milwaukee Downer and Kalamazoo, few students took advantage of this offering as a degree did not seem necessary. Therefore, most students received highly specialized training with no liberal arts input and received a diploma in occupational therapy in three years. Beginning in 1932, certificate programs for persons with bachelor's degrees were given at Boston, Philadelphia, and St. Louis. These courses required one-year didactic preparation plus nine months of hospital practice. Graduates of the certificate program were permitted to become registered occupational therapists. There was no thought of graduate degrees in the field at this time and there seemed to be no desire on the part of practitioners to write or publish literature for the field.[47] These schools graduated a total of 100 qualified therapists per year.

By 1938, 13 percent of the hospitals approved by the American Medical Association had qualified occupational therapists on their staffs. The majority of therapists were employed in mental hospitals.[50] The impetus given to the treatment of physical dysfunction through occupational therapy by World War I had diminished. The profession had been from its inception primarily one for women, and only one school, the St. Louis School of Occupational Therapy, accepted male students. Thus, only about 2½ percent of qualified therapists were men and they were employed primarily in mental institutions, tuberculosis sanitoria, and penal institutions.[55,56] A few occupational therapists were in private practice in 1939 and five cities, Philadelphia, Hartford, Detroit, Milwaukee, and St. Louis, had visiting therapists, similar to visiting nurses, working the homebound.[50]

In 1939 the first formal subjective registration examination developed by a committee of therapists was given, permitting those who failed to register on the basis of experience to become registered. About 1944, examinations were developed by each school and submitted for approval to the Registration Committee of the American Occupational Therapy Association.

DURING WORLD WAR II AND IMMEDIATELY FOLLOWING

World War I had given impetus to the new field of occupational therapy but its development after the war was slow. After World War I, occupational therapy programs and personnel in all Army hospitals had been reduced to a minimum. There were five permanent Army General Hospitals, only three of which had an occupational therapist employed.[57] At the beginning of World War II the total number of practicing occupational therapists in the United States was less than was needed by the military hospitals alone.[58]

Because of the need for therapists in both military and civilian hospitals a number of new schools were organized. The number of approved schools increased from 5 in 1940 to 18 in 1945. At the request of the Surgeon General's Office, war emergency courses were started in a number of schools and prepared over 500 qualified therapists for duty in the Army hospitals. These schools met American Medical Association minimum standards since they were intensive one-year courses for college graduates who had basic psychology and at least 20 semester hours of fine, applied, or industrial arts, or home economics. The course consisted of four months of theory in the civilian occupational therapy schools and eight months practical application and training under registered occupational therapists in Army hospitals.[59] Registration was acquired through passing of the Registration Examination approved by the American Occupational Therapy Association.

The critical personnel needs of the armed forces

and war industries demanded maximum conservation of manpower. Thus a reconditioning program in the Armed Forces was established to

> accelerate the return to duty of convalescent patients in the highest state of physical and mental efficiency consistent with the capabilities and the type of duty to which they are being returned . . . or to provide for their return to civilian life in the highest possible degree of physical fitness, well oriented in the responsibilities of citizenship and prepared to adjust successfully to social and vocational pursuits.[60]

The reconditioning program included a coordinated program of educational reconditioning, physical reconditioning, and occupational therapy. Occupational therapists were civilians appointed to Army hospitals by the Surgeon General's Office. They supervised both the treatment programs and the volunteer Red Cross Arts and Skills, Recreational, and Diversional Programs.

By the end of World War II over a thousand occupational therapists were providing services in the military hospitals in the United States and abroad. Occupational therapists had to be prepared to work with persons having psychological and psychiatric problems as well as those having orthopedic and neurological problems. Techniques were developed for rapid total rehabilitation of patients in order to return them physically and mentally fit for service or work. The war had expanded the techniques and knowledge in occupational therapy, especially in the area of the treatment of the physically disabled.

In February 1947 the first National Objective Registration Examination was given. Very few men worked in the profession of occupational therapy so it was looked upon as a woman's field. From 1941 to 1946 the number of registered occupational therapists almost doubled, going from 1144 to 2265,[61] but the number of men in the profession remained at about 2½ percent of the total, or about 50 men.

Clare S. Spackman—Restoration of Physical Function

Because of increase in medical knowledge, discovery of new drugs, and improved medical care after World War II, the population of patients to be treated changed and increased. This placed new demands on therapists and required that new treatment procedures be developed. Other specialities were developed to satisfy unmet needs, i.e., recreational therapy, educational therapy, and corrective therapy. Occupational therapists became specialized in treatment of certain types of disabilities such as peripheral nerve injuries and amputations. This added to the base of knowledge and improved treatment techniques for these areas of practice.[62]

Occupational therapists had to be skilled in using constructive activities for treatment and also were required to utilize as treatment activities of daily living (ADL), work simplification, rehabilitation techniques for the handicapped homemaker, and training in the use of upper extremity prostheses. This expansion in techniques and knowledge in the area of physical dysfunction required extensive reorganization in the curricula of the accredited schools of occupational therapy. In order to assist schools in providing this new information to students, the first textbook in the United States on occupational therapy written primarily by occupational therapists, edited by Helen S. Willard and Clare S. Spackman, was published in 1947.[63] Spackman provided detailed information in this volume on the evaluation and treatment of patients with physical dysfunction.

Spackman felt that the exact function of occupational therapy in the treatment of physical dysfunction should be specifically defined. In an article in which she traced the history of occupational therapy practice for restoration of physical function she says

> Occupational therapy treats the patient by the use of constructive activity in a simulated, normal living and/or working situation. This is and always has been our function. Constructive activity is the Keynote of occupational therapy. . . . True occupational therapy cannot be used until the patient is capable not only of performing a given motion but of utilizing it to carry out a constructive activity. Occupational therapy's value lies in teaching the patient by use of constructive activities to transfer the motions and strength gained by corrective exercise in physical therapy into coordinated activity which will enable the patient to become personally independent and economically self-sufficient.[62]

Spackman made an impact on the treatment of patients physically disabled by disease or injury through publication of the book on occupational therapy and by the education of students utilizing the principles of evaluation and treatment.

Spackman represented the United States when the World Federation of Occupational Therapists was founded in 1954. She was elected to the position of Assistant Secretary-Treasurer at its first meeting, served as President of the organization from 1957 to 1962, and was Secretary-Treasurer from 1964 to 1972. Her interest and involvement with the World Federation did much to develop good relationships with member countries and encouraged expansion of the profession into many underdeveloped countries.

Formation of the World Federation of Occupational Therapists

The aftermath of World War II led to the rapid growth of allied medical services in many countries throughout the world. There was a need for exchange of information in regard to new methods of treatment and many foreign therapists were seeking admission to take the registration examination of the American Occupational Therapy Association. The International Society for the Rehabilitation of the Disabled, concerned with the establishment of rehabilitation programs throughout the world, encouraged the formation of an International Association of Occupational Therapists which would establish international standards for education and practice. In April 1952 representatives of six countries met in Liverpool, England, and drafted a constitution including qualifications of member associations and proposed "Minimum Educational Standards for Occupational Therapists" (revised in 1963). The American Occupational Therapy Association became one of the ten founding members of the World Federation of Occupational Therapists. The six countries represented at the founders' meeting were Canada, Denmark, Great Britain (England and Scotland), South Africa, Sweden, and the United States. Australia, New Zealand, Israel, and India were represented by written opinion and thus were included as founding members.

The first congress met in Edinburgh, Scotland, in 1954. Four hundred representatives from ten countries attended. The organization continued to grow and by its second congress in 1958 there were 750 representatives from 38 countries.[64] In 1959 the World Federation of Occupational Therapists joined the World Health Organization and established a roster of expert advisors to work with countries trying to establish or develop their own occupational therapy programs. This roster has been maintained and continues to be used when therapists are needed to assist developing programs.

In 1960 the World Federation of Occupational Therapists formulated a code of "Ethics for Occupational Therapists" and "Functions of Occupational Therapy" (revised in 1962). The American Occupational Therapy Association also worked with the World Rehabilitation Fund, the Peace Corps, and the International Cooperation Administration. By the early 1960s there was an active exchange of therapists among countries. Many American therapists worked abroad and therapists from member countries worked in the United States. Members from countries meeting World Federation of Occupational Therapists standards were permitted to take the registration examination of the American Occupational Therapy Association.[64]

MOVE TOWARD AN "EXACT" SCIENCE

The 1950s saw an increase in the development of rehabilitation techniques in physical dysfunction. The use of more exact methods of measuring physical function initiated a movement to make occupational therapy a more exact science. Advances were made in medical science for the control of diseases including poliomyelitis and tuberculosis. This caused a shift in emphasis in occupational therapy of physical dysfunction to the chronic conditions of arthritis, heart disease, stroke, traumatic injuries, and congenital defects. Federal legislation and the interest of insurance carriers and federal and state rehabilitation agencies gave added stimulus to the growth of occupational therapy in the treatment of physical dysfunction. New techniques were developed by therapists and biomedical engineers, and these new techniques influenced the procedures used in occupational therapy. The emphasis of treatment was to reduce defects related to the patient's pathological condition and to allow the individual to function at the highest level of which he or she was capable.[62] The occupational therapist functioned as a member of a team dedicated to the rehabilitation of the disabled.

During this period the treatment of the psychiatric patient was also being examined by occupational therapists with an increasing emphasis being made on the social adaptation of the patient or client and the individual's return to functioning in family and community. The concept of the "therapeutic use of self" became the primary focus of treatment and utilized psychotherapeutic techniques. This concept used social interactions as the tool for helping patients or clients to deal with their emotional responses and with both the human and nonhuman environment.[65]

Gail S. Fidler—Psychiatric Occupational Therapy

The first comprehensive book on psychiatric occupational therapy was published in 1954. This book, *Introduction to Psychiatric Occupational Therapy*, by Gail S. Fidler and Jay W. Fidler, M.D., gave impetus to the psychodynamic approach to occupational therapy.[66] The Fidlers presented occupational therapy as a collaborative effort between the occupational therapist and the psychiatrist. Occupational therapy was the laboratory in which the patient or client could experiment in handling emotions and developing living skills through the use of productive activity. Guidelines for detailed activity analysis were developed. The book presented a process in which groups could be used to facilitate treatment; it also encouraged the study of projective techniques. In 1963, a second textbook on psychiatric occupational therapy was published by the Fidlers, *Occupational Therapy—A Communication Process in Psychiatry*. This book presented occupational therapy as an important communication tool because activities could provide a means for understanding individuals through nonverbal communications during the activity process.[67]

From 1963 to 1964 Gail Fidler presented graduate courses in Occupational Therapy Supervision in Psychiatry at Columbia University. In 1967 she developed the masters program in Psychiatric Occupational Therapy at New York University, where she encouraged use of the scientific method in occupational therapy. Some of the leaders in the practice of psychiatric occupational therapy today are graduates of these programs.

Fidler has continued to be involved in clinical, academic, and administrative affairs of the profession because she sees importance in maintaining competence as an occupational therapist in all of these areas.

New Levels in Occupational Therapy Education

In spite of the fact that there was an increase in the number of occupational therapy schools, there continued to be a lack of qualified occupational therapists to fill the vacancies in both psychiatry and physical disability therapy. By 1960 there were 24 accredited schools of occupational therapy, all located in university settings giving bachelor's degrees in conformance with the "Essentials" as revised in 1949.

With the dearth of qualified personnel, employers began to utilize persons trained in other fields to fill vacancies, thereby giving impetus to the expansion of related therapeutic groups such as recreational therapy, art therapy, music therapy, vocational rehabilitation counselors, manual arts therapists, and educational therapists. Development in these fields and the overlapping of roles caused some occupational therapists to question whether the profession was operating without a theoretical base.[68,69]

In 1947 the first program leading to a master's degree in occupational therapy was established at the University of Southern California. This course was for those persons who were registered occupational therapists who had bachelor's degrees. Later in the same year New York University began a similar graduate program. These programs were developed for therapists desiring advanced work in clinical specialty areas such as clinical psychopathology, physical disabilities, vocational rehabilitation, and special education.[47] It was hoped that graduate study on the part of occupational therapists would promote research, which was recognized as essential for increasing the knowledge and theoretical base of the profession.

At this same time the profession began to examine the possibility of training a technical level person to work as an assistant to the occupational therapist, thereby providing for the lack of manpower in the field.[70] Criteria for the educational programs were determined and standards for training assistants for general practice were implemented in October 1960.[71]

CHANGES IN FOCUS—1960s AND 1970s

During the 1960s psychiatric occupational therapists began to examine their role and function. Grant funded consultants were hired by the American Occupational Therapy Association to help these therapists look at the impact of their treatment. Workshops were conducted throughout the country in group techniques and object relations. These workshops led psychiatric occupational therapists to examine neurobehavioral orientation to treatment, thus adding the dimension of perception to psychiatric treatment, which had previously had only a social and emotional base.[72]

During this same period the basic master's program was introduced as a means of educating persons with bachelor's degrees in other fields to the basics of occupational therapy with advanced level work in research methodology for the profession. The first program was a two-year course conducted at the University of Southern California in 1964. Shortly thereafter basic master's programs were begun at other universities: Boston University and Virginia Commonwealth University. These courses encouraged students to conduct research in the profession and to publish the results. This caused a gradual change in the articles published in the *American Journal of Occupational Therapy* and encouraged therapists to become involved in clinical research.

A. Jean Ayres—Neurobehavioral Orientation

A. Jean Ayres became interested in neurophysiological and developmental approaches to occupational therapy through her contacts with Margaret S. Rood, an occupational therapist and physical therapist who had investigated literature in these areas and developed the following basic principles:

1. Motor output is dependent upon sensory input. Thus sensory stimuli are utilized to activate and/or inhibit motor response.
2. Activation of motor response follows a normal developmental sequence. . . .
3. Since there is interaction within the nervous system between somatic, psychic and autonomic functions stimuli can be used to influence one or more directly or indirectly.[73]

In the early 1960s A. Jean Ayres began conducting research that laid the foundation for a neurobehavioral orientation to occupational therapy. The basis of her work "is the recapitulation of the sequence of development."[74] This orientation was consequently termed "sensory integrative therapy" and accepted developmental stage concepts. Ayres proposed that the "principles that determined the direction of evolutionary development are manifested in the principles that govern the development of the capacity to perceive and learn by each child today." Therapy is based on the premise that the brain is a "self-organizing system" which integrates or coordinates "two or more functions or processes in a manner which enhances the adaptiveness of the brain's responses" and the fact that "one of the most powerful organizers of sensory input is movement which is adaptive to the organism." Treatment is based upon purposeful movement that causes the individual to respond adaptively and requires a response which represents a "more mature or integrated action than previous performance."[75]

Mary Reilly—Occupational Behavior Orientation

In the 1960s Mary Reilly suggested that the concern of occupational therapy should be patient achievement since we are dealing with behavior that is subject to maturation and regression of illness. She suggests that we use the work-play continuum because "the play of childhood . . . contains a critical ability to transmit the adaptive skills necessary for complex work technology and urban living of today." Thus, it would seem that Reilly is reemphasizing the need for habit training along with reduction of incapacity.[76]

Reilly's orientation indicates recommitment to Meyer's and Slagle's philosophy of occupational therapy. Reilly stresses the importance of "examining the various life roles of the population relative to community adaptation, to identify the various skills that support these roles, and to create an environment where the relevant behavior could be evoked and practiced."[77] The occupational therapist's role is to facilitate achievement of competence. Emphasis is placed on the patient's or client's ability to cope with the community and with changes in life situations. Interpersonal relationships are essential factors in this process.

Wilma West—Prevention and Community Occupational Therapy

In 1966 Wilma West stated that the shift from medical to health concerns had implications for occupational therapy. She said that the profession must be involved in the new emphasis of "maintaining optimum health rather than an intermittent treatment of acute disease and disability" and that "health and medical care in the future . . . will emphasize human development by programs designed to promote better adaptation, rather than technologically oriented programs offering specific solutions to specific difficulties."[78] She described four emerging roles for the occupational therapist that would create new dimensions of function. These were evaluator, consultant, supervisor, and researcher. She suggested that the occupational therapist, to fulfill these roles in the prevention of disease, must move into and work in community settings.

Anne Cronin Mosey—Frames of Reference for Psychiatric Occupational Therapy

In 1970 Anne Mosey said that occupational therapy in psychiatry appeared to be functioning on the basis of intuition and without a theoretical base. She felt there should be a "conscious use of theoretical frames of reference as the basis for the treatment of psychosocial dysfunction." She categorized the three frames of reference available as analytical, acquisitional, and developmental. She said the *analytical* base "describes man as striving for need fulfillment, expression of primitive impulses or control of inherent drives." She described dysfunction as "symptom-producing unconscious content." Therapy attempts to bring the symptom-producing unconscious content to consciousness and integrate it with conscious content.

The *acquisitional* base "focuses upon the various skills or abilities which the individual needs for adequate and satisfactory interaction in the environment." Human abilities are viewed as qualitative and nonstage specific. Dysfunction is described in terms of what behavior must be eliminated and what must be added in order for an individual to function in a normal environment.

The *developmental* base is similar to the acquisitional in that it specifies the various skills and abilities which the individual needs for satisfactory interaction in the community. However, the abilities are considered to be interdependent, qualitative, and stage specific. The developmental base "assumes that the individual must go through incompleted stages in order to function in a mature manner." The individual's current adaptive skill, learning, and the expected environment must all be evaluated.[79] Mosey's developmental base is drawn from the theoretical formulations developed by Ayres.

In 1974 Mosey proposed an orientation to occupational therapy as an alternative to the medical and health model. She called it the "biopsychosocial model." She said this model "directs attention to the body, mind and environment of the client. It takes these facets into consideration without any sense of wellness or sickness on the part of the client." This model focuses on the individual as a "biological entity; a thinking and feeling person and a member of a community of others."[80] Although this model is described as an alternative, it seems to have been drawn from all previous orientations to occupational therapy.

CHANGES WITHIN THE ASSOCIATION—1960s AND 1970s

During the 1960s the American Occupational Therapy Association was called upon by its members to perform new functions such as providing administrative guidelines, suggesting treatment and consultative rates, and sponsoring a lobbyist for health legislation. These activities endangered the status of the professional organization as one established for "charitable, scientific, literary and educational nature." Therefore in 1965 the American Occupational Therapy Foundation was established under the laws of the state of Delaware as a philanthropic organization "to administer programs of a charitable, scientific, literary and educational nature." Its work aimed at "advancing the science of occupational therapy, supporting the education and research of its practitioners and increasing the public knowledge and understanding of the profession." This move then allowed the American Occupational Therapy Association to serve as a "business league" and perform the requested noneducational activities.[81]

The emphasis on accountability to consumers caused the national association to develop new standards for education and practice. In 1970 "Standards and Guidelines for an Occupational Therapy Affiliation Program" were drawn up.[82] In 1972 a new definition and statement of function was developed for the profession.[83] In 1973 "Standards for Occupational Therapists Providing Direct Service" were developed and published in the official journal of the association.[84] That same year the revised "Essentials of the Accredited Educational Programs for the Occupational Therapist" were adopted by the American Occupational Therapy Association and the House of Delegates of the American Medical Association.[85] These "Essentials" were approved by the Representative Assembly of the American Occupational Therapy Association in 1977.

The "Essentials of an Approved Educational Program for the Occupational Therapy Assistant" were developed and adopted by the Council of Education of the American Occupational Therapy Association in 1975.[86] These were adopted by the Representative Assembly in 1977.

Since 1972 the Association has adopted numerous position papers including those on consumer involvement,[87] aging,[88] national system of certification for allied health personnel,[89] and national health issues.[90] In October 1975 the Delegate Assembly adopted a resolution authorizing the development of a certification examination for occupational therapy assistants[91] and in April 1976 the Assembly passed a resolution authorizing the use of the certification examination as a partial fulfillment for certification of occupational therapy assistants.[92] The first certification examination was given in June 1977.

In September 1976, new bylaws were adopted by the Association and became effective in November 1976.[93] These bylaws made many changes in the structure and organization of the total Association. They identify the Representative Assembly as the policy-making body, which elects its own officers, with representatives from each state, the Association officers, the second delegate of the World Federation of Occupational Therapists, and the president of the Student Association as voting members of the Assembly. The executive board became the management body with Association officers, Representative Assembly officers, a World Federation delegate, and the president of the Association of Affiliate Presidents as members. The purpose of changes in the bylaws was to make the Association more responsive to the membership and their needs and concerns.

In April 1977, the Representative Assembly adopted a "Definition of Occupational Therapy" for the purpose of licensure. This is to be used as a legal document and not as a philosophical definition for the profession (see Appendix 1). At this same meeting, the Representative Assembly adopted the "Principles of Occupational Therapy Ethics" (see Appendix 2). The ethics statements are to be used as guides for the profession and its practitioners but are not to be used as standards of care expected.

SUMMARY

Although the focus within the profession of occupational therapy has changed, it is evident that there are at least four common propositions that have characterized the profession throughout its history:

1. The use of occupation or purposeful activity can influence the state of health of an individual. Stated another way, people have a need to self-actualize through work or leisure activities; occupational therapy's goal has remained to correct or ameliorate whatever prevents self-actualization.
2. Individuals and their total functioning must be viewed in respect to their own environment and remediation must take into consideration all the physical, psychological, and social factors.
3. Interpersonal relationships are an important factor in the occupational therapy process.
4. Occupational therapy is an adjunct to and has its roots in medicine and must work in cooperation with medical professionals and other persons involved as health care providers to assure maximum benefits for clients.

Being founded on the principles and practices of moral treatment that valued the quality of daily life of disabled people, occupational therapy has focused from its beginning on health and function.

REFERENCES

1. Taylor, G.: Pioneer for Social Justice, 1851–1938; Louise C. Wade. Chicago: University of Chicago Press, 1964, p. 170.
2. Levin, H. L.: Occupational and recreational therapy among the ancients. Occup. Ther. Rehabil. 17:311–316, 1938.
3. Ibid., p. 312.
4. Licht, S.: Occupational Therapy Source Book. Baltimore: Williams & Wilkins Co., 1948, p. 1.
5. Haas, L. J.: Practical Occupational Therapy. Milwaukee: Bruce Publishing Company, 1944, p. 6.
6. Licht: Source Book, p. v.
7. Pinel, P.: Medical philosophical treatise on mental alienation, Paris, 1801. In Licht: Source Book, p. 19.
8. Dunton, W. R., Jr.: Reconstruction Therapy. Philadelphia: W. B. Saunders Co., 1919, p. 20.
9. Licht: Source Book, p. 8.
10. Reil, J. C.: Rhapsodies on the psychic treatment of the insane, Halle, 1803. In Licht: Source Book, pp. 25 and 27.
11. Tuke, S.: Description of the Retreat, an institution near York, for insane persons, York, 1816. In Licht: Source Book, pp. 41–56.
12. Leuret, F.: On the moral treatment of insanity, Paris, 1840. In Licht: Source Book, p. 63.
13. Ibid., p. 9.
14. Haas: Practical Occupational Therapy, p. 11.
15. Kirkbride, T. S.: Report of the Pennsylvania Hospital for the Insane for the years 1841, 1842, and 1843, Philadelphia. Published by order of the Board of Managers, Pennsylvania Hospital, 1841, 1842, 1843.
16. Dunton, W. R., Jr., and Licht, S.: Occupational Therapy, Principles and Practice, ed. 2. Springfield IL: Charles C Thomas, 1957, p. 11.
17. Haas: Practical Occupational Therapy, p. 13.
18. Meyer, A.: The philosophy of occupational therapy. Arch. Occup. Ther. 1:1–10, 1922.
19. Ibid., p. 5.
20. Chicago School of Civics and Philanthropy Yearbook and Bulletin. August 1908–July 1911, p. 98.
21. Tracy, S. E.: Studies in Invalid Occupations—A Manual for Nurses and Attendants. Boston: Whitcomb and Barrows, 1910.
22. Dewey, J.: The School and Society. Chicago: University of Chicago Press, 1900. Paperback ed. 1956, pp. 132–133.
23. Tracy, S. E.: Flier on occupation course offered at Experiment Station for the Study of Invalid Occupations, Jamaica Plains MA, 1914.
24. Hall, H. J.: Occupational Therapy, A New Profession. Concord: The Rumford Press, 1923.
25. Hall, H. J.: Work cure, a report of five years experience at an institution devoted to the therapeutic application of manual work. J.A.M.A. 54:12, 1910.
26. Hall, H. J., and Buck, Mertice, M. C.: The Work of Our Hands—A Study of Occupations for Invalids. New York: Moffat, Yard and Co., 1915.
27. Loomis, B., and Wade, B. D.: Chicago. Occupational Therapy Beginnings: Hull House, The Henry B. Favill School of Occupations and Eleanor Clark Slagle. Special Improvement Grant, U.S. Public Health Services, Allied Health 50579-01, 1973, p. 2.
28. Slagle, E. C.: Occupational therapy. Trained Nurse Hosp. Rev. April 1938, p. 380.
29. Experience of Eleanor Clark Slagle, 1910–1922. Document from Archives, American Occupational Therapy Association, Bethesda MD.
30. Slagle, E. C.: Training Aides for Mental Patients. Papers on occupational therapy. Utica NY: State Hospital Press, 1922, p. 40.
31. Slagle, E. C., and Robeson, H. A.: Syllabus for Training of Nurses in Occupational Therapy. Utica NY: State Hospital Press, 1933, p. 10.
32. Bing, R.: William Rush Dunton, Jr.—American Psychiatrist, a Study in Self. Unpublished doctoral dissertation, University of Maryland, 1961.
33. Dunton, W. R., Jr.: Occupational Therapy—A Manual for Nurses. Philadelphia: W. B. Saunders Co., 1915.
34. Barton, G. E.: Teaching the Sick, A Manual of Occupational Therapy as Re-education. Philadelphia: W. B. Saunders Co., 1919, p. 60.
35. Constitution of the National Society for the Promotion of Occupational Therapy. Baltimore: Sheppard Hospital Press, 1917, p. 1.
36. Historical Documents and Letters, Archives, American Occupational Therapy Association, Bethesda MD.
37. Proceedings of the National Society for the Promotion of Occupational Therapy: First Annual Meeting. Catonsville MD: Spring Grove State Hospital, 1917.
38. Dunton, W. R., Jr.: Occupational therapy. In Barr, D. P.: Barr's Modern Medical Therapy in General Practice, Vol. 1. Baltimore: Williams & Wilkins Co., 1940, p. 697.
39. Dunton, W. R., Jr.: Credo. In Reconstruction Therapy. Philadelphia: W. B. Saunders Co., 1919, p. 10.
40. Then and Now, 1917–1967. American Occupational Therapy Association, 1967.
41. History. Occup. Ther. Rehabil. 19:32, 1940.
42. Circulation of information concerning employment of reconstruction aides. Washington: Medical Department, U.S. Army, January 22, 1918–March 27, 1918.
43. Subjects and lectures for the first class (Reconstruction aides) April 24, 1918 to July 13, 1918. Historical documents from Archives, Boston School of Occupational Therapy, Boston, 1918.
44. Historical documents from Archives, American Occupational Therapy Association, Bethesda MD.
45. Baldwin, B. T.: Occupational Therapy Applied to Restoration of Function of Disabled Joints. Washington DC: Walter Reed Monograph, April 1919, pp. 5–6.

46. Minimum standards for courses of training in occupational therapy. Arch. Occup. Ther. 3:295–298, 1924.
47. Greenman, N. B.: The influence of the university setting on occupational therapy education. Unpublished master's thesis, Tufts College, Boston, 1953.
48. Bowman, E.: Psychology of occupational therapy. Arch. Occup. Ther. 1:172, 1922.
49. Principles of Occupational Therapy. AOTA Bulletin No. 4, 1923.
50. Stern, E. M.: The work cure. Survey Graphic April 1939, pp. 1–4.
51. Personal discussion with Clare S. Spackman and Helen S. Willard.
52. Report of the Committee on Teaching Methods. Occup. Ther. Rehabil. 7:287, 1928.
53. Elwood, E. S.: The National Board of Medical Examiners and medical education and the possible effect of the Board's program on the spread of occupational therapy. Occup. Ther. Rehabil. 6:341–348, 1927.
54. J.A.M.A. 104:1632–1633, 1935; 105:690–691, 1935; 107:683–684, 1936.
55. Fish, M.: Occupational therapy in American colleges. J. Am. Assoc. Collegiate Registrars, October 1945, pp. 21–32.
56. Historical documents from Archives, American Occupational Therapy Association, Bethesda MD.
57. Kahmann, W. C., and West, W.: Occupational therapy in the United States Army hospital, World War II. In Willard, H. S., and Spackman, C. S. (eds.): Principles of Occupational Therapy. Philadelphia: J. B. Lippincott Co., 1947, p. 330.
58. Barton, W. E.: The challenge to occupational therapy. Occup. Ther. Rehabil. 22:262, 1943.
59. Barton, W. E.: Training programs for occupational therapists in the U.S. Army. Occup. Ther. Rehabil. 23:282, 1944.
60. Occupational Therapy. War Department Training Manual 8-291. Washington DC: U.S. Government Printing Office, 1944, p. 1.
61. Cobb, M. R.: Report of the Executive Secretary to the twenty-sixth Annual Meeting of the American Occupational Therapy Association, August, 1946. Occup. Ther. Rehabil. 25:259, 1946.
62. Spackman, C. S.: A history of the practice of occupational therapy for restoration of physical function: 1917–1967. Am. J. Occup. Ther. 22:68–71, 1968.
63. Willard, H. S., and Spackman, C. S. (eds.): Principles of Occupational Therapy. Philadelphia: J. B. Lippincott Co., 1947.
64. Spackman, C. S.: The World Federation of Occupational Therapists 1952–1967. Am. J. Occup. Ther. 21:301–309, 1967.
65. Semrad, E. V.: The emotional needs of the disabled person. Proceedings of the Occupational Therapy Institute, New York. American Occupational Therapy Association, 1956, pp. 28–38.
66. Fidler, G. S., and Fidler, J. W.: Introduction to Psychiatric Occupational Therapy. New York: Macmillan Publishing Co., 1954.
67. Fidler, G. S., and Fidler, J. W.: Occupational Therapy —A Communication Process in Psychiatry. New York: Macmillan Publishing Co., 1963.
68. Gilette, N. R.: Changing methods in the treatment of psychosocial dysfunction. Am. J. Occup. Ther. 21:230, 1967.
69. West, W.: Professional responsibility in times of change. Am. J. Occup. Ther. 22:9, 1968.
70. Final Report, Project Committee on Recognition of Occupational Therapy Assistants. Am. J. Occup. Ther. 13:269, 1958.
71. Crampton, M. W.: Educational upheaval for occupational therapy assistants. Am. J. Occup. Ther. 21:317, 1967.
72. Mazer, J.: The occupational therapist as consultant. Am. J. Occup. Ther. 23:417–421, 1969.
73. Willard, H. S., and Spackman, C. S. (eds.): Occupational Therapy, ed. 4. Philadelphia: J. B. Lippincott Co., 1971, p. 380.
74. Ayres, A. J.: The development of perceptual motor abilities: a theoretical basis for treatment of dysfunction. Eleanor Clark Slagle Lecture presented at AOTA Conference, October 1963, St. Louis. Am. J. Occup. Ther. 17:221, 1963.
75. Ayres, A. J.: Sensory Integration and Learning Disorders. Los Angeles: Western Psychological Services, 1972, p. 8.
76. Reilly, M.: The educational process. Am. J. Occup. Ther. 23:303, 1969.
77. Laukaran, V. H.: Toward a model of occupational therapy for community health. Am. J. Occup. Ther. 31:71, 1977.
78. West, W.: The occupational therapist's changing responsibility to the community. Am. J. Occup. Ther. 21:312, 1967.
79. Mosey, A. C.: Three Frames of Reference for Mental Health. Thorofare NJ: Charles B. Slack, 1970, pp. v., 15–17.
80. Mosey, A. C.: An alternative: the biopsychosocial model. Am. J. Occup. Ther. 23:140, 1974.
81. American Occupational Therapy Foundation—The First Decade 1965–1975. Am. J. Occup. Ther. 29:636, 1975.
82. Standards and guidelines on occupational therapy affiliation program. AOTA Committee on Basic Professional Education. Am. J. Occup. Ther. 25:314–316, 1971.
83. Occupational therapy: its definition and functions. Am. J. Occup. Ther. 26:204–205, 1972.
84. Standards for occupational therapists providing direct service. Am. J. Occup. Ther. 28:237. 1974.
85. Essentials of an accredited educational program for the occupational therapist. Am. J. Occup. Ther. 29: 485–496, 1975.
86. Essentials of an approved educational program for the

occupational therapy assistant. Am. J. Occup. Ther. 30:245–261, 1976.
87. Position paper on Consumer Involvement. Am. J. Occup. Ther. 27:48, 1972.
88. Position paper on Aging. Am. J. Occup. Ther. 28:564, 1974.
89. National system of certification of allied health personnel. Am. J. Occup. Ther. 30:50, 1976.
90. Policy statement on national health issues. Delegate Assembly Minutes. Am. J. Occup. Ther. 31:110, 1977.
91. Resolution #465-75. Delegate Assembly Minutes. Am. J. Occup. Ther. 30:177, 1976.
92. Resolution #471-76. Delegate Assembly Minutes. Am. J. Occup. Ther. 30:587, 1976.
93. AOTA Bylaws. Am. J. Occup. Ther. 31:111–118, 1977.

Part Two

Theory and Philosophy

2

Current Basis for Theory and Philosophy of Occupational Therapy

Helen L. Hopkins

Occupational therapy is the art and science of directing man's participation in selected tasks to restore, reinforce and enhance performance, facilitate learning of those skills and functions essential for adaptation and productivity, diminish or correct pathology, and to promote and maintain health. Its fundamental concern is the capacity, throughout the life span, to perform with satisfaction to self and others those tasks and roles essential to productive living and to the mastery of self and the environment.[1]

Throughout its history the focus of the occupational therapy profession has been on the nature of the individual in relation to society and the world in which the person lives. The body of knowledge in occupational therapy is drawn from several broad scientific areas including biological and behavioral sciences, sociology, and anthropology. Knowledge in these areas is continually expanding and being modified, making it mandatory that occupational therapy be responsive and change. Occupational therapy uses the broad knowledge areas as its theoretical underpinnings and can be effective only in proportion to the accuracy of these knowledge bases. Theoretical propositions presently are being built upon these broad knowledge areas to form the beginning of occupational therapy's unique body of knowledge. Theoretical propositions by Ayres, Reilly, and Mosey are among the propositions that can be identified as occupational therapy's beginning knowledge base.

Occupational therapy's concern still is for the health and function of each individual within his or her own environment. It is committed to the uniqueness of the individual and fosters the growth and development of each person. Using both medical and social vantage points, the occupational therapist is committed to providing for development and maintenance of the highest potential in the biological, psychological, and social functioning of each individual. It is also recognized that there is a function-dysfunction continuum that must be considered. Occupational therapy provides intervention to alleviate dysfunction and to maintain the highest level of function in all aspects of living through the use of purposeful activity.

Because occupational therapy is concerned with

both human function throughout the life span and the uniqueness of the individual, it is essential that practice be based on the normal development process. The nature of the individual and the function-dysfunction continuum, along with pathological processes that may impinge on function, must be understood so that appropriate occupational therapy intervention procedures may be determined. The impact of purposeful activity on the human organism must be understood so that age-appropriate activities may be utilized in the intervention process.

The occupational therapy process requires problem identification, data collection, and provision of various options for intervention depending on pathological or psychosocial problems, the stage of development, and individual preferences, interests, and expertise. On the basis of data collected and options available, choices must be made and programs implemented for the resolution of problems. Thus it would seem that the occupational therapy process may be one of inductive reasoning or reasoning based on deriving conclusions on the basis of data gathered. There are many decisions, however, that are made on the basis of deductive reasoning or making inferences from general principles that have been learned. Whether the decision making done during the intervention process is based on inductive or deductive reasoning, it can be assumed that occupational therapy is a problem-solving approach to intervention.

The profession as a whole has not identified the characteristics of occupational therapy which make it unique. No single perspective has been identified and accepted by the total profession. Several theoretical vantage points have been identified and are being used. These include several *developmental approaches*, i.e., Ayres' sensory integrative approach, Mosey's developmental approach, and Rood's neurophysiological approach; *rehabilitation/habilitation approach*, and Reilly's *occupational behavior approach*. Each approach is still in the process of being researched and developed in order to provide regulation and validation. Each approach is attempting to identify a valid theoretical base for occupational therapy. These approaches may change as research validates, negates, or challenges them. Developments and changes in these occupational therapy approaches, and changes in the broad knowledge bases on which we build will provide for new options and new intervention possibilities.

Any specific intervention approach, if it is to be considered occupational therapy, must be in synchronization with the basic premises of the profession. In trying to equate the basic premises of the profession with schools of philosophical thought it would seem that the profession is eclectic in its philosophy.[2,3] Since the profession is committed to the uniqueness of individuals and fosters the growth and development of each person, one of its bases must be the *human development* process with examination of all aspects that make individuals unique. The profession is also concerned with human nature, the function-dysfunction continuum, and pathological processes and other problems that impinge on function; thus occupational therapy has a *medical base*. Since occupational therapy practice is based on occupying those we work with in activity to prevent regression and enhance function, occupational therapy includes the impact of activity on the human organism; thus the *activity process* becomes one of the required bases of the profession. This then requires three bases of knowledge for the profession—*the human development process, the medical base*, and *the activity process*. These three bases will be discussed in depth in the remainder of Part 2.

REFERENCES

1. Occupational therapy: Its definition and function. Am. J. Occup. Ther. 26:204, 1972.
2. Dunning, R. E.: Philosophy and occupational therapy. Am. J. Occup. Ther. 27:18–23, 1973.
3. Owen, C. M.: An analysis of the philosophy of occupational therapy. Am. J. Occup. Ther. 22:502–505, 1968.

3

The Human Development Process

section 1 / Human Development / Mary Margaret Daub

INTRODUCTION

What Is Human Development?

Human beings grow and mature, fulfilling their needs and striving to interact with their environment. They gain competence from this process of interaction and adaptation, gradually building a realistic sense of self-worth. Thus, each person becomes a unique individual with the potential of self-actualization.

Human development can be defined as changes in the structure, thought, or behavior of a person which occur as a function of both biological and environmental influences.[1] These changes may be quantitative or qualitative. Quantitative changes, such as height, physical skills, and vocabulary are easily understood and measured. Qualitative changes are not so easily measured because they include a subjective element; there is no scale on which to weigh the influence of social interactions, the significance of dreams, or the level of a child's self-awareness.

This quantitative and qualitative development involves an ongoing, orderly process that continues from conception to death.

How Is Human Development Studied?

Human development can be studied from many perspectives. Biologists, psychologists, epistemologists, anthropologists, and others investigate the principles and processes of human development but from varied points of view.

Methods of study also differ. We can study and experiment with animal behavior and draw implications concerning human behavior. We can study human behavior in an experimental setting and draw conclusions from controlled situations. We can do a longitudinal study (observation of the same individual over an extended period of time) or a cross-sectional study of behavior (observation of different individuals of different ages at one time. We can follow a specific trait or pattern of behavior in various cultures and construct cross-cultural hypotheses concerning development.

For our immediate purposes, we will view the following developmental aspects of a person which contribute and interrelate to make him or her such a miraculous and complex entity: physical, sensory, perceptual, emotional, cognitive, cultural, and social. As the individual grows, these aspects mature and expand along a developmental continuum. Although the aspects are distinct from each other at one level, they are dynamically interrelated and interdependent.

Why Study Human Development?

Occupational therapists work with individuals who have had an interruption in one or more areas of development somewhere along the life continuum. In order to provide a meaningful service to these individuals, the therapist must understand the underlying principles of man's growth and function and the sequences of growth and behavior that are somewhat predictable for normal human development. (For our purposes, normal is determined by that wide range of data collected for a particular population within a given time and culture referring to a specific area or segment of development.)

The occupational therapist is an agent of change. The client, often against severe odds, must change and adapt within his or her life situation. The therapist can directly influence the quality of that change. Therefore, the therapist must know the range and potential for change available and must have a working knowledge of those concepts of change and adaptation inherent in the study of human development.

The primary motivation is pragmatic; the normal must be learned in order to assist clients with a disruption in the normal pattern of development. But a second motivation inevitably lures us—the age-old curiosity about who I am, how I began, and how I can grow and change. The study of development sheds light on these questions.

Factors that Influence Human Development

Biological and environmental influences act upon each individual making up the individual's unique gestalt. Biological influences include stages of growth, maturation, and aging. Growth is increase in size, function, or complexity up to some point of optimal maturity. Maturation is the emergence of an organism's genetic potential; it consists of a series of preprogrammed changes which comprise alterations not only in the organism's structure and form but also in its complexity, integration, organization, and function. Aging is biological evolution beyond the point of optimal maturity.[2]

Environmental influences touch everyone at each moment of the day. Sensory input and interpersonal interactions within the home and community can create physiological and emotional stress or comfort. These major influences will be studied further as they relate to learning and the developmental process.

General Principles of Human Development

There are some general principles and issues of human growth and development that must be understood before looking closer at specific areas of normal human growth.

1. *Development is orderly, predictable, sequential, and cumulative.* Even though an individual is unique, each possesses particular patterns of behavior following a definite sequence. For example, a child is capable of rolling over before sitting, sitting before standing, and standing before walking. With maturation, development expands by building on previous acquisitions. Developed behaviors continue to influence the future functioning of the emerging being. Since development is cumulative, a child's experiences may have definitive effects on his behavior in adult life.

2. *Each child develops at a different pace.* There is a wide range of individual differences along the normal continuum. Normative data show, for example, that by 26 months a child should be able to combine two words. In reality, some children are speaking by that time, some are not. For example, at two years, Megan is happily combining words into phrases and short sentences: "Me go store," "Mommy give candy." However, Megan's friend Mike speaks only when his need is pressing and then only the short effective word or syllable: "wawa" when he wants a drink, "bye" when he would like to go outside. This does not necessarily mean that Mike has a developmental problem. Other operant factors may be: (1) amount of stimulation in the home environment and (2) amount and intensity of physical or psychological stress he may be encountering. These factors may cause only a temporary delay in the development of a particular function. Perhaps Mike's assumed hesitant speech fol-

lows a recent bout with measles. Once his health and confidence are restored, he may quickly return to a more age-appropriate pattern of speech.

3. *The expectation of others affects a child's behavior.* Mike's parents, for example, may value verbal expression and expect Mike to be more verbal than he is. On the other hand, his sister and brother (siblings) anticipate his needs and often do not allow Mike the opportunity to verbalize his requests.

4. *At any one stage of development a child might be placing particular emphasis on one aspect at the expense of another.* For example, a 3-year old may be developing gross motor skills in play and doing little in the area of fine motor skills. This emphasis may be a function of maturation, the desire to learn a specific skill, or a result of environmental/cultural influences. Chess proposes eight areas[3] in which individual differences are most conspicuous:

> *Activity level.* Children vary in their level of movement and activity (even when asleep).
>
> *Regularity.* Children have different "biological clocks" in terms of self-imposed schedules and their daily demands of themselves and others.
>
> *Adaptability to routine changes.* Some children readily accept changes in schedules; others bitterly resist the new and different.
>
> *Level of sensory threshold.* Some children can sleep through a thunderstorm while others awake at the slightest noise.
>
> *Positive or negative mood.* Some children appear either happy or sad no matter what the situation.
>
> *Intensity of response.* Some children's responses are always noisy, bellowing, and active (high energy level); some have mild responses even when angry (low energy level).
>
> *Distractibility.* Some children study with radio and television blaring; some require almost absolute quiet in order to study effectively.
>
> *Persistency.* Some children just sit for hours and refuse to give up until the task is finished or solved. Some leave trails of unfinished tasks and are always looking for something new.

5. *The behavior of a child does not consistently "improve"; it seems to alternate between periods of equilibrium (a good balance) and disequilibrium (less balance) (Fig. 3-1).* The level of balance a child

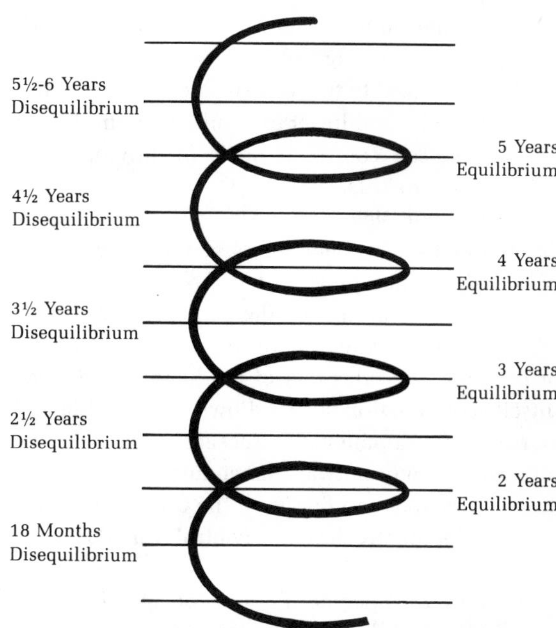

FIGURE 3-1. Spiral of equilibrium and disequilibrium. From Ames, L. B.: Child Care and Development. Philadelphia: J. B. Lippincott Co., 1970, p. 5. Used with permission.

reaches is dependent on his/her stage of maturation and on effective interaction within the environment.

The question then arises: How do I know when a child has a developmental delay?

1. Be a keen observer. Observational skills can be learned. Train yourself to become more aware of your human and nonhuman environment.
2. Know the normal sequences of maturation and the resultant behaviors.
3. Know the extremes of the normative scales, since they may be indicators of a delay or dysfunction.
4. Look at the child as a *total* being.

A person's action or reaction is not a function of any one aspect of human development; rather, it is a function of the relationships of all areas of development at any given point in his or her life span.

Principles of Maturation

There are certain principles of maturation that tend to be relatively independent of environmental influences. They are:

1. *Cephalocaudal Pattern of Development.* Muscular development, control, and coordination progress from the head to the feet. Head control precedes that of the trunk and lower extremities. A child must have good head control if he is to develop other *effective* motor skills.

2. *Proximal-Distal and Medial(Rostral)-Lateral Patterns of Development.* Parts of the body closest (proximal) to the spine tend to be controlled in a coordinated manner before the parts farthest (distal) away from it. Coordination of shoulder musculature, for example, precedes that of the hand and fingers. Muscle coordination also follows a medial-lateral course of development: it proceeds from the midpoint of the body outward (anatomical position). A child is able to grasp first with the ulnar side of his hand, and gradually develops control from the radial side.

3. *Mass to Specific Pattern of Development.* Initially much of the motor activity of the infant consists of whole body movement. With maturity, these undifferentiated and generalized mass responses become more specific. At first the neonate moves his arms freely in no specific pattern; in a few months he will be able to grasp an object.

4. *Gross Motor to Fine Motor Pattern of Development.* Since control of proximal musculature precedes that of distal musculature, it follows that mastery of the larger muscles precedes mastery of the smaller muscles. This mastery must then become even more refined and definitive to allow for the acquisition of skills.

These four principles governing growth are not static but are continuously influencing motor development.

THEORETICAL FOUNDATIONS

Learning Theory

Learning is the basic developmental process by which an individual's behavior is changed by the environment. Learning is relatively permanent change in behavior or in the capacity for behavior resulting from either experience or practice.[4] This change occurs through experience and repetition. Psychologists have developed theories and paradigms to account for an individual's ability to adapt within his or her life space. Their theories serve as a framework for understanding varied aspects of human development.

Behavioral Theory

Some learning theorists view the individual as a purely responsive being, a mechanistic result of present and past environments. They observe the individual making responses to stimuli but give little regard to interpreting underlying reasons for those responses. Learning theorists view mankind within narrow parameters, assuming that behavior is a function of immediate stimuli. For them, learning takes place via respondent (classical) and/or operant conditioning.

In *classical conditioning:* (1) Two stimuli are presented *at the same time.* One is reinforcing (e.g., food); the other is irrelevant (e.g., sound of refrigerator door). This leads to: (2) The expectation of reinforcement, and concomitant automatic response (e.g., salivation), are associated with the irrelevant stimulus. (*Learning has taken place.*) Thus: (3) The irrelevant stimulus is presented without the reinforcing stimulus and there is a response.

In *operant conditioning:* (1) Reinforcement (e.g., praise or candy) is presented *following* behavior. Therefore: (2) Reinforcement is associated with the behavior. (*Learning has taken place.*) Thus: (3) Behavior is repeated.

For the learning theorists, learning is a direct result of one or the other of these processes. In reality, even within the limitations of this theory, most learning would probably combine the two processes.

Social Learning Theory

The social learning theory is an outgrowth of learning theory. Its proponents believe that most learning takes place through observing behavior and the effects of behavior. They attempt to explain why mankind uses models to learn social traits and how a socially acceptable repertoire of behaviors is developed. Research in this area proves to be very interesting. In 1963 Bandura, Ross, and Ross[5] showed children films that demonstrated levels of aggressive behavior. One group saw this behavior rewarded, another saw it punished, another saw nonaggressive play, and still another saw no film. Results indicated that children who saw aggressive behavior rewarded were more aggressive in play, while those who saw it punished tended to avoid aggressive play.

Although the learning theorists have given developmentalists volumes of empirically based research explaining human behavior, the types of behavior that lend themselves to experimental methods are limited. These theorists cannot explain complex qualitative behaviors such as emotions or individual differences. Thus the social learning theory is best applied to specific behaviors rather than to the total area of development.

Psychoanalytical Theory

Sigmund Freud, Erik Erikson, the NeoFreudians, and the ego psychologists deal primarily with emotional and personality development.

Sigmund Freud

Freud looks at the unconscious biological drives as the primary forces behind human behavior. Personality development, according to Freud, occurs in five psychosexual stages. The first three, *oral stage*, *anal stage*, and *phallic stage*, center around areas of the body which at each stage become a center for pleasure. These stages are followed by the *latency* and *genital stages*, during which the personality is influenced by degrees of sexual interest, socialization, and an evolving focus on life goals. Freud sets the stage for the explanation of development of an individual's unconscious mind and its relationship to the ability to function.

Erik Erikson

A NeoFreudian, Erikson expands Freud's theory to include the societal environment. He focuses on human psychosocial development. Erikson sees personality development as progressively unfolding throughout the life cycle. He does not place paramount importance on childhood experiences as did Freud. His eight stages of development are delineated by eight emotional crises or issues that must be resolved by the person (Table 3-1).

Table 3-1. Erikson's eight emotional issues.

Stages	*Ages*
Trust—Mistrust	0– 1
Autonomy—Shame	1– 3
Initiative—Guilt	4– 5
Industry—Inferiority	6–11
Identity—Role Diffusion	12–18
Intimacy—Isolation	young adult
Generativity—Stagnation	middle age
Ego Integrity—Despair	aging

The resolution of these issues is the balance between the negative and positive poles of each stage. This resolution and its importance at any one point in life is a function of the individual's relationship to his place in his social and cultural environment. How a person resolves a crisis directly affects the quality of his or her ability to deal with a subsequent developmental issue. Further, Erikson believes that these crises may emerge throughout life.

The basic strength of theorists such as Freud and Erikson is their willingness to look at the whole person and at the conscious and unconscious factors of emotional development. They deal with interpersonal relationships particularly as they relate to childhood experiences.

The weakness of psychoanalytical theory lies in the difficulty of defining parameters of development and of validating research. Most data is gleaned from adults whose subjective reconstruction of their childhood experiences may lead to invalid or vague conclusions.

Cognitive Theory

Jean Piaget

Piaget, biologist-epistemologist, investigates the origin, nature, methods, and limits of human knowledge (Table 3-2).

In contrast to the learning theorists, Piaget sees the human being as active, alert, and capable. A person processes information rather than merely receiving it. He does more than respond to stimuli; he gives structure and meaning to stimuli. Piaget postulates that until a certain age, children form judgments via their perceptual world rather than via principles of logic: "What you see is what you get." If the child's perceptions and experiences (schemata—methods of processing information) fit a structure within his mind they are assimilated or understood. If the information received does not fit

Table 3-2. The continuum of cognitive development.

Modality of intelligence	*Phases*	*Stages*	*Approximate chronological age*
Sensorimotor intelligence	Sensorimotor Phase	1. Use of reflexes	0 to 1 month
		2. First habits and primary circular reactions	1 to 4½ months
		3. Coordination of vision and prehension, secondary circular reactions	4½ to 9 months
		4. Coordination of secondary schemata and their application to new situations	9 to 12 months
		5. Differentiation of action schemata through tertiary circular reactions, discovery of new means	12 to 18 months
		6. First internalization of schemata and solution of some problems by deduction	18 to 24 months
Representative intelligence by means of concrete operations	Preconceptual Phase	1. Appearance of symbolic function and the beginning of internalized actions accompanied by representation	2 to 4 years
	Intuitive Thought Phase	2. Representational organizations based on either static configurations or on assimilation to one's own action	4 to 5½ years
		3. Articulated representational regulations	5½ to 7 years
	Concrete Operational Phase	1. Simple operations (classifications, seriations, term-by-term correspondences, etc.)	7 to 9 years
		2. Whole systems (Euclidian coordinates, projective concepts, simultaneity)	9 to 11 years
Representative intelligence by means of formal operations	Formal Operational Phase	1. Hypothetico-deductive logic and combinatorial operations	11 to 14 years
		2. Structure of "lattice" and the group of 4 transformations	14 years—on

From Maier, Henry W. (ed.): *Three Theories of Child Development: The Contributions of Erik H. Erikson, Jean Piaget and Robert R. Sears,* revised ed. New York: Harper & Row, Publishers, 1969, p. 155. Reprinted with permission. The source was Piaget's paper: Les Stades du Developpement intellectuel de l'Enfant et de l'Adolescent (1956). Adapted from Table 1, Intelligence is an ultimate goal, in Décarié, T. G.: *Intelligence and Affectivity in Early Childhood.* New York: International Universities Press, 1965, p. 15. Reprinted with permission.

existing structure, the mind must change in order to accommodate to the new experience. The schemata of a child expand as he/she grows. A person continuously adjusts his or her schemata in order to assimilate and accommodate new information. The human mind seeks equilibrium between assimilation and accommodation just as the human body seeks biological homeostasis.

As the child grows, his structural abilities to accommodate to new information grow also. Piaget sees this as occurring in four major steps. The steps and mode of learning for each follow:

1. Sensorimotor Period—body and movement
2. Preoperational Period—imagery
3. Concrete Operational Period—concrete human/nonhuman environment
4. Formal Operational Period—abstraction

Jerome Bruner

Bruner, also a cognitive theorist, investigates the individual as an artist (aesthetic being) and as a scientist (problem solver). Like Piaget, he sees the qualitative changes in the cognitive structures corresponding to biological growth. Both see the mind developing in stages. Bruner describes three stages and the modes of learning:

1. Enactive Stage—the infant learns through action

2. Iconic Stage—the use and development of imagery
3. Symbolic Stage—the use of language to relate

Piaget and Bruner differ on the role of language in development. Piaget views thought as preceding language skill while Bruner sees language as a causative factor in acquiring problem-solving ability.

Unlike learning theorists, cognitive theorists attempt to explain that the individual is motivated by his or her own basic competence and not merely by a stimulus-response reaction.[6] They also account for the role of such things as values, beliefs, and attitudes.

The major concern of cognitive theory is intellectual development; it does not explain all of human behavior (for example, social, emotional, and personality development). However, some of its proponents are now investigating these areas.

Humanistic Self-Theory of Self-Development

Humanistic psychologists react to the environmental determinism of learning and psychoanalytic theorists. Their primary focus is the individual's concept of *self*. They see man as self-determining and creative. Their aim is to maximize human potential. These theorists view each individual optimistically as a function of the individual's self. "Man experiences himself as well as others as spontaneously self-determining and creatively striving toward a goal."[7]

Abraham Maslow

Maslow stresses that each person has an innate need for self-actualization. It is possible to attain this innate goal only when a well-integrated individual has satisfied "lower needs" such as safety, love, food, and shelter.

Carl Rogers

Rogers, another humanist, is concerned with helping each individual realize his/her own potential by creating an interpersonal climate for growth with characteristics such as empathy, unconditional willingness to accept a person as he or she is, and a genuine involvement in the person's growth. The strength of this relatively new approach to human development is its concern with real-life situations. Humanistic theory is becoming an important consideration in educational programs for children although its primary concern is adult adjustment. It does not, however, incorporate a method for achieving self-actualization.

Ethology

Ethologists study humans and animals in their natural environments and view them as having evolved similar behavior traits. They think it possible that humans, like other animals, have inherited behavior patterns. Ethologists do not ignore the history and the situation of behavior patterns, but essentially they are looking at behavior in terms of preserving the individual or the species within the evolution of civilization.

Confronted with the situation of a child crying, an ethologist considers four components: *immediate cause*—hunger; *historical cause*—child was fed when she cried in the past; *adaptive cause*—cry triggers an alarm for the mother to get food; *evolutionary cause*—child is immobile, she cannot run to her mother, and so crying is a dominant response.

Ethology is an interesting and relatively new way of studying human behavior. It presupposes that animal behavior is a valid indicator of human behavior. A growing interest in its methods and principles indicates that ethology will play an increasing role in the study of human development.

Maturational Theory

Arnold Gesell

Gesell purports that the baby's behavior is modified as a consequence of physiological maturation. He feels that the child requires only general support and attention from the outside environment in order to develop normally. Gesell emphasizes the stability and conservatism of growth. "All things considered, the inevitableness and surety of maturation are the most impressive characteristics of his early development. It is the hereditary ballast which conserves and stabilizes the growth of each individual infant."[8]

Gesell developed normative data about a child's gross motor, fine motor, adaptive skill, language, and social development as they relate to maturation of the central nervous system. He provides actual chronological scales for the parameters of normal development against which possible developmental delays can be detected. Such scales may serve the occupational therapist as a base line for setting occupational therapy goals and plans. Data collected from a large population of children evaluated by such scales may serve as a basis for research in child development.

Normative data are and must be updated continually. Scales must be used cautiously. A therapist has to know the type of population on which the scale was standardized and when it was developed. Many scales are not done cross-culturally and may be invalid for certain groups of children.

Why Theories of Human Development Are Important to the Occupational Therapist

1. Theories serve as an organizing mechanism. They attempt to sort out some of the complex factors in development.
2. Theories provide a basis for frames of reference from which one can develop therapeutic program objectives and treatment.
3. Theories are a basis for the generation of research that is needed in the field of occupational therapy.
4. Knowledge of different theories extends insight into human behavior, presenting alternative explanations of behavior on which to base treatment goals.
5. Theories provide the bases for justification and accountability. In essence, a theory becomes the rationale for our treatment process.

If adhering to a single theory to the exclusion of others the therapist must keep in mind that:

1. No one theory accounts for each and every aspect of the developmental process; therefore, the therapist must fully understand the parameters of any chosen theory.
2. The therapist must be able to translate the theory effectively into occupational therapy application.
3. Strict adherence to just one theory does not always allow for individual differences.
4. A single-theory approach may narrow a therapist's perspective and limit professional growth potential.

On the other hand, when a therapist chooses an eclectic approach, that is, bases a rationale on varied sources or theories, caution is advised because:

1. In order to be truly eclectic, the therapist must be thoroughly versed in each theory. "A little knowledge" here can be truly dangerous.
2. The therapist must know the advantages and limitations of these theories so as to present a clearly defined rationale for client treatment.

No matter which approach is chosen, it is imperative that everyone involved in the treatment process (1) know what rationale is being used, (2) understand how the rationale can be translated into occupational therapy practice, (3) be clear about how this treatment can be adapted to the individual client's needs, and (4) concur with the adoption of this rationale as a basis for treatment.

PRENATAL DEVELOPMENT

Aristotle observed the growth of the chick embryo. He surmised that the embryo was a mixture of seminal fluid and menstrual blood and that the embryo carried in the female was stimulated into growth by the male. Five hundred years later Galen purported a different theory. He believed that a miniature baby was encased in the egg, to be "uncased" by the male before growth could begin. This imaginative theory dominated scientific thought for 1500 years.

In 1677 Van Leewenhoek observed the movement of the male sperm. This discovery led to two major theories of prenatal development in the seventeenth and eighteenth centuries. The *ovists* believed that a prefabricated baby was contained in the mother's egg, to be stimulated into growth by the sperm. The *homunculists* believed that a baby was formed in the tip of the sperm, the womb serving as the incubator environment for growth.

These theories prevailed until 1759 when Wolff postulated that both the male and female contributed equally to the growth of the human organism. Approximately 50 years later the human ovum was seen under the microscope. It was not until 1930, however, that the ripened human egg and sperm were observed. Finally, in 1944, scientists witnessed the union of the egg and sperm. Since that time a myriad of knowledge about prenatal development has been accumulated, so that now we have a clear picture of human development from a single cell to a person.

Periods of Prenatal Development

Following fertilization of the ovum, there is a gestation period of 266 days (with a grace period of 11 days). The first phase (2 weeks) of prenatal growth is the *germinal period*. This is primarily a time of cell division and differentiation. Once the growing cell is fully implanted in the wall of the uterus, the *embryonic period* begins. During the embryonic period (8 weeks), structures and organs are formed and differentiated. Approximately twelve weeks following conception the *fetal period* begins: the first bone cells are developed, and growth continues until birth.

These first several weeks of development are marked by the emergence of physical characteristics. Approximately twenty-six days following conception a body form is evolving and there is the beginning of arm and leg buds. Two days later the arms are developing at a greater rate than the legs. By the end of the first month, the details of the head with rudimentary eyes, ears, mouth, and brain are seen faintly. The brain already shows primitive specialization. There is also a primitive heart and umbilical cord as well as such organs as the liver, kidney, and stomach. The primitive embryo is now ¼ to ½ inch long, the size of half a pea. In one month's time the embryo is 10,000 times larger than the fertilized egg.[9]

By the end of the second month the embryo has familiar features: face, eyes, ears, nose, lips, tongue, muscles, and finally skin covering. Flanagan states that the developing arms are no bigger than exclamation points, but they have discernible fingers and thumbs. The legs have knees, ankles, and toes. All organs in the body are formed. The brain sends out impulses, the muscles and nerves are working together, and the heart is beating regularly and steadily. The endocrine system is functioning and so are the stomach, liver, and kidneys. Even isolated reflexes can be elicited. In several months these primitive systems will be truly functional.

The third month after conception traditionally marks the beginning of the fetal period. By the end of this month the fetus has become active. It can kick, turn, close fingers, move its thumb into opposition, and open its mouth, although its eyelids are still closed. This period is marked by refinements of facial and extremity features. The palate and lips are formed and fused. Sexual differentiation is beginning.

The fourth month is a period of growth in which the lower body parts develop more rapidly. The fetus weighs approximately 4 ounces and is 6 inches long. Its muscles and reflexive capabilities are maturing. The mother can now feel a "quickening" movement.

The fifth month is a stage of continued refinement. There is an increase in spontaneous activity. Its movements are markedly perceived by the mother. The fetus sleeps and wakes. However, its respiratory system is still too immature for life outside the uterus.

In the sixth month the eyelids of the fetus open. Its eyes are formed and capable of movements (lateral and vertical). Taste buds have developed, as have eyelashes and brows. The fetus has a marked grasp reflex. It now weighs approximately 1½ pounds and is 12 to 14 inches long. But its breathing patterns are irregular; it can usually survive for only twenty-four hours outside the womb.

During the seventh month the cerebral hemispheres cover almost all the brain and the organism can make specialized responses. If born now, the child can survive in a sheltered environment.

The eighth and ninth months are periods of refinement of function. The immune system of the fetus matures, enabling it to sustain independent life more safely when it is born.

During gestation, the fetus has grown from 1 to 200 million cells and its weight at birth is 600 billion times greater than its conceptual weight.[10] (If we were to continue to grow at our prenatal rate until adulthood, we would be 20 feet tall and our weight would exceed the earth's weight by many million times.)

Given this brief account of normal prenatal activity, we must consider those factors of heredity and environment which may affect and/or alter normal growth and development.

Inherited and Environmental Influences

Although the uterus is a relatively safe and stable environment, it is not immune to environmental factors. The seriousness of the effect of these factors depends on (1) the type of influence, (2) the intensity of the influence, and (3) the time the influence was introduced.

Since the germinal and embryonic stages are formation and differentiation periods, this first trimester of pregnancy (first 12 weeks) is critical in development. If normal growth is interrupted during this time, defects can originate. Major environmental influences include:

1. Ingestion of certain agents or drugs.
2. Factors in maternal health and nutrition such as vitamin deficiency or excess, endocrine levels, exposure to roentgen rays, exposure to virus and bacteria, emotional state of the mother (brings about chemical changes that may cross the placental barrier), Rh factor, composite factors, and cultural influences.

Hereditary factors also contribute to the integrity of the growing organism. It is imperative that the therapist understand (1) the basis of genetic functioning, (2) implications of genetic malfunctioning on the developing organism, and (3) those dysfunctions that are a direct result of genetic inheritance.

Scientists have researched DNA (deoxyribonucleic acid), the complex molecules which make up the genes. They have shown how the information transmitted by the genes determines the functions of the body. The increased knowledge in this area has shed light on those developmental traits that have specific hereditary components. These components are dependent on one's autosomal, dominant, and recessive inheritance, sex-linked inheritance, and chromosomal integrity. Genetic make-up delineates the parameters for development. Environmental factors influence the quality and extent to which heredity affects the potential for growth.

The nature/nurture controversy or the relationship and extent of hereditary and environmental factors on the individual continues. In a classic article on the nature/nurture question Anastasi says "the nature and extent of the influence of each type of factor depends on the contribution of the others."[11]

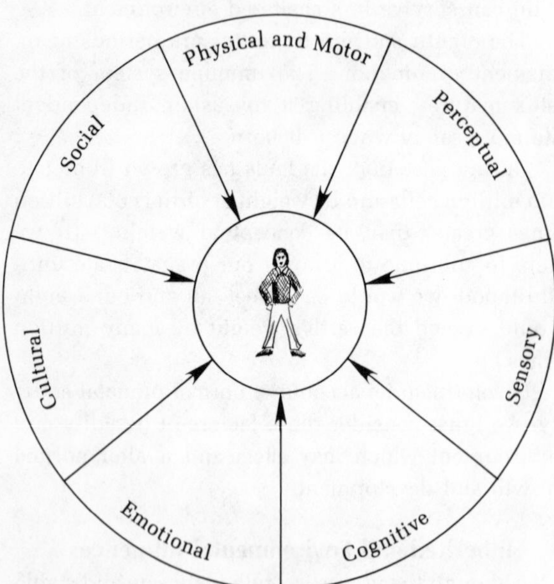

FIGURE 3-2. The developmental wheel.

THE DEVELOPMENTAL CONTINUUM

Fifteen or twenty years ago an infant was considered a dependent creature who could not see, hear, or interact within the environment. Today we know that the infant and growing child possesses a vast repertoire of capabilities.

This section presents an overview and appreciation of a normal child's development from birth to adulthood, based on major developmental aspects (Fig. 3-2). Not all aspects will be considered at each milestone of growth, only those considered most significant for that stage.

To enliven this study, we will observe an imaginary child, Leslie, with her family and friends. Leslie, the typical child, is a prototype of any normal child traversing the developmental continuum.

Infancy

The Neonate

Early one morning, Leslie abandons the warm, dark, comfortable womb of her mother and struggles her way into a cool, bright, noisy, and expectant world. Her lusty protests elicit smiles of relief from her waiting audience but add little to her red scrunched-up cheese-coated natural beauty.

The difficult trip down the birth canal leaves most neonates looking a little the worse for wear. The head may be somewhat misshapen as a result of pressure and/or forceps delivery. Face and eyes are usually puffy and the limbs, particularly the feet, may be in an awkward position. The newborn must adjust to several drastic changes in life style: a drop in body temperature, an external mode of nourishment, a different metabolic system, and a redirection of oxygen flow. (Adjustment to change in oxygen concentration is as great as that experienced by a mountain-climber descending from Mt. Everest to Katmandu.)

Leslie is a full-term neonate; she measures 20 inches and weighs 7 pounds. (Normal range: 19 to 22 inches; 5½ to 9½ pounds.) Before she is five minutes old, her general health is evaluated by the Apgar Test (see Table 3-3). Other similar tests may be used. Special attention is given to general reflex response, heart rate, muscle tone, and color. A score of 7 or more indicates that her health is within normal limits.[12]

Leslie can see within an 8 to 12 inch range and soon after birth prefers complex patterns to simple ones. She may show a preference for the human face and for clear rather than blurred images.

Fantz, among others, has made marvelous discoveries about the visual ability of infants. In one test he presented simple pattern stimuli to infants and found there was significant preference for the complex pattern. He also presented three different oval images to forty-nine infants ranging in age from four days to six months. The images included (1) a stylized human face, (2) the same features of the stylized face in a scrambled pattern, and (3) an oval with a solid dark patch at one end. All the infants tested showed a definite preference for the human face. Further studies found that the infants selectively focus on the eye region of the face before encompassing the entire face.[13]

Leslie can detect changes in temperature and distinguish tastes. Even as early as the third or fourth day she demonstrates a preference for sweet and a dislike for bitter flavors.[14]

Leslie can also smell and discriminate between odors. Lipsitt has shown that newborns can not only distinguish between two smells, but they may actually despise foul odors.[15] He also discovered that infants as little as fifty-five hours old can differentiate smells with no rehearsals. When introduced to a strong odor, the babies startle and cry. As they grow older, the babies tend to get used to the strong odors if provided in small doses.

Leslie also seems to have an amazing auditory ability. She demonstrates preference for certain sounds and volume as well as an ability to localize those sounds.

An experiment by Lipsitt and Siqueland[16] demonstrated the one-day-old infant's ability to hear and learn. They paired (1) the sound of a bell and a bottle on the child's right side and (2) the sound of a buzzer and a bottle on the child's left side. Infants tested were able to distinguish the buzzer from the bell, right from left, and most important, they understood the contingency between the sound and reward. Scientists have also found that infants seem to prefer high-pitched sounds to low-pitched sounds. This poses an interesting question: Since the mother's voice is usually higher pitched, is there an inborn preference for her voice? Other studies have already confirmed the soothing effect on the infant of its mother's heartbeat.

Leslie responds favorably to rocking and bottom-

Table 3-3. Apgar test—an objective test for evaluating a newborn's health.

Test	*Scores* 0	1	2
Heart rate	Absent	Less than 100	More than 100
Breathing	Absent	Slow (irregular)	Strong cry
Muscle tone	Decreased (floppy)	Some flexion of extremities	Active movement
Reflex response	Absent	Grimace	Vigorous cry
Color (Nonwhite child alternative test of mucous membranes, palms, and soles are used)	Blue, pale	Body pink, extremities blue	Completely pink

Adapted from Apgar.[12]

patting. Her contemporary in another culture is content when completely swaddled. No matter which system is employed, babies react favorably to the combination of light touch, warmth, and pressure, and mothers rely heavily on the touch system for peace in the nursery. Touch has been called the communication system of infants, and more and more studies are emphasizing the importance of tactile stimulation in the neonatal period. Frank's studies[17] with institutionalized babies indicate that infrequent handling can lead to delayed development.

Leslie's motor development at this period is primarily reflexive (see reflex development, Table 10-4); *her nonreflexive motor activity is gross and random.* She responds with total body movements to sudden changes within her environment. She typically lies on her tummy in a flexed position with fisted hands, but she has a variety of both fine and gross motor movements.

In observing the neonate it is important to consider the state of consciousness or *state* of the infant. Reactions to stimuli must be interpreted within the context of the presenting state of consciousness, since reactions may vary markedly as the infant passes from one state to another. State depends on physiological variables such as hunger, nutrition, degree of hydration, and the time within the wake-sleep cycle of the infant. The pattern of states and the movement from one state to another appear to be important characteristics of infants in the neonatal period. This kind of evaluation may be the best predictor of the infant's receptivity and ability to respond to stimuli in a cognitive sense.[18] In addition, the neonate's use of a state to maintain control of reactions to environmental and internal stimuli is an important mechanism and reflects the neonate's potential for organization.[19]

An example of a sleep state would be "deep sleep, with regular breathing, eyes closed, no spontaneous activity except startle or jerky movements at quite regular intervals; external stimuli produce startles with some delay; suppression of startle is rapid, and state changes are less likely from other states; no eye movement."[20]

During the first month of life, Leslie displays undifferentiated crying. Early crying is a reflexive form of communication. Although we often think of it as a reaction to discomfort, we cannot determine anything definite about it at this stage.

Leslie assimilates her environment according to her organic demands, building confidence in it as these demands are met.

To Piaget, the first phase of cognitive development is the sensorimotor phase and the first stage of intelligence is via the use of reflexes (birth to 3 months). By their very nature, a child's reflexes (the spontaneous repetition resulting from internal or external stimulation) provide the necessary experience for future sequential function. Repetition and experience produce regularity, order, and rhythm. Piaget feels that repetitive use of reflexes, combined with neurological and physical maturation, tend to form habits. Repetition and accident lead to new experiences and these new experiences allow for continued adaptation (assimilation and accommodation) with the environment. For example, Leslie possesses a repertoire of reflexes that support her survival. Her rooting and sucking reflexes meet the need for nourishment. Initially, she does not recognize the breast as the source of nourishment but, with time and repetitive use of the two reflexes, she learns to go right to the source.

Erikson's view of personality development in the infant period centers around acquiring a sense of *trust versus mistrust* (birth to 12 months). This first phase is the foundation for subsequent psychosocial development. For the neonate a sense of trust requires a feeling of physical comfort. If this feeling is given to the child she will extend it to new experiences. If it is not given, the child will have a sense of mistrust arising from unfulfilled physical and psychological needs. Leslie as an infant has her needs met through loving care and attention. Her later outlook on the world will reflect the sense of trust formed in this first stage of development. When an issue relating to trust emerges later in the developmental process, she will resolve it because of her previous positive experience.

According to Freud, a child is in the oral stage of development from birth to 12 to 18 months, her id is striving for immediate gratification of her oral needs. During this stage Leslie gains gratification from sucking, most obviously during feeding. This stage has two substages: (1) oral dependent, when a child can do nothing more assertive than cry to be fed, and (2) oral aggressive, when a child is teething and can achieve gratification by biting as well as sucking.

Behavioral theorists look beyond maturation and environment in order to explain the competency of the infant. Through experimentation with newborns, they conclude that the infant learns through two processes: reward and deprivation. Researchers Kalnins and Bruner[21] wanted to know if infants could control sucking when they were rewarded with something other than food. Pacifiers were wired to slide projectors. When the infants sucked the slide was brought into focus; when they did not suck the picture was blurry. The infants were also able to learn to focus the picture if the process for focusing it was reversed. Their only reward was a clear rather than blurred picture.

Behaviorists believe that once the child has learned a specific response to a particular stimulus via reinforcement, he or she can become accustomed to the stimulus and no longer respond to it. This demonstrates another learning phenomenon—*habituation*. Papousek[22] taught infants to turn on a light by movement of the head to the left. The infants turned on the light several times in a short period. Then they stopped, as if they were bored with it all. When the process was reversed (light activated from the right) interest was revived, only to be short lived. This supported not only the competency rather than reward theory of learning, but it indicated that infants (3 weeks old) could habituate. Behaviorists infer from this experiment that infants' sensory capabilities and perceptual processes are more highly developed than was previously thought. It may even imply that children learn best from moderately novel events!

In 1937 an ethologist, Lorenz[23] described *imprinting*, the process by which animals develop a social attachment for a particular object. Later studies of imprinting imply that the innate instinctual rapid form of learning social behavior common to animals seems evident in human infant/mother relationships as well. Harlow's monkey study[24] is a classical example of imprinting research.

Harlow delineated a number of factors that seem to be important in forming the essential bond between mother and child. He separated baby monkeys from their mothers 6 to 12 hours following birth and raised them with surrogate mothers: one was a terry-cloth-covered mother, the other was a wire-mesh mother. The babies were fed by a bottle attached to each mother. When the monkeys were allowed to spend time with either mother, the babies clung to the cloth mother even if they had been fed by the wire mother. When the baby monkeys were placed in an unfamiliar environment, those babies raised by the cloth mother showed more interest in exploring the surroundings. Following a separation from the mothers for one year, those babies raised by cloth mothers remembered and related to the cloth surrogate and those raised by the wire mother showed virtually no interest in the wire surrogate.

More recent studies of infant-mother bonding by Klaus and Kennell[25] corroborate our understanding of this very important aspect of development. They expound on maternal and paternal behavior in human beings, extrapolating and expanding observations made on a wide range of animal species. This area of study is interesting, and it may be relevant to extrapolate animal studies to human behavior. However, it must be remembered that human beings rely less on instinctual behavior than do lower animals.

Leslie initiates a social interaction formed with her mother from birth. A social attachment refers to an active, affectionate, reciprocal relationship between two persons as distinguished from all other persons. The interaction between the two individuals continues to strengthen their underlying social bond. The bond between Leslie and her mother seems to be a function of the quality and reciprocity of their initial interaction.

Leslie is also affected, right from the start, by cultural and societal influences. They would include such factors as (1) mothering styles, (2) the role of the father in child rearing, (3) feeding schedules, (4) bottle versus breast feeding, and (5) differences in treatment of male and female infants.

There are many interesting cross-cultural and sub-cultural studies regarding racial differences and motoric behavior in infants.[26,27,28,29] It appears that black babies may be more advanced in motor development, at least during the first fifteen months of life. Further study is indicated in order to discover more about the interrelationship between hereditary and environmental influences relating to racial differences in motor development.

Leslie at One Month

Leslie is a child of movement and continues to demonstrate reflex postures (see Section 2 of this chapter). She may lift her head briefly but, when unsupported, she still shows definite head lag. When supported in sitting, she may hold her head in line with her back (Fig. 3-3).

Leslie's visual acuity, coordination, and perceptions are evolving. Her eye coordination is better developed. She fixates on her mother's face in response to a smile and stares at Mommy for a long time, especially during feeding. She follows a toy from the side to the center of her body. She focuses on objects as long as they are in her direct line of vision. When she sees a person or toy she gets excited and responds with total body movement. Leslie prefers visual patterns to any kind of color or brightness. She cries deliberately when needing assistance and makes small throaty sounds. Leslie now recognizes her parents' voices.

Her physiological state is more stable. According to Dr. Peter H. Wolff, a month-old baby sleeps more than he or she is active and divides the short time awake between drowsiness and alertness.[30]

Leslie expects feedings at certain times, although her daily routine is still somewhat disorganized.

Cultural influences that dominate now include parenting style, schedules and routine, breast or bottle feeding, and amount of handling.

Leslie at Three Months

Leslie now has an increased capacity to show delight in her world with vocalization, smiling, and increased responsiveness. She is gaining motor function; reflexive postures are decreasing. When picked up, Leslie shows good body alignment. On her tummy (prone), she lifts her head and may be able to maintain that position for a few minutes.

When sitting with support she can assist in holding that position with little head bobbing. Her hands begin to swipe at objects but often do not reach the target. Usually Leslie attempts to reach for an object with arms starting at her side and closing in front of her.

Her language is a delight; her vocabulary consists of one-syllable vowel sounds (ooh, ah, ee). She squeals, gurgles, whimpers, and coos in response to someone's voice or smile.

Visually Leslie is able to follow a toy past the midline. Her facial expression toward the toy may be evident. She may also stare at a picture or toy, glancing from one to another. She prefers three-dimensional to two-dimensional pictures. She looks at the rattle in her hand and may accidentally play with it. She explores her face, eyes, and mouth with her hand and repeats an action for its own sake. She virtually searches for a sound and may even stop sucking to search for it. Leslie combines movement and vision more actively within her environment. These behaviors are the precursors of adaptive behavior. According to Piaget,[31] learning now takes place via primary circular responses (1 to 4 months).

A *primary circular response* is an active effort to reproduce a response that was first achieved by accident. The response is repeated purely for the pleasure of the action. This is the beginning of the coordination of sensory information. Leslie, for example, has had the sucking reflex since birth, then one day purely by accident she puts her thumb in her mouth. She sucks her thumb and enjoys it.

Leslie at Seven Months

Leslie moves from a period of total dependence on gravity to a period of emerging control against gravity which ultimately results in postural stability. She sits for several minutes without support, her hands free to hold an object. She can hold two blocks (one in each hand) and can transfer (shift) a block from one hand to the other. She enjoys banging objects.

Her creeping is improving and she goes forward most of the time. She now begins to practice crawling. Leslie puts weight on the palms of her hands and knees and rocks back and forth for hours, never quite "getting off." Her seven-month-old friend Andrew demonstrates a variation on this theme. He crawls around using one arm for pulling and one leg for pushing (army crawl). He is very active and even tries pulling himself to standing. In play, both Leslie and Andrew are usually seen with a toy or block in one hand or the other. They love to play with such things as a bunch of keys—shaking, rattling, and

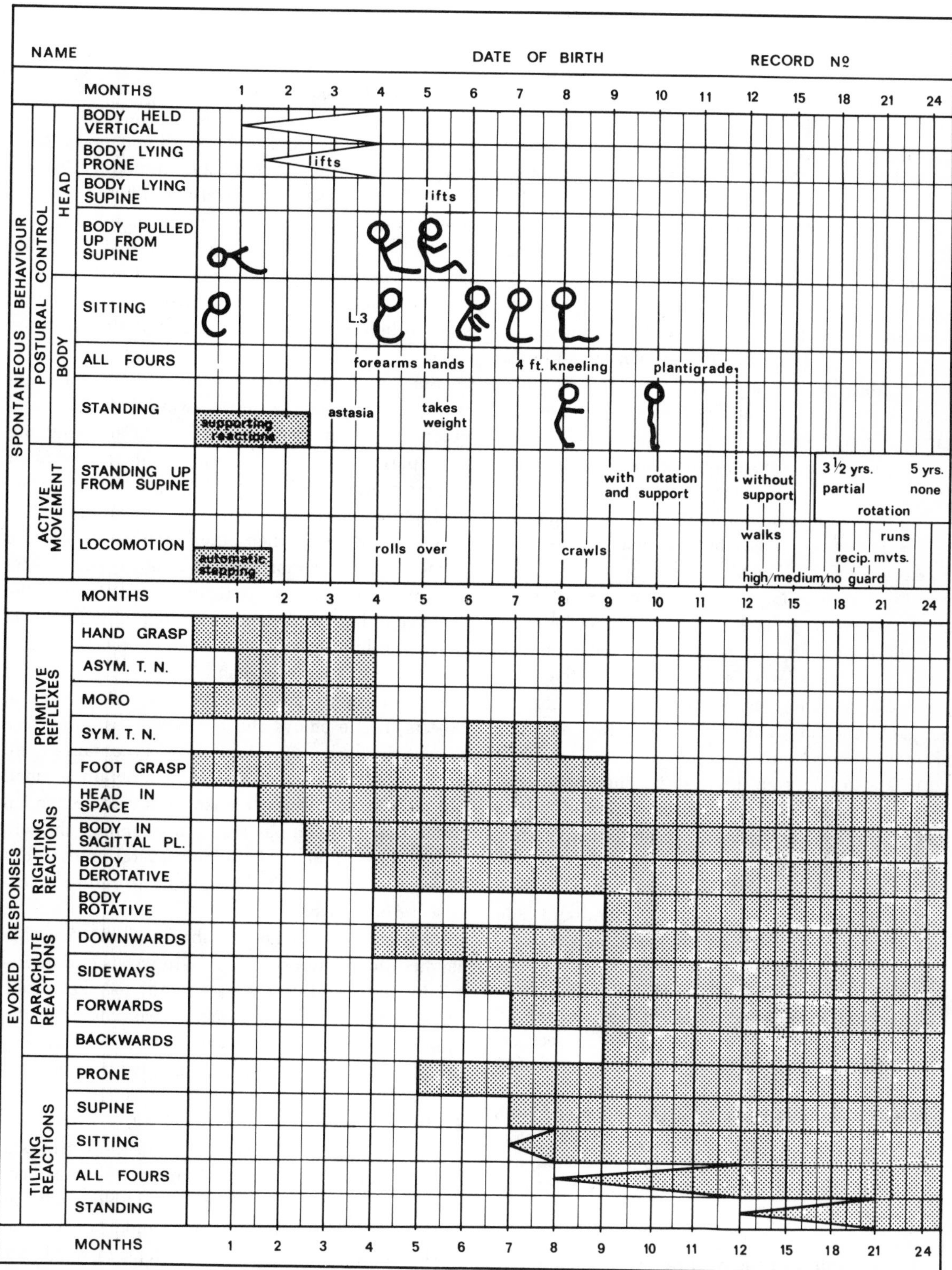

FIGURE 3-3. Developmental chart. Reprinted with permission from Milani Comparetti A., and Gidoni, E. A.: Routine developmental examination in normal and retarded children. Dev. Med. Child Neurol. 9:766, 1967.

mouthing them. They usually prefer larger to smaller objects and can pick up toys with thumb and first finger (thumb opposition).

With her increased dexterity and movement, Leslie loves to explore. She scoots around mouthing, poking, and peering at everything. This sudden new freedom of movement exposes her to increased stimulation and she may have difficulty adapting. She may even experience a period of disequilibrium, temporarily becoming more dependent and fearful of separation, particularly from Mommy. She enjoys interaction, is delighted with her own image in the mirror, and displays a delightful sense of humor. Grown up enough to join the family for dinner, she happily finger feeds in her high chair.

Leslie now attempts to imitate sounds. She often puts her favorites together in one breath (for example, ma-mu-di-ba), fooling her vulnerable parents into believing they really hear ma-ma, da-da.

According to Piaget,[32] the child at this age is learning via *secondary circular reactions*. Although new patterns of behavior continue to occur accidentally during random movements, Leslie now repeats them in order to see what results they will bring. She becomes interested in her effect on external objects and events. This stage is the beginning of intentional action.

It is also important because it ushers in the beginning of *object permanence*. This concept tells us that objects exist outside of perceptual experience; they are separate entities and continue to exist even if they cannot be seen. Piaget conducted the following experiment to see if his 7-month-old son, Laurent, had the schema of the permanent object:

> At the time of his feeding I show him the bottle, he extends his hand to take it, but, at that moment, I hide it behind my arm. If he sees one end sticking out he kicks and screams and gives every indication of wanting to have it. If, however, the bottle is completely hidden and nothing sticks out, he stops crying and acts for all we know as if the bottle no longer existed, as if it had been dissolved and absorbed into my arm.[33]

Mothers all over the world play peek-a-boo with their infants, who find the game delightful. This activity focuses on the emergence of object permanence.

Leslie at Ten Months

Leslie's struggle against gravity continues; she has gained control of her head, trunk, and arms and is now getting her legs underneath her for support. She is attempting to stand and hesitantly cruises (holds on to objects while walking) around a room. She gets down from a chair or stair now but is cautious of distances, distrusting her visual cues. She carries two small objects in one hand and is beginning to differentiate use of her hands. For example, she can hold with one while manipulating with the other.

Socially, Leslie begins to show moods and emotions as she becomes more aware of herself and others. Social approval and imitation are emerging as important facets of behavior. Imitative behavior centers around previous experiences. (For example, Leslie attempts to feed others at the dinner table.) She shows delight when others imitate her posture or movements. Memory of past behavior and objects out of sight (representational memory) and the understanding of distance and depth help Leslie imitate and understand the nature of objects. In play Leslie reaches for toys behind her without seeing them. She continues to learn about properties of objects. Leslie enjoys shaking boxes, listening to a watch tick. She will look into a container and grasp small objects. If she cannot obtain a small object, she usually will poke at it with extended index finger. If she has seen a toy hidden, she will search for it. If the toy is hidden several times in different places, Leslie will continue to return to the first hiding place.

While playing, Leslie jabbers away. She has learned the relationship of certain words and appropriate gestures (for example, "no"—shakes head; "bye"—waves). She says one or two words besides ma-ma and da-da and she can understand and obey simple commands (for example, "give it to me").

Leslie at One Year

Leslie is ready to forge ahead in the world; she has overcome the bondage of gravity. She has been standing and walking with assistance. Now, with increased trunk rotation and eye-hand coordination, Leslie takes her first unsteady steps forward. She walks with her hands raised and a wide-base gait. She meanders forward looking like a somewhat clumsy, baggy-legged sailor, supremely pleased with her accomplishment. However, when visiting unfamiliar places, Leslie still prefers to crawl.

Her hand control and dexterity is improving. She loves to pick up both small and large objects and can hold many toys at one time. At Harvard's Center for Cognitive Studies, visiting infants showed their end-of-the-year dexterity by pushing up and holding a sliding see-through door with one hand and retrieving a toy with the other.[34]

Leslie's conversation has intonation patterns and she produces sounds specific to her parents' language. She practices her words (two to eight words) such as "bye," "ma-ma," "da-da," "no," "hi." She can imitate sounds of objects (bow-wow). (See Sequences of Language Development.)

SEQUENCES OF LANGUAGE DEVELOPMENT*

Prelinguistic Speech

Before a child says his first real word, he goes through the following six, and perhaps seven, stages of speech:

1. *Undifferentiated crying*. With "no language but a cry," babies come into this world. Early crying is a reflexive reaction to the environment produced by the expiration of breath.
2. *Differentiated crying*. After the first month of life (and of crying), the close listener can often discriminate a difference between a baby's cries and their causes.
3. *Cooing*. At about six weeks, chance movements of the child's mechanisms produce a variety of simple sounds called cooing. These squeals, gurgles, and bleats are usually emitted when he is happy and contented. The first sounds are vowels, and the first consonant is h.
4. *Babbling*. These vocal gymnastics begin at about three or four months, as a child playfully repeats a variety of sounds. Again, he is most likely to babble when he is contented and when he is alone. As he lies in his crib or sits in his infant seat, he loquaciously, and often loudly, spouts forth a variety of simple consonant and vowel sounds: "ma-ma-ma-ma-ma," "da-da-da-da-da," "bi-bi-bi-bi-bi," and so forth. While most children babble, a few seem to skip this stage. Deaf children babble normally for the first few months of life, but then appear to lose interest when they cannot hear themselves.
5. *Lallation or imperfect imitation*. Sometime during the second half of the first year, a child seems to become more aware of the sounds around him. He will become quiet as he listens to some sound. When it stops, he babbles in excitement, accidentally repeating the sounds and syllables he has heard. Then he imitates his own sounds.
6. *Echolalia or imitation of the sounds of others*. At about the age of nine or ten months, a child seems to consciously imitate the sounds made by others, even though he still does not understand them.
7. *Expressive jargon*. During the second year, many children use *expressive jargon*. This term, coined by Gesell, refers to a string of utterances that *sound* like sentences, with pauses, inflections, and rhythms. However, speech is not yet communicated verbally on a consistent basis.

Linguistic Speech

1. *One-word sentence (holophrase)*. At about a year, a child points to a cracker, a toy, a pacifier, and says "da." His parents correctly interpret the command as "Give me that" or "I want that." He points to the door and says, "out." His single word thus expresses a complete thought, even though his listeners may not always be able to divine what that complete thought may be.
2. *Multiword sentence*. Some time about the age of two, a child strings together two or more words to make a sentence. When he wants to feed himself with no interference, he says imperiously, "Mommy 'way."

The child may develop a combination of sounds that mean something to him but may not necessarily be understood by the listener. Usually this communication style occurs at the time the child is learning nouns. The sounds or syllables are attached to the newly learned nouns.

The earliest multiword sentences are combinations of nouns and verbs. Other parts of speech, such as articles, prepositions, and adjectives, are lacking. Although these sentences are far from grammatical, they do communicate. This is *telegraphic speech*; it contains only words that carry meaning.

3. *Grammatically correct verbal utterances*. At about the age of three, the child has an impressive command of the language. He now has a vocabulary of some 900 words; he speaks in longer sentences that include all the parts of speech; and he has a good grasp of grammatical principles. His grammar is not the same one used by adults because he makes little allowance for exceptions to the linguistic rules he has assimilated. So, he says, "We goed to the store."

*Adapted from Eisenson,[35] Lenneberg,[36] and Clifton.[37]

With her peers she engages in parallel play but, while she is on her own, Leslie loves to investigate objects. She has the concept of container and contained. She shakes toys, puts blocks in and out of a box, unwraps toys, and delights in looking for a hidden toy, even if she did not see it hidden.

Cognitively, during the first year the child begins to differentiate and generalize experiences. Each experience has signs which evoke a different set of action sequences. Once the child can perceive actions beyond his sensorimotor capabilities, intelligence emerges. The discovery of objects as objects introduces the awareness of spatial relationships. For example, Leslie is putting blocks in a box. She turns them, examines their shapes, and then puts them in the box. For her they occupy space and have dimension. Leslie is also beginning to realize that *she* is doing something that she is the determiner of some of the events in her environment.

Leslie begins to experience by observation. She lets things happen and observes results. This discovery of new means through active experimentation is referred to by Piaget[38] as *tertiary circular reactions*.

Cultural and societal influences become more diverse. Leslie's learning experiences from now on will be affected more by such cultural factors as

1. parental attitudes toward activity and their willingness and ability to provide varied learning experiences
2. schedules and routine
3. an opportunity for movement and exploration
4. sexual differences and parental attitudes about them
5. the type and quality of toys and play the child is allowed to experience.

Preschool Years

Leslie's friends Kim (18 months), Billy (2 years), and Joan (3 years) demonstrate the preschool milestones of behavior.

Eighteen-Month-Old Kim

Kim is entering the toddler phase—a period of harrowing impulsiveness. He is walking along as are most of his peers, continuing a wide stance gait that lacks a true sense of balance. He may be able to take a few steps backward, but as yet he is unable to kick a ball forward or climb stairs in a smooth coordinated manner. This is due primarily to his immature equilibrium responses and maturation. He enhances his support system by holding onto objects, and he enjoys pushing and pulling toys. He concentrates on and practices his new-found abilities. For example, Kim has just mastered climbing over the front doorsill and, much to his mother's chagrin, he keeps going in and out of the door.

In fine motor development, he scribbles spontaneously with a crayon, builds a tower with blocks (two to four blocks) and is able to handle small objects.

At home he is able to bring a cup to his mouth and drink. He can fill his spoon but has difficulty inserting it into his mouth; there is considerable spilling. He attempts to do simple undressing, proudly taking off his hat and socks.

Socially he enjoys other children but his play is still parallel play. Each child does his/her own thing.

Play at this age is still largely gross motor. The child likes to pull little carts and wagons or carry a favorite doll, teddy bear, or blanket around with him all day. Sensory play is important at this age (for example, sand and water play, pounding and banging pots and pans).

With an increased tone, range, and vocal pitch, Kim enjoys humming and dancing with his whole body. He also enjoys listening to short catchy rhymes, especially if they are action-oriented.

He interacts freely within his environment. Since he is emerging from a relatively dependent phase, Kim cannot always differentiate between what he should and should not do. He forges ahead with great abandon toward autonomy. His feelings about his parents are evolving. His loving attachment continues, but he is beginning to feel and see them as being restrictive and frustrating. For the first time Kim encounters a myriad of external limitations.

Kim's vocabulary consists of approximately three words other than ma-ma and da-da. He still communicates primarily by gestures.

According to Erikson,[39] the child is entering Crisis II: Autonomy versus Shame (18 months to 3 years). This stage corresponds to Freud's Anal Period. With the establishment of a sense of trust in his mother and in the world, Kim is developing a sense of self. At the same time, he realizes the limits impinging on him as he begins to assert himself. This push to autonomy is partly maturational. His new-found motor and functional capabilities coupled with increased ability to express desires impel Kim to expand the boundaries of his world. If he is thwarted in this expansion, he may begin to doubt his ability to become autonomous, eventually developing a sense of shame and doubt, but, encouraged to explore (with secure limits or under supervision), his competence will evolve and with it a positive sense of self-worth.

According to Piaget,[40] Kim continues in the Sensorimotor Period (18 months to 2 years), inventing new means through mental combinations. He now has the ability to picture events in his mind; experimentation is not necessary. In effect, he can try out new solutions in his mind and discard solutions that don't work. For example, Kim picks up the plug to the vacuum and toddles over to the socket. Then he remembers (mentally pictures) his mother saying "hot, don't touch." He sits, plug in hand, seriously repeating the warning, "hot, hot, hot." He is also able to imitate actions even when his model is no longer in front of him. The concept of object permanence is fully developed.

Kim now understands visible and invisible displacements. When he looks for a toy that had been hidden in several consecutive places, he will now look for it in the last hiding place. This is an improvement over the previous ability to search for a toy in its first hiding place.

Two-Year-Old Billy

Billy at two is just beginning to break through into new skill areas and accomplishments. He walks, runs, jumps in place, and climbs stairs. He crawls into, under, around, and over objects. In play he can kick forward and throw a ball overhand.

In fine motor development, he is capable of building a tower of four to eight cubes and can make a horizontal bridge of three blocks. His spontaneous block play shows matching of simple shapes and symmetry.

Billy's sensory and perceptual abilities are improving. He is beginning to have good color sense and by approximately thirty months will be able to match primary colors. His visual focus is good and he can recognize objects 8 millimeters in diameter; but his visual-motor coordination is still rudimentary.

Billy's auditory acuity is double that of a year-old child and his auditory discrimination has improved.

With increased postural integration, his equilibrium improves and his sense of position in space becomes more accurate.

Emotionally, Billy must learn to deal with a host of feelings such as joy, affection, anger, fear, and frustration. All of these feelings are just as real to a two-year old as they are to an adult. He must cope with his new autonomy, with its advantages and limitations.

Autonomy, mastery, and competence refer to slightly different drives but they are all part of the same motivational and behavioral complex which plays an important part in determining actions throughout life.[41,42,43]

The "terrible twos" are a time of manifestation of autonomy. Billy must constantly test his new self-image and his hitherto undreamed of powers, sometimes to the destruction of family tranquility.

In play Billy enjoys rhythmical activities. He dances with *great* movement—bouncing, swaying, and tapping his feet. He likes to fill containers with things such as stones and dirt.

PLAY BEHAVIOR*

Unoccupied Play Behavior. The child seems not to be playing but watches momentarily activity in the environment. When not attending, the child plays with his/her body, engages in gross motor behavior (e.g., climbing up or down from chairs, following people around) or just sits looking around the room.

Onlooker Play. The child watches others play and engages in conversation with those playing. He/she definitely is observing the children rather than events, although he/she does not engage in actual play.

Solitary Independent Play. The child pursues play activities alone and independently from the other children playing. Although the child often positions himself close to others, he/she makes no reference to what they are doing.

Parallel Play. The child plays with toys similar to those used by other children near him/her, but the child plays beside rather than with the children.

Associative Play. The child plays with others. There is no organization of play activities in his/her peer group, no division of labor, and no product. Each child acts individually; his/her interest focusing on the association rather than the play activity.

Cooperative or Organized Supplementary Play. The child plays with other children in an organized manner for a purpose (e.g., making something, formal games). There is a marked sense of belonging to the group, which is now directed by one or two leaders. Each child finds some role in the new organization, his efforts augmented by the other members of the group.

* Adapted from Parten.[44]

At bath time you can hardly see Billy for the boats and toys, and he loves to play in the water. When wielding a crayon he gingerly experiments with vertical, horizontal, and circular motions but tends to extend his colorful patterns to his hands, clothes, table, and wall. This is partly due to his lack of fine motor control and partly to his easy distractibility.

Billy also likes to engage in imaginative play, particularly when it involves imitating (playing house, Mommy, Daddy).

At home, Billy can now drink from a small glass. He continues to need supervision when eating and shows definite food preferences. Billy helps dress himself, usually by thrusting his arms into arm holes. He tries to wash and dry his hands but often fails miserably.

"No" becomes his favorite word. He can now combine two words and asks questions such as "What's that?" Billy can verbalize immediate experiences and can talk and play at the same time. He refers to himself "Me Billy."

Between the ages of two and three (in contemporary American culture) Billy is probably introduced to toilet training. His control of elimination relies on maturational readiness, but he must learn a great deal before training can be initiated. He must know what is expected of him and have some concept of his own capabilities.

Much controversy has raged regarding when and how toilet training should be initiated. Two points must be emphasized: (1) the child must be maturationally ready and (2) whatever method is chosen, it must be carried out in a clear and consistent manner.

To Freud, the child now enters the Anal Period (12/18 months to 3 years). He obtains pleasure from the ability to control his bowels. Freud feels that the way in which toilet training is handled determines the effective resolution of this stage of development.[45]

Societal and cultural influences are of paramount importance to the child at this time. They include:

1. Toilet training. There are cross-cultural attitudes and methods for this training. Parent attitudes, particularly in relationship to punishment, may have a marked influence on the child.

2. Parenting style. There are definite cross-cultural and subcultural differences in "mothering" styles.

3. The father's role in childrearing. Rebelsky and Hanks[46] made 24-hour tapes of father-baby interaction for a group of ten lower middle class to upper middle class fathers of infants. The average father in the group spent 37.7 seconds per day doing things with or for his baby; the most devoted spent less than 10 minutes a day with his baby.[46] Initially these men spent more time talking to their infant daughters but, by the time the babies were three months old, the sons were getting more attention. By the end of the study, the fathers were spending less time talking to their babies than they had in the beginning, especially their baby daughters. Other studies have found this to be the reverse of mother-baby interactions.

4. Absence of either the mother or father in childrearing.

5. Presence of/and relationship to other siblings.

6. Reaction to peers and strangers.

Three-Year-Old Joan

She has grown four inches taller in the last year and her motor skills have definitely improved. One minute she is standing on one foot (momentarily) in dancing school; the next she is running, turning, climbing, and riding her tricycle. Her eye-hand coordination has also improved. She can copy a circle with a crayon, pour milk from a pitcher, and button and unbutton clothes.

Imitation and dramatic play are an important part of the three-year-old's play repertoire. If you were to observe Joan in school she would still be engaged in parallel play. Each child in Joan's group continues to show egocentric behavior. Let's listen to a typical conversation between Joan and her playmate Jon as they play house.

> *Joan:* I am pretty like my mommy.
> *Jon:* I like cookies. I want them.
> *Joan:* I have pink toe shoes.
> *Jon:* I want coffee and cookies.

In preschool activities, the "threes" happily engage in many activities: building blocks, puzzles, finger painting, clay, puppets, dolls, simple musical games. They love "grown up" projects like making vegetable soup with the help of their teacher, who bravely issues plastic knives, carrots, potatoes, and onions to her energetic helpers.

Of greatest delight, however, is gross motor play —jungle gyms, sliding boards, swings, sandbox, and the baby pool.

At home Joan does uncomplicated dressing and undressing, although she has a tendency to look a bit disheveled. She may also develop wardrobe favorites and be hard to dissuade from her favorite Wonder Woman T-shirt. Toilet training is complete with rare accidents at night.

Joan helps with simple chores such as picking up toys, dusting, or working in the garden, mostly when the activity has some special appeal (like "helping daddy").

Emotionally, Joan is learning to control her drives and develop socially acceptable behaviors (sublimation). Her parents, family, and teacher are setting new limits, which she cannot always comprehend or obey.

All these new experiences may put Joan, by 3½, in a state of temporary disequilibrium. Her delightful sense of joy, affection, and curiosity may dissolve quickly into periods of irritability, anger, and sometimes even temper tantrums. For example, Joan comes running into the house with a rock she found while playing. She quizzes her mother about where it came from, what it was made of. She plays with it, giving it magical properties. Then suddenly reality rears its head; dinner is ready and her mother asks her to wash her hands. Joan doesn't seem to hear her. After some prodding, she retorts with an angry "No!" and throws the rock on the floor.

Joan cannot yet accurately differentiate between reality and fantasy. She thinks and learns by recalling "reality sequences in her head just as she might do overt action."[48] For example, Joan spends a day at the zoo. When asked later what she saw, she recalls only one or two highlights. It is difficult to relive a whole day in her mind!

Joan cannot at this time grasp the concept of reversibility. For instance, if you ask if she has a sister she replies "yes," but if you ask her if her sister has a sister she says "no."

The three-year-old's concepts are preconcepts. They are active and concrete. They do not allow the child to recognize[49]

1. an object and/or person under different circumstances. For example, Joan may not recognize her mother who is wearing huge *new* sunglasses but, once the glasses are removed, she exclaims, "There's my mommy.

2. different objects and/or persons of the same type as anything but one and the same. For example, Joan sees a butterfly and calls it *the* butterfly. She thinks that each butterfly she sees is *the* original butterfly.

The child goes from one particular of a situation to another rather than from a particular to the whole (centering). It will be another three or four years before Joan will have the ability to think in a more sophisticated manner. As a "pre-operational" child, Joan still focuses on successive states and cannot make transformations from one state to another. For example, when equal amounts of water are poured into two different containers (one tall and thin, one short and wide) she invariably says that the taller one has more water because of its height (concept of conservation). When asked who is older, mommy or daddy, she says daddy because he is taller. Because of centering, Joan cannot accommodate to transformations. This type of associative thought process is known in piagetian terms as *transductive reasoning.*

SUMMARY OF KOHLBERG'S SIX STAGES OF MORAL REASONING*

Level I

Pre-Moral (4–10 yrs.). Primary emphasis is on external control and ideas of others. These standards are followed either to avoid punishment or gain reward.

Type I—Punishment and obedience. The child obeys to avoid punishment.

Type II—Naive instrumental hedonism. Conformity to rules is out of self-interest.

Level II

Morality of Conventional Role Conformity (10–13 yrs.). The child wishes to please others and internalizes some of the standards of those persons deemed important to him or her. The child now decides if some action is good by his or her standards.

Type III—Maintaining approval of others. The child judges the intentions of others and yields an opinion.

Type IV—Authority maintaining morality. The child shows respect for authority and maintenance of social order.

Level III

Morality of Self-Accepted Moral Principles (13 to adulthood). True morality. The individual recognizes the possible conflict between standards. He/she realizes that conduct and reasoning about right and wrong are a result of internal control.

Type V—Morality of contract, of individual rights, and of accepted democratic law. People think in logical terms, valuing the will of society as a whole. These values are for the most part substantiated by obeying the law.

Type VI—Morality of individual principles of conscience. The individual does what he/she thinks is right as a result of his/her internalized values.

* Adapted from Kohlberg.[47]

School Years

Five-Year-Old Sam

For Sam, just entering kindergarten, five is a golden age. In general, Sam is self-contained and friendly, both at home and at school. He is just barely discovering the actual world. The five-year old gives the impression of competency and stability. He is not overly assertive and enjoys small responsibilities as opposed to hard challenges. Sam likes to fit into his culture; he is eager to please others and to conform to social boundaries. This period of calm and conformity does not mean he is highly socialized. He does engage in cooperative play, usually in small groups (one to three peers). But even in group play he is primarily concerned with his own activity.

In his gross motor activities, Sam displays excellent equilibrium on the balance beam, he skips well and plays a fair game of ball. His fine motor activity has markedly improved. Sam is now definitely right-handed. He can draw recognizable objects from memory, including a fair representation of a man. He can also copy a square as well as some capital letters. Sam can handle small objects fairly dexterously. He uses children's scissors competently and performs most of his activities of daily living. He now dresses and undresses with little or no assistance, although it might be a while before he ties his shoelaces.

Sam likes to finish what he starts. He enjoys most of the kindergarten play materials: paints, crayons, blocks, workbooks, tracing figures, and basic math games. Outdoor play consists of tree climbing, jumping, and acrobatics. Imitative play is becoming more reality-oriented. Kindergarteners play house, doctor, school, and so forth. This type of accurate imitation yields a more extensive comprehension of cultural mores and values.

By the middle of his kindergarten year, Sam tends to gravitate to all-boy play groups. The unspoken patterns of sex-role behavior are becoming more evident. Sam's new-found chauvinism is much more vociferous (girls are yukky) when bolstered by his pals. Alone, he may forget it entirely and enjoy playing with his girlfriend next door.

Five-year-olds have already spent several years acquiring behaviors and attitudes regarded by their culture as characteristically masculine or feminine (sex typing).[50] The extent to which male and female behavior is biologically or culturally determined continues to be a great controversy. Despite evolving traditional male-female roles, most children develop specific sex-appropriate behavior. Recent studies confirm this. Greenberg and Peck showed one hundred twenty preschool children (three to six years) pictures of boys and girls and asked which of the picture-children would grow up to be a teacher, doctor, and so forth. The children were also tested for IQ. All the children gave stereotyped responses: the brightest giving the most traditional answers—boys seen as doctors, girls as teachers, and so forth.[51,52]

Sam's communication has expanded; he now has a 2000 word vocabulary and has abandoned most of his infantile speech. He employs egocentric speech and often uses words without fully understanding their meaning.

According to Erikson, the preschool child (three to six years) is in Crisis III, Initiative versus Guilt. Sam is turning from total attachment to his parents to identification with them. He is eager to plan and execute activities but is limited partly by the Oedipal complex and partly by a developing conscience (superego). Guilt arises if rules and regulations are perceived as too restrictive. The child's own superego may be harder on him than his parents in a given situation (Table 3-4). He must learn to regulate these two parts of his personality so that he will develop a balance between a sense of moral responsibility and joie de vivre.

Seven-Year-Old Jim

Jim, a second grader, takes in more of his environment than he gives back, mulling over his new impressions in a kind of reflective fantasy. Although he has a tendency for self-absorption, Jim is interested in others (parents, teacher, and friends) and is increasingly sensitive to their attitudes. He is becoming more detached from mother, developing new attachments outside the home.

Jim is prone to sudden bursts of very active behavior. His strength is increasing and he is learning to inhibit his motor activity. He repeats activities over and over in order to master them. In school, Jim is writing less painstakingly. His letters are becoming more uniform and his drawings of a man are

Table 3–4. A child's view of rules.

Practice of rules	*Thinking about rules*
Stage I: Motor Activity A child manipulates objects in an individual way to see what he/she can do with them.	*Stage I: Absolutism* (from 4 to 7) Rules are considered as interesting examples, but not reality. A child considers rules sacred, although in practice the child is willing to accept changes in the rules because he/she recognizes them as changes.
Stage II: Egocentrism (from 2 to 5) The child has a general idea of rules and believes he/she is playing by the rules. Actually the child engages in play via idiosyncratic systems and changes the rules to fit his/her needs.	*Stage II: Morality of Constraint* (from 7 to 10) The child is limited by respect for adults and older peers. Authority is absolute; the child refuses to accept any change in rules.
Stage III: Incipient Cooperation (about 7 or 8) The child tries to win and wants to play by a set of rules. Ideas are vague and each child playing the game will give an individual or different account of the rules.	*Stage III: Morality of Cooperation* (from 10 on) The child sees rules as laws resulting from mutual consent. Most children no longer accept parents and others as the authority figures without question. They see themselves as equals; since people make the rules, people can change them.
Stage IV: Codification (about 11 or 12) The child knows every detail of procedure. The group knows and plays by the same rules.	

Adapted from Papalia and Olds.[53] Original source Piaget (1932).

more accurate in relation to size. Usually a good listener, he loves a story, though his own reading abilities are still in the labored phonetic stage.

Jim is eager to please his teacher and with her support grows more confident of his abilities. The teacher realizes that her children need speech to clarify their thoughts and develop their social contacts. By establishing empathetic two-way relationships, she can foster self-reliance and encourage independence.

Language at this age is increasingly interposed between thought and action. *When* verbal mediation comes into play is much debated, partly as a corollary to the question of whether language must precede the formulation of certain cognitive concepts. Verbal mediation involves the use of verbal links between the overt stimulus and the final result[54] (Jim thinks before he acts).

Jim is gradually developing a sense of time and space orientation. In preschool and kindergarten he had the notion of "before and after"; he understood time differences in relationship to spatial distances. Now he is becoming more independent of sequential and perceptual data. He can read the clock, tell you the month, and identify seasons of the year. Jim will not fully understand the time concept until he can coordinate the concepts of equal distance and speed. By the time he is a young adolescent he will be able to explain that time has equal duration regardless of the content of that time.[55]

Jim's cognitive growth may be indicated by the increasing predictability of his adult IQ (see Chapter 24). While there is only minimal correlation between a person's IQ at two and his adult IQ, there is a highly significant correlation between his test scores at seven and his adult IQ.[56] Psychologists dispute the underlying causes of cognitive changes, but generally they believe that the seven-year old increasingly resorts to rule-controlled thought, although simple association remains an important part of his mental process. His thought tends to be deliberate and reflective rather than impulsive.

Piaget characterizes the four- to seven-year-old age span as the Intuitive Phase. The intuitive child relies heavily on immediate perception and on direct experience rather than on logical operation. He centers on one dimension or feature at a time (centering), he views the world from his own point of view (egocentric), and he tends to be static and irreversible in his thinking. Toward the end of this stage, the rigid, static, and irreversible qualities of intuitive thought begin to "thaw out," becoming more reversible and flexible. This emerging ability to go beyond the immediate self with mental leaps and bounds is the precursor of systematic reasoning.

Jim is now emerging into what Piaget terms the Concrete Operational Phase (seven to nine and one-half years), determining relations through a process of trial and error. He can now coordinate inverse relations as well as understand the concept of conservation. His inner and outer world are going through complex change. At home, he not only handles his own self-care activities, but is expected to meet increasing household demands and responsibilities. In school, he is learning more complex concepts and is becoming more aware of structure and rules.

At play, Jim is inclined to be obsessive in his interests. For instance, he develops a passion for models often to the exclusion of other activities. In gross motor activities, he is cautious but not fearful. He enjoys his bike and rides it on the sidewalk, he climbs trees, he likes to play ball (although he is better at batting than catching). Jim is also taking an interest in swimming and skating. The group games he now enjoys are much better defined and realistic. He gradually abandons the concepts of animism and artificialism and becomes interested in cooperation and competition. His ability to cooperate and compete is tentative. When playing a game, he knows the rules but still likes to add his own—and he loves to win.

Freud views personality development of the school-age child as being in the Latency Period. By six, the child has a functioning superego that allows him to internalize the morals and ethics of society. He has resolved his Oedipal conflicts and sex role and now turns his attention to the acquisition of facts, skill, and cultural attitudes. (This does not imply that sexual interest is absent.) It is also during his school-age years that a child develops defense mechanisms to uphold the strength and integrity of his ego and self-concept.

Erikson sees the school-age child as entering Crisis IV, Industry versus Inferiority. This is the age where productivity is important. The school years are critical for the development of self-esteem because the child must gain a sense of mastery over the tools of his culture and society. If he perceives himself as failing, he may feel hopelessly inadequate.

Maier explains Erikson's view of the school-age child as follows:

> The latent child continues to invest as much of himself and libidinal energy as he did before, and works incessantly on his bodily, muscular and perceptive skills as well as on his growing knowledge of the world which becomes increasingly important to him. Above all, he concentrates on his capacity to relate to and to communicate with individuals who are most significant to him—his peers. A sense of accomplishment for having done well, being the strongest, best, wittiest or fastest are the successes toward which he strives. The child wards off failure at almost any price. As long as ego tasks are mastered within the sphere of his age group, the id and the superego remain unchallenged and within safe boundaries . . . He senses that if he proves his skills within the area of his best competence, his successful future will be assured.[57]

Cultural influences are of paramount importance in the early school years. They include

1. parenting style; for example, permissive versus authoritarian
2. type of school program
3. differentiation of sex roles and/or sex typing
4. emphasis and types of play available

Ten-Year-Old Laura

Laura refines her skills: she thoroughly enjoys her friends and family and experiences a period of relative equilibrium as she stands on the threshold of adolescence. Her individuality is well defined. Still in the phase of concrete operations, her industry is directed at refining the skills she has mastered. Since her energies and motor functions are better organized and executed, she is freer to interact within her environment. This new relaxed attitude makes Laura more responsive to social influences. She is beginning to make comparative judgments based on her own observations of home, school, family, and peers as well as on her developing sense of fairness.

Laura's peer group is the testing ground for parent-derived attitudes as well as a forum for development of social skills. As a group member, she is learning to adjust to the needs and desires of others. Peer groups at this age tend to be homogeneous according to sex, race, economic status, and general interest. Laura, for example, belongs to a club, The Butterflies. Members share such common interests as hiking and playing ball. They have special meetings and enjoy sharing secret experiences.

Bronfenbrenner made a study of American and Russian twelve-year olds and their responsiveness to peer and adult influences. Dramatic cultural differences were displayed:

> The children were confronted with thirty hypothetical situations involving their readiness to cheat, steal, play a practical joke on a teacher, neglect homework, and go against parental wishes in several specific ways. Some children were told that their classmates would see their answers, some that parents and teachers would see them, and some that no one but the researchers would see them. Both Russian and American children gave more socially approved responses when they thought adults would see their answers, although the Russian children were influenced more by adults and the Americans more by peers. Furthermore, the effects of peer-group pressures took different directions for the two groups of children. In Russia, peer-group pressure influenced children toward adult standards of behavior, while just the opposite held true in the United States. American children who thought their friends would see their answers were more likely to show a willingness to go against adult-approved standards.[58]

Adolescence

Adolescence is derived from a Latin word meaning "to come to maturity." It begins at pubescence, a period of about two years prior to the onset of puberty. Pubescence is a time of physiological changes: a growth spurt, a synchronous growth of body systems, and increased hormonal activity which triggers the emergence of primary and secondary sex characteristics[59] (Table 3-5). Pubescence culminates at puberty, when sexual maturity and reproductive capacity are complete.

Table 3-5. Emergence of sex characteristics.

Girls	*Boys*
PRIMARY SEX CHARACTERISTICS	
ovaries	testes
fallopian tubes	penis
uterus	organs that transmit sperm from testes to penis
vagina	
SECONDARY SEX CHARACTERISTICS	
breasts	facial hair
pubic hair	pubic hair
axillary hair	axillary hair
increased width and depth of pelvis	body hair
	voice change

It is not as easy to determine when adolescence ends and adulthood begins. This depends on a combination of physical, emotional, social, legal, and cultural determinants.

Theories of Adolescence

Anthropologist Margaret Mead believes that physiological factors underlie adolescent changes but that cultural factors determine the quality of these changes. If a society decrees a smooth transition from one developmental period to another, the adolescent experiences little or no conflict.

Freud's view of adolescence centers on the *genital stage,* that point of mature adult sexuality when reawakened sexual urges are directed in socially approved channels. Although his theory of adolescent behavior is sketchier than his explanations of earlier development, he does emphasize achievement of identity in respect to career choice, cultural values, and ethics.

Erikson sees adolescence as Crisis V, Identity versus Role Confusion. The adolescent's rapid physical maturation implies that adulthood is approaching and an adult role must soon be assumed. Establishing an identity in his or her life career as well as establishing meaningful psychosocial relationships help the adolescent define and clarify his adult role.

Puberty sees the full development of a system of cognitive thought. Inhelder and Piaget[60] characterize the adolescent's formal operational thought process as follows:

1. The capability of dealing logically with many factors at once.

2. The ability to utilize a secondary system, for example, trigonometry. The ability to manipulate symbols makes the adolescent's thought processes more flexible. He is now able to introspect and reflect upon his own mental capacities.

3. The ability to construct ideal or contrary-to-fact situations.

4. The ability to deal with the possible as well as the real.

These components comprise the basis for hypothetical problem solving, a necessary adult tool.

In *pre- and early adolescence*, physiological changes coupled with emerging cognitive abilities lay the foundation for the establishment of identity. This tumultuous period often finds the adolescent moody, sensitive, and ambivalent about identity and role.

Mid-adolescence centers around a struggle for autonomy and a continued search for self and vocational identity. Pressure to make a vocational choice is mounting. From a developmental point of view, the choice of career has been going on since childhood, beginning with parental modeling and identification. Besides his parents' values, a child's own needs for creativity, sharing, and self-expression provide a further base for assuming various role behaviors. He explores future vocational aspirations through play activities. During youth and adolescence exposure to "real" jobs allows the young person a pragmatic testing ground for such things as sex-peer group interaction, specific interests and capabilities, attitudes, and patterns of work behaviors.

Despite the ability to conceptualize, the mid-adolescent may manifest lingering egocentrism. He realizes that other people have their own thoughts and perceptions, but his self-preoccupation persuades him that their thoughts are focused on him. Elkind[61] describes manifestations of this egocentrism as follows:

1. *Imaginary audience.* The adolescent is constructing or reacting to an imagined audience. For example, when the student catches the eye of the teacher he wonders what the teacher is thinking about him at that moment.

2. *Personal fable.* The adolescent imagines that because so many people are interested in him, he must be very special. For example, the adolescent knows that "no one ever has felt the way I do."

During *late adolescence* the focal point of behavior is increased autonomy and a more realistic approach to vocational choice. With increased cognitive ability, the adolescent is better able to view alternatives and can more easily evaluate himself in relationship to future life goals.

As adolescence comes to a close, the young person, forced to adapt to the realities of adult life, begins to engage in productive work. He also reassesses the adult world as well as his own limitations and becomes more accepting of both.

Adult Life

An individual's developmental progression throughout the lifespan reaches its height in adulthood. Continuing up the life line one refines his self-image, develops sexual and psychosocial intimacy, becomes productive and effective in the world of work and family, and finally reaches an integrity and a sense of fulfillment which affirms his life as a meaningful adventure.

The complexity of the modern world, society, and culture inhibit the smooth resolution of many issues of adulthood. There is no ideal. But as Horace (Epistles) said, "He has half the deed done, who has made a beginning."

Chapter 17 covers in detail the later years of the adult developmental continuum.

REFERENCES

1. Craig, G. J.: Human Development, Englewood Cliffs NJ: Prentice-Hall, 1976, p. 11.
2. Ibid., p. 11.
3. Ames, L. B.: Child Care and Development. Philadelphia: J. B. Lippincott Co., 1970, pp. 15–17.
4. Craig: Human Development, p. 12.
5. Bandura, A., Ross, D., and Ross, S. A.: Vicarious reinforcement and imitative learning. J. Abnorm. and Soc. Psych. 66:601–607, 1963.
6. Craig: Human Development, p. 32.
7. Severin, F. T.: What Humanistic Psychology is About. Newsletter Feature Supplement. San Francisco: Association of Humanistic Psychology, 1974.
8. Gesell, A., and Thompson, S.: The Psychology of Early Growth. New York: Macmillan Publishing Co., 1938, p. 198.

9. Flanagan, C.: The First Nine Months of Life. New York: Simon & Schuster, 1960, p. 34–36.
10. Ibid, p. 81.
11. Anastasi, A.: Heredity, environment and the question of "how?" Psycholo. Rev. 65:197–208, 1958.
12. Apgar, V.: Proposal for a new method of evaluating the newborn infant. Anesth. Analg. 32:260–267, 1953.
13. Fantz, R.: The origin of form perception. Scientif. Am. May 1961, pp. 66–72.
14. Pratt, K. C., Nelson, A. K., and Sun, K. H.: The Behavior of the Newborn Infant. Columbus: Ohio State University Press, 1930.
15. Lipsitt, L. P., Engen, T., and Kaye, H.: Developmental changes in the olfactory threshold of the neonate. Child Develop. 34:371–376, 1963.
16. Lipsitt, L. P., and Siqueland, E. R.: Conditioned head turning in human infants. J. Exper. Psychol. 3:356–376, 1966.
17. Frank, L.: On the Importance of Infancy. New York: Random House, 1966.
18. Brazelton, T. B.: Neonatal Behavior Assessment Scale. Philadelphia: J. B. Lippincott Co., 1973, p. 5.
19. Brazelton, T. B.: Psychophysiologic reactions in the neonate. I. The value of observation of the neonate. J. Pediatr. 58:508, 1961.
20. Brazelton: Neonatal Scale, p. 5.
21. Kalnins, J. V., and Bruner, J. S.: The coordination of visual observation and instrumental behavior in early infancy. Perception 1974.
22. Papousek, H.: Conditioned head rotation reflexes in infants in the first months of life. Acta Paed. Scand. 50:565–576, 1961.
23. Lorenz, K.: The companion in the birds' world. Auk 54:247–273, 1937.
24. Harlow and Zimmerman: Affectional responses in infant monkeys. Science 1959.
25. Klaus, M. H., and Kennell, J. H.: Maternal-Infant Bonding. St. Louis: C. V. Mosby Co., 1976.
26. Mead, M.: Sex and Temperament in Three Primitive Societies. New York: Morrow, 1935.
27. Bayley, N.: Comparisons of mental and motor test scores for age 1–15 months by sex, birthorder, race, geographic location and education of parents. Child Develop. 36:379–411, 1965.
28. Geber, M., and Dean, R. F. A.: The state of development of newborn African children. Lancet 1:1216–1219, 1957.
29. Tronick, E., Koslowski, B., and Brazelton, T. B.: Neonatal Behavior among Urban Zambians and Americans. Presented at the Biennial Meeting of the Society for Research in Child Development, Minneapolis MN, April 1971.
30. Caplan, F.: The First Twelve Months of Life. New York: Grosset and Dunlap, 1973, p. 132.
31. Maier, H.: Three Theories of Child Development. New York: Harper and Row Publishers, 1969, pp. 105–107.
32. Ibid., pp. 107–112.
33. Piaget, J.: The Construction of Reality in the Child. New York: Basic Books, 1954, p. 32.
34. Caplan, F.: First Twelve Months, p. 241.
35. Eisenson, J., et al.: The Psychology of Communication. New York: Appleton-Century-Crofts, 1963.
36. Lenneberg, E. H.: Biological Function of Language. John Wiley & Sons, 1967.
37. Clifton, C.: Language acquisition. In Spencer, T. D., and Kass, N. (eds.): Perspectives in Child Psychology: Research & Review. New York: McGraw-Hill Book Co., 1970.
38. Maier: Three Theories, pp. 112–115.
39. Erikson, E.: Childhood and Society. New York: W. W. Norton & Co., 1963, pp. 251–254.
40. Maier: Three Theories, pp. 115–118.
41. Erikson, E.: Childhood and Society, pp. 255–257.
42. Murphy, L. B.: The Widening Mastery World of Childhood: Paths Toward Mastery. New York: Basic Books, 1962.
43. White, B.: Motivation reconsidered: the concept of competence. Psycholog. Rev. 66:297–333, 1959.
44. Parten, M. B.: Social play among pre-school children. J. Abnorm. Soc. Psychol. 27:243–269, 1932.
45. Papalia, D., and Olds, S.: A Child's World: Infancy Through Adolescence. New York: McGraw-Hill Book Co., 1975, p. 224.
46. Rebelsky, F., and Hanks, C.: Fathers' verbal interaction with infants in the first three months of life. Child Develop. 42:63–68, 1972.
47. Kohlberg, L.: The child as a moral philosopher. Psychol. Today 2:25–30, 1968.
48. Flavell, J.: The Developmental Psychology of Jean Piaget. New York: Van Nostrand Co., 1963.
49. Papalia and Olds: Child's World, p. 280.
50. Ibid., p. 343.
51. Ibid., p. 351.
52. Kirchner, E. and Vondracek, S.: What do you want to be when you grow up? Vocational choice in children aged three to six. Paper presented at the Biennial Meeting of the Society for Research in Child Development, 1973.
53. Papalia and Olds, p. 427.
54. Craig: Human Development, p. 298.
55. Maier: Three Theories, p. 141.
56. Bayley, N.: Consistency and variability in the growth of intelligence from birth to eighteen years. J. Genet. Psychol. 75:165–196, 1949.
57. Maier: Three Theories, p. 54–55.
58. Bronfenbrenner, U.: Responses to pressure from peers versus adults among Soviet and American school children. In Papalia and Olds: Child's World.
59. Papalia and Olds: Child's World, p. 538.
60. Inhelder, B., and Piaget, J.: The Growth of Logical Thinking from Childhood to Adolescence. New York: Basic Books, 1958.
61. Elkind, D.: Egocentrism in adolescence. Child Develop. 38:1025–1034, 1967.

BIBLIOGRAPHY

Ames, L. B.: Child Care and Development. Philadelphia: J. B. Lippincott Co., 1970.

Bernard, H. W.: Human Development in Western Culture, ed. 4. Boston: Allyn & Bacon, 1975.

Craig, G. J.: Human Development. Englewood Cliffs NJ: Prentice-Hall, 1976.

Developmental Psychology Today. Del Mar CA: CRM Books, 1971.

Gesell, A., and Armatruda, C.: Developmental Diagnosis. New York: Harper & Row Publishers, 1967.

Hurlock, E. B.: Developmental Psychology, ed. 4. New York: McGraw-Hill Book Co., 1974.

Kaluger, G., and Kaluger, M. F.: Human Development: The Span of Life. St. Louis, C. V. Mosby Co., 1974.

Kopp, C. B. (ed.): Reading in Early Development: For Occupational and Physical Therapy Students. Springfield IL: Charles C Thomas, Publishers, 1971.

Lovell, K. and Elkind, D.: An Introduction to Human Development. Glenview IL: Scott, Foresman and Co., 1971 (paperback).

Mussen, P. H. (ed.): Carmichael's Manual of Child Psychology, ed. 3., Vol. I. New York: John Wiley & Sons, 1970.

Mussen, P. H., and Conger, J. J.: Child Development and Personality, ed. 4. New York: Harper & Row Publishers, 1974.

Spencer, T. D., and Kass, N. (eds.): Perspectives in Child Psychology: Research and Review. New York: McGraw-Hill Book Co., 1970.

Talbot, T. (ed.): The World of the Child: Clinical and Cultural Studies from Birth to Adolescence. New York: Jason Aronson, 1967.

Wendell, J. E. (ed.): Child Development, Vol. 44, No. 2. Chicago: University of Chicago Press, June 1973.

White, R. W.: The urge towards competence. Am. J. Occup. Ther. 25:271–274, 1971.

Theoretical Foundations

Baldwin, A. L.: Theories of Child Development. New York: John Wiley & Sons, 1967.

Beard, R. M.: An Outline of Piaget's Developmental Psychology for Students and Teachers. New York: Basic Books, 1969.

Erikson, E.: Childhood and Society. New York: W. W. Norton & Co., 1964 (paperback).

Flavell, J. H.: The Development Psychology of Jean Piaget. New York: Van Nostrand Co., 1973.

Freud, S. (Strachey, J., translator): Totem and Taboo. New York: W. W. Norton and Co., 1952 (paperback).

Ginsburg, H., and Opper, S.: Piaget's Theory of Intellectual Development: An Introduction. Englewood Cliffs NJ: Prentice-Hall, 1969.

Hall, C.: A Primer of Freudian Psychology. New York: New American Library: W. W. Norton & Co., 1973.

Hilgard, E. R., and Bower, G. H.: Theories of Learning, ed. 4. New York: Appleton-Century-Crofts, 1974.

Hill, W. F.: Learning: A Survey of Psychological Interpretations, rev. ed. Corte Madera CA: Chandler & Sharp, Publishers, 1971.

Maier, H.: Three Theories of Child Development, ed. 2. New York: Harper & Row Publishers, 1969.

Piaget, J.: The Origins of Intelligence in Children. New York: International Universities Press, 1952.

Prenatal Development

Developmental Psychology Today. Del Mar CA: CRM Books, 1971.

Flanagan, G.: The First Nine Months of Life. New York: Simon & Schuster, 1962.

Hooker, D.: The Pre-Natal Origin of Behavior. New York: Hafner Press, 1969.

Ingelman-Sundberg, A., and Wirsen, C.: A Child Is Born: The Drama of Life Before Birth. New York: Dell Publishing Co., 1966.

Rugh, R., et al.: From Conception to Birth: The Drama of Life's Beginnings. New York: Harper & Row Publishers, 1971.

Infancy and Childhood

Aldrich, M., and Anderson, C.: Babies Are Human Beings. London: Collier and Macmillan, 1967.

Babcock, D. E.: Introduction to Growth, Development, and Family Life. Philadelphia: F. A. Davis Co., 1972.

Beadle, M.: A Child's Mind. Garden City NY: Anchor Books, Doubleday & Co., 1971.

Bettelheim, B.: The Children of the Dream. New York: Macmillan Publishing Co., 1971.

Brazelton, T. B.: Infants and Mothers: Individual Differences in Development. New York: Dell Publishing Co., 1969.

Brazelton, T. B.: Neonatal Behavioral Assessment Scale. Philadelphia: J. B. Lippincott Co., 1973.

Caplan, F. (ed.): The First Twelve Months of Life: Your Baby's Growth Month by Month. New York: Grossett & Dunlap, 1973.

Castle, P., Held, R., and White, B. L.: Observations on the development of visually-directed reaching. Child Develop. 35:349–364, 1964.

Connolly, K. J. (ed.): The Growth of Competence. New York: Academic Press, 1974.

Cottle, T. J.: Time's Children: Impressions of Youth. Boston; Little, Brown, & Co., 1971.

Dekaban, A.: Neurology of Early Childhood. Baltimore: Williams & Wilkins Co., 1959.

Elkin, F., and Handel, G.: The Child and Society: The Process of Socialization. New York: Random House, 1972.

Elkind, D.: Children and Adolescents, Interpretive Essays on Jean Piaget, ed. 2. New York: Oxford University Press, 1974.

Elkind, D.: A Sympathetic Understanding of the Child: Birth to Sixteen. Boston: Allyn & Bacon, 1974.

Fraiberg, S.: The Magic Years. New York: Charles Scribner's Sons, 1968.
Furth, H. G., and Wachs, H.: Thinking Goes to School: Piaget's Theory in Practice. New York: Oxford University Press, 1975.
Gesell, A.: The First Five Years of Life. New York: Harper & Row Publishers, 1940.
Gesell, A., and Ilg, F. L.: The Child from Five to Ten. New York: Harper & Row Publishers, 1946.
Goethals, G. W., and Klos, D. S. (eds.): Experiencing Youth: First Person Accounts. Boston: Little, Brown, & Co., 1970.
Hartley, R. E., and Goldenson, R. M.: The Complete Book of Children's Play, rev. ed. New York: Apollo Editions, 1963.
Hartley, R. E., et al.: Understanding Children's Play. New York: Columbia University Press, 1952.
Held, R., and White, B. L.: Plasticity of sensorimotor development in the human infant. In Rosenblith, J. F., et al. (eds.): Causes of Behavior: Readings in Child Development and Educational Psychology. Boston: Allyn & Bacon, 1966.
Kennell, J., and Klaus, M. H.: Maternal Infant Bonding. St. Louis: C. V. Mosby Co., 1976.
McGraw, M.: The Neuromuscular Maturation of the Infant. New York: Hafner Press, 1963.
Millar, S.: The Psychology of Play. Baltimore: Penguin Books, 1968.
Mussen, P. H., and Conger, J. J.: Child Development and Personality, ed 4. New York: Harper & Row Publishers, 1974.
Peiper, A.: Cerebral Function in Infancy and Childhood. New York: Plenum Publishing Corp., 1964.
Piaget, J.: Construction of Reality in the Child. New York: Basic Books, 1954.
Piaget, J.: Play, Dreams and Imitation in Childhood. New York: W. W. Norton & Co., 1951.
Piaget, J.: The Moral Judgment of the Child. New York: Macmillan Publishing Co., 1932.
Piaget, J.: The Origins of Intelligence in Children. New York: International Universities Press, 1966.
Piaget, J., and Inhelder, B.: The Psychology of the Child. New York: Basic Books, 1969.
Prechtl, H.: A Neurological Examination of the Full Term Newborn Infant. London: Spastics International Medical Publishers, 1964.
Reilly, M.: Play as Exploratory Learning. Beverly Hills: Sage Publications, 1974.
Schaefer, C. (ed.): The Therapeutic Use of Child's Play. New York: Jason Aronson, 1975.
Smith, D. W., and Bierman, E. L. (eds.): The Biologic Ages of Man: From Conception Through Old Age. Philadelphia: W. B. Saunders Co., 1973.
Stone, J., et al.: The Competent Infant: Research and Commentary. New York: Basic Books, 1974.
Talbot, T.: The World of the Child: Clinical and Cultural Studies from Birth to Adolescence. New York: Jason Aronson, 1967.
White, B. L.: Human Infants: Experience and Psychological Development. Englewood Cliffs NJ: Prentice-Hall, 1971.

Adolescence

Adams, J. F.: Understanding Adolescence: Current Developments in Adolescent Psychology, ed. 2. Boston: Allyn & Bacon, 1973.
Alexander, T.: Children and Adolescents: A Biological Approach to Psychological Development. Chicago: Aldine Publishing Co., 1969.
Bronfenbrenner, U.: Two Worlds of Childhood: U.S. and U.S.S.R. (Touchstone Edition) New York: Simon and Schuster, 1972.
Cantwell, Z., and Svajian, P. (eds.): Adolescence: Studies in Development. Itasca IL: Peacock Publishers, 1974.
Caplan, G., and Lebovici, S. (eds.): Adolescence: Perspectives. New York: Basic Books, 1965.
Conger, J. J.: Adolescence and Youth: Psychological Development in a Changing World. New York: Harper & Row Publishers, 1973.
Dragastin, S. E., and Elder, G. H., Jr. (eds.): Adolescence in the Life Cycle: Psychological Change and the Social Context. New York: Halsted Press, 1975.
Elkind, D.: Children and Adolescents: Interpretive Essays on Jean Piaget. New York: Oxford Press, 1974.
Erikson, E. H.: Identity: Youth and Crisis. New York: W. W. Norton & Co., 1968.
Feinstein, S. C., and Giovaccini, P. (eds.): Adolescent Psychiatry, Vol. IV. New York: Jason Aronson, 1975.
Friedenberg, E. Z.: Coming of Age in America. New York: Random House, 1965.
Friedenberg, E. Z.: The Vanishing Adolescent. New York: Dell Publishing Co., 1962.
Garrison, K. C., and Garrison, K. C., Jr.: Psychology of Adolescence, ed. 7. Englewood Cliffs NJ: Prentice-Hall, 1975.
Grinder, R. E. (ed.): Studies in Adolescence, ed. 3. New York: Macmillan Publishing Co., 1975.
Inhelder, B., and Piaget, J.: The Growth of Logical Thinking: From Childhood to Adolescence. New York: Basic Books, 1958.
James, M., and Jongeward, D.: Born to Win: Transactional Analysis with Gestalt Experiment. Reading MA: Addison-Wesley Publishing Co., 1971.
Josselyn, I. M. (ed.): Adolescence: A Report. New York: Harper & Row Publishers, 1971.
Kohen-Raz, R.: The Child from Nine to Thirteen. New York: Jason Aronson, 1974.
Mead, M.: Culture and Commitment. Garden City NJ: Natural History Press, Doubleday & Co., 1970.
Muuss, R.: Theories of Adolescence, ed. 2. Gloucester MA: Peter Smith Publisher, 1975.
Rogers, C.: On Becoming a Person. Boston: Houghton Mifflin Co., 1970.
Shamsie, S. J.: Youth: Problems and Approaches. Philadelphia: Lea and Febiger, 1972.

Talbot, N. B.: Raising Children in Modern America. Boston: Little, Brown, & Co., 1976.

Winder, A.: Adolescence, ed. 2. New York: Van Nostrand Reinholt Co., 1974.

Adulthood

Beauvoir, S. de: The Coming of Age: The Study of the Aging Process. New York: Putnam & Sons, 1972.

Bowlby, J.: Separation: Anxiety and Anger. New York: Basic Books, 1973 (children and adult).

Clausen, J. A. (ed.): Socialization and Society. Boston: Little, Brown, & Co., 1969.

Clayre, A.: Work and Play. New York: Harper & Row Publishers, 1975.

Duvall, E. M.: Family Development, ed. 4. Philadelphia: J. B. Lippincott Co., 1971.

Jung, C. G.: The stages of life. In Campbell, J. (ed.): The Portable Jung. New York: Viking Press, 1971.

Kimmel, D. C.: Adulthood and Aging. New York: John Wiley & Sons, 1974.

Klein, C.: The Single Parent Experience. New York: Walker and Co., 1973.

Leshan, E.: The Wonderful Crisis of Middle Age. New York: David McKay, 1973.

McFadden, M.: Bachelor Fatherhood: How to Raise and Enjoy Your Children as a Single Parent. New York: Walker and Co., 1974.

Neugarten, B. L.: Dynamics of transition of middle age to old age. J. Geriatr. Psychiatr. 4:1, 1970.

Neugarten, B. L. (ed.): Middle Age and Aging: A Reader in Social Psychology. Chicago: University of Chicago Press, 1968.

Neugarten, B. L., and Doroty, N.: The Middle Years. American Handbook of Psychiatry, March 3, 1972, (1) pt. 3.

Parker, S.: The Future of Work and Leisure. New York: Praeger Publishers, 1972.

Puner, M.: To the Good Long Life: What We Know about Growing Old. New York: Universe Books, 1974.

Schlesinger, B. (ed.): The One Parent Family: Perspectives and Annotated Bibliography, ed. 3. Buffalo: University of Toronto Press, 1975.

Sears, R. R., and Feldman, S. S. (eds.): The Seven Ages of Man. Los Altos CA: William Kaufmann, 1974.

Sheehy, G.: Passages: Predictable Crises in Adult Life. New York: E. P. Dutton & Co., 1976.

Terkel, S.: Working. New York: Pantheon Books, 1974.

White, R.: The Enterprise of Living: Growth and Organization. New York: Holt, Rinehart, & Winston, 1972.

ACKNOWLEDGMENTS

Thanks to my colleagues, Gundega Berzins, O.T.R., Margaret Fatula, O.T.R., Marie Marchant, O.T.R., Elizabeth Tiffany, M.Ed., O.T.R., and Gail Tower, M.S., L.P.T., for their direction and support, Ruth E. Levine, M.Ed., O.T.R., for her artistic developmental wheel, the faculty and students of Temple University, and my family for their encouragement and patience. A special thanks to Virginia Alpaugh, who made the children real.

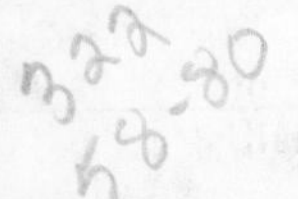

section 2 / Posture and Movement/

Elnora M. Gilfoyle and Ann P. Grady

> It is the child who makes the man, and no man exists who was not made by the child who once he was.[1]

Certain aspects of the theory and philosophy of occupational therapy are based upon the process of human growth, development, and maturation. Throughout the human developmental process, posture and movement serves as a background for an individual's life activities. The acquisition of posture and movement evolves from the early reflex/reaction patterns of the fetus and neonate. In this chapter we present our theory regarding the developmental process of posture and movement and provide a theoretical framework for the application of the process. The theory and framework is related to aspects of dysfunction/disability and to an occupational therapy service program. For further clarification regarding the roles and functions of the occupational therapist as related to the theoretical framework presented in this chapter, the reader is referred to Chapter 14, Minimal Brain Dysfunction.

THEORY OF SPATIOTEMPORAL ADAPTATION

Development results from interaction of the child with his world. Interaction is a spatiotemporal adaptation process by which the child discovers and absorbs the environment. Spatiotemporal adaptation is the continuous, ongoing state or act of adjusting those bodily processes required to function within a given space and at a given time. The process of spatiotemporal adaptations has a developmental sequence and matures with the alteration or modification of performance, which in turn enhances growth, maturation, and development.[2]

Growth is defined as the biological/structural changes of the body (i.e., skeletal/muscular), maturation as the modification within the individual's neurophysiological systems, and development as the modification of the bodily processes in order to perform spontaneous behaviors and adapt to the environment. Although each term has a distinct meaning there is a constant interrelationship among growth, maturation, and development. The interrelationship affects spatiotemporal adaptation and contributes to the uniqueness of each person's developmental process. The developmental process, or the manner, rate, and sequence of acquiring behaviors, results from the transaction between the child and his environment. The term environment, as used in reference to adaptation, is all inclusive. Environment is the complete setting or surrounding, that is, the milieu, including the self, other persons, objects, the earth, space, and the relationship within space. Thus, environment is everything with which an individual interacts.

The spatiotemporal adaptation process of environmental interaction has four components: assimilation, accommodation, association, and differentiation. *Assimilation* is the sensory process of taking-in or receiving information that is external to and/or within the self-system (e.g., a ball is seen as coming toward oneself, and the hands are perceived as being inside one's pockets). *Accommodation* is the response or the motor process of adjusting the body to react to the incoming stimulation (e.g., as the moving ball is perceived the body posture is modified; the hands come out of the pockets and are directed in front of the body in preparation to catch the ball). *Association* is the organized process of relating the sensory information with the motor act and of relating present and past experiences with each other (e.g., relating the perception of the moving ball with the accommodation of the body, the perception of the contact of the body with the ball in space and time, and the present act of catching the ball with a past experience of ball catching). *Differentiation* is the process of discriminating those essential elements of a specific behavior that are pertinent to a given situation, distinguishing those that are not and thereby modifying or altering the behavior in some manner (e.g., discriminating the degree of the forearm pattern that is used to catch the ball, distinguishing the amount of elbow flexion and supination necessary, and thus modifying the forearm position for more efficient ball catching).

Inherent in the spatiotemporal adaptation process is the integration of the sensory input, the motor output, and the sensory feedback. The assimilation component is the sensory input, the accommodation is viewed as the motor output, and the association-differentiation components are the vital parts of sensory feedback that occur as one functions within the environment. The sensory-motor-sensory process of adaptation is integrated by the self-system. Through integration the child organizes for use the information from his environment.[3,4,5] Integration is the child's "inner path" to discovery.

As the child discovers the world, the environment provides the stimulation for new experiences. A child will adapt to the new experience using an older acquired behavior that is a part of his or her self-system.[6] The nervous system integrates the sensory feedback from the new experience with the older acquired behavior that was used to adapt to the new experience. The sensory feedback from the new experience is associated and differentiated, thus facilitating a higher level adaptation.[7,8]

The integration of the new with the old is dependent upon and results in the modification of the nervous system. Therefore, maturation of the nervous system and the resulting enhancement of higher level behaviors results from sensory-motor-sensory (SMS) integration, an inherent process of adaptation.

The term sensory-motor-*sensory* emphasizes the importance of the sensory feedback integration with the initial sensory input and motor accommodation.[9]

The SMS integrative process of spatiotemporal adaptations can be illustrated by the ever-widening and upward continuum of a spiral (Fig. 3-4). The continuum illustrates the ongoing process of development, while the spiral effect emphasizes the integration of the old with the new. The spiraling continuum illustrates and emphasizes that behaviors are modified and expanded by environmental inter-

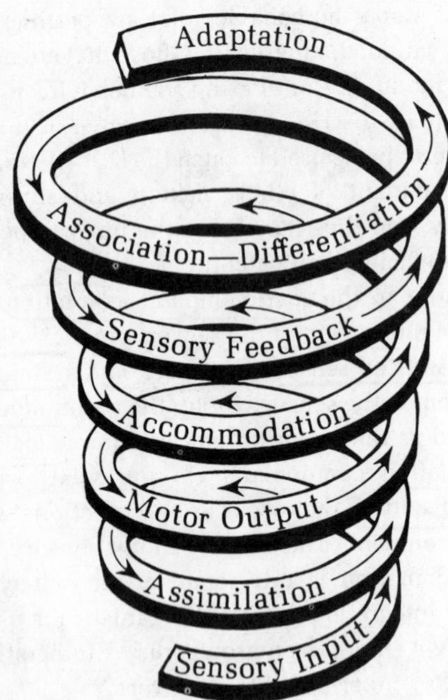

FIGURE 3-4. Spiraling continuum of spatiotemporal adaptation.

actions and nervous system integration to eventually encompass the highest levels of complex functioning.[10]

The spiraling continuum of spatiotemporal adaptation emphasizes three important points:

1. Adaptation to new experiences are dependent upon past acquired behaviors.
2. With the integration of past experiences with new experiences, the past behaviors are modified in some manner and result in a higher level behavior.
3. The integration of higher level behaviors influences and increases the maturity of the lower level behaviors.

Throughout the developmental process, a network of spontaneous SMS behaviors occurs with additional environmental experiences. These observable behaviors, which result from SMS integration and modification of the earlier lower level reactions, are functional expressions of a child's SMS integration. The lower level reactions are integrated into the ontogenic sequence to the extent that they may lose their original identity but their trace effects contribute to the higher level spatiotemporal adaptations. For example, the foot contact reflexes that facilitate total flexion and extension of the legs of the neonate are modified throughout the developmental process to form higher level patterns of reciprocation. The spiraling continuum framework illustrates the theory that a child does not acquire totally new behaviors but rather behaviors are modifications of the older lower level reactions. Modifications enhance and expand one's performance into high level complex skilled behaviors.[11,12]

With the spiraling process of SMS integration, the association of the old with the new and the new with the old provides the basis for perception. Perception is here defined as the sensory judgment and feeling given to one's experiences and environment. Perception requires thought and memory and as such cannot be separated from the cognitive processes of development. The ability to perceive is dependent upon the process of integrating the sensory input, both external and internal to the body, with the motor act; and then associating and differentiating the new experience with the older past-acquired behaviors. The importance of sensory feedback becomes more apparent when one considers that, without association/differentiation, sensory input would remain at a receptive level. Thus perception is basic to an individual's spatiotemporal adaptations and results from the inner-path of SMS integration.

As a child interacts, the challenge of the environment may exceed his or her functional capacity to adapt and the child will experience spatiotemporal stress. In the stress situation, certain aspects of lower level SMS behaviors will be utilized to adapt to the environmental demands. For example, in patterns of early sitting and walking, shoulder retraction and elbow flexion, an aspect of the lower level pivot-prone posture, can be observed (Fig. 3-5). The child adapts with this lower level pattern in order to facilitate the spinal extension necessary for maintaining the vertical posture. As the vertical sitting and walking experiences are repeated, the lower level reactions are associated and differentiated so that the essential elements are integrated to form higher level adaptations. With the above example, the essential elements of the postural extensor tone are differentiated from the shoulder-retraction/elbow-flexion pattern of the pivot-prone posture. Through SMS

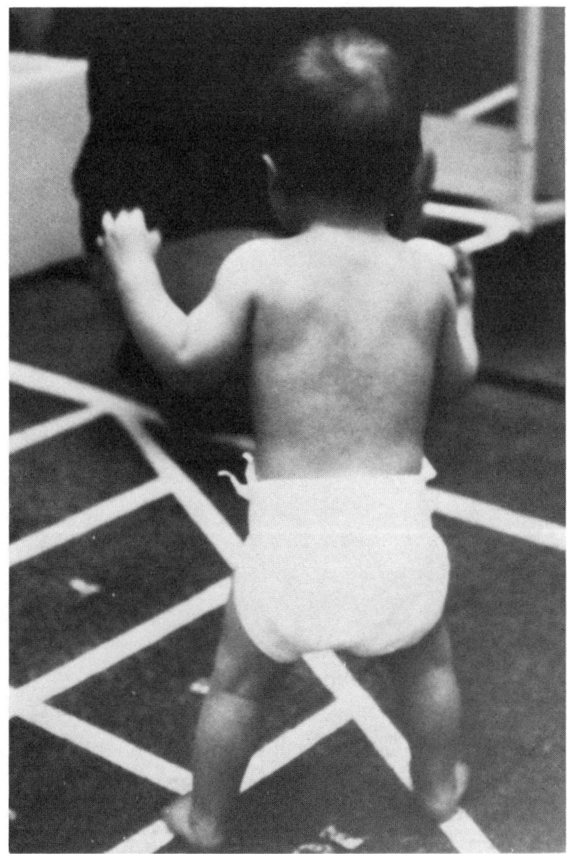

FIGURE 3-5. Early walking pattern illustrating shoulder retraction to facilitate spinal extension.

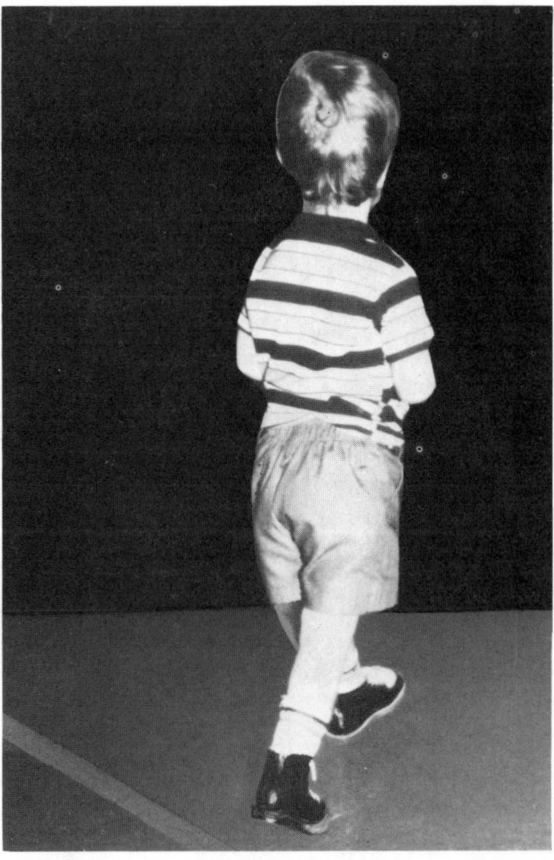

FIGURE 3-6. Mature postural pattern illustrating trunk stability in walking.

experiences and the adaptation process, the child modifies the lower level pattern utilized for trunk stability into a higher level vertical posture (Fig. 3-6).

The effects of stress upon a child's spatiotemporal adaptation are further illustrated in Figures 3-7 through 3-10. In these figures, the child's sensory integration has been temporarily altered. Figure 3-7 illustrates the child adapting with a beginning form of the Landau reaction. When deprived of vision, as in Figure 3-8, the child's sensory integration has changed and the midline stability of the Landau reaction is interrupted. The child adapts to this stress situation with a lower level pattern of asymmetrical stability.

A five-year-old boy demonstrates the stress phenomenon on a higher level in the next two illustrations. While walking with his eyes open on a balance beam he utilizes a mature equilibrium adaptation with his upper extremities (Fig. 3-9). Compare the equilibrium reaction in Figure 3-9 with Figure 3-10, where the child walks on a balance beam with eyes closed. Note the lower level immature equilibrium adaptation. The changing integration that occurs with vision occluded results in spatiotemporal stress and the child adapts with a more primitive pattern.

Spatiotemporal stress is a natural phenomenon that frequently is observed during the developmental process. A child appears to regress downward on the spiral to utilize the more familiar lower level behavior when adapting to new situations. Through the association/differentiation component of adaptation, the child integrates and perceives the aspects of lower level behaviors that are essential for perform-

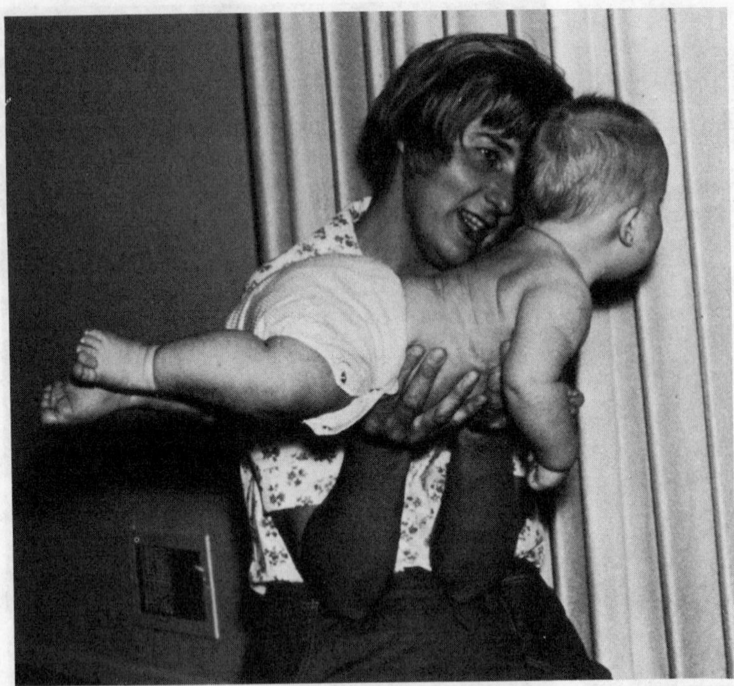

FIGURE 3-7. Adaptation with midline holding pattern.

ance and thus modifies the more primitive behavior in some manner. The modification results in a higher level adaptation, performance behaviors are enhanced, and the child's functional capacities expand.[13]

When the nervous system cannot differentiate the essential elements from lower level behaviors and integrate these elements into higher level reactions, a child will repeatedly adapt with the more primitive SMS behavior. If the lower level primitive reaction persists and is repeatedly elicited, the persistent primitive behavior will interfere with the individ-

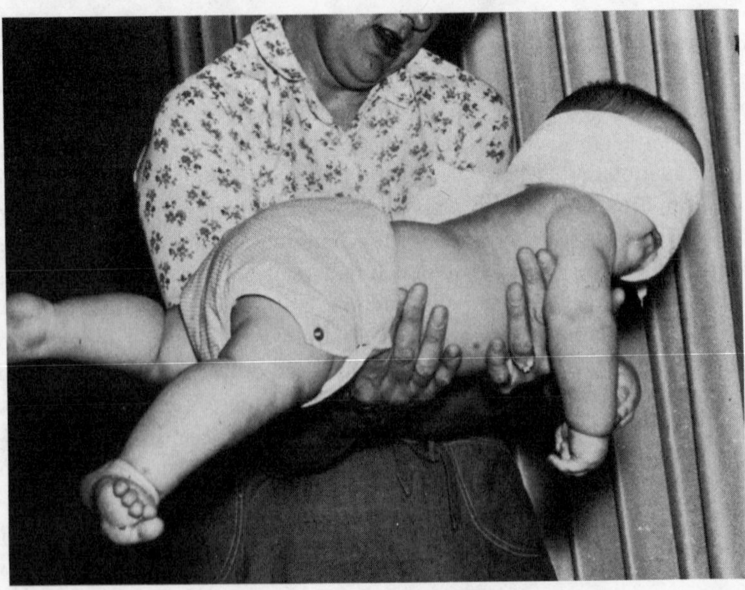

FIGURE 3-8. Under stress the child adapts with a lower level asymmetrical posture.

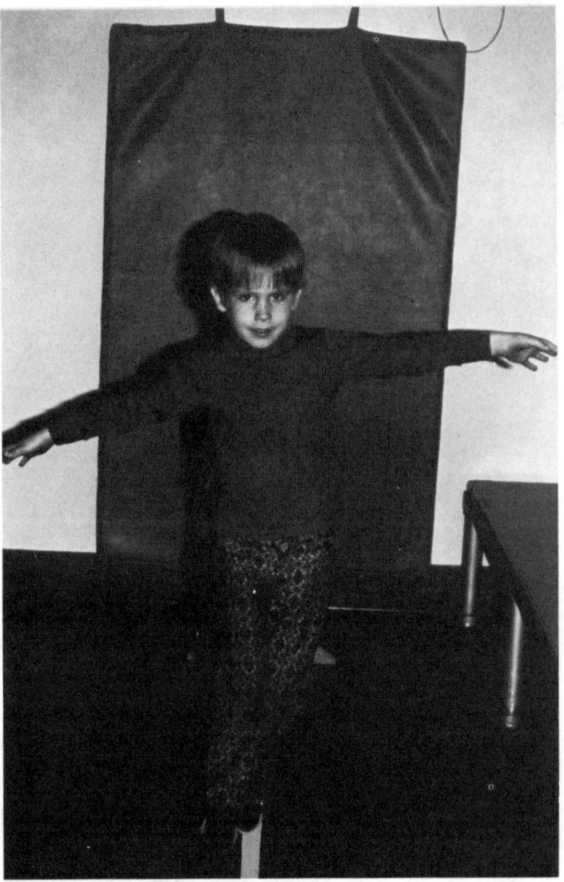

FIGURE 3-9 Adaptation with mature midline stability and equilibrium.

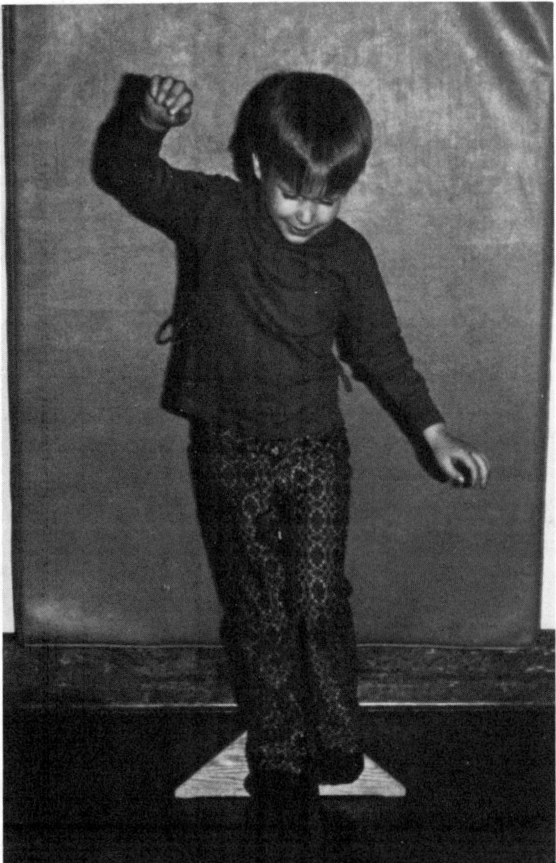

FIGURE 3-10. Under stress the child adapts with immature, assymetrical patterns.

ual's adaptation to space. When the lower level behavior persists, a developmental deviation occurs and dysfunction results.[14]

Dysfunction is defined as the inability effectively to perform and interact with the environment. The spatiotemporal adaptation process and the inherent SMS integration is affected, resulting in a developmental disability. Developmental disability is the result of any condition, trauma, deprivation, or disease (congenital, acute, progressive, or chronic) which interrupts or delays the sequence and rate of normal growth, development, and maturation. The interruption or delay of the developmental sequence perpetuates further dysfunction.

During the developmental process the therapist may observe dysfunction and/or disability of two main types:[15]

1. Dysfunction with primitive patterns of posture and movement.
2. Dysfunction with pathological patterns of posture and movement.

Primitive dysfunction is characterized by the influence of primitive, lower level behaviors being utilized repeatedly to adapt to the environment. The patterns are described as clumsy, awkward, uncoordinated, and immature (Fig. 3-11). The patterns are similar to those observed with younger children during the normal developmental process; however, they reflect a stronger influence of primitive generalized reactions. There is the clumsy, awkward quality that is not present with the child during a course of normal development.

Pathological dysfunction may also represent

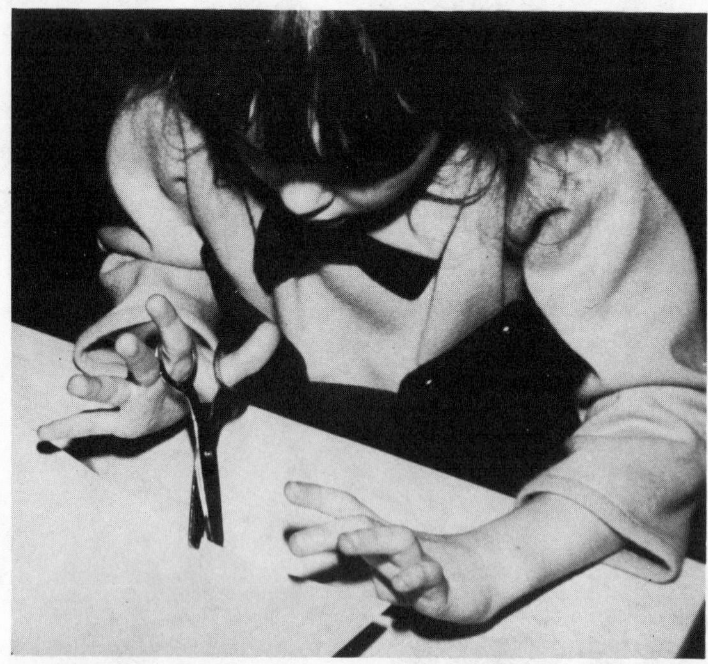

FIGURE 3-11. Dysfunction illustrated by primitive finger extension and associated movements.

many primitive patterns of posture and movements; however, pathological patterns are accompanied by abnormal muscle tone and abnormal reflexive behaviors that control the posture and movement of the child (Fig. 3-12). A pathological pattern may include hypertonicity and/or hypotonicity, abnormal stretch reflexes, and involuntary athetoid movements. Primitive patterns of dysfunction frequently are associated with children diagnosed as minimal brain dysfunction, while pathological patterns are associated with cerebral palsy.[16]

Developmental disability or dysfunction is neither a single diagnosis nor a disease but a condition which may result from a variety of etiological factors. Diagnostic categories which are frequently characterized by developmental deviations and have been classically serviced by an occupational therapy program are given in Table 3-6. Children with diagnostic labels listed in the chart frequently manifest dysfunction, either primitive or pathological. Further information regarding dysfunction and developmental disabilities will be presented in following chapters.

In summary, the theory of the development of posture and movement is based upon a child's spatiotemporal adaptation process. The process has a hierarchical organization and is illustrated by a spiraling continuum model. The spiral emphasizes that adaptation of new environmental experiences is dependent upon past behaviors and that, with the introduction of new experiences, higher level adaptations of the past behaviors result. The development of spatiotemporal adaptation is dependent upon and results in the maturation of the nervous system. The theory is based on eight assumptions:

1. Sensory-motor-sensory behaviors are functional expressions of a child's integration.
2. Sensory-motor-sensory integration, an adaptation process, is dependent upon the interaction between nervous system maturation and environmental experiences.
3. Sensory-motor-sensory development is hierarchical with increasingly higher level behaviors gradually emerging from the lower level behaviors as a result of continual environmental contact.
4. Perception results from the integration of new adaptations becoming associated and differentiated with past behaviors.
5. Lower level sensory-motor-sensory behaviors will emerge when the environmental demands exceed the functional capacities of a child.

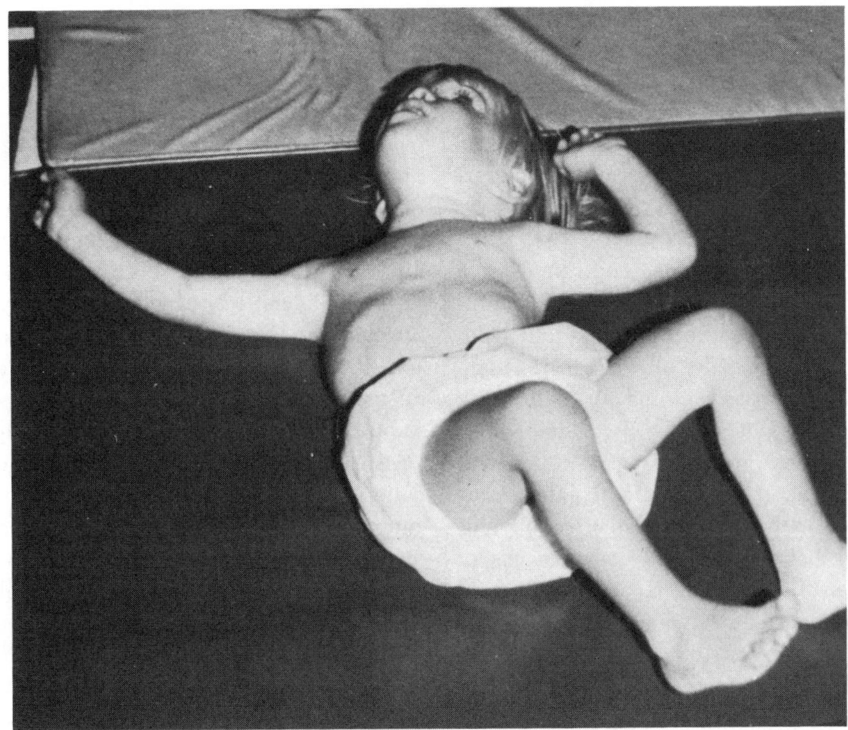

FIGURE 3-12. Dysfunction illustrated by pathological asymmetrical posture and abnormal muscle tone.

Table 3-6. Pathological categories associated with developmental dysfunctions.

Congenital-Developmental Deviations	*Acquired-Regressed Development and/or Developmental Deviations*
Cerebral palsy	Aphasia
Childhood aphasia	Asthma/Allergies
Down's syndrome	Arthritis
Epilepsy	Autism
Ego deviations	Behavior disorders of childhood and adolescence
Hydrocephalus	Cerebrovascular disease
Infantile autism	Encephalitis
Minimal brain dysfunction	Ego deviations
Spina bifida	Child abuse/Battering
Tay-Sachs disease	Meningitis
Turner's syndrome	Multiple sclerosis
Congenital amputee	Muscular dystrophy
	Spinal cord injuries
	Schizophrenia
	Organic brain syndrome with psychosis
	Neoplasms of brain

6. If lower level behaviors persist, a developmental deviation occurs and dysfunction/disability results.
7. Dysfunction/disability delays and interferes with the process of growth, maturation, and development.
8. Dysfunction/disability is characterized by immature spatiotemporal adaptation with primitive and/or pathological patterns of posture and movement being enhanced.

These assumptions are utilized in the construction of a framework for the developmental process. The theoretical framework can be utilized as the foundation for the occupational therapy service programs.

THEORETICAL FRAMEWORK

Occupational therapy is concerned with the development and/or restoration of occupational performance skills. Occupational performance skills include self-help, school/work, and play/leisure activities. The occupational therapist's knowledge of the SMS integrative processes which contribute to occupational performance skills provides a framework for evaluation and remediation of developmental deviations and dysfunction. The therapist can assess an individual's abilities and determine deficits by considering the SMS processes underlying skill performance and dysfunction in performance.

Knowledge of the process also contributes to a frame of reference for treatment planning and progression when therapeutic intervention is indicated. A therapeutic program can be planned to facilitate the normal SMS processes required for skill while the individual is simultaneously engaged in skill performance activities. For example, a child with dysfunction may react to an oncoming ball by covering his face with his hands in a protective manner, he may lose his balance and fall over because of postural instability, or he may respond with nondirected or random arm movement, recognizing that arm movement is necessary to catch a ball but lacking the control and direction to contact the ball accurately. All of these responses are reflective of normal reactions to a moving ball for children of younger ages. The child described above manifests a deficit. Performance expectations for him indicate that he should have developed an SMS integrative process which allows him to:

1. maintain postural stability in space automatically.
2. respond to a moving ball by timing and directing arm movements toward the ball.
3. concentrate his attention toward the objective of the performance skill—catching the ball.

Postural stability and controlled, directed movement should have developed to the extent that they are automatic reactions elicited by association with visual perception of the oncoming ball. The exact postural set and series of movements is differentiated from the generalized response and is determined by the specific location and speed of the ball. The responses described, such as protection, loss of balance, or random movements, indicate that the child has not sufficiently developed automatic posture and movement reactions within his nervous system and/or integrated those reactions with his visual perception of his environment. A therapeutic program and progression may include facilitation by the therapist of basic postural stability of the body to maintain and move from different positions securely. In addition, the therapist can facilitate the control, direction, and timing of movement in appropriate response to stationary and moving objects. The child may be engaged in the developmental steps of catching a ball: handling it, rolling it, picking it up and receiving it as it approaches, first slowly, then faster. Throughout the therapeutic progression the child achieves a goal related to the ball. He is simultaneously facilitated to acquire automatic postural stability and control of movement, or postural patterns, timing and direction of movement, i.e. skill patterns of movement. The child associates the use of automatic responses with his visual perceptions of the object and performance of an activity. He integrates internal (his body) and external (space and objects) sensory assimilations with his motor accommodations and feedback from the achievement of a goal. He develops SMS skill patterns, which can be differentiated, to perform a wide variety of activities. The process can be modified for catching, hitting, bouncing or kicking a ball, or relating to other similarly moving objects.

An occupational therapy program, based upon the theoretical framework, has four basic objectives:

1. To provide sensory input that facilitates the development of automatic postural patterns underlying occupational performance skills.
2. To develop specific motor output by engaging the child in a developmental sequence of activities or components of activities that facilitate skill patterns in relation to space and objects.
3. To facilitate SMS integration of automatic postural and skill patterns through association of feedback from achievement of the goal.
4. To adapt the SMS process to a wide variety of sequential activities for repetition and differentiation of automatic patterns of posture and movement necessary for spatiotemporal adaptation.

The occupational therapist is uniquely qualified to assess and remediate SMS integrative dysfunction. The therapist's knowledge of normal development, with emphasis on the specific components of neuromusculoskeletal functions underlying SMS integration, together with knowledge of the sequential acquisition of skills, provides a framework to analyze the deficits in performance and facilitate both the automatic and voluntary components of skill.[17]

Neuromusculoskeletal Function Underlying SMS Integration

The SMS integrative process is manifested by neuromusculoskeletal functions. Neuromusculoskeletal (NMS) function describes the coordinated actions of the nervous, muscular, and skeletal systems. The structures and functions of these systems provide the means by which a person interacts with his environment. Sensory assimilations are received through these systems, motor accommodations are expressed by postures and movements dependent upon these systems, and sensory feedback is transmitted from and by these systems.[18]

Primitive NMS functions exist in utero and are present at birth. By means of the SMS process (i.e., assimilation, accommodation, association, and differentiation) primitive structures and functions are modified, expanded, coordinated, and differentiated. For example, a localized response such as head turning associated with the rooting reflex[19] is expanded to a more generalized response, such as head turning causing total trunk rotation or complete rotation pattern for early rolling. Total patterns are differentiated so that the essential function can be combined with other functions, such as combining partial body rotation with sitting posture so the child can maintain sitting, turn head and upper trunk toward one side, pick up a toy, return to the original sitting posture, and play (Fig. 3-13). Primitive structures and functions of the fetus and neonate are changed by maturation, development, and growth which is facilitated by the SMS process and results in spatiotemporal adaptation to the environment.[20,21]

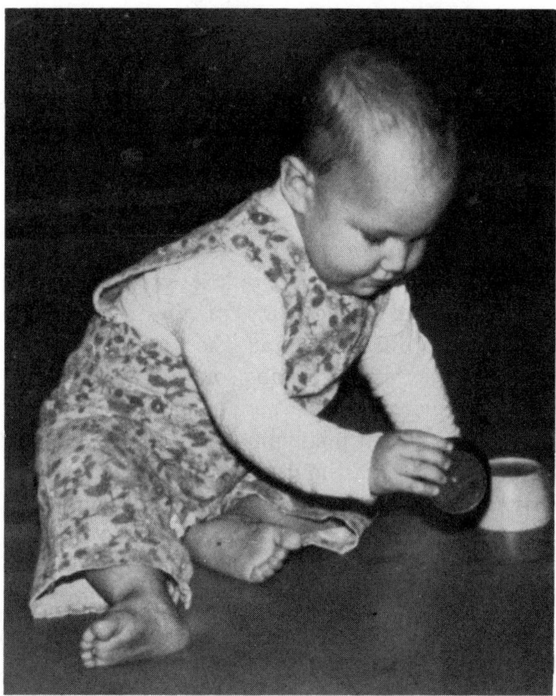

FIGURE 3-13. Child functioning with controlled posture and movement.

The basic functions of the neonate are integrated at the subcortical level since most of the cortex is not functioning as a control for behavior during the first few months of life.[22] As the cortex matures and the infant's environmental experiences expand, primitive responses are modified and integrated under cortical control. Reflexes and reactions which are mediated in the central nervous system mature according to specific functions.[23] Muscles and muscle groups develop specific patterns of mobility and stability. The skeletal system grows to support neuromuscular action. Automatic CNS reflexes and reactions, transmitted by nervous pathways, facilitate appropriate muscle contraction and inhibition, skeletal alignment and realignment, and feedback from the body and the environment. Integration of maturation, development, and growth of the neuromusculoskeletal systems progress according to an orderly sequence that can be analyzed and utilized to evaluate normal and abnormal functioning. The evaluation of NMS function serves as the foundation to plan remediation of dysfunction. The following section describes the theoretical framework of spatiotemporal adaptation by:

1. relating the SMS integrative process to the development of neuromusculoskeletal function.
2. identifying the reflex/reaction maturation components of NMS function.
3. identifying the stability-mobility developmental components of NMS function.

Reflex and Reaction Maturation

Automatic reflexes and reactions are functions of the central nervous system. They are neurological mechanisms that are manifested as predictable patterns of posture and/or movement. The terms "reflex" and "reaction" are used to describe specific responses or series of responses to particular sensory input or to a combination of sensory stimuli. "Reactions are distinguished from reflexes by their greater complexity and inconstancy of the response."[24] According to this distinction, the term "reflex" is probably preferred to describe some of the fetal and neonatal responses that are simple, more predictable, and probably result predominately from one or two sources of sensory stimulation such as tactile and vestibular. The term "reaction" probably applies to more complex responses that develop from infancy and may be retained in maturity, for example, the parachute reaction. Reactions usually develop from integration of simultaneous sensory stimuli such as tactile, vestibular, visual, and auditory. (This text will generally follow these distinctions in terminology unless the accepted term for the particular response differs in most of the literature, e.g., positive supporting reaction.

Reflexes and/or reactions develop through three phases: primitive, transitional, and mature. The primitive phase encompasses phasic and tonic reflexes, the transitional phase includes vertical and rotational righting reactions, and the mature phase consists of midline stability and equilibrium reactions.

Primitive Phase: Phasic and Tonic Reflexes and Reactions

Primitive reflexes and reactions seem to serve two basic purposes in development of NMS function. One purpose is to provide the stimulus for movement so that muscles can begin to develop by activation through a range of motion. Activation of muscles through a range of motion initiates mobility functions of muscles. In addition, sensory assimilations which initiate some of the reflexes provide exteroceptive feedback from the periphery to the central nervous system. Sensory assimilation increases the baby's awareness of both self and environment. The reflexive motor accommodation provides additional feedback about the body in motion.

A second purpose is to provide preliminary fixation of body segments and temporary cessation of movement which may contribute to the development of postural stability. Preliminary fixation and cessation of movement distribute muscle tone in patterns related to stability functions of muscle groups. The baby receives feedback from specific muscle groups activated for fixation. As he or she moves from one primitive stability posture to another, feedback is received about changes in the distribution of muscle tone. Patterns of primitive distribution of tone may be adapted to background postural tone at higher levels of functioning. There are also other influences on the infant's movement and cessation of movement. The baby moves or is quiet in response to sight or sound or moves spontaneously in a variety of unpredictable patterns.

Primitive reflexes and reactions can be classified as phasic reflexes/reaction, which contribute to mobility function, and tonic reflexes/reactions, which contribute to stability development.[25] These two classifications may not be mutually exclusive but the reflexes/reactions are classified according to their apparent purpose.

Phasic reflexes/reactions originate from many kinds of sensory assimilations. The assimilations may be exteroceptive, proprioceptive, or interoceptive. Phasic reflexes are observable movements in response to a touch, pressure (Fig. 3-14), or movement of the body or sight or sound received. Some phasic reflexes such as rooting, sucking, and swallowing are related to survival.[26] Other phasic reflexes are related to protection, causing withdrawal from a stimulus, such as avoiding and flexor withdrawal reflexes.[27] Some phasic reflexes possess the essential elements for reciprocal activity of the limbs, such as crossed extension reflex,[28] primary crawling reflex,[29] and stepping reflex.[30] These reflexes activate the limbs in a reciprocal type of flexion-extension pattern on opposite sides of the body. The reciprocal patterns may be adapted to later crawling, creeping, and walking. In general, phasic reflexes tend to affect the limbs and it is the limbs which will be most mobile in later development of skill. During the spiraling process of adaptation the phasic reflexes will be modified. Some primitive survival reflexes will be modified to more refined patterns such as chewing and swallowing.[31] Some protective reflexes

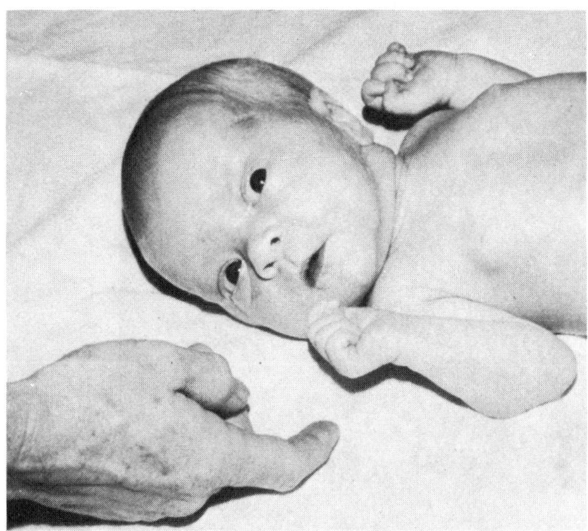

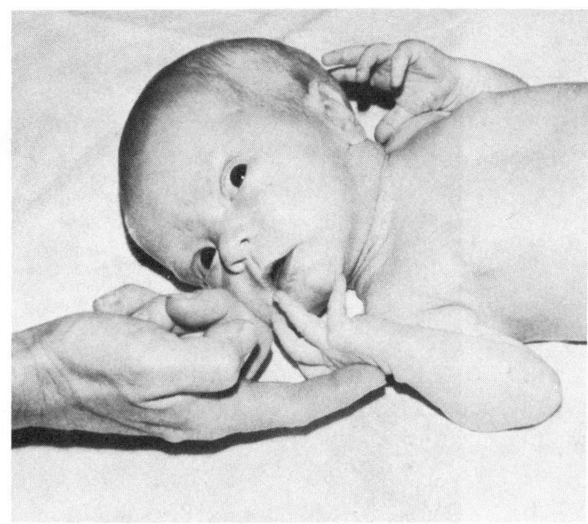

FIGURE 3-14. *Left,* Primitive grasp pattern; *Right,* Finger extension pattern facilitated by touch/pressure.

will be modified when the baby can discriminate between noxious stimuli which require withdrawal and pleasurable stimuli which encourage reaching out for interaction. During the adaptation process essential elements of primitive mobilization, such as reciprocation, will be differentiated and integrated with stability patterns to control and direct reciprocal functioning of the limbs. Higher level CNS reactions, such as righting and equilibrium, will contribute to the development of coordinated sequences of movement.

Tonic reflexes/reactions originate from exteroceptors, proprioceptors, or interoceptors.[32] They are observed as a posture of the body in response to the position of the head and trunk in space or in relation to each other.[33] Tonic reflexes/reactions distribute muscle tone for specific postural patterns (Fig. 3-15). For example, primary standing reflex[34] and positive supporting reaction[35] of the lower extremities distribute lower extremity muscle tone in extension which will be adapted to standing. The asymmetrical tonic neck reflex[36] distributes flexor and extensor tone in opposite patterns on either side of the midline and the symmetrical tonic neck reflex[37] distributes tone in opposite patterns in the upper and lower segments of the body. The stabilization of body segments in specific patterns on either side of the midline or waistline may be adapted to higher level stabilization of one body segment in order to control mobility of an opposite segment (e.g., maintaining stable sitting posture while rotating the upper body to reach for an object). The grasp reflex facilitates flexor tone in the hand[38] which will be adapted to later grasping and holding patterns. Most tonic reflexes/reactions affect parts of the body which will eventually require stabilization to support posture and control movement, such as midline and proximal limb segments, or to control highly-skilled movement, such as hand function.

Phasic and tonic reflexes/reactions influence primitive patterns of movement and distribution of postural tone. Primitive patterns of posture and movement are modified as the nervous system matures and the infant's environmental experiences expand. The essential elements of phasic and tonic reflexes are adapted to higher level righting reactions.

Transitional Phase: Vertical and Rotational Righting Reactions

The development of righting reactions facilitates blending of mobility and stability patterns which were initiated during the primitive phase. Righting reactions[39] adapt the primitive mobility and stability of reflex behavior to total muscle synergies which begin to move the body in space. Righting reactions integrate simultaneous sensory assimilations from tactile, vestibular, visual, and/or auditory recep-

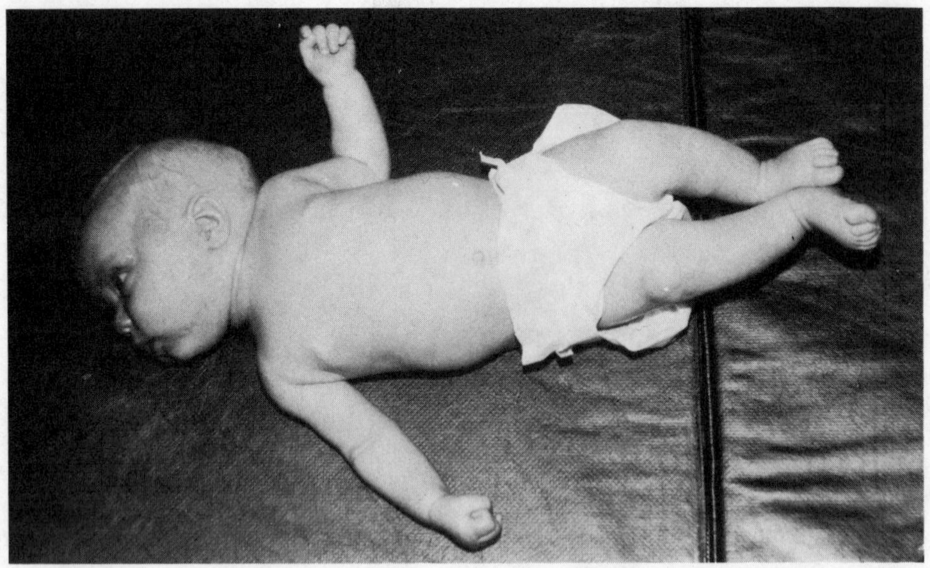

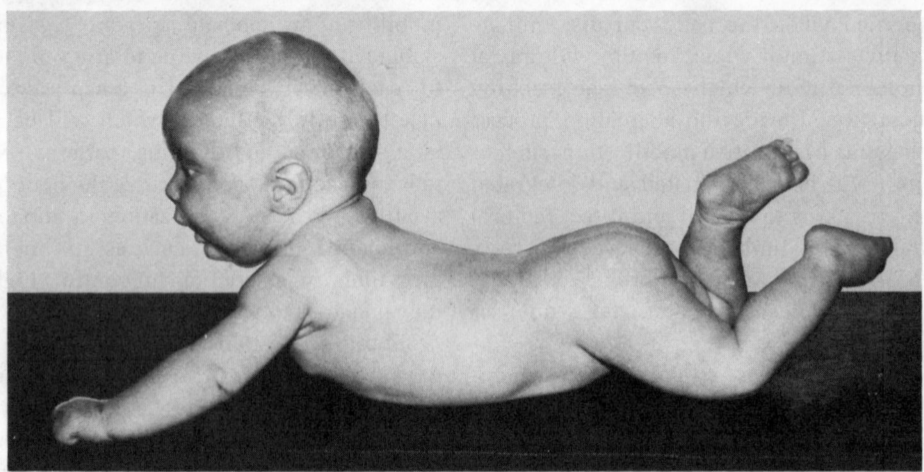

FIGURE 3-15. *Above,* Assymetrical tonic neck reflex; *Below,* Symmetrical tonic neck reflex.

tors.[40] Combined sensory reception stimulates muscle groups which facilitate body alignment and movement from one position to another. The purpose of righting reactions is the distribution of muscle tone in total synergies. The reactions cause the head and other body segments to align in space and with each other,[41] by facilitating vertical or rotational patterns of movement. For example, as an infant raises his head toward vertical from prone-lying, the trunk and limbs tend to follow the head and lift off the supporting surface. Or, as the infant turns his head, the rest of the body tends to rotate with the head and initiate rolling. Righting reactions control the position of the head and body in space and facilitate movement from one position to another during early stages of development. The infant uses righting reactions to sequence movement and maintain postural control when beginning to move between supine and prone, creeping and sitting, and pulling to stand.

Righting reactions can be classified into two groups according to the type of body alignment and direction of movement which characterizes the reaction. The two groups are vertical and rotational righting reactions. The essential differences between the two are the direction of movement and the groups of muscles facilitated by the reaction. Vertical righting reactions move the midline of the body into alignment with the center of gravity and mobilize muscle groups which will be adapted to maintain a vertical posture (Fig. 3-16). Rotational righting reactions move the body around the central axis and mobilize muscle groups which will be adapted to regain vertical postures when the center of gravity is disturbed (Fig. 3-17). During the spiraling continuum, vertical and rotational righting reactions are differentiated and integrated so the infant can combine vertical and rotational body alignment and movement to assume higher level postures. For example, the baby can rotate from prone into sitting, rotate from sitting to creeping, and pull to stand. Integrated vertical-rotational righting reactions automatically facilitate the sequential patterns of mobility and stability.

Vertical righting reactions include labyrinthine righting acting on the head,[42] optical righting,[43] and body righting acting on the head.[44] The individual reactions are termed according to the sensory receptors which are assumed to be primarily responsible for the reaction. Vertical righting is probably initiated by labyrinthine receptors during early stages, but labyrinthine reception is rapidly integrated with input from touch, pressure, and visual receptors. Vertical righting reactions begin with head raising from prone, supine, and lateral positions. With further maturation, the trunk follows the head in a chain reaction, as noted in pull to sit or on-elbows position.[45] The term "chain reaction" is used to describe the tendency for one body segment to follow the movement of an adjacent segment in order to maintain the normal alignment of body parts. Chain reactions facilitate sequences of movement.

Neck and trunk muscles develop in flexion, extension, and lateral flexion. When these muscle groups are fully activated through full range of motion they are prepared to contract simultaneously. Flexors and extensors are activated in a shortened range around the midline and proximal joints to stabilize these body segments. Vertical righting reactions facilitate movement into vertical postures and stabilize body segments to maintain vertical postures.

Rotational righting reactions include neck righting[46] and body righting on the body.[47] The individual reactions are termed according to whether the reac-

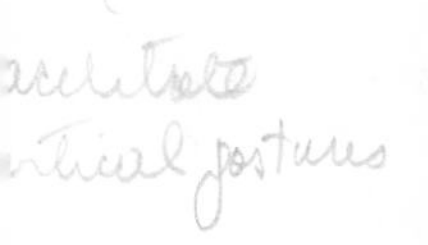

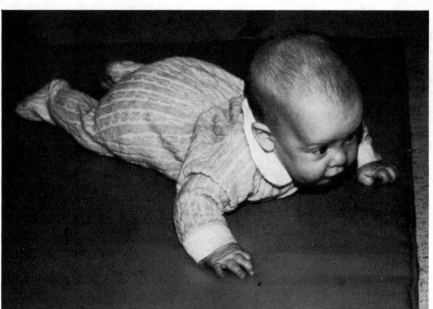

FIGURE 3-16. Vertical righting reaction in prone position.

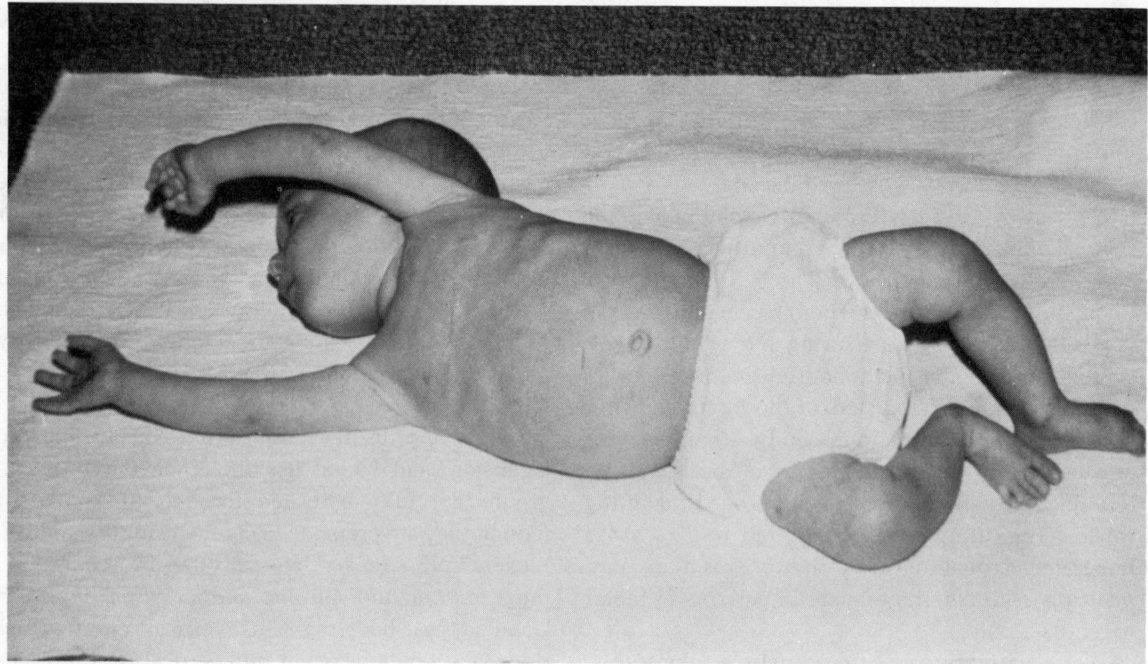

FIGURE 3-17 Rotational righting reaction for rolling.

tion is initiated by the neck or trunk and limbs. Tactile, vestibular, visual, and auditory assimilations are integrated to initiate rotational righting. Rotational righting begins with neck righting—the head turns and the rest of the body follows automatically to roll to sidelying and maintain normal alignment of body segments.[48] With further maturation the trunk segments are differentiated to move independently of each other. Head turning is automatically followed by upper trunk rotation, and upper trunk rotation rotates the lower trunk in a chain reaction and completes a rolling pattern. Rotation between individual body segments allows body righting on the body to develop. The child can initiate rolling with head and neck, upper trunk, or lower trunk.[49]

The child can rotate one body segment in one direction and interrupt the complete rotation pattern by rotating another segment in the opposite direction. Muscle groups are activated through full range of motion in complete rotational synergies and counter-rotational synergies. Rotational muscle action allows the baby to shift weight and free one extremity for reaching out for objects or moving the body in space. Rotational righting reactions are adapted to equilibrium reactions since rotation and counter-rotation are necessary to maintain and regain balance.

Mature Phase: Midline Stability and Equilibrium Reactions

Midline stability and equilibrium are integrated components of mature mobility and stability. They are automatic reactions underlying the child's ability to maintain and regain balance. These reactions integrate the essential elements of head and trunk control from righting reactions with automatic reactions of the extremities. Midline stability and equilibrium are automatically sequenced in an infinite variety of individual patterns to ensure control of posture and movement.

Midline stability reactions are defined as invisible or barely discernible changes in postural stability tone necessary to maintain vertical postures. Muscle groups are coactivated around the midline of the body and proximal limb segments in response to the influence of gravity on stretch receptors and in response to touch-pressure from the supporting surface. The child responds with constant, but barely observable, changes in muscle tone in order

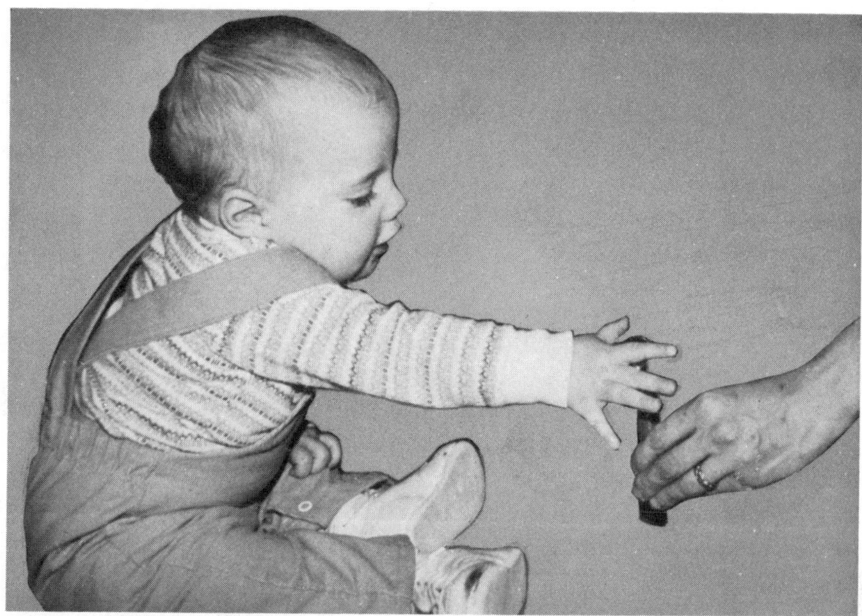

FIGURE 3-18. Midline stability combined with reaching in sitting.

to maintain alignment of the midline of the body with the center of gravity (Fig. 3-18). Midline stability contributes to the child's ability to maintain vertical postures independently.

Equilibrium reactions[50] are compensatory movements to regain midline stability when the alignment of the midline of the body and the center of gravity is sufficiently disturbed. Movement of the body toward the center of gravity is observable. The tactile, vestibular, visual, and auditory receptors receive input for equilibrium reactions. Rotation and counter-rotation of body segments are activated for equilibrium. If the head and upper trunk rotate away from the center of gravity (e.g., reaching from a sitting position), the lower trunk rotates toward the center of gravity to control the upper body and maintain balance (Fig. 3-19). To regain vertical sitting posture, the upper trunk rotates back toward the center and the lower trunk counter-rotates to control the degree of rotation. In addition, if movement away from the center of gravity is rapid, as in loss of balance, the extremities may extend and abduct toward the center of gravity to assist the head and trunk to regain balance. The opposite extremities may extend and abduct to protect the body if balance is lost. Equilibrium reactions are used to maintain and regain balance for all activities.

In summary, automatic reflexes and reactions develop in three phases as the child's CNS matures and his environmental experiences require more complex postures and movements. The essential elements of primitive reflexes are differentiated and adapted to higher level righting, and equilibrium reactions. Reflexes/reactions are simultaneously integrated with other aspects of neuromusculoskeletal function to control posture and movement.

Stability and Mobility Development

Stability, or the ability to maintain or regain equilibrium, is a dynamic process underlying postural control and controlled movement. Stability provides a constantly changing but stable background of normal postural tone that is sufficient to maintain a position while simultaneously allowing movement in the position or from one position to another.[51] Stability is responsible for alignment of body segments at rest or in motion. In addition, stability provides fixation of body segments as a reference point for the initiation and control of movement. The role of stability is less visible to the

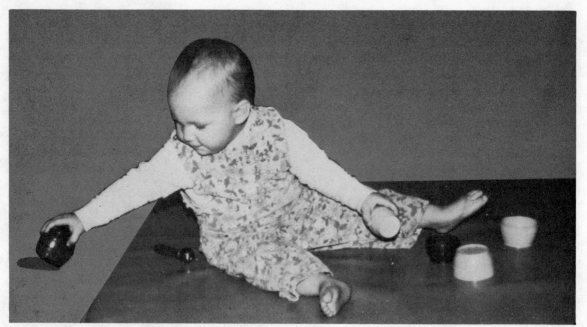

FIGURE 3-19. Rotation and counter-rotation maintains body alignment during reaching.

observer of performance of complex skills which require movement. However, stability is a necessary element for control of purposeful movement. Dysfunction that results in movement disorders may be caused by insufficient stability to control movement or increased stability interfering with the flow of movement.

Mobility, or movement is essential to man's functioning and is the means by which a person interacts with and controls the environment. Movement is necessary for survival since many bodily functions, including breathing and feeding, are dependent on movement. In addition, movement is basic for protection as such actions as withdrawing or fleeing from danger demonstrates, for performance or physical skills requiring mobile action in space or manipulation of objects, for communication through gesture or language, for social interaction as in gathering with others and sharing in activities, and for a variety of ways in which emotion is expressed.[52]

Mobility function is basic to complex sequences of movements which occur in an infinite variety as one movement flows into another.[53] Movement sequences are visible in the performance of most skills. Sequences are combined and modified according to the requirements for specific interaction with space, such as running, jumping, or skipping and/or specific interaction with an object to be manipulated, such as a ball, pencil, or scissors. Dysfunction in skill performance may occur if there is a lack of or interruption of development of smooth sequential movements which flow from one pattern to another while the performer attends to the objective of the skill.

Stability and mobility muscle function is dependent on physiological development of specific muscles and muscle groups, as well as differentiation of muscle groups, according to their primary function, i.e. stability or mobility. Some muscle groups, especially muscles used for skill activities, function primarily as mobilizers. These muscles are characterized by their ability to act with range, speed, and accuracy.[54] Some muscle groups, especially more proximal muscles, function primarily as stabilizers. These muscles readily respond to constant stimuli from gravity and from the supporting surface. Stabilizers maintain contraction in shortened ranges of motion at the midline and around proximal joints for postural stability and control of movement.[55] Some mobilizing muscles develop through a phase of stabilization in order to develop control of movement. For example, certain muscles of the upper extremities function as stabilizers when the baby supports himself in the creeping position. When the baby assumes independent standing, the upper extremities are freed from their support role. The upper extremities can function to protect the body from falling and be utilized in mobility patterns for environmental interaction.[56]

Proximal stability gained from supporting functions allows more controlled or skill patterns of the distal limb segments. According to the spiraling continuum of adaptation, the child develops primitive stability and mobility first. The primitive patterns are modified, differentiated, and blended to perform specific functions, first proximally, then distally, until mature postural patterns and skill patterns are available for purposeful activities.

The neonate begins extrauterine life with primitive mobility patterns which were activated in utero by fetal reflex activity.[57,58,59] The infant is dependent upon the environment for stability. An infant's posture is supported by external sources such as the crib, floor, or his mother's arms. He begins to move in an environment which includes gravity as a force to move against and initiates movement from the surface which gives support as a source of stability. The infant's body constantly interacts with the supporting surface and gravity. It develops musculature that provides internal stability to support posture independently and control movement functionally.

From birth onward, muscles and muscle groups develop stability and mobility functions through four phases:[60]

1. Activation of muscles and muscle groups (Fig. 3-20).
2. Coactivation of agonists and antagonists (Fig. 3-21).
3. Combined stability-mobility actions (Fig. 3-22).
4. Stability and mobility functions (Fig. 3-23).

Activation of Muscles and Muscle Groups

The activation phase of muscle development includes primitive mobility, chain reaction mobility, and primitive stability. During this phase muscles and muscle groups are activated through a complete physiological shortening of agonists and lengthening of antagonists in order to develop the ability to move through a complete range of motion. Reciprocal innervation for contraction of agonist and inhibition of antagonist is facilitated by full shortening and lengthening. Primitive mobility is observed as actual movements of total flexion, extension, or rotation of body segments. The neonate receives feedback about his body parts in motion. Movements for primitive mobility are stimulated by specific phasic reflexes and/or spontaneous behaviors which stimulate full range of body segment movement. Examples of primitive mobility are the flexor withdrawal reflex which causes full flexion of the

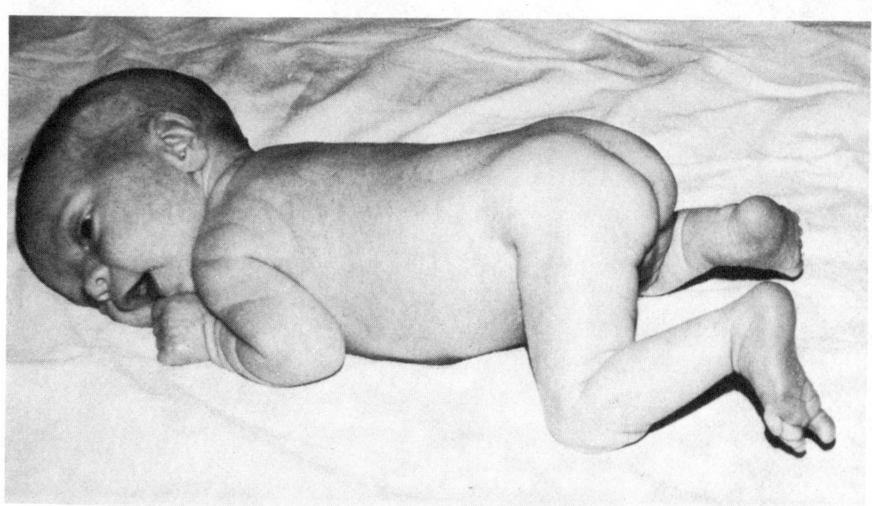

FIGURE 3-20. Activation of flexor muscle groups in prone position.

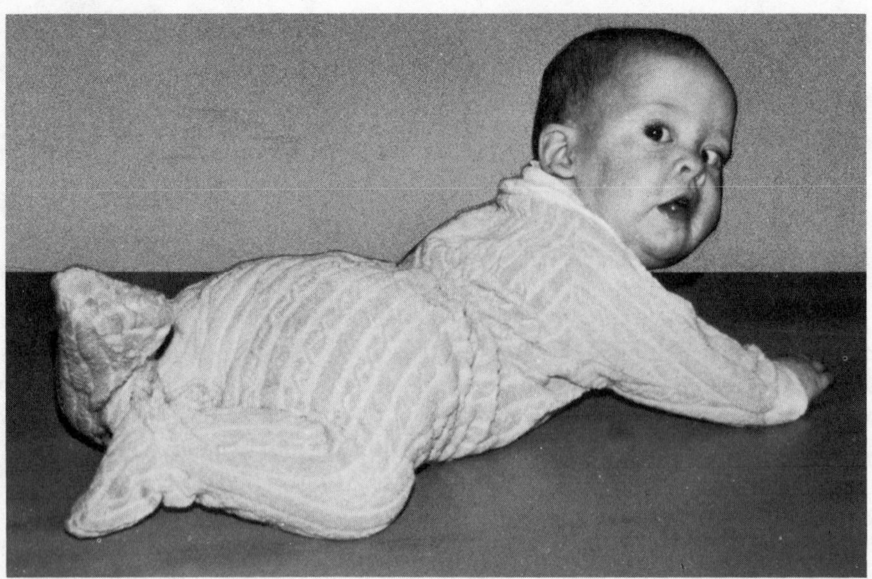

FIGURE 3-21. Coactivation of upper extremity muscle groups for support in prone position.

lower extremity, the avoiding reflex which causes full extension of fingers, and the rooting reflex which causes full rotation of neck.

Muscle activation for mobility is expanded by maturation of righting reactions. Muscle groups are activated in flexion, extension, or rotation synergies which affect the body as a whole. The baby moves into different positions and experiences movement through space and change of body position. Righting reactions activate neck muscles to function

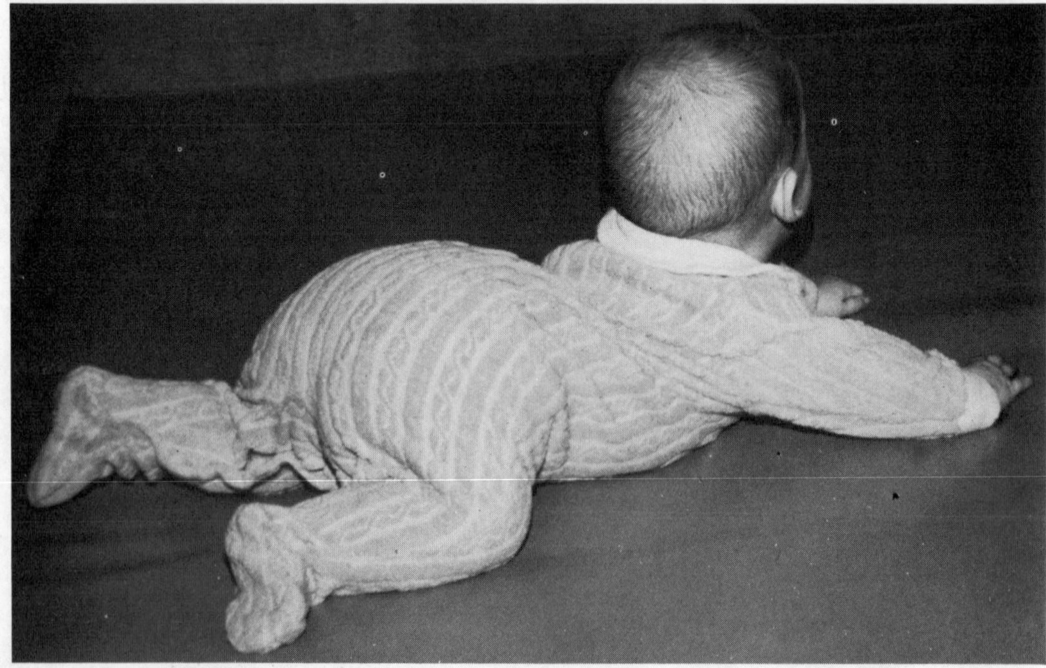

FIGURE 3-22. Combined stability-mobility muscle action to move body in prone position.

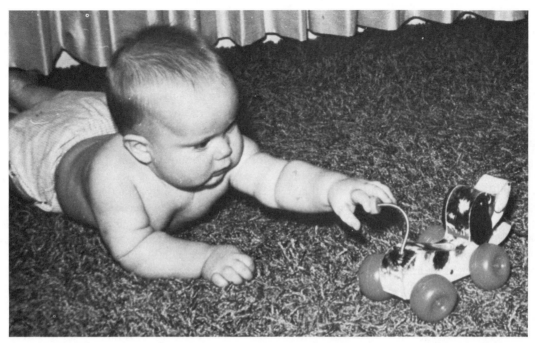

FIGURE 3-23. Dynamic stability and controlled mobility for skill.

against gravity. Neck muscles facilitate trunk and proximal joint muscles by chain reactions; thus synergistic patterns of flexion, extension, and rotation develop. Chain reactions activate flexion mobility patterns when the baby is pulled to sit, extension mobility patterns when he assumes pivot prone extension, and rotation mobility patterns when he rolls over completely. Muscle groups mobilized in flexion, extension, and rotation patterns will be differentiated and blended for flexion-rotation and extension-rotation patterns of movement at higher levels of stability-mobility development.[61]

Primitive stability is observed as specific postures which the baby assumes with support from the environment. Muscle groups are activated in shortening and lengthening contractions for temporary static positions. Tonic reflexes and/or spontaneous behavior facilitate primitive stability. The neonate moves into and from specific postures and experiences cessation of movement associated with primitive distributions of muscle tone. He receives feedback from primitive stability which may serve as a reference point to initiate spontaneous movement. Muscle functions for stability will be expanded during the coactivation phase of muscle development.[62]

Coactivation of Agonists and Antagonists

The initial coactivation phase of muscle development includes midline holding stability and support stability. During the early development of this phase, muscles which have been fully activated are prepared to contract at any point of shortening or lengthening. Coactivation initially develops with simultaneous contraction of agonists and antagonists around joints in order to stabilize joint movement. Muscle groups around the midline of the body are coactivated to facilitate midline holding stability. Midline holding stability maintains head and trunk alignment against gravity when the head and trunk are no longer supported by external sources of stability.

Muscle groups around proximal joints of the body are coactivated for extremity support stability. Extremity support stability allows weight bearing on extremities to support head and trunk in new positions. First the upper extremities, then upper and lower extremities together, and finally lower extremities alone provide contact with the supporting surfaces. The infant develops the ability to move away from total support to extremity support with the advent of righting reactions. Flexors, extensors, and rotators, which are activated by righting reactions and allow the infant to assume new positions against gravity, are coactivated to allow the baby to maintain new positions against gravity. Coactivation of agonists and antagonists initiates the development of internal stability for later development of independent postural and skill patterns. Initial coactivation of muscle groups allows the baby to maintain postures. In order to further develop coactivation, stability function gained from coactivation of muscles in a shortened range will have to be blended with mobility function gained from activation of muscles through the complete range.

Combined Stability-Mobility Actions

The purpose of combining mobility from activation phase with stability from coactivation phase is to develop internal stability for background postural tone which allows the baby to maintain stable postures and retain stable continuity when moving into and out of positions. By blending muscle actions, initial coactivation action, which appears relatively static, is modified into a dynamic process. Mobility which moves the body or body segments is blended with stability which supports posture.[63]

Blended muscle actions develop in a proximal to distal sequence. Patterns of mobility and stability are blended around the midline and proximal segments with the distal limb segments supporting the body in weight-bearing positions. Mobility and stability of the flexor groups and extensor groups are blended in bilateral weight bearing when the baby pushes back and pulls forward in the on-elbows position, while he rocks back and forth in creeping and squat positions, and while he bounces up and down in the standing position.[64] The distal segments of the extremities support the body and movement occurs in the proximal segments.

Muscle actions are further blended when the baby shifts weight from side to side in on-hands position, creeping, squat, and standing. As he shifts weight, he begins to rotate upper and lower body segments in relation to each other. Rotator muscle groups are combined with flexor-extensor groups. Rotation combined with flexion-extension differentiates the total patterns which are developed by means of chain reactions. The baby can extend and rotate the body from prone when pivoting in a circle or pushing up from prone to sit or flex and rotate as he moves from sitting to prone with upper extremity support. Blending flexion, extension, and rotation actions around the midline and proximal segments prepares for adaptation of midline holding patterns to more dynamic midline stability reactions at higher levels of independent postural control. Rotation for weight shift prepares the baby for unilateral weight bearing, which will free one extremity for controlled movement in space.

Stability and Mobility Functions

Specific stability and mobility functions are differentiated from combined stability-mobility actions for independent control of posture and movement. Dynamic stability functions of muscles around the midline and proximal joints are adapted from bilaterally supported postures to unilaterally supported postures in prone, creeping, sitting, kneeling, and standing as well as to vertical postures with upper extremities free in sitting, kneeling, and standing. Stability functions contribute to background postural tone, which is necessary to maintain these positions with midline stability reactions, and, together with mobility functions, to change or regain positions with equilibrium reactions.[64] Stability muscle groups are comprised of muscles which respond to gravity by maintaining sufficient tone to support posture and also allow movement. When mobility muscle groups (agonists) are activated to change or regain positions in space, stability groups (antagonists) are activated to help regulate postural adjustments and changes. The child's posture is secure and he or she can freely engage in skill activities.

Controlled mobility of the extremities for skill performance develops with postural stability. Unilateral weight bearing frees opposite extremities for skill and lower extremity weight bearing frees both upper extremities for skill. Unilateral weight bearing allows the child to reach out and move his body by crawling, creeping, kneel-walking, and walking or reach out to grasp and manipulate objects.[65] Vertical postures allow the child to use his or her hands together or separately for manipulative or nonmanipulative skills such as coloring or ballplaying. Lower extremities develop coordination for skills requiring movement of the body through space such as running, skipping, and hopping.

Free movement of the upper extremities for nonmanipulative activities and all movement of the lower extremities is controlled and directed by stability from the more proximal joints. Agonist-antagonist actions of adjacent extremity segments regulate range, speed, and accuracy of movement in relation to the purpose of the activity.

The upper extremities develop a higher level of skill through the manipulation of objects. Moving and directing an object, such as a pencil or a scissors as an extension of moving and directing one's hand, requires additional control. The child reinforces proximal stability and gains some distal stability when he grasps or prehends an object. By fixing the hand on the object, additional muscle groups are recruited for stabilization required to perform fine movement. Rotation and counter-rotation patterns of the arm and thumb are blended with stabilization to direct the hand as well as the object for smooth sequencing of movements.

In summary, stability and mobility functions develop in four spiraling phases as the muscles and muscle groups develop physiologically and are modified and differentiated to function together for specific purposes. Neuromusculoskeletal function develops with the maturation of reflexes and reactions, the development of stability and mobility patterns, and skeletal growth. The development of neuromusculoskeletal function has an underlying spiraling process. Automatic reactions which are integrated within the nervous system, together with the child's spontaneous interaction with the environment, facilitates progressively higher levels of stability-mobility function. Concurrently, the development and coordination of stability-mobility muscle groups support more complex automatic reactions and a variety of behaviors.

Primitive reflexes and reactions activate primitive flexor, extensor, or rotator stability and mobility patterns, which provide a transitory type of posture and movement control, further adapted by righting reactions to assume more mature postures. New postures facilitate the complex righting and equilibrium reactions which are integrated with combined flexion-extension-rotation patterns and are differentiated in supported and independent postures.

The child relies less on the supporting surface; he has developed his own internal stability and mobility functions, which are coordinated by automatic reactions and available for performance of complex skills (Fig. 3-24).

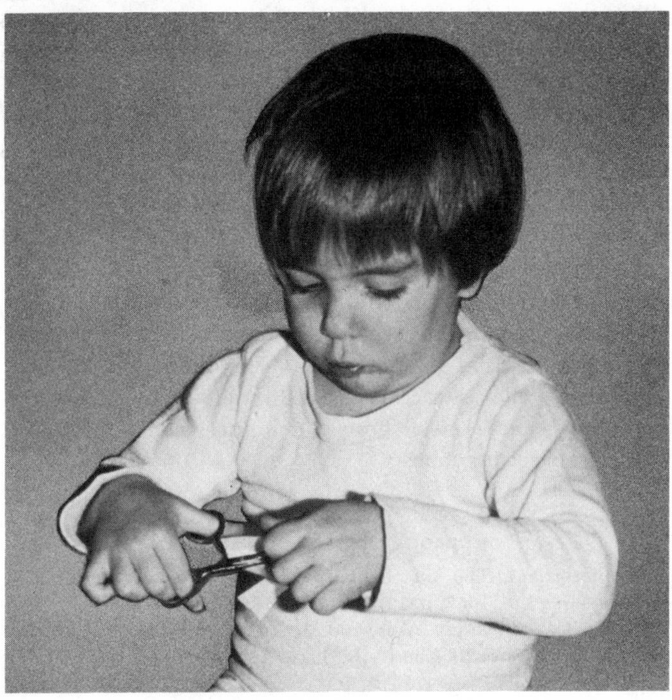

FIGURE 3-24. Posture and movement adapted to complex skills.

As neuromusculoskeletal functions develop, the child is able to move about and explore his environment of space and objects, expanding his perceptions of himself and his world. The child integrates feedback from internal receptors, which tell him about his position in space and his own movement, with information from his external receptors, which tell him about himself in relation to space and objects and objects in relation to space or each other. Internal and external information is associated, differentiated, and integrated through the SMS process. The child develops integrated sequences of movement which can be readily elicited and accurately timed and directed toward the objective of skill performance activities.

SUMMARY

The content of this section provides a theory and a theoretical framework for the development of posture and movement. The developmental theory presented by the authors is based upon the spiraling process of assimilation, accommodation, association, and differentiation. These four components comprise spatiotemporal adaptation, a continuous transaction of the child with the environment. Inherent within the spatiotemporal adaptation theory is the integration of sensory input, motor output, and sensory feedback. Through the spiraling continuum of sensory-motor-sensory integration, higher level behaviors emerge. The spiraling model illustrates that the development of posture and movement patterns are modifications of the lower level primitive behaviors.

The framework for the spatiotemporal adaptation theory is the spiraling continuum of reflexes/reactions, the development of mobility and stability muscle patterns, and skeletal growth. The interrelationships of reflexes/reactions, mobility and stability patterns, and skeletal growth comprise neuromusculoskeletal functions.

REFERENCES

1. Montesorri, M.: The Absorbent Mind. New York: Dell Publishing Co., 1967, p. 15.
2. Gilfoyle, E. M., Grady, A. P., and Moore, J.: Children Adapt. Thorofare NJ: Charles B. Slack, 1978.
3. Ibid.
4. Ayres, J.: Sensory Integration and Learning Disorders. Los Angeles: Western Psychological Services, 1972.
5. Flavell, J.: The Developmental Psychology of Jean Piaget. Princeton: Van Nostrand, 1963.
6. Ibid.
7. Ibid.
8. Gilfoyle, Grady, and Moore: Children Adapt.
9. Ibid.
10. Ibid.
11. Ibid.
12. Flavell: Developmental Psychology of Piaget.
13. Gilfoyle, Grady, and Moore: Children Adapt.
14. Ibid.
15. Bobath, B., and Bobath, K.: Motor Development in the Different Types of Cerebral Palsy. London: W. Heinemann Medical Books, 1975.
16. Ibid.
17. Gilfoyle, Grady, and Moore: Children Adapt.
18. Moore, J.: Neuroanatomy Simplified. Dubuque IA: Kendall/Hunt Publishing Co., 1968.
19. Peiper, A.: Cerebral Function in Infancy and Childhood. New York: Consultants Bureau, 1963.
20. Gilfoyle, Grady, and Moore: Children Adapt.
21. McGraw, M.: The Neuromuscular Maturation of the Human Infant. New York: Hafner Press, 1966.
22. Ibid.
23. Gilfoyle, Grady, and Moore: Children Adapt.
24. Thomas, A.: The Neurological Examination of the Infant. Clin. Develop. Med. 1. London: W. Heinemann Medical Books, 1964, p. 1.
25. Fiorentino, M. R.: Reflex Testing Methods for Evaluating C.N.S. System Development. Springfield IL: Charles C Thomas, Publishers, 1965.
26. Peiper: Cerebral Function.
27. Fiorentino: Reflex Testing Methods.
28. Ibid.
29. Peiper: Cerebral Function.
30. Ibid.
31. Ibid.
32. Gilfoyle, Grady, and Moore: Children Adapt.
33. Fiorentino: Reflex Testing Methods.
34. Peiper: Cerebral Function.
35. Fiorentino: Reflex Testing Methods.
36. Ibid.
37. Ibid.
38. Twitchell, T.: Attitudinal Reflexes, The Child with Central Nervous System Deficit. Children's Bureau, Publication No. 432, 1965.
39. Fiorentino: Reflex Testing Methods.
40. Gilfoyle, Grady, and Moore: Children Adapt.
41. Fiorentino: Reflex Testing Methods.
42. Ibid.
43. Ibid.
44. Ibid.
45. Holt, K. (ed.): Movement and Child Development. Clin. Develop. Med. 55. Philadelphia: J. B. Lippincott Co., 1975.

46. Fiorentino: Reflex Testing Methods.
47. Ibid.
48. Ibid.
49. Ibid.
50. Ibid.
51. Bobath and Bobath: Motor Development.
52. Holt: Movement and Child Development.
53. Bobath and Bobath: Motor Development.
54. Pearson, P., and Williams, C. (eds.): Physical Therapy Services in Developmental Disabilities. Springfield IL: Charles C Thomas, Publishers, 1972.
55. Ibid.
56. Fiorentino: Reflex Testing Methods.
57. Flavell: Developmental Psychology of Piaget.
58. McGraw: Neuromuscular Maturation.
59. Twitchell: Attitudinal Reflexes.
60. Pearson: Physical Therapy Services.
61. Bobath and Bobath: Motor Development.
62. Pearson: Physical Therapy Services.
63. Ibid.
64. Bobath and Bobath: Motor Development.
65. Pearson: Physical Therapy Services.

4
Scientific and Medical Bases

section 1/Anatomy and Physiology/Helen D. Smith

Anatomy, physiology, neuroanatomy, neurophysiology, kinesiology, psychology, psychiatry, and pathology are considered basic areas of study for the occupational therapist. Each area is a course in itself; thus, it is not my intent to include extensive information in these areas. The intent is to give a brief overview of each area and to provide references for more in-depth study.

ANATOMY

Anatomy is the study of body structures and systems. Actually, the word anatomy is derived from two Greek words: *ana* meaning "up" and *temnein* meaning "to cut." Dissection of cadavers and/or prosected materials have always been used to facilitate understanding of the relationships of anatomical parts.

There are four general areas of human anatomy: *microscopic anatomy* (histology), a study of anatomical structures with the aid of a microscope; *gross anatomy*, a study of structures that are visible to the eye; *embryology*, a study of the origin and development of an organism; and *neuroanatomy*, a study of the nervous system.

In order to understand and discuss anatomical structures and systems and how parts relate to one another, basic terminology must be clarified. Anatomical position refers to the body in an upright, standing position, face forward, upper extremities at the side, forearms supinated, and palms facing forward. The cardinal planes of the body are sagittal, frontal, and transverse. A midsagittal plane is a vertical plane through the longitudinal axis which divides the body down the middle into left and right sections. Any plane parallel to this line is a sagittal plane. A frontal or coronal plane is a vertical plane at right angles to the sagittal plane and divides the body into ventral (front or anterior) and dorsal (back or posterior) sections. The transverse or horizontal plane is at right angles to the sagittal or frontal planes and divides the body into top and bottom sections. The point at which these planes intersect is the center of gravity. The terms cranial or superior indicate toward the head and caudal or inferior indicate toward the tail. The use of proper terminology is imperative when describing or defining anatomical structures and systems in order to visualize, discuss, and define relationships of one area to another.

PHYSIOLOGY

Physiology is the study of body functions. The word physiology is derived from the Latin word *physiologia* meaning "the study of nature." The body systems, structures, and functions work in an integrated manner in order to maintain a state of homeostasis. When one system is in a dysfunctional state all systems are affected.

The human body is comprised of a skeleton, 206 bones, 8 systems, over 600 muscles, and cells, protoplasm, tissues, nerves, skin, organs, and fluids. The cell is the basis of the life process. A cell arises from a preexisting cell by mitosis (indirect cell division) or amitosis (direct cell division). The number of cells increases as the human body grows and develops. In addition to cell division, the process of differentiation must occur where each cell develops into a specific type of cell such as a muscle cell or nerve cell. These cells make up the human body systems.

BODY SYSTEMS—STRUCTURE AND FUNCTION

Musculoskeletal System

The musculoskeletal system is made up of muscles and bones. Both the skeleton and the muscles act to give the body support and movement. Body movement results when muscles attached to bones pull against these bones. There are three types of muscle tissue: (1) striated or skeletal muscle under voluntary control, which functions to move body parts and to help maintain body posture; (2) smooth muscle not usually under voluntary control, which is found in the respiratory, circulatory, and digestive systems; and (3) cardiac or heart muscle, which is not under voluntary control.

Respiratory System

The lungs, pleura, bronchi, trachea, pharynx, larynx, and nose make up the respiratory system. Respiration or breathing allows the body to take in oxygen and expel carbon dioxide, elements which pass through tissues to and from the blood stream by a process called diffusion. Respiraton or breathing is vital to life and, should disease or injury cause this system to malfunction, the act of respiration must be sustained by outside means if life is to continue.

Gastrointestinal System

The mouth, the salivary glands, pharynx, esophagus, stomach, and large and small intestines comprise the gastrointestinal system. Food which is eaten is broken down, undergoes chemical changes, and then is distributed by the circulatory system and absorbed by the body cells as nourishment.

Endocrine System

The endocrine system's main function is "to regulate the metabolic activities of the various organ systems in such a manner as to maintain homeostasis."[1] This system is comprised of ductless glands which secrete hormones into the blood and lymph. These secretions are then carried to all parts of the body where they are designed to have a specific effect on a specific organ or tissue. The endocrine organs are the hypothalamus, pituitary, thyroid, parathyroid and adrenal glands, and the gonads.[2]

Urogenital System

The urogenital system includes the urinary organs (kidneys, ureter, bladder, and urethra), which excrete waste materials from the body and the male and female reproductive organs.

Circulatory System

Both the cardiovascular system and the lymphatic system are included in this category. Both function as transportation systems.

The cardiovascular system is comprised of the heart and the blood vessels. The heart pumps the blood throughout the body via the blood vessels. The arteries carry blood away from the heart and the blood returns through the veins. At rest, each half of the heart pumps approximately 5 liters of blood per minute. During exercise this simultaneous pumping is increased to 25 liters per minute.[3]

The heart is divided into four chambers: the right and left atrium and the right and left ventricles.

Blood returns from the body through the superior and inferior vena cava, passes into the right atrium through the tricuspid valve, and into the right ventricle. Blood leaves the right ventricle through the pulmonic valve and flows into the lungs, where blood loses carbon dioxide and gains oxygen. The oxygen-enriched blood then returns to the heart through the pulmonary veins and flows into the left atrium, passes through the mitral valve, and then into the left ventricle. The aorta (the major artery) carries the blood from the heart to all parts of the body. The blood returns to the heart through the superior and inferior vena cava.

The lymphatic system is also a transport system. It carries tissue fluids which are waste products away from the tissues and back to the blood. When a malfunction takes place and extra fluid remains in the tissues, edema occurs. All organs of the body have a lymphatic system except for the eye, inner ear, and central nervous system.

Nervous System

The central and peripheral nervous systems comprise the human nervous system. The functions of this system range from "simple reflex control of muscles to the enormously complex phenomena of language, learning and memory."[4]

The central nervous system comprises the brain and spinal cord. The cranial nerves and spinal nerves are part of the peripheral nervous system and the autonomic nervous system.

The cerebrum, cerebellum, and brain stem are the main divisions of the brain. The cerebrum is further divided into two cerebral hemispheres. Each hemisphere has four lobes: occipital, temporal, parietal, and frontal. The medulla, pons, and midbrain make up the brain stem. The cerebellum lies dorsal to the pons and medulla. The chief function of the cerebellum is the coordination of muscular actions.

The spinal cord is approximately 18 inches long in the adult human. The vertebral column acts as a protective covering. Information moving to and from the brain is transmitted via the spinal cord.

The peripheral nervous system is divided into an afferent system and an efferent system. The efferent system is further subdivided into the somatic and autonomic nervous systems. The efferent fibers of the somatic system go "from the central nervous system to skeletal muscle cells."[5] The autonomic nervous system is a regulatory system and is subdivided into sympathetic and parasympathetic components. The autonomic nerves are usually involuntary motor nerves. These fibers innervate cardiac and smooth muscle or glands. The sympathetic component is used in stressful situations and provides a fright or flight response. The parasympathetic component is responsible for functions such as digestion and urination. Usually both branches of the autonomic system innervate each organ. This provides for control; one system is depressed when the other is activated.

The cranial nerves have both sensory and motor fibers. The twelve cranial nerves originate either in the brain or in the brain stem. They are referred to by Roman numerals, I to XII (Table 4-1).

The spinal nerves have both afferent (sensory) and efferent (motor) fibers and originate in the cord. The 31 pairs of nerves take their name from the nearest vertebra. There are 8 cervical, 12 thoracic, 5 lumbar, 5 sacral, and 1 to 3 coccygeal vertebra. The spinal nerves give rise to (1) cervical plexus and nerves innervating muscles and skin of the shoulder and neck area, (2) branchial plexus and nerves innervating muscles and skin of the upper extremity; and (3) lumbosacral plexus and nerves innervating the lower extremity muscles and skin.

For a more detailed explanation of the central nervous system, please refer to the bibliography at the end of this part and Section 3 of this chapter.

KINESIOLOGY

Kinesiology, which is the study of human motion, is vital to the analysis and understanding of body movement. The study of normal motions is emphasized as a base for understanding abnormal movement patterns. Kinesiologic concepts must be understood in order to analyze an activity for the motions involved. This information, then, is utilized in planning and implementing treatment both for individuals who have reversible dysfunction and for those who may have to live with permanent disability. The therapist must therefore understand basic mechanical concepts, the effects of exercise on the body, the function of muscles during activity, the types of

Table 4-1. Cranial nerves.

	Nerve	Type	Function
I	Olfactory	sensory	smell
II	Optic	sensory	vision
III	Oculomotor	motor	eye movements
IV	Trochlear	motor	eye movements
V	Trigeminal	mixed	mastication
VI	Abducens	motor	eye movements
VII	Facial	mixed	facial expression, taste
VIII	Auditory	sensory	hearing
IX	Glossopharyngeal	mixed	swallowing, taste
X	Vagus	mixed	swallowing, taste, and visceral functions
XI	Spinal accessory	motor	shoulder and head movement
XII	Hypoglossal	motor	tongue movements

Adapted from Noback.[6]

muscle contractions, and the influence of gravity and resistance on movement during performance of an activity.

In discussing movement, anatomical position and the planes of the body are used as points of reference. These were discussed earlier under anatomy. It is also necessary to understand the terms used to describe joint motions.

Flexion—a decrease in the angle of a joint as it is being moved.
Extension—a return from flexion.
Hyperextension—a movement beyond extension and past anatomical position.
Abduction—a movement away from the midline of the body.
Adduction—a movement toward the midline of the body and a return from abduction.
Internal rotation—a rotation toward the midline.
External rotation—a rotation away from the midline.
Supination—with elbow positioned at 90 degrees, the palm is turned up.
Pronation—with elbow positioned at 90 degrees, the palm is turned down.
Ulnar deviation—in anatomical position, a movement at the wrist toward the midline.
Radial deviation—in anatomical position, a movement at the wrist away from the midline.
Circumduction—a combination of movements: flexion, abduction, hyperextension, adduction, and extension.
Inversion—turning the sole of the foot toward the midline.
Eversion—turning the sole of the foot away from the midline.

Types of Muscle Contraction

A contraction refers to the development of tension in a muscle. *Concentric contraction* is a shortening contraction. The muscle shortens, moving its attachments closer together. For example, when picking up a 10-pound weight from a table the biceps contracts concentrically.

Eccentric contraction is a lengthening contraction. The distance is increased between the two attachments and is a controlled return of a muscle to its starting position. This can be illustrated by the controlled lowering of the 10-pound weight to the table. The biceps muscle still performs the action but it now contracts eccentrically.

In *static contraction* of a muscle there is no change in the relationship of the two attachments. The length remains the same. Frequently agonist and antagonist contract together to provide stability. For example, when using the hands to type, wrist flexors and extensors contract statically to maintain a stable position allowing freedom of finger movement.

Isotonic contraction is a shortening contraction and is often used interchangeably with concentric contraction.

Isometric contraction is a contraction of a muscle

in which there is no change in length. For example, a physician often instructs a patient in a long leg cast to statically contract the quadriceps muscle to prevent atrophy.

Role of Muscles During Purposeful Activity

During activity the body muscles can assume several roles depending on the action being performed. A muscle may act as a *prime mover,* in which case the muscle has the major responsibility for the motion. An *assistant or secondary mover* is a muscle that contracts to assist in performance of a movement when increased resistance requires additional power. An *agonist* muscle performs the desired movement and may be a prime mover. An *antagonist* muscle performs the opposite motion to the agonist. A *fixator or stabilizer* muscle contracts statically and performs a stability function.

Synergism means working together. The word comes from the Greek *sun* meaning "together" and the word *ergon* meaning "work."[7] Synergistic muscle may be used to prevent an unwanted movement, thus assisting in performance of a task. Forcefully gripping a tool will be used to illustrate this concept: the long finger flexors cross more than one joint and have the potential to act on each joint they cross. Forceful gripping of a tool would cause the wrist to flex if the wrist extensors did not contract synergistically to prevent this unwanted motion.

Influence of Gravity on Motion

Gravitational force tends to pull all matter towards the center of the earth, thus exerting a constant downward pull. When performing an activity the weight of the body part in relation to the pull of gravity must be overcome. The effect of gravity can be eliminated or used to assist movement by careful positioning. For example, a patient or client with limited muscle power in elbow extensors would be assisted by gravity while sanding a board if positioned so that the sanding was performed down an incline. However, it must be remembered that, in returning to starting position, the elbow flexors must be strong enough to be able to overcome gravity, the weight of the body part, plus the weight of the implement being used for sanding.

Levers

The principle of levers from physics can be applied to the human body. In the body the bones become the levers, the muscles provide the force and the joints become the axis or fulcrum. The lever principle states that when the force times the length of the force arm equals the resistance times the length of the resistance arm, the force will balance the resistance.

$$\textit{force} \times \textit{force arm} = \textit{resistance} \times \textit{resistance arm}$$

There are three types of levers (Fig. 4-1). In a *first class lever* the axis or fulcrum is between the force and the resistance. An example is a seesaw. The first class lever gives the advantage of either power or speed and excursion depending upon the placement of the axis. In a *second class lever* the resistance is between the axis and the force. A wheelbarrow is an example of this type of lever. The second class lever gives a power advantage. In the *third class lever* the force is between the axis and the resistance. An example is a door closed by a spring. A third class lever gives the advantage of excursion and speed, thus providing for speed in movement.

There are few first class levers in the body. One example is the head flexion and extension on the neck. According to Brunnstrom[8] and Wells[9] the existence of second class levers in the body is debatable. When an example is given, rising on the toes is often used to explain a second class body

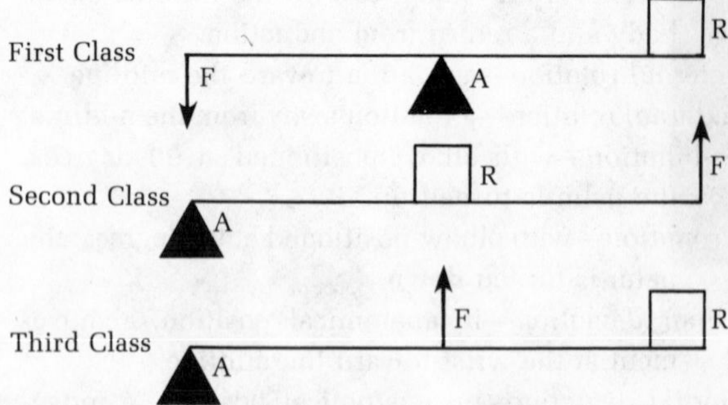

FIGURE 4-1. Relationship of force (F), axis (A), and resistance (R) in first, second and third class levers. An example of first class is a seesaw; an example of the second class is a wheelbarrow; and an example of the third class is a spring closing a door.

lever. Most levers in the body are third class levers. One example of a third class lever is flexion of the elbow. The joint axis becomes the axis or fulcrum, the force is located at the insertion of the biceps muscle, and the resistance is the forearm and the hand.

The lever principles as utilized in the body are important concepts and must be understood in order to understand muscle action and body movement. Understanding the concept of levers, how muscles contract, the effect of muscle pull on body parts, and the effect of resistance allows the therapist to determine which muscles must contract to perform a particular activity. The accompanying example of a kinesiologic activity analysis utilizes these principles.

KINESIOLOGIC ACTIVITY ANALYSIS

Activity:

Position of activity and/or patient or client:

Component parts of the activity:

	Motion	*Muscles utilized*	*Type of contraction*	*Gravity or resistance force*
Scapular				
Glenohumeral				
Elbow				
Wrist				
Fingers				
Thumb				
Hip				
Knee				
Ankle				
Foot				

Summary and Application:

Goals, diagnosis, and adaptation of positioning relative to patient or client or activity:

Adaptations:

PHYSICAL PATHOLOGY

Occupational therapists must have an in-depth knowledge of normal structures and functions in order to understand the effect of disease or injury on the human body.

The study of disease or dysfunction, its causes, processes, development, and consequences makes up the study of pathology. The word pathology is derived from the Greek words *pathos* and *pathologia* meaning "suffering" or "the study of emotion."[10] Causes of disease include bacteria, viruses, poisons, system malfunctions, and injury.

Physical pathology is the study of dysfunction in the major body systems. Some conditions studied include disturbances of the circulatory system (coronary artery disease and congestive heart failure); the respiratory system (pulmonary emphysema); the musculoskeletal system (arthritis, bursitis, and low back pain); the nervous system (multiple sclerosis, spinal cord injury, and cerebral vascular accident). Other areas of dysfunction include metabolic disturbances such as diabetes mellitus; physical injury including fractures and contusions; thermal injuries or burns; skin and connective tissue problems such as systemic lupus erythematosus. These are but a few of the medical, neurologic, and orthopedic conditions studied by the occupational therapist.

Treatment of these conditions includes, but is not limited to, surgery, chemotherapy, occupational therapy, physical therapy, and speech therapy. Not all causes of disease can be treated or eliminated. Therefore treatment is sometimes geared to reducing the discomfort or disability caused by the disease. For example, neither surgery nor drugs can cure arthritis. The occupational therapist's goals, based on pathology, would include reducing disability through (1) the use of splints to prevent deformity and (2) instruction in joint protection measures when the individual is engaged in daily living activities.

The use of chemotherapy, the treatment of disease by drugs, is prevalent. Chemotherapy has revolutionized medicine and many individuals living today owe their recovery or maintenance to drugs. Problems do exist, however. Drugs are not always effective. An organism can change and develop a resistance to a specific drug, and the medication that once helped loses its effectiveness. There is the potential for side effects—toxicity, autonomic disturbances such as sweating and blurred vision, neurological reactions such as tremors and vertigo, gastrointestinal complications such as nausea and diarrhea, skin rashes,behavioral disturbances, and depression.[11]

In order to plan and carry out an effective treatment program with realistic goals, the etiology, symptoms, treatment, prognosis, and potential drug side effects must be understood by the therapist.

Information on pathology as it relates to specific diseases or injury has been included in appropriate chapters throughout this book.

REFERENCES

1. Selkurt, E. E. (ed.): Basic Physiology for the Health Sciences. Boston: Little, Brown, & Co., 1975, p. 279.
2. Ibid.
3. Vander, A. J.: Human Physiology—The Mechanics of Body Function, ed. 2. New York: McGraw-Hill Book Co., 1975, p. 231.
4. Selkurt: Basic Physiology, p. 89.
5. Vander: Human Physiology, p. 163.
6. Noback, C.: The Human Nervous System. New York: McGraw-Hill Book Co., 1967, p. 122.
7. Morris, W. (ed.): The American Heritage Dictionary of the English Language. New York: American Heritage Publishing Co., 1969, p. 1305.
8. Brunnstrom, S.: Clinical Kinesiology, ed. 3. Philadelphia: F. A. Davis Co., 1972, p. 21.
9. Wells, K. F.: Kinesiology, ed. 5. Philadelphia: W. B. Saunders Co., 1971, p. 55.
10. Morris: American Heritage Dictionary, p. 961.
11. Lyght, C. E. (ed.): The Merck Manual, ed. 11. Rahway NJ: Merck Sharp & Dohme Research Laboratories, 1966.

BIBLIOGRAPHY

Arnold, M.: Reconstructive Anatomy. Philadelphia: W. B. Saunders Co., 1968.

Barr, M.: The Human Nervous System, ed. 2. Hagerstown: Harper & Row Publishers, 1974.

Chusid, J. Correlative Neuroanatomy and Functional Neurology, ed. 14. Los Altos, Lange Medical Publications, 1970.

Dean, W. B., Farrar, G. E., and Zoldos, A. J.: Basic Concepts of Anatomy and Physiology, A Programmed Study. Philadelphia: J. B. Lippincott Co., 1966.

Ellis, H.: Clinical Anatomy, ed. 3. Oxford England: Blackwell Scientific Publications, 1974.

Everett, N. B., Sundsten, J. W., and Lund, R.: Functional Neuroanatomy, ed. 6. Philadelphia: Lea and Febiger, 1971.

Goss, C. M. (ed.): Gray's Anatomy of the Human Body, ed. 28. Philadelphia: Lea and Febiger, 1966.

Grant, J. C.: An Atlas of Anatomy, ed. 5. Baltimore: Williams & Wilkins Co., 1962.

Minckler, J., et al. (eds.): Pathobiology—An Introduction. St. Louis: C. V. Mosby Co., 1971.

Nilsson, L.: Behold Man. Boston: Little, Brown, & Co., 1974.

Pansky, B., and House, E. L.: Review of Gross Anatomy, ed. 3. New York: Macmillan Publishing Co., 1975.

Rasch, P. J., and Burke, R. K.: Kinesiology and Applied Anatomy. Philadelphia: Lea and Febiger, 1963.

Snell, R. S.: Clinical Anatomy for Medical Students. Boston: Little, Brown, & Co., 1973.

Wells, B. B., and Halsted, J. A.: Clinical Pathology/Interpretation and Application, ed. 4. Philadelphia: W. B. Saunders Co., 1967.

section 2/Psychopathology and Clinical Psychology/

Elizabeth G. Tiffany

The *Diagnostic and Statistical Manual of the American Psychiatric Association* (DSM-II) lists ten major categories of psychiatric disorders. These classifications are in standard use in recording the diagnoses of individuals who are hospitalized in psychiatric facilities throughout the country. The DSM-II has undergone revision and is being coordinated with a new edition of the *International Classification of Diseases* (ICD-9).

The major categories of mental disorder currently identified are (1) mental retardation, (2) organic brain syndrome, (3) functional psychoses, (4) neuroses, (5) personality disorders, (6) psychophysiological disorders, (7) special symptoms; (8) transient situational disturbances, (9) behavior disorders of childhood and adolescence, and (10) nonspecific conditions or social maladjustment without manifest psychiatric disorder.

Mental retardation subsumes a number of categories which are dealt with in Chapter 19. The primary problems of the mentally retarded are associated with their levels of intellectual functioning. There are, however, some forms of psychiatric disorder associated with certain kinds of mental retardation.

Organic brain syndrome includes categories of psychiatric disorder associated with the actual impairment of brain tissue function. Symptoms include problems in judgment, memory, orientation, and general cognitive functioning. There may be emotional lability or shallowness of affect. There is a distinction between acute or reversible conditions and those which are chronic and irreversible. The psychotic forms of organic brain syndrome include senile and presenile dementia, alcoholic psychoses, psychoses associated with intracranial infection such as syphilis or encephalitis, and psychoses associated with other cerebral or physical conditions such as epilepsy, brain trauma, metabolic or endocrine disturbances, and drug or poison intoxication. There are also nonpsychotic forms of organic brain syndrome associated with most of the above causes and with intracranial neoplasms, circulatory disturbances, degenerative central nervous system diseases, and other physical conditions.

The *functional psychoses* or "psychoses not attributable to physical conditions listed previously"[1] include two large categories—the schizophrenias and the affective disorders—and two smaller categories—paranoid states and psychotic depressive reaction. (The fact that there is research in process to determine the etiologies of the psychoses, especially of schizophrenia, accounts for the vague wording of this category in the DSM-II.) The subcategories of schizophrenia are simple, hebephrenic, catatonic, paranoid, acute schizophrenic episode, latent, residual, schizo-affective, childhood, and chronic undifferentiated types. The major affective disorders include involutional melancholia and the manic-depressive illnesses (manic, depressed, and circular types). True paranoia, involutional paranoid, and other paranoid states are described in the paranoid category. All of the divisions described in the DSM-II include a category of "other," perhaps reflecting the fact that not all functional psychoses fit comfortably into the categories which have been defined.

Neuroses generally refer to nonpsychotic disorders which are characterized by symptoms such as anxiety, depression, phobias, obsessions, and compulsions. They include anxiety neurosis, hysterical (conversion and dissociative types), phobic, obsessive-compulsive, depressive, and neurasthenic types of neuroses, and symptoms of depersonalization and hypochondriasis.

Personality disorders include paranoid, cyclothymic, schizoid, explosive, obsessive-compulsive, hysterical, asthenic, antisocial, passive-aggressive, and inadequate types; forms of sexual deviation including disturbances of sexual orientation, fetishism, pedophilia, transvestitism, exhibitionism, voyeurism, sadism, and masochism; and addictions such as alcoholism and drug dependence.

Psychophysiological disorders include the wide range of physical problems which have often been referred to as "psychosomatic." These are conditions which may occur in any bodily part or system but which are clearly caused by emotional factors.

The *special symptoms* category covers a small number of problems usually occurring in childhood or in adolescence, such as anorexia nervosa, sleep disorders, certain psychomotor conditions, speech and learning disturbances, enuresis, and encopresis. Generally these are conditions that are quite specific but important enough not to be listed as symptomatic of a different major category.

Transient situational disturbances include the adjustment reactions of infancy, childhood, adolescence, adulthood, and later life. They occur in people who have had no previous history of psychiatric disorder and usually occur as reactions to overwhelming environmental stress. They are indeed transient, usually lasting for only a short time.

The *behavior disorders of childhood and adolescence* are those conditions that are psychoses, neuroses, or adjustment reactions. They include reactions described as hyperkinetic, runaway, withdrawing, overanxious, unsocialized, aggressive, and group delinquent.

The final category, *nonspecific conditions*, accounts for problems which occur in psychiatrically "normal" individuals in response to a variety of problems in life, such as marital discord or occupational maladjustment. The problems are felt severely enough that these individuals may seek psychiatric help.

There is some controversy about the usefulness of diagnostic labels when one is working with people in a treatment context. The practice raises the issue of depersonalization or of predisposing the professional to perceive a classical picture or fantasy patient rather than a unique human being with a personal *gestalt* which is different from that of any other person's. On the other hand, a diagnosis represents a compilation of research and experience with large numbers of people over a long period of time, and, as such, presents important guidelines for understanding the disease process, methods for treating it and certain expectations regarding its prognosis. It is a professional responsibility for mental health professionals to recognize both aspects of this issue and to seek to achieve a balance in their use of diagnosis which will serve their clients best.

Psychiatry has had a stormy history in the years since it has become recognized as a field of medical concern. Lacking concrete, definable, and measurable variables, psychiatry, by its very nature, has never been able to subject all of its hypotheses to rigorous scientific research.

Table 4-2 represents some of the major streams of thought which have dominated psychology and psychiatric practice during the past century. An examination of their premises reveals some of the differences among them.

Early psychiatric theory was based on empirical data, most of which was collected under the highly variable conditions of clinical practice. As a result, psychiatry, more than any other branch of medicine, has been and continues to be subject to controversy about such basic issues as the nature of mental illness, etiology, prognosis, and treatment methods. Perhaps the problem is that "mental illness" is a general and vague term similar to the term "physical illness."

We have come to understand that the term covers a wide range of clinical entities, which have many different etiologies and for which varying treatment approaches are viable. No single frame of reference for treatment works for all mental illnesses or all psychiatric problems. Some of the clinical entities defined as mental illness are, in fact, diseases, while others may be problems in adjustment or the effects of developmental lags, genetic deficits, or the results of pathological social patterns of the culture. Developing the data and the criteria on which to base clinical differentiations is a core concern of the research efforts in psychiatry at the present time.

REFERENCES

1. American Psychiatric Association Diagnostic and Statistical Manual (DSM-II). Washington DC: American Psychiatric Association, 1968, Category III.
2. Millon, T.: Theories of Psychopathology and Personality. Philadelphia: W. B. Saunders Co., 1973.
3. Freedman, A. M., Kaplan, H. I., and Sadock, B. J.: Modern Synopsis of Comprehensive Textbook of Psychiatry/II. Baltimore: Williams & Wilkins Co., 1976.

BIBLIOGRAPHY

Feighner, J. P., et al.: Diagnostic criteria for use in psychiatric research. Arch. Gen. Psychiatr. 26:57, 1972.

Table 4-2. Major streams of thought in psychiatry.

School of thought	*Basic ideas*	*Major proponents*	*Treatment modes*
Biophysical	Biophysical defects; deficits in anatomy, physiology, biochemistry, genetics, and metabolism.	Emil Kraepelin Eugen Bleuler Franz Kallman William Sheldon Ernst Kretschmer Kurt Goldstein	Psychopharmacology, insulin and electric shock, psychosurgery. Nutritional and special dietetic concerns. Emphasis on present.
Psychoanalytic intrapsychic	Unconscious processes and conflicts (repressed material) in early years of life. Defense mechanisms may be maladaptive or inadequate. Concepts of id vs. superego. Disruptions or trauma in sequence of development lead to pathology. There are many variations on this original theme.	Sigmund Freud Anna Freud Carl Jung Karen Horney Harry Stack Sullivan Otto Rank Alfred Adler Erich Fromm Franz Alexander Frieda Fromm-Reichmann Sandor Ferencz Paul Schilder Sandor Rado Theodor Reik Melanie Klein Wilhelm Reich	Psychoanalytic therapy. Psychotherapy. Use of free association, dreams, and projective techniques to uncover unconscious material. Support for ego functions. Reconstruction through catharsis, insight, use of transference phenomena. Exploration of the past.
Behavioral	All behavior is learned. Reinforcements shape behavior. Differences explained in terms of reinforcement patterns.	B. F. Skinner John Dollard Neal Miller H. J. Eysenck Joseph Wolpe	Behavior therapies: operant conditioning; reciprocal inhibition; desensitization.
Phenomenological	Individual's perception of the world is warped, distorted. Experience leads to self-concept. Loss of personal potentials, feelings and values (self-ness) in assuming others externally imposed. Social isolation in "mass" society.	Rollo May Carl Rogers Viktor Frankl R. D. Laing Albert Ellis Frederick Perls Eric Berne William Glasser	Existential analysis. Rational therapy. Gestalt therapy. Transactional analysis. Reality therapy. Some exploration of past but emphasis on present.
Sociocultural	Community, culture, social forces of primary importance.	Thomas Scheff Erving Goffman Maxwell Jones	Milieu therapy. Prevention programs. Community psychiatry. Emphasis on present.
Integrative biopsychosocial	Biological and psychological unity. Psychological processes are multidetermined, multidimensional, include social, and cultural processes and development.	Adolf Meyer Roy Grinker Paul Meehl	Focus on coping strategies, competence. A great variety of treatment modes and development of understanding about all factors. Emphasis on present.

Adapted from Millon[2] and Freedman, Kaplan, and Sadock.[3]

section 3/Neuroanatomy and Neurophysiology/

A. Joy Huss

In order to understand human behavior and function it is necessary to have a basic knowledge of the structure and function of the nervous system. This system is responsible for control not only of the skeletal and smooth muscles but also of the emotions, memory, and intellect. Thus it becomes important for the occupational therapist, regardless of specialty area, to have a basic understanding of the nervous system. Since knowledge of the nervous system is not yet complete, it is the professional's responsibility to stay abreast of current information.

BASIC CONCEPTS

The nervous system is divided arbitrarily into three divisions: the central nervous system (CNS); the peripheral nervous system (PNS); and the autonomic nervous system (ANS) which in turn has two subdivisions, the sympathetic (SNS) and parasympathetic (PSNS).

The CNS consists of those structures located inside the skull and vertebral column: the brain and spinal cord. The PNS structures are located outside of the bony cavities and carry sensory and motor information from and to the peripheral structures and sensory information from smooth and cardiac muscles and glands to the CNS.

The ANS is an efferent (motor) system supplying information to the smooth muscles, cardiac muscle, and glands. The SNS (thoracolumbar system) is located at spinal cord levels T_1 to L_2. The PSNS anatomically surrounds the SNS being found in cranial nerves, 3, 7, 9, and 10 and in sacral levels 2, 3, and 4 (craniosacral system). The SNS supplies both axial and appendicular structures, while the PSNS supplies only axial structures. Thus axially the two systems work synergistically. The SNS provides an adrenalin response which is a generalized, fast acting, excitatory reaction. The PSNS is a specific, slower acting system which tends to conserve energy. In the appendicular areas the SNS provides its own synergistic action. For example, it can either increase or decrease the blood flow to the extremities depending on the needs of the organism.

Functionally all three divisions (CNS, PNS, ANS) are interrelated and cannot be isolated. What occurs in one division will have an effect on the other divisions. Even though a given treatment approach may be said to affect a certain part of the system, it will ultimately have an effect, either positive or negative, on the entire system and thus on the individual's behavior because the nervous system functions holistically.

The CNS contains more than twenty billion plus neurons of varying sizes, cell body sizes and shapes, and degrees of axonal myelination. Generally, the larger the axon diameter the more heavily myelinated it becomes with nervous system maturation and the faster it will conduct an impulse. Conversely, the smaller the axonal diameter, the less myelin and the slower the conduction rate will be. Neurons can thus be classified according to axon diameter and myelin covering (Table 4-3). Although the smallest fibers are classified as nonmyelinated, a single Schwann cell may envelop several of these fibers with a single layer of myelin. The heavier the myelin sheath the longer it takes to develop. Therefore it may be years before full functional capacity is reached. Generally, the larger fibers process the more discriminative, exploratory, or epicritic functions, while the intermediate size fibers process the protective or protopathic functions and the smaller fibers process the more primitive functions of the ANS and reticular formation.

In the spinal cord the A fibers (largest) are found predominately in the dorsolateral portion and will cross over in the medulla. These include such functions as conscious proprioception, discriminatory tactile, two-point discrimination, vibratory sense, and voluntary motor activity. The B fibers (intermediate) are found predominately in the ventrolateral portion of the spinal cord and cross at spinal levels. Functions served include pain, temperature, light touch, vibratory sense, and nonvoluntary motor activity. The C fibers (smallest) are generally found in the area surrounding the gray matter of the cord and will have a bilateral effect.

Table 4-3. Nerve fiber classification in descending order of myelin thickness and conduction velocity.

General classification	*Dorsal root classification*	*Ventral root classification*
A		
alpha (α)	I. 70–120 m/sec. Ia—primary sensory ending from neuromuscular spindle Ib—from Golgi tendon organ II. 30–70 m/sec. secondary sensory ending from neuromuscular spindle cutaneous touch-pressure joint receptors dermal receptors	Motoneurons to somatic muscles (extrafusal) 15–120 m/sec.
beta (β)		Few in number. Innervate both extrafusal and intrafusal fibers
gamma (γ)		Motoneurons to intrafusal fibers of neuromuscular spindles 10–45 m/sec.
delta (δ)	III. Free nerve endings. 12–30 m/sec.	
B		Preganglionic autonomic fibers. 3–15 m/sec.
C	IV. Unmyelinated fibers. Probably serve all sensory modalities. 0.5–2 m/sec.	Postganglionic sympathetic axons of ANS. 0.7–2.3 m/sec.

Adapted from Barr[1] and Noback.[2]

Phylogenetically, the nervous system has developed from the most primitive, bilateral functions such as ANS and reticular, referred to as *archi*, to intermediate protective functions known as *paleo*, to the discriminative functions called *neo*. The neo functions, because they involve larger cell bodies and nerve fibers which require more oxygen, are thus more vulnerable to trauma while the archi systems are the least vulnerable. Although it depends to some degree on the location and nature of the trauma, the nervous system tends to protect the archi systems the longest. This, then, has implications for rehabilitation. If the system has been damaged one should first integrate the archi systems, progress through the paleo functions and finally attempt to rehabilitate the neo functions such as speech and fine manipulation. It is extremely difficult, for example, to use the hands for fine control if the background base of postural stability is deficient.

At birth the individual operates on an excitatory basis. The slightest stimulus sets off a mass reaction. At this time the nervous system is basically immature. With maturity of the system a base of inhibition is laid down because of the myelination of higher centers that are inhibitory in function. Normal functioning is dependent on a balance of excitatory and inhibitory influences on the lower motoneurons of the spinal cord and cranial nerves. In order for excitation and inhibition to be mediated by the CNS there are two basic types of neurons: excitatory and inhibitory. Histologically, the two are similar. The difference is the chemical secreted at the synapse and the effect of that chemical on the postsynaptic neuron. Since a given neuron can have synaptic input from 1000 to 100,000 other neurons, whether or not the firing threshold is reached for propagation of an impulse depends on the total balance between excitatory and inhibitory synapses. For example, if the ratio is 2:1 inhibitory/facilitory, then the excitatory impulse will be blocked. If the total system balance is more towards excitation, then the clinical picture may be one of hyperactivity or hypertonicity. If the balance is more towards inhibition, then the clinical picture will be hypotonicity. Depending on the area of trauma and the moment-to-moment state of the individual, which is based in part on the amount and type of sensory input being received and processed, the tonal picture may fluctuate. One can see such fluctuations even in the normal individual.

Excitation and inhibition within the CNS is a complex interaction of presynaptic and postsynaptic inhibition via interneurons and inhibitory centers. For a more thorough understanding of this process, two of the better references are Noback[3] and Williams and Warwick.[4]

The balance of excitation and inhibition ultimately affects the threshold levels of postsynaptic neurons within the CNS and the lower motoneurons. Generally speaking, the normal resting threshold is −70 mV and the firing potential is −50 mV. With repeated excitation the resting potential may shift toward a −60 mV which means that a lesser amount of additional excitation is needed to reach firing potential. On the other hand, if the system is receiving more inhibitory overlay the resting potential may be close to −80 mV so that additional excitation is needed to reach the firing potential. The hypertonic or hyperactive individual may have an overall balance of too much excitation so that resting potentials are very close to firing potentials while, conversely, the hypotonic individual may have a greater discrepancy between resting and firing potentials. The aim of treatment thus becomes an *appropriate* use of sensory input to change the overall balance of the system toward a more normal range of −70 mV resting potential.

One way this can be accomplished is through the use of the sensory receptors. *Exteroceptors* are located in the skin, eyes, and ears. They respond to changes in the external environment such as the general senses of pain, temperature, light touch, and light pressure and the special senses of vision and hearing. *Proprioceptors* are concerned with vibration, deep pressure, and the position and movements of the body. These receptors are located in the muscles (neuromuscular spindles), tendons (Golgi tendon organs), fascia, joint capsules, ligaments, and the vestibular or equilibrium mechanisms of the inner ear. *Interoceptors,* also called visceroceptors, mediate sensations from the viscera. They play a role in digestion, control of blood pressure, cardiac function, respiration, and so forth. The sensations of fullness of stomach and bladder or pain from excessive distention are the result of stimulation of these receptors. Visceral sensations are diffuse and poorly localized. The sensations of olfaction and taste have been variously classified as exteroceptors or interoceptors.

Since the nervous system acts as a sensorimotor-sensory feedback system with integration provided by the CNS, various treatment approaches, discussed later in this book, have been developed to excite or dampen these sensory receptors which in turn will have an effect on motor control. If the system is deprived of appropriate sensory input and its integration, disorganized behaviors will result. Sensory deprivation affects synaptic growth and development as well as delaying myelination. An enriched environment will have the opposite effect. Appropriate input includes not only stimulation of the suitable receptors, whether they be exteroceptors, proprioceptors, and/or interceptors, but it also must be meaningful to the individual's system, be of correct intensity and duration, and be applied with tender loving care (TLC) for concurrent emotional integration.

Each of us is bombarded constantly with a multiplicity of sensory input, most of which does not evoke a response at a conscious level but is filtered by the reticular system and integrated subcortically. The reticular system extends throughout the spinal cord, brainstem, and diencephalic nuclei of the thalamus and hypothalamus with indirect connections with the cerebral cortex and limbic system.[5] The entire system is polysynaptic.

The reticular activating system (RAS), or ascending portion, provides a generalized bombardment of the cerebral cortex for the purposes of providing the level of consciousness or "awakeness" and the level of alertness to that which is most important in the environment. Olfactory and cutaneous stimuli have a profound effect on the level of consciousness. Psychic, auditory, and visual stimuli affect the level of alertness and attention. Damage to this system may result in prolonged coma.[6]

The descending fibers of the reticular system, having received information from the motor centers of the cortex, basal ganglia, and cerebellum, play a major role in influencing the threshold levels of both alpha and gamma motoneurons of the spinal cord and cranial nerves. Since the nuclear centers of this system in the brainstem consist of both excitatory and inhibitory centers, the effect on the motoneurons can be either facilitory or inhibitory. Control centers of the ANS of the brainstem are also affected by this system with effects on respiration, circulation, and heart rate.[7,8,9]

This entire reticular system thus has implications for treatment not only of the individual with CNS dysfunction but also for those with other types of problems, as well as for dealings with students, peers, and others. The type and amount of stimuli being received in relation to the individual's present state will have an effect on his responses to the environment and his ability to learn.

The limbic system consists of structures found on the medial surfaces of the cerebral hemispheres such as the cingulate, hippocampal, and parahippocampal gyri, the mammillary bodies of the hypothalamus, the fornix, the uncus, and amygdala, and the medial aspect of the thalamus. According to Moore,[10] the limbic system, because of its location and structures involved, serves to integrate the older sensorimotor, visceral, and reticular systems with the newer, higher level cognitive functions. In lower animals these structures serve the olfactory functions.

Moore indicates that in human beings the limbic system is that which drives us to act for survival as individuals and as a species. She uses the mnemonic word *MOVE* to outline the functions. The *M* stands for *memory*. Although memory is probably stored in many areas of the CNS, certain parts of the limbic system such as the hippocampus and mammillary bodies appear to be a necessary part of the circuitry for both long term and short term memory.

The *O* stands for *olfaction*. Although man no longer depends on the sense of smell for survival, it still has an influence on the sense of taste, recall of past experiences, emotional responses, and visceral functions.

The *V* stands for *visceral* functions related to behavior in conjunction with sensorimotor, cognitive, and emotional responses. The system helps to maintain the homeostatic balance. Excessive emotional or physical stress may disturb this balance with resultant alerting of the SNS for "fight or flight" responses. If continued for too long the response to fear may disturb the entire balance of the nervous system, leading to disintegration of the individual's behavior.

The *E* stands for the individual's basic *emotional* tone or drive. These have been referred to as the "3 Fs" of feeding, fighting, and reproduction.[11] The feeding drive consists not only of the necessity of food, water, and air for physical survival but also, and probably even more important, of the need for love or TLC or, as Broadbent[12] has called it, the "belonging instinct." This drive must be met in order to assure the survival of the individual and the species.[13,14,15]

Since the limbic system is very complex, made up of fiber connections not only within the system itself but also with adjacent areas including the reticular system, any stimulation causes long-lasting afterdischarges. Many of its pathways are circular in nature as well as reciprocal. Thus stimulation of one area has an effect on all other areas which then give feedback both directly and indirectly to the site of original stimulation. Emotional learning thus has strong reinforcement. We are all familiar with an event or song that continually replays itself within our own mind and with the patient with a cerebrovascular accident who still retains emotional language such as swearing, singing, laughter, and crying although the higher cortical functions of language are lost.[16] Therefore as therapists we cannot ignore the effects of what we do on the limbic system and the implications for affecting the entire balance of the client.

The corticobulbar system, which innervates the motor nuclei of the cranial nerves, and the corticospinal system, both of which are commonly referred to as the pyramidal system, originate in several areas of the cortex. The figures vary from author to author,[17,18,19] but, contrary to popular belief, this system does not originate in only Brodmann's area 4 or motor strip of the frontal lobe. Noback[20] indicates that approximately 60 percent of the fibers originate in areas 4 and 6 of the frontal lobe, while the remaining 40 percent come from areas 3, 1, 2, and 5 of the parietal lobe. Barr[21] indicates that 40 percent are from area 4, 20 percent from 3, 1, and 2, and the remainder are predominantly from 6 and 8 of the frontal lobe and the rest from areas 5 and 7 of the parietal lobe.[22] Approximately 90 percent of the fibers in this system are small fibers with 2 to 3 percent being the large fibers from the Betz cells of area 4. Of the more than one million fibers making up the corticospinal system, 85 to 90 percent cross over in the medullary pyramidal decussation to form the lateral corticospinal tract. Most of the remaining fibers, which do not cross over, make up the anterior corticospinal tract while a few enter the ipsilateral lateral corticospinal tract. Most of these uncrossed fibers, however, do cross in the spinal cord at their level of function. The lateral corticospinal tracts extend throughout the spinal cord. Approximately 50 percent of the fibers terminate in the cervical region, 20 percent in the thoracic area, with the remaining 30 percent extending to the lumbosacral segments.[23] Barr's figures are 55, 20, and 25 percent respectively.[24] The anterior corticospinal tracts terminate primarily in the cervical area.

Both the corticobulbar and corticospinal fibers traverse the posterior portion of the internal capsule which is supplied primarily by branches of the middle cerebral artery. This is probably the most common area of occlusion in a cerebral vascular accident. Also traversing this area of the internal capsule are sensory projection fibers from the thalamus to the parietal lobe and fibers from the optic and auditory radiations.

At spinal cord levels it is estimated that at least 90 percent of the corticospinal fibers synapse with interneurons before exerting their influence on both alpha and gamma motoneurons. Some fibers may synapse directly on alpha motoneurons, especially for fine control of the digits. The remainder of the fibers synapse via interneurons in the sensory relay nuclei of the posterior horn of the spinal cord and the brainstem nuclei for the pathways of conscious proprioception.[25,26]

Thus the pyramidal system which was once thought to be *the* direct, monosynaptic pathway for voluntary control of all musculature is now thought by some observers to be a system for control of speed and agility of voluntary movement and especially significant in the ability to use the digits independently for fine skill.[27]

The extrapyramidal system includes all of the motor systems other than the corticobulbar and corticospinal (pyramidal) system. The extrapyramidal system originates from the same cortical areas as well as the basal ganglia of the telencephalon, red nucleus, reticular system, substantia nigra of the brainstem, and certain thalamic nuclei of the diencephalon. There is considerable interaction between the pyramidal and extrapyramidal systems via collaterals and feedback circuits. Thus the extrapyramidal system also plays a role in voluntary movement as well as possibly providing the background base necessary for postural control.[28,29] With a pure lesion of the pyramidal system, which is relatively rare, there will be flaccidity. However, if any extrapyramidal areas are also involved, there will be hypertonicity. The automatic components of movement and posture are controlled subcortically while the volitional component is controlled primarily at the cortical level. It is difficult, if not impossible, to control on a cortical level more than one act at a time. Therefore it is necessary for these two systems to act together in order that one may perform a skilled activity on a solid postural base. For example, one can consciously direct the necessary finger movements to perform a Beethoven sonata but the necessary wrist, forearm, arm, shoulder, trunk, and lower extremity movements are directed simultaneously by subcortical extrapyramidal centers. It is probable that more than 90 percent of the activities that one performs daily are subcortically controlled.

The circuitry is extremely complex and a breakdown in one area will affect the functioning of other areas. Thus the clinical picture will vary considerably from one individual to another. This also makes it extremely difficult to localize the exact area of trauma based on the clinical picture.

The connections and pathways of the vestibulocochlear system are many and very intricate. Any of the newer neuroanatomy texts review this information. At one time the vestibular or equilibrium mechanisms were considered to be separate from the cochlear or auditory processes. The newer evidence from both the clinical and laboratory research areas now indicates that there are many interactions between these two senses. Enhancement of one will affect the other. Input to this total system has been shown to assist in the integration of brain stem functions,[30] which then releases the higher centers to more adequately perform their functions. Vestibular therapy is now an accepted method of treatment. However, its various methods and effects, both positive and negative, should be understood by the clinician before being used with any client. Ayres is an excellent reference for this understanding.[31] Basically any movement that is done slowly and repetitively will dampen the system, while movement that is rapid will enhance the system. Many techniques based on this premise are discussed later in this book.

As research continues into the structure and function of the neuromuscular spindle and the neurotendinous organ (Golgi tendon organ, GTO), these sensory receptors become more complex and thus more difficult to understand. Moore[32] updated this complexity. At the present time it appears that the primary sensory ending of the neuromuscular spindle is highly sensitive to vibration, which is why vibrators are being used in treatment. Bishop[33,34,35] has written three articles on this subject. Noback[36] provides an understanding of the structure and possible functions of both of these sensory receptors.

It is important to remember that stimulation of these sensory organs is only *one* way to provide input to the CNS and *may* be an appropriate treatment technique if used in conjunction with other types of input. Used in isolation it may not be appropriate.

Basic information at this time seems to indicate that the neuromuscular spindle provides autogenic excitation, while the neurotendinous organ provides autogenic inhibition. These two structures work very closely together and are influenced by higher CNS structures as well as the present state of the individual.

REFERENCES

1. Barr, M. L.: The Human Nervous System, ed. 2. New York: Harper & Row Publishers, 1974, pp. 29–30.
2. Noback, C. R., and Demarest, R. J.: The Human Nervous System: Basic Principles of Neurobiology. New York: McGraw-Hill Book Co., 1975, pp. 83–85.
3. Ibid., pp. 387, 388, 408.
4. Williams, P. L., and Warwick, R.: Functional Neuroanatomy of Man. Philadelphia: W. B. Saunders Co., 1975, pp. 750, 751, 768, 775, 832.
5. Ibid, pp. 888–890.
6. Barr: Human Nervous System, p. 148.
7. Ibid.
8. Noback: Human Nervous System, pp. 274–275.
9. Williams and Warwick: Functional Neuroanatomy, p. 890.
10. Moore, J. C.: Behavior, bias, and the limbic system. Am. J. Occup. Ther. 30:11–19, 1976.
11. MacLean, P. D.: The limbic system with respect to self-preservation and the preservation of the species. J. Nerv. Ment. Dis. 127:1–11, 1958.
12. Broadbent, W. W.: How To Be Loved. Englewood Cliffs NJ: Prentice-Hall, 1976, pp. 175–184.
13. Ibid.
14. Moore: Behavior, bias, and the limbic system.
15. Huss, A. J.: Touch with care or a caring touch? Am. J. Occup. Ther. 31:11–18, 1977.
16. Moore: Behavior, bias, and the limbic system.
17. Noback: Human Nervous System, p. 175.
18. Barr: Human Nervous System, p. 321.
19. Clark, R. G.: Manter and Gatz's Essentials of Clinical Neuroanatomy and Neurophysiology, ed. 5. Philadelphia, F. A. Davis Co., 1975, p. 20.
20. Noback: Human Nervous System, p. 175.
21. Barr: Human Nervous System, p. 321.
22. Ibid.
23. Noback: Human Nervous System, pp. 176–177.
24. Barr: Human Nervous System, p. 234.
25. Ibid.
26. Noback: Human Nervous System, p. 177.
27. Barr: Human Nervous System, p. 324.
28. Ibid, p. 325.
29. Noback: Human Nervous System, p. 422.
30. Ayres, A. J.: Sensory Integration and Learning Disorders. Los Angeles: Western Psychological Services, 1972, p. 57.
31. Ibid.
32. Moore, J. C.: The Golgi tendon organ and the muscle spindle. Am. J. Occup. Ther. 28:415–420, 1974.
33. Bishop, B.: Vibratory stimulation I. J. Am. Phys. Ther. 54:1273–1282, 1974.
34. Bishop, B.: Vibratory stimulation II. J. Am. Phys. Ther. 55:28–34, 1975.
35. Bishop, B.: Vibratory stimulation III. J. Am. Phys. Ther. 55:139–143, 1975.
36. Noback: Human Nervous System, pp. 70, 71, 165–170.

BIBLIOGRAPHY

Andrew, B. L. (ed.): Control and Innervation of Skeletal Muscle. Dundee, Scotland: D.C. Thomson & Co., 1966.

Angel, R. W., and Eppler, W. G.: Synergy of contralateral muscles in normal subjects and patients with neurological disease. Arch. Phys. Med. 48:233–239, 1967.

Ashworth, B., Grimby, L., and Kugelberg, E.: Comparison

of voluntary and reflex activation of motor units. J. Neurol. Neurosurg. Psychiat. 30:91–98, 1967.

Banker, R. J., et al. (eds.): Research in Muscle Development and the Muscle Spindle. Amsterdam: Excerpta Med. Found. 1972.

Basmajian, J. V.: Control and training of individual motor units. Science, 1963.

Bekesy, G. von: Sensory Inhibition. Princeton NJ: Princeton University Press, 1967.

Brooks, V. B., and Stoney, S. D.: Motor mechanisms: The role of the pyramidal system in motor control. Ann. Rev. Physiol. 33:337–392, 1971.

Calne, D. B., and Pallis, C. A.: Vibratory sense: A critical review. Brain 89:723–746, 1966.

Carmon, A.: Disturbances of tactile sensitivity in patients with unilateral cerebral lesions. Cortex 7:83–97, 1971.

Chase, M. H., et al.: Somatic reflex response—reversal of reticular origin. Exp. Neurol. 50:561–567, 1976.

Cook, W. A., and Gangiano, A.: Presynaptic and postsynaptic inhibition of spinal motoneurons. J. Neurophysiol. 35:389–403, 1972.

Crosby, E. C., et al.: The alterations of tonus and movements through the interplay between the cerebral hemispheres and the cerebellum. J. Comp. Neurol. Suppl. 1:1–91, 1966.

Denny-Brown, D.: The Cerebral Control of Movement. Liverpool: Liverpool University Press, 1966.

Denslow, J. S., and Gutensohn, O. R.: Neuromuscular reflexes in response to gravity. J. Appl. Physiol. 23:2:243–247, 1967.

Dimitrijevic, M. R., and Nathan, P. W.: Studies of spasticity in man. 3. Analysis of reflex activity evoked by noxious cutaneous stimulation. Brain 91:349–368, 1968.

Engberg, I., Lundberg, A., and Ryall, R. W.: Reticulospinal inhibition of transmission in reflex pathways. J. Physiol. (Lond.) 194:201–223, 1968.

Engberg, I.: Reticulospinal inhibition of interneurons. J. Physiol. (Lond.) 194:225–236, 1968.

Ermolaeva, V. Y., and Ermolenko, S. F.: Reciprocal connections between the first and second somatosensory cortical areas and the caudate nucleus. Neuroscience Behav. Physiol. 6:325–331, 1973.

Gellhorn, E.: Principles of Autonomic-Somatic Integrations. Minneapolis: University of Minnesota Press, 1967.

Gordon, B.: The superior colliculus of the brain. Scientif. Amer. 227:72–82, 1972.

Granit, R. (ed.): Nobel Symposium I—Muscular Afferents and Motor Control. New York: John Wiley & Sons, 1966.

Granit, R.: Receptors And Sensory Perception. New Haven CN: Yale University Press, 1955.

Granit, R.: The functional role of the muscle spindles—facts and hypotheses. Brain 98:531–556, 1975.

Grimby, L., and Hannerz, J.: Recruitment order of motor units in voluntary contraction: Changes induced by proprioceptive afferent activity. J. Neurol. Neurosurg. Psychiatr. 1968.

Grimby, L., et al.: Disturbances of voluntary recruitment order of low and high frequency motor units on blockades of proprioceptive afferent activity. Acta Physiol. Scand. 96:207–216, 1976.

Hagbarth, K. E., et al.: Effects of the Jendrassik manoeuvre on muscle spindle activity in man. J. Neurol. Neurosurg. Psych. 38:1143–1153, 1975.

Hall, V. E. (ed.): Annual Review of Physiology. Palo Alto: Annual Reviews, Inc., published yearly.

Harris, F. A.: The brain is a distributed information center. Am. J. Occup. Ther. 24:264–268, 1970.

Hinoki, M., et al.: Optic organ and cervical proprioceptors in maintenance of body equilibrium. Acta Otolaryngol. (Suppl) 330:164–184, 1975.

Houk, J., and Simon, W.: Responses of Golgi tendon organs to forces applied to muscle tendon. J. Neurophysiol. 30:6, 1967.

Howard, I. P., and Templeton, W. B.: Human Spatial Orientation. New York: John Wiley & Sons, 1966.

Hunt, C. C., and Ottoson, D.: Initial burst of primary endings of isolated mammalian muscle spindles. J. Neurophysiol. 39:324–330, 1976.

Iggo, A. (ed.): Handbook of Sensory Physiology. Vol. II, Somato-Sensory System. New York: Springer-Verlag, 1973.

Jansen, J. K. S.: Spasticity—functional aspects. Acta Neurol. Scand. 1962.

Jasper, H. (ed.): Reticular Formation of the Brain. Boston: Little, Brown, & Co., 1958.

Jones, B.: The importance of memory traces of motor efferent discharge for learning skilled movements. Dev. Med. Child. Neurol. 16:620–628, 1974.

Kenshalo, D. R. (ed.): The Skin Senses. Springfield, IL: Charles C Thomas, Publisher, 1968.

Kimble, D. P. (ed.): The Anatomy of Memory, Learning, Remembering and Forgetting. Palo Alto: Science & Behavior Books, 1965.

Kimura, D.: The asymmetry of the human brain. Scientif. Amer. 228:70–78, 1973.

Knighton, R. S., and Dumke, P. R. (eds.): Pain. Henry Ford Hospital International Symposium. Boston: Little, Brown, & Co., 1966.

Kots, Y. M., and Zhukov, V. I.: Supraspinal control over segmental centers of antagonistic muscles in man. III. Tuning of spinal reciprocal inhibition system during organization preceding voluntary movement. Neuroscience Behav. Physiol. 6:9–15, 1973.

Luria, A. R.: Human Brain and Psychological Process. New York: Harper & Row Publishers, translated 1966.

Magni, F., and Willis, W. D.: Cortical control of brain stem reticular neurons. Arch. Ital. Biol. 102:418–433, 1964.

Magni, F.: Afferent connections to reticulo-spinal neurons. Prog. Brain Res. Elsevier, 12:246–258, 1964.

Magni, F.: Subcortical and peripheral control of brainstem reticular neurons. Arch. Ital. Biol. 102:434–438, 1964.

Magoun, H. W.: The Waking Brain, ed. 2, Springfield IL, Charles C Thomas, Publisher, 1963.

Moore, J. C.: Concepts From The Neurobehavioral Sciences. Dubuque: Kendall-Hunt, 1973.

Moore, J. C.: Neuroanatomy Simplified. Dubuque: Kendall-Hunt, 1969.

Morin, C., et al.: Role of the muscular afferents in the inhibition of the antagonist motor nucleus during a voluntary contraction in man. Brain Res. 103:373–376, 1976.

Neff, W. D. (ed.): Contributions to Sensory Physiology, ed. 2. New York: Academic Press, 1967.

Piercey, M. F., and Goldfarb, J.: Discharge patterns of Renshaw cells evoked by volleys in ipsilateral cutaneous and high threshold muscle afferents and their relationship to reflexes recorded in ventral roots. J. Neurophysiol. 37:294–302, 1974.

Rispal-Padel, L., et al.: Relations between the ventrolateral thalamic nucleus and motor cortex and their possible role in the central organization of motor control. Brain Res. 60:1–20, 1973.

Ruch, T. C., et al.: Neurophysiology, ed. 2. Philadelphia: W. B. Saunders Co., 1966.

Rushworth, G.: Some aspects of the pathophysiology of spasticity and rigidity. Clin. Pharmacol. Ther. 1964.

Schultz, D. P.: Sensory Restriction—Effects on Behavior. New York: Academic Press, 1965.

Sherrington, C.: The Integrative Action of The Nervous System. New Haven CN: Yale University Press, 1961.

Speyer, K. M., Ghelarducci, B., and Pompeiano, O.: Gravity responses in main reticular formation. J. Neurophysiol. 37:705–721, 1974.

Tokizane, T., Shimaza, H.: Functional Differentiation of Human Skeletal Muscle. Tokyo: Tokyo University Press, 1964.

Wagman, I. H., Pierce, D. S., and Burger, R. E.: Proprioceptive influence in volitional control of individual motor units. Nature (Lond) 7:957–958, 1965.

Wolstencroft, J. H.: Effects of afferent stimuli on reticulospinal neurons. J. Physiol. 1961.

Woodburne, L. S.: The Neural Basis of Behavior. Columbus: Charles E. Merrill Publishing Co., 1967.

Yahr, M. D., and Purpura, D. D.: Neurophysiological Basis of Normal and Abnormal Motor Activities. New York: Raven Press, 1967.

ACKNOWLEDGMENT

My appreciation to Josephine C. Moore, Ph.D., O.T.R., for her continuing efforts to assist all of us in the understanding of the neuroanatomical and neurophysiological aspects of human function.

5

The Activity Process

Helen L. Hopkins, Helen D. Smith, and Elizabeth G. Tiffany

The things human beings do and the objects human beings make provide a bridge between their inner reality and their external world. In their activities they show their concern with how to survive, be comfortable, have pleasure, solve problems, express themselves, and be related with others and the wider world of society. They experience themselves and come to know their strengths and weaknesses or limits through the things they do. The roles they assume have inherent functions, skills, and behaviors which are necessary to support them. There are, for example, characteristic activities that are necessary for the student, parent, store manager, beach bum, and so forth. It is probably for these reasons, more than for any others, that occupational therapy, with its emphasis on the use of activity to promote function, came into being.

CHARACTERISTICS OF OCCUPATIONAL THERAPY ACTIVITY

The term "occupation" in occupational therapy "is in the context of man's goal-directed use of time, energy, interest and attention."[1] Thus occupation is used in the context of being occupied productively in activities that "are primary agents for learning and development and an essential source of satisfaction."[2] Activities as used in occupational therapy should have at least eight characteristics:

1. *Be goal directed.* Activities should have some purpose or reason for their use to be considered occupational therapy activity. "Busy work," in its keeping hands occupied, may be of some value to the client but generally is not chosen with a specific goal in mind.
2. *Have significance at some level to the client.* Activities should have some value and usefulness to the client, even though the value may be one that will be realized only at some future date. This indicates that the activity may seem to have no immediate value in reaching a specified goal but will make it possible to reach that goal in a week, a month, or sometime later. The activity should have some relationship to the roles the individual plays in society.
3. *Require client involvement at some level* (either mental or physical). Activities require "doing" or participation on the part of the client. The

individual engaged in the activity should be involved in the process of determining the activity as well as in the performance of it and thus receives self-gratification from the results. He or she is not a recipient but rather a participant. Participation may be active or passive.

4. *Be geared to prevention of malfunction and/or maintenance or improvement of function and quality of life.* The choice and type of activity is dependent upon the client level of function and ability to participate; however, the goal is clear.

5. *Reflect client involvement in life task situations* (ADL, play, work). Activities are used to acquire or redevelop those skills essential for fulfillment of life roles. Activities provide for development of competence in the performance of those tasks essential to the life roles of each individual.

6. *Relate to the interests of the client.* Involvement in the choice of activity is vital. Commitment to the tasks will be attained only if client goals and interests are considered and are met.

7. *Be adaptable and gradable.* Activity must be age appropriate, be able to be increased or decreased in complexity, and be graded in time and strength required.

8. *Be determined through occupational therapist's professional judgment based on knowledge.* Knowledge of human development, medical pathology, interpersonal relationships, and value of activity to the person are required to make the match between client problems and the activities that will be most meaningful and serviceable in reaching the therapeutic goals of the occupational therapy process.

FACTORS TO BE CONSIDERED IN SELECTION OF APPROPRIATE ACTIVITIES

Activities must be selected for their properties that are most applicable to the treatment of the individual problem. In conditions involving physical dysfunction the activities are selected for their physical restorative powers as well as for their psychological and psychosocial properties. They must be constructive as well as provide the desired exercise. This enables the client to translate the motion, strength, and coordination gained to normal activity, thus providing the additional psychological value of success in achievement. Activities used for treatment of physical disabilities must be adaptable so they can provide specific exercise for affected joints or muscles. Activities used should be in accord with the following criteria to meet physical restoration requirements[3]:

1. *Provide action rather than position.* Activity should provide for alternate contraction and relaxation of muscles. Activities should be analyzed from a kinesiological point of view to determine components of the activity, motions required to perform the activity, muscle power required, and the range of motion and strengthening the activity can provide.

2. *Require repetition of the motion.* Activity should permit repetition of the desired motion for an indefinite but controllable number of times.

3. *Permit gradation in range of motion, resistance, and coordination.* Activity should allow a greater range of motion than is permitted by the limitation found in the joint so the activity can allow for increase of *joint range.* Resistance is required in order to strengthen a muscle. Thus the activity should be gradable in the amount of resistance it provides so that resistance can be increased as power returns. When *coordination* is affected, the activity should be graded so that it provides exercise requiring gross coordination and working toward fine coordination. The activity may also be varied or adapted through positioning or by changing the way the task is performed.

In psychiatric conditions, activities must be selected for their psychosocial or psychodynamic properties as well as their physical value. Some of the aspects that must be considered include[4]:

1. Property of materials resistive, pliable, controlled, or messy, as well as the sensory input they provide (tactile, auditory, olfactory, visual, proprioceptive).

2. Complexity of the activity—number of steps in the activity, repetition required.

3. Preparation required—prearrangement of supplies, adaptation of environment.

4. Amount and type of directions—verbal or written directions, diagrams, demonstration.

5. Structure and controls (rules) inherent in the activity.

6. Predictability of results.
7. Type of learning required—old learning, adapted old learning, or new learning.
8. Decision making required on part of patient.
9. Attention span—minutes or hours.
10. Interaction—solitary, parallel, interaction with peers, small group, large group, cooperation.
11. Communication—nonverbal, little, oral directions, reading, writing.
12. Motivation—creative, gratifying, intellectually challenging, affect on others, relevance to life space and roles.
13. Time—completion of activity in one session or sessions, quick success, delayed gratification.

In working in the field of pediatrics, a combination of psychosocial, psychodynamic, physical, and developmental factors must be considered. The activities may be required to provide specific aspects relating to normal growth and development, must be age appropriate in complexity and dexterity required, yet may need to provide some aspects which promote physical function and promote psychological well-being.

Prevocational activities are selected on the basis of their ability to contribute to work-related skills. They must be selected for their relationship to the components of the actual work requirements. These include such aspects as physical performance, coordination required, concentration needed, speed and accuracy involved, endurance needed, routinization and boredom factors, initiative and decision making required.

For individuals with sensory-integration problems (cognitive-perceptual-motor dysfunction), sensory stimuli presented by the activity must be analyzed along with the "intersensory-integrative mechanisms involved and the motor response required."[5] Thus tactile, kinesthetic, visual, auditory, and olfactory sensory modalities must be analyzed for each activity along with the type of response required including motor, visual, and verbal. Activity analysis in this area requires the analysis of the neurological integration of input from the senses and the muscular response to this stimulation and integration and is therefore called the neurobehavioral approach to activity analysis. Activities must be analyzed with all the components in mind in order to choose the most appropriate one to meet all therapeutic requirements.[6]

In selecting an activity to be used in the therapeutic process, the therapist must answer five basic questions:

1. *How* do you do the activity? The therapist must know the basic components of the activity, the process involved, the tools, equipment, and supplies needed, and must know how to do it well enough to be able to teach it successfully.
2. *What* activity is most appropriate to meet the requirements of the situation? The therapist must assess the problems involved, the needs, interests, and preferences of the patient/client, and, with the individual, must determine the activity that best meets the requirements for therapeutic intervention.
3. *Why* was a specific activity chosen? The therapist must be able to determine the reason for the choice of activity on the basis of a rationale for this choice which is consistent with the overall treatment rationale.
4. *Where* will the activity be performed? The therapist may be constrained in the choice of an activity because of the location or situation within which the activity will be carried out. For example, if the activity is to be done by an individual in bed, it cannot be too messy or require large tools or equipment.
5. *When* will the activity be carried out? The time of day or season of the year may influence the type of activity that is relevant. For example, self-care activities are most logically carried out at the time of day when they are usually done, i.e., bathing and dressing before breakfast. Activities that are relevant may be dictated by the time of year, i.e., making decorations or presents at Christmas.

ACTIVITY ANALYSIS

The therapist's skill in activity analysis is critical in determining the validity of his or her use of activities. There are many approaches used in occupational therapy to analyze activities. The nature of activity analysis used will be influenced by the therapist's frame of reference for treatment. Some occupational therapists have undertaken the task of analyzing the major activities which are used and keeping these analyses on file for reference when doing treatment planning. In some instances, activity analyses have been adapted to record evaluative data acquired in the use of specific activities as evaluation.

The accompanying sample form is one form of activity analysis, focusing on the skills requirements of the activity and built on the concept of the developmental wheel described in Chapter 3 (see Fig. 3–1). This analysis may easily be adapted to record evaluative data.

ACTIVITY ANALYSIS FORM

Activity analyzed:
Average time required for completion:
Average number of sessions required to complete:
Brief description: (include criteria for determining success)

Activity Characteristics	*Explanations*		
A. MOTOR 1. Position: a. activity b. patient/client 2. Motion(s) components a. joints involved b. motion(s) involved 3. Muscles utilized 4. Direction of resistance			
	Skill required √	Degree Low Medium High	Is activity gradable? How?
5. Action rather than position 6. Repetition of motion(s) 7. Rhythm developed 8. Maintained contraction (static) 9. Manual dexterity 10. Gross motor 11. Fine motor 12. Bilateral 13. Unilateral 14. Endurance 15. Rate of performance 16. Grading adaptability a. R.O.M. b. resistance c. coordination d. substitution			
B. SENSORY 1. Visual 2. Auditory (impact on) 3. Gustatory 4. Olfactory 5. Tactile a. temperature of material b. texture of material c. heavy to light touch			
C. COGNITIVE 1. Organizational ability 2. Problem solving ability a. planning b. trial and error			

Activity Characteristics	Skill required ✓	Degree Low Medium High	Is activity gradable? How?
3. Logical thinking			
4. Concentration			
5. Attention span			
6. Written/oral/demonstration directions			
a. complex			
b. simple			
7. Reading			
8. Seriation			
9. Interpret signs & symbols			
10. Multiple processing/steps involved			
11. Creativity			
12. Use of imagination			
13. Establish goal & carry out means to attain it			
14. Causal relationships involved (perceive cause & effect)			
15. Centering			
16. Perceive viewpoint of others			
17. Test reality			
D. PERCEPTUAL			
1. Sensory integration required			
2. Differentiation			
a. Figure-ground			
b. Space relationships			
c. Object constancy			
d. Kinesthesia			
e. Proprioception			
f. Stereognosis			
g. Form constancy			
h. Color perception			
i. Auditory perception			
3. Tactile integration			
4. Motor planning			
5. Bilateral integration			
6. Body scheme			
7. Vestibular			
E. EMOTIONAL			
1. Passive or aggressive motion			
2. Destructive			
3. Gratification			
a. immediate			
b. delayed			
4. Structured			
5. Unstructured			
6. Allows control			
7. Success/failure possibility			
8. Independence			
9. Dependence			
10. Symbolism involved			
11. Reality testing			
12. Handle feelings			
13. Impulse control			
F. SOCIAL			
1. Interaction required			
2. Isolating activity			
3. Group activity			

Activity Characteristics	Skill required ✓	Degree Low Medium High	Is activity gradable? How?
4. Competition 5. Responsibility involved 6. Communication necessary 7. Work in small groups 8. Work in large groups 9. Work with one other person 10. Test reality 11. Control—lead 12. Follow—cooperate			

G. CULTURAL
1. Relevancy to personal
   a. Value system
   b. Life situations

H. COMMON TO ALL
1. Age appropriateness
2. Safety precautions & hazards
3. Sexual identification
4. Space required
5. Equipment needed
6. Vocational application
7. Cost
8. Adaptability

REFERENCES

1. Occupational therapy—its definition and functions. Am. J. Occup. Ther. 20:204–205, 1976.
2. Ibid.
3. Willard, H. S., and Spackman, C. S. (eds.): Occupational Therapy, ed. 4. Philadelphia: J. B. Lippincott Co., 1971, pp. 171–182.
4. Activity analysis. Occupational Therapy Dept., Norristown State Hospital, Norristown PA, 1977.
5. Llorens, L.: Activity analysis for cognitive-perceptual-motor dysfunction. Am. J. Occup. Ther. 27:453–456, 1973.
6. Ibid.

Part Three

Occupational Therapy Approaches for Intervention

6

Occupational Therapy—A Problem Solving Process

Helen L. Hopkins and Elizabeth G. Tiffany

The occupational therapy process is one which utilizes problem solving methods for finding the best, most appropriate means of helping those individuals requiring occupational therapy intervention reach their highest potential for function in their own roles within their own environments. Occupational therapists must approach each new situation as an opportunity or challenge to find meaningful solutions to the problems facing the patients or clients with whom they are working.

Occupational therapists must become skilled in problem identification, using astute observation and the many evaluation procedures available to them. In this way a data base can be established which will identify the real problems. Once general problems are identified, they can be broken down into subproblems that guide the therapist in determining the goals of treatment or intervention. Alternative approaches for solving the problems must be identified and a plan of action is chosen that seems to be promising for resolution of the problem.

The patient or client must be involved in the process of problem identification so that assets as well as liabilities may be determined. The goals that are established, the alternative chosen, and the plan of action must reflect what is desired by and acceptable to the patient or client. In order to be successful, the plan of action and the approach chosen must also be in synchronization with those of the family and other professionals working with the individual.

Once a plan of action is chosen, it must be examined for its probable value and the potential outcomes of treatment or intervention. If the plan appears to be feasible and is a promising solution, it can be implemented. Long term goals which can be broken down into short term goals or manageable elements should be included. There must be periodic reevaluation to determine progress, goals reached, and problems solved. It may be necessary to make modifications or adapt goals and plans as changes occur. There are occasions when abandonment of an unsuccessful plan is necessary, requiring determination of another course of action from the alternatives available. As new knowledge develops and new viewpoints evolve, new alternatives arise that provide different approaches for intervention in occupational therapy.

Use of the problem solving process in occupational therapy requires creativity and imagination on the part of the therapist. The therapist must use knowledge, skills, and good professional judgment in order to find the best possible solution for each patient or client.[1,2]

APPROACHES TO INTERVENTION

In occupational therapy today there are several alternative approaches to intervention that may be chosen by practicing therapists depending on their orientation and their rationale for treatment. Each approach has a specific knowledge base, is built on stated concepts, and utilizes a rationale which places constraints on the occupational therapy program specifying the type of activities appropriate for occupational therapy intervention.

The approaches which are used in current occupational therapy practice fall into three categories:

1. Developmental Approach
2. Rehabilitation/Habilitation Approach
3. Occupational Behavior Approach

Each of these approaches is discussed in another chapter (7, 8, and 9).

Although each approach to occupational therapy intervention is based on specific knowledge and concepts there may be varying frames of reference that may be utilized by individual therapists or agencies all functioning under the same approach. The experience, values, sociocultural assumptions, individual points of view, and the subjective reality within the individual or inherent in an agency's philosophy may cause them to choose a specific frame of reference within which to function.[3] For example, within the developmental approach, one occupational therapist, group of therapists, or agency may use a neurodevelopmental perspective for treatment of children with cerebral palsy and choose to utilize the Bobath frame of reference for treatment. Another therapist, group of therapists, or agency may use the developmental approach with a neurophysiological perspective for treatment of children with cerebral palsy and choose to utilize a Rood frame of reference for treatment.

In some situations, although operating under the developmental approach, more than one frame of reference may be utilized according to the varying conditions of the clients, the philosophy of the agency, and the preferences, biases, and expertise of the therapists. Some agencies may use more than one approach to intervention depending on the type of clients as well as on the preferences, biases, and expertise of the therapists, thus increasing the possibility of the number and variety of frames of reference that may be used. The rationale and basis for choosing an approach and frame of reference must be understood by the therapist along with the knowledge base and concepts inherent in that approach.

The occupational therapy intervention process will differ according to the approach and frame of reference chosen, but the overall goals of the process can be described as *prevention* of conditions causing or resulting in loss of function, *remediation, treatment* or *rehabilitation* for restoration of function and performance, and *maintenance* of health and the ability to function in all aspects of living. Depending upon the conditions and problems involved, any or all of these goals may be appropriate in the intervention process for a patient or client at any time along the developmental continuum from conception to death.

Certain educational requirements must be met in order to be able to practice in occupational therapy. The "Essentials of an Accredited Educational Program for the Occupational Therapist"[4] delineates the required knowledge areas. The areas include knowledge about the basic human sciences, including physical, psychological, and social aspects; the human development process; specific life tasks and activities; the health-illness-health continuum; and occupational therapy theory and practice. The relationship between education and practice components of the occupational therapy process and the developmental continuum are shown in Figure 6-1.

BASIS FOR TREATMENT APPROACHES

The Four Elements

What are the organizing principles which have given occupational therapy its essence? Occupational therapists have been concerned with maintaining, improving, and restoring the patient's or client's ability to function in his or her own world. They have been aware, with varying degrees of

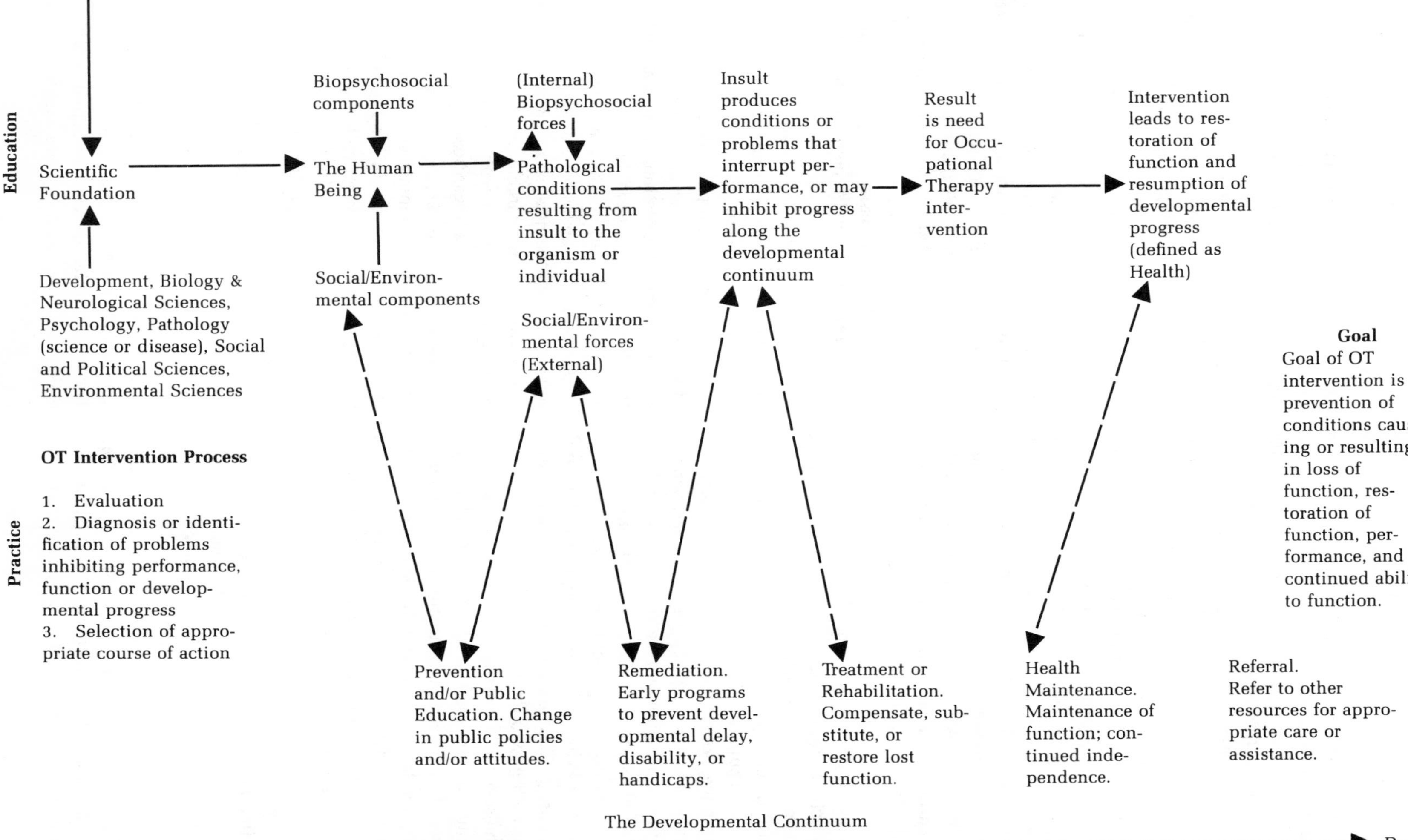

FIGURE 6-1. The occupational therapy process and developmental continuum. Adapted from Johnson, J. A., Delegate Assembly Address.[5]

interest and levels of sophistication, that human beings are complex and whole. Therapists' work has been based on four components: the *patient or client, the therapist and therapeutic relationship,* the *activity,* and the *context or setting for treatment.* The therapeutic process, implemented formally or informally, has been one of evaluation, treatment planning, and treatment implementation. Therapists have collaborated with other people and shared plans and observations. Through all of the changes, increased knowledge, and new approaches that have taken place over the years, these principles have continued to guide the practice of occupational therapy. The struggle, as reflected in the 1976 Mental Health Task Force Report,[6] has been to acquire a strong, current, and valid knowledge base and effective skills and then public recognition to permit their use.

The drawing together of the client, the therapist, and the activity represents an exceedingly complex and dynamic situation. When confronted with providing valid and effective treatment for the disabled client, the occupational therapist must address a number of questions: On what basis do I understand this person? How do I conceptualize human personality, human behavior, physical function, and the ways in which human beings learn, grow, and change? How do I understand pathology or the disease process? What about its etiological factors and its prognosis? What do I know about the external factors which now impinge upon this person? What about the social and work worlds in which he or she must function now and in the future? What do I know about the methods of treatment or frames of reference for treatment currently being used with this person? How can I best communicate with this person so that we build a mutual understanding of reality that is as clear as possible?

The Patient or Client

It is important to understand the human elements involved—the patient or client, the therapist, and other significant people. There are a great many ways in which human personality and behavior may be conceptualized. For the purpose of establishing a baseline, we will consider here a few of the factors which are especially salient for the occupational therapy process. These are in no way exclusive, and the reader is referred to the bibliography and encouraged to search the literatures of the social and biological sciences for other perspectives.

STRESS. Any consideration of disability or dysfunction must include attention to the role that stress plays in the development and exacerbation of problems. In 1956 Hans Selye wrote a book, *The Stress of Life,*[7] in which he described the interrelationships of the body systems and the extensive effects of stress upon the whole. In the years which have followed the publication of Selye's work, interest in the nature of stress has spurred a great deal of research as well as much public speculation about the subject. In the 1960s and 1970s in the technological advances, ideas, and new awarenesses described by Toffler in *Future Shock*[8] we have seen a proliferation of interest in popular movements and literature dealing with methods for coping with stress and tension.

Coleman broadly defines stress as the "adjustive demands made upon the individual."[9] He points out that stress may occur on physiological or psychological levels. On the physiological level, examples of stressors which make adjustive demands upon the individual are a broken limb, the invasion by a virus, the ingestion of a poison, blood sugar imbalance, or an arthritic condition. On the psychological level, stressors may be the loss of a loved one, failure in an important test, the necessity of making a choice between two highly desirable (or undesirable) alternatives, or bombardment with too many things to do. The effects of stress, regardless of the original stressful event, are felt in varying degrees throughout the system. Data on autonomic system responses, cortical changes, muscle tension, and the client's subjective experience have been collected and measured. These data indicate clearly that mind, emotions, and body are inseparably involved in their reactions to stress.

Coleman further points out that the severity of stress depends upon three factors: (1) the characteristics of the adjustive demand; (2) the characteristics of the individual; and (3) the external resources and supports available to the individual. Adjustive demands may be very brief or very long in duration. The threat to the individual's actual survival may in reality be very great or very small. The stressful event may occur alone or may occur in combination with a number of other stressful factors. Stressful reactions may predispose an individual to further negative stress reactions.

According to Coleman, the longer stress continues the more severe it becomes. Many small stresses occurring together at the same time may subject the individual to stress overload, and the gradual building up of insignificant events over a long period of time may add up to greater stress than a single severe incident.

On the other hand, stress, as "the adjustive demands made upon the individual," may be viewed as having the potential for positive effects. It is in the second two factors mentioned by Coleman—the characteristics of the individual and the external resources and supports available—that there exist possibilities for change, growth, and strengthening of coping mechanisms to deal with inevitable future life stresses. One is reminded that the Chinese character for "crisis" is a combination of two elements meaning "danger" and "opportunity." Recognition of these possibilities is important in occupational therapy.

According to Piaget[10] adaptation and the continual interplay between disequilibrium and equilibrium are the major ways in which human beings comprehend their world. Consider this possibility: periods of disequilibrium represent stresses and, when these stresses are dealt with positively, equilibrium is achieved and growth has taken place.

Characteristics of the individual include genetic predispositions such as innate intelligence; temperament; body type; structural strengths and weaknesses of the body systems; basic environmental influences such as nutrition, clothing, and housing; parental nurturance; discipline; the cumulative effects of interactions with significant people in school, church and the neighborhood; and the mores and cultural factors that impinge upon the development of personality. The individual is a total being, a composite of physical, sensory, perceptual, emotional, cognitive, social, and cultural learned behaviors and skills. The extent to which this composite is elastic (able to rebound), flexible (able to bend, compromise, and change), and strong (able to stand firm) is significant in determining the extent to which the individual can meet the adjustive demands made upon him or her. The characteristics of the individual, although basically determined by adulthood, may be considered as dynamic and alterable in some measure throughout life. If this were not so there would be no reason for therapy.

External resources for coping with stress are multi-dimensional—factors such as the family, the neighborhood, the church, friends, money, educational opportunities, the possibility of a vacation, and even the climate.

For the health professional whose commitment is to facilitate competence on the part of the dysfunctional, the careful consideration of Coleman's three aspects is essential. It is important to be sensitive to the possibility that stress, regardless of its nature, may be responsible for regression and a lessened ability to perceive realistically or to behave adaptively. This in itself contributes to further stress and further regression and a vicious downward spiral has been started. On the other hand, true coping behavior in which an individual is able to feel competent and to experience success or mastery seems to lead to further strengths, more adaptive skills, and successes.

MOTIVATION. The key to success in a program of occupational therapy often lies in the extent to which the patient or client may be motivated to participate in it. Human motivation has been a much studied personality variable and seems to be one of the most important areas to which the occupational therapist should give attention. Motivation may be defined as an arousal to action, initiating, molding, and sustaining specific action patterns.[11] The task of the occupational therapist requires that the client be motivated, first, to participate in treatment and, second, to sustain the healthy patterns hopefully established in the process.

One may consider that behavior is motivated by principles of drive-reduction, need satisfaction, and the pleasure principle. The role of reinforcement as a basic motivator has been much studied and one needs to look carefully at the many aspects of reinforcement and aversive conditioning approaches to achieving motivation. Other theories suggest that behavior beyond that which is related to issues of survival is motivated, in addition, by innate curiosity and a need to interact with the environment.[12]

The examination of the range of "normal" behavior reveals that people are motivated by many factors, e.g., novelty, complexity, surprise, competition, and cooperation. Personality types have been characterized in terms of dominant social motivational patterns: (1) *affiliation*—liking people; (2) aggression—moving against people; (3) *dominance*—drive to dominate people; and (4) *cognizance*—exploring and asking questions.

McClelland has studied factors related to "need for achievement" which was defined as the extent to which a person could enjoy competition against a standard of excellence. Individuals may be characterized as falling somewhere along a continuum with regard to this variable. At the low end the individual tends to prefer to be involved in no risk situations where competition is minimal and either success or failure at a given task will be dependent upon his or her performance. This personality variable appears to be dynamic and powerful and appears also to be set at a very early age.[13]

Related to achievement motivation as a personality factor is the issue of field dependence. Some people demonstrate unique, integrated, individual, internal schemes; those who do tend to be less conforming to social pressure and seem to behave more in conformity to standards which are internalized and personal. Such individuals are characterized as field-independent. Those individuals who seem to be highly motivated to conform to standards or pressures which are external are characterized as field-dependent.[14]

Another related and powerful factor is locus of control. Locus of control refers to the extent to which individuals perceive that the events and situations of their lives are controlled by themselves or by chance or luck. This variable is, again, measured on a continuum which goes from an extreme internal locus of control to an extreme external locus of control. Internals perceive themselves as responsible and able to direct and control their life situations while externals see themselves as the recipients or victims of fate. Extremes in either direction, obviously, are unrealistic.[15,16,17]

Two factors may be critical in determining the nature of one's orientation with regard to achievement motivation, field dependence, and locus of control. First, there are the quality and quantity of experiences that growing children have and the extent to which they are experienced as pleasurable, reinforcing, or satisfying. Second, and perhaps more basic, is the consideration of the individual's ability to process the information which is received from the world. Both of these considerations appear to be of great importance, and there is need for continuing research into their complex relationships with human motivation and basic self-concept.

Piaget[18] and White[19] have spoken eloquently of the importance of the experience of success in promoting feelings of efficacy and motivation for further performance. What seems to be of great importance is that the individual very clearly understands, experiences, and owns the behaviors and their effects. Those situational variables which are not, in fact, related to an individual's behavior or control need to be understood as such. Another factor, which is very powerful in determining motivation, is anxiety. Anxiety may be a strong motivator for performance up to a point, a factor which varies from individual to individual and with situations. Beyond that point, anxiety becomes an inhibitor to motivation, tends to render the individual rigid and unable to adapt to new situations, and results in a decrease in integrative mechanisms.

All of these considerations are of great importance to the occupational therapist because of the need to elicit the active cooperation and participation of the patient or client. The results of illness and disability may be perceived differently by different individuals with regard to their sense of responsibility and efficacy. The extent to which standards of achievement must be internalized to be motivating to an individual varies. Clarity of feedback, awareness of anxiety levels, and the ability to identify what may be uniquely reinforcing to an individual may be critical to determining the success or failure of a treatment program.

THE NONHUMAN WORLD. From the moment of birth, human beings become part of a world of things to be experienced—to be seen, felt, heard, smelled, tasted, feared, and enjoyed. There is controversy about whether very young infants experience differentiation between themselves and the external objects of their world and about whether they are able to distinguish between animate and inanimate objects.[20,21,22] For infants and growing children, however, the human and nonhuman objects of their worlds are crucial in determining the kinds of people they will become. For the occupational therapist, understanding of the ways in which a person interacts with the nonhuman world is important. Harold Searles, in his book *The Nonhuman Environment*,[23] explores in depth the kinds and qualities of meanings that human beings invest in their worlds of things, places, and spaces. He refers to kinds of relationships that characterize human interactions with their nonhuman worlds as they grow up. Mankind is able to use the nonhuman world to give a sense of stability and continuity, to practice skills in relating, to assuage strong feelings, to foster self-realization, to deepen the awareness of reality, and to foster appreciation and acceptance of fellow human beings.

The healthy adult has learned to live in some degree of adaptation with the things and places of his or her world. What is the range of feelings inherent in the experiences of the nonhuman world? Some are experiences of pride in fixing the engine of a car, pleasure in baking a cake, excitement in riding a roller coaster, frustration in coping with a machine that won't work, discomfort of being wet and cold in a storm, power in moving a heavy object, helplessness in not being able to move a heavy object, catharsis in housecleaning, wholeness in being beside the ocean, or comfort in a warm bed on a cold night.

The things and places of the world offer sources of pleasure and pain, opportunities to practice skills and to express ourselves, challenges to survive, and chances to live well. There is a continual and intimate relatedness with the nonhuman world.

The arts and artifacts which human beings come to treasure become symbolically invested with the values of the people who produce and use them. This goes far beyond things like dishes, vases, furniture, books, toys, and paintings. It goes into the uses of space and the kinds of personal privacy that may be fostered and the extent to which the world of nature is regarded and incorporated into an individual's living space.

What does all this mean to the occupational therapist? It has everything to do with attention to the potential meanings of the tools and materials of the activities used in treatment and the kinds of environments in which the therapist practices. It means the therapist can help the patient or client develop ways of trusting and *using* the nonhuman worlds; that this may have primary importance all by itself. The use of the nonhuman world is significant in providing a bridge for human relationships. It means the articles used and treasured by a person give clues not only to that person's private gestalt but also to the culture of the society in which he or she lives. It means that when a patient or client has permitted himself to invest in creating or producing something tangible or ideational in occupational therapy, the therapist needs to respect the person's ownership of that product.

CULTURAL IMPLICATIONS. Much is said about the need to understand the family and community to which each patient or client belongs. The rich literatures of sociology and anthropology on the subject of cultural influences are worth study by health professionals. There is little doubt that social systems are a powerful, although often subtle, influence on basic ways of perceiving, thinking, feeling, and behaving. Learning begins at conception and continues through interactions with both human and nonhuman environments; therefore cultural values, biases, and customs are powerful in the formation of personalities. The kinds of toys, games, foods, and other objects that are presented, the kinds of music and stories, the humor, the behavior that is encouraged and the behavior that is discouraged, the quality and quantity of parenting experienced and the amount of touching and closeness between people are just some of the ways in which children are influenced by the culture of their families. Cultural influences are deep. As Edward Hall says,

> Most of culture lies hidden and is outside voluntary control, making up the warp and weft of human existence. Even when small fragments of culture are elevated to awareness, they are difficult to change, not only because they are so personally experienced but because people cannot act or interact at all in any meaningful way except through the medium of culture.[24]

Both the therapist's perceptions and behavior and the client's perceptions and behavior are filtered through the screen of culture.

The occupational therapist must be concerned about values. Values determine how the individual feels about people, ideas, and things and how he acts toward them. Value conflicts, both within self and between individuals and groups, are responsible for many of the difficulties which are part of everyone's living experience. In today's society, with rapid mass communication and mobility, the potential for value conflicts seems to be increased.

Among the daily behaviors to be considered are the ways in which a client views and manages time, space (personal distance and territory), objects, dress, daily self-care activities, money, work, play, and study. How does the client respond to pain, loss, illness, and death? What is considered rude? How important is the family? What constitutes friendship? What about religious beliefs, rituals, and observances? Is anxiety handled by laughing and talking or by withdrawing? What is the significance of food and mealtimes? How is anger dealt with? What are the characteristic support systems of the group?

A gypsy queen was hospitalized in a large metropolitan hospital and the gypsy band literally camped at the doorsteps, keeping close to their queen in all possible ways. In no way would the staff of the hospital wish to chase them away or diagnose the queen's use of their support as pathological dependency. Certain oriental groups laugh when they are confronted with danger. Some groups consider manual occupations degrading. The average American is more scheduled and time-bound than the individuals from most cultural groups.

In a culturally heterogeneous population there will be a wide range of behaviors and life styles which may be considered normal. To help the client function within his own world, the therapist needs to understand that world.

The Therapist

The therapist in a treatment setting is, by definition, a helper. The roles a therapist assumes may vary. The therapist may legitimately be a teacher or a facilitator who brings knowledge and skills to the patient/client's unique situation.

The most important prerequisite to being an effective helper is self-knowledge. The helper needs to be aware of his or her own needs, perceptual biases, and capabilities.

The relationship that is established between the therapist and the patient/client may well determine the success or failure of the treatment plan. The establishment of effective and clear communication both ways is the first essential part of the relationship. Sensitivity to the level and mode of communication that will work with a given patient/client and skill in using this knowledge may be the critical factor in the establishment of a therapeutic relationship. For example, if a patient/client is functioning on a pre-verbal level of understanding, one must think of nonverbal ways of communicating meaning. If a patient or client thinks in concrete terms and understands only tangible things, one must think of concrete and tangible ways to explain feelings, meanings, and actions. With a patient/client who is severely regressed, it may be important to use the process of *naming* and showing, as the purposes and processes of the activities are explained.

Frank has pointed out that one must be aware, also, that in any encounter between two people, there may be at least six selves who are communicating: each party possessing an idealized self, a self perceived by the other person, and the actual self.[25] The transactional analysis model describes the parent self, child self, and adult self. Discrepancies between the individuals' perceptions of one another lead to complex distortions. Transference and countertransference phenomena may also be encountered. When one is working within the psychoanalytic frame of reference, these phenomena are recognized and used as part of the therapeutic process. Most other frames of reference used in the occupational therapy process, however, tend to deemphasize transference when it occurs and work toward the conscious perception of the therapist as a new person, different from past significant persons. The therapist can accomplish this by acting as a "total, reacting, feeling person."[26]

Without the establishment of trust between the patient/client and therapist it is unlikely that a truly collaborative effort will be possible. For some people, the trust issue may be powerful and the establishment of trust may take a long time. The

Communication Trust

therapist's own self-confidence, the therapist's ability to be honest and open in the relationship, and the extent to which the therapist is able to communicate "unconditional positive regard" and empathy for the patient/client will affect the patient/client's ability to invest trust in the relationship.[27]

Purtilo[28] has identified some of the issues and factors which are vital in the therapeutic relationship. Some of her practical guidelines for the professional therapeutic relationships follow.

The Personal-Professional Self*

He decides whether to use the first or last name of each new patient; he is cautious knowing the casual use of the first name may be harmful; he is relaxed in using the last names of patients.

He incorporates actions that communicate caring into the patient-health professional interaction; he recognizes efficiency as a trait which can express caring when it does not impose rigid limits on the interaction.

He recognizes that wearing a uniform does not necessarily make a patient feel *less* cared for nor does the more casual appearance of street clothes make a patient feel *more* cared for.

He combines a pleasant approach with professional competence.

He is interested in the patient as a person with values, needs and beliefs, but does not encourage a relationship that will lead to overdependence (detrimental dependence).

He is respected by the patient who recognizes his integrity. He acknowledges that complete, open, mutual sharing with each other is not conducive to the functioning of a public-sector relationship.

He maintains a balance between sound health care and effective patient-health professional interaction.

He does not need to overprotect himself or to take unnecessary risks; he knows his limits.

*From Purtilo, R.: The Allied Health Professional and the Patient © 1973 by W. B. Saunders Co., Philadelphia PA. Reprinted with permission.

Interpersonal issues such as dependency, aggressiveness or passivity, and personal need gratification or control are often challenges to the therapeutic relationship. They need to be identified for what they are and resolved as realistically and honestly as possible. When these kinds of behaviors emerge they are usually manifestations of the maladaptive modes of thinking, feeling, and acting which have interfered with the person's ability to function. If efforts between the therapist and client to identify and change what may be occurring are unsuccessful, the therapist may wish to find another professional with whom to discuss and objectify the situation.

One of the ways of conceptualizing the progress of a therapeutic relationship is to think in terms of phases. The first phase is an affective one in which the therapist elicits the trust of the client by demonstrating empathy or understanding for his or her feelings and plight. This, depending on the client's need state, or pathology, may be accomplished in a few words, a nod, or touch of the hand. It may, however, take a long time.

The second phase is one of gathering facts and information, identifying the problems to be solved, and sorting out the realistic levels of solution that may be worked toward.

In the third phase, the period of developing an action plan to work on resolving the problems, some form of contract or agreement is made with the patient or client. This is implicit in what has been, on some level at least, a cooperative effort. The contract is an understanding on the part of both the therapist and the patient/client of what the process will be and of what expectations each person may have of the other.

In the fourth phase, the period of implementation of the plan, the conditions of the contract are tested. The issues of trust may emerge again and it is important for the therapist to meet his or her responsibilities as planned and to communicate clearly the expectation that the patient or client will follow through in meeting his or her responsibilities also.

In the final phase, the termination period, when separation becomes imminent, new issues may arise. If the therapeutic relationship has been important and helpful, the termination of the relationship may feel difficult to both the therapist and the patient/client. On the other hand, all of the focus of treatment in occupational therapy has been directed toward increasingly independent functioning and, thus, the termination of treatment may call for celebrative feelings.

The Activity

Activities are used as facilitators for transactions between people. The focus on doing, not merely talking, is useful in both one-to-one and group interactions. It allows for nonverbal communication, confrontations around interpersonal issues, and safe withdrawal when needed.

Activities within a behavioral modification milieu provide a natural and relatively easily controlled vehicle for reinforcement or extinction of behaviors.

The activities with which occupational therapy is primarily concerned are those which help to promote competence and achievement in the patient's or client's ability to function in his/her own world. The three categories of self-care, work, and play, and the maintenance of a healthy balance in the individual's activity life, are an important focus of occupational therapy. This emphasis requires consideration of the client's developmental levels of functioning and the demands of daily living, as these are expressed in their activity lives.

Activities used as treatment are limited only by constraints of the treatment context, which includes time, space, cost, the support of other team members, and the preferences and skills of the therapist.

Achieving a scientific understanding of the nature of activities and their ability to promote performance is a monumental task and continues to be a major challenge to occupational therapy. We have intuitive notions about activities and have experienced some degree of empirical success in their use through the years, but hard, scientific research data still are lacking. The importance of understanding the elements of activity cannot be overemphasized.

CHOICE OF ACTIVITIES. The art of occupational therapy with the disabled is in finding and using activities which are relevant to meeting the treatment objectives and which have meaning to the patient or client. It seems a simple, almost glib, statement to say that one matches the activity (which has been carefully analyzed) with the needs of the patient or client (who has been carefully evaluated). This process is far from simple. The choice of activity, within the scope and limitations of a program, remains crucial to the success of treatment in occupational therapy. Decisions need to be made centering around whether the activity should be done on a one-to-one basis or in a group. How important is the process and how important is an end product? How much of the activity should rely on verbal communication? How much physical or sensory involvement should be planned? What is the range within which time requirements may be graded? In what ways will the patient or client experience exploration, mastery, and achievement?

To use crafts or not to use crafts? The early occupational therapists used a wide range of activities of which crafts were an important part. In more recent times, except in some segments of the population, crafts became less well respected and less well used. The basket-weaver image of the occupational therapist was a ludicrous one which ignored the fine possibilities for learning and growth which were part of the potential in crafts and ignored very basic anthropological and physiological data relating hand use with cognitive functioning. From the perspective of modern mechanistic achievement and production-oriented society, simple handcrafts were viewed as quaint, childish, or primitive. This attitude is a pervasive one and affects how both therapist and patient or client may feel about a given craft activity. Crafts, however, offer a highly flexible, easily controlled modality, through which an individual may explore, practice, and develop a wide range of basic physical, perceptual, and cognitive skills. One may experience the tools and materials through the senses and one may experience the effects of one's actions on something that is visible and tangible. For the patient or client who is unable to cope with many social variables or verbal interactions, the craft still may be the modality of choice.

The Context or Setting

When we speak of the context for treatment, we mean much more than merely the setting in which treatment is to take place. Context here has a dimension of time, including today with an awareness of yesterday and a deliberate plan for tomorrow. In terms of place, it includes all those areas which a treatment plan includes, e.g., a shop, a ward, a home, a work setting, Main Street, and the baseball diamond. It also includes some sense of the overall treatment objectives and plan and the efforts and thinking of all of the other people, the professional team, and even the family and friends of the patient or client, engaged in the helping process. The context for treatment has parts which are controllable and parts which are not controllable. In proceeding with treatment, we may wish to move from a highly controlled context (e.g., in the hospital, with a professional team, planned treatment procedures, set schedules) to a gradually less controlled and more realistic context (e.g., in the community with semi-autonomy to in the home and autonomy). In modern occupational therapy, contexts for treatment have become highly varied and far more complex than they were when occupational therapy began.

Factors which are considered in identifying contexts for treatment include:

1. The client population—their issues, needs, and objectives.
2. The kind of setting and its means of support.
3. Frames of reference for treatment and the nature of the treatment team.
4. Kinds of evaluative procedures that are used.
5. Kinds of treatment objectives that are set.
6. Kinds of treatment plans that are developed.
7. Kinds of records and reports that are made—to whom the treatment team is accountable and how this is accomplished.

Developing Objectives

When initial evaluation has been concluded, the therapist should have a clear picture of the client, of his or her assets and limitations, and of realistic expectations for future performance. In the evaluation process, there should have been certain basic ingredients contributing to setting both long and short term goals for treatment.

1. *The patient's or client's needs and personal goals.* However obliquely they may have been communicated, the wishes and needs of the patient or client are there. Unless the goals of treatment are mutually understood by therapist and patient/client on some level, they probably cannot be achieved.

2. *The treatment goals, the treatment approach, and frame of reference for treatment of the total team.* Again, coherence between the patient/client's own goals and those of the team is important. The goals of occupational therapy must fit with both.

3. *Knowledge of the individual's disease process and the possible residual physical or psychological limitations.*

4. *Knowledge of the treatment methods and approaches being used.* What medications is the patient receiving?

5. *Knowledge about the world in which the patient/client may be expected to live.* The skills needed to cope with the demands of life at home, in the community, at work, at play, or in the institution.

6. *Knowledge about the patient/client's value system and what is important to him/her.*

The therapist takes the evaluation data and analyzes its many pieces in the light of the potential situation for treatment in occupational therapy. What does the therapist know about the prognosis for recovery or maintenance of function for people diagnosed as having a specific disease? Who are the other members of the treatment team and what is the potential for collaborative efforts among them? Can the therapist expect professional and/or community support for efforts made in occupational therapy? What are the realistic limits of the occupational therapy setting? To what extent will it be possible to manipulate objects and the environment to provide the best opportunities for the patient to grow and function to maximum capabilities? In what ways can we measure the success of the plan? These are hard, but vital, questions that must be faced in the process of setting objectives and planning treatment.

Long term objectives in occupational therapy usually represent a piece of the long term treatment objectives of the team. A long term objective may be stated, "the patient will be able to function well enough to go back to his job." A long term objective related to this in occupational therapy might be stated, "the patient will be able to organize his thoughts and actions to carry out a task from beginning to end." Short term objectives are designed to contribute to the achievement of long term objectives. A short term objective related to the above might be stated, "the patient will be able to maintain attention to a given task for fifteen minutes." Short term objectives then represent the steps of achievement which will facilitate the ultimate attainment of the long term objective (Fig. 6-2).

Depending upon the treatment situation and the pathology of the client, there may be either multiple or single sets of objectives for treatment. The results of the evaluation may also indicate that occupational therapy is not needed or relevant with a client at a given time. If viable treatment objectives for occupational therapy cannot be determined, it is probably not appropriate for the client to be referred to occupational therapy.

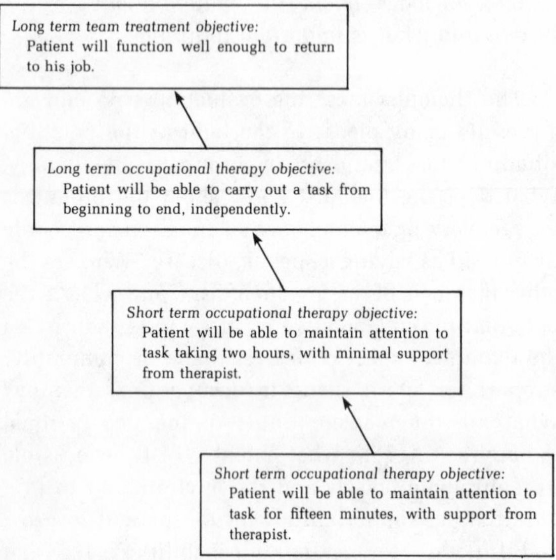

FIGURE 6-2. Simplified representation of treatment objectives.

The Treatment Plan

A description of the methods that are used to meet the treatment objectives constitutes the treatment plan. Just as the treatment objectives represent an action-oriented summary of the evaluation of the patient or client, the treatment plan represents a synthesis of the therapist's knowledge of the potential of activities and relationships as facilitators of growth and performance. It is a "nuts and bolts" statement of such things as the tools, materials, and equipment, the kinds of direction or guidance, the structure of the activity, the times and places in which the activity will take place, whether treatment will be accomplished individually or in a group, and the extent to which the family or the community are to be involved. A treatment plan is first stated in reference to each short term objective and needs to be flexible enough to permit changes if reevaluation suggests that the plan is not working.

It is probably in the development of a treatment plan that the therapist is most often faced with the responsibility for sound professional judgment. The plan needs to be reasonable and possible and show a clear relationship to the objectives of treatment.

Implementation of treatment consists of three distinct phases: (1) the orientation phase when the therapist and patient or client define the parameters and expectations of the activities which will be used and the therapist may describe or demonstrate the procedures which are involved; (2) the development phase during which the therapist guides the patient/client through exploration or practice in doing the activities; and (3) the termination phase when the patient or client has completed the plan, reevaluation takes place, and the need for further objective setting is considered.

During the development phase there should be a process of ongoing evaluation to check on the effectiveness of the plan and the relevance of the objectives. During this time it is very likely that new objectives and new treatment plans will evolve.

In reality, the termination phase is not always achieved for a variety of reasons. Patients or clients may be discharged before objectives are met. In some situations, particularly with chronically ill patients, the treatment goal is maintenance of function and, therefore, short term objectives are so numerous that the occupational therapy process may continue for a long period of time. In other situations the occupational therapy process is limited to evaluation only. The total occupational therapy process is outlined in Table 6-1.

As occupational therapists move increasingly in the direction of home and community treatment, it becomes increasingly important to conceptualize ways for treatment plans to be implemented in contexts other than the original setting where evaluation may have taken place.

Table 6-1. The occupational therapy process.

RECORDS		AND		REPORTS →	
Initial evaluation →	*Treatment objectives* →	*Treatment plan* →	*Treatment implementation* ⟷	*Periodic or ongoing evaluation* →	*Treatment termination*
Baseline of data —reflects scope of occupational therapy and knowledge base.	Synthesis of data obtained and therapist's professional knowledge and judgment.	Action plan for meeting objectives.	Carrying out the treatment plan with the patient.	Reassessment of patient's status and objectives.	Discharge of patient from occupational therapy.
DESCRIBES patient through objective data about patient: skills, history, developmental level, social and cultural world, value systems as well as pathology and its effect on the patient's life.	NAMES reasonable predicted outcomes of the occupational therapy process. STATES long and short term goals that can realistically be attained in occupational therapy and can be clearly measured and/or observed. ESTABLISHES contract or mutual understanding between patient and therapist.	DESCRIBES the way in which long and short term objectives may be accomplished, the activities to be used, therapeutic relationship, and context for treatment.	CONNECTS action and performance of activities with meeting the objectives of treatment. ACTS upon the implicit contract between therapist and patient.	ASSESSES the efficacy of the treatment plan and process. DETERMINES the need for changes of approach. DETERMINES when treatment may be terminated.	AFFIRMS the success (or failure) of the occupational therapy process in helping the patient meet objectives.

REFERENCES

1. Marshall, E.: A problem solving method of learning, measured against a rote memory method. Am. J. Occup. Ther. 19:60–64, 1965.
2. Parnes, S. J.: Creative Behavior Guidebook. New York: Charles Scribner's Sons, 1967.
3. Conte, J. R., and Conte, W. R.: The use of conceptual models in occupational therapy. Am. J. Occup. Ther. 31:262–265, 1977.
4. Essentials of an accredited educational program for the occupational therapist. Am. J. Occup. Ther. 29: 485–496, 1975.
5. Johnson, J. A.: Delegate assembly address—April 19, 1976. Am. J. Occup. Ther. 30:449, 1976.
6. Preliminary report: Mental health task force. Occup. Ther. Newspaper 30:4, 1976.
7. Selye, H.: The Stress of Life. New York: McGraw-Hill Book Co., 1956.
8. Toffler, A.: Future Shock. New York: Random House, 1970.
9. Coleman, J. C.: Life stress and maladaptive behavior. Am. J. Occup. Ther. 27:169–179, 1973.
10. Piaget, J.: The Origins of Intelligence in Children. New York: International University Press, 1952.
11. Cratty, B. J.: Movement Behavior and Motor Learning. Philadelphia: Lea and Febiger, 1967.
12. Piaget: Origins of Intelligence.
13. McClelland, D.: The Achieving Society. New York: Free Press, 1967.

14. Rotter, J. B.: Clinical Psychology. Englewood Cliffs NJ: Prentice-Hall, 1971.
15. Ibid.
16. Ducette, J., and Wolk, S.: Cognitive and motivational correlates of generalized expectancies for control. J. Personal. Soc. Psychol. 26:420–426, 1973.
17. Wolk, S., and Ducette, J.: The motivating effect of locus of control on achievement motivation. J. Personal. 41:59–70, 1973.
18. Piaget: Origins of Intelligence.
19. White, R. W.: The urge towards competence. Am. J. Occup. Ther. 25:271, 1971.
20. Hartmann, H.: Ego Psychology and the Problem of Adaptation. (tr. by David Rapaport). New York: International University Press. 1953.
21. Werner, H.: Comparative Psychology of Mental Development, ed. 2. NY: International U. Press, 1957.
22. Mahler, M. S.: Autism and symbiosis. Internat. J. Psychoanal. 39:77–83, 1958.
23. Searles, H.: The Nonhuman Environment. New York: International University Press, 1960, pp. 78–120.
24. Hall, E. T.: The Hidden Dimension. Garden City NY: Doubleday & Co., 1966, p. 188.
25. Frank, J.: The therapeutic use of self. Am. J. Occup. Ther. 12:215, 1958.
26. Mosey, A. C.: Three Frames of Reference for Mental Health. Thorofare NJ: Charles B. Slack, 1970, p. 23.
27. Rogers, C.: Client Centered Therapy. Boston: Houghton Mifflin Co., 1951.
28. Purtilo, R.: The Allied Health Professional and the Patient. Philadelphia: W. B. Saunders Co., 1973, p. 125.

7

Developmental Approaches

section 1 /The Developmental Treatment Approach: Cognitive, Social, and Emotional Aspects/Elizabeth G. Tiffany

The developmental approach to treatment in occupational therapy is one which is applied both generally and specifically. In the general sense it is important for anyone, whose professional commitment is to help people to function, to have the knowledge of the continuum of learning and maturation through which human beings develop and an understanding of the conditions which foster or impede that process.

The developmental approach is applied more specifically in a number of therapeutic situations: (1) with infants and children where there is evidence of a delay or interruption in the normal process of development; (2) with psychiatrically ill clients whose behaviors show regression to earlier stages of adaptation; (3) with the mentally retarded; and (4) with any clients who, because of the stress of physical pain, illness, loss of function, or some disabling condition, may be unable to think, feel, or act at a normal level.

Briefly described, the developmental approach is based on the following premises:

1. Human beings normally develop in a sequential way.
2. Each new gain in structure (physical or mental) enables the individual to gain in function.
3. Each new gain in functional ability makes further development possible.
4. Physical, sensory, perceptual, cognitive, social, and emotional aspects of the individual are intimately connected and affect the developmental state of the *whole* individual.
5. Conditions of stress cause the stressed individual to regress to earlier levels of adaptation.
6. Successful experiences foster a sense of wholeness. Human beings tend to be facilitated toward positive development or reintegration of their adaptive abilities when their experiences are successful ones.

In 1968 Mosey described seven adaptive skills in the developmental approach.[1] Adaptive skills, as Mosey defined them, are learned abilities which enable human beings to satisfy their needs and meet environmental demands.[2] A chart based on her descriptions accompanies this section. The subskill components which make up each of the adaptive skills are listed hierarchically. Mosey postulated that each subskill must be learned in proper

SEVEN ADAPTIVE SKILLS

1. Perceptual-Motor Skill: The ability to receive, integrate, and organize sensory stimuli in a manner which allows for the planning of purposeful movement.

   The subskills required are the abilities
   a. to integrate primitive postural reflexes, to react appropriately to vestibular stimuli, to maintain a balance between the tactile subsystems, to perceive form, and to be aware of auditory stimuli.
   b. to control extraocular musculature, to integrate the two sides of the body, and to focus on auditory stimuli.
   c. to perceive visual and auditory figure-ground, to be aware of body parts and their relationships, and to plan gross motor movements.
   d. to perceive space, to plan fine motor movements, and to discriminate auditory stimuli.
   e. to discriminate between right and left and to remember auditory stimuli.
   f. to use abstract concepts, to scan, integrate, and synthesize auditory stimuli, and to give auditory feedback.

2. Cognitive Skill: The ability to perceive, represent, and organize objects, events, and their relationships in a manner that is considered appropriate by one's cultural group.

   The subskills required are the abilities
   a. to use inherent behavioral patterns for environmental interaction.
   b. to interrelate visual, manual, auditory, and oral responses.
   c. to attend to the environmental consequence of actions with interest, to represent objects in an exoceptual manner, to experience objects, to act on the bases of egocentric causality, and to seriate events in which the self is involved.
   d. to establish a goal and intentionally carry out means, to recognize the independent existence of objects, to interpret signs, to imitate new behavior, to apprehend the influence of space, and to perceive other objects as partially causal.
   e. to use trial-and-error problem solving, to use tools, to perceive variability in spatial positions, to seriate events in which the self is not involved, and to perceive the causality of other objects.
   f. to represent objects in an image manner, to make believe, to infer a cause given its effect, to act on the bases of combined spatial relations, to attribute omnipotence to others, and to perceive objects as permanent in time and space.
   g. to represent objects in an endoceptual manner, to differentiate between thought and action, and to recognize the need for causal sources.
   h. to represent objects in a denotative manner, to perceive the viewpoint of others, and to decenter.
   i. to represent objects in a connotative manner, to use formal logic, and to work in the realm of the hypothetical.

3. Drive-Object Skill: The ability to control drives and select objects in such a manner as to ensure adequate need satisfaction.

   The subskills required are the abilities
   a. to form a discontinuous, libidinal object relationship.
   b. to form a continuous, part, libidinal object relationship.
   c. to invest aggressive drive in an external object.
   d. to transfer libidinal drive to objects other than the primary object.
   e. to invest libidinal energy in appropriate abstract objects and to control aggressive drive.
   f. to engage in total and diffuse libidinal object relationships.

4. Dyadic Interaction Skill: The ability to participate in a variety of dyadic relationships.

   The subskills required are the abilities
   a. to enter into association relationships.
   b. to interact in an authority relationship.
   c. to interact in a chum relationship.
   d. to enter into a peer, authority relationship.
   e. to enter into an intimate relationship.
   f. to engage in a nurturing relationship.

5. Group Interaction Skill: The ability to be a productive member of a variety of primary groups.

   The subskills required are the abilities
   a. to participate in a parallel group.
   b. to participate in a project group.
   c. to participate in an egocentric-cooperative group.
   d. to participate in a cooperative group.
   e. to participate in a mature group.

6. Self-Identity Skill: The ability to perceive the self as an autonomous, whole, and acceptable person with permanence and continuity.

   The subskills required are the abilities
   a. to perceive the self as a worthy object.
   b. to perceive the assets and limitations of the self.
   c. to perceive the self as self-directed.
   d. to perceive the self as a productive, contributing member of a social system.
   e. to perceive the self.
   f. to perceive the aging process of the self in a rational manner.

7. Sexual Identity Skill: The ability to perceive one's sexual nature as good and to participate in a sexual relationship that is oriented to the mutual satisfaction of sexual needs.

   The subskills required are the abilities
   a. to accept and act upon the bases of one's pregenital sexual nature.
   b. to accept sexual maturation as a positive growth experience.
   c. to give and receive sexual gratification.
   d. to enter into a sustained sexual relationship.
   e. to accept physiological and psychological changes that occur at the time of the climacteric.

Adapted from Mosey: *Three Frames of Reference.*[2]

sequence before mastery of the next subskill may be achieved. Learning of several subskills within one adaptive skill may, however, occur simultaneously. An individual may also be working on the achievement of mastery in more than one adaptive skill at any given time. Failure to master any part of an adaptive skill results in difficulty when the individual attempts to undertake a task at a higher level. Treatment then is aimed at helping the individual to experience personal, social, and task demands which will facilitate mastery of each subskill.

The developmental approach to treatment requires that the therapist assess and understand the levels of adaptation on which his or her client is functioning, and, as much as possible, the conditions which tend to make the client function at the highest and at the lowest levels. The therapist then needs to think in terms of providing opportunities for the client to have experiences that (1) provide success experiences by meeting his/her levels of adaptation; (2) encourage "safe" exploration and practice as he or she becomes enabled to move to more mature levels of adaptation; and (3) provide opportunities for challenge, surprise, and novelty when the client is ready.

Chapter 3 on human development provides important background and resource suggestions for understanding developmental levels of function. For in-depth knowledge, the reader is referred especially to the writings of Jean Piaget, Erik Erikson, Sylvano Arieti, and Harold Searles. Chapter 12, Psychiatry and Mental Health, provides background on the developmental levels of activities and their application as treatment.

REFERENCES

1. Mosey, A. C.: Recapitulation of ontogenesis. Am J. Occup. Ther. 22:426–438, 1968.
2. Mosey, A. C.: Three Frames of Reference for Mental Health. Thorofare NJ: Charles B. Slack, 1970.

BIBLIOGRAPHY

Arieti, S.: The Intrapsychic Self. New York: Basic Books, 1967.

Bearison, D. J.: The construct of regression: A Piagetian approach. Merrill-Palmer Quart. 20:21–30, 1974.

Erikson, E.: Childhood and Society. New York: W. W. Norton & Co., 1950.

Gillette, N.: Occupational therapy and mental health. In Willard, H., and Spackman, C. (eds.): Occupational Therapy, ed. 4. Philadelphia: J. B. Lippincott Co., 1971.

Llorens, L.: Facilitating growth and development: The promise of occupational therapy. Am. J. Occup. Ther. 24:93–101, 1970.

Mosey, A. C.: Activities Therapy. New York: Raven Press, 1973.

Piaget, J.: The Origins of Intelligence in Children. New York: International Universities Press, 1952.

Reilly, M.: Play as Exploratory Learning. Beverly Hills: Sage Publications, 1974.

White, R. W. Motivation reconsidered: The concept of competence. Psychol. Rev. 66:297–333, 1959.

section 2/Sensorimotor Approaches/A. Joy Huss

This section provides an historical overview of the various sensorimotor approaches, their current status, a statement regarding the application of these principles to occupational therapy, and a bibliography of greater depth for those interested. It is not an exposition in depth but rather an additional tool for the beginner or the uninitiated.

OVERVIEW

Fay-Doman-Delacato: Neuromuscular Reflex Therapy

Temple Fay, neurosurgeon, was the forerunner of sensorimotor approaches, beginning in the early 1940s. For nearly two decades he observed, discussed, demonstrated, and wrote about neuromuscular reflex therapy, which he defined as the "utilization of reflex levels of response to the highest level possible."[1] Much of his work was done prior to the present knowledge and understanding regarding the central nervous system and was based on the work of Sherrington. His basic premise was that ontogeny recapitulates phylogeny. Therefore an individual's neurological development parallels the evolution from fish to amphibian, to reptile, to anthropoid. Since human movement is based on patterns of muscle activity, not on individual muscle response, he believed that if reflex patterns were elicited and utilized properly, functional movement could be established. As a result his treatment program involved the following six concepts[2]:

1. After careful observation of the patient's level of functioning, including existing reflexes and automatic responses, treatment began with simple patterns of movement utilizing these reflexes.

2. Since in normal development each stage lays the foundation for the next stage, so in treatment it is essential that lower levels of mobility be developed before expecting higher levels.

3. Reflexes in and of themselves are not abnormal, but may indicate pathology if they interfere with refined coordinated movement. Therefore reflexes can be utilized to develop muscle tone, inhibit antagonists, and lead to higher levels of coordinated movement.

4. Passive exercise patterns which involve the total extremity, not isolated joints, can enhance the sensory feedback mechanisms important for movement.

5. Active or passive patterns done repeatedly will in time lead to the spontaneous development of higher level patterns.

6. The patterns utilized are prone patterns of forward propulsion that can be observed in normal human infants as well as in amphibian and reptilian life forms.

The three basic patterns used are homologous (bunny hop), homolateral (camel walk), and crossed-diagonal (reciprocal).

Homologous is a bilateral-symmetrical pattern. With the head in midline with extension of the neck, the upper extremities are flexed at the shoulder while the lower extremities are extended at the hip. The extremities are then reversed rhythmically with neck flexion. In prone this is not too effective for propulsion but in the all-fours position it is commonly called the bunny hop.

Homolateral is an ipsilateral pattern with the head, thorax, and pelvis turned toward the flexing upper and lower extremities with extension of the contralateral extremities. The pattern is then reversed leading with the head. In the all-fours this provides a gait similar to that of a camel.

Crossed-diagonal is a more highly integrated pattern with flexion of the upper extremity and extension of the lower extremity on the face side with extension of the upper limb with flexion of the lower limb on the opposite side. In the all-fours this provides the typical reciprocal gait pattern seen in higher mammals and human infants.

Following the prone position are the all-fours (hands and knees), plantigrade (hands and feet), and erect postures. All three patterns are utilized in the first three positions. Homolateral and crossed-diagonal are utilized in the erect position. Depending on the level of development, patterns are done passively, active-assistively, or actively. The key elements in determining the program planned for a patient are intellectual and functional motor development levels. Chronological age is less important.

Fay's work has provided the basic foundation for the approach now advocated by Carl Delacato, Ed.D., Robert Doman, M.D., and Glenn Doman, physical therapist. The same patterns of movement are utilized. In addition the program includes selective use of sensory stimulation procedures such as heat, cold, brushing, and pinching to establish hand dominance and a breathing exercise routine to increase the vital capacity.

The program for any given patient is administered at least four times per day for five minutes, seven days a week. Each treatment requires at least three adults because each extremity must be manipulated smoothly and rhythmically in the proper pattern.

Bobath: Neurodevelopmental Treatment Approach

The neurodevelopmental treatment approach has been developed in England by Berta Bobath, physical therapist, and Karel Bobath, neuropsychiatrist. Their work was begun in the 1940s with the cerebral palsied and adult-acquired hemiplegics. The treatment, however, is appropriate to a wide variety of other dysfunctions of the central nervous system. Treatment foundations are based on the experimental works of Magnus, Sherrington, deKleijn, Rademaker, Schaltenbrand, Walshe, and Weisz.

The concept of neurodevelopment treatment is based on two fundamental principles about the nature of the central nervous system dysfunction:

(1) the arrest, or retardation, of normal movement is caused by the interference with normal brain maturation resulting from brain lesion, and (2) the resultant release of abnormal, or immature, postural reflex activity causes the observed abnormal patterns of posture and movement. On the basis of these concepts, treatment techniques have been developed by the Bobaths and others and are continually being added to and refined. Kong, Quilan, Finnie, Mueller, Reye, and Morris are names often associated with neurodevelopmental treatment.

The primary aim of treatment handling is the inhibition of abnormal movement patterns with the simultaneous facilitation of normal righting and equilibrium reactions and other appropriate normal movement patterns. The patient is so handled that the abnormal patterns are blocked and higher level reactions are elicited to give the patient more normal sensory experience. The therapist takes the patient through a series of graded sensory and motor experiences which set the stage for learning new, less stereotyped movement patterns. Through "preparation" activities the therapist normalizes the muscle tone (increasing it in the individuals or body parts where tone is too low and decreasing it in the individuals or body parts where it is too high), moves the patient passively to provide sensory experience to unfamiliar movement patterns, encourages active movement from the patient while still providing guidance control and, eventually, encourages the patient to move actively without control. This sequence may all take place in one treatment session or may involve weeks or months of therapy.

Movement is a physiological necessity. It allows us to maintain normal muscle tone and yet to be prepared to instantaneously change that tone in response to environmental demand. Movement is the primary modality of treatment in neurodevelopmental treatment. Normal movement inhibits abnormal movement, thus normal movement becomes both the process and the goal of therapy. Key points of control are used to influence the movement and balance of tone in the rest of the body. Key points of control are body parts, usually proximal; for example, the trunk and shoulders may be used to prepare the arms for weight bearing and the rest of the body for side-sitting. In addition to facilitation of movement, techniques of tapping, placing, and holding, and compression may be used to change the muscle tone when appropriate.[3]

The primary success of neurodevelopmental treatment is contingent on the therapist's ability to make changes in the muscle tone. Prolonged bracing, extensive surgery, and static positioning are usually incompatible with this treatment because they do not allow for changes in muscle tone.

As in all good systems of therapy, a thorough initial assessment and frequent reassessment are necessary. The evaluation includes the following: type, strength, and distribution of muscle tone in all positions; abnormal patterns of posture and movement; basic automatic (normal) reactions; general stage of development with awareness of important gaps; contractures and deformities; and other associated handicaps. Readers not familiar with the basic reflex and developmental information are referred to Bobath, Fiorentino, Gesell, and Peiper. On the basis of the initial assessment, a plan of therapy is individualized appropriate to the present level of development and needs of the patient.

Teamwork among occupational therapist, physical therapist, speech therapist, physicians, classroom teacher, and parents is considered an essential aspect of treatment. Therapy is a twenty-four hour a day process when the whole patient and his/her perceptual systems, learning capabilities, personality, and motor system are influenced by the damage to the central nervous system. Close communication and cooperation in the whole treatment plan are essential to prevent disagreement in approach and confusion for the patient and his/her family.

Rood: Neurophysiological Approach

Margaret S. Rood, occupational therapist and physical therapist, frustrated by the slow improvement of patients with cerebral palsy, began to study the neurophysiological and developmental literature in the late 1930s. Based on the works of Sherrington, Gesell, Denny-Brown, Eldred, Hooker, Magoun, Cooper, Boyd, and others a method of treatment has evolved since the 1940s. The basic principles utilized are as follows[4]:

1. Motor output is dependent upon sensory input. Thus sensory stimuli are utilized to activate and/or inhibit motor responses.

2. Activation of motor responses follows a normal developmental sequence. All muscles progress through the following stages of development:

a. Full range of shortening and lengthening with the antagonist. Phasic movement—reciprocal innervation.
b. A pattern of co-contraction in which antagonistic muscles of one or more joints work together for a holding action. Stability-tonic postural set.
c. A pattern of heavy work movement superimposed on the co-contraction. Movement in weight-bearing position.
d. Skill or coordinate movement. Movement in nonweight-bearing position with stabilization at the proximal joints.

3. Since there is interaction within the nervous system between somatic, psychic, and autonomic functions, stimuli can be used to influence one or more directly or indirectly.

This treatment approach can thus be defined as "the activation, facilitation, and inhibition of muscle action, voluntary and involuntary, through the reflex arc."[5]

This treatment approach assumes that an exercise per se is not treatment unless the pattern of response is correct and results in feedback which enhances learning of that response. Treatment or therapy is not in the form of a motor act alone, but rather is the application of stimuli to activate a response, followed by sensory input from a correct response with additional stimuli given to facilitate or inhibit elements in the pattern. The use of stimuli is an integral part of treatment, since sensory factors are essential for the achievement and maintenance of normal motor functions.[6]

Developmental sequences are outlined in Tables 7-1 and 7-2. These patterns are used to evaluate the patient's level of development which determines the level of treatment.

Sensory stimulation is provided first for the proprioceptors, utilizing vibration, rubbing pressure into the muscle bellies, joint compression, quick stretch of the muscle to be facilitated, and appropriate vestibular input. If necessary this is followed by exteroceptive input of light touch and/or rapid brushing. Ice, if used at all, is applied with great caution and only to the extremities. If exteroceptive input is used there should be a careful follow-up of the patient by the therapist for several hours. Since cutaneous stimuli have a profound effect on the reticular system there may be adverse rebound effects if exteroceptive stimulation is not used appropriately.

Inhibitory procedures used by Rood include slow stroking, neutral warmth, and slow rolling for over-

Table 7-1. Skeletal developmental sequences.

Reciprocal innervation	*Stability or co-innervation*	*Movement superimposed on stability*	*Skill*
1. Withdrawal: total flexion in supine	4. Co-contraction of neck with vertebral extension		
2. Roll over: flexion top side, extension bottom side	5. Prone on elbows static holding with co-contraction neck and shoulder	6. Push back	
		7. Pull forward	8. Belly crawling
3. Pivot prone: total extension in prone except for elbows, which are flexed with arms adducted	9. All-fours: static holding	10. Shifting weight backward-forward, side-to-side, alternate arm-leg	11. Creeping: homologous, homolateral, reciprocal
	12. Standing: static	13. Shifting weight backward-forward, side-to-side	14. Walking: must analyze stance, push off, pick up, and heel strike

Table 7-2. Vital function developmental sequences.

Reciprocal innervation	*Stability or co-innervation*	*Movement superimposed on stability*	*Skill*
1. Inspiration			
2. Expiration	3. Sucking	4. Swallowing fluids	5. Phonation
		6. Chewing	
		7. Swallowing solids	8. Speech

all relaxation and pressure to the muscle insertion for specific relaxation. Slow stroking is an alternate stroking of the posterior primary rami with a firm but light pressure. One hand starts at the cervical area and progresses to the lower lumbar region. As the first hand finishes, the second hand starts. Thus there is always contact with the patient. This is done for no more than three minutes. If the hair growth pattern is irregular this may be irritating to the patient. Neutral warmth is the wrapping of part or all of the patient in a cotton towel or blanket until the appropriate amount of relaxation is observed. Slow rolling from supine to side and return is also generally inhibitory. The rolling continues until relaxation is seen.

Depending on the type of muscle tone and developmental level of the patient, a treatment program may be all-inhibitory, inhibitory and facilitory, or all-facilitory.

Cortical demand for voluntary effort on the part of the patient is directed through activities that utilize the patterns that have been stimulated. The patient's attention is thus directed to the activity and not to specific movement or stabilizing patterns.

Kabat-Knott-Voss: Proprioceptive Neuromuscular Facilitation

Around 1946, Herman Kabat, physiatrist and neurophysiologist, began the development of a therapy system based on neurophysiological principles outlined by Sherrington, Coghill, McGraw, Gesell, Hellebrandt, and Pavlov. The major emphasis is stimulation of the proprioceptors with active participation by the patient. These principles were expanded and utilized in treatment by Margaret Knott and Dorothy Voss, both physical therapists. "Proprioceptive neuromuscular facilitation enlists the less involved parts, to promote a balanced antagonism of reflex activity, of muscle groups and of components of motion."[7]

As stated by Knott and Voss in the second edition of *Proprioceptive Neuromuscular Facilitation,* the philosophy of treatment is

> . . . based upon the ideas that all human beings respond in accordance with demand; that existing potentials may be developed more fully; that movements must be specific and directed toward a goal; that activity is necessary to the best development of coordination, strength, and endurance; and that the stronger body parts strengthening weaker parts through cooperation lead toward a goal of optimum function.[8]

The technique is therefore defined as "methods of promoting or hastening the response of the neuromuscular mechanism through stimulation of the proprioceptors."[9]

There has been a gradual evolution of the technique since the 1940s. Initially greatest emphasis was placed on the use of maximal resistance throughout the range of motion. Patterns of movement were utilized which allowed action at two or more joints and required two component actions of a given muscle. Other factors considered important were stretch for proprioceptive stimulation, positioning to enhance contraction, motion beginning in the strongest part of the range progressing to the weaker part, incorporation of reflexes, and reinforcement through resistance.

In 1949, based on Sherrington's law of successive induction, rhythmic stabilization and slow reversal procedures were added to enhance facilitation of the weaker muscles. In 1951 the patterns of movement were analyzed more thoroughly. In order to apply stretch to maximally elongated muscles it was found that patterns that were spiral and diagonal were most effective and that they also corresponded more nearly to normal functional patterns of movement.

Since that time the above principles have been incorporated into mat, gait, and self-care activities to assist in motor learning and the development of strength and balance.

Current techniques being used are maximal, but not overpowering resistance; quick stretch; postural and righting reflexes; mass movement patterns with spiral and diagonal components; reversal of antagonists (rhythmic stabilization and slow reversal); and ice (generally used for inhibition and occasionally for facilitation).

The patient is evaluated developmentally and treatment begun appropriately. In all cases, beginning treatment utilizes the strongest groups of muscles and the most coordinated movements the patient has for reciprocal innervation, irradiation, and summation. Movement patterns are reinforced through simple verbal commands which utilize the patient's voluntary control.

Brunnstrom

Around 1951, Signe Brunnstrom, physical therapist, became concerned with the lack of rehabilitation of the upper extremity in acquired hemiplegia. She studied the research on reflex responses in decerebrate cats and hemiplegia in man. From the research efforts of Riddoch and Buzzard, Magnus and deKleijn, and Simons, Brunnstrom selected the effects of associated reactions initiated either by voluntary effort on the noninvolved side or by reflex stimulation, postural reactions resulting from tonic neck and tonic labyrinthine reflexes, and the flexion and extension synergies. After careful observation of over 100 hemiplegic patients she delineated the stages of recovery and techniques to facilitate the patient's progression from one stage to the next. Thus treatment consists of developing the potential for "coordinate movement with reflexlike mechanisms, sensory cues, volitional effort and gradation of demand through the stages of recovery."[10]

The stages of recovery follow a definite sequence and the patient never skips a stage. However, he or she may plateau at any one of the following six stages:

1. Immediately following the vascular insult there appears to be flaccidity with no voluntary movement in the affected extremities.
2. Spasticity begins to develop. The flexion and extension synergies can be stimulated reflexively. They first appear with co-contraction but gradually become more distinct with the flexion synergy dominating the upper extremity and the extension synergy dominating the lower extremity.
3. Spasticity becomes quite severe. However, the synergies can now be voluntarily initiated with some range of motion. Any attempt to use the extremity voluntarily results in a synergy pattern.
4. Spasticity begins to decrease. Simple uncoordinated movements which differ from the basic synergies can be performed slowly and deliberately. Also reciprocal movements within the synergies are beginning to develop.
5. Spasticity continues to decrease to the point that the patient can perform some functional activities although still slowly and deliberately without eliciting synergies. Some independence of the synergy patterns is achieved, and isolated individual joint movement is possible.
6. Spasticity has almost disappeared. Individual joint motion is freer and has controlled speed and direction. With rapid, reciprocal movement some incoordination may still be present.

Because of the degree of cortical control necessary for hand control, recovery of function in the hand is more difficult and less predictable. Mass grasp does precede mass extension and thumb motion precedes finger motion.

After evaluation of the patient's stage of recovery and sensory status, treatment aimed at reflex training follows. The steps of treatment are:

1. Motion synergies are elicited on a reflex level. Reflexes used include
   a. tonic neck reflex
   b. tonic labyrinthine reflex
   c. tonic lumbar reflex
   d. resistance to voluntary contraction of noninvolved limb*
   e. Sensory stimulation includes quick stretch, passive movement, tapping over a muscle

* It is important to note that in the upper extremities resistance to flexion of the noninvolved extremity facilitates flexion in the involved extremity and vice versa. In the lower extremities resistance to flexion in the noninvolved extremity facilitates extension of the involved extremity and vice versa.

belly, surface stroking, positioning, and pressure on muscle belly or tendon.

2. Motion synergies are captured, i.e., an effort is made to establish voluntary control of the synergies. This is accomplished by utilization of the following stages:

a. repetition using facilitation
b. repetition without using facilitation
c. working from proximal to distal, concentrating on various components of the synergy with and without the use of facilitation. Reciprocal motion between the two synergies is started with a goal of diminishing the time lag between contraction and relaxation of antagonistic muscles.

3. Motion synergies are conditioned by combining elements of antagonistic synergies starting with the stronger components. At this point, time is also spent on muscles which do not participate in the synergies, such as the serratus anterior and the peroneal muscles. As progress occurs, more complex motions with rapid reciprocation are initiated.

4. The most difficult step is the elicitation of voluntary hand and finger function. Maneuvers such as Souque's phenomenon and imitation synkinesis are helpful.[11]

Postures and positions used during treatment include supine, sitting, and standing. Visual and verbal cues are used throughout. Volitional effort and functional activities are initiated early and are considered necessary if there is to be carry-over by the patient.

Ayres: Sensory Integration Approach to Learning Disorders

A. Jean Ayres, Ph.D., O.T.R., began her studies of children with learning disabilities in the 1950s. She and others observed that the cognitive approach to treatment of such children had led to dissatisfaction of skill training as an end in and of itself because too many children were still unable to generalize and respond adaptively to their environment. Study of the approaches of Knott, Bobath, Fay, and especially Rood for the physically handicapped, which placed an emphasis on integration of the nervous system at subcortical levels, seemed to have some application to those with learning problems.

Ayres' intensive and extensive research studies of these latter problems along with intense study of the integrative functions of the nervous system led to her present and still evolving theoretical framework from which treatment procedures are devised. This is discussed further in the next section of this chapter.

Fuchs: Orthokinetics

Julius Fuchs, orthopedic surgeon, dissatisfied with the static approach of braces, casts, and splints, created devices that provided immediate mobilization as well as support. His work was done in the 1920s and was published in German in 1927; however, a description in English was not published until 1951. The principles originally were applied to fractures, scoliosis, and other orthopedic problems. The application to neurological and arthritic dyskinesias was made in the 1950s by Manfred Blashy, physiatrist, and Elsbeth Harrison and Ernest Fuchs, both occupational therapists.

The basic idea in orthokinetics is the use of a segment or cuff composed of elastic and inelastic parts. Several of these put together form the orthokinetic tube. The inelastic or inactive fields cover those parts where support and muscle inactivity are desired. The elastic or active fields cover those parts where muscle activity is desired. The inactive field, thus, becomes the inhibitory field and the active field the facilitory field.

Originally these cuffs were made of leather and molded directly to the patient. Currently they are made of Ace bandages or sewing elastic 1 to 6 in. wide, depending on the size of the area of application. The device is usually two or three layers thick for the active field and three to four layers thick in the inactive field. The layers are stitched firmly together to provide the inactive field and left free for the active field. The cuff can be fastened with Velcro.

Among the results claimed by Fuchs and others are (1) rapid relief of pain, (2) increase of muscle strength, (3) increase of range of motion, (4) muscle re-education, and (5) improvement of coordination. I have also noted an increase in girth as muscle bulk fills in.

The cuffs are worn repeatedly to increase the effects. They can be worn all day while the individual is active. This provides continuous sensory input. The greater the imbalance initially between agonist and antagonist muscle groups the quicker the effects will be noticed.

This is an effective, inexpensive procedure which supplies continuous input when the patient is not "in therapy." It should be further investigated by occupational and physical therapists as to its value as an adjunct to treatment.

SUMMARY

In looking at the various sensorimotor treatment approaches it is helpful to place them in a continuum of control needed by the patient.

The Fay-Doman-Delacato approach is initially one of passive movement superimposed upon the patient; only later does this call for active participation on the part of the patient.

Rood uses a strong mixture of exteroceptive and proprioceptive input in developmental patterns followed by activity utilizing the stability and mobility of the patterns. The individual's attention is directed to the activity and not to the patterns per se.

Orthokinetics provides a continuous exteroceptive input followed by proprioceptive feedback as muscles are facilitated and inhibited. The individual is able to use the resultant muscle function in activities of daily living.

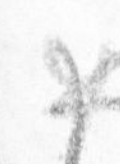

Bobath inhibits primitive patterns and then facilitates righting and equilibrium reactions, controlling at key points, so that the nervous system receives feedback only from more normal movement. Whenever possible, cortical control of movement is demanded.

Brunnstrom uses the initial synergy patterns seen in recovery from cerebral vascular insult on both a reflexive level and with conscious control by the patient. Using exteroceptive and proprioceptive input as well as cortical control these patterns are then broken up and lead to functional movement.

Kabat-Knott-Voss place primary emphasis on proprioceptive input reinforced by visual and verbal cues, which demand cortical control by the patient. Exteroceptive stimulation is considered primarily in the placement of the therapist's hands.

Thus when the patient is at a level in which cortical control hinders movement, approaches such as Rood, Fuchs, Bobath, and Fay can be utilized. Once cortical control begins to develop and strengthening is needed, Brunnstrom and Kabat-Knott-Voss approaches become appropriate.

Many of the techniques of the various approaches are quite similar. Often it is feasible to employ techniques from various approaches at any given time with any individual. The therapist must know and understand normal human development, neurophysiology, and techniques of evaluation in order to use effectively these treatment approaches.

REFERENCES

1. A. J. Phys. Med. NUSTEP, p. 816, 1967.
2. Ibid., p. 817.
3. Manning, J.: Facilitation of movement—the Bobath approach. Physiotherapy (Eng.) 58:403–408, 1972.
4. NUSTEP, p. 900–954.
5. Rood, M. S.: Unpublished class notes, 1958, 1959, 1970, and 1975.
6. NUSTEP, p. 903.
7. Knott, M., and Voss, D. E.: Proprioceptive Neuromuscular Facilitation: Patterns and Techniques, ed. 2. New York: Harper & Row Publishers, 1968, p. 14.
8. Ibid., p. 3.
9. Ibid., p. 4.
10. NUSTEP, p. 794.
11. Ibid.

BIBLIOGRAPHY

Ayres, A. J.: Occupational therapy for motor disorders resulting from impairment of the central nervous system. Rehab. Lit. 21:10, 1960.

Ayres, A. J.: Perceptual-Motor Dysfunction in Children. Monograph from Greater Cincinnati District, Ohio Occupational Therapy Association Conference, 1964.

Ayres, A. J.: Sensory Integration and Learning Disorders. Los Angeles: Western Psychological Services, 1972.

Banus, B. S.: The Developmental Therapist. Thorofare NJ: Charles B. Slack, 1971.

Bishop, B.: Vibratory stimulation. Part I—Neurophysiology of motor responses. J.A.P.T.A. 54:1273–1281, 1974.

Bishop, B.: Vibratory stimulation. Part II—Vibratory stimulation as an evaluation tool. J.A.P.T.A. 55:28–34, 1975.

Bishop, B.: Vibratory stimulation. Part III—Possible applications of vibration in treatment of motor dysfunction. J.A.P.T.A. 55:139–143, 1975.

Blashy, M.: Manipulation of the neuromuscular unit in the periphery of the central nervous system. J. So. Med. Assoc. 54:873–879, 1961.

Blashy, M., and Fuchs, R.: Orthokinetics: A new receptor facilitation method. Am. J. Occup. Ther. 13:226–234, 1959.

Blashy, M., Harrison, H. E., and Fuchs, E. M.: Orthokinetics—a preliminary report on recent experiences with a little known rehabilitation therapy. V. A. Bull., 1955.

Bobath, B.: Abnormal Postural Reflex Activity Caused by

Brain Lesions. London: Wm. Heinemann Medical Books, 1965.
Bobath, B.: Adult Hemiplegia: Evaluation and Treatment. London: Wm. Heinemann Medical Books, 1974.
Bobath, B.: Motor development, its effect on general development, and application to the treatment of cerebral palsy. Physiotherapy (Eng.) 57:526–32, 1971.
Bobath, K.: The motor deficit in patients with cerebral palsy. Clin. Develop. Med. 23:1966.
Bobath, K., and Bobath, B.: The facilitation of normal postural reactions and movements in the treatment of cerebral palsy. Physiotherapy (Eng.) 50:246–262, 1964.
Bobath, K., and Bobath, B.: The importance of memory traces of motor efferent discharges for learning skilled movements. Dev. Med. Child. Neurol. 16:837–838, 1974.
Brunnstrom, S.: Movement Therapy in Hemiplegia: A Neurophysiological Approach. New York: Harper & Row Publishers, 1970.
Child With Central Nervous System Deficit—Report of Two Symposiums. Washington DC: U.S. Dept. of Health, Educ. & Welfare, 1965.
Dayhoff, N.: Rethinking stroke: soft or hard devices to position hands. Am. J. Nurs. 7:1142–1144, 1975.
Doman, G., and Delacato, C.: Children with severe brain injuries. J.A.M.A. 174:257–267, 1960.
Eviatar, L., Eviatar, A., and Naray, I.: Maturation of neurovestibular responses in infants. Dev. Med. Child. Neurol. 16:435–446, 1974.
Fay, T.: Basic considerations regarding neuromuscular and reflex therapy. Spastics Quart. 3, 1954.
Fay, T.: Neuromuscular reflex therapy for spastic disorders. J. Florida Med. Assoc. 44, 1958.
Finnie, N.: Handling the Young Cerebral Palsied Child at Home. London: Wm. Heinemann Medical Books, 1968.
Fiorentino, M.: Reflex Testing Methods For Evaluating C.N.S. Development, ed. 2. Springfield IL: Charles C Thomas Publishers, 1976.
Fox, J.V.D.: Improving tactile discrimination of the blind: A neurophysiological approach. Am. J. Occup. Ther. 19:5–7, 1965.
Fox, J. V. D.: The olfactory system: Implications for the occupational therapist. Am. J. Occup. Ther. 20:173–177, 1966.
Friedlander, B. Z., Sterritt, G. M., Kirk, G. E. (eds): Exceptional Infant: Assessment and Intervention, Vol 3. New York: Brunner/Mazel, 1975.
Gesell, A.: The First Five Years of Life. New York: Harper & Row Publishers, 1940.
Goff, B.: The application of recent advances in neurophysiology to Miss M. Rood's concept of neuromuscular facilitation. Physiotherapy (Eng) 58:409–415, 1972.
Griffin, J. W.: Use of proprioceptive stimuli in therapeutic exercise. J.A.P.T.A. 54:1072–1079, 1974.
Harris, F. A.: In defense of facilitation techniques. Arch. Phys. Med. Rehab. 51:438–441, 1970.
Harris, F. A.: Multiple-loop modulation of motor outflow: A physiological basis for facilitation techniques. J.A.P.T.A. 51:391–396, 1971.
Hellmuth, J. (ed.): Exceptional Infant, 1, The Normal Infant, New York: Brunner/Mazel, 1967.
Huss, A. J.: Application of Rood technique to treatment of the physical handicapped child. In West, W. (ed.): Occupational Therapy for the Multiply Handicapped Child. Chicago: University of Chicago, 1965.
Huss, A. J.: Clinical Application of Sensorimotor Treatment Techniques in Physical Dysfunction, Controvery and Confusion in Physical Dysfunction Treatment Techniques—Clinical Aspects, Expanding Dimensions in Rehabilitation. Springfield IL: Charles C Thomas Publishers, 1969.
Johnston, R. M., Bishop, B., and Coffey, G. H.: Mechanical vibration of skeletal muscles. J.A.P.T.A. 50:499–505, 1970.
Kabat, H.: Central facilitation; the basis of treatment for paralysis. Permanente Fnd. Med. Bull. 10, August 1962.
Knott, M.: Bulbar involvement with good recovery. J.A. P.T.A. 42:38–39, 1962.
Knott, M.: Neuromuscular facilitation in the child with central nervous system deficit. J.A.P.T.A. 46:721–724, 1966.
Knott, M.: Neuromuscular facilitation in the treatment of rheumatoid arthritis. J.A.P.T.A. 44:737–739, 1964.
Knott, M., and Voss, D. E.: Proprioceptive Neuromuscular Facilitation, ed. 2. New York: Harper & Row Publishers, 1968.
Koczwara, H.: Use of a vibrator to facilitate motor and kinesthetic behavior in children. J.A.P.T.A. 55:510, 1975.
Kottke, F. J.: Neurophysiologic therapy for stroke. In Licht, S. (ed.): Stroke and Its Rehabilitation. New Haven: Elizabeth Licht Publishers, 1975.
Lindblom, U.: On the treatment of spastic paresis. J. Swed. Assoc. Reg. Phys. Ther. 27, Reprint, 1969.
Loomis, J.: Facilitation techniques in hemiplegia—treatment of the arm. J Can. Physiother. Assoc. 25:283–285, 1973.
Neeman, R.: Techniques of preparing effective orthokinetic cuff. A.O.T.A. Bull. 6:1, 1971.
Norton, Y.: Neurodevelopmental and sensory integration. Am. J. Occup. Ther. 29:93–100, 1975.
Ohwaki, S., et al.: Preference for vibratory and visual stimulation in mentally retarded children. Am. J. Ment. Def. 77:733–736, 1973.
Oster, C.: The neurophysiologic treatment of hemiplegia. J. Am. Osteopath. Assoc. 74:124–130, 1974.
Pearson, P. H., and Williams, C. E. (eds.): Physical Therapy Services in the Developmental Disabilities. Springfield IL: Charles C Thomas Publishers, 1972.
Peiper, A.: Cerebral Function in Infancy and Childhood. New York: Consultants Bureau, 1963.
Piercy, J. M.: The place of facilitation in non-neurological problems. Physiotherapy (Eng): 59:2–6, 1973.

Reuck, A. V. S. and de Knight, J. (ed.): Myotatic, Kinesthetic and Vestibular Mechanisms. London: Churchill, 1967.

Rood, M. S.: Proprioceptive neuromuscular facilitation and demonstration physiotherapy and occupational therapy. South Africa Cerebral Palsy J. 13:3, 1969.

Rood, M. S.: Use of Reflexes as an Aid in Occupational Therapy. Speech delivered at World Fed. of O.T., Copenhagen, Denmark, August, 1958.

Sattely, C. (ed.): Approaches to the Treatment of Patients with Neuromuscular Dysfunction. Dubuque IA: William C. Brown, 1962.

Schwartzman, R. J., and Bogdonoff, M. D.: Behavioral and anatomical analysis of vibration sensibility. Exp. Neurol. 20:43–51, 1968.

Semans, S.: Physical therapy for motor disorders resulting from brain damage. Rehab. Lit. April, 1959.

Shepherd, R. B.: Physiotherapy in Pediatrics. London: Wm. Heinemann Medical Books, 1974.

Smith, K. U.: Delayed Sensory Feedback and Behavior. Philadelphia: W. B. Saunders Co., 1962.

Smith, K. U., and Smith, W. M.: Perception and Motion. Philadelphia: W. B. Saunders Co., 1962.

Troyer, B.: Sensorimotor integration: A basis for planning occupational therapy. Am. J. Occup. Ther. 15:51–54, 1961.

Voss, D. E.: Proprioceptive neuromuscular facilitation: Application of patterns and technics in occupational therapy. Am. J. Occup. Ther. 13:191–194, 1959.

Voss, D. E., and Slatinsky, J. P.: Textured cane handle. J.A.P.T.A. 53:1295, 1973.

West, W. (ed.): Occupational Therapy for the Multiply Handicapped Child. Chicago: University of Chicago Press, 1965.

Whelan, J. K.: Effects of orthokinetics on upper extremity function of the adult hemiplegic patient. Am. J. Occup. Ther. 18:141–143, 1964.

Yamanaka, T.: Effects of High Frequency Vibration on Muscle Spindles In The Human Body. Zhiba Igakkai Zasshi 40, 1964.

Zamir, L. J. (ed.): Expanding Dimensions in Rehabilitation. Springfield IL: Charles C Thomas Publishers, 1969.

section 3/Sensory Integrative Theory/Mary Silberzahn

This summary of literature on the theory of sensory integration as it has been constructed and published by A. Jean Ayres is intended to introduce the reader to selected basic concepts of the theory. The therapeutic application of this body of knowledge requires in-depth study of the theory as cited in the original works of the author. Omitted from this summary is the extensive research underlying the theoretical construction.

THE SENSORY INTEGRATION PROCESS

A theoretical model of the process of sensory integration has been constructed by Ayres. The theory, built on both brain and behavioral research, was developed as a guide to improve neurological dysfunction and promote learning ability. The research underlying the theory focuses on the development of sensory integrative mechanisms and identification of irregularities in the learning disabled child. "The theory is not considered final: rather, it is seen as a continually evolving formulation of ideas to incorporate information from neurobiological research."[1]

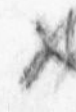

Sensory integration is the neurological process of organizing and processing, or perceiving, sensations for use. The organization of events between the sensation and the response is dependent upon the brain's ability to filter, sort, and integrate a mass of sensory information. The manner in which these events can be influenced is a major concern of the theory.

The objective of the sensory integrative approach to the treatment of learning disabilities is to enhance the brain's ability to develop the capacity to perceive, remember, and motor plan in order to provide a basis for mastery of all academic and other tasks rather than a focus on specific content. The therapeutic approach is directed towards controlling sensory input in order to activate brain mechanisms. Therapy in some but not all learning disabled children results in a reduction of the severity of the difficulty and allows specific skills to be learned more rapidly. Thus it "is considered a supplement, not a substitute to formal classroom instruction or tutoring."[2]

NEUROPHYSIOLOGICAL CONSTRUCTS

The understanding of certain basic principles of brain function on which sensory integrative theory is constructed is essential to the implementation of a therapeutic approach to learning disabilities.

Intermodality Association

The convergence of sensory input on a common neuron or larger structure is one method by which the brain associates sensory input from various sensory modalities. Implications for the therapeutic process lie in the premise that some neurons require convergence of many impulses for discharge. Thus the summation of stimuli from various sensory modalities, when directed toward a specific response, may be more effective than input from one modality alone.

Sensory Feedback

Awareness from action or feedback from the somatosensory and vestibular systems is essential to organizing and using sensory input for motor performance. For example, appropriate adaptive responses are impossible if the child does not know if he is falling and in which direction he will fall. "The problem is not one of loss of sensation but of inadequate discrimination of the temporal and spatial qualities which, presumably, results in 'hazy' or vague feedback."[3] The therapist should utilize procedures and activities that emphasize the processing of accurate discriminative information. Selection of activities that have simple motor demands and require integrative responses are preferable to more complex motor activities requiring a great many responses that cannot be adequately integrated.

Centrifugal Influence

The ability to suppress part of the sensory flow and prevent sensory overload is an important regulatory function of the central nervous system. The influences operate in a direction away from the cerebral cortex and toward the periphery to regulate the sensory flow. "Some of the disinhibited behavior, hypersensitivity to sensation, deficient perception and clumsiness can be linked, in one way or another to inadequate centrifugal influences from cortical or subcortical levels."[4] Therapy should be directed toward providing sensory input which is designed to enhance influences operating in a direction away from the cerebral cortex and toward the periphery.

Movement

"One of the most powerful organizers of sensory input is movement which is adaptive to the organism."[5] The theory proposes that the brain will tend to organize itself in response to functional environmental demands resulting in integrative responses. The therapeutic procedure should be concerned with the selection of activities that require organization of a more complex response than previously made.

Developmental Sequence

The importance of the developmental sequence to sensory integration is viewed in terms of phlogeny, ontogeny, and neurodevelopment and developmental stages. "In children, intersensory integration follows a developmental sequence with the most rapid maturation of the function occurring before eight years of age."[6]

The progress of evolution of the brain is, at least in part, a result of the organizing of successful or adaptive responses to environmental demands. "The therapeutic situation attempts to modify both the child's capacity and the environmental demands to make it possible for the child to succeed in organizing a response and thus to proceed with the developmental sequences that eventually result in the capacity for academic learning."[7]

Levels of Brain Function

The concept of levels of function, derived mainly from brain evolution, is that lower structures of the brain are phyletically less complex and develop before the higher and more complex structures.

The importance of the brain stem is particularly critical to sensory integrative theory because it evolved earlier, is an important area for convergence of sensory input, and has widespread influence over the rest of the brain. It is concerned primarily with total massive patterning involving overt responses of the entire body, determined by a relatively simple integration. It contributes to visual perception, especially to the development of an environment scheme or map to which the body relates. The cerebral hemispheres evolved later, enabling more discrete, individualistic motor patterns based on more precise interpretation of sensory information. A general principle of brain function is that higher levels do not function optimally without adequate lower function. Similarly, higher structures never quite lose their dependence on lower structures. "The course of therapy follows a progression similar to that of the developmental course of brain function. Enhancing maturation at the lower, less complex levels of environmental-response function enables a child to become more competent at the higher, more complex levels."[8] Thus, a great deal of the therapeutic emphasis is placed on organization of sensory-integrative mechanisms at the brain stem level.

Sensory Modalities

Knowledge of sensory modalities in terms of neural pathways, intersensory influences, developmental sequence, and contribution to sensory integration is basic to evaluation and treatment of sensory integrative dysfunction. The theory proposes hypotheses of neural functioning as suggestions for exploring therapeutic procedures or as providing tentative explanations for their apparent effectiveness. Because vestibular, tactile, and proprioceptive sensory systems mature earliest they have received the greatest emphasis in theory development. These modalities have pervasive influence on brain function, mature early, and are important to survival. They provide input from the body for unconscious neural control of sensorimotor activity and to convergent neurons for intersensory association. They contribute to perceptual-motor development including body scheme, motor planning, motor and academic skill development, and psychosocial development. The therapeutic use of motor activity is important to sensory integrative development because of the input to the tactile, vestibular, and other proprioceptive systems. Visual and auditory functions mature later and are seen as end products of sensory integration.

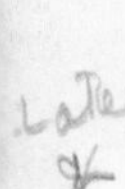

EVALUATION

Evaluation of sensory integrative dysfunction is both objective and subjective; standardized tests are used to strengthen and increase clinical impressions.

The Southern California Sensory Integration Tests and the Southern California Postrotary Nystagmus Test, a battery of 18 tests, were constructed by Ayres "to detect and to determine the nature of sensory integrative dysfunction."[9] The tests measure parameters statistically identified as related to learning disabilities, which include tactile, kinesthetic, vestibular, and visual senses and aspects of motor planning and motor coordination. The total test battery should be administered to obtain adequate reliability. Dysfunction can be detected by comparing standard scores of a child's performance with the expected performance derived from the normative sample. The nature of sensory integrative dysfunction can be identified by comparing one area of performance which comprises a meaningful cluster (e.g., visual) with other areas of performance (e.g., tactile). The appropriate use of these tests "is dependent upon wide background knowledge of neurobiology, especially that related to sensory integration and processing, and extensive experience with children who have sensory integrative problems."[10] (The reader is referred to the *Southern California Sensory Integration Tests Manual*, the *Southern California Postrotary Nystagmus Test Manual*, and the *Southern California Sensory Integration Interpretation Manual* for extensive coverage of evaluation procedures.)

Subjective assessment relies heavily on the understanding of postural mechanisms and sensory systems in relation to sensory integrative development and function.

Postural Mechanisms

Postural responses, elicited by gravity and movement, influence the sensory integrative process at the brain stem level and contribute to neural integration required for academic learning. Principles and functions underlying the therapeutic approach to enhancing postural mechanisms include the antigravity nature of these responses, the brain stem level of organization, the developmental sequence, the relationship to muscles and muscle receptors and to extraocular muscle control.

The ability to assume and maintain a prone extension and a supine flexion position is considered to be an indicator of one aspect of sensory integrative development. The tonic labyrinthine reflex (TLR), activated by change of position of the head in space, biases postural changes in the neonate in the direction of gravity. As the more mature antigravity responses develop, the child can assume and maintain the basic motor patterns of flexion when supine and extension when prone. The child who demonstrates an inadequate response will need to be provided with opportunities for a more mature level of response. The prone extension pattern may be reflexively facilitated by riding a scooterboard down an incline in a prone extension position. If this position has previously been difficult, the nervous system may need to be prepared to make an appropriate response. Therapeutic procedures such as brushing, quick stretch, and vibration may be employed previous to the scooter ride.

The tonic neck reflex (TNR), which originates from receptors in the joints and ligaments of the first three cervical vertebrae, reflexively orients the limbs in relation to the head-body angle. The ability of the head to move freely on its axis indicates integration of the primitive TNR and, as such, is another indicator of sensory-motor development. A proposed remedial procedure is for the child to assume and maintain an anti-tonic neck position, a reverse position of the head and forearms in relation to the head.

The integration of primitive reflexes is mainly dependent upon adequate vestibular and proprioceptive functions, the righting reactions involve receptors from several sensory modalities—visual, tactile, proprioceptive, and vestibular.

The righting reactions, including the neck-righting reflex, triggered by sensory input to neck receptors for automatic body turning, represent a more mature response, integrating the TNR and eliciting rotation on the longitudinal axis. Activation of the neck-righting reflex is best promoted by rolling activities replicating the early rolling patterns of the developing infant.

Activities designed to elicit equilibrium reactions in prone, quadruped, and sitting and the protective extension responses are introduced as part of the developmental sequence. These activities should involve trunk and extremities in an attempt to attain and maintain balance. The development of kneel and squat patterns should be encouraged. It is recommended that standing balance not be emphasized in the therapeutic process until the earlier developmental steps have been achieved.

Therapeutic procedures for developing postural mechanisms are described in *Sensory Integration and Learning Disorders* by Ayres.

SENSORY SYSTEMS

Integration of the tactile, proprioceptive, and vestibular systems are considered of primary importance because of their contribution to generalized neurological integration and to enhanced perception in other sensory systems. The planning and controlling of sensory input for facilitation of neural development in as near normal sequence as is possible is an important therapeutic consideration.

Tactile System

It is hypothesized that the tactile system has a pervasive, primal, and preparatory influence on generalized neurological integration. It is a primal source of input to the reticular formation by way of both ascending and descending fibers. It has a generalized effect on the neuromuscular system as well as a specific facilitory effect on a given muscle. It is quite probable that tactile input may be facilitory to the cortex. Early maturation of this system is further evidence of its importance to the sensory integrative process.

Because of the prolonged effect and primacy of the tactile system it is suggested that treatment sessions be initiated with tactile stimulation. It is estimated that a barrage of tactile stimuli will exert a major influence on the nervous system for approximately half an hour. The quality and quantity of the stimuli administered is guided by the child's response. Positive responses are generally considered to be integrating. If overstimulation results in undesired arousal and negatively affects sleep patterns and attention, this response is interpreted as an inability to organize this stimuli adequately, rather than a lack of need of this type of input. It may be advisable to use alternate procedures for a while. The general level of reticular excitation may be inhibited by touch pressure and slow vestibular stimulation. Light touch, especially when applied directly over the muscle belly, may elicit phasic contraction. The neuromuscular system may be counterbalanced by vestibular stimulation to elicit a tonic response in the muscles.

Vestibular System

The early normalization of vestibular functions provides a background for skill development. Vestibular input is important to the integration of many postural responses and to other types of sensory integrative processes and should be introduced early in the treatment program.

The child may be involved passively for generalized stimulation or actively to elicit adaptive responses that tend to have an organizing influence.

Vestibular stimulation may be excitatory or inhibitory to the central nervous system. Excitatory, such as that which occurs from rapid spinning without an adaptive response, may be disorganizing. The child should be carefully observed. Inhibitory influence may be elicited by slow, rhythmical movements. This type of stimulation may inhibit the brain stem centers governing vital functions such as respiration. An activity that demands an adaptive response tends to normalize the sensory input. If the child demonstrates a hypo-responsiveness to vestibular stimulation the therapeutic approach may be to bombard the system through the many different vestibular receptors. If the child shows anxiety and a hyper-responsive reaction to vestibular stimulation the therapist may need to employ a slow, safe, nonthreatening approach to the introduction of vestibular stimulation.

Different receptors are stimulated by different planes of movement and different head positions. The horizontal position is considered optimal for horizontal semicircular canal input and more effective for activating the otoliths than the upright position.

Other Proprioceptive Stimuli

Proprioceptive input from joints, bones, and muscles may contribute to sensory integration through organization of locomotion and visual input at the brain stem level. Proprioception is enhanced through muscle contraction, especially against resistance. The therapeutic procedure should include activities such as riding a scooter prone which requires maintained or static contraction. The sensory input is tonic, influencing secondary afferents from the muscle spindle rather than phasic action which affects the primary afferents. Input to the proprioceptors through joint compression or approximation and traction may increase kinesthesia or the conscious sense of joint movement or position. Methods of increasing sensory feedback to proprioceptors may include use of weights for traction or rapid alternating resistance to antagonistic muscles for contraction. Vibration may be used to excite muscles under contraction or to inhibit and lower the central excitatory state over muscles not contracting.

Adaptive Response

Activities that require purposeful, goal-directed actions, or adaptive responses add functional meaning to motion and enhance the sensory integrative process. The therapeutic value of the motor response is dependent upon the accuracy of the somatosensory and vestibular feedback. When combined with emotional involvement and effort, a motor response which requires a level of response more complex than previously demonstrated is considered an adaptive response and integrating to the central nervous system.

Precautions

The therapist must be constantly alert to the potential dangers in providing therapy. Consideration must be given to general safety precautions as well as those incurred in the therapeutic procedure such as tone increase in irregular and hypertonic muscles, sensory overload, over-inhibition, and seizure precipitation. Vestibular stimulation is a particularly powerful therapeutic tool. Its influence on the autonomic nervous system may be recognized by flushing, blanching, perspiring, nausea, or yawning. These signs are indicators that, at least temporarily, the amount of stimulation should be reduced.

SYNDROMES OF DYSFUNCTION

Test data were subjected to factor analysis as a method of investigating, identifying, and clarifying the nature of different types of sensory integrative dysfunction. The relationships of test parameters yielded through repeated studies led to hypothesizing syndromes, or constellations of symptoms, characteristic of dysfunction. Types of neural system disorders are not clear cut, nor consistently defined, but are sufficiently independent to contribute to theory construction from which therapeutic procedures were derived.

A brief description of two types of sensory integrative dysfunction—deficit in hemispheral function and developmental apraxia—is presented. A third type, a deficit in form and space perception, has not been included because, in this theoretical model, it is considered to be an end product of the integration of vestibular, kinesthetic, and tactile stimuli. Treatment procedures are therefore based on concepts of treatment for vestibular, kinesthetic, and tactile dysfunction.

Deficit in Interhemispheral Function

The theory proposes that hemispheric specialization of function is important for greater adaptiveness and specificity of cortical function. The neural basis for learning is considered optimal when language functions are lateralized in the left hemisphere and visuo-spatial functions are in the right hemispheres (in right-handed people).

> Central to the theory and treatment of this syndrome is the postulate that the brain stem interhemispheral integrating mechanism is functionally associated with the brain stem postural reflexes and reactions and, furthermore, that inadequate maturation of the brain stem mediated postural reactions interferes with maturation of the interhemispheral integrative mechanism at that level. The resultant dysfunction interferes with the development of specialization of function in the cerebral cortex.[11]

Lack of integration of function of two sides of the body is the most characteristic symptom of a deficit in interhemispheral function. It is hypothesized that the neural mechanisms involved in bilateral integration are directly related to learning problems, especially reading problems. A disorder in the neural system subserving interhemispheral integration includes "disorder in postural and ocular mechanisms, and usually, but not invariably, auditory-language problems, poor right-left discrimination, and deficits in visual form and space perception."[12]

Clinical findings include poorly integrated TLR and TNR, immature righting and equilibrium reactions, and poor eye pursuits. Hypotonic musculature and diminished co-contraction and inadequate postural adjustments such as protective extension, poor weight shift, and poor trunk rotation are frequently observed. There is a tendency toward ipsilateral hand usage and avoidance of midline crossing, difficulty using two hands together in a coordinated manner and, frequently, poorly established hand dominance. The child may appear to be clumsy and lack flexibility of movement.

Treatment procedures are designed to normalize postural reactions and develop the capacity to motor plan. It is proposed that function of the two sides of the body will automatically begin to integrate functions. Treatment steps should follow the developmental sequence as much as possible. The treatment program should

1. normalize the tactile and vestibular systems through activities that provide general stimulation of these sensory systems
2. utilize neurophysiological procedures and activities to elicit a more mature level of response which encourages integration of primitive reflexes; develop supine flexion and prone extension patterns
3. provide activities that elicit a postural response such as protective extension and postural background movements
4. assimilate TNR and activate neck-righting reflex
5. develop more mature postural reactions through activities that elicit equilibrium reactions in prone, quadruped, and sitting postures
6. develop eye and neck musculature
7. enhance bilateral coordination
8. develop visuo-spatial perception

Specific procedures are cited in the original publications.

Developmental Apraxia

Developmental apraxia is defined as "a disorder of sensory integration interfering with the ability to plan and execute skilled or non-habitual motor tasks."[13] The dysfunction is characterized by a clumsiness in motor activity, a lack of knowing how to go about executing an unusual motor task, reduced quality of oral motor proficiency, and inadequate extraocular control. Although skill development usually is slower than age expectation, the child can and does learn splinter skills. Dressing, constructive manipulation, drawing, cutting, pasting, assembling, and learning to write are frequently difficult for an apraxic child.

The somatosensory input that contributes to development of body scheme is inadequate. As a result the child has difficulty in associating the different anatomical elements of the body and how they work together. He has not developed a sensorimotor awareness of body parts and their potential motions, especially in relation to each other as a basis for motor planning.

Sensory integrative therapy for the apraxic child focuses on "specificity versus non-specificity of sensory process and excitation versus inhibition of sensation."[14] The treatment principles that guide the therapeutic procedure are:

1. enhance sensory integration at the brain stem level; provide generalized tactile, vestibular, and other proprioceptive input
2. activate joint receptors for enhancement of kinesthesia
3. develop postural mechanisms
4. develop the basic motor repertoire: basic gross motor patterns of flexion in supine and extension in prone, portions of the basic flexion and extension synergies, gross diagonal patterns
5. provide an opportunity for a variety of activities to promote growth of sensory integration in general and to develop a generalized ability to motor plan
6. require an adaptive motor response to promote organization of the sensory input.

SUMMARY

The theory of sensory integration extends the body of knowledge which focused primarily on motor function to a body of knowledge which considers the interaction between sensory and motor. Procedures such as therapeutic exercise and neuromuscular facilitation may contribute to sensory integrative therapy when they enhance neural integration. Sensory integration cannot, therefore, be considered in isolation. This theoretical model will extend and expand as knowledge increases.

REFERENCES

1. Ayres, A. J.: Sensorimotor foundations of academic ability. In Cruickshank, W., and Hallahan, D. (eds.): Perceptual and Learning Disabilities in Children, Vol. 2. Syracuse University Press, 1975, p. 36.
2. Ayres, A. J.: Sensory Integration and Learning Disorders. Los Angeles: Western Psychological Services, 1972, p. 2.
3. Ibid., p. 33.
4. Ibid., p. 32.
5. Ibid., p. 36.
6. Ibid., p. 28.
7. Ibid., p. 11.
8. Ibid., p. 12.
9. Ayres, A. J.: Southern California Sensory Integration Tests Manual. Los Angeles: Western Psychological Services, 1972, p. 1.
10. Ayres, A. J.: Southern California Sensory Integration Interpretation Manual. Los Angeles: Western Psychological Services, 1977, p. 1.
11. Ayres: Sensorimotor foundations. In Cruickshank and Hallahan (eds.): Perceptual Learning Disabilities, p. 342.
12. Ibid., p. 336.
13. Ayres: Sensory Integration, p. 165.
14. Ibid., p. 176.

8

Rehabilitation Approach

Helen L. Hopkins, Helen D. Smith, and Elizabeth G. Tiffany

REHABILITATION AND HABILITATION

The term "rehabilitation" in its broadest sense means restoration of or return to ability. In 1947 the National Council on Rehabilitation defined rehabilitation as "the restoration of the handicapped to the fullest physical, mental, social, vocational and economic usefulness of which they are capable."[1] Procedures were developed to accomplish this purpose.

Medical care is not considered to be complete until each individual with a residual disability has been trained to live and work with his or her remaining capabilities. A vital factor in rehabilitation is motivation or "the will to get well" and to return to society and the community.

Children born with or acquiring disability shortly after birth have not had the opportunity to develop ability to function. The term "rehabilitation" is not appropriate in their cases. Therefore a different term, "habilitation," is used to indicate development of the ability to function regardless of the disability and the process of learning to live and work with one's capabilities.

Philosophy of Rehabilitation/Habilitation

The philosophy of rehabilitation/habilitation requires that the total capabilities of each individual must be considered. This includes physical, emotional, cognitive, social, cultural, vocational, and economic factors. In 1953 Whitehouse stated that rehabilitation is a social problem whose roots are in the life of a community. He said the rehabilitation center exists for the client and centers around the client's needs. Thus rehabilitation must be dynamic and keep step with both scientific advances and changes in society. Rehabilitation includes the concept of prevention or of the exacerbation of dysfunction in all aspects of human activity, thus requiring an ongoing process of assessment with follow-up being a necessity.[2]

Rehabilitation is concerned with the intrinsic worth and dignity of the individual. It is therefore committed to the restoration of the disabled to a life that is purposeful and satisfying, one that allows each individual the opportunity to function adequately as a family member and as a member of society with the capabilities to meet the responsibilities of that society.[3]

Government Involvement in Rehabilitation/Habilitation

The United States has had state and federal programs of vocational rehabilitation since 1920. Early programs were limited to guidance, vocational training, and placement of the physically handicapped. Training was focused on working around the disability with no concern being given to alleviating or reducing the effect of the disability on the physical and mental capabilities of the individual.

It was not until 1943 when Public Law 113 (Barden-LaFollette Act) was passed that federal and state laws were amended to allow for the provision of medical rehabilitation services. It was recognized at that time that medicine as a whole, using the skills of all those specialized in patient care, must be applied through a team approach to assure restoration of both the physically and the mentally disabled to their highest potential in all aspects of function. To assure the alleviation or reduction of the effect of disability as well as reaching of the highest potential for each individual, rehabilitation became the concern of the physician with the nurse, occupational therapist, physical therapist, speech therapist, psychologist, vocational counselor, and prosthetist/orthotist as members of the rehabilitation team.[4] The client had to be involved in the decision-making processes and thus was also a member of the rehabilitation team. The client's participation helped promote the development of maximum commitment and optimum function.

In 1954, through Public Law 565, federal laws were expanded to include payment for the training of rehabilitation personnel, expansion of rehabilitation facilities, and support of research.[5] This law helped to alleviate the shortage of qualified personnel and caused the development and expansion of rehabilitation centers throughout the country to meet the growing demands for rehabilitation services.

In 1965 a federal law established a National Commission on Architectural Barriers under the Rehabilitation Services Agencies; in 1968 a federal law was passed to eliminate architectural barriers from all governmentally funded buildings. These laws brought to public consciousness the architectural requirements of the physically disabled. As a result, many public places are accessible to handicapped individuals today. Much still needs to be done to make total communities accessible.

In 1973 a law was passed giving the handicapped equal access to schools and jobs. In April 1977, because of non-enforcement of the 1973 law, there were numerous demonstrations by the handicapped who claimed infringement on their civil rights. Thus, Health, Education, and Welfare Secretary, Joseph Califano, Jr., signed regulations for elimination of discrimination in health insurance and government contracts to assure the handicapped of equal access to schools and jobs.[6]

REHABILITATION OF THE PHYSICALLY HANDICAPPED

World War II precipitated many advances in medicine which preserved the life of many severely disabled individuals. Changes in industrial technology also made it possible for the employment of many of these persons. Manpower shortages gave these individuals the opportunity to demonstrate their productivity and value to the economy.[7] In order to meet the needs and demands of the physically disabled, the dynamic process of rehabilitation was developed. This process viewed each individual as a total person and was not concerned with illness or disability alone but with restoration of the person's total capabilities as well. This approach allowed the individual to participate in his or her own rehabilitation, to communicate with others, and to adapt his/her physical environment to meet his/her physical and energy requirements. In this way the person was able to resume his/her self-care, work, and leisure activities by utilizing maximum physical, intellectual, social, and vocational potential.[8]

Rehabilitation centers for the physically disabled were developed immediately after World War II. The first outpatient rehabilitation center was the Institute for the Crippled and Disabled in New York City, which opened under the direction of George G. Deaver, M.D., in 1946. The five objectives for treatment at this center[9] were for the client to

1. gain maximum independence in bed and wheelchair activities
2. gain maximum use of hands
3. be able to ambulate and elevate

4. achieve maximum ability in communication (hear and speak)
5. function in as nearly normal manner as possible.

To achieve these goals, underlying pathology had to be assessed along with the chances of overcoming disability. Deaver said, "Rehabilitation is the medical management of physical disability." He described rehabilitation medicine as active rather than reactive, for it focused on the patient and the patient's function and relationship with others, especially family and community members, rather than solely on treatment of the disease.[10]

The first inpatient rehabilitation center was established at New York City's Bellevue Hospital in 1946 under the direction of Howard A. Rusk, M.D.[11] Subsequently rehabilitation centers were established throughout the United States, many independent and many affiliated with hospitals with both inpatient and outpatient facilities. In the 1960s many general hospitals throughout the United States established Rehabilitation Centers or Physical Medicine and Rehabilitation departments within their facilities, for it was recognized that to ignore a disability was far more costly than to start rehabilitation early in an individual's hospital stay.[12] It is now the practice in many general hospitals, whether or not they have rehabilitation centers, to begin rehabilitation of physically disabled individuals as soon as the acute phase of the disease or injury is past. Insurance carriers, federal and state rehabilitation agencies, parents, and patients added impetus to the development of this practice.

OCCUPATIONAL THERAPY IN REHABILITATION OF PHYSICALLY DISABLED

Rehabilitation/habilitation as a treatment approach in occupational therapy means a dual approach to problems: (1) helping clients increase the functioning of disabled extremities and overcome disturbances in the ability to function and (2) helping clients utilize remaining capabilities to reach their highest potential in meeting the demands of daily living. This treatment approach attempts to overcome dysfunction resulting from disease or injury and to enhance the ability to function and better utilize remaining capabilities. This approach uses constructive activity, which is guided by the therapist to achieve the desired physical and psychological results.[13]

Occupational therapy must begin with assessment of capabilities to determine a baseline of function. A treatment plan is established in conjunction with the rehabilitation team and client, keeping in mind the client's goals. The treatment program is then planned so as to eliminate or diminish disability through the use of activity while focusing on the individual's capabilities in all aspects of function. Activities utilized include exercise that can be translated into useful activity, self-care activities (ADL—activities of daily living), expressive or creative activities, intellectual or educational activities, play or leisure activities, pre-vocational activities, and simulated or actual vocational activities including homemaking and other work tasks. Energy conservation, joint protection, and work simplification techniques should be included in the rehabilitation program. Reassessment of capabilities and progress must be continued on a regular basis to determine gains made and to prevent problems from developing. Preventive measures such as splinting and positioning must be utilized to eliminate contractures, deformity, skin breakdown, or other secondary problems.

The client's family should be involved in the total process of rehabilitation if there is to be a smooth transition from living in the rehabilitation center to successful integration into the home and community. There must be an increase of independence on the part of the client and less dependence on rehabilitation personnel.

The family must be counselled regarding the role it must play in helping the disabled individual attain maximum capability and independence. Visits to the client's home before discharge, when possible, may assist families in eliminating architectural barriers and making the transition from rehabilitation facility to home easier. Follow-up through reevaluation within the rehabilitation facility, through home visits, and through utilization of services of community agencies is required for the total success of the rehabilitation process.

Rapid change in society and health care now requires that rehabilitation services be provided at the convenience of the consumer. Rehabilitation services once housed only within a rehabilitation center are now becoming a part of and are available within the community.[14] Many professionals are providing services in such institutions as schools and community centers as well as in the client's home.

PSYCHIATRIC OCCUPATIONAL THERAPY AND REHABILITATION

In the years since the advent of the use of drugs to control the symptoms of mental illness, there has been a marked increase in the kinds of occupational therapy programs that may be defined as rehabilitative. There have been both subtle and dramatic changes in attitudes about mental illness both in society at large and on the part of the providers of services. As mental illness came to be viewed as reversible, the mentally ill person came to be considered as a possible participant in a rehabilitation program. A shift in the emphasis and context of treatment came with the community mental health movement of the 1960s. The patient who previously had been regarded as having potential for only marginal adjustment to the sheltered life of the institution now began to be viewed as potentially able to return to life and productivity "on the outside." Efforts began to be directed toward minimizing the length of the institutional stay of acutely ill people and toward the development of outpatient treatment facilities.

Rehabilitation in psychiatry refers to the development of skills that will enable the individual to return to function successfully in the world outside the institution. This includes being competent in caring for one's daily living needs and adapting to the demands of work and social life. Rehabilitation becomes the focus after the major treatment effort has taken place. Rehabilitation is differentiated from treatment in that its concern is no longer the interruption of or direct intervention in the pathological process of the illness but the improvement and organization of existing strengths and skills of the client and on the development of competence in handling the demands of everyday living. Much of modern psychiatric occupational therapy is directed toward rehabilitation. The differentiation between treatment and rehabilitation in psychiatry itself, however, tends to lack clarity. Perhaps one of the characteristics of work with the mentally ill is that treatment and rehabilitation may need to be, in some cases, continuous and reciprocal.[15]

The psychiatric occupational therapist, working within a rehabilitation context, must first be able to identify clearly the client's existing assets and liabilities and the internal and external areas that may be developed, improved, or changed through the occupational therapy process. Second, the occupational therapist must know the kinds of skills that will be required for the client to function in his/her social and work community. The occupational

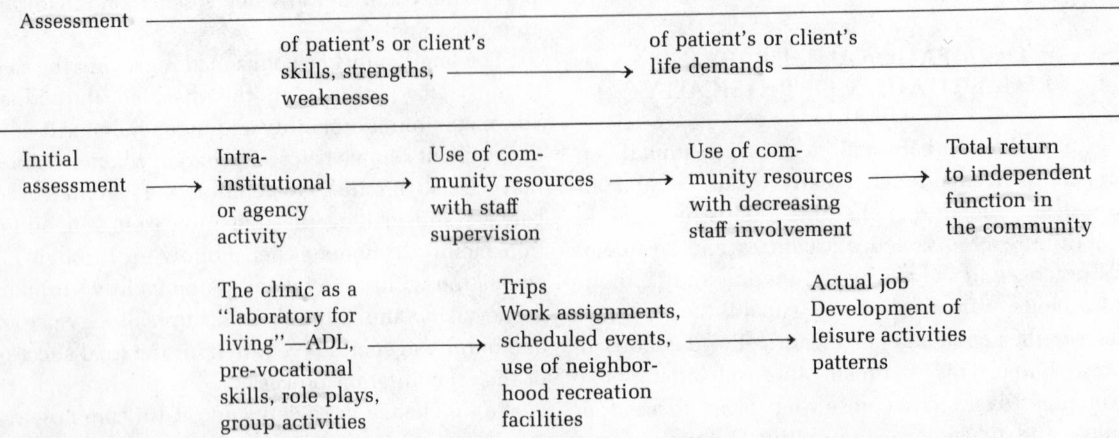

FIGURE 8-1. Suggested steps in psychiatric rehabilitation in occupational therapy.

therapy process, then, is geared to providing experiences and opportunities that are oriented realistically and directly to improving those skills. An important goal of rehabilitation underlying all other goals is for the client to achieve the ability to know his or her own strengths, limitations, and needs and to have a sense of ways to use the strengths, minimize limitations, and seek to satisfy real needs. In this process, the participation of the occupational therapy staff decreases as the client's ability to assume autonomy increases in the following areas: (1) self-assessment; (2) management of life activities so that a healthy balance of work, play, rest, and sleep is achieved; (3) management of the time requirements of life-schedules, appointments, and pacing oneself through being able to predict how long a given activity may take; and (4) handling of the problem-solving and decision-making demands that present themselves.

A sequence of steps that may be followed in psychiatric rehabilitation in occupational therapy is suggested in Figure 8-1.

REFERENCES

1. Reggio, A. W.: Rehabilitation—what is it? Am. J. Occup. Ther. 1:149–151, 1947.
2. Whitehouse, F. A.: The rehabilitation center—some aspects of a philosophy. Am. J. Occup. Ther. 7:241, 1953.
3. Licht, S.: Rehabilitation and Medicine. Baltimore: Waverly Press, 1968, pp. 1–13.
4. Rusk, H. A.: Rehabilitation Medicine, ed. 3. St. Louis: C. V. Mosby Co., 1971, pp. 1–8.
5. Ibid.
6. Boston Globe, April 29, 1977.
7. Licht: Rehabilitation and Medicine, pp. 1–13.
8. Ibid.
9. Ibid.
10. Ibid.
11. Rusk: Rehabilitation Medicine, pp. 1–8.
12. Licht: Rehabilitation and Medicine, pp. 1–13.
13. Spackman, C. S.: A history of the practice of occupational therapy for restoration of physical function: 1917–1967. Am. J. Occup. Ther. 22:67, 1968.
14. Hightower, M. D.: Rehabilitation—a part of the community or apart from the community. Am. J. Occup. Ther. 28:296–298, 1974.
15. Fidler, G. S., and Fidler, J. W.: Occupational Therapy: A Communication Process in Psychiatry. New York: Macmillan Publishing Co., 1963, p. 27.

9

Occupational Behavior Approach

Helen L. Hopkins and Elizabeth G. Tiffany

In spite of the fact that rehabilitation, as a philosophy, requires that the total capabilities of each individual be considered, the rehabilitation approach as it has been practiced has been classified with the medical model of treatment and thus has been identified as an approach whose major emphasis has been on the reduction of deficits through direct cause and effect treatment procedures. In the 1960s Reilly proposed a new approach, which dealt with the social nature of the individual, and suggested that the original life space and life style concepts of Adolf Meyer and Eleanor Clark Slagle be revived. The occupational behavior approach indicates that interdisciplinary knowledge in which each person is viewed as a biosocial being must be utilized. Problems of disrupted roles are dealt with in order to enable the individual to gain skills and habits for socialization and adaptation for adequate functioning in his or her family, neighborhood, and community.[1]

All human beings, growing up in society, learn to function within a number of systems. In each system there are definable roles whose functions support it. Some of the roles that can be examined are preschool child, student, worker, mother, father, homemaker, and wage earner. Human society has been structured in such a way that there are basic expectations regarding behavior and functions within the roles. The systems will break down if these basic expectations are not met.

The examination of the functional skills components of the roles that are assumed by patients in their lives has heuristic value for occupational therapy. Most human roles fall into the categories of play, self-care, and work; the skills required for each of these categories have been studied and designated as part of the occupational therapy process almost from the beginnings of occupational therapy as a profession. Proponents of the occupational behavior approach have analyzed with great care the kinds of skills that are required in society and the experiences that tend to promote successful performance. The play behavior of the infant and child is seen as the prototype for adult functional behavior. The leisure-play experiences of the adult are seen to support the more demanding components of the learning situation provided and to support the need for balance in the life activities of the patients. It is important to know the opportunities and demands made upon the patient in the past and to have a sense of the ways in which he or she met them; it is equally important to have a sense of the opportunities and demands characteristic of the patient's future plans. Then, in the treatment situation, it will be possible to plan realistically for the restoration or development of the skills necessary to function.[2,3]

Exploration of play behavior in children has yielded important theoretical ideas about what underlies the development of effective functional behavior. Reilly refers to three hierarchical stages of play,[4] each progressing to a higher level of excitement and requiring greater control:

1. Exploratory behavior characterizes the earliest kind of play behavior, beginning early in infancy and continuing throughout life, whenever an event is new or very different from the familiar. Motivated by curiosity and by interest in novelty, the individual "plays" with the many aspects of an experience or an object. In the process, one learns not only about the objects of the exploration, but about one's own capabilities and limits as well.

2. Competency behavior is the stage in which the individual wishes to influence the environment and to be influenced by it. In this stage one practices the newly acquired skills in an effort to achieve mastery —a sense of using one's capabilities with competence.

These first two stages may be considered as *intrinsically motivated*—behavior engaged in for itself and for the pleasure of the doing.

3. Achievement behavior builds upon the previous two stages. At this point the individual is engaged in interacting with the environment with an emphasis on performance, using an external standard of excellence. It appears that there is a shift in this stage from intrinsic to *extrinsic motivation*.

In this analysis of play behavior, which parallels the work of Erikson and Piaget, White, and others, occupational therapy finds some new guidelines for its total process. In an achievement-oriented society, it may be critical to plan for environments that can first promote exploration and competence.

Thus, the occupational behavior treatment approach provides or creates an environment that allows the individual to perform and practice various skills and relevant behaviors that are required for the roles he/she must perform in society.

REFERENCES

1. Kielhofner, G.: The Evolution of Knowledge in Occupational Therapy: Understanding Adaptation of the Chronically Disabled. Unpublished master's thesis. Los Angeles, California. University of Southern California, 1975.
2. Reilly, M.: A psychiatric occupational therapy program —a teaching model. Am. J. Occup. Ther. 20:66–67, 1966.
3. Matsutsuyu, J.: Occupational behavior: A perspective on work and play. Am. J. Occup. Ther. 25:291–294, 1971.
4. Reilly, M. (ed.): Play as Exploratory Learning. Beverly Hills: Sage Publishing Co., 1974, pp. 117–149.

Part Four

Evaluation Process and Procedures

10

Assessment and Evaluation

section 1/Evaluation Overview/Helen D. Smith and Elizabeth G. Tiffany

In 1971 Gillette referred to the evaluation process as a professional responsibility. She defined the functions of the evaluation process [1] as (1) determining the baseline for objectives and providing the foundation for a treatment program, (2) identifying which problems can and cannot be mediated in the occupational therapy process, (3) giving some indication of the potential for change, (4) enlisting the cooperation of the client in beginning to assess his or her capabilities and dreams, and (5) helping the client begin a course of action designed to master some of the difficulties he or she has previously tried to master alone.

> Evaluation also serves the purpose of keeping the therapist's work current, for it is a spiral, building process. Each treatment session should be assessed and each target area reviewed, in order to determine the effectiveness of the activity process and to revise the objectives as they are mastered or found to be unreachable. Treatment should not persist in a straight line. It is the system of evaluation which is built into the treatment process which ultimately determines the effectiveness of treatment.[2]

In occupational therapy, evaluation is a process of collecting and organizing the relevant information about a patient or client so that the therapist will be able to plan and implement a program of treatment that can be meaningful and effective. Several steps are involved in the process:

1. *The collection of data.* This includes the selection and use of tools and methods by which information is obtained. The frame of reference for treatment will determine the kinds of data which will be sought. Critical to the success of the program is the participation of the client in this process.
2. *The organization of the data* into a meaningful, dynamic description of the client's strengths and weaknesses with a focus on those areas in which the occupational therapy process can be of help. This description must be one that can be understood by both the client and the therapist at some level. It must also be one that can be readily communicated to others.
3. *The setting of treatment objectives.* This involves the use of clinical judgment and predictive assumptions on the part of the therapist and must be

based on the accumulated data, including the client's goals, the therapist's knowledge about the clinical pathology, and the treatment frame of reference.

4. *Commitment to continuing evaluation* as the occupational therapy plan is carried out for reassessment of the original objectives and treatment plan. Changes in the occupational therapy plan are dependent upon the results of ongoing reevaluation.

There are two keys to successful evaluation: skill in observation and skill in gaining the trust of the client so that a truly cooperative effort takes place.

TYPES OF EVALUATION

Medical Records

The medical record provides valuable information about the client and gives indications for precautions that must be considered when planning and carrying out treatment. Information gleaned from the medical record adds to the baseline information necessary for effective treatment planning.

The past and present medical history, written by the physician, gives the therapist information on patient or client health status, former medical problems, present medical or physical findings, diagnoses, precautions, and prognosis. Daily physician and nursing notes list medications and treatments being given and patient or client responses. Reports and/or evaluations from other specialties are also included: x-ray, dietary, social service, psychiatry, psychology, physical or speech therapy, vocational and/or rehabilitation counselling. With information from medical records as background, the therapist is ready to move on to the next step in the evaluation process.

Observation

A key to successful evaluation lies in the therapist's skills in observation. The ability to see and to listen well must be accompanied by the ability to sort through the mass of perceptual and conceptual data which may be presented and to focus on what is relevant to the process. Human beings communicate information about themselves in a great many ways.

There is verbal communication—the choice of words and sentences and their meanings and the quality of tone and inflection with which the words are said. There are the paralinguistic and nonverbal behaviors that accompany verbal communication—facial expression, gestures, posture, and body movements. Attention to nonverbal communication is especially important to the occupational therapist inasmuch as a large part of the occupational therapy process is doing, not talking. Nonverbal expressions in human beings are established earlier in life than verbal ones and rely upon older neurophysiological structures.[3] A third mode of communication is the written form. It can be assumed that the written work has been, in some ways, more carefully considered and censored and is less spontaneous than the spoken, although this is not necessarily true. What an individual writes about him or herself may be useful as a representation of a desired or ideal self. The organization and form of the handwriting and placement on the page have been considered as clues to personality, feelings, and cognitive functioning at the time of the writing. Closely related to writing are other forms of psychomotor projection through which communication takes place—the behaviors connected with the use of media and the choice of clothing, colors, and objects an individual has made. Over a longer period of time, an individual communicates much information by the total effect of behavior, especially small, unconscious, and automatic behaviors in a variety of circumstances.

It is in the communication process between the patient or client and the therapist that the foundations for rapport and trust are laid. The client needs to feel that communications have been heard and understood by someone who has not only some empathy but also some knowledge and skill. The therapist's confidence in his or her abilities and in the profession may be crucial in setting the tone for all future transactions with the client. Four filters affect interactions between people and are significant in their potential for distortion of the observation process[4]:

Perceptual—how sensory stimuli such as color of clothing or perfume affect the way the other person is perceived.

Conceptual—the knowledge base which is brought to the interaction.

Role—the way each person perceives the role to be played in the interaction.

Self-esteem—the way each person feels about himself or herself.

It is useful for the therapist to consider these filters and the ways in which they might affect objectivity in observation.

The occupational therapist is in a position to observe the patient or client in a variety of structured and unstructured situations. The interview, formal testing procedures, and planned activities represent structured opportunities for observation. These usually involve some elements of prediction or expectation on the part of the therapist and will be discussed in the next sections.

The therapist's opportunities to see and interact with clients in situations that are less planned will vary depending upon the setting. If it is possible for the therapist to interact informally and spontaneously with patients in situations where role differentiation may be less clear, information may be available which otherwise might be difficult to obtain. Different perspectives on values, interests, and functional levels, for example, may be gained by seeing the patient in the local snack shop, in the elevator, or at recreational activities. It is desirable when possible to build into the evaluation process some opportunities for informal contact away from the occupational therapy context.

Interview

There are occasions when a health professional may wish to interview a client formally or informally. Probably the most important occasion is the initial interview, undertaken as part of the process of evaluation. The initial interview serves several vital purposes. It provides for (1) collection of information about the client to help develop objectives and a plan for treatment, (2) establishment of understanding on the part of the client about the role of the therapist and purposes of the occupational therapy process, and (3) opportunity for the client to discuss and reflect about his or her situation and to think about plans for change.

Benjamin in the *The Helping Interview*[5] refers to both external and internal factors that are important and need careful consideration in preparing for an interview. The external factors refer to such things as the room in which the interview is to take place and the extent to which the place will be private, free of interruptions and other distractions. Internal factors are the attitudes, knowledge, and feelings that the interviewer brings to the interview. It is important for the therapist to be clear about the purpose of the interview, to know specifically the kinds of information desired, to be self-trusting, and to be honest.

Allen, in a paper presented at the American Occupational Therapy Association Annual Conference in October 1976,[6] points out there are two essential requirements for the therapist to be able to conduct a successful interview with a patient: a solid knowledge base and skills in active listening. These requirements are not simple. They necessitate study, preparation, and practice. The solid knowledge base must underly the therapist's selection of questions or areas to be covered in the interview. It is important that the interview reflect what the therapist knows and cover areas that will be relevant to treatment in occupational therapy. Active listening means that the interviewer plays a vital, deeply involved role, which demonstrates genuine respect for the patient or client.

Benjamin[7] delineates three parts to an interview: initiation, development, and closing. In the initiation phase the interviewer explains the purpose of the interview and his or her role in relation to the person interviewed, and begins to establish some level of mutual trust and understanding. It is during the initiation phase that the interviewer should define the parameters of the interview—the amount of time it should take, the kind of material to be discussed, and the uses to be made of the information.

During the development phase the interviewer seeks information and explores issues with the person interviewed. The occupational therapist doing an initial interview as an evaluation procedure should bring some form of outline or a list of planned questions to the interview to be certain that information vital to the future process of setting objectives and treatment planning will be covered. The kinds of questions the occupational therapist may ask should allow the patient to respond with more than a simple "yes" or "no" answer. The occupational therapist needs to have skill in asking one question at a time, tolerating silence, listening carefully, observing both verbal and nonverbal responses, restating or clarifying questions when needed, and encouraging the client to continue or to stay on the track.

Clues marking the end of the interview are either the end of the time as defined in the beginning of the interview or the end of the list of questions or issues to be explored. It is important for both the therapist and the client to know that the interview is coming to a close. No new material should be brought up at this point. It is best to plan another time and place to discuss new material. Summarizing the material which has been discussed may be a useful way to terminate the interview as well as to double-check on the accuracy of information gained.

The therapist will need to make notes unless he or she has an unusual memory and time to record the interview later. The purpose of writing notes (or using a tape recorder) should be explained to the client at the beginning of the interview. The client should also be told that he or she may read the notes or listen to the tape and that their sole purpose is to provide valid guidelines for the occupational therapy process.

Sometimes it is useful to have clients answer a simple questionnaire before coming to the interview. The use of the questionnaire has some advantages. It may save time in situations where setting aside thirty to forty-five minutes for personal interviewing of each client initially is not feasible. It can provide information about the client's ability to read and to respond in an organized fashion in writing. The disadvantage is that some of the richness of detail and interaction will be lost. A written questionnaire can never completely replace a face-to-face interview.

The kinds of information which are best gained through an interview may vary somewhat according to the kind of population and the general context for treatment. In general the occupational therapist may learn about education; work experience; leisure interests and pursuits; the way patients' balance their work, sleep, and play and manage time; the quality and extent of their care for their own personal needs (grooming, nutrition, laundry, housekeeping, hygiene); the families or significant people in households; friends or other family members who are supportive; the communities in which they live; their values and familiar objects; their own assessment of their current situations and problems; their own personal goals; and current housing situations including potential architectural barriers.

Knowledge about the success or failure of the patient's early skills in fulfilling roles of his or her life contains important clues to the kinds of experiences which should be provided in occupational therapy. The importance of collecting information about the history has been outlined by Moorehead:

> In gathering occupational history, the investigator is concerned with discovering how and under what conditions the individual patient has learned to approach tasks and role expectations as he does; and whether he was ever more competent than he now appears. Can the therapist expect that the patient will be able to improve his role skills, and if so, how much? In other words, the investigator asks what a patient's particular life style is in terms of occupational function, so that therapy can be structured for him to build upon his experiences for improved function.[8]

A terminal interview, undertaken just before the client leaves treatment, serves other important functions. It gives the client and therapist an opportunity to look together at what has taken place and to identify some of the things that have been learned in the process. Often the occupational therapy experience may be significant in helping the patient know how to balance activities at home. He/she learns what activities provide exercise or energy conservation or are integrative and provide energy release. A final interview helps to reinforce this learning.

Inventories and Check Lists

An adjunct to the interview is the check list, in which the client is asked to respond on paper to questions regarding interests, hobbies, and desires. One such list, which was developed by Janice Matsutsuyu[9] has been widely adapted and used (Table 10-1). When play is considered as the ground from which work behaviors emerge and as a clue to the adult activities that are experienced as integrative and pleasurable, this kind of data can be exceedingly useful. Another inventory which is useful is the Activities Configuration developed by Sandra Watanabe (Table 10-2). This may be used to identify the qualitative aspects of the ways in which a person meets his or her needs in life.

Table 10-1. Interest check list.

Name: ....Unit: ....Date: ....

Please check each item below according to your interest.

Activity	*Interest*		
	Casual	*Strong*	*No*
1. Gardening			
2. Sewing			
3. Poker			
4. Languages			
5. Social Clubs			
6. Radio			
7. Bridge			
8. Car Repair			
9. Writing			
10. Dancing			
11. Needlework			
12. Golf			
13. Football			
14. Popular Music			
15. Puzzles			
16. Holidays			
17. Solitaire			
18. Movies			
19. Lectures			
20. Swimming			
21. Bowling			
22. Visiting			
23. Mending			
24. Chess			
25. Barbecues			
26. Reading			
27. Traveling			
28. Manual Arts			
29. Parties			
30. Dramatics			
31. Shuffleboard			
32. Ironing			
33. Social Studies			
34. Classical Music			
35. Floor Mopping			
36. Model Building			
37. Baseball			
38. Checkers			
39. Singing			
40. Home Repairs			
41. Exercise			
42. Volleyball			
43. Woodworking			
44. Billiards			
45. Driving			
46. Dusting			
47. Jewelry Making			
48. Tennis			
49. Cooking			
50. Basketball			
51. History			
52. Guitar			
53. Science			
54. Collecting			
55. Ping Pong			
56. Leatherwork			
57. Shopping			
58. Photography			
59. Painting			
60. Television			
61. Concerts			
62. Ceramics			
63. Camping			
64. Laundry			
65. Dating			
66. Mosaics			
67. Politics			
68. Scrabble			
69. Decorating			
70. Math			
71. Service Groups			
72. Piano			
73. Scouting			
74. Plays			
75. Clothes			
76. Knitting			
77. Hairstyling			
78. Religion			
79. Drums			
80. Conversation			

Please list other special interests:

Table 10-2. Activity configuration.

Weekly Schedule of:____________________ Therapist: ____________________

Typical week at home:_____ in hospital:_____ in day care:_____

Part I

Directions: List in detail *all* activities which are a part of your day.

Morning	*Mon.*	*Tues.*	*Wed.*	*Thurs.*	*Fri.*	*Sat.*	*Sun.*
7:00– 9:00 9:00–11:00 11:00– 1:00 Afternoon							
1:00– 3:00 3:00– 5:00 5:00– 7:00 Evening							
7:00– 9:00 9:00–11:00							

Part II

Directions: List each activity (once) that you included in Part I. Use as many sheets as necessary. Rate all activities according to the rating scale attached.

List Activities	**Function** A	**Autonomy** B_1	 B_2	**Adequacy** C

Rating Scale

A. Function
1. Work
2. Chore
3. Education
4. Skill practice
5. Exercise
6. Recreation
7. Social activity
8. Rest
9. Therapy
10. Your own designations

B_1. Autonomy
1. Have to do it
2. Want to do it
3. Both

B_2. Autonomy
1. IG—I want to do this and I think this is good
2. IN—I want to do this and I think this is not good
3. OG—Others make me do this and I'm glad they do
4. ON—Others make me do this and I wish they didn't

C. Adequacy
1. I do this very well
2. I do this well enough
3. I don't do this well enough

Adapted by Sandra Watanabe from materials from the 1968 Regional Institute on the Evaluation Process sponsored by the American Occupational Therapy Association. Final Report RSA-123-T-68, New York, 1968, pp. 46–47. Reprinted with permission of Sandra Watanabe.

Object History

One useful way of learning about a patient's or client's values and the cultural system to which he or she belongs is the object history. It is a flexible evaluation tool and may be incorporated into the formal interview, into informal conversations, or in written form. It may be done individually or in a group and often serves the purpose of establishing a rapport between the individuals involved by permitting exploration of mutualities in background and experience. It may also provide some important clues about the early beginnings of the patient's pathology. The object history simply asks the client to try to remember something that was important or that he or she valued at earlier periods of life and to explain why it was important or valued. For example, a young man recalled a bush in front of his house where he went to hide as a child whenever he was scolded. In this statement one can learn that the world of nature may represent refuge to him. Another person recalled an erector set with which he felt he could build anything mechanical in the whole world. Thus one can learn that mechanical things represent pleasure in accomplishment for him. A young woman recalled a stereo set to which she used to dance. In this one can learn that social dancing once was important to her. Through the exploration of important nonhuman objects the therapist may learn both the kinds of things that might be integrative to the client and the ability that the client has had in the past to use the nonhuman world to meet emotional needs.

SUMMARY

Evaluation of the patient's or client's physical or psychological condition is indicated when a suspected or obvious problem exists. Those procedures chosen depend upon the diagnosis, medical reports, interview, patient or client life style, interests and needs, observations made by the therapist, and checklists previously prepared by the patient/client. Special areas such as perceptual-motor function, activities of daily living, or prevocational evaluation, and others may also be indicated. The remainder of this chapter deals with specific evaluation procedures utilized by occupational therapists in problem identification.

REFERENCES

1. Gillette, N.: Occupational therapy and mental health. In Willard, H. S., and Spackman, C. S. (eds.): Occupational Therapy, ed. 4. Philadelphia: J. B. Lippincott Co., 1971, p. 79.
2. Ibid.
3. Freedman, A., Kaplan, H., and Saddock, B.: Modern Synopsis of Comprehensive Textbook of Psychiatry/II. Baltimore: Williams & Wilkins Co., 1976, p. 146.
4. Fidler, Gail S.: Talk given at Medical College of Georgia. Augusta, Georgia, 1976.
5. Benjamin, A.: The Helping Interview. Boston: Houghton Mifflin Co., 1974.
6. Allen, C.: The Performance Status Examination. Paper presented at the American Occupational Therapy Association Annual Conference, San Francisco, October 1976.
7. Benjamin: Helping Interview.
8. Moorehead, L.: The occupational history. Am. J. Occup. Ther. 23:331, 1969.
9. Matsutsuyu, J.: The interest checklist. Am. J. Occup. Ther. 23:323–328, 1969.

BIBLIOGRAPHY

Garrett, A.: Interviewing: Its Principles and Methods. New York: Family Service Association of America, 1972.

Hurff, J.: A play skills inventory. In Reilly, M. (ed.): Play as Exploratory Learning. Beverly Hills, Sage Publications, 1974.

Knox, S.: A play scale. In Reilly, M. (ed.): Play as Exploratory Learning. Beverly Hills, Sage Publications, 1974.

Llorens, L.: Projective techniques in occupational therapy. Am. J. Occup. Ther. 21:266, 1967.

Takata, N.: The play history. Am. J. Occup. Ther. 23:314–318, 1969.

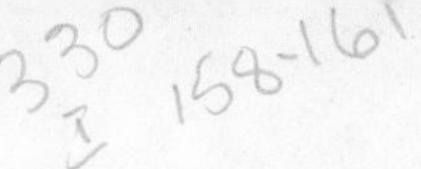

section 2/Specific Evaluation Procedures/Helen D. Smith

MANUAL MUSCLE TESTING

Manual muscle testing (M.M.T.) is a procedure which determines the strength of a muscle through manual evaluation. Rating is done by having the patient or client move the part through its full range against gravity and then against gravity and resistance. When the patient or client cannot perform the motion against gravity the part is positioned to eliminate gravity and then the muscle power is reevaluated. Manual muscle testing should not be used when spasticity is present since the increased tone invalidates the results.

Procedure

1. Check the client's passive range of motion (R.O.M.) before beginning M.M.T.
2. Position patient or client so that the muscle will be tested against gravity.
3. Stabilize the joint above the one being tested to prevent substitution of incorrect muscles.
4. Have client perform the motion and observe the performance.
5. Palpate muscle performing the motion to be sure it is contracting.
6. Apply resistance into the opposite motion of the one being performed. (Resistance should be applied before the extreme end of the R.O.M.)
7. Grade the muscle strength.
8. In order to maintain reliability and accuracy, the same therapist should repeat this test on the patient or client at the same time of day.
9. Enter the results of each test, sign and date.

Grading Scale

N Normal—complete R.O.M. against gravity with full resistance.
G Good —complete R.O.M. against gravity with some resistance.
F Fair —complete R.O.M. against gravity.
P Poor —complete R.O.M. with gravity eliminated.
T Trace —evidence of contractility on palpation. No joint motion.
0 Zero —no evidence of contractility.

See Figure 10-1 for sample form for manual muscle testing.

JOINT RANGE OF MOTION—GONIOMETRY

Joint range of motion (R.O.M.) is measured to determine existing freedom of motion at a joint. This is either done passively (part moved by an outside force) or actively (part moved by muscle contraction, i.e., muscle power.) Causes of decreased R.O.M. can be spasticity, weakness, or a bone block. When a difference is noted between active and passive R.O.M. in the same joint it is an indication of muscle weakness.

Types of Motion

Passive Motion is movement performed by an outside force. No muscle contraction can be seen or palpated. *Active Motion* is movement performed independently by the individual.

Measurement Tool

The goniometer (Fig. 10-2) is the most frequently used tool for measurement of joint motion. Other methods used either alone or in conjunction with the goniometer are a ruler to measure distance (used especially in hand evaluation); photographs of the client performing the motion(s); outline drawings, for example, tracing the fingers while in abduction; and hand prints made by inking hands on a stamp pad and pressing on paper.

Procedure

1. To maintain reliability and accuracy each time the same therapist should measure the client using the same method at the same time of day.
2. When measuring the upper extremity use anatomical position as a starting position when pos-

CLINICAL RECORD—MANUAL MUSCLE EVALUATION

Name ____________________

Age ____________________

Diagnosis ____________________

LEFT | RIGHT

Examiner's Initials

Date

	ACTION	PRIME MOVERS	INNERVATION	SP. C. LEVEL	
NECK					NECK
	Flexion	STERNOCLEIDOMASTOID	Spinal Accessory,	C 2-3	
	Extension	EXTENSOR GROUP	Spinal Accessory,	C 1-8	
TRUNK	Flexion	RECTUS ABDOMINUS		T 5-12	TRUNK
	Rotation	EXTERNAL OBLIQUE		T 5-12	
		INTERNAL OBLIQUE		T 5-12	
	Extension	Thoracic	Post. Rami Spinal Nerves		
		Lumbar			
	Pelvic Elevation	QUADRATUS LUMBORUM		T 12 L 1-3	
HIP	Flexion	ILIOPSOAS	Femoral	L 2-4	HIP
		SARTORIUS	Femoral	L 2-4	
	Extension	GLUTEUS MAXIMUS	Inf. Gluteal	L 5 S 1-2	
	Abduction	GLUTEUS MEDIUS	Superior Gluteal	L 4-5 S 1	
		TENSOR FASCIA LATAE	Superior Gluteal	L 4-5 S 1	
	Adduction		Obturator	L 2-4	
	External Rotation			L 3 S 3	
	Internal Rotation			L 4 S 1	
KNEE	Flexion	BICEPS FEMORIS	Sciatic	L 5 S 1-2	KNEE
		SEMITENDINOSUS SEMIMEMBRANOSUS	Tibial	L 5 S 1-3	
	Extension	QUADRICEPS	Femoral	L 2-4	
ANKLE	Inversion	ANTERIOR TIBIALIS	Deep Peroneal	L 5 S 1-2	ANKLE
		POSTERIOR TIBIALIS	Tibial	L 4-5 S 1-2	
	Eversion	PERONEUS LONGUS	Sup. Peroneal	L 4-5 S 1	
		PERONEUS BREVIS	Sup. Peroneal	L 4-5 S 1	
	Plantar Flexion	GASTROCNEMIUS	Tibial	S 1-2	
		SOLEUS	Tibial	S 1-2	
TOES	Flexion	DIGITORUM LONGUS	Tibial	L 5 S 1-2	TOES
		DIGITORUM BREVIS	Tibial	L 5 S 1-2	
	Extension	DIGITORUM LONGUS & BREVIS	Deep Peroneal	L 4-5 S 1	
HALLUX	Flexion	HALLUCIS LONGUS	Tibial	L 5 S 1-2	HALLUX
		HALLUCIS BREVIS	Tibial	L 5 S 1-2	
	Extension	HALLUCIS LONGUS	Deep Peroneal	L 4-5 S 1-2	

KEY:

5	N	NORMAL	Complete range of motion against gravity with full resistance
4	G	GOOD	Complete range of motion against gravity with some resistance
3	F	FAIR	Complete range of motion against gravity
2	P	POOR	Complete range of motion with gravity eliminated
1	T	TRACE	Evidence of slight contractility. No joint motion
0	0	ZERO	No evidence of contractility

FIGURE 10-1. Manual muscle evaluation form. Printed with permission of Moss Rehabilitation Hospital, Department of Physical Therapy, Philadelphia PA.

CLINICAL RECORD—MANUAL MUSCLE EVALUATION (Cont.)

Name ______________ Age ______ Diagnosis ______________

LEFT				ACTION		PRIME MOVERS		INNERVATION	SP. C. LEVEL		RIGHT		
			Examiner's Initials										
			Date										
				ACTION		PRIME MOVERS		INNERVATION	SP. C. LEVEL				
			SCAPULA	Elevation		UPPER TRAPEZIUS		Spinal Accessory	C 3-4	SCAPULA			
				Adduction		MID TRAPEZIUS		Spinal Accessory	C 3-4				
						RHOMBOIDS		Dorsal Scapular	C 4-5				
				Abduction		SERRATUS ANTERIOR		Long Thoracic	C 5-7				
				Depression		LOWER TRAPEZIUS		Spinal Accessory	C 3-4				
			SHOULDER	Flexion		ANTERIOR DELTOID		Axillary	C 5-6	SHOULDER			
				Abduction		MIDDLE DELTOID		Axillary	C 5-6				
				Horizontal Adduction		PECTORALIS MAJOR Clavicular		Ant. Thoracic	C 5-8				
						Sternal			C 5 T 1				
				Extension		LATISSIMUS DORSI		Thoracodorsal	C 5-8				
				Horizontal Abduction		POST. DELTOID		Axillary	C 5-6				
				External Rotation					C 5-6				
				Internal Rotation					C 5-8				
			ELBOW	Flexion		BICEPS		Musculocutaneous	C 5-6	ELBOW			
						BRACHIALIS		Musculocutaneous	C 5-6				
						BRACHIORADIALIS		Radial	C 6				
				Extension		TRICEPS		Radial	C 5-8				
			FORE ARM	Supination		SUPINATOR		Radial	C 6	FORE ARM			
				Pronation		PRONATOR TERES		Median	C 6				
			WRIST	Flexion		CARPI RADIALIS		Median	C 6	WRIST			
						CARPI ULNARIS		Ulnar	C 8				
				Extension		CARPI RADIALIS L. & BREV.		Radial	C 6-7				
						CARPI ULNARIS		Radial	C 7				
			FINGERS	Flexion MP joint		LUMBRICALES	1,2	Median	C 7-8	FINGERS			
							3,4	Ulnar	C 8				
				Prox.	IP joint	DIG. SUBLIMUS		Median	C 7 T 1				
				Dist.	IP joint	DIG. PROFUNDUS	1,2	Median	C 8 T 1				
							3,4	Ulnar	C 8 T 1				
				Extension		DIG. EXT. COMMUNIS		Radial	C 6				
				Adduction		INTEROSSEI		Ulnar	C 8 T 1				
				Abduction		INTEROSSEI		Ulnar	C 8 T 1				
				Abduction, digit 4		DIGITI QUINTI		Ulnar	C 8				
				Opposition, digit 4		OPPONENS DIGITI QUINTI		Ulnar	C 8				
			THUMB	Flexion	MP joint	POLL. BREV.		Median	C 6-8	THUMB			
					IP joint	POLL. L.		Median	C 8 T 1				
				Extension	MP joint	POLL. BREV.		Radial	C 7				
					IP joint	POLL. L.		Radial	C 7				
				Adduction		ADDUCTOR POLLICIS		Ulnar	C 8				
				Abduction		POLL. L.		Radial	C 7				
						POLL. BREV.		Median	C 6-7				
				Opposition		OPPONENS POLLICIS		Median	C 6-8 T 1				

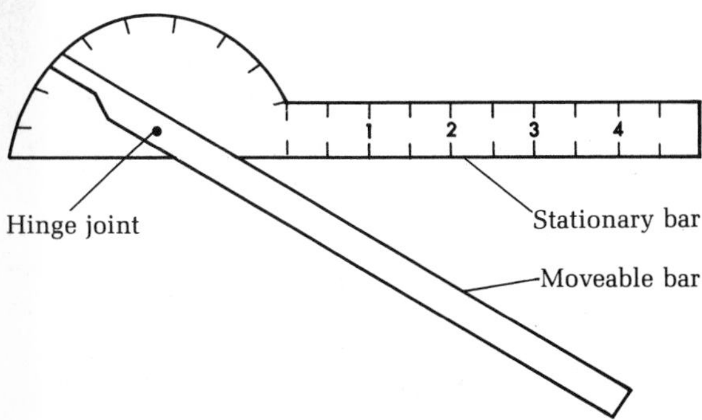

FIGURE 10-2. Goniometer.

sible. The starting position is recorded as zero degrees. Some exceptions to starting in anatomical position are shoulder internal and external rotation and forearm supination and pronation.

3. Prevent substitution by positioning and stabilizing the joint proximal to the joint being measured.

4. Check both passive and active R.O.M. when indicated.

5. Align the stationary bar parallel to the long axis of the stationary bone.

6. Align the movable bar parallel to the long axis of the movable bone.

7. The axis of the goniometer should be aligned with the joint axis.

8. Measure both the starting position and the maximum range. This indicates the arc through which the part moves thus giving the freedom of motion at the joint.

9. Compare with opposite extremity or, if amputee, compare with a chart giving average joint R.O.M.

10. Indicate whether active or passive motion is being measured.

11. Record degrees of motion on a R.O.M. form (see Figs. 10-3 and 10-4).

12. When a patient or client is unable to reach zero degrees starting position (the normal position for that joint), indicate by stating number of degrees of motion from zero (Example: −10 degrees of elbow extension).

13. Indicate if any pain, swelling, or spasticity is present.

14. Enter the results of each test, sign, and date.

SENSORY TESTING

Sensory testing is performed when the therapist suspects that a sensory problem might exist. A client with neurological disease or damage should always be tested for sensory loss. The following areas are usually examined: tactile sense, temperature, proprioception (position sense), and stereognosis.

General Procedure

1. Explain the test procedure to the client. Ask for feedback to be sure instructions are understood.

2. Occlude vision of the patient or client with a blindfold, if acceptable, a shield, or have him or her voluntarily close eyes.

3. Test distally to proximally.

4. Enter the test results, date, and sign.

Specific Procedure

1. *Tactile sense:* Test for recognition and localization of sharp and dull stimuli using a pencil or a safety pin. Test two point discrimination using a compass. Texture discrimination is tested using smooth and rough objects.

2. *Temperature:* Test for the recognition of hot and cold using test tubes filled with hot and cold water.

3. *Proprioception* (position sense): Move body part up or down. Have the client indicate up or down or duplicate the motion with the opposite extremity.

4. *Stereognosis:* Familiar objects of various size, shape, and weight are placed individually into the palm of the client who is to indicate what object was placed in the hand. If the object cannot be manipulated, the therapist manipulates the object making sure contact is made with the fingers and thumb. If the client cannot communicate verbally, an alternative is to have him/her point to the object. Familiar objects such as a coin, key, pencil, or safety pin are examples of objects that are frequently used.

Sample Rating Scale

Intact—A quick, correct response
Impaired—An incorrect or delayed response
Absent—No response

Joint Range of Motion: Upper Extremity

Patient: Age: Diagnosis:

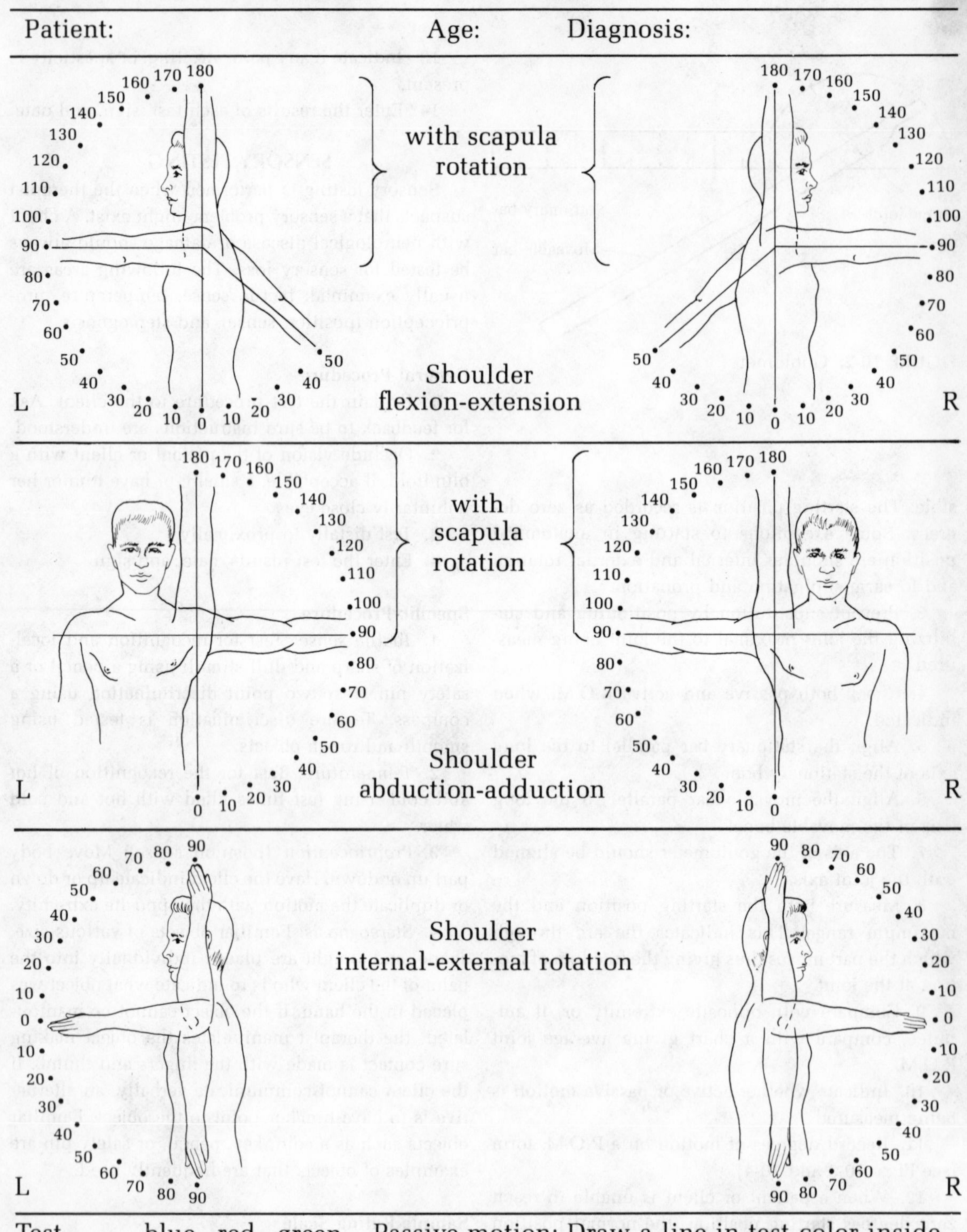

Test	blue red green	Passive motion: Draw a line in test color inside the arc
Date		
Therapist		Active motion: Mark the degrees in test color outside the arc

FIGURE 10-3. Form for measurement of joint range of motion, upper extremity. Redrawn and printed with the permission of Moss Rehabilitation Hospital, Department of Physical Therapy, Philadelphia PA.

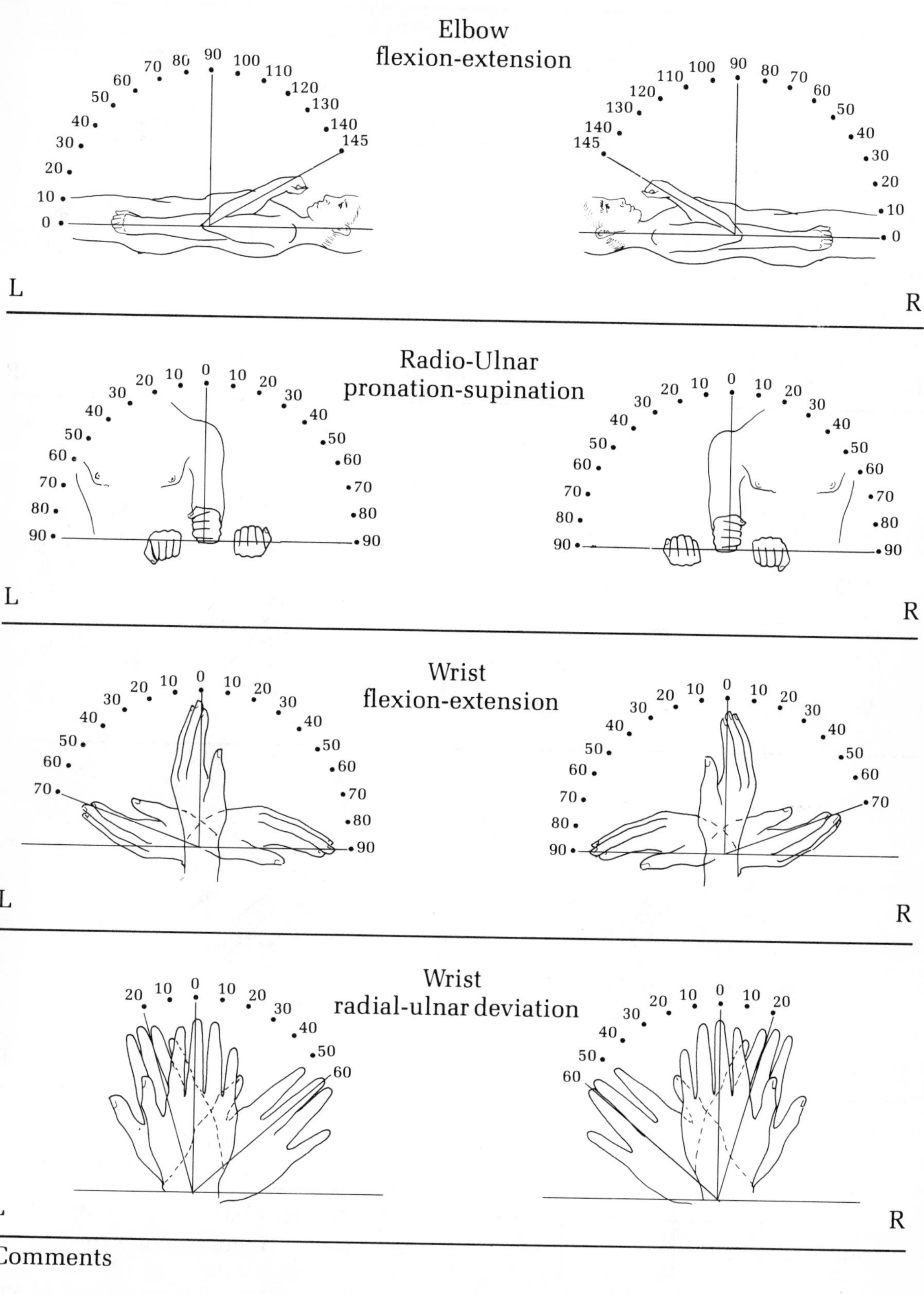
Elbow
flexion-extension
L
R
Radio-Ulnar
pronation-supination
L
R
Wrist
flexion-extension
L
R
Wrist
radial-ulnar deviation
L
R
Comments

Joint Range of Motion: Lower Extremity

Patient: Age: Diagnosis:

Hip flexion-hyperextension (straight knee)

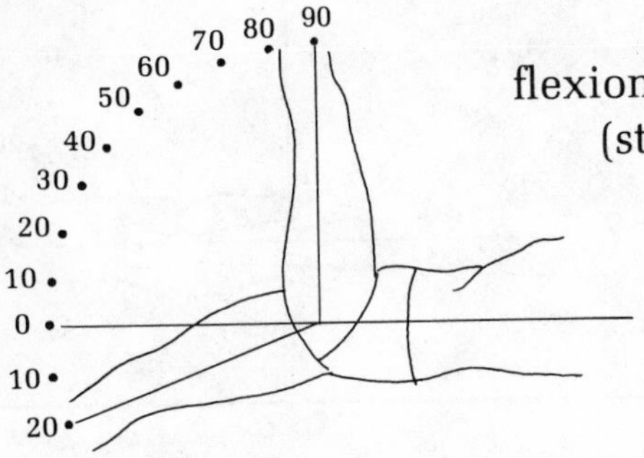

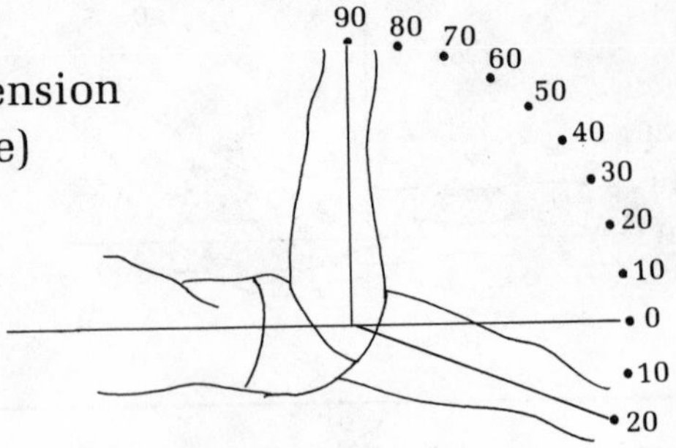

L: 90, 80, 70, 60, 50, 40, 30, 20, 10, 0, 10, 20

R: 90, 80, 70, 60, 50, 40, 30, 20, 10, 0, 10, 20

Hip flexion-(bent knee)

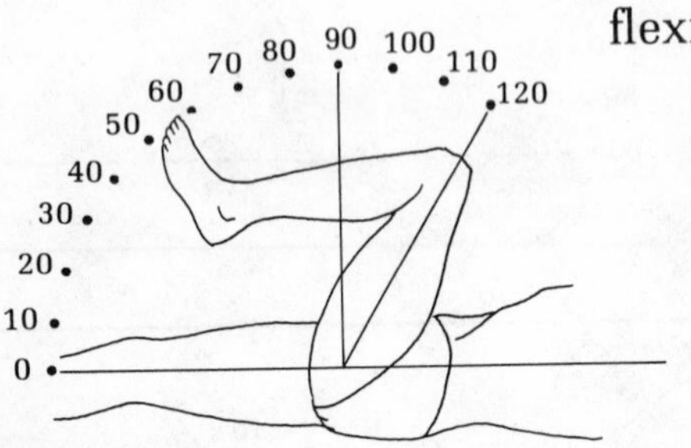

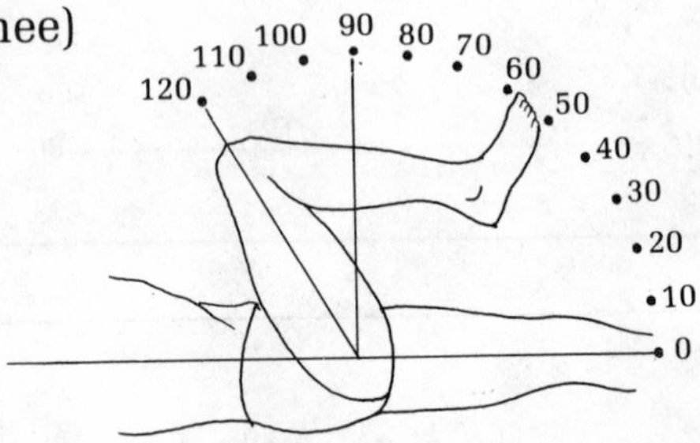

L: 120, 110, 100, 90, 80, 70, 60, 50, 40, 30, 20, 10, 0

R: 120, 110, 100, 90, 80, 70, 60, 50, 40, 30, 20, 10, 0

Hip abduction-adduction

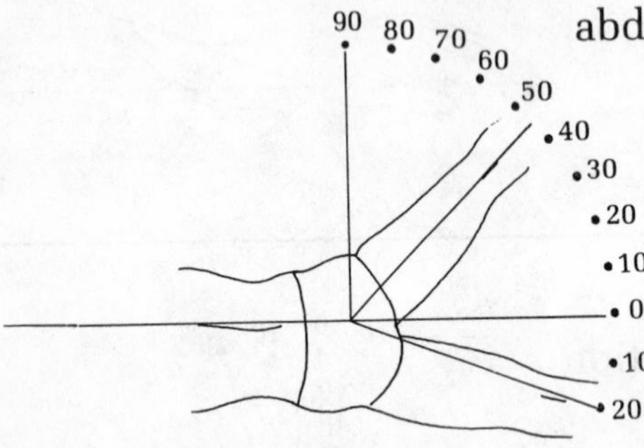

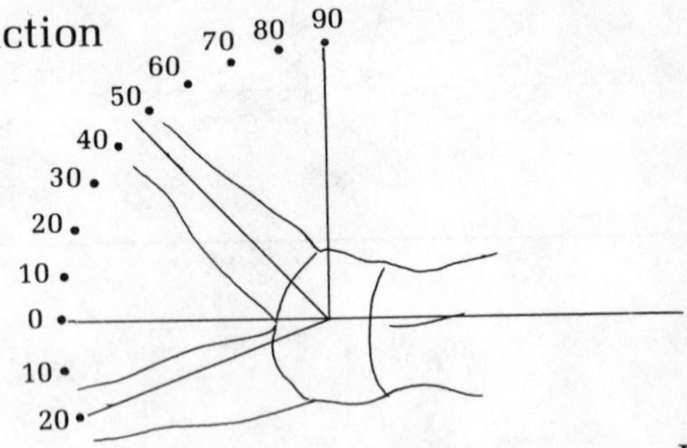

L: 90, 80, 70, 60, 50, 40, 30, 20, 10, 0, 10, 20

R: 90, 80, 70, 60, 50, 40, 30, 20, 10, 0, 10, 20

Test	blue	red	green
Date			
Therapist			

Passive range: Draw a line in test color inside the arc

Active range: Mark the degrees in test color outside the arc

FIGURE 10-4. Form for measurement of joint range of motion, lower extremity. Redrawn and printed with the permission of Moss Rehabilitation Hospital, Department of Physical Therapy, Philadelphia PA.

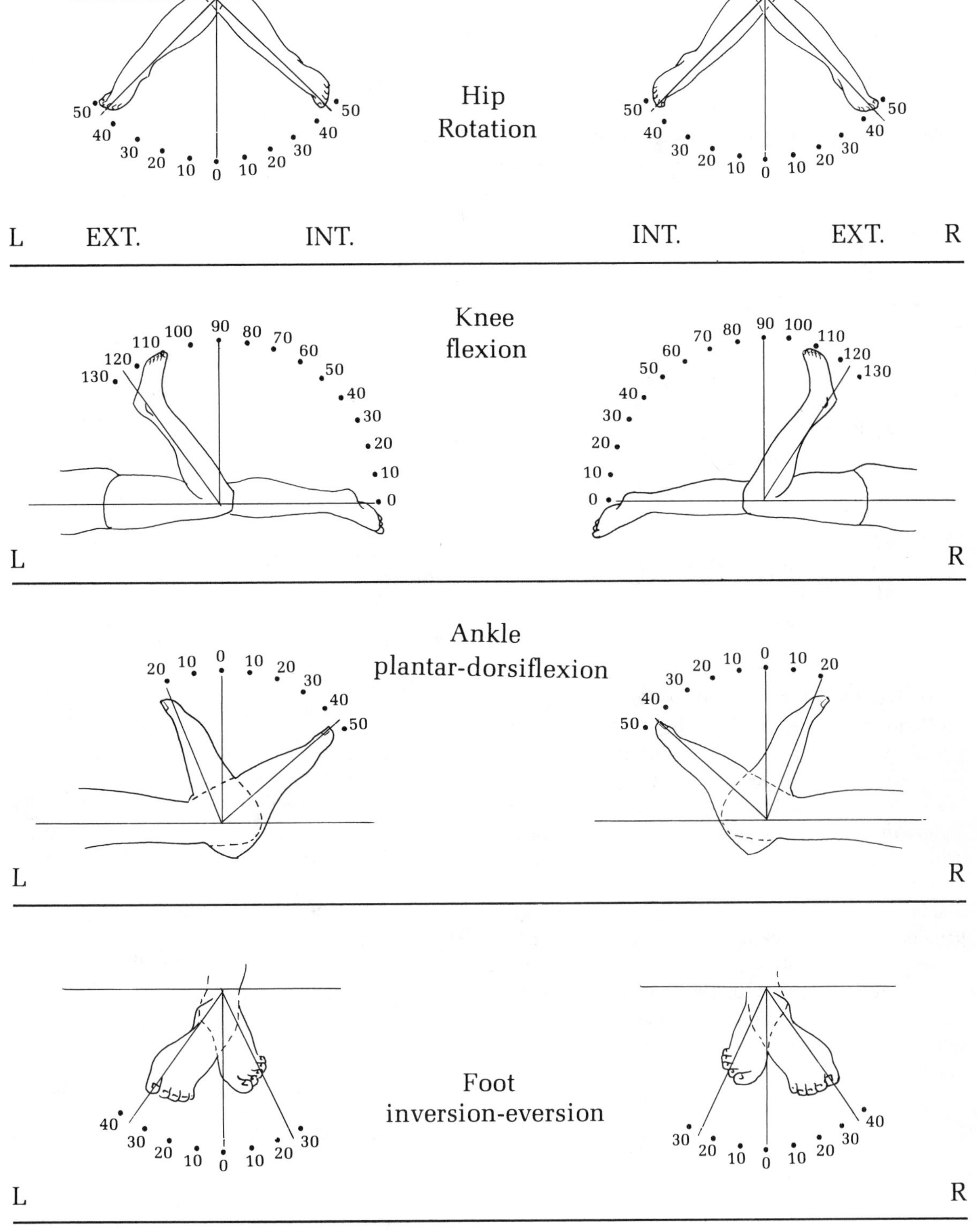

Hip
Rotation
50 40 30 20 10 0 10 20 30 40 50
50 40 30 20 10 0 10 20 30 40 50
L EXT. INT. INT. EXT. R
Knee
flexion
130 120 110 100 90 80 70 60 50 40 30 20 10 0
0 10 20 30 40 50 60 70 80 90 100 110 120 130
L R
Ankle
plantar-dorsiflexion
20 10 0 10 20 30 40 50
50 40 30 20 10 0 10 20
L R
Foot
inversion-eversion
40 30 20 10 0 10 20 30
30 20 10 0 10 20 30 40
L R

Comments

COGNITION

Cognition is the mental process by which knowledge is acquired; it is the ability to think and reason. Following disease or injury in which impairment of cognitive functioning is suspected, the following should be evaluated:

1. Ability to follow simple or complex instructions.
2. Ability to carry over learned skills from one day to the next.
3. Ability to attend to a task (attention span).
4. Ability to follow numerous steps in a process.
5. Ability to understand cause and effect.
6. Ability to problem solve.
7. Ability to concentrate.
8. Ability to perform in a logical sequence.
9. Ability to organize parts into a meaningful whole.
10. Ability to interpret signs and symbols.
11. Ability to read.
12. Ability to compute.

HAND AND PINCH STRENGTH TESTING

Hand strength is measured by the client's gripping a dynamometer. The dial is calibrated in either pounds or kilograms and the indicator will stay at the highest reading until reset manually. An added feature in some dynamometers is an adjustable hand grip.

Pinch strength is measured on a pinch gauge. The dial is calibrated in pounds and measures finger prehension force. A quick reading of the dial must be made if the indicator on the dial does not stay at the highest reading point. Both the dynamometer and the pinch gauge can be purchased through suppliers of physical medicine and rehabilitation equipment.

ENDURANCE TESTING

The patient or client is often tested for the ability to reach or maintain the necessary energy output required to perform an activity. This is especially important in activities of daily living, homemaker retraining, and work-related activities. The amount of work and the time required to do the work are carefully noted, and work output and time are carefully increased according to the tolerance of the client until either the desired level is reached or the client reaches his or her maximum.

STANDARDIZED TESTS

Standardized tests of hand function, motor ability, intelligence, learning disability, development, sensorimotor ability, and personality have been incorporated into Table 10-3. Most information was obtained from Buros in *Mental Measurement Yearbooks*[1–5] with additional material from sources indicated in the table. The tests mentioned in the table are referred to in various chapters of this book. This table is not intended to be a complete listing of all tests used by occupational therapists.

REFERENCES

1. Buros, O. K. (ed.): The Seventh Mental Measurement Yearbook. Highland Park NJ: Gryphon Press, 1972.
2. Buros, O. K. (ed.): The Sixth Mental Measurement Yearbook. Highland Park NJ: Gryphon Press, 1965.
3. Buros, O.K. (ed.): The Fifth Mental Measurement Yearbook. Highland Park NJ: Gryphon Press, 1959.
4. Buros, O. K. (ed.): The Fourth Mental Measurement Yearbook. Highland Park NJ: Gryphon Press, 1953.
5. Buros, O. K. (ed.): The Third Mental Measurement Yearbook. Highland Park NJ: Gryphon Press, 1949.
6. Jebsen, R., et al.: An objective and standardized test of hand function. Arch. Phys. Med. Rehabil. 50:311, 1969.

BIBLIOGRAPHY

Specific Procedures

Daniels, L., Williams, M., and Worthingham, C.: Muscle Testing, ed. 3. Philadelphia: W. B. Saunders Co., 1972.

Joint Motion: Method of Measuring and Recording. Chicago IL: American Academy of Orthopaedic Surgeons, 1965.

Kellor, M., et al.: Hand strength and dexterity. Norms for clinical use, age and sex comparisons. Am. J. Occup. Ther. 25:77–83, 1971.

Moberg, E.: Emergency Surgery of the Hand. London: E. S. Livingston Ltd., 1967.

Weiss, M. W., and Flatt, A. E.: A pilot study of 198 normal children: Pinch strength and hand size in the growing hand. Am. J. Occup. Ther. 25:10–12, 1971.

Werner, J. L., and Omer, G. E.: A procedure—evaluating cutaneous pressure sensation of the hand. Am. J. Occup. Ther. 24:347–356, 1970.

Willard, H. S., and Spackman, C. S. (eds.): Occupational Therapy, ed. 4. Philadelphia: J. B. Lippincott Co., 1971.

Table 10-3. Sampling of tests used in evaluation.

Name	*Type*	*Description*	*Features*	*Source*
		MANUAL DEXTERITY AND MOTOR FUNCTION TESTS		
Jebsen-Taylor Hand Function Test[6]	Individual test to evaluate functional capabilities.	Seven subtests measure major aspects of hand function often used in activities of daily living. Equipment needed: stopwatch	Standardized tasks, objective measurements taken with stopwatch. Norms (360 normal subjects) included. Easy to administer. Test equipment and material are either made or easily available. Subtests are writing, card turning, picking up small objects, simulated feeding, stacking checkers, picking up large light objects, picking up large heavy objects. Time: 12–15 min. Age: Child–adult	Jebsen, R. et al.: Arch. Phys. Med. Rehab. 50:311, 1969. Sand. P.: Am. J. Occup. Ther. 28:87, 1974.
Purdue Pegboard	Individual test to aid selection of employees for industrial jobs requiring manipulative dexterity.	Measures both gross movements of arms, hands, and fingers and fingertip dexterity. Equipment: stop watch	Two operations: rapid placing of pins in pegboard, assembly of pins, washers, and collars. Norms for male industrial applicants, veterans, college students, female college students and industrial applicants Time: 12–15 min. Has Face Validity, Low acceptable reliability	Science Research Associates, Inc., 259 East Erie St., Chicago IL, 60611
Minnesota Rate of Manipulation Test	Individual test of manual dexterity.	Designed to measure dexterity of individuals grade 7 to adult.	Five operations resulting in five scores: placing, turning, displacing, 1-hand turning and placing, and 2-hand turning and placing. Form board used—wells and round discs. Time: 30–50 min.	American Guidance Service, Inc., Publishers Bldg., Circle Pines MN, 55014.
(Oseretsky Tests of Motor Proficiency) Revised: The Lincoln-Oseretsky Motor Development Scale	Scale of motor development. Individual test for hand and arm movements measuring speed, dexterity, coordination, and rhythm.	First published in Russian, 1923. Portuguese adaptation, 1943. English translation, 1946. Sloan adaptation, 1948. Items sample variety of motor performances.	Items arranged in order of difficulty. Instructions concise, scoring is specific. Correlations of each item score with age and tentative percentile norms. Separately and combined scores given for sexes. Validated in relation to changes with age.	C. H. Stoelting Co., 424 N. Hohman Ave., Chicago IL, 60624

Table developed from Buros[1–5] and miscellaneous sources.

Table 10-3. Sampling of tests used in evaluation *(continued)*

Name	Type	Description	Features	Source
MANUAL DEXTERITY AND FUNCTION TESTS				
Pennsylvania Bi-Manual Work Sample	Individual test of bi-manual dexterity: Finger dexterity of both hands, gross movements of both arms, eye-hand coordination, and indication of use of both hands.	Selection of a bolt with one hand and a nut with the other, assembling the two objects and placing in a receiving hole. Norms given for age, sex, blind and partially blind.	First part—assembly of 100 nuts and bolts. Second part—dissassembly of nuts and bolts. Two scores—one for each operation. Time: 10 min. assembly and 5 min. disassembly. Reliable. Validity not indicated.	Educational Test Bureau American Guidance Service, Inc., Publishers Bldg., Circle Pines MN, 55014
Crawford Small Parts Dexterity Test	Individual measure of fine eye-hand coordination and manipulation of small hand tools.	10-inch square board. Round wells for parts to be manipulated, i.e., pins, collars, and screws; a metal plate containing 42 unthreaded and 42 threaded holes; two metal trays beneath the plate to receive the pins and screws. Tools: a tweezer and a small screwdriver.	*Part I*—Examinee picks up pin with tweezer, inserts in small hole in metal plate and places collar over it using preferred hand. *Part II*—Examinee picks up screw, starts it in threaded hole with the fingers, then screws through metal plate with screwdriver, using both hands in operation. 6 practice trials. Scored by time required. Time: *Part I*—5 min. *Part II*—10 min. High reliability Face Validity	Psychological Corporation, 304 East 45th St., New York, NY, 10017
DEVELOPMENTAL TESTS				
Bayley Scales of Infant Development	Individual scales of infant development.	A three-part evaluation of a child's development in relation to other children of the same age. Scales include mental, motor, and behavior ratings.	Well standardized. No data on validity of motor scale or predictive validity of mental scale. Reliability is satisfactory. Testing Time: 45–90 minutes. Age: 2–30 mo.	Psychological Corporation, 304 East 45th St., New York, NY, 10017
The Gesell Developmental Tests	Individual scale of developmental levels.	Scale of behavioral observations by age level (5–10) of the mental growth of the child to aid in determining school readiness.	Qualitative measure of motor development, adaptive behavior, and personal-social behavior. Present functional level is evaluated. Time: 20–30 min.	Programs for Education, Box 85, Lumberville PA, 18933

Brazelton Behavioral Assessment Scale	Individual score of infant interactive behavior.	Evaluates the neonate's reaction to stimuli and responses to the environment.	Best performance is scored. Photographs of testing procedures are included. Testing time: 20–30 min. Research in progress on test reliability and validity.	J. B. Lippincott Co., East Washington Square, Philadelphia, PA, 19105 4 training films: Educational Development Corp., 8 Mifflin Place, Cambridge MA, 02138
Callier-Azusa Scale (1975)	Individual developmental scale for assessment of deaf, blind, and multi-handicapped children.	Designed to be used in a classroom, this scale is divided into five subscales: motor development, perceptual development, daily living skills, language development, and socialization. Subscales are made up of sequential steps describing developmental milestones.	Examples of behavior are provided for many items. (Behaviors were observed on deaf-blind children.) Lists criteria. Observation period to extend over a 2-week period. Reliability information available from author.	Robert Stillman, PhD, Callier Center for Communication Disorders, University of Texas/ Dallas, 1966 Inwood Rd., Dallas TX, 75235
Denver Developmental Screening Test	Individual formalized observations of normal developmental behavior of infants and children.	A screening tool for detecting infants and children with developmental delays. Areas evaluated: gross motor, fine motor, language, and personal-social development.	Standardized on children age 2 wk–6.4 yr. in Denver. High percentage came from professional families. Inexpensive, quick, easy to use. Uses common items. Manual and scoring guide are clear. Reliability and validity vary with age groups.	Ladoca Project and Publishing Foundation, Inc., East 51st Ave. & Lincoln St., Denver CO, 80216
Developmental Screening 0–5 Years	Individual screening inventory of abnormal development.	History and observation ratings in five areas: adaptive, gross motor, fine motor, language, and personal-social. (Selected items were used from the Gesell Developmental Schedules)	Age: 1 yr.–18 mo. No reliability data available. Testing time: 5–30 min.	Knobloch, H., et al.: A developmental screening inventory for infants. Pediatrics 38:1095, 1966.
		SENSORY INTEGRATION TESTS		
Developmental Test of Visual-Motor Integration (Berry, K.)	Test to detect children with problems in visual-motor integration.	Subject is presented with 24 geometric forms arranged in order of increasing difficulty which are then copied into a test booklet.	Standardized test that can be group administered. Emphasis is on preschool group. Directions are clear. Separate age norms for each sex. Two Forms: ages 2–15 (long form), ages 2–8 (short form). Reliability and validity information does not appear complete. Time: 10 min.	Follett Educational Corporation, 1010 W. Washington Blvd., Chicago IL, 60607

Table 10-3. Sampling of tests used in evaluation (*continued*)

Name	*Type*	*Description*	*Features*	*Source*
		SENSORY INTEGRATION TESTS		
Marianne Frostig Developmental Test of Visual Perception	Individual and group test measuring visual perception.	Five subtests of visual perception: eye-motor coordination, figure-ground, constancy of shape, position in space, and spatial relations.	Five areas relate to preschool and early elementary academic performance. Group administration possible. Norms for ages 3–8 yr. Reliability appears adequate. Validity information does not appear to be complete. Testing Time: Individual, 30–45 min.; Group, 40–60 min.	Consulting Psychologists Press, Inc., 577 College Ave., Palo Alto CA, 94306
The Imitation of Gestures: A Technique for Studying the Body Schema and Praxis of Children Three to Six Years of Age.	Individual test of perceptual motor function.	Berges, J., and Lezine, I.: Clin. Develop. Med., No. 18. Spastic Society Medical Education and Information Unit. London: W. Heinemann Medical Books Ltd., 1965.		Medical Market Research Inc., 227 South 6th St., Philadelphia PA, 19105
Perceptual Forms Test	Individual and group testing for perceptual and readiness evaluation and training.	Two Parts: perceptual forms test and incomplete forms in which subject is required to complete partial drawings. Visual-motor coordination is required. Test used to identify children who might have problems in school achievement.	Geometric forms are copied. Templates are used. Formal scoring on the perceptual form test but not on the incomplete forms. Age: 5–8 yr. Reliability and validity information not complete.	Winter Haven Lions Research Foundation, Inc., P.O. Box 111, Winter Haven FL, 33880
The Purdue Perceptual Motor Survey	Individual test of perceptual motor abilities.	Identifies children with perceptual motor problems that could interfere with learning of academic skills. Eleven subtests: rhythmic writing; walking board; jumping; identification of body parts; imitation of movements; obstacle course; chalkboard; Kraus-Weber; angels-in-the-snow; ocular pursuits; developmental drawing.	Test based on theory. Easy to administer and instructions and scoring keys are adequate. Reliability and validity information are said to be good. Age: 6–10 yr. Time: 20 min.	Charles E. Merill Publishing Co., 1300 Alum Creek Drive, Columbus OH, 43216
Southern California Sensory Integration Tests	Individual tests of perceptual motor development. A series of separate tests.	See individual test listings.		Western Psychological Services, 12031 Wilshire Blvd., Los Angeles CA, 90025

Southern California Figure-Ground Visual Perception Test	Individual test of figure-ground.	Assessment of visual perception of a foreground figure superimposed on a background.	Instructions are well done, scoring is simple. Norms available for children 4–10 yr. Test has face validity. Reliability information is questionable. Time: 5–20 min.
Southern California Kinesthesia and Tactile Perception Tests	Individual evaluation of dysfunction in somesthetic perception.	Six subtests: kinesthesia; manual form perception; finger identification; graphesthesia; localization of tactile stimuli; double tactile stimuli perception.	Verbal responses are not required. Studies have shown girls tend to score higher than boys. Norms available for 6-mon. intervals from age 4–0 to 8–6. Reliability and validity are said to be moderate. Time: 15–20 min.
Southern California Motor Accuracy Test	Individual test of motor accuracy.	Assesses the degree of sensorimotor involvement of the CNS in a motor planning task. Involves eye-hand coordination using sensory information from eyes, touch, and proprioceptors.	Requires child to cross midline of body. Both upper extremities are tested and scores are recorded for most accurate and least accurate hand. Norms available for ages 4–0 to 7–11. Reliability and validity are said to be high. Time: 10 min.
Southern California Perceptual-Motor Tests	Individual evaluation of perceptual motor function.	Six subtests: imitation of posture; crossing midline of body; bilateral motor coordination; standing balance with eyes opened and closed.	Verbal responses not required except for two items in right-left discrimination. Manual and protocol sheet can easily be followed. Test administration is not difficult. Norms for ages 4–8 yr. No validity data at this time. Time: 20 min.
Southern California Postrotary Nystagmus test	Individual test of the duration of nystagmus or reflexive eye response to rotary movement	Passive rotation of S sitting in cross-legged position with head in 30° of flexion on freely turning board 10 times in 20 sec. to the left, stop abruptly, and time duration of involuntary eye movement to the nearest sec.; observe excursion of eye movements. Repeat procedure to the right.	Standardized test. Time: 20 sec. to left 10 sec. between 20 sec. to right 50 sec. total Reliability: 0.834 Standard error: Boys—3 sec. Girls—2.6 sec. Reliability coefficient: 0.485

Table 10-3. Sampling of tests used in evaluation *(continued)*

Name	*Type*	*Description*	*Features*	*Source*
		SENSORY INTEGRATION TESTS		
Ayres Space Test	Individual measure of space relations.	Measures speed of perception of stimuli: position in space or directionality and space visualization.	Test consists of 60 items. Form and two blocks presented each time. Difficulty increases throughout test. Norms available from age 3–11 yr. Validity and reliability information appears incomplete. Time: 20–30 min.	
Illinois Test of Psycholinguistic Abilities (I.T.P.A.)	Individual test of cognitive functioning.	A test of language perception and short term memory abilities to assist in diagnosing learning problems.	Visual and auditory channels are used for input. Vocal and motor channels are used for output. Norms on children from slightly above average homes, age 2–10 yr. Reliability is said to be moderate. Time: 45–50 min.	University of Illinois Press, Urbana, IL, 61801
Meeting Street School Screening Test	Individual test to determine children with learning difficulties.	Short battery for children, kindergarten to first grade. Four scores: motor patterning; visual-perceptual motor; language; total score.	No reading required. Reliability and validity data do not appear to be complete. Time: 15–20 min.	Crippled Children and Adults of Rhode Island, Inc., Meeting Street School, 333 Grotto Ave., Providence RI, 02906
		INTELLIGENCE TESTS		
Peabody Picture Vocabulary Test	Individual test of verbal intelligence.	Untimed test which estimates verbal intelligence by measuring hearing vocabulary. Subject chooses one of four pictures after hearing a word.	No reading required. Standardized age range 2.5–18 yr. Content and item validity are good and reliability is said to be adequate.	American Guidance Service, Inc., Publishers Bldg. Circle Pines MN, 55014
Goodenough-Harris Drawing Test	Individual or group test of conceptual and intellectual maturity.	Tests accuracy of observation and development of conceptual thinking, The subject draws a picture of a man, woman, and a self-portrait.	A simple nonverbal test. Norms were established on children 5–15 yr. from four major geographical areas representative of various occupations. Reliability and validity information are said to be adequate. Time: 10–15 min. Age: 3–15 yr.	Harcourt Brace Jovanovich, Inc. 757 3rd Ave. New York, N.Y. 10017

PSYCHOLOGICAL TESTS

Adaptive Behavior Scales	Individual scale assessing adaptive behavior of the mentally retarded and emotionally maladjusted individual.	Evaluation of subject's effectiveness to cope with environmental demands. Twenty-four areas of social and personal behavior are covered.	Easy to administer but hand-scoring is complex. Norms based on institutionalized retardates beginning at age 3. Has face validity but no data on reliability. Time: Children, 20–25 min; Adults, 25–30 min.	American Association on Mental Deficiency, 5201 Connecticut Ave. N.W., Washington DC, 20015
Vineland Social Maturity Scale	Individual performance scale of social maturity	Behavioral observations of self-help, self-direction, locomotion, occupation, communication, and social relations. Provides an evaluation of subject's social competency.	Useful tool for evaluating mentally retarded individual. Includes 117 items. Age: birth to maturity. Time: 20–30 min.	Educational Test Bureau, American Guidance Service, Publishers Bldg., Circle Pines, MN, 55014
Bender-Gestalt Test	Individual or group projective evaluation of personality dynamics.	Measure nonverbal gestalt functioning in perceptual motor area. The subject copies designs.	Evalutes perceptual motor functioning, neurological impairment and maladjustment. Scoring system quantified and objective. Most validity research done on scoring system. No data on reliability. Time: 10 min. Age: 4 and over.	American Orthopsychiatric Association, Inc., 1790 Broadway, New York, NY, 10019
H-T-P, House-Tree-Person Projective Techniques	Individual and group projective test of personality appraisal.	Freehand drawing by subject of a house, tree, and person. Notes are made by tester of behavior of subject.	Quantitative and qualitative scoring. Achromatic and chromatic drawings. Eight assorted color crayons are used. Ages: 5 and over. No norms for ages 5–14. Time: 60–90 min.	Western Psychological Services, 12031 Wilshire Blvd., Los Angeles CA, 90025
Minnesota Multiphasic Personality Inventory (MMPI)	Individual and group nonprojective test measuring psychopathology.	Assesses the type and degree of emotional dysfunction in adults.	Spanish edition is available. Normative and reliability data has not been changed since 1951. Time: Individual, 30–90 min.; Group, 40–90 min. for complete form and 40–75 min. for short version.	The Psychological Corporation, 304 East 45th St., New York NY, 10017

Table 10-3. Sampling of tests used in evaluation (*continued*)

Name	*Type*	*Description*	*Features*	*Source*
		PSYCHOLOGICAL TESTS		
Nurses' Observation Scale for Inpatient Evaluation (NOSIE)	Nonprojective individual rating scale measuring behavioral status and change.	Highly sensitive ward behavior scale which assesses subject's status and change over time.	Seven scores: competence, social interest, personal neatness, irritability, manifest psychosis, and retardation. Easy to use. Norms based on adult male schizophrenics age 55–69. Validity and reliability appear to be adequate. Time: 3–5 min.	Behavior Arts Center, 90 Calla Ave., Floral Park, New York NY, 11001
		OTHER		
Parachek Geriatric Rating Scale	Geriatric rating scale.	Designed to help in planning treatment programs for the geriatric patient. Areas rated: physical capabilities; self-care skills; social-interaction skills.	Items arranged and rated in developmental sequence. A treatment manual is attached. Time: 3–5 min. once a month.	Greenroom Publishing Co., 8512 East Virginia, Scottsdale AZ, 85257

General

Ayres, A. J.: Interrelationships among perceptual-motor functions in children. Am. J. Occup. Ther. 20:68–71, 1966.

Bell, E., et al.: Hand skill measurement, a gauge for treatment. Am. J. Occup. Ther. 30:80, 1976.

Brayman, S.: Measuring device for joint motion of the hand. Am. J. Occup. Ther. 25:173, 1971.

Brazelton, T. B.: Neonatal Behavioral Assessment Scale. Philadelphia: J. B. Lippincott Co., 1973.

Denhoff, E., et al.: Developmental and predictive characteristics of items from the Meeting Street School Screening Test. Develop. Med. Child Neurol. 10:220, 1969.

DeVore, G. L., and Hamilton, G.: Volume measuring of the severely injured hand. Am. J. Occup. Ther. 22:16, 1968.

Fiorentino, M.: Reflex Testing Methods for Evaluating C.N.S. Development, ed. 2. Springfield IL: Charles C Thomas, 1965.

Hasselkus, B. R., and Safrit, M. J.: Measurement in occupational therapy. Am. J. Occup. Ther. 30:429, 1976.

Hurt, S. P.: Considerations in muscle function and their application to disability evaluation and treatment—joint measurement. Am. J. Occup. Ther. (Part 1—1:209, 1947; Part 2—1:281, 1947; Part 3—2:13, 1948.)

Llorens, L.: An evaluation procedure for children 6–10 years of age. Am. J. Occup. Ther. 21:64, 1967.

MacBain, K., and Hill, R.: A functional assessment for juvenile rheumatoid arthritics. Am. J. Occup. Ther. 26:326, 1973.

McNary, H.: Keynote address—A look at occupational therapy. Am. J. Occup. Ther. 12:203, 1958.

Milani-Comparetti, A., and Gidoni, E.: Routine developmental examination in normal and retarded children. Develop. Med. Child Neurol. 9:631, 1967.

Sand, P., et al.: Hand function in children with myelomeningocele. Am. J. Occup. Ther. 28:87, 1974.

Sand, P., et al.: Hand function measurement with educable mental retardates. Am. J. Occup. Ther. 27:138, 1973.

Skerik, S. K., et al.: Functional evaluation of congenital hand anomalies, Part 1. Am. J. Occup. Ther. 25:98, 1971.

Smith, H. B.: Smith hand function evaluation. Am. J. Occup. Ther. 27:244, 1973.

Von Prince, K., and Butler, B.: Measuring sensory functions of the hand in peripheral nerve injuries. Am. J. Occup. Ther. 21:385, 1967.

Weiss, M. W., and Flatt, A. E.: Functional evaluation of the congenitally anomalous hand, Part 2. Am. J. Occup. Ther. 25:139, 1971.

Zimmerman, M.: The functional motion test as an evaluation tool for patients with lower motor neuron disturbances. Am. J. Occup. Ther. 23:49, 1969.

section 3/Selected Developmental Reflexes and Reactions—A Literature Search/Gail Tower

One purpose of the profile given in Table 10-4 is to acquaint the reader with basic reflexes and reactions that are of particular relevance to the therapist. Another equally important purpose, however, is to stress the tremendous variation found within the normal limits of development during the first year of life. Average ages, regarding the time of initial appearance (emergence) and the time when a particular response is fading out of the infant's consistent behavioral repertoire (integration), are available from most of the authorities cited in this literature search. However, the normal age suggested by one authority may vary by as much as six months (in the extreme case, three years) from another authority. This is essential to remember when reflex testing is being used to contribute to a diagnosis of normal or abnormal during the infant's first year of life. There are tremendous variations among normal infants. In fact, deviations from average seem to be the rule rather than the exception. For this reason, the variations encountered in the literature are encompassed in the profile.

The shaded areas of the profile represent the normal time cited most frequently in the literature during which the response was most consistently active. The solid arrows pointing right encompass the youngest age given when a reflex begins to fade (tail of arrow) and the oldest age for normal integration (point of arrow). The wavy arrows pointing left include the youngest age at which a reaction begins to appear (point) and the oldest age for normal appearance (tail).

Despite the accepted fact that obligatory occurrence of a reflex past its expected normal time

Table 10-4. A literature search for a profile of selected developmental reflexes and reactions.

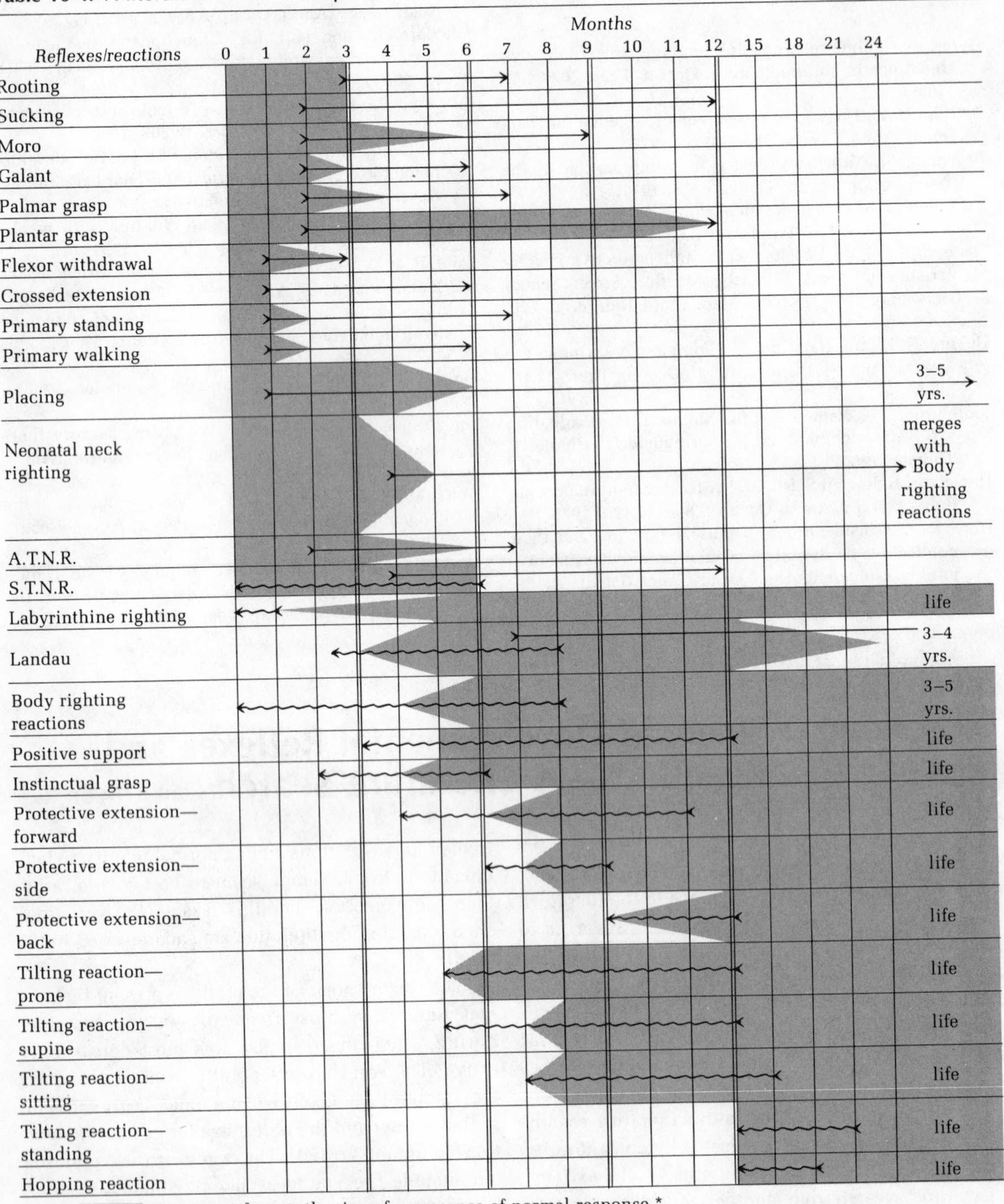

KEY: [shaded] Time most frequently given for presence of normal response.*
[straight arrow] Spans age ranges given for reflex normally fading.
[wavy arrow] Spans age ranges given for response normally emerging.

* With the exception of the last few reactions, there are approximately four references among those listed after each reflex/reaction (see descriptions) which discuss the test and response but do not list definite ages.

may be indicative of central nervous system (CNS) deficit,[1–5] the novice to reflex testing should be aware that reflexes do not just disappear. In many instances (e.g., rooting, sucking, the A.T.N.R., palmar grasp) reflex response is gradually superseded by voluntary willed movement yet remains within the response repertoire of the CNS, either to contribute to normal muscle tone and movement[6,7] or to emerge in some cases of CNS damage at a later time in life.[8] It is also important to note that a positive reflex response at any given time is dependent upon the central state of the nervous system. In other words, the preoccupation or activity of motor neurons at the moment of testing will influence the response seen. This is vividly illustrated in neonatal testing where there are at least four factors having direct bearing upon the testing.

1. The reflex response of the neonate is best determined two or three days postnatally when he has had some time to adjust to the change in his environment and the new demands placed upon him. Responses within those first days are usually characterized as being highly irregular.
2. The physiological and behavioral state of the infant may directly influence whether or not a response is obtained.[9,10]
3. The amount and type of analgesic or anesthetic, especially CNS depressants, used upon the mother during the labor-delivery process may affect the reflex response of the infant.[9,11]
4. The reflexes present in the newborn actually emerge at various times during the gestational period and thus can be used by the physician to help determine the maturity of a premature infant.[12]

An outlined description of each reflex/reaction given in Table 10-4 follows. The reflexes or reactions in parentheses following the name of the response being described refer to those tested in the same way as that presented or to a response so similar to that being elicited that, in the author's opinion, it was testing the same area of integrity.

The references were selected on the basis of clinical relevance and research integrity and as occupying the time-tested position of national or international authority. It is not, however, an exhaustive list.

DESCRIPTIONS

Rooting Reflex

(Reaction of the four cardinal points)[4,5,9,12–20]

Procedure: Place infant supine with head in midline and hands secured against chest. Examiner uses a finger to lightly stroke the perioral skin at the corners of the mouth and the middle of the upper and lower lips.

Response: "After stimulation of the corners of the mouth, there is directed head turning towards the stimulated side. With stimulation of the upper lip there is opening of the mouth and retroflexion of the head. Following stimulation of the lower lip, the mouth opens and the jaw drops. In all instances the infant tries to suck the stimulating finger."[21]

Comments:

1. The tongue generally seeks the stimulus also.
2. This response may be difficult to elicit in satiated or occupied (crying, defecating, etc.) infants who may turn away from the stimulus.

Sucking Reflex[4,5,9,10,12,15,17,18]

Procedure: With the infant supine and head in midline, the examiner inserts a fingertip or nipple into the infant's mouth.

Response: The infant will suck vigorously and rhythmically.

Comments:

1. The soft palate is probably the most sensitive area for eliciting sucking followed by the inside of the mouth and the lips.[9]
2. Sucking may be depressed in infants whose mothers received CNS depressants during the labor-delivery process.[11]
3. Only three of the references[4,5,15] include an age of integration and they vary from two months to one year.

Moro Reflex[1,2,4,5,10,12–15,17–19,22–31]

Procedure: The examiner holds the infant in a semi-seated position, supporting the head in midline with one hand and the back with the other. The infant's hands should not be grasping anything and the neck muscles should be relaxed. Let the head drop a few centimeters before stopping it.

Response: Initially the arms abduct at the shoulders and extend at the elbows and fingers, and the back may arch. This is followed by an adduction-flexion movement back toward the midline. Response in the legs is varied depending upon their initial starting position.

Comments:

1. The Moro reflex is considered one of the most consistently seen and one of the easiest responses to elicit in a normal neonate.
2. A normal response is very sudden in nature so the test should be carried out more than once to observe all response components.
3. An absent or asymmetrical response is generally considered to be indicative of some abnormality, e.g., fractured clavicle, cerebral hemorrhage.
4. A Moro reflex may be seen in response to several different stimuli. Another commonly used stimulus is to slap the table on either side of the supine lying infant's head so as to jar the head.

Galant Reflex (Incurvation reflex)[4,5,10,14,17–19]

Procedure: The infant is placed in prone and the examiner runs a fingernail from shoulder to buttocks about 3 cm. lateral from the vertebral column on either side in turn.

Response: The trunk briskly curves away from the stimulus producing folds in the skin.

Comments:

1. This reflex is considered one of the most constant in the neonatal state.
2. Stimulation of the lateral portion of the trunk produces a greater response than close to the midline.

Palmar Grasp (Hand grasp, tonic finger flexion, tonic grasp)[2,4,5,8,10,12–19,23,26,27,29,31]

Procedure: With the infant supine, head in midline, the examiner inserts his index fingers into the infant's hands from the ulnar side and presses against the palmar surface.

Response: The infant's fingers will strongly flex around the examiner's fingers.

Comments:

1. Sucking facilitates the response.
2. Light contact on the dorsum of the hand inhibits the response and facilitates opening of the hand: the avoidance reaction.
3. Some authorities feel this reflex must be inhibited before voluntary grasp may be developed,[14,17] while others feel there is no definitive relationship between the disappearance of the palmar grasp and the appearance of the voluntary grasp.[31,32]

Plantar Grasp (Tonic reaction of the toe flexors, tonic plantar grasp, foot grasp)[3,5,8,10,14,15,17–19,25,27,29]

Procedure: With the infant supine the examiner presses the shaft of one finger along the metatarsophalangeal groove of the soles of the feet.

Response: There is a strong flexion of the toes as if to grasp the finger.

Comment: The response is strongest with the foot in dorsiflexion.

Flexor Withdrawal (Withdrawal reflex, defense reflex)*[5,10,12,14,15,17,18,24,25,33]

Procedure: Place the infant supine with head in the midline and legs relaxed, i.e., semiflexed. The examiner applies a noxious stimulus, e.g., pinprick, to the sole of each foot in turn.

Response: There is abrupt flexion of the hip and knee and dorsiflexion of the foot on the stimulated side resulting in withdrawal of the leg.

Comments:

1. The response may be diminished in a normal neonate born breech with extended legs.
2. Only three of the references[5,24,25] include an age of integration.

Crossed Extension*[2,3,5,10,12,14,15,17,19,24,25,33]

Procedure: With the infant relaxed in supine, head in the midline, the examiner extends one leg, holds it down, and pricks the sole of the extended leg with a pin.

Response: There is a slow flexion of the unstimulated free leg followed by extension and finally adduction.

Primary Standing (primary righting, neonatal righting)[2–5,12–15,18,20,25,27–29,33]

Procedure: The examiner suspends the infant vertically by supporting the trunk under the axilla. The soles of the infant's feet are then brought into firm contact with the table top.

*Although ages of integration are given for these reflexes, all nociceptive and protective responses are present for life.

Response: There is a general mobilization of extensor tone in the legs and trunk for partial, flat-footed weight bearing. The neonate does not, however, extend hips and knees or trunk fully as later in the positive support reaction.

Comment: An infant may continue to bear weight on his legs in this position throughout the course of development until the positive support for normal standing is fully developed. However, an infant may pass through a period referred to as astasia abasia, refusing to take any weight on the legs (astasia) or step (abasia) until the positive support emerges for standing.

Primary Walking (Stepping response, automatic walking, reflex stepping, walking reflex)[2,3,4,5,10,12–15,17–19,20,25,26,28]

Procedure: The examiner supports the infant under the arms and holds the infant in a standing, weight-bearing position on the table. Tip the trunk slightly forward and gently move the infant forward.

Response: The infant will rhythmically step, alternating legs, in a heel-toe gait. The hips and knees remain in some flexion during this walking.

Comments:

1. It is not true walking because there is little participation of the trunk and only partial weight bearing.
2. The legs may adduct or even cross in the normal neonate.
3. This may be absent in infants born of breech delivery.

Placing (Proprioceptive placing, limb placement reflex, tactile placing)[1,2,4,5,10,12,14,17–19,25,28,33,34]

Procedure: The examiner suspends the infant vertically by supporting the trunk under the axilla. The infant is then moved so the dorsum of the foot makes contact with the under edge of a table.

Response: The infant will flex hip and knee, lifting the foot above the table and then extend the leg, placing the foot firmly on the table top.

Comments:

1. This response is usually tested one foot at a time. If both feet are simultaneously touched, the normal infant will often place one leg before the other.
2. Vision is not required for this response. Visual placing of the limbs occurs at a later date.
3. The times reported in the literature for integration of this reflex vary from one month to five years.
4. The same reflex is present in the hands.[2,5,13,24]

Neonatal Neck Righting[2,5,17,18,24–26]

Procedure: Place the infant supine with head and trunk symmetrical. The examiner passively rotates the infant's head fully to one side.

Response: The trunk rotates as a whole in the direction of the head.

Comment: Some references do not distinguish between the trunk rolling as a whole seen in the neonate and young infant and the segmental rolling seen later in response to the same procedure.[5,18] Many more references are available regarding the latter response. (See Body Righting Reactions.)

Asymmetrical Tonic Neck Reflex (A.T.N.R.)[1,2,5,7,10,14,15,17,18,23–25,27–29,34,35]

Procedure: Place the infant supine with the head in midline, shoulders horizontal. The examiner passively laterally rotates the head to one side and holds the head in that position while observing the response. Repeat to the other side.

Response: Rotation of the head produces extension of the "face" arm and leg and flexion of the "skull" arm and leg. The legs often participate less vigorously than the arms.

Comments:

1. Infants may assume this position by actively turning their heads.
2. This response is never consistently obligatory in a normal infant.
3. There may be a response delay of many seconds in infants with CNS pathology.
4. The response may be manifested only through distribution of muscle tone which the examiner must then feel by passively moving the extremities.

Symmetrical Tonic Neck Reflex (S.T.N.R.)[1,2,5,17,24,25,27]

Procedure: Place the infant on hands and knees or prone over examiner's knees if unable to assume the quadriped position. Passively extend and flex the head.

Response: Extension of the infant's head results in extension of the arms and flexion of the legs. Flexion of the head results in flexion of the arms and extension of the legs.

Comments:

1. As with the A.T.N.R., the response may be manifested more by tone changes in the extremities than by actual movement.
2. There is a paucity of information in the literature regarding this reflex in the human. In addition, there is *considerable* variance regarding time of appearance and of integration.

Labyrinthine Righting (Otolith righting)[2,4,5,13–15,17,18,20,23–25,27,34]

Procedure: Suspend the infant vertically, supporting under the axilla. Tilt the body anteriorly, posteriorly, and laterally to each side.

Response: The infant will right the head to vertical from all of the positions.

Comments:

1. Vision is not required so the infant may be blindfolded to eliminate its effects.
2. It is generally felt that the response is first manifested in the prone position at birth or shortly after, then in the upright by 3 to 4 months and finally in supine by about 6 months, yielding normal head control. Several of the references do not differentiate the position of the infant but generally state that the reaction begins at a given time and persists throughout life.

Landau Reflex (Horizontal or prone suspension in space)[2,4,5,14,15,17–19,24,25,27,29]

Procedure: The examiner supports the infant prone in space so the trunk is resting on the examiner's hands (arms) with the infant's head and hips free of support.

Response: The head extends to above the horizontal, extensor tone in the back increases, and the back arches and the hips extend.

Comments:

1. There is great variance in the literature regarding the length of time that this response persists (past six to eight months) in the normal infant.
2. The Landau reflex probably is a combination of righting reactions and tonic reflex activity.[5,18,36]

Body Righting Reactions (Rotative neck righting, body righting on head, body righting on body)[2,3,5,6,15,17,18,24,26–29,33,34,37]

Procedure: (a) Place the infant supine with head and body symmetrical. The examiner passively flexes the infant's leg and then adducts it across the infant's body, thereby rotating the pelvis or (b) the examiner passively rotates the infant's head to one side.

Response: Depending upon the body part passively rotated, the infant will actively, segmentally rotate the rest of the trunk, i.e., in (a) above, the infant's shoulders will rotate followed by the head and in (b) above, the infant's shoulders will rotate after the head followed by the hips.

Comment: There is more reference in the literature to the righting reactions in animals than in humans[33,37] where the body righting reactions are separated into neck righting (see Neonatal Neck Righting), body righting on the body, and body righting on the head.

Positive Support[2–5,14,15,18,19,23,26–29,33–35]

Procedure: The examiner supports the infant under the axilla, suspends the infant vertically in space and lowers the infant so the soles of the feet firmly contact the floor.

Response: The infant will bear full body weight with knees, hips, and trunk extended.

Comment: An infant who is pulling himself or herself to standing exhibits a positive support reaction.

Instinctual Grasp (Voluntary grasp)[4,5,8,13–15,17,23,29,38,39]

Procedure: With the infant in any position in which the arms and hands are free, the examiner lightly strokes any portion of the infant's hand.

Response: The infant will grope after the stimulus and grasp it.

Comments:

1. Vision does not play a role in this response.[5,8,39] Some authorities describe visually directed grasp which is not generally considered to be

reflexive in nature.[35,40] Other authorities simply speak of the development of voluntary grasp without specifically referring to vision.[4,13–15,17,23,29,38] These references were included because there appeared to be general agreement regarding age of emergence with the references to instinctual grasp.[5,8,39]

2. As the instinctual grasp is emerging, a response can only be obtained by contacting the radial portion of the hand which results in supination.
3. Be aware of the avoiding response which is withdrawal (and opening) of the hand from a lighter contactual stimulus than the instinctual grasp requires and is part of the normal reflex repertoire of an infant. It is most easily elicited between 3 and 8 weeks of age.[39]

Protective Extension—Forward (Parachute, supporting response)[1–5,13–15,17,18,19,22,24,25,27–29,33]

Procedure: The examiner suspends the infant horizontally in space by supporting under the axilla. The infant is lowered head first at moderate speed toward a flat surface.

Response: As the infant approaches the surface, the upper extremities are extended in front of him as if to break the fall. The wrists extend and fingers extend and abduct when the reflex is fully developed.

Comments:

1. Vision is not required for a positive response.
2. The functional interpretation of this reaction is that it is needed for the infant to be able to support himself in sitting. Only one authority, however, differentiated a forward response in sitting from that described above. The child is tipped forward to elicit the response rather than the downward plunge.[27]

Protective Extension—Side (Lateral propping)[2,5,14,19,27]

Procedure: Place the infant on a flat surface in a symmetrical sitting position with the legs out in front and hands and arms free. Push the child on either shoulder in turn with enough force to cause the infant to lose his or her balance. Guard the infant against falling in the event that the response is not developed.

Response: The infant will stop the fall by rapid abduction of the arm and extension of elbow, wrist, and fingers resulting in a weight-bearing (support) reaction against the flat surface.

Comments:

1. Many authors do not test separately from the protective extension—forward reflex for this response although three of the four references state that this reaction develops later than the protective extension forward.
2. The range of the five authors was 6 to 9 months for time of emergence so this range is used as the average time on the chart.

Protective Extension—Back (Posterior propping)[2,5,14,27]

Procedure: Place the infant on a flat surface in a symmetrical sitting posture with his legs out in front and his hands and arms free. Push the infant backward with enough force to cause a loss of balance. Guard the infant against falling in the event that the response is not developed.

Response: The infant will stop the fall by rapidly extending both arms behind him, resulting in a weight-bearing (support) reaction against the flat surface.

Comment: "The full reaction is backward extension of both arms, but more frequently an element of trunk rotation comes in and the reaction is seen in one arm only."[27]

Tilting Reaction—Prone[2,3,5,24,25,27,41]

Procedure: Place the infant prone on a tiltboard so that he or she may be tipped from side to side. Tip the infant slowly to one side and then the other, guarding against his or her falling off the board.

Response: The infant's trunk will curve, concavity of the spine toward the elevated side of the board, the upper arm and leg abduct and the lower arm and leg increase in support tone (extension).

Comment: While this reaction is emerging the infant may only be able to respond to a slow tilt but when fully developed the infant should respond to a faster tilt.

Tilting Reaction—Supine[2,3,5,24,25,27,41]

Procedure: Place the infant supine on a tiltboard so that he or she may be tipped from side to side.

Tip the infant slowly to one side and then the other, guarding against his or her falling off the board.

Response: The infant's trunk will curve, concavity of the spine toward the elevated side of the board, the upper arm and leg abduct, and the lower arm and leg increase in support tone (extension).

Comment: While this reaction is emerging the infant may only be able to respond to a slow tilt, but when fully developed the infant should respond to a faster tilt.

Tilting Reaction—Sitting[2,5,19,24,25,27,41]

Procedure: Place the infant sitting symmetrically on a tiltboard. Slowly tilt the board to either side of the infant and then in an anteroposterior direction.

Response: "To lateral tilt, the body remains upright, and is flexed against the tilt with the concavity of the spine upward, the neck is flexed laterally and the head slightly rotated with the face toward the upper side. The arm and leg on the upper side are abducted while those on the lower side are adducted and extended. To anterior tilt, the body remains upright, the spine extends and the limbs are retracted. To posterior tilt the body remains upright with the spine flexing and the limbs are advanced."[42]

Comment: While this reaction is emerging the infant may only be able to respond to a slow tilt but when fully developed the infant should respond to a faster tilt.

Tilting Reaction—Standing[2,5,27,41]

Procedure: Place the infant standing in the center of the tilt board. Tip the infant to either side and then anteroposteriorly.

Response: To a lateral tilt the body is flexed against the tilt with the concavity of the spine upward. The upper leg is flexed and the upper arm is abducted. The lower leg is extended and strongly braced. To an anterior tilt the infant leans back, the legs extend, and the arms extend and retract. To a posterior tilt the child leans forward, legs extend, and the arms are flexed at the shoulders and extended at the elbows.[5]

Comments: While this reaction is emerging the infant may only be able to respond to a slow tilt but when fully developed the infant should respond to a faster tilt.

Hopping Reaction (Stagger reactions, shifting reaction, see-saw reaction)[2,5,6,24,34,41]

Procedure: While the child stands on the floor the examiner pushes the child forward, to the sides, and backward.

Response: The child protects himself against falling by making the appropriate correcting movements of flexion, extension, abduction, or adduction of the legs to restore his or her center of gravity.

Comment: Although all of the above named reflexes are not tested for exactly as described above, they all test the child's ability to withstand passive displacement of the body in a horizontal plane.

REFERENCES

1. Bleck, E. E.: Locomotor prognosis in cerebral palsy. Develop. Med. Child Neurol. 17:18–25, 1975.
2. Bobath, B.: Abnormal Postural Reflex Activity Caused by Brain Lesions. New York: Wm. Heinman Medical Books, 1975.
3. Bobath, B., and Bobath, K.: Motor Development in the Different Types of Cerebral Palsy. New York: Wm. Heinman Medical Books, 1975.
4. Fiorentino, M. R.: Normal and Abnormal Development, The Influence of Primitive Reflexes on Motor Development. Springfield IL: Charles C Thomas, Publisher, 1972.
5. Heriza, C., and Wilson, J.: Reflex Developmental Evaluation Research Form. Presentation, American Physical Therapy Association National Convention, New Orleans, 1976.
6. Martin, J. P.: The Basal Ganglia and Posture. London: Pitman Publishing Co., 1967.
7. Parr, C., et al.: A developmental study of the asymmetrical tonic neck reflex. Develop. Med. Child Neurol. 16:329–339, 1974.
8. Seyffarth, H., and Denny-Brown, D.: The grasp reflex and the instinctive grasp reaction. Brain 71:9–183, 1948.
9. Brazelton, T. B.: Infants and Mothers, Differences in Development. New York: Dell Publishing Co., 1969.
10. Prechtl, H., and Beintema, D.: The Neurological Examination of the Full Term Newborn Infant. Spastics International Medical Publications. New York: Wm. Heinman Medical Books, 1964.
11. Kron, R., Stein, M., and Goddard, K.: Newborn sucking behavior affected by obstetric sedations. In Stone, L. J., Smith, H., and Murphy, L. B. (eds.): The Competent Infant, Research and Commentary. New York: Basic Books, 1973.
12. Saint-Anne Dargassies, S.: Neurological maturation of the premature infant of 28–41 weeks gestational age. In Falkner, F. (ed.): Human Development. Philadelphia: W. B. Saunders Co., 1966.

13. Andre, T., and Autgaerden, S.: Locomotion from pre- to post-natal life. Clin. Develop. Med., No. 24, Spastic Society Educational and Informational Unit. New York: Wm. Heinman, 1966.
14. André-Thomas, Chesni, Y., and Saint-Anne Dargassies, S.: The Neurological Examination of the Infant. Clin. Develop. Med., No. 1. Spastics International Medical Publications. New York: Wm. Heinman, 1966.
15. Dekaban, A.: Neurology of Early Childhood. Baltimore: Williams & Wilkins Co., 1970.
16. Humphrey, T.: Some correlations between the appearance of human fetal reflexes and the development of the nervous system. In Progress in Brain Research 4. New York: Elsevier Publishing Co., 1964.
17. Illingsworth, R. S.: The Development of the Infant and Young Child. New York: Churchill Livingstone, 1974.
18. Peiper, A.: Cerebral Function in Infancy and Childhood. New York: Consultants Bureau, 1963.
19. Saint-Anne Dargassies, S.: Neurodevelopmental symptoms during the first year of life. Develop. Med. Child Neurol. 14:235–246, 1972.
20. Twitchell, T. E.: Normal motor development. In The Child with Central Nervous System Deficit, Report of Two Symposiums. Washington DC: U. S. Dept. of Health, Education, and Welfare, 1965.
21. Prechtl and Beintema: Neurological Examination, p. 39.
22. Bench, J., et al.: A comparison between the neonatal sound-evoked startle response and the head drop (Moro) reflex. Develop. Med. Child Neurol. 17:18–25, 1975.
23. Caplan, F.: The First Twelve Months of Life. New York: Grossett & Dunlap, 1973.
24. Fiorentino, M. R.: Reflex Testing Methods for Evaluating CNS Development. Springfield IL: Charles C Thomas, Publisher, 1965.
25. Hoskins, T., and Squires, J.: Developmental assessment: A test for gross motor and reflex development. Phys. Ther. 53:117–126, 1973.
26. McGraw, M. B.: The Neuromuscular Maturation of the Human Infant. New York: Hafner Press, 1963.
27. Milani-Comparetti, A., and Gidoni, E. A.: Routine developmental examination in normal and retarded children. Develop. Med. Child Neurol. 9:631–638, 1965.
28. Paine, R. S., et al.: Evolution of postural reflexes in normal infants and in the presence of chronic brain syndromes. In Kopp, C. (ed.): Readings in Early Development for Occupational and Physical Therapy Students. Springfield IL: Charles C Thomas, 1971.
29. Paine, R. S., and Oppe, T. S. E.: Neurological Examination of Children. Philadelphia: J. B. Lippincott Co., 1966.
30. Parmalee, A. H.: A critical evaluation of the Moro reflex. Pediatr. 33:773–788, 1964.
31. Touwen, B. C. L.: A study on the development of some motor phenomena in infancy. Develop. Med. Child Neurol. 13:435–446, 1971.
32. Twitchell, T. E.: Attitudinal reflexes. In The Child with Central Nervous System Deficit, Report of Two Symposiums. Washington DC: U. S. Dept. of Health, Education, and Welfare, 1965.
33. Rushworth, G.: On postural and righting reflexes. In Kopp, C. (ed.): Readings in Early Development for Occupational and Physical Therapy Students. Springfield IL: Charles C Thomas, Publisher, 1971.
34. Twitchell, T. E.: Variation and abnormalities of motor development. In The Child with Central Nervous System Deficit, Report of Two Symposiums. Washington DC: U. S. Dept. of Health, Education, and Welfare, 1965.
35. Gesell, A., and Amatruda, C. S.: Developmental Diagnosis. New York: Harper & Row Publishers, 1974.
36. Cupps, C., Plescia, M., and Houser, C.: The Landau reaction: A clinical and electromyographic analysis. Develop. Med. Child Neurol. 18:41–53, 1976.
37. Roberts, T.: Neurophysiology of Postural Mechanisms. London: Butterworths, 1967.
38. Humphrey, T.: Postnatal repetition of human prenatal activity sequences with some suggestions of their neuroanatomical basis. In Robinson, R. J. (ed.): Brain and Early Behavior. New York: Academic Press, 1969.
39. Twitchell, T. E.: Reflex mechanisms and the development of prehension. In Connolly, K. (ed.): Mechanisms of Motor Skill Development. New York: Academic Press, 1970.
40. White, B., Castle, P., and Held, R.: Observations on the development of visually directed reaching. In Kopp, C. (ed.): Readings in Early Development for Occupational and Physical Therapy Students. Springfield IL: Charles C Thomas, Publishers, 1971.
41. Weisz, S.: Studies in equilibrium reaction. J. Nerv. Mental Dis. 18:150–162, 1938.
42. Heriza and Wilson: Reflex developmental research, p. 13.

section 4/Life Works Tasks/Maude H. Malick and Bonnie Sherry

ACTIVITIES OF DAILY LIVING

The concept of Activities of Daily Living (ADL) has always encompassed feeding, dressing, and personal hygiene activities which are basic to an individual's independence. The loss of independence in these basic activities has a traumatic effect on body image and may also affect those persons associated with the patient. Therefore careful assessment, goal setting, planning, and training programs can be geared for accomplishment of short- and long-term goals that aim at self-sufficiency for a patient who is either temporarily or permanently disabled. Dependency in self-care is often the first sign of depression or the major cause of depression. Therefore early recognition of patient needs and ADL training are essential, especially in acute care settings. Conversely, a chronically disabled person who can be independent in self-care activities requires far less custodial care and thus can be cared for in a more independent unit in a community setting.

The traditional program of ADL has been an integral part of all occupational therapy programs no matter what the setting, disability, or age group. Assessment and training can take place in the home, school, acute care hospital, rehabilitation center, special school, institution, long-term care agency, or nursing home. Many tests are available for self-care assessment with simple grading forms providing ready reference to the nursing and health team. Cognition and judgment should enter into the assessment process. Merely accomplishing a task does not constitute competency. In many cases simple self-help devices are useful but should not be used unless essential. Devices such as built up handles, attachments to faucet handles, reachers, overhead rings, and mats to anchor plates and tableware are very simple aids that can make a great difference in independence. Simple energy saving techniques and planning can also change dependence to independence. In all cases, safety should be a prime concern.

ADL in its broadest sense encompasses independence in the home, at work, and in the community. In this sense the individual should be assessed regarding ability to make judgments, function in a community setting, communicate with others, carry out acceptable social behavior, and manage his or her own life style financially, socially, vocationally, and avocationally.

A grant to develop "Rehabilitation Indicators: A Method for Enhancing Accountability" was awarded New York University Medical Center, Institute of Rehabilitation Medicine, in 1976, with Doctors Diller, Fordyce, and Jacobs as codirectors. An ADL Task Force chaired by Carl Granger, M.D., developed and explored levels of ADL performance indicating the scope of skills assessed under activities of daily living. As a result of this task force meeting and others throughout the country, rehabilitation indicators (RI), which describe a client's behavior and environment, were developed. Four types of RIs have been developed: status, activity pattern, skill, and environment. Phrases have been written to describe what clients actually do, what clients demonstrate they can do, and what clients plan to do. The field testing of this project has not yet been completed; thus a full report or description is premature.*

A health/disability scale used to delineate the aspects of ADL function is given in Table 10-5. In many cases substitution using strengths in one area to compensate for deficits in another area can be effective. For example, speech and communication skills can supplement writing skills.

Assessment and training techniques described by Lawton in 1963[1] are as valid today as when they were written. Zimmerman,[2] writing on ADL in the previous edition of this book, developed an analysis of motion and self-help aids used in eating and writing (Tables 10-6 and 10-7).

HOMEMAKER REHABILITATION

Homemakers constitute the largest group among the disabled. With current figures exceeding 10

* Further information can be obtained from Margaret Brown, Project Coordinator, New York University Medical Center, Institute of Rehabilitation Medicine, 400 East 34th Street, New York NY 10016.

Table 10-5. Health/disability scale determining illness and dependency or health and independence.

	Internal limitations (Basic survival)	External obstacles/adaptations (Role identification)
Bodily functions	Self-care	Household tasks
Mobility in space	Mobility	Use of transportation
Communication	Speech, hearing, vision	Aids, equipment, devices, etc.
Social	Appropriateness and self-presentation	Social competence in confronting and using support systems
Cognitive	Orientation, problem solving, etc.	Management of personal affairs
Emotional	Tolerance of psychological stress, orientation to goals, phobias, anxiety, depression	Acting out behaviors, motivation

million, it is essential both socially and economically that the rehabilitation process be utilized in helping the individual reestablish his or her place in family, home, and community. Physical rehabilitation services encompass those techniques that are instrumental in developing physical residual capabilities, whether it be by training or reeducation, with emphasis on modifications of performance or task completion. The home economist introduces to rehabilitation a set of tools that can be utilized in the development of a comprehensive homemaker rehabilitation program.

The recent metamorphosis of "homemaking" into "homemaker rehabilitation" has necessitated a broadening of the definition to be in tune with the emerging holistic concerns of rehabilitation. It is essential in any program to incorporate methods for coping with the individual's physical, personal, and social needs while putting emphasis on promoting self-integration as well as integration into family and society.

The rehabilitation process must include provisions for the personal and social needs, goals, and resources of each potential homemaker. According to Switzer[3]:

> Homemaking activities—whether carried out by men, women or children—contribute to the welfare and stability of the family and to its economic productiveness and well-being. Homemaking itself is a composite of physical tasks, managerial functions, spirit, emotional climate that holds the family or personality together and fosters development. Damage to this process at any point weakens its total capacity to function. Where possible, the damage must be repaired; where this is not possible, other measures must be taken. Perhaps the environment can be changed so that the function can continue; perhaps the other areas of the complex must be brought to greater prominence and use; perhaps the very depths of personality must be touched and a new role learned.

The Rehabilitation Act of 1973 and the Social Services Act of 1974 emphasize the pertinence and urgency of developing comprehensive programs for enabling the homebound individual to realize his or her potential. Homemaking is now a viable occupation and should be considered as such when funding is necessary for implementing the rehabilitation process. Schwab[4] says disabled homemakers with a recent rehabilitation experience exhibit positive changes in self-perception in relation to household tasks. The self-respect and self-confidence derived from this experience can transfer to other activities, which may make the individual more productive, even in terms of competitive employment.

Homemaking programs traditionally have encompassed the teaching and assessment of basic work skills. These programs include the utilization of work simplification techniques to promote time and energy conservation concurrently providing therapeutic exercise, teaching the use of prostheses or orthotic equipment, promoting psychological gains through satisfactory performance, and assisting constructive planning for home adjustment. However, a homemaker by definition is "one who manages his or her own household." Thus the inclusion of the management factor in the process of home-

Table 10-6. Analysis of motions used in eating with one arm only.

Body part	*Motion*	*Purpose*	*Substitution*	*Loss*	*Device used to compensate*
Hand	*Pick-up* palmar prehension *Holding* lateral prehension to middle finger (modified lateral pinch)	Pick up and hold utensil	1. Lacing spoon between fingers 2. adduction of fingers 3. Hook grasp	Minimal Moderate Severe Complete	1. Utensil interlaced in fingers (some shaping may be necessary) 2. Moleskin or tape over handle to prevent slipping 3. Built-up handle (wood, sponge or other material) 4. Grip-shaped handles 5. Handle with horizontal and vertical dowels (pegged handle) 6. Handle with finger rings 7. Warm Springs type short opponens with C-bar and utensil attachment 8. Plastic and metal holder 9. ADL (universal) cuff 10. Prehension orthosis—manually operated —power operated
Wrist	Stabilization (slight flexion and extension or radial and ulnar deviation normally used depending on whether grasp is hook or pinch)	Positioning of hand for optimal function (to prevent wrist flexion)	1. Use of finger or thumb extensors	Partial stability Complete	1. ADL wrist support, dorsal (leather with spring steel insert) 2. Flexible, adjustable nylon wrist support or Klenzac joints 3. Tubular spring-clip (ADL) orthosis 4. Cock-up splint, rigid, palmar 5. Warm Springs type long opponens
Forearm	Pronation	Pick up food on utensil	1. Shoulder abduction and internal rotation 2. Raise forearm to vertical position and then rotate	Partial or complete	1. Swivel spoon 2. Bent fork or spoon
	Supination	Keep utensil level while putting food in mouth to avoid spill	1. Shoulder adduction and external rotation		1. Swivel spoon 2. Placing fork or spoon over thumb, use thumb extensors
Elbow	Flexion of forearm Extension	Raising hand to mouth Lowering hand to plate	1. Use of knee 2. Shoulder abduction 3. Trunk flexion 4. Rock forearm on edge of table	Partial or complete	1. Balanced Forearm Orthosis (ball bearing feeder) 2. Overhead sling with 'feeder' attachment 3. Overhead sling with built-up lapboard 4. Long handled utensil 5. Functional arm orthosis
Shoulder	Stabilization against hyperextension and internal rotation in position of —Slight flexion —Slight abduction plus slight active [illegible]	Provides positioning and assists in raising hand to level of mouth	1. Trunk flexion 2. Prop elbow on table	Partial or complete	1. Pillow behind upper arm 2. Overhead sling 3. Balanced Forearm Orthosis (BFO) 4. Functional arm orthosis with hyperextension stop

Table 10-7. Analysis of motions used for writing using right hand only.

Method and position	*Body part*	*Motion*	*Purpose*	*Devices used to compensate*
Commonly used method ——— Sitting with arm on writing surface	Hand	Opposition of thumb to index finger and lateral opposition to middle finger (modified palmar prehension) Flexion and extension of middle phalangeal joints and/or	Provides grasp Moves pencil	1. Built-up pencils, diameter increased 2. Spring-clip holder (used in ADL cuff) 3. Leather holding device 4. Clothespin holder with pegs 5. Holder with finger rings or finger bands 6. Adjustable holder (used with ADL cuff) 7. Fiberglas cuff 8. Prehension orthosis— —manually operated —power operated
	Wrist	Slight flexion and extension . . . . or . . . . stabilization in neutral or slight cock-up position	Moves pencil Provides positioning	1. ADL wrist support, dorsal (leather with spring steel insert)—flexible 1. Anterior cock-up, rigid 2. Long opponens orthosis 3. ADL orthosis
	Forearm	Stabilization in approximate mid-position	Provides positioning	1. Supination assist
	Elbow	Stabilization in approximately 90° flexion	Provides positioning	1. Overhead sling 2. Balanced Forearm Orthosis 3. Functional arm orthosis
		Alternating action of —flexors	Lifts weight of arm from writing surface	1. Overhead sling 2. Foot operated cable control to elbow of functional arm orthosis
		—extensors	Provides pressure during writing	1. Soft lead pencil (needs less pressure) 2. Certain pens, ball point pens, felt-tip pens 3. Elastic strap from hand to forearm on anterior surface (substituting wrist flexors for elbow extensors)
		Slight flexion and extension with ↓	Moves hand across paper	1. Ball caster support 2. Powder on board, formica surface or teflon covered arm (elbow) cuffs
	Shoulder	Slight internal and external rotation	Moves hand across paper	1. Overhead slings 2. Rotation mechanism on functional arm orthosis
		Stabilization in position of slight flexion and abduction	Provides positioning and	1. Overhead slings 2. Balanced Forearm Orthosis (BFO) 3. Functional arm orthosis
		Minimal synergistic action of shoulder girdle muscles	Minimum motion and pressure	

maker training is essential. Educational programs that aid the homemaker in developing managerial expertise strengthen the entire rehabilitation process. Although the actual managerial processes remain unchanged, disability may alter the individual's goals or resources and the demands on those resources.

Management is the means by which an individual uses available assets to accomplish a goal. The concept is easy for the disabled homemaker to comprehend as well as implement. As an essential part of the rehabilitation team, the homemaker is responsible for assisting in the development of her own program and, primarily, for setting her own goals.

Management means not only the performance of tasks but also control. It is essential that the homemaker does not feel out of control.

Physical or mental disability necessitates many changes. Because of accident or illness the homemaker may have to cope with changes that are out of his or her realm of control, and he or she may be unable to set realistic goals freely. It is the therapist's role to assist the homemaker in using management skills to bring about the change in an orderly way. This involves the homemaker's adapting to alternatives and finding outside resources in the family. Although functioning may be limited in one area, resources can be channeled in new directions. Tasks do not need to be limited to one member of the family. All family resources must be considered when faced with decision making.

Sometimes the disabled homemaker is so distraught by the changes in herself or himself that he or she may bypass an essential step in the decision-making process and therefore must be given guidance. The process involved in decision making is relatively simple. It is as follows:

1. State the problem.
2. Seek and explore alternatives.
3. Discuss possible solutions.
4. Choose one alternative.
5. Accept the responsibility for the decision made.

The working through of this process provides the family with a better communication system, which in turn leads to greater satisfaction with the ultimate decision.[5]

The managerial aspects of the homemaker training program necessarily affect all other areas of concentration. Possessing rehabilitative skills, the homemaker needs to explore all areas in which he or she will be involved, either as a participant or as a manager. The rehabilitation home economist is trained specifically in these areas, which so frequently elude the therapist. With a strong background of knowledge in family relationships, foods and nutrition, clothing and textiles, child development, equipment, family economics, home management and housing, the home economist proves to be an essential member of the rehabilitation team and one who can be instrumental in the development of a truly comprehensive homemaker rehabilitation program.

Today's homemaker rehabilitation programs have grown and expanded in many new and exciting directions, all aimed towards the goal of producing home managers who are functioning to their capacity in all areas. Among the most important areas of concentration is the fulfillment of nutritional needs. This includes basic food preparation skills with emphasis on planning, purchasing, and serving nutritious meals that meet all dietary needs. Assistance with financial management, and information on budgeting, spending, and saving can be incorporated in the basic program. Selection, care, and adaptation of clothing is yet another facet of the program which can make the handicapped homemaker a more effective and efficient home manager. Child care can consume a good portion of the homemaker's day. With instruction on purchasing functional equipment and clothing as well as techniques regarding actual feeding, dressing, and bathing of children, the handicapped homemaker can resume many tasks that previously were allocated to other family members or to hired help.

Today's homemaker training programs are the keystone in the structure of rehabilitation that enables the disabled person to build a new life with an emphasis on ability and not disability.

RECORDING AND SCORING OF FUNCTION IN ADL AND HOMEMAKING

Because the entire rehabilitation process is directed towards change in the total patient profile—

change in attitude, ability, activity, awareness, and aptitude for the program—it is necessary to record changes and use these records in the upgrading of the client's program. It is essential to establish a scale of performance and a code for noting the levels of performance before an evaluation begins. There are potentially as many scales and codes as there are therapists. Experimentation may be necessary to find one that is flexible and functional for use in various treatment settings. However, all therapists in a department should use the same recording system or patients functioning at the same level may receive differing reports from various therapists. This can be confusing, especially when reporting to other treatment departments. Several ADL and homemaking charts with codes are included as examples (Figs. 10-5 to 10-9).

In order to note a change, a baseline, that is, a point of reference or the initial evaluation, is needed. It is from this that the program develops. The information gleaned from the initial evaluation should be used in setting the goal towards which the therapist and patient will be working. The general levels of functioning, tolerance, and attitude are to be determined. Once a program is established, it is of paramount importance to note daily changes and periodic differences in levels of improvement. These are easily coded and marked on the scales. A progress chart frequently provides some motivation for the patient as a visual and concrete indication that he or she is improving.

Daily reports often take the form of short notes which include activity performed; level of success; tolerance; attitude; pertinent observations including physical limitations such as perceptual, visual, and hearing deficits; use of adapted or standard equipment; ability to solve problems, read, and follow directions; mental reliability (e.g., disorientation or hallucination); and general method of approaching the activity (e.g., precise or careless). Positive or negative changes noted on the chart are indicators of a need for program adaptation. Retraining may be indicated or, possibly, the program may need to be accelerated. It often is helpful for the family to see the coded scales when the therapist explains alterations in the program. Carry-over on home visits generally is greater when the family is aware of the exact level of functioning that can and should be expected.

Not all information relating to progress or condition can be included on a checklist based on observations or testing. Many factors not able to be coded and scaled will influence the patient's performance. These should not be neglected. Each chart should include space for impressions and subjective observations. Records should be accurate and concise but contain all pertinent information. The treatment goals should be noted. In most cases the physician will make referrals indicating general treatment procedures.

The final report, usually a discharge summary, should include the results of the initial evaluation, the treatment procedures, the results of the final evaluation, the final level of functioning, the achievement of goals, prognosis, and recommendations for maximal carry-over upon discharge. This final report often goes to the sponsoring agency and to agencies that may be working with the patient on an outpatient or home program.

CASE STUDY

Susan A. is a spry, spunky, 82-year-old widow. She had been living alone in a high rise for the elderly not far from the business district of a small milltown in Pennsylvania. Although she has had two strokes, the most recent one and a half years ago, and has a history of heart trouble, she has returned to independent living following a 6-week stay at a comprehensive rehabilitation center.

Susan tells her story:

"I was always a busy lady, active with my family and at church. My husband was hurt badly in a mill accident just after we were married. We had to live some way, so I turned our house into a guest home. My whole life was spent making people comfortable and happy. It wasn't easy. I've had heart trouble for about 30 years now and then I got a stroke on my left side about 18 years ago. My daughter died of rheumatic heart disease. She left a wonderful husband and two sons. The boys still see me often and send money if I need it.

"After my husband died, about 10 years back, I sold the house and moved into this apartment near my sisters. The place is really nice—we have elevators, a laundry room, even grab bars in the bathroom for us old folks.

"Just over a year ago, I fell down getting out of bed. By crawling across the floor, I finally got to the phone for help. An ambulance took me to the hospi-

(Case study is continued on 199.)

TEST FOR ACTIVITIES OF DAILY LIVING

Mr.
Miss
Name: Mrs. ____________ Age: ________ Room # ________ Date of Initial Test ____________ Patient In Out
M.D. ____________

Address: ____________ Vocation: ____________

Onset Date: ________ Lesion: ____________ flaccid spastic Admission Date: ____________

Disability: ____________

Cause: ____________

Decubiti: ____________

Surgery: ____________

METHOD OF RECORDING TEST AND PROGRESS
SYMBOLS for GRADE

√—patient can perform activity independently
S—patient needs supervision
A—patient needs assistance
L—patient has to be lifted
X—activity is not indicated

1. *At initial testing:* use *BLUE PENCIL:*
   Enter grade symbol in column G/1 and your initials in column 1.
   The initial date appears at top of page.

2. *Progress* is recorded with *RED PENCIL:*
   Enter grade symbol in column G/2 and your initials in column 1.
   Date in column "Date."

If there is more than one method or item listed with an activity, circle which indicated

BED ACTIVITIES	G/1	G/2	Date	1
Moving in bed: lying, sitting				
Roll to right: to left				
Turn on abdomen				
Manage: pillows, blankets				
Sit up				
Reach objects on night table				
Operate signal light				

FIGURE 10-5. Activities of daily living checklist. From Institute of Rehabilitation Medicine, New York University Medical Center, New York, 1957. Reprinted with permission.

WHEELCHAIR ACTIVITIES	G/1	G/2	Date	1
Propel: forward, backward, turn				
Open, through, and close door				
Up, down ramp				
Bed to wheelchair				
Wheelchair to bed				
Wheelchair to straight chair				
Straight chair to wheelchair				
Wheelchair to easy chair, couch				
Easy chair, couch to wheelchair				
Wheelchair to toilet (high toilet seat, regular seat)				
Toilet to wheelchair				
Adjust clothing				
Wheelchair to tub				
Tub to wheelchair				
Wheelchair to shower (chair in stall shower, or tub)				
Shower to wheelchair				
TRAVEL: Wheelchair to car—on curb				
Car to wheelchair—on curb				
Wheelchair to car—no curb				
Car to wheelchair—no curb				
Place wheelchair in car—on street				

SELF-CARE ACTIVITIES

HYGIENE (TOILET ACTIVITIES)	G/1	G/2	Date	1
Comb, brush hair				
Brush teeth				
Shave (electric razor, safety razor), put on make up				
Turn faucet				
Wash, dry hands and face				
Wash, dry body and extremities				
Take bath (wheelchair, walking)				
Take shower (wheelchair, walking)				
Use urinal, bedpan				

EATING ACTIVITIES	G/1	G/2	Date	1
Eat with spoon				
Eat with fork				
Cut meat				
Handle: straw, cup, glass				

DRESSING ACTIVITIES	G/1	G/2	Date	1
Undershirt—bra				
Shorts—panties				
Slip-over garment				
Shirt—blouse				
Slacks—dress				
Tying neck tie—bow				
Socks—stockings				
Shoes (laces, buckles, slip-on)				
Coat, jacket				
Braces, prosthesis, corset				

MISCELLANEOUS HAND-ACTIVITIES	G/1	G/2	Date	1
Write name and address				
Manage: watch				
match or cigarette lighter				
cigarette				
book, newspaper				
handkerchief				
lights; chain, switch, knob				
telephone: receiver, dial, coins				
handle: purse, coins, paper money				

WALKING ACTIVITIES	G/1	G/2	Date	1
Open, go through, and close door				
Walking outside				
Walking carrying				

STANDING UP AND SITTING DOWN	G/1	G/2	Date	1
Up from wheelchair				
Down on wheelchair				
Up from bed				
Down on bed				
Up from straight chair				
Down on straight chair				
Up from straight chair at table				
Down on straight chair at table				
Up from easy chair				
Down on easy chair				
Up from center of couch				
Down on center of couch				
Up from toilet				
Down on toilet				
Adjust clothing				
Into car, on curb, up curb				
Out of car				
Down on floor				
Up from floor				

CLIMBING AND TRAVELING ACTIVITIES	G/1	G/2	Date	1
Up flight of stairs (railing, no railing)				
Down flight of stairs (railing, no railing)				
Into and out of car, taxi				
Walk one block and back				
Down curb, cross street, on curb				
Into bus				
Sit down, get up from bus seat				
Out of bus				

FIGURE 10-5. *(continued)*

ACTIVITIES OF DAILY LIVING EVALUATION

NAME: ______________________ AGE: __________ CASE #: __________

DIAGNOSIS: ______________________ PRECAUTIONS: ______________________

CODE

PERFORMANCE SCALE

I *Independent*—Patient can accomplish activity consistently without assistance or supervision.

A *Assistance*—Patient can accomplish activity with some level of physical assistance.
A-1 Assistance Minimum
A-2 Assistance Moderate
A-3 Assistance Maximum

S *Supervision*—Patient requires supervision of another person due to either physical or mental limitations.
S-V Verbal Cueing
S-G Gestural Cueing
S-P Physical Cueing

D *Dependent*—Patient unable to help in activity.

PLACE OF ACTIVITY

C Regular Chair
W Wheelchair
B-1 Bed—Sitting on edge
B-2 Bed—Sitting up
B-3 Bed—Supine

TIME

N Within normal limits
X Excessive

THERAPIST:

DATES										COMMENTS (EQUIP.)
	Perf.	Place	Time	Perf.	Place	Time	Perf.	Place	Time	
UPPER TRUNK & ARMS										
SHIRT/BLOUSE—ON/OFF										
BRA/UNDERSHIRT—ON/OFF										
SWEATER/COAT—ON/OFF										
SPLINT/PROSTHESIS—ON/OFF										
LOWER TRUNK, LEGS & FEET										
TROUSERS/SLACKS—ON/OFF										
SHORTS/PANTIES—ON/OFF										
SOCKS/HOSE—ON/OFF										
SHOES—ON/OFF										
PROSTHESIS/ORTHOSIS—ON/OFF										
SHOE LACES										
MISC. ARTICLES										
FEEDING										
PERSONAL HYGIENE										

FIGURE 10-6. From the Harmarville Rehabilitation Center, Pittsburgh PA. Reprinted with permission.

HOMEMAKING EVALUATION AND TREATMENT

Name: Age: Date Referred:

Address: Visual Difficulty:

Disability:

Mobility Status: ________ independent ________ W/C ________ cane ________ crutches ________ walker

Dominant Hand: R L Limitations:

Goal: Special Diet:

Discharge Plans:

Household members and ages:
1.
2.
3.
4.
5.

Available help within or outside of family:

Description of home or apartment: ________ floors ________ stairs ________ rooms

Are bath facilities functional? ________ kitchen facilities functional? ________

(X) Patient formerly responsible for:

( ) Patient wants to return to doing:

( ) ( ) Food preparation
( ) ( ) Serving and cleaning
( ) ( ) Washing dishes
( ) ( ) Grocery shopping
( ) ( ) Meal planning
( ) ( ) Budgeting
( ) ( ) Child care
( ) ( ) Bed making
( ) ( ) Laundry—facilities in home ________
( ) ( ) Ironing
( ) ( ) Cleaning
( ) ( ) Sewing

SKETCH PROBLEM AREA

Special problems:

Special interests:

Patient's attitude toward homemaking:

Family's attitude toward patient's role as homemaker and toward family help:

FIGURE 10-7. (Legend on facing page)

(Illustration on facing page.)

FIGURE 10-7. Code used when stating goals for homemaker evaluation. Goals are established after the patient has been interviewed and is seen working in the area. At the time of discharge from the area, it is determined whether or not he has reached the set goal.

A Independent Homemaker—Patient appears capable of performing all homemaking activities without assistance or supervision.

B Independent Light Homemaker—Patient appears capable of performing all light homemaking activities without assistance or supervision.

C Good Partial Homemaker—Patient appears capable of performing most light homemaking activities independently. May require assistance with some heavier or very complex tasks.

D Partial Homemaker—Patient appears capable of performing some light homemaking activities independently or with minimal assistance with heavy or complex activities. May be limited in performing certain activities by physical inadequacy.

E Partial Homemaker with Assistance—Patient appears capable of performing many light homemaking activities but requires assistance in at least one aspect of most of these activities. May be limited by tolerance or mental ability.

F Partial Homemaker with Supervision—Patient appears to require general supervision while performing most homemaking activities but physically performs well.

G Simple Partial Homemaker—Patient appears capable of performing simple, repetitive homemaking activities without supervision or assistance. May need to be set up at an activity but able to follow through.

H Simple Partial Homemaker with Supervision—Patient appears to require supervision to perform even simple repetitive tasks.

I Not Feasible—Patient did not appear capable of working on a homemaking evaluation at the time as a result of either physical or mental insufficiency.

J Incomplete—Homemaking evaluation had been initiated but not completed because of medical problems, early discharge, or referral to another program.

K Refused—Patient was referred to the Homemaking area for an evaluation but refused to attend the program.

From the Harmarville Rehabilitation Center, Pittsburgh PA. Reprinted with permission.

HOUSEHOLD ACTIVITIES PERFORMANCE EVALUATION

MEAL PREPARATION ACTIVITIES	Perf.	Place	Time	Perf.	Place	Time	Perf.	Place	Time	Perf.	Place	Time	Perf.	Place	Time	COMMENTS Equip. & Devices
DATE																
1. Turn on water																
2. Turn on stove																
3. Pour hot liquid																
4. Open package																
5. Open jars																
6. Use can openers																
7. Use refrigerator																
8. Bend to low cupboards																
9. Reach high cupboards																
10. Peel vegetables																
11. Use sharp tools																
12. Measures																
13. Use oven																
14. Use range																
15. Stir against resistance																
16. Use electric mixer																
17. Cut with shears																
18. Read directions																
19. Follow directions																
MEAL SERVICE																
1. Set and clear table																
2. Carry items to table																
3. Wash dishes																
4. Dry dishes																
5. Clean area																
6. Wring out dishcloth																
CLEANING ACTIVITIES																
1. Retrieve objects from floor																
2. Wipe up spills																
3. Make bed																
4. Use dust mop																
5. Vacuum																
6. Use dust pan																
7. Clean bathtub																
8. Sweep with broom																
9. Dust high surfaces																
10. Dust low surfaces																
11. Clean refrigerator																

FIGURE 10-8. From Harmarville Rehabilitation Center, Pittsburgh PA. Reprinted with permission.

	Perf.	Place	Time	Perf.	Place	Time	Perf.	Place	Time	Perf.	Place	Time	Perf.	Place	Time	
LAUNDRY ACTIVITIES																
1. Sort clothes																
2. Wash lingerie																
3. Iron																
4. Fold clothes																
5. Set up board																
6. Use washing machine																
SEWING ACTIVITIES																
1. Thread needle																
2. Make a knot																
3. Sew buttons																
4. Use machine																
5. Diversional activity																
MARKETING ACTIVITIES																
1. Make out list																
2. Put groceries away																
CHILD CARE ACTIVITIES																
1. Bathe																
2. Dress																
3. Feed																

CODES

Performance
- X—unnecessary
- A—independent
- B—with assistance
- C—impossible
- D—training needed

Place
- W—wheelchair
- O—ambulatory
- Ө—ambulatory with assistive devices

Time
- N—within normal limits
- X—excessive

HOMEMAKING FOLLOW-UP QUESTIONNAIRE

Please complete and return this form in the enclosed, stamped, self-addressed envelope.

1. What are your present living arrangements? (where and with whom)

2. Have you made any changes to your home since you left the Rehabilitation Center? (grab bars, ramp, moved)

3. Did you make any changes before leaving the Center?

4. Are there any changes that need to be made in your home that we can assist you with?

5. Do you do most of your work from the wheelchair, with a walker, crutches, quad cane, conventional cane, or walking independently?

   What were you using when you left the Rehabilitation Center? ______________________

   ____

	ALWAYS	SOMETIMES	NEVER
6. Do you prepare your own meals?	______	______	______
7. Do you do your own dishes?	______	______	______
8. Do you do your own dusting?	______	______	______
9. Do you do your own vacuuming?	______	______	______
10. Do you do your own mopping?	______	______	______
11. Do you do your own laundry?	______	______	______
12. Do you fold the laundry?	______	______	______
13. Do you do your own bedmaking?	______	______	______

14. List any other homemaking activities that you do. ______________________

    ____

15. Do you use any special homemaking equipment, such as spike board, rubber placemat, etc? ______

16. Could you benefit from the use of any equipment you had used in the Homemaking area at the Rehabilitation Center? ______________________ Which ones? ______________________

17. Do you receive help with any of your homemaking activities?

    Which jobs? ______________________

    How often? ______________________

    By whom? ______________________

18. What is the most difficult homemaking activity that you try to do?

19. Do you receive help for any of your personal care?

    What type? (Grooming, dressing, bathing, toilet, eating, etc.)

    How often? ______________________

    By whom? ______________________

FIGURE 10-9. From Harmarville Rehabilitation Center, Pittsburgh PA. Reprinted with permission.

20. Are you presently receiving services from a community agency? ______
If yes, which one: (VNA, Home Health Care, Outpatient Treatment)

21. Are you on a special diet? ______
If so, what kind? ______
Have you lost weight? ______ If so, how much? ______
Have you gained weight? ______ If so, how much? ______

22. What activities are you involved with outside your home: (such as shopping, visiting, driving, church or other)

23. Are you satisfied with the progress you have made since leaving the Center? Comments.

24. Would a home visit from one of our Rehabilitation Home Economists be of help to you now? ______
For what purpose?

25. Do you have any questions, comments, or special problems?

Name:
Address:
Phone:

(continued from page 189.)

tal. It was another stroke, on the left side again. I could shrug my shoulder but couldn't move my hand at all. Two people had to hold me to let me walk. For the first time I was really afraid. There was no one who could take care of me and I surely couldn't do much for myself. Although I could feed myself a little I couldn't fix my hair or put on my bra, panties, or slacks. Couldn't tie my shoes either. Housework was unthinkable with one hand. I thought they'd make me go to some home for old people. Just to get better and go back to my apartment was all I wanted.

"My doctor thought I could make some progress at a rehabilitation center. I'm sure glad I went. They had special groups for discussion about strokes. I got to talk to a lot of people who were in the same shape as I was. They gave me therapy on my arm and showed me how to walk with a cane. A lady from ADL worked with me and showed me how to dress and feed myself. I got my hair cut on beauty shop day so I could take care of it myself.

"One of my other classes was homemaking. I told them I didn't need any cooking lessons, but they showed me how to cook my favorite meals with one hand, even how to peel potatoes. I was supposed to be on a 2 gram sodium diet, but I had never followed it because I didn't know what it was. At homemaking they showed me how to eat what I like and still stay on my diet. I learned lots of tricks too, so I wouldn't get so tired doing my work. I used to think it was lazy to sit to work but it's just plain smart!

"I never had much money. I was a regular tightwad. The rehabilitation home economist showed me how to save money in many ways. Now I have a little left over to save for my old age. We went grocery shopping too. My sisters thought it was too hard for me to walk and push a cart too, but I did it.

"The therapists got me in pretty good shape at the rehabilitation center but I was still a little leery about going home to stay by myself. Oh, I wanted to but, with my stroke, wasn't sure I could. My sisters wanted me to move in with them, but at my age it's better to live by yourself.

"The rehabilitation center had an apartment right in the building. I didn't want to stay there; my doctor had other ideas. I think he thought I couldn't do it—I showed him. I stayed there just like I was at home by myself. I washed and dressed myself, took my pills, made the bed, cooked my meals, did laundry, and dusted around the apartment. I did my exercises and had my social worker in for tea. I thought I could do it, but it sure gave me confidence to know for sure. It gave me a real big lift—I was ready to go home.

"My sisters insisted that I get meals-on-wheels. I did for a few weeks, but the food wasn't so hot. I started cooking on my own again. The spikeboard I made in occupational therapy was a big help.

"After I was home for a few weeks the homemaking therapist came to see me. She brought the long-handled sponge and long shoehorn I had asked for. She showed me how to arrange things in the kitchen to make it easier for me to reach. I showed her how I fixed my calendar so I don't get mixed up about when to take my pills. I learned how to get in the tub at the center so I bought those stick on flowers so I don't slip. I think the therapist was surprised at how well I was doing. Guess I surprised myself too."

Six months later Susan was evaluated on an outpatient visit. Because of her persistence in doing the prescribed exercises and wearing her cock-up splint, she was gaining function in her left hand. Ambulation status was independent. She reported actively participating in apartment activities and utilizing Adult Services for transportation to visit and shop. Figure 10-10 shows Susan's chart.

Discharge Summary

Mrs. Susan A was referred to the Occupational Therapy Department for a homemaking evaluation by Dr. Jones. She was initially seen in the area in her wheelchair and progressed to ambulation with a one-point cane. Balance appeared good. Tolerance was within normal limits. She appeared alert and oriented to time, person, and place. She was pleasant, cooperative, and very well motivated to work in the area and to resume independent living.

GOAL: Good partial homemaker. This goal was achieved.

OCCUPATIONAL THERAPY DEPT.—ADL PROGRAM

NAME ______________________ Independent X blue

Admitted ______________________ Some Help //// yellow

Discharged ______________________ All Help XXX red

	1/8/78	1/15/78	1/23/78	2/1/78	2/7/78
Comb Hair	////	X	X	X	X
Brush Teeth	X	X	X	X	X
Shave					
Dress Self					
Undershirt—bra	XXX	////	////	X	X
Shirt	////	X	X	X	X
Shorts—Pants	////	////	////	X	X
Trousers	////	////	////	////	X
Dress	////	X	X	X	X
Socks—Stockings	////	////	X	X	X
Shoes	////	X	X	X	X
Ties Laces	XXX	////	////	////	X
Braces					
Feed Self	////	////	X	X	X
Cut Meat	XXX	XXX	////	X	X

FIGURE 10-10. Sample form for case study.

Mrs. A's program included:

1. Vegetable preparation—used spikeboard safely and appropriately.
2. Food preparation—successfully read and followed directions, opened packages, used range, oven, and refrigerator while ambulating.
3. Dishwashing—worked with no apparent difficulty from standing position.
4. Bedmaking—balance and tolerance appeared good. Works neatly and efficiently.
5. Vacuuming—difficulty was noted when patient attempted to move furniture.
6. Laundry—effectively used coin operated facilities.
7. Received instruction in work simplification techniques and management principles. Comprehension appeared good.
8. Received instruction on 2 gm. Na diet and meal planning.
9. Completed 48 hour apartment living experience with excellent results.

Mrs. A was discharged from the program on 2/10/77. At this time she appeared capable of living independently in her apartment in a high rise for the elderly. She will receive homemaker services once every 2 weeks to assist with heavy homemaking tasks. She appeared determined to utilize skills developed in program. A home visit is planned for 2 weeks post-discharge. She will be seen for outpatient evaluation at 3-month intervals.

Jane Doe
Rehabilitation Home Economist

INITIAL INTERVIEW: 1/27/77
DATE DISCONTINUED: 2/10/77
THERAPY SESSIONS: 20
EQUIPMENT: Long sponge, rubber mat, spikeboard

REFERENCES

1. Lawton, E. B.: Activities of Daily Living for Physical Rehabilitation. New York: McGraw-Hill Book Co., 1963.
2. Zimmerman, M. E.: Occupational therapy in the A. D. L. program. In Willard, H. S., and Spackman, C. S. (eds.): Occupational Therapy, ed. 4. Philadelphia: J. B. Lippincott Co., 1971, pp. 217–256.
3. Switzer, M. W.: Foreword. In Rehabilitation of Physically Handicapped in Homemaking Activities. Proceedings of a Workshop, Highland Park IL, 1963. U.S. Department of Health, Education and Welfare.
4. Schwab, L. O.: Self Perception of Physically Disabled Homemakers. Ed.D. Thesis, University of Nebraska, 1966.
5. Gross, I., and Crandall, E. W.: Management for Modern Families. New York: Appleton-Century-Crofts, 1963.

BIBLIOGRAPHY

Barrier-Free Site Design. HUD Publication, 1974. Available from Superintendent of Documents, U.S. Government Printing Office, Washington DC.

Barton, D. H.: Self-help clothing. Harvest Years, March 1973, pp. 19–23.

Beppler, M. C., and Knoll, M. M.: The disabled homemaker: Organizational activities, family participation, and rehabilitation success. Rehab. Lit. 35:200–206, 1974.

Botwinick, J.: Cognitive Processes in Maturity and Old Age. New York: Springer Publishing Co., 1967.

Bryce, T. E.: A home economist on the rehabilitation team. Am. J. Occup. Ther. 23:258–262, 1969.

Clothes for the Physically Handicapped Homemaker. Agricultural Research Service, U.S. Department of Agriculture, Home Economic Research Report #12, June 1971, Washington DC.

Clothing for Wheelchair Users, 1971. Disabled Living Foundation, 346 Kensington High Street, London W14.

Clothing for the Incontinent Older Child, 1972. Disabled Living Foundation, 346 Kensington High Street, London W14.

Cookman, H., and Zimmerman, M. E.: Functional Fashions for the Physically Handicapped. New York Institute of Physical Medicine and Rehabilitation, New York University Medical Center, 1961.

Diffrient, N., Tilley, A. R., and Bardagiy, J. C.: Humanscale 1/2/3. Designer: Henry Dreyfuss Associates. Cambridge MA: M.I.T. Press, 1974.

Ford, J., and Duckworth, B.: Physical Management for the Quadriplegic Patient. Philadelphia: F. A. Davis Co., 1974.

Friend, S. D., Zaccagnine, J., and Sullivan, M.: Meeting the clothing needs of handicapped children. J. Home Economics, May 1973.

Further Action Needed to Make All Public Buildings Accessible to the Physically Handicapped. Report to the Congress by Comptroller General of the United States, July 15, 1975.

Goldsmith, S.: Designing for the Disabled, ed. 2. New York: McGraw-Hill Book Co., 1967.

Harkness, S. P., and Groom, J. N., Jr.: Building Without Barriers for the Disabled. The Architect Collaborative Inc., Whitney Library of Design, Cambridge, Massachusetts, 1976.

Harmarville Rehabilitation Center, Inc., "Handicapped Homemaker Follow-Up Study," P.O. Box 11460, Guys Run Road, Pittsburgh, PA 15238, 1972.

I.C.T.A. Information Center, Bromma, Sweden.

Jay, P. E.: Help Yourselves—A Handbook for Hemiplegics and Their Families. London: Butterworths, 1966.

Johannsen, W. J., and Thill, J. D.: Effectiveness of homemaking training for hemiplegic patients. *Arch. Phys. Med. Rehabil.* 47:1967.

Koch, A. R.: Significance and Scope of Rehabilitation in Homemaking Activities. Rehabilitation of the Physically Handicapped in Homemaking Activities, Vocational Rehabilitation Administration, Washington DC, 1963, pp. 7–16.

Kliment, S. A.: Into the Mainstream: A Syllabus for a Barrier-Free Environment. Prepared under a grant to the American Institute of Architects by the Rehabilitation Services Administration of the Department of Health, Education, and Welfare, Washington DC, 1975.

Klinger, J. L.: Self Help Manual for Arthritic Patients. New York: The Arthritis Foundation, 1974.

Klinger, J. L., Friedman, F. H., and Sullivan, R. A.: Mealtime Manual for the Aged and Handicapped. New York: Simon and Schuster, 1970.

Knoll, C. S., and Schwab, L. O.: The outlook for homemaking in rehabilitation. J. Home Economics, January 1974, pp. 39–41.

Krusen, F. H.: Handbook of Physical Medicine and Rehabilitation. Philadelphia: W. B. Saunders Co., 1971.

Kubler-Ross, E.: On Death and Dying. New York: Macmillan Publishing Co., 1969.

Lowman, E. W., and Klinger, J. L.: Aids to Independent Living: Self Help for the Handicapped. New York: McGraw-Hill Book Co., 1970.

Making Facilities Accessible to the Physically Handicapped. New York State University Construction Fund, Albany, 1974.

Malick, M.: Manual on Dynamic Hand Splinting. Harmarville Rehabilitation Center, Pittsburgh PA, 1974.

Malick, M.: Manual on Static Hand Splinting. Harmarville Rehabilitation Center, Pittsburgh PA, 1970.

May, E. E., and Waggoner, N. R.: Work Simplification in Child Care. Teaching Materials for the Rehabilitation of Physically Handicapped Homemakers, University of Conn., School of Home Economics, Storrs CN, 1962.

May, E. E., Waggoner, N. R., and Hotte, E. B.: Independent Living for the Handicapped and the Elderly. Boston: Houghton, Mifflin Co., 1974.

McGowan, J. F., and Gust, T.: Preparing Higher Education Facilities for Handicapped Students. Columbia, University of Missouri, Services for the Handicapped, Columbia, 1968.

McHugh, H. F.: The 1977 Family as Consumers. J. Home Economics, January 1977.

Morgan, M.: Beyond disability: A broader definition of architectural barriers. A/A Journal 65:50–54, 1976.

Mondale, W. F.: Government policy, stress and the family. J. Home Economics, November 1976.

Nau, L.: Why not family rehabilitation? J. Rehabil. 39:14–17, 1973.

Newton, A.: Clothing: A rehabilitation tool for the handicapped. J. Home Economics, April 1973, p. 2.

Olson, S. C., and Meredith, D. K.: Wheelchair Interiors. National Easter Seal Society for Crippled Children and Adults, Chicago, 1973.

Rednick, S. S.: The Physically Handicapped Student in the Regular Classroom. A Guide for Teaching Housing and Home Care. Danville IL: Interstate Printers and Publishers, 1976.

Reference List on Self Help Devices for the Handicapped. National Easter Seal Society for Crippled Children and Adults, Chicago, 1972.

Rehabilitation of the Physically Handicapped in Homemaking Activities. Proceedings of a Workshop. U.S. Department of Health, Education and Welfare, Washington DC, 1963.

Rusk, H. A.: Manual for Training the Disabled Homemaker. Rehabilitation Monograph VII, Institute of Rehabilitation Medicine, New York, 1970.

Rusk, H. A.: Rehabilitation Medicine, ed. 3. St. Louis: C. V. Mosby Co., 1971.

Schwab, L. O.: Rehabilitation of physically disabled women in a family oriented program. Rehabil. Lit. 36:34–47, 1975.

Schwab, L. O., and Fadul, R.: Are we prepared for the new rehabilitation legislation? J. Home Economics, March, 1975, pp. 33–34.

Slater, S. B., Sussman, M. B., and Straud, M. W.: Participation in household activities as a prognostic factor in rehabilitation. Arch. Phys. Med. Rehabil. 51:1970.

Smith, C. R.: Home planning for the severely disabled. Medical Clinics N. Am. 53:703, 1969.

Shattel, F. M.: Workshop on Rehabilitation of the Physically Handicapped in the Homemaking Activities. Sponsored by AHEA, OVR, U.S. Department of Health, Education and Welfare, January 1963.

Steinke, N., and Erickson, P.: Homemaking Aids for the Disabled. 1963. Available at American Rehabilitation Foundation, 1800 Chicago Avenue, Minneapolis MN 54404.

Straus, R.: Social change and the rehabilitation concept. In Sussman, M. B. (ed.): Sociology and Rehabilitation. Cleveland OH: American Sociological Association, 1965.

Suchman, E. A., "A model for research and evaluation on rehabilitation. In Sussman, M. B. (ed.): Sociology and Rehabilitation. Cleveland OH: American Sociological Association, 1965.

Technical Handbook for Facilities Engineering and Construction Manual. Section 4.12: Design of Barrier-Free Facilities. U. S. Department of Health, Education, and Welfare, Washington DC, 1974.

Waggoner, N. R., and Reedy, G. N.: Child Care Equipment for Physically Handicapped Mothers, Suggestions for Selection and Adaptation. University of Connecticut, School of Home Economics, Storrs CN, 1961.

Watkins, S. M.: Designing functional clothing. J. Home Economics, November, 1974, pp. 33–38.

Wedin, C. S., and Nygren, L. G. (eds.): Housing Perspectives, Individuals and Families. Minneapolis: Burgess Publishing Co., 1976.

Wheeler, V. H.: Planning Kitchens for Handicapped Homemakers. Rehabilitation Monograph 27. Institute of Rehabilitation Medicine, New York, 1966.

Zimmerman, M. E.: Homemaking training units for rehabilitation centers. Am. J. Occup. Ther. 20:226, 1966.

section 5/Prevocational and Vocational Assessment/Dorothy L. Kester

Prevocational Evaluation. Vocational Evaluation. Work Evaluation. What are they? What is their purpose? Who is involved? Are these terms synonymous? Do some people use one term to mean different things, or do some people use different terms to mean one thing?

The use of the work potential evaluation has become a logical and necessary step in the rehabilitation process of many disabled persons. These persons need to define and refine their knowledge of their abilities, disabilities, potentials, behaviors, interests, and job requirements. Such knowledge is also needed by vocational rehabilitation counselors, job trainers, and employers who are working with clients towards vocational success. Evaluation of work potential developed in order to help clients obtain this knowledge. Different types of evaluations vary as to breadth and depth of investigation.

The *prevocational evaluation* focuses on areas determined by the occupational therapists providing the service. Major factors evaluated include activities of daily living (ADL), educational abilities, and physical capacities and deficits. *Work evaluation* assesses vocational strengths and weaknesses through the utilization of real or simulated work. *Vocational evaluation* involves the assessment of pertinent medical, psychological, educational, social, environmental, cultural, and vocational factors. In other words, all factors that could affect successful employment are evaluated. This is an interdisciplinary assessment coordinated by the vocational counselor.

The vocational counselor needs definitive information about the client. The scope of the necessary information is far-ranging because of individual client problems and needs. The counselor wants assistance in differentiating the client who will benefit from remediation before evaluation, the one who requires only evaluation to determine feasibility of placement on, or return to, a specific job, the one who is ready for a full vocational evaluation to determine vocational potentials, and the one who does not have vocational potential.

The counselor needs to receive precise information about the client's strengths and weaknesses in such areas as dexterity, discrimination, work speed, quality of work, short and long term memory, ability to understand written and verbal instructions, and job skills. This information, however, can be of no benefit or be misleading to the counselor if other factors affecting employment are not also reported. These factors include interpersonal relationships with coworkers and supervisors, work behavior, motivation, interests in addition to those enumerated in interest tests, work readiness, health, self-care, transportation problems, or family concerns such as need for day care for children or unwillingness to leave the children or a disabled spouse.

No matter how well informed the counselor becomes, there are times when counseling and planning with clients can fail if the clients do not have sufficient self-knowledge or an awareness of their potentials and the world of work. If the evaluation system provides experiences that the client can easily relate to real jobs (*vocational exploration*) and the client is provided with input regarding performance, then the client and the counselor can choose a placement more accurately. This increases the probability of successful employment. This is especially true if the client must develop completely new skills, whether because of a catastrophic disability, long term illness, institutionalization, or lack of work experience. Clients need to "see for themselves" that they can do the job.

To be most effective the evaluation must provide information to the counselor in as many areas as possible and increase the client's knowledge in areas of personal and vocational exploration. Such evaluation speeds the client's return to employment, ensures client and employer satisfaction, and eliminates trial-and-error methods that are costly in time, money, and self-confidence for both the client and the counselor.

HISTORY

No special methods were utilized in determining vocational placement for the handicapped throughout most of recorded history. Handicapped individuals were on their own, as was anyone else seeking employment. People tried their parents' occupation or what appeared to be something they could do. If failures occurred other jobs were chosen by trial-and-error until the individual succeeded or became too frustrated to do anything.

It was not until the twentieth century, especially during World War I, that any attempt at systematic placement assistance was made. The first method was trial in several trade training classes in order to select the course in which the person was interested and had shown potential. The first objective method involved analyzing and charting the specific demands of jobs such as physical, visual, auditory, verbal, and environmental factors. Clients were evaluated for their capacity to fulfill the same list of demands. By comparing the client's checklist to those of a variety of jobs, some job might be found that the individual was capable of performing well. Consideration was given to skill factors in this method, but consideration of interest was minimal.

World War I appears to have been the impetus for the broadening of psychometric testing, which increased consideration of interests, skills, and potentials. Job performance tests, which developed during World War II, further broadened the scope of these evaluations.

In 1936 the Institute for Crippled and Disabled (I.C.D.) recognized that traditional psychometric and employment batteries utilized for able-bodied job applicants were not suitable for the majority of persons with physical disabilities. Although these batteries provided some of the necessary information, more in-depth information, closely related to actual work, was needed by both the counselors and the clients. However, it was not until 1953 that the move to develop actual tasks finally gained widespread acceptance and broadened to include both physical and psychological disabilities. Since then techniques for evaluation have undergone many changes and will continue to do so.

In 1954 new laws were written stating that the minimum vocational requirement could be met only if a prevocational evaluation unit with sufficient space, equipment, and personnel was available as part of the vocational rehabilitation process.

In the late 1950s the majority of evaluators were occupational therapists but now evaluators from other disciplines are in the majority. Several universities have developed departments for the education and training of vocational evaluators.

THE OCCUPATIONAL THERAPIST IN WORK EVALUATION

For many occupational therapists, the evaluator's role, which helps finalize the client's rehabilitation, is rewarding. The goals of occupational therapy programs, by their very nature, should always be aimed towards furthering vocational goals. Work evaluation is a specialty directly related to occupational therapy, with its primary emphasis geared to discovering appropriate vocational goals. Skills already acquired by occupational therapists must be enhanced and some new skills learned in order to do work evaluations. The personal and professional knowledge relevant to occupational therapy are already pertinent to work evaluation.

The occupational therapist is interested in working with people. The therapist must develop an ability to observe and perceive, learn how to analyze what was seen and heard, and relate this knowledge to a patient's problems and goals. When this is combined with an ability to learn the techniques and tool-handling skills of a wide variety of tasks, the therapist has achieved a versatility essential to a work evaluator.

Other factors that give the occupational therapist the capability of performing work evaluations include knowledge of disabling conditions and the problems involved, focus on minimizing the problems and maximizing the assets, knowledge of methods for achieving a therapeutic relationship, and skill in techniques for motivating and teaching "problem" patients.

The need to relate *with* patients and clients and educate them is present in both occupational therapy and vocational evaluation. Behavioral techniques must be developed and the job market in the community must be investigated in depth. Reality must be emphasized when working with a client and in reporting. Although Tender Loving Care (TLC), motivational techniques, and so forth play an important role with many clients, it is essential that the client knows the "cold facts" of reality before the end of the evaluation.

VOCATIONAL EVALUATION— AN OVERVIEW

The comprehensive vocational evaluation includes a complete spectrum of factors that might affect the client's vocational placement and success and involves persons who are not always housed in the same facility. The work evaluations vary in nature and may be performed in a variety of situations. The type of evaluation used varies with the comprehensiveness of the centers, the clients served, the informational needs of the counselors, and the backgrounds of the evaluators.

Timing for these evaluations vary to some extent but, to be most effective, the client should be at or near his maximal potential prior to evaluation. Information from other disciplines, prior contacts, counseling, testing, and rehabilitation should be utilized. Examples are counselor intake interview, contacts, and counseling; medical evaluation and pertinent treatment; psychological testing; physical or psychiatric rehabilitation; and work and personal adjustment.

Reports of the evaluation should not repeat information previously known to the counselor but should confirm or refute continuation of previously noted problems and assets.

An effective aid in job placement is the Dictionary of Occupational Titles (D.O.T.). This multivolume publication indexes, cross indexes, and describes tasks of and trait requirements of all jobs.

Work Sample Evaluations

These evaluations consist of samples of actual job tasks or a simulation of actual tasks used to determine job skills or isolated traits such as finger dexterity. They are used in settings such as rehabilitation centers, vocational rehabilitation centers, special schools, hospitals, and other institutions.

Situational or Simulated Job Tryout

In this evaluation the client is placed in actual work situations in a sheltered workshop, institution, or other appropriate place.

Job Tryout

In this vocational evaluation the client is placed on an actual job in industry. Prior evaluation has not always taken place.

COMMERCIAL SYSTEMS OF EVALUATION*

The number of commercially available evaluation systems is increasing. Some of the main systems are included here.

McCarron-Dial Work Evaluation System

This system was developed by Lawrence T. McCarron and Jack G. Dial for use with the mentally retarded and chronically mentally ill. It involves seventeen widely accepted instruments based on five neuropsychological factors: verbal-cognitive, sensory, fine and gross motor abilities, emotional, and integration-coping. The first three factors involve instruments that are primarily psychometric in nature, require a formal testing site, and can be performed in one day. The last two factors involve specific instruments and systematic observation in a work situation such as a sheltered workshop and require two weeks of testing.

Few tasks are timed; the emphasis in scoring is on quality of performance. The combined scores for each task area are converted to percentile and plotted on a profile sheet. Work performance as well as work and personal behaviors are included in the scoring, utilizing five-point scales. The final report format includes a profile, narrative summaries for each of the five factors, and recommendations.

No data are available regarding reliability and data on validity is insufficient.

This system attempts to combine useful psychometric testing with performance and behavior observation in one prediction tool. No clear guidelines are given for cutoff points. It is available from:

Commercial Marketing Enterprises
Department: MDWES
11300 North Central, Suite 105
Dallas, Texas 75231

Philadelphia Jewish Employment and Vocational System

This system was originally designed for the disadvantaged and is now being adapted for the dis-

* Information has been adapted from *A Comparison of Seven Vocational Systems* by K. F. Bottenbusch and A. B. Sax.

abled. The twenty-eight work samples are based on the Worker Trait Group Organization of the D.O.T. and are arranged in ten worker trait groups. Each work sample is packaged individually. The work samples are administered in order of difficulty. Client-evaluator contact is minimized and feedback on performance and behavior follows the evaluation process.

The final report utilizes standardized forms for work sample recording, daily observational summaries, and a feedback report. This includes a ranking of work sample performance, recommended worker trait groups with rationale and space for extensive written comments on performance and behavior. Because of the correlations with the D.O.T. many kinds of jobs are covered in the recommendations, which could be broadened further by the counselor familiar with the D.O.T.

No data are available regarding reliability and results of studies done by the U.S. Department of Labor on validity have not been released to the public.

This is a well-integrated highly-standardized system, which emphasizes accurate observation and recording of pertinent information. A major problem is the abstract nature of many of the work samples, which affects the client's ability to relate them to real jobs. This system is available from:

Vocational Research Institute
Jewish Employment and Vocational Service
1913 Walnut Street
Philadelphia, Pennsylvania 19103

Singer Vocational Evaluation System

Developed by Singer Education Division, this system has an unspecified target group and basis. There are twenty groupings of work samples, each located in a separate carrel, the order of administration being left to the discretion of the evaluator. Client-evaluator contact is close as a result of frequent checkpoints. A system is included for self-ratings of interest and performance. Audiovisual instruction, with a controllable rate of advancement, is utilized for all the work samples; written material occasionally supplements the program. The client is able to gain a fairly high degree of vocational exploration because of the format of the work samples.

Scoring focuses on timing intervals, work behaviors, work performance, error, and quality, with the emphasis on quality. Five-point scales are used and forms are provided. It is recommended that the final report include the forms and a narrative report.

No data is available for reliability, validity, or group norms used.

The twenty work samples in this system include mostly skilled trades. The built-in career exploration and occupational information are strong points of this system, but this information is often gained at the expense of increased knowledge of the client's potential. Many of the procedures are not clarified in the manual. Information is available from:

Singer Educational Division
Career Systems
80 Commerce Drive
Rochester, New York 14623

Talent Assessment Programs

There is no specific target group for this system. It is based on occupational clusters of related jobs. The eleven tests are geared to assess perceptions and dexterities. Each work sample is independent and packaged individually. Three of the samples must be given at specified times, the others are interchangeable. The instructions are given orally and no reading is required but, because of the nature of the tests, there is little client-evaluator contact. The battery can be administered in about two and one-half hours. Scoring for errors is not completely defined in the manual; the emphasis is on time which is converted to a percentile. Behaviors do not appear to be rated. The final report includes a profile sheet, a form for recording job possibility clusters, and space for a narrative report and recommendations.

This system does not provide any direct vocational information to the client. It was normed against seven groups, primarily young people. Reliability is stated but no data is available on validity.

Although this system is accepted for specific factors, it is not a system that provides a true vocational evaluation. The developers suggest that other assessment devices be used as well. Information may be obtained from:

Talent Assessment Programs
7015 Colby Avenue
Des Moines, Iowa 50311

Tower System

The tower system is an outgrowth of a system developed by the Institute for Crippled and Disabled (I.C.D.) in 1936. It contains ninety-three work samples arranged into fourteen job training areas. The samples are grouped by area and are not individually packaged.

Administration of the tests takes three weeks. It is progressive within each area, but choice of areas is at the discretion of the evaluator. A realistic work setting and atmosphere is stressed. Instructions are written but should be supplemented as needed before the client proceeds. Client-evaluator contact is not specified but is taken for granted. The client is exposed to many training areas and can be given additional specific occupational information.

In scoring this system, time and work quality are given equal weight, criteria are carefully defined, and scoring aids are extensive. Scoring is on a five-point scale. Work factors and work behaviors are mentioned minimally and are not specifically defined.

Standardized forms are utilized for recording and reporting each work sample and job area but apparently are not included in the final report. A narrative summary utilizes both a standardized outline and a section giving global ratings directly related to the work samples.

This system, based on job analysis, is very useful in evaluating clients, but applies only to a narrow group of jobs unless the counselor utilizes the D.O.T. to broaden the scope. Precise definitions of performance and behaviors and lack of adequate norms are the major weaknesses of the system. Information is available through:

I. C. D. Rehabilitation and Research Center
340 East 24th Street
New York, New York 10010

Valpar Component Work Sample Series

Developed by Valpar Corporation for industrially injured workers, the Valpar component work sample series involves a worker trait and work factor approach based on task analysis. There are presently twelve work samples, which are used individually rather than as a group. Each sample is self-contained, mostly in lockable cases.

The order of administration is at the discretion of the evaluator, as is feedback on performance. The time required is not given but is estimated at twelve to fifteen hours. Instructions are given orally and by demonstration; reading is not required unless inherent to the task.

Scoring emphasizes time and quality, equally; then scores are converted to percentiles and combined to provide total performance scores. Seventeen work behaviors are rated on a five-point scale. The samples are each rated on standard forms, but no combined final report form is used.

Reliability estimates are fairly high, although no data is available for validity.

This series is well designed, appealing to clients, easy to administer, and combines well with another system, but many aspects of an integrated system are lacking. As a consequence of the abstract nature of the samples, vocational exploration is limited. Since this series was not developed as an evaluation system, the manuals indicate areas for further evaluation. Contact may be made with:

Valpar Corporation
655 N. Alvernon
Suite 108
Tuscon, Arizona 85716

Wide Range Employment Sample Test

This test, developed by Guidance Associates of Delaware, Inc., does not have a designated target group. The samples were developed for a sheltered workshop dealing with mentally retarded and physically handicapped. The ten samples are fairly low level. Each sample is independent in nature, but the samples are not individually packaged. They are administered in numerical order and it is assumed that there is little client-evaluator involvement. Administration time is about one and one-half hours for one client and two hours for small groups. Instructions are oral with demonstration; no reading is required.

The samples are timed by stopwatch and times are rated on a nineteen-point scale. Errors are checked against clearly defined criteria, totaled for all ten tasks, and compared to a norms table. There is no indication that work performance and behaviors are observed. The final report combines a summary of results form with narrative commentary.

Some reliability estimates are given but the

methodology is questioned; no data are available for validity.

This system appears to be most appropriate for determining assignments for clients new to a sheltered workshop, and an emphasis on retesting should determine the client's ability to improve with practice. The major problems include lack of behavioral observations and failure to relate results to the competitive job market. The samples are not appropriate for adding to the client's job awareness. Tests may be obtained from:

Guidance Associates of Delaware, Inc.
1526 Gilpin Avenue
Wilmington, Delaware 19806

PHYSICAL AND FUNCTIONAL EVALUATION

This evaluation requires a maximum of one day and is designed primarily for two purposes: it helps eliminate the client who really cannot be helped because of severe physical limitations and who cannot perform any of the more sedentary tasks because of educational and/or mental deficits, and it is geared to discovering the client who has employment potential despite limitations.

A standardized test battery is utilized to analyze the ability to perform and tolerate physical activities such as sitting, standing, walking, lifting, and handling. Tasks are used to provide basic information about potential skill levels. For example, math, reading, and mechanical skills can be tested concurrently with sitting tolerance. This knowledge can be utilized for planning during further testing if employment potential is indicated.

A sample form is shown in Figure 10-11. Norms have not been filled in since they vary depending on the tasks in the individual center's test battery. The norms are recorded for comparison with the client's actual tolerances and strengths which are entered in the limits column. A narrative section includes observations, a summary, and recommendations. The report should define the limitations created by the disability and the capacities remaining despite the disability.

CASE HISTORY

Mr. L. D. was sixty years of age and mildly retarded with minimal schooling. He had a lumbar disk problem and ulcers for 35 years, osteoarthritis, parkinsonism, emphysema, hypertension, history of alcoholism, loss of memory, and personality disorder. His work history included farming, labor force, and truck driving. He is now unable even to help around the house.

Because of legal technicalities, further evaluation was required to prove lack of work potential.

Mr. D. tolerated sitting for 5-minute periods of time and standing for 1 minute. He required 45 seconds to walk 80 feet with rests, and he was breathing heavily before he had reached 40 feet. He braced his hand on the table during the standing and on the second attempt hand tremor was so great that the table shook. Strength of grip was only 10 pounds unless he stabilized his arm against his side. Scores for all capacities were in the zero column.

WORK TOLERANCE EVALUATION

This evaluation includes a physical and functional evaluation with special emphasis on tolerances for those actions and capacities required for a specific job or type of job. For the client who has been unemployed for some time as a result of illness or injury, it also includes an evaluation of ability to perform a full day's work. The length of the evaluation varies with the length of lay-off and severity of the problem but should always be longer than one day because the client can frequently tolerate much more for one day than he can on a sustained basis.

The battery used varies with the goals for the individual client, but the closer the activities relate to the job the more effective the evaluation. In many cases, if the requirements of the activities are graded for stress, tolerance increases as the evaluation proceeds.

CASE HISTORY SUMMARY

On Mr. F.J.'s stock clerk job a bicycle was used on level ground for delivering some of the materials; activity was intermittent. Items were stored at all heights, but none weighed more than 25 pounds. After recovery from a posterior myocardial infarction, he required nitroglycerine infrequently. His physician and his counselor were positive that he could safely return to his job but the employer was reluctant.

Mr. F. J. was admitted for an evaluation of his tolerance for activity and was seen for two successive days.

On the first day, periods of active tasks were alternated with more sedentary ones. The active tasks included:

Bicycling—15 min.—no resistance—no pulse change, some shortness of breath.

PHYSICAL CAPACITIES EVALUATION

Name: ______________________________ Date: ______________________

	NORMS	N	G	F	P	O	LIMITS	COMMENTS
1. Sitting								
Standing								
Walking								
Stooping								
Kneeling								
Crouching								
Crawling								
2. Climbing								
Balancing								
3. Lifting (Unilateral)								
Lifting (Bilateral)								
Carrying								
Pushing								
Pulling								
4. Reaching								
Handling								
Fingering								
Feeling								
Placing								
5. Talking								
Hearing								
6. Seeing								
a. Acuity								
b. Depth perception								
c. Field of vision								
d. Accommodation								
e. Color vision								

FUNCTIONAL TOLERANCES

	NORMS	N	G	F	P	O	LIMITS	COMMENTS
1. Standing								
2. Sitting								
3. General mobility								
4. Fine work								
5. Rapid work								
6. Repetitive work								
7. Sequential work								
a. Short cycle								
b. Long cycle								
8. Stamina								

Norms are based on D.O.T. Standards

KEY: O—Unable to perform, or impractical
P—Performed with assistance, improvement needed
F—Performed without assistance, but improvement needed to be adequate
G—Adequate for practical performance even though affected by disability
N—Performance not affected by disability

FIGURE 10-11. Sample form for a physical functional evaluation. From Delaware Curative Workshop, Wilmington. Reprinted with permission.

Lifting—41 lb. from floor to waist height 1 time
37 lb. from chair to head height 1 time
37 lb. from floor to head height 11 times—some shortness of breath noted.
Stair climbing—7 round trips on 8 steps with a pulse increase from 72 to 104.

The other tasks on the check sheet were performed as a group without a rest period.

On the second day, two sedentary tasks were performed and the active tasks were performed without rest periods. Printing was done on a hand press on which the handle must be raised in an arc (up and away from the body) from waist height to head height; graded springs were used to resist raising the handle. The schedule followed was:

Printing—15 min.—30 lb. handle on the right
15 min.—25 lb., no symptoms
Bicycling—15 min.—28 lb. resistance, no symptoms
Lifting—3 min.—61 lb. 1 time from 12 in. to waist height
53 lb. 6 times—pulse increased from 72 to 80. (Normal increase can be up to 30 units)
Sedentary task—7 min.
Lifting—6 min.—41 lb.—10 times from 12 in. to waist height—pulse increased to 92
Sedentary task—15 min.
Bicycling—15 min.—40 lb.
Printing—15 min.—50 lb. resistance

Mr. F. J. was able to perform resistive tasks for a 2-hour period with minimal rest and minimal symptomatology. Shortness of breath or pulse rise was noted only with repetitive stairclimbing and repetitive lifting of more than 30 pounds to head height or more than 50 pounds to waist height.

This was adequate tolerance for the intermittently active type of job described. The actual report provided sufficient evidence that the employer allowed him to return to work.

SPECIFIC VOCATIONAL EVALUATION

This evaluation is designed to determine ability to perform a specific new job or type of work, to analyze ability to return to a prior employer in a previous or new job, to substantiate or repudiate prior information, or to help the client realize his potential (or lack of potential) for that specific work.

The process involves appropriate commercial work samples, if available, augmented by increasingly definitive tasks. A physical and functional evaluation and at least pertinent aspects of a tolerance evaluation should be included. This evaluation varies in length from one to several days.

CASE HISTORY SUMMARY

Mr. M. C. was 41 years old. His physical condition following an accident at work had deteriorated. When admitted he required two canes and had a body posture that placed stress on his hands and arms to the extent that his sense of touch was being affected. His hands were large and heavy.

His only vocational interest was to be a locksmith, which all previous testing ruled out as a possibility. He was admitted for a Specific Work Evaluation to determine his aptitude for this. Emphasis was placed on testing general physical tolerance, manual dexterity, and mechanical comprehension. His overall endurance and lower extremity and trunk strength were poor. He leaned heavily on his canes when ambulating and had considerable difficulty moving from a sitting to a standing position.

His manual dexterity proved to be higher on functional tasks than on tests, varying from below average to well above the norm. For example, his scores on the Crawford Small Parts Dexterity Test ranged from the eighth to the forty-third percentiles. When given actual job-related tasks such as simple lock or cigarette lighter repair, he performed at a higher level of manual skill, handling small parts, springs, and so forth in the usual manner or finding a method which counterbalanced the largeness of his fingers.

Scores on the Bennett Mechanical Comprehension Tests, added to give a complete picture of his potential, were in the eightieth percentile when compared to industrial applicants. Actual work samples were satisfactorily completed well within required standards.

This job-relevant information provided his counselor with specific information and a correspondence course was purchased for him. Before he had finished the course, Mr. C was semiemployed by a locksmith near his home and, after completion, he opened his own shop.

SENSORY MOTOR EVALUATION

The sensory motor evaluation, either partial or complete, is given to persons of all ages on the same basis that it is used for children. For example, those who have had difficulty learning, cannot function to expected capacities, appear to have visual or coordination problems, and poor visual or physical tolerance not from obvious causes, and/or have hyper or hypoactive behavior can undergo the evaluation. In other words, it is given to those who should benefit from training or further education but seem unable to do so.

The purposes are to diagnose any perceptual dysfunction, whether primary or secondary in nature, and to assist with planning by analyzing the effect of any dysfunction on vocational potentials.

The battery consists of a standardized sensory motor battery, which includes all levels of perceptual development plus age-appropriate vocationally-oriented tests that provide perceptual information. This evaluation has been utilized during the process of other evaluations or as a separate entity for clients who are having unexpected difficulties in training programs.

Since scoring is available only for children and has no real meaning to the counselors, it is necessary to convert the information to the age level at which the clients are functioning in the different perceptual areas and to include the more meaningful vocational test scores. The narrative part of the report is used to educate the counselors and the training personnel and to relate the problems to vocational potentials as well as to the difficulties that are being seen.

CASE HISTORY SUMMARY

O. B. was a husky 16-year old who looked older. His speech development was slow and he had received therapy. He participated in sports, apparently doing well, but had problems with his peers. He had a long history of school-related problems. These problems were increasing, as were family tensions and pressures. Testing placed his grade levels at 5 for reading, 3.5 for spelling, and 7 for math. He avoided fine tasks, was heavy handed, and his family perceived him as careless, lazy, unwilling to stick to a task, and poorly motivated.

Test results and observations made during the evaluation indicated that perceptual dysfunction played a major role in many of his problems. The asymmetrical tonic neck reflex and tonic labyrinthine response were incompletely integrated, crossing of the midline was avoided, vision was used minimally to assist balance, and laterality was not completely automatic.

Reception and interpretation of tactile stimuli were more highly developed on the left and symptoms of tactile sensitivity and poor tolerance became increasingly more pronounced as testing progressed. In order to provide auditory reinforcement his handling of the pieces on the Minnesota Rate of Manipulation Test and The Minnesota Spatial Relations Test became increasingly heavy as his tactile tolerance was reached. He also became more careless, barely raising the pieces if they could be slid into place. The effects of the preceding problems were most pronounced on tasks requiring combined gross and fine motor functions and/or bilateral use of the hands.

Much manipulation of body and materials was noted during visual-motor tasks, minimal shoulder motion was used on the right and midline crossing was avoided, especially by the left hand. When copying designs he demonstrated difficulty with closure, directionality and crossing of any previously drawn lines.

The major factors affecting visual ability were poor visual memory, visual tolerance, and figure ground perception. Convergence was poor and near focus was inadequate. Perseveration was noted on visual and visual-motor tasks.

Auditory discrimination, selective attention, sequential memory, translation from sounds to symbols, and processing were deficient.

(Although nowhere near an ideal solution, in some cases evaluation alone can produce results. Confirmation that there is a basis for many of the problems can ease the pressures, producing a more relaxed attitude which in itself allows the persons to function at a higher level.) With this client much more was attained even though he could not attend the remediation program. He was provided with a home program which he *did* follow with the help of his family.

His mother observed the evaluation; her observations and discussions with the evaluator provided an understanding of the depth of his problems. She was able to relate what she saw and heard to problems seen at home and in school. Notes she took during this time enabled her to communicate her new knowledge and understanding to the rest of the family and to relate remediative suggestions on the home program list to activities done by him at home.

Communication from the mother was fairly frequent until the family moved out of state. Each telephone call provided further evidence of increase in O. B.'s ego strength and family togetherness in solving this problem.

SUMMARY

As a summary to this section, the best way to demonstrate the value and use of work evaluations is to present a case study in which all levels of evaluation and some aspects of adjustment were required.

CASE STUDY

Mrs. H. H. was seen over a period of 3 months. Her major disability was a psychoneurotic disorder with depressive reaction, but hypertensive vascular disease, alcoholism, and a long medical history contributed. Discomfort from a previously fractured coccyx limited sitting tolerance. Educational level was high average except for math which tested at the 7th grade; intellectual potential was superior. She had checked hats in a hotel for 10 years.

Mrs. H. H. was admitted for a work evaluation. She was given a commercial work sample battery, a partial perceptual battery, and a physical and functional evaluation. Extra time was taken for this because of her depression and poor self-esteem.

She complained of arthritis, primarily in her right hand and buttocks, and had high blood pressure. The only vocationally limiting physical factor was poor tolerance for continuous standing or sitting. She was a perfectionist who did not believe she had any saleable abilities. Reaction to even minor failures was exaggerated and resulted in temporary increase in her depression. She had the additional pressure of her son's return home with all of the problems of the younger generation, including drug addiction.

On admission, she worked slowly, neatly, methodically, and carefully. On most tasks quality was average to superior but speed was inferior. She found unexpected abilities as the evaluation progressed. Her confidence and speed increased while her depression decreased and her blood pressure lowered. Originally she required a fairly high amount of T.L.C. and a great deal of flexibility in length of time given for a specific task. Some flexibility in stated standards for tasks during the first week also added to her self-confidence.

Perceptions were average or above, stereognosis was within normal limits although sensation was slightly diminished in the right hand, and motor planning was above average.

Mrs. H. H. did well on all types of tasks involving precision such as drafting, lettering, copying, paper cutting, printing on a hand press, and electronics other than cable tying. Clerical work was average or above except for mathematics, spelling was superior, and use of English was above average. She had some difficulty learning to use new tools, but once she learned the basic techniques she was able to amplify them.

At first she had difficulty concentrating in noisy surroundings but later was able to work both alone or among others. She was able to teach other clients jobs with which she was familiar.

She discovered an interest and ability in artistic work, especially copying. Her work was precise, her sense of color good, and the work was calming to her. She also demonstrated an interest and ability in food preparation, but her tolerance for continuous standing was too limited for many jobs in this area.

Considering the overall picture, it was felt that work in an art, printing, or layout department would be the best vocational choice. It was also felt that Mrs. H. H. would have difficulty learning in a formal setting but would be able to function, at this stage, in a more sheltered training situation. Some degree of T.L.C. was still required.

A conference was held including the evaluator, the vocational rehabilitation counselor, and two people from the sheltered workshop which could provide layout training. As a result of this, a specific work evaluation and tolerance (emotional, in this case) evaluation were begun at the center. A second purpose for this method of evaluation was to acquaint her with her future supervisor while still in a familiar setting. A second report was written concerning a conference with the workshop personnel so as to put into the records her need for financial assistance for medical purposes. Actual work was brought and demonstrated to her, and results were discussed with her.

The transition was made to the sheltered workshop; she was hired after a period of on-the-job training and, before long, she was capable of teaching other trainees new work as she learned it herself.

Mrs. H. H. was made aware of her capabilities through the evaluation. This, and the adjustment techniques that were used, provided her with the confidence needed for success.

Summarizing the Physical Capacities Evaluation*

In writing the summary of a client's physical capacities, one should try to summarize the client's ability, endurance, speed, safety, and strength in all of the activities tested. The activities which the client was unable to perform can be listed and, in the test, it can be stated why he was unable to perform each activity. The length of time the test took, the frequency of rest periods, any appliances used, the amount of pain or discomfort, and the client's overall work endurance should be stated. The client's emotional reactions, including his emotional tolerance, ability to follow directions, appearance, and cooperativeness might also be stated. An example outline follows:

* This evaluation procedure is based upon the physical capacities requirements of the *Dictionary of Occupational Titles* (D.O.T.), U.S. Department of Labor. It was adapted from the physical capacities evaluation developed at The Woodrow Wilson Rehabilitation Center, Fisherville, Virginia, by Susan L. Smith, New Orleans LA. It is reprinted with the permission of Ms. Smith.

1. Emotional picture
   A. Appearance
   B. Attitude and cooperativeness
   C. Emotional reactions
   D. Amount of pain
   E. Evidence of visual or speech defects
II. Physical performance
   A. Limitations and achievements in:
      1. Ability (including strength and safety)
      2. Endurance (specifically in each test)
      3. Speed
   B. Activities client unable to perform
   C. Additional tests if pertinent
   D. Overall time test completed in and frequency in rests
   E. Overall work endurance

PHYSICAL CAPACITIES EVALUATION

Administrator's Guide for Physical Capacities Evaluation

Performance Rating:
Within Normal Range (W.N.R.)
Fair
Poor
Unable
Not appropriate (N.A.)

"Comment" space to be used only for:
Reason unable to perform
Other significant performance

Use of exercise mats:
"Kneeling" and/or "Crawling" if client's knees are tender
"Reclining" if floor too hard

Standard of comparison:
"Walking": Army Regulation—66 seconds per 100 yards
"Climbing" (stairs): Average time between 3 and 5 seconds each way

---

Walking:
Request:
1. To walk as ordinarily 100 yd. on rubber tiled flooring.
   A. Performance:
      a. Type of gait:
      b. Appliances used:
      c. Endurance:
      d. Safety:
2. The client's estimate of distance and length of time he is able to walk.
   A. Estimate:
      a. Distance inside:
      b. Distance outside:
      c. Time inside:
      d. Time outside:

Comment: ____________________

____

Running
Request:
1. To run 30 yds on rubber tiled flooring.
   A. Performance:
      a. Endurance:
      b. Type of gait:
      c. Safety:

Comment: ____________________

____

Jumping:

Request:

1. To jump from a 19 in. & 30 in. high platform onto rubber tiled flooring landing on both feet.
   A. Performance:
      a. Balance: 19″: ______ 30″: ______
      b. Ability: 19″: ______ 30″: ______
      c. Safety: 19″: ______ 30″: ______

Comment: ______

Climbing

Request:

1. Ramp (8′ × 12° textured brick tile surface): To walk up and down five consecutive times.
   A. Performance:
      a. Gait:
      b. Endurance:
      c. Use of handrail:
      d. Use of appliance:
2. Stairs: (10 steps, 7 in. rise, steel and stone tread) to walk up and down once.
   A. Performance:
      a. Safety:
      b. Endurance:
      c. Speed:
      d. Use of handrail:
      e. Use of appliances:
      f. Foot-over-foot: Foot-by-foot:
3. Curbs: (9 in. and 14 in. high) To climb and descend curbs once.
   A. Performance in reference to public transportation:
      a. Ability: 8″ ______ 14″ ______
      b. Use of appliances:
      c. Safety:
4. Straight ladder (8 rungs, 10 ft. high): to climb up and down five consecutive times.
   A. Performance:
      a. Foot-over-foot: Foot by foot:
      b. Hand-over-hand Hand on rail:
         Hand-by-hand:
      c. Balance:
      d. Safety:
5. Step Ladder. (6 ft. 10 in. rise): To climb up and down once carrying a 10 lb. paint pail in one hand.
   A. Performance:
      a. Foot-over-foot: Foot-by-foot:
      b. Balance:
      c. Safety:

Comments: ______

Crouching:

Request:

1. To work in a squatting position for 3 minutes placing 1½ lb. cans (4″ × 8″) from the floor to a 19″ high shelf.
   A. Performance:
      a. Ability to carry out task:
      b. Ability to assume position:
      c. Ability to regain standing:
      d. Balance:
      e. Endurance:

Comments: ______

Lifting:
Request:
1. Left Hand—To lift maximum weight from floor to a waist-high surface five consecutive times.
   A. Performance:
      a. Number of lb.:
      b. Ability:
      c. Balance:
      d. Endurance:
2. Right Hand—Same as left
   A. Performance:
      a. Number of lb.:
      b. Ability:
      c. Endurance:
      d. Balance:
3. Both hands—To lift maximum in weighted box from floor to a waist high surface five consecutive times.
   A. Performance:
      a. Ability:
      b. Balance:
      c. Endurance:
      d. Number of lbs.:

Comments: ____

____

Carrying:
Request:
1. To bilaterally carry maximum weight in weighted boxes 25 yd. while walking on rubber tiled flooring.
   A. Performance:
      a. Number of lb.:
      b. Ability:
      c. Endurance:
      d. Balance:

Comments: ____

____

Handling:
Administrator's estimate of the maximum weight the testee is able to handle comfortably.
1. Estimate:

Comments: ____

____

Pushing: Push—Pull
Request:
1. To push a wheelbarrow (heavy duty with inflated rubber tire) for 25 yd. on rubber tiled flooring with maximum load.
   A. Performance:
      a. Ability:
      b. Endurance:
      c. Balance on turning:
2. To alternately push and pull bilaterally to arm's length the maximum in a weighted box on a waist high rough wooden surface, ten times, both from standing and sitting positions.
   A. Performance:
      a. Number of lb. ____________ Standing: Sitting:
      b. Ability:

Comments: ____

____

Pulling:

Request:

1. To pull in a hand-over-hand fashion the maximum weight on a single pulley (¾ in. cotton rope) ten consecutive times.
   A. Performance:
      a. Number of lb.:
      b. Ability:
      c. Endurance:
      d. Balance:

Comments: ____

____

Stooping:

Request:

1. To perform in 3 min. standing and stooping repeatedly while placing 5 lb. cans (4 in. × 8 in.) from the floor to a 48 in. high shelf.
   A. Performance:
      a. Ability:
      b. Endurance:
      c. Ability to grasp— Right hand: Left hand:

Comments: ____

____

Reaching:

Request:

1. Overhead—from a standing position to bimanually reach a 10 lb. box from an overhead shelf; return it to position. To reach with separate hands small objects from the same shelf.
   A. Performance:
      a. Ability: 10 lb.: Right: Left:
      b. Range of motion
      c. Balance:
      d. Coordination: Grasp:
2. Forward: Standing—To reach forward and pick up a 10 lb. box from a table with both hands.
   A. Performance:
      a. Balance: Both: Right: Left:
      b. Coordination: Both:
      c. Grasp: Right: Left:
      d. Range of motion: Both: Right: Left:
3. Forward: Sitting—To reach forward for a small object on the table with separate hands, both directly and across the body.
   A. Performance:
      a. Balance: Both: Right: Left:
      b. Coordination: Both:
      c. Grasp: Right: Left:
      d. Range of motion: Both: Right: Left:
4. Low: Standing—To pick up small objects on floor from front position with both hands. To pick up same object on right and left sides with separate hands both directly and across body.
   A. Performance:
      a. Balance: Both: Right: Left:
      b. Coordination: Both:
      c. Grasp: Right: Left:
      d. Range of motion: Both: Right: Left:
5. Sitting—To reach directly for small object on floor with separate hands at the right, left, and front positions.
   A. Performance:
      a. Balance: Right: F. Right: F. Left:
      B. Range of motion:
      c. Grasp: Right: Left: F. Right: F. Left:

Comments: ____

____

Kneeling:

Request:

1. To assume a kneeling position on a rubber tiled floor and maintain it for a 1 min. period.
   A. Performance:
      a. Ability to assume position:
      b. Ability to regain standing:
      c. Balance:
      d. Endurance:

Comments: ______________________________

____

Crawling:

Request:

1. To crawl on rubber tiled flooring 8 ft. forward and then backward with head and shoulders down.
   A. Performance:
      a. Type crawl: 4-point: 3-point: Other:
      b. Speed:
      c. Agility:

Comments: ______________________________

____

Reclining:

Request:

1. To assume a backlying position on rubber tiled flooring. When in position.
   A. Performance:
      a. Ability to assume position:
      b. Ability to regain standing:
      c. Ability to turn: Right: Left: Face:
      d. Comfort on: Right: Left: Face: Back:

Comments: ______________________________

____

Turning:

Request:

1. To lift maximum weight in box from the floor, to turn trunk only and place it to the right at waist level and back to floor. Repeat for left side.
   A. Performance:
      a. Ability to: Right: Left:
      b. Balance: Right: Left:
      c. Endurance:

Comments: ______________________________

____

Balancing:

Request:

1. To one-leg stand on individual legs for 30 sec. each.
   A. Performance:
      a. Ability: Right: ______________ Left: ______________
      b. Endurance: Right: ______________ Left: ______________
      c. Leg dominance: Right: ______________ Left: ______________

Comment: ______________________________

____

Sitting:

With what ability is the client able to get in and out of a straight-backed chair? For an estimated period how long could he sit comfortably and with what type posture?

1. Ability to sit:
2. Ability to rise:
3. Estimated time:
4. Type of posture:

Comment: ______________________________

____

Standing:

What type of posture and stance does the client exhibit? Client's estimate of time he can stand.

1. Posture:
2. Stance:
3. Estimate of time:

Comment: ______________________________

____

Hand Grasp:

As measured with a dynamometer, the strength of the client's hand grasp.

1. Broad grasp: Right: ________ Left: ________
2. Tight grasp: Right: ________ Left: ________
3. Hand dominance: Right: ________ Left: ________

Comment: ______________________________

____

BIBLIOGRAPHY

Brewer, E., Miller, J., and Ray, J.: The effect of vocational evaluation and work adjustment on clients' attitude toward work. Voc. Eval. Work Adjustment Bull. 8:18–25, 1975.

Bottersbusch, K. F., and Sax, A. B.: A Comparison of Seven Vocational Systems, Materials Development Center, Stout Rehabilitation Institute, University of Wisconsin, Menomonie WI, 1976.

Dinneen, T.: Work Evaluation as a technique for improving self-concept. Voc. Eval. Work Adjustment Bull. 8:28–34, 1975.

Granofsky, J.: A Manual for Occupational Therapists on Prevocational Exploration. Dubuque IA: W. C. Brown Book Co., 1959.

Hoffman, P. R.: Work evaluation, an overview. Work Evaluation in Rehabilitation, Reprint Series RS-70-2, 3–18, 1969.

Olshansky, S.: Reply to Kopstein and Lores. Rehabil. Lit. 36:142, 1975.

Raymond, E.: Measuring the interpersonal aspects of work behavior. Voc. Eval. Work Adjustment Bull. 8:19–23, 1975.

Roberts, C. L.: Definitions, objectives and goals in work evaluation. Work Evaluation in Rehabilitation, Reprint Series RS-70-2, 19–30, 1969.

Part Five

Treatment Process and Procedures

11

Treatment Process and Procedures

section 1/Therapeutic Application of Activity/Helen L. Hopkins

Therapeutic application of activity to meet the specific needs of each client requires that the choice of activity be made on the basis of those activity properties that seem to have an impact on the previously identified problems. Consideration must be given to all factors that may have an impact on the individual's ability to function, including physical, psychosocial, cultural, and economic factors. The activity may need to be adapted in order to provide the desired amount of complexity, the correct exercise, or the desired amount of social interaction. Successful completion of the activity chosen promotes development of competence. Client interest and involvement may be enhanced by providing feedback on progress. Some activities, utilized in the treatment of physical dysfunction, allow the use of biofeedback as a means of providing an indication of correct use of muscles and adequate performance. Interaction between the therapist and the client, which provides reassurance and encouragement as well as accurate perception of function, is vital to the therapeutic process.

In order to use activity as therapeutic intervention, each occupational therapist must become adept in giving individuals or groups instructions in the processes involved. Therapists must also learn to make astute observations regarding how the activity is approached, the way it is carried out, and the work habits exhibited in the performance of the activity. These nonverbal cues can assist the therapist in determining the actual functional level of the individual.

METHODS OF INSTRUCTION

Occupational therapists must know how to teach the processes involved in an activity so that the client understands clearly what is to be done yet requires a minimum amount of correction and supervision. The better the instruction the more chance of successful accomplishment. The more successful the experiences the more competency gained. It is therefore vital that the therapist determine the complexity of the activity so that it is within the ability of the individual to assure successful accomplishment.

Preparation for Instruction

Successful instruction is dependent upon preparation done by the therapist before instruction begins. The therapist should analyze the processes and the steps involved in the procedure along with the key points involved in the performance of the activity. This is called the *breakdown of the activity*. The *important steps* are the component parts of the total activity, while the *key points* are the specific steps involved in performance of the activity (Table 11-1).

The therapist should have the proper tools, necessary materials, and equipment ready for use before beginning instruction. The work area should be arranged properly with a minimum amount of clutter so that work can be conducted with safety and without strain. Before beginning, consideration must be given to how much of the total activity may be accomplished in one session. A simple activity with few steps or component parts may be taught in a half-hour session while a more complex activity with many steps may require several sessions to accomplish. The activity of typing, for example, with three steps, may be accomplished in one session with many individuals and might be considered to be one unit of learning. However, becoming adept in typing could not be completed in one session and will require additional learning units to acquire skill. Activities such as dressing may have several units of learning such as (1) put on shirt and button, (2) put on slacks and fasten, (3) put on socks, and (4) put on shoes and tie. Each unit may need to be taught in one or more sessions with repetition required for competence.

Steps in Instruction

After the therapist has made all preparations, instruction may begin using a combination of verbal directions and demonstration. There are four basic steps used in instruction: (1) preparation of the patient/client, (2) presentation of the activity, (3) try out performance, and (4) follow-up.

Step 1. Preparation of the Patient/Client

1. Establish rapport between the therapist and individual to be instructed in order to allay fear and encourage participation.

2. Find out how much the individual knows about the activity so that instruction may be geared accordingly.

3. Involve the individual in the activity in order to assure interest in it. Be sure the individual understands the purpose and value of performance of the activity.

4. Place the individual in comfortable and correct position for performance of the activity. When demonstrating, work at side of the individual so that process may easily be seen. Do *not* work opposite or a reverse mental image may be developed. (When teaching an individual with hand dominance differ-

Table 11-1. Example of breakdown of an activity.

Activity: Typewriting on Standard Typewriter

Important steps	*Key points*
1. Insert paper in typewriter	1. Pick up paper 2. Insert paper at back of platen 3. Pull paper release lever forward 4. Slide paper to typing level and adjust 5. Snap paper release into place
2. Type	1. Place fingers on "home" keys 2. Type to end of line 3. Push carriage return lever to return carriage which moves paper to next line
3. Take paper out of typewriter	1. Pull paper release forward 2. Remove paper 3. Snap paper release into place

ent from that of the therapist, it may be appropriate to instruct while sitting opposite the individual.)

Step 2. Presentation of the Activity

1. Give verbal directions as well as demonstration of the process. Written directions and diagrams may be helpful depending on the complexity of the activity and the learning ability and preferences of the individual.

2. Present instruction slowly and patiently.

3. Teach process step by step, stressing key points.

4. Teach no more than can be mastered at one time.

Step 3. Try out Performance

1. The individual should perform the activity either step by step with the therapist or immediately after being shown.

2. Correct errors as they occur. If possible they should be anticipated so they can be avoided.

3. Have individual explain process.

4. Have individual repeat activity several times to be sure individual knows it and can perform it correctly.

Step 4. Follow-Up

1. Put the individual on his or her own. Allow individual to work independently.

2. Designate the person who can help if difficulties arise.

3. Check progress frequently to correct errors and assure success in performance. Less frequent checks are sufficient as competence increases.

Adaptation in Instruction

Adaptation in the method of instruction and preparation for instruction may be required for persons having special problems. The visually handicapped, for example, must have the work area precisely and consistently arranged, with every tool or piece of equipment in the same place for each session. Since use of sensation is vital to learning with the visually handicapped, opportunity must be provided and emphasized for tactile input in every step of the process. Verbal instructions must be more specific and very clearly stated.

Individuals with cognitive problems, or those having difficulty following directions, require modification in the instructions in order to be able to perform. The activity must be simplified as much as possible so that only one or two step operations are required. Directions must be given one step at a time and must be clear, concise, consistent, and concrete.

Special adaptations must be made for those individuals having any specific physical dysfunction. For example, an individual who can use only one hand should be instructed by the therapist who demonstrates using only one hand. This requires that the therapist must learn to do the activity successfully with one hand in order to demonstrate adequately.

BIBLIOGRAPHY

Willard, H. S., and Spackman, C. S.: Occupational Therapy, ed. 4. Philadelphia PA: J. B. Lippincott Co., 1971, pp. 43–50.

section 2/Activities of Daily Living and Homemaking/Maude H. Malick and Bonnie Sherry

ACTIVITIES OF DAILY LIVING (ADL)

Numerous techniques for training in activities of daily living (ADL) have been explored and devised but the primary component for success always is the patient's motivation. The patient must understand what his or her needs and deficits are and understand the purpose and goal of the training. The patient will then be more cooperative and more willing to follow through with personal care. The therapist and patient must assess abilities and determine together which accomplishments are best done in bed, in a chair, in a wheelchair, or standing.

Often simple assistive devices such as grab bars, an overhead ring, or sliding board can aid in gross positioning. These devices (easily constructed) are not orthotic devices but can make the difference between independence and dependence. An overhead ring or a braided rope attached to the foot of the bed can permit a patient to pull himself up to a sitting position and comfortably transfer with or without a sliding board to a wheelchair or glide-about chair. Once trunk balance can be maintained, a patient may proceed with self-care activities in a chair.

In any disability group it is important that the patient reach maximum physical strength, balance, and skill through a structured exercise and activity program. The occupational therapist should work closely with the physical therapist in developing maximum muscle and joint function so that the patient can be trained to use the maximum of his or her abilities and substitute for any deficits. In the case of the spinal cord injured patient, the development of muscle strength in the upper extremities is vitally important in order to do useful transfers and self-care activities.[1] At the same time energy conservation and fatigue must be considered, especially when scheduling a patient for training.

ADL is of primary concern when priorities must be set. Muriel Zimmerman states there is a direct corollary in planning physical therapy and occupational therapy activities. "Mat exercises, for instance, precede and coincide with sitting up in bed and transferring from the bed to the wheelchair. However, the needs and interest of the individual patients should always be considered. Independent eating may be started as soon as a patient can sit comfortably in bed or in a wheelchair, and in some instances it may be started while the patient is being tilted on tilt-bed or tilt-board."[2] "After the initial test, the patient is scheduled for training sessions in activities in which he is deficient and which are deemed suitable. He may merely need a few practice periods, with or without special guidance or equipment, or he may need carefully planned and supervised methods of procedure, such as sequence of performance, and the placement of the body or the hands, with repeated practice."[3]

In all self-care and dressing procedures there are some basic considerations which should be employed.

1. The bed, chair, or wheelchair should be positioned properly. All pieces of clothing and self-care items should be placed within easy reach of the patient and stored in a convenient location.
2. Patients should be encouraged to do tasks independently as much as possible. The patient's own ingenuity is an important factor.
3. Little or no adaptive equipment should be used unless it is absolutely necessary and then primarily for safety or to reduce energy and time consumption.
4. All safety precautions should be observed, especially when the patient's stability is in question. The wheelchair should be locked while transferring and during dressing procedures. For example, the patient himself may need to be stabilized by hooking his arm over the wheelchair back if necessary.

Physical disability may be increased when edema and loss of sensation exist. The therapist must instruct the patient to prevent injury from burns or trauma to the affected extremity through use of vision and by placing the extremity in a comfortable, anatomically-sound position. When training a patient, the treatment plan must include precautions if there is a loss of depth perception or if there is hemianopsia or stereognosis.

Independence without assistive devices is most desirable, but many patients cannot manage without some special equipment or even start without an aid. Assistive devices, when wisely selected and designed, can provide independence and often increase safety, speed, and group acceptance. ADL training can be started with an assistive device and later, as physical gains are made, the device can be discarded. Perhaps one of the simplest devices is a built-up handle for an eating utensil or a simple spoon holder with the spoon fitting into a pocket of a simple elastic band (Fig. 11-1). When insufficient wrist stability exists, a simple ADL splint can be made either volarly or, as in Figure 11-1, dorsally. These are most frequently used with the quadriplegic, multiple sclerosis, or muscular dystrophy patient. A clamp or plate guard and a dycem place mat are frequently used to give better food and plate control (Fig. 11-2).

Many ADL techniques for the physically handicapped have been developed. We recommend the

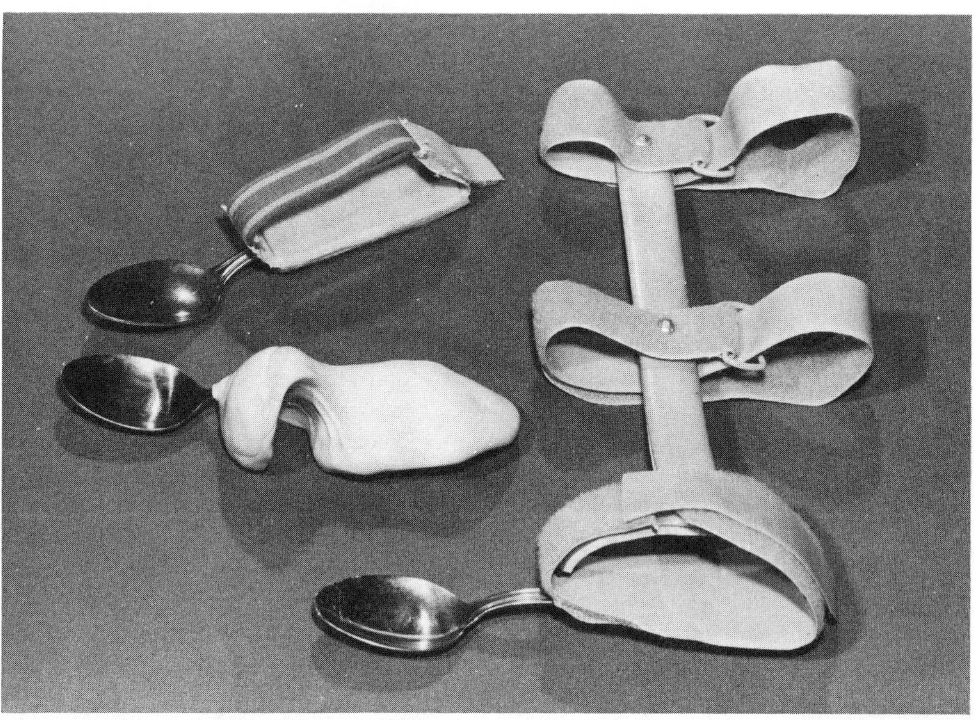

FIGURE 11-1. Assistive devices to aid in holding eating utensils.

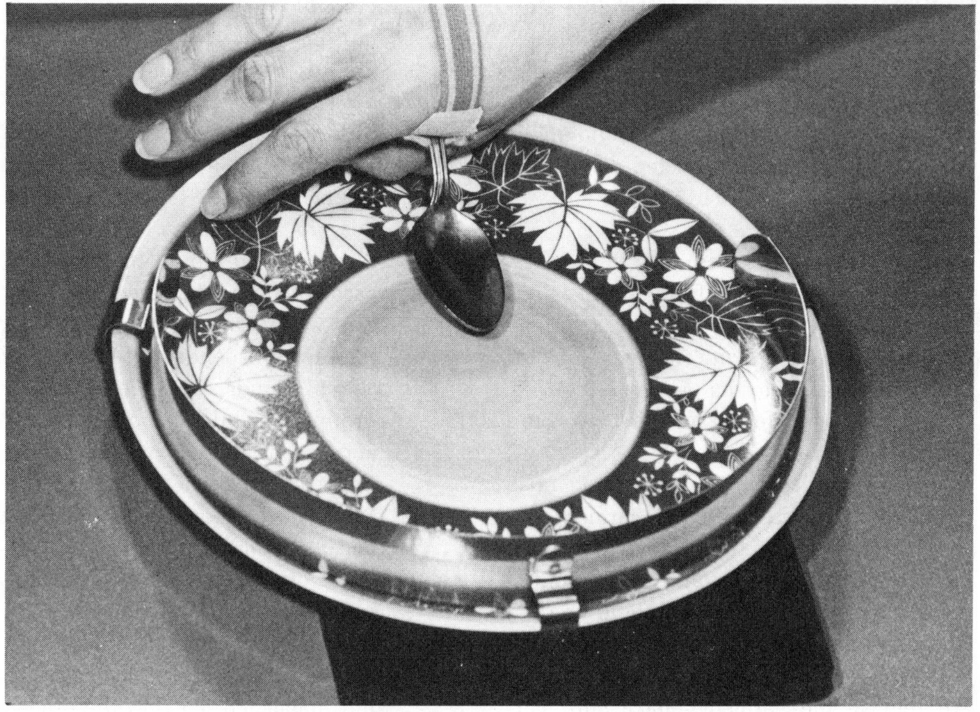

FIGURE 11-2. A dycem plate mat and plate guard used to stabilize the plate and control food spillage.

techniques that follow. Many of these, additionally, are outlined and illustrated in *Physical Management for the Quadriplegic Patient.*[4]

ADL for the Hemiplegic Patient

Feeding. A rocker knife allows the individual to cut food with one hand.

Dressing Techniques.

I. Shirts, pajama jackets, robes, and dresses opening completely down the front.

Recommended Style:

a. Action-back blouses.
b. Polyester-cotton, nylon, or seersucker.
c. Full skirts on dresses so they slip easily over the hips.
d. Loosely fitting sleeves.
e. Garments should be loose fitting.
f. Clothes fastening in the front.

Procedure:

Method A:

1. Put garment on affected arm first, working sleeve on completely.
2. Pull material over affected shoulder and throw it around to the back. "Walk" unaffected hand around collar and slip shirt over unaffected side.
3. Put the unaffected arm in the armhole and adjust (arm should be directed downward rather than over the head).
4. Button.
5. Remove from unaffected arm first, then from shoulder, and last from affected arm.

Method B:

1. Position shirt on lap with inside of shirt up and collar closest to the patient.
2. Put garment on affected arm first, working sleeve up over the elbow.
3. Put unaffected arm into sleeve, then raise the unaffected arm and let the garment slip over head and down the back. (With a shirt, gathering the garment up the middle of the back from hemline to collar or holding onto tail may make it easier to guide over the head.)
4. To remove the garment—make sure garment is free in back, with unaffected arm gather the garment up in back of neck (or take hold of collar), pull over the head, and remove first from the unaffected arm and then from the affected arm.

Comments:

1. Sleeve on unaffected side should be buttoned before garment is put on. Button can be secured with elastic thread if cuff is too tight.
2. Button hook may be helpful.

II. Men's trousers and shorts, women's underwear and slacks.

Recommended Style:

a. Boxer style may be easier to manage than zipper. A loop may be attached to zipper to help pull up.
b. Trousers should be loose fitting.

Procedure:

Method A (Sitting Position):

1. Sit on side of bed or in straight arm chair or wheelchair.
2. Cross hemiplegic leg over good leg. Balance is best maintained if the good leg is brought to a point directly in front of the midline of the body.
3. Slip trouser onto hemiplegic leg, uncross the leg.
4. Slip on opposite trouser leg and work trousers up to the hips.
5. Wiggle from side to side, pulling the pants over the hips, or
6. Place affected arm in the pocket to prevent garment from dropping to the floor while the patient stands up to pull trousers over the hips. Suspenders, if fastened before the patient stands, will prevent trousers from dropping, while the patient gets his balance. (Alternative method is to slip the finger into the belt loop.)
7. Sit down to fasten the front or side opening.

Method B (Lying Position):

1. Put clothing on affected leg first and remove from unaffected leg last.
2. Bend affected leg at the knee and hip using unaffected hand. Slip on the pant leg, then put unaffected leg into the other pant leg.
3. Work over the hips either by rolling from

side to side or hiking the hips with the uninvolved knee and hip bent.

III. Slips and dresses for women and undershirts and pullover shirts for men.

Recommended Style: Garments should be loose fitting. Dacron and nylon jersey are preferable.

Procedure:

Method A:

1. Position clothing on lap with neck of garment at the knees and back of garment on top.
2. Put affected arm through strap or sleeve.
3. Put unaffected arm through strap or sleeve.
4. Slip garment over the head.

Method B:

1. Gather clothing in unaffected arm and slip over affected arm.
2. Slip over head.
3. Put unaffected arm through strap or sleeve.

Method C:

1. Drop slip over head to the waist.
2. Pull strap over the affected arm and then over the unaffected arm.

IV. Stockings.

Recommended Style:

a. Stockings with tight elastic bands are to be avoided.

b. Stretch stockings are recommended. (They are more difficult to apply but eliminate wrinkles.)

c. Avoid sheer stockings, which are easily snagged.

Procedure:

1. Sit on edge of bed or in a straight chair with arms.
2. Cross affected leg over good leg or prop on a stool.
3. Open top of stocking by inserting the thumb and first two fingers near the cuff and spreading the fingers apart.
4. Put the great toe in first and work over the rest of the foot, alleviating all wrinkles.

Comments: Stockings must be kept free from wrinkles, which may cause pressure areas.

V. Brassieres.

Recommended Style: Front opening style may be easiest to apply.

Procedure:

Method A (Conventional Style):

1. Anchor bra strap with thumb of affected hand, pull around to front.
2. Hook bra in front at the waist and slip around to the back.
3. Place affected arm through the shoulder strap and then place the unaffected arm through the other strap.

Comments: Elastic may be added to the straps for ease in applying.

VI. Shoes and short leg braces.

Procedure:

Method A:

1. Apply the brace while in bed if balance is poor.
2. Sit on the edge of the bed or in a chair if balance is good.
3. Cross hemiplegic leg over unaffected leg. Balance is best maintained if the unaffected leg is brought to a point directly in front of the midline of the body.
4. Slip the toes into the shoe while holding the short leg brace in the unaffected hand by the metal bar. Insert toes sideways first, then slip the shoe around to the correct position to avoid catching the toes on the outer edge of the shoe.
5. Place the shoehorn, long-handled if necessary, into the shoe from the side to the back.
6. Frequently the back of the shoe will buckle and the broad part of the shoehorn will be under the heel. Place affected leg on floor or a stool, place pressure on the knee with the unaffected hand, and put weight on the affected foot. The shoehorn is now in a position where the patient's heel is pressing on it.
7. Bring the shoehorn up slowly, flat against the heel and inside the back of the shoe, but do not pull out.
8. Continue to press on knee and put weight on the foot, intermittently moving the

shoehorn until the foot slips into shoe and the back of the shoe is straight.

9. Remove the shoehorn and lace the shoe. Elastic shoe laces can be used if the patient has difficulty tying a bow using the one-handed shoe tie method.
10. Press the Velcro closure together or fasten the buckle to stabilize the brace to the leg calf.

Hygiene and Grooming

Recommended Equipment:

a. Electric razor for safety. (Norelco is suggested.)
b. Long-handled bath sponges with a place in the sponge for soap permits the patient to reach nearly all parts of the body.
c. Use bath tub stools or chair inside tub for safe transfers and use hand held shower hose for bathing.
d. Suction cups attached to handbrushes are recommended to enable patient to scrub nails and hand on unaffected side. These brushes are also used for washing dentures (place a wash rag in the sink basin for safety).
e. Bath mitt with soap pocket.
f. Mirror fastening around neck or on knee.
g. Nail file secured to table with masking tape or adhesive.
h. Long lipsticks may be easier to manage.
i. Rubber spool or Velcro hook curlers can be applied with one hand.
j. Toilet articles packaged under pressure or in plastic bottles, such as spray deodorant, are easier and safer to use than those in screwtop glass jars.
k. Combs with long or built-up handles may be of value.

ADL for the Paraplegic Patient

Dressing.

I. Shirts, pajama jackets, robes, and dresses opening completely down the front.

Recommended Style:

a. Material should be wrinkle-resistant, smooth, and durable.
b. Action-back blouses, roomy sleeves, full skirts that slip easily over the hips.

Procedure:

1. Balance body by putting palms of hands on mattress on either side of body.
2. Seek assistance or elevate bed backrest if balance is poor. With backrest elevated, both hands are available.
3. Method of putting clothing on does not usually create a problem; however, if difficulty is encountered, the following method is suggested: With garment open on the lap, collar toward patient's chest, put arms into sleeves and pull up over elbows. Then, holding on to the shirt tail or back of dress, pull over head, adjust, and button.

II. Men's trousers and shorts, women's underwear or slacks.

Recommended Style:

a. Slacks are easier to fasten if they have a front zipper closure. However, in some instances, zippers in the side seams are easier to apply over braces.
b. Wear loose fitting clothes for ease in getting over braces.
c. If the patient is incontinent, pants should close with snap opening in front.

Procedure:

1. Sit on bed and pull knees into a flexed position.
2. Hold the top of the trousers and flip the pants down to the feet.
3. Work pant legs over the feet and pull up to the hips.
4. Roll from hip to hip in a semi-reclining position and pull up the garment.

III. Slips and skirts.

Recommended Style:

a. Loose fitting half slips.
b. Full skirts for ease in pulling over hips and for better appearance over braces.

Procedure:

1. Sit on bed, slip garment over head, and let it drop to waist.
2. Roll from hip to hip in a semi-reclining

position and pull the garment down over the hips and thighs.

IV. Shoes.

Recommended Style: Shoes should be of oxford type if braces are to be attached.

Procedure:

Method A:

1. Pull one knee at a time into flexed position with hands while in sitting position on bed and, supporting leg with upper arms, slip on shoe.

Method B:

1. Sit on edge of bed or in wheelchair for back support.
2. Bend one knee to a flexed position, supporting leg with upper arm, and slip shoe on.

Method C:

1. Patient sits on edge of bed or in wheelchair for back support.
2. Patient crosses one leg over the other and slips shoe on.

V. Stockings.

Recommended Style:

a. Socks with tight elastic bands should be avoided.
b. Service-weight nylons are recommended for women.
c. Stockings should fit smoothly since any wrinkles may cause pressure areas.

Hygiene and Grooming.

1. A spray hose is helpful in bathing. The patient should keep a finger over the spray to determine sudden temperature change in water.
2. Long-handled bath brushes with soap insert are helpful for ease in reaching all parts of the body.
3. Soap bars attached to a cord around the neck may be helpful.

ADL for the Quadriplegic Patient

Dressing Activities. These suggestions depend on the level of lesion of the patient.

1. Zippers and Velcro fastenings facilitate dressing.
2. Blouses should be cut with extra length.
3. Garments should be loose fitting.

Feeding. It may be helpful to have:

1. Leather or plastic cuff with a pocket to hold fork or spoon.
2. Combination spoon-fork (spork).
3. Plate guard to aid in getting food on spoon.
4. Double suction cup or dycem plastic mat to stabilize plate.
5. Long plastic straw.

Grooming.

1. ADL splint attachments help in using razor, toothbrush, and comb. When an Engen reciprocal wrist orthosis or wrist-driven flexor-hinge hand splint is used, few assistive devices are needed.
2. A cigarette holder or a robot smoker for safety and a mouth stick for turning pages, painting, typing, writing, and dialing the telephone can be made if needed.
3. Bath tub bench or chair for safe bath tub transfers and hand held shower for bathing can be used.
4. Sliding board for transfer to wheelchair, bath tub or car is helpful.

In the case of a C_4-level quadriplegic, sophisticated environmental control systems can be made using electronic techniques and utilizing external power sources (Fig. 11-3). Battery power sources have been far more successful than carbon dioxide power. Powered wheelchairs and mobile carts have been perfected and are easily available. They should be prescribed carefully because many options are available. The telephone companies have many options in communication aids available for the handicapped, such as push button dialing, voice controls, and amplifiers. These may vary depending on the region or country in which the patient lives.

ADL for Patients with Limited Range of Motion

Generally there are no standard procedures for activities of daily living for patients with limited

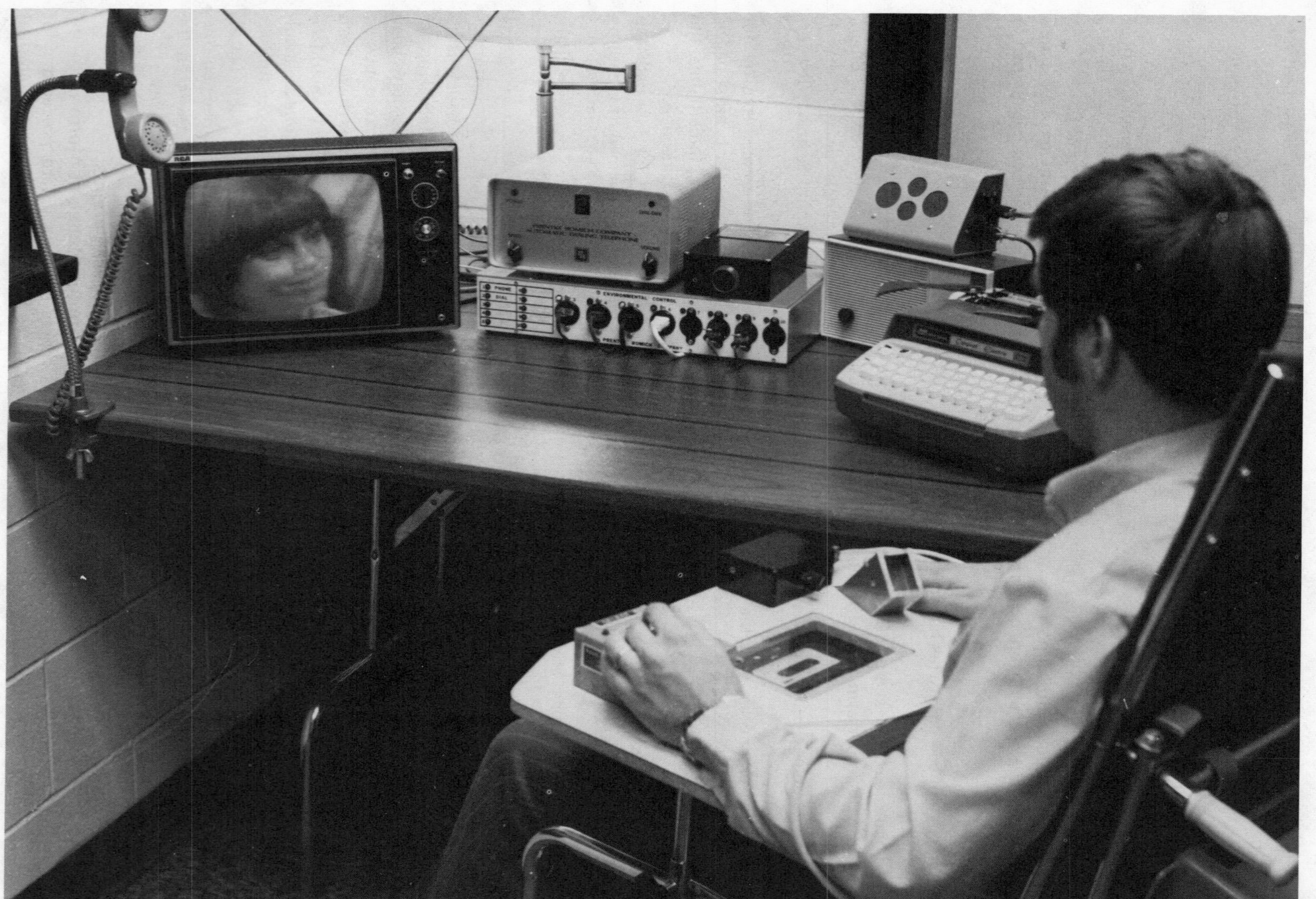

FIGURE 11-3. Environment control for the severely disabled. Subject can operate household appliances (telephone, lamp, intercom, radio) through environmental control packages. He controls powered wheelchair, onboard tape recorder, lights, horn, power recline, and remote control table top appliances through DU-IT wheelchair control system. (Prentke Romich Co. and Romich, Berry and Bayer, Inc.)

range of motion (ROM). However the following adaptations may prove helpful.

Dressing Activities.

1. Larger size clothing, made of materials which may have some stretch.
2. Adapted styles of clothing.
3. Larger buttons or zippers with a loop on the pull tab.
4. Long shoehorn.
5. Reaching tongs of all types.
6. Elastic shoe laces.
7. Stocking aids: garter attached to string, garters sewn on wooden hoop at end of straps, commercial aids.
8. Tabs sewed on clothing to facilitate use of hook on a long handle.

Feeding.

1. Built-up handles on utensils.
2. Elongated handles.
3. Plastic straw if ROM is limited in shoulder and when it is difficult to pick up a glass or cup.

Hygiene and Grooming.

1. Hand-held shower for bathing or shampooing hair.
2. Reachers to hold washcloth, powder puff, and so forth.
3. Long-handled combs, toothbrush.
4. Long lipstick.
5. Long-handled bath brush with soap container.
6. Extended handle for safety on electric razor.
7. Spray type deodorant.
8. Extended or built-up handles on water faucets.

HOMEMAKING

Energy Saving Techniques

The current definition of homemaker rehabilitation reflects the blending of the traditional treatment procedures with contemporary managerial techniques and philosophies. Without losing sight of the holistic approach to homemaker rehabilitation, it is necessary to consider the actual treatment methods involved in each area. The introduction of basic energy saving techniques is of prime importance regardless of disability (Fig. 11-4).

The homemaker must be made aware of new demands or limitations placed on his or her energy. Use of a wheelchair or walking device requires an extra expenditure of energy. Cardiac problems or arthritis may necessitate stopping or altering some activities. One of the most difficult areas of homemaker rehabilitation is that of helping the patient feel comfortable with and accepting the new rate and method of work. Many individuals become frustrated with initial attempts at activity. Frustration, fear, and mental stress can drain energy faster than the actual performance of some tasks. Efforts should be made to provide an atmosphere for training and evaluation that is pleasant, conducive to learning, and allows for exhibition of maximum performance.

Decision making is an integral part of work simplification. The decisions made may indicate role reversal, hiring help, compromise of priority, or modifications in the home. Many homemakers see work simplification techniques as the lazy way to work and are very uncomfortable with accepting new methods, products, or equipment. If the attitude cannot be changed, these feelings should be respected and, if at all feasible, alternate methods that are acceptable to the homemaker in meeting her standards should be instituted. Efficiency may suffer but the degree of carry-over at home will be increased. Making the homemaker aware of results of time and motion studies and demonstrating analysis of activity may build a discriminating attitude toward expenditures of energy.

The homemaker should first question the reason for doing each task. Is it necessary? Many tasks or at least portions of tasks can be eliminated. Is the homemaker best suited to do this task? Many family members may be capable of assuming the responsibility. The homemaker may, in turn, assume activities more in tune with present abilities. It is important to consider when a task must be completed in relation to other planned activities (Fig. 11-5). It may be necessary to alternate the tasks of a passive nature with more active tasks. Discussion of how a task should be completed will provide an opportunity to introduce convenience foods and appropriate

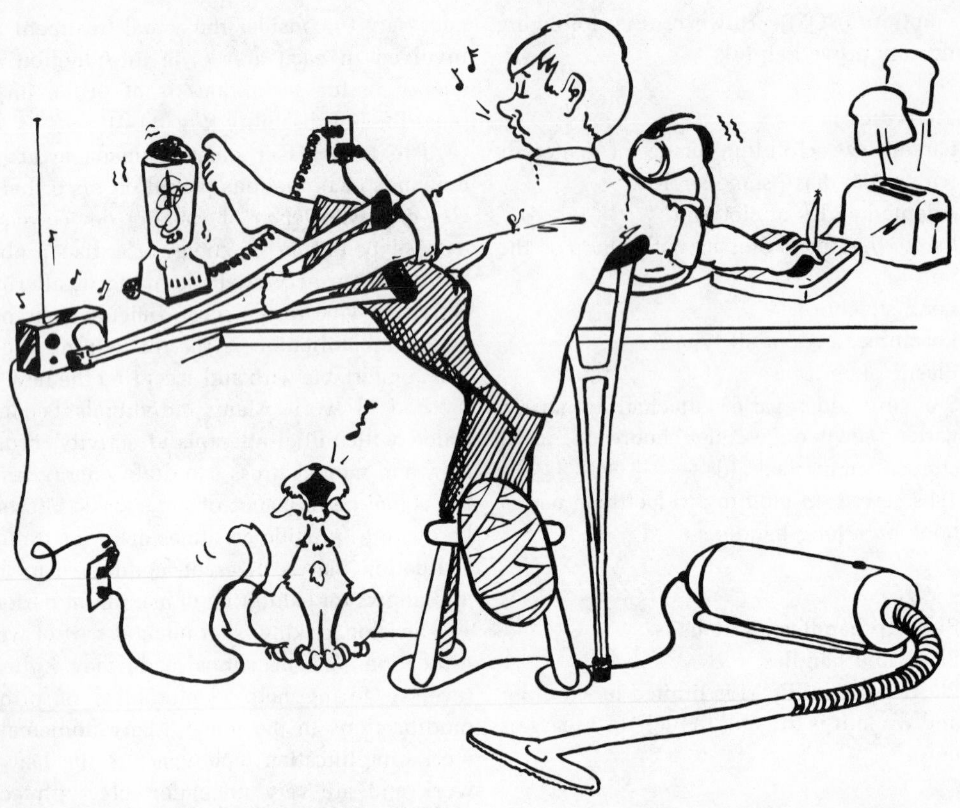

FIGURE 11-4. Combine tasks to conserve energy.

small appliances or assistive devices. Many individuals are concerned with excessive cost but, in terms of the cost of time and energy saved, the homemaker cannot afford to limit herself to old methods or equipment. *Rehabilitation Monograph VIII*[5] offers assistance in developing an improved method in work simplification techniques and principles:

1. Use both hands to work, in opposite and symmetrical motions if possible, smooth flowing path motions in a curve with no angles such as dusting and washing windows.
2. Lay out work areas within normal reach. Work where the areas of both hands overlap and arrange supplies in a semicircle within normal reach.
3. Slide—don't lift and carry. Slide pots from sink to range. Use a wheeled table where work surfaces are broken.
4. Fixed work stations. Have a special place to do each job so that supplies and equipment may always be kept there ready for immediate use.
5. Select equipment that may be used for more than one job; eliminate unnecessary motions. Use recipes that emphasize the "one bowl method" and quick mixing.
6. Avoid holding—use utensils with a flat base, suction cups, rubber mats or electric mixers to free both hands.
7. Let gravity work—a laundry chute, a pan below the level of the cutting board.
8. Pre-position tools. Store small tools in such a way that they are in the right position to grasp and start work immediately. Hang utensils separately within sight.
9. Locate machine control and switches within easy reach. Select household appliances with control located within easy reach for standing or sitting, depending on which position will be used. Change the location of switches if possible or insert switches in electric cord for easier use.
10. Sit to work whenever possible. Sit to iron, work at the sink, prepare vegetables, mix foods. Find a comfortable chair and adjust the workplace height

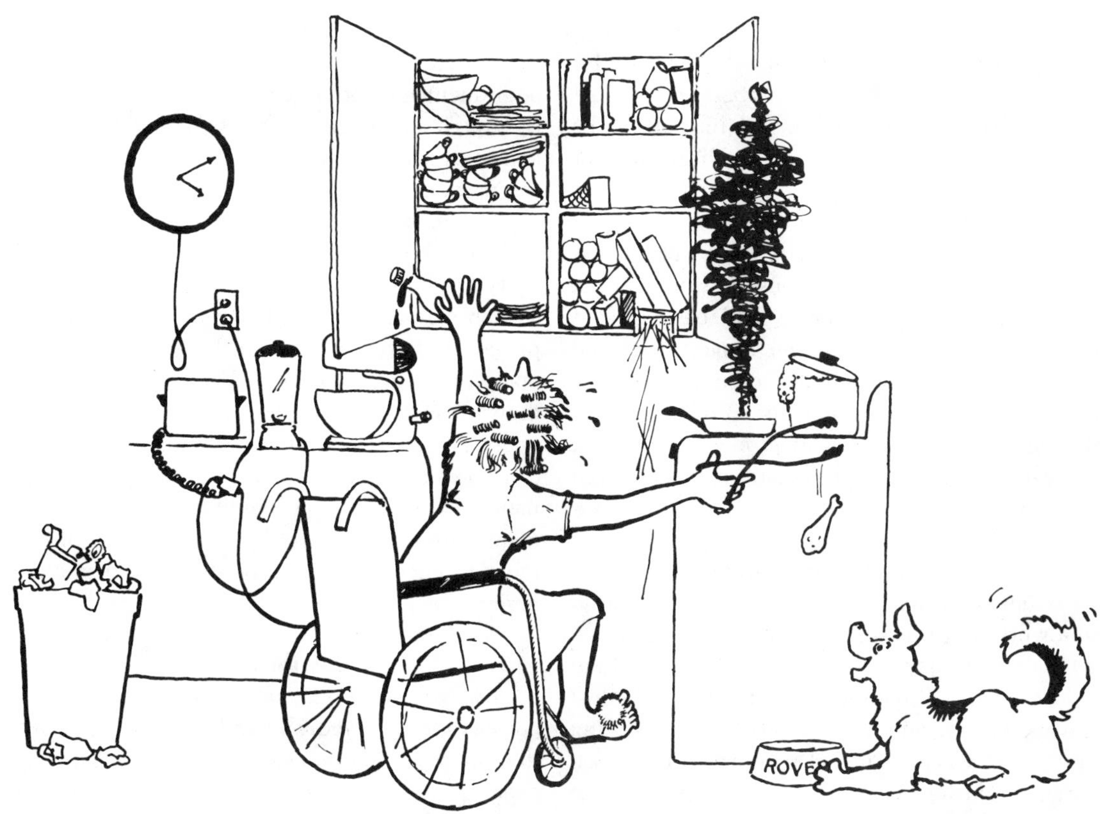

FIGURE 11-5. Organize tasks in order of importance.

to it or if this cannot be changed fit the chair to the workplace.

11. Select work place height appropriate for the worker and for the job. The jobs requiring hand activity will need a higher work surface than those requiring arm motion or pressure. There are no "standard heights," as body proportions differ.

12. Working conditions. If the surrounding conditions are good, the job will be pleasanter and less tiring. Good light, directed toward the work, good ventilation, comfortable clothing, pleasing colors, and order set the stage for work without strain.*

Incoordination

Incoordination can be caused by a variety of diseases or conditions such as Parkinson's disease, multiple sclerosis, and cerebral palsy. Regardless of the specific cause, it is necessary to attempt to use the affected extremity to develop coordination. Homemaking tasks may provide a productive form of exercise.

Before introducing specific techniques, it is especially important to allay any of the patient's fears that could aggravate the coordination problem or hinder safe functioning. Fatigue, also, can influence the degree of spasticity or incoordination. In order to promote working in a relaxed, rested manner at home the patient should be made aware of factors that could influence performance.

Energy saving techniques are an essential part of any program, and management of time and energy should be practiced with all activities. Convenience foods that eliminate the need for extensive cutting, chopping, or mixing should be recommended. Easy open packages and containers are helpful. Substitution of a technique such as sliding instead of lifting or the use of equipment such as a wheelchair lap

---

* This list is from Rusk, H. A.: Manual for Training the Disabled Homemaker, Rehabilitation Monograph VIII. Institute of Rehabilitation Medicine, New York University Medical Center, New York, 1967. Reprinted with permission.

tray or wheeled cart will promote safer functioning. Weighted utensils and items with double handles that can be gripped easily will partially counteract the affects of the incoordination. Stabilization can be achieved by utilizing a spikeboard, rubber mats, or sponges. Blenders, crockpots, and electric skillets are often essential kitchen aids when placed at appropriate heights on stationary work surfaces. A coffee urn can be utilized as a constant source of hot water for instant soups, cereals, and beverages; it negates the need for using the range. Oversized bowls can contain food which would normally be spilled by extraneous movements. Long mitts promote oven safety. Meals which meet nutritional needs yet simplify the food preparation process can be planned.

One-Handed Techniques

It is important for the one-handed individual to plan a work schedule that allows for periods of rest and for alternating heavy and light tasks. The patient should organize all equipment and supplies, adjust the work height, and use the utility cart, sliding technique, or wheelchair tray to assist in transporting items. Consider convenience foods and the use of small equipment to assist in any activity. If difficulty is noted in reading or following directions, it may be necessary to enlarge print or simplify instructions. If hemianopsia is a problem, compensation as well as general awareness of the affected extremity should be taught for safety's sake. Lack of sensation in the affected extremity can be extremely dangerous, particularly when the task involves use of a knife, hot liquids, or appliances. If poor balance is noted, suggest sitting to work, especially when attempting to use oven or refrigerator. The use of long tongs and proper storage techniques can eliminate some problems caused by inadequate balance. Organizational ability can be easily assessed in such simple activities as setting the table or separating utensils in a silverware drawer. Many homemakers may acquire good return of affected extremities but still experience difficulty in using good judgment or in problem solving. This can create more difficulties than the physical dysfunction.

Emphasis should be placed on activities that the patient can complete easily and safely. Families should be made aware of all limitations as well as abilities. Self-help catalogs have many gadgets for the individual with the use of one hand. While some equipment may be necessary for independent functioning, it should be stressed that most homemaking activities can be completed with nothing more than the proper technique.

A spikeboard, two aluminum or stainless steel nails on a board, becomes a second hand to stabilize everything from potatoes to cupcakes to meat. A rubber mat can be used to hold bowls, pans, or plates. Packages or jars can be stabilized for easy opening by using the knees or a partially opened drawer. Teeth or scissors are helpful in opening many types of packaging. Jar openers and electric can openers are also useful aids that promote independence. Each person should be allowed to experiment with various techniques and pieces of equipment to encourage the problem solving method at home.

The Arthritic Patient

The arthritic homemaker may find it crucial to conserve energy and protect his/her joints from undue stress. Some homemaking tasks provide good exercise and actually may be beneficial. All activities must be monitored with regard to joint stress produced, amount of time required in one position, and contribution to general fatigue. It is important to emphasize the following:

1. Sit when possible but not for prolonged periods of time.
2. Use fingers in extension whenever possible, i.e., in dishwashing and dusting.
3. Stress should not be put on the thumb or fingers. Utilize palms or wrist and attempt to distribute the weight of an object evenly. Use both hands when possible.
4. Utilize proper work height. Avoid tasks that put undue stress on joints such as scrubbing, wringing, or opening jars.
5. Slide equipment and supplies when possible rather than carrying them. Use the utility cart.
6. Prevent lifting of heavy items, bending, and reaching by careful storage. Use of light weight bowls, utensils, and appliances is recommended.
7. Avoid prolonged holding of a book, needlework, pencil, or telephone.

The arthritic homemaker, attempting to function at home, will be well aware of his/her limitations. Adapted equipment may be required in addition to demonstration and training in proper techniques. A few well-chosen items early in the treatment program may eliminate the need for restriction of activity or increase in the number of devices necessary as the disease progresses. The homemaker must fully understand the reasoning behind the instructions being given, or he/she may perform activities in a manner which could be detrimental. *The Self-Help Manual for Arthritic Patients* from the Arthritis Foundation[6] answers many questions on equipment needs and specific task techniques.

Because of the general nature of the progression of arthritis, the homemaker may have psychological problems of varying degrees. The therapist may be instrumental in easing psychological problems as well as easing pain and increasing function in the affected joints.

The Quadriplegic Patient

A quadriplegic individual functioning effectively in the home provides a study in management principles.

Brain power, not manpower, must be emphasized. The quadriplegic patient must be equipped with knowledge and skills to organize and manage effectively. Introduced in the early stages of rehabilitation, basic management skills can help allay the feelings of total helplessness. Financial management, childrearing theories, diet instructions, and meal planning are mental tasks which can be accomplished to provide positive reinforcement and increase motivation. With use of telephone and typing skills, manually or by mouth, it is possible to assume tasks such as ordering groceries, paying bills, and being the family's social secretary. It is important that families be involved, especially when role reversals or modifications are indicated.

The subject of home modification can be approached when both the patient and family exhibit signs of acceptance of the disability and an understanding of the permanence of the situation. Although the rehabilitation process for quadriplegic patients generally is lengthy, the extent of home modification may necessitate early initiation. Weekend visits will be more pleasurable and better indicators of post-discharge success if the home is adequately modified. The degree of modification indicated is dependent on the functional level of the patient. Possibly the home would best be designed for the ease of the attendant or the family caring for the patient. *Building Without Barriers for the Disabled*[7] is one of many possible sources of information relating to home modification. Home-planning consultants and rehabilitation home economists are being utilized by innovative rehabilitation facilities to work with the patient and families in the planning process.

For those quadriplegics (generally C_5 and below) who will be assuming some or most homemaking tasks, special attention should be given to equipment selection and utilization of work simplification techniques (Figs. 11-6 and 11-7). The use of such small appliances as electric skillet, can opener, coffee urn, toaster-oven, or slow cooker can provide a great degree of independence (Fig. 11-8). Convenience foods provide a simple but adequate source of nutritional needs. *Mealtime Manual for the Aged and Handicapped*[8] offers specific suggestions for use and selection of adapted equipment and appliances. Because of the patient's loss of sensation, safety should be a prime consideration, especially with use of heat or sharp objects.

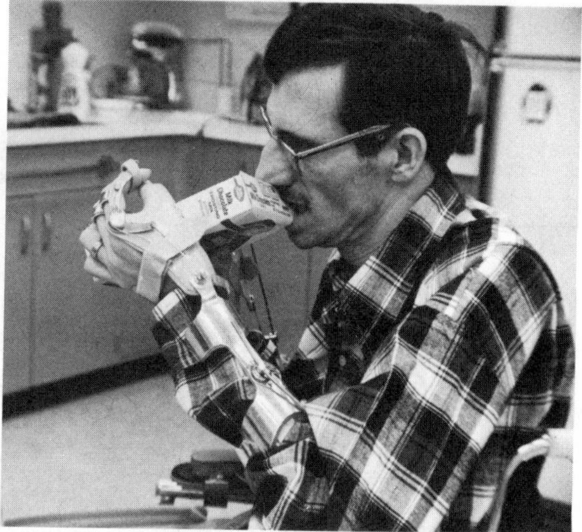

FIGURE 11-6. Teeth and tenodesis splints work together effectively to open packages.

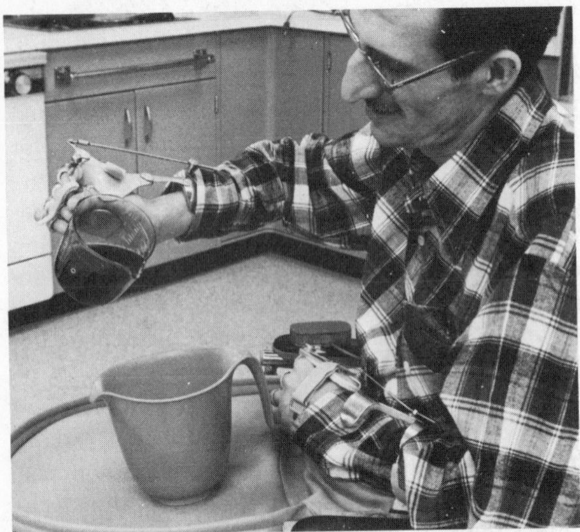

FIGURE 11-7. A light-weight measuring cup, bowl with a handle, and vinyl lap tray promote independence for the quadriplegic patient with natural or mechanical tenodesis functioning.

Clothing

A large portion of the activities of daily living program is directed towards gaining independence in dressing. It is obvious that certain types of clothing may be more comfortable, safer, easier to care for or provide for a greater degree of independence. Many sources illustrate styles of clothing particularly suitable for different disabilities. One such source is *Independent Living for the Handicapped and the Elderly.*[9] Clothing does more than merely cover the body. It can provide a method of self-expression and promote confidence and acceptance in society. Personal preferences vary. This must be considered when making recommendations. General considerations include that clothing:

1. be strong enough to take abrasion caused by orthotic devices or sliding transfer techniques to a wheelchair.
2. have openings which are easily accessible and fasteners which are operable by individuals with limited arm movement or poor hand coordination.
3. provide for ease of movement in a wheelchair or with assistive devices for ambulation.
4. be attractive as well as functional.

The homemaker may have actual experience in adapting clothing to make it more functional or to conceal a deformity or device. Basic safety precautions should be taken with persons having decreased reaction time, incoordination, or assistive devices.

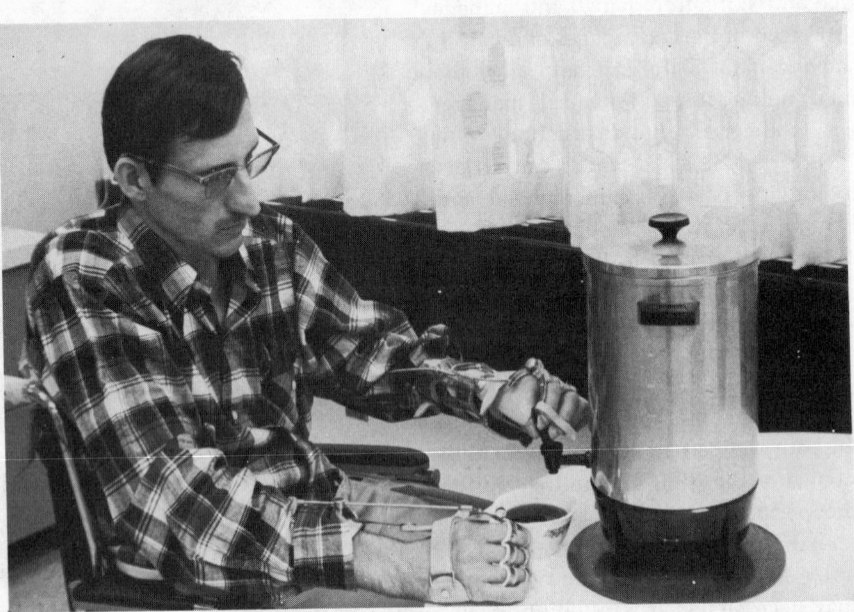

FIGURE 11-8. An urn, stabilized with a rubber mat, provides a constant source of hot water for instant cereals, soups, and beverages.

Discourage the wearing of loose-sleeved garments over open flame or near equipment. Keep slacks and skirts of appropriate length and width to allow ambulation with assistive devices or safe use of a wheelchair. Fireproof garments are recommended.

Emphasis should be placed on the type of fabric selected. Consideration should include allergy or irritations, washability (especially where incontinence is a problem), required ironing, wrinkling, absorption of or resistance to perspiration, and colorfastness. Laundering techniques which are proper for varying types of garments and fabrics include type of detergent, water temperature, use of softener and prewash soaks. These may reduce amount of time and energy expended by the homemaker. Proper technique for laundering slings or support garments will lengthen the life of these costly items.

Care should be taken, especially in selection of undergarments. They must be functional for the wearer and permit independence in dressing and toileting. Fit should not interfere with circulation nor cause skin breakdown by binding or rubbing. A fabric that absorbs perspiration is generally most comfortable. Certain garments may be adapted or eliminated entirely for comfort or ease in dressing—quadriplegic males frequently find undershorts restrictive and nonfunctional for them. The Fashion Able Company offers a wide selection of adapted undergarments and swimwear.

Child Care Techniques

Many disabled persons find themselves responsible not only for their own care but also for that of small children. Modern technology has lightened the task with the advent of disposable diapers and bottles and with premixed formulas. However, the greatest problem is the fear and uncertainty surrounding the resumption of this responsible role. Children also are capable of sensing the confidence, or lack of it, and will respond accordingly.

The introduction of the parents or grandparent to child care techniques is an integral part of the program that can make the transition to home easier and more comfortable for the entire family. A weighted doll can be utilized in developing basic skills of dressing, feeding, and bathing. The homemaker should be made aware of products on the market that make child care easier. Even if some items are costly, it may be more economical monetarily and psychologically than hiring an assistant. Use of these products save time and energy and allow the parent to spend time with the child. A severely disabled person can offer much to the development of a child by offering love and by teaching, playing, and helping the child develop self-confidence and skills. It may be necessary to introduce some basic considerations for selection and use of equipment.[10]

1. Is the equipment manageable within physical limitations?
2. Can height be adjusted easily?
3. Can equipment be moved easily?
4. Are controls easily used?
5. Can it be cared for and cleaned easily?
6. Is it sufficiently sturdy and durable?
7. Is it multipurpose and able to be used over a long period of time?
8. Is it adapted to growth of the child?
9. Is it safe for the child as well as the parent?
10. Will it promote early independence in children?

Children can learn at an early age to assist with dressing and feeding. With well-selected self-help clothing, supervision, and encouragement, they soon become independent. Usually around four years of age children express interest in helping and should be given the opportunity to be contributing members of the household. The homemaker's management principles may come into use here, with the utilization of family resources.

The disabled parent should be forewarned that discipline of small children may be a problem. However, children generally respond best when they have responsibility in accord with their age and have rules and standards for behavior. A parent's tone of voice or look can be a sufficient indicator of displeasure. Children are by nature flexible beings who can adapt to almost any situation if given proper guidance and stimulation. Guiding a child's development can be a rewarding experience for any homemaker.

Dietary Considerations

The incorporation of nutrition principles is an essential part of any homemaker rehabilitation program. Nutritional needs are established and prescribed by the physician or dietitian but the homemaker rehabilitation area provides a natural area for testing, training, and explaining dietary plans. The American Dietetic Association offers many audiovisual aids, posters, and pamphlets which are helpful in teaching nutrition.

New demands are being placed on the homemaker's body; the patient must realize this. Depending upon one's level of activity, wheelchair use may indicate an increase or decrease in caloric needs for the day. Age is another determining factor. Many patients experience weight gains during long periods of inactivity during hospitalization. The homemaker can better comprehend the need for a change in diet if he or she understands the reasons for these changes.

Excess weight is a factor that severely limits a handicapped homemaker in reaching his or her potential. Transfers are more difficult and dressing problems are increased. More energy is required to ambulate or perform other physical activity. General tolerance is reduced. Prostheses, if used, often do not fit correctly. Weight control is especially crucial for the cardiac patient or the patient with pulmonary problems. Diabetic diets are prevalent among the amputee population. Many are so frightened by diabetes that they no longer enjoy food. Practice in planning and preparing meals can alleviate the fear and offers a better chance for effective carry-over.

Introduction of new food preparation methods may be helpful. For example, teach broiling instead of frying foods or introduce new products such as sugar substitutes. Take a diet history, if possible, including premorbid eating patterns. Using this as a guide, assist the homemaker in planning nutritious meals. In explaining a diet it often is necessary to go beyond the general exchange list given by the doctor or dietitian. Cultural, religious, and family customs must be taken into consideration as well as cost and nutritional needs. Emphasis should be placed on planning foods that are not only relatively easy to prepare but also are nutritious (Fig. 11-9).

Basic nutrition principles are essential not only for the homemaker but also for the family. Often it is necessary to emphasize the manner in which the

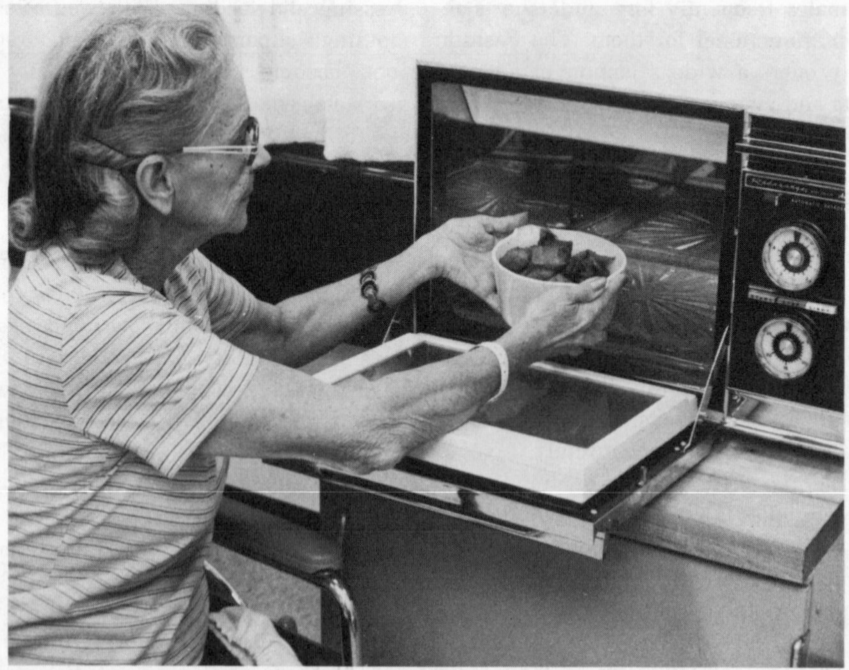

FIGURE 11-9. Fast, no mess cooking in a microwave oven can encourage those who live alone or are on modified diets to prepare meals that meet their nutritional needs.

patient's dietary restrictions can be coordinated with family food planning. A trip to the grocery store, in addition to enabling the therapist to determine tolerance, the patient's use of money, and social interactions, also gives the homemaker a practical experience of reading food labels and seeing products on the market which are permitted by the diet. Many special diet foods are expensive and not necessarily indicated. Effective substitutes should be noted for those people on limited budgets. The use of food stamps or other government-sponsored assistance programs should be explained and the homemaker may be referred to the appropriate agency if indicated. Successful carry-over is predictable if the patient is made aware of the extent of assistance available.

Financial Management

Frequently, because of circumstances surrounding an accident or illness, a family discovers that its previous financial plan is no longer adequate. In planning for disposition of the patient, the therapist and family may find it helpful to go over the new demands on financial resources. Arrangements may have to be made for home modifications, special equipment, nursing care, household help, a new vehicle or means of transportation, tutors for children, or medical expenses and supplies.

For a budget to be flexible and functional it is necessary to involve the entire family. Budgeting is not easy but, when seriously undertaken, should result in a realistic plan for utilization of family financial and other related resources. Five basic steps are needed:

1. Record items and services required by the family for the allotted portion of time.
2. Estimate the cost involved and total each category.
3. Estimate anticipated income.
4. Bring anticipated income and anticipated expenditures into balance.
5. Evaluate plans for realistic chance of success.

Gross and Crandel's *Management for Modern Families*[11] can serve as a guide for budget preparation. A budget cannot be made *for* a family; the therapist can only *guide* the family in devising a plan that is suitable for its own needs and flexible enough to change with its needs. Once the budget is established, the homemaker, though limited physically, may be responsible for keeping the family's records, paying bills, and determining need for future expenditures or changes in the budget.

Training Apartment

In addition to the basic homemaker training and evaluation center, a training apartment provides an essential setting for an important portion of the evaluation process (Figs. 11-10 and 11-11). According to the Procedures and Policies established for the use of the Harmarville Rehabilitation Center apartment,[12] the purposes of a trial stay in the training apartment are:

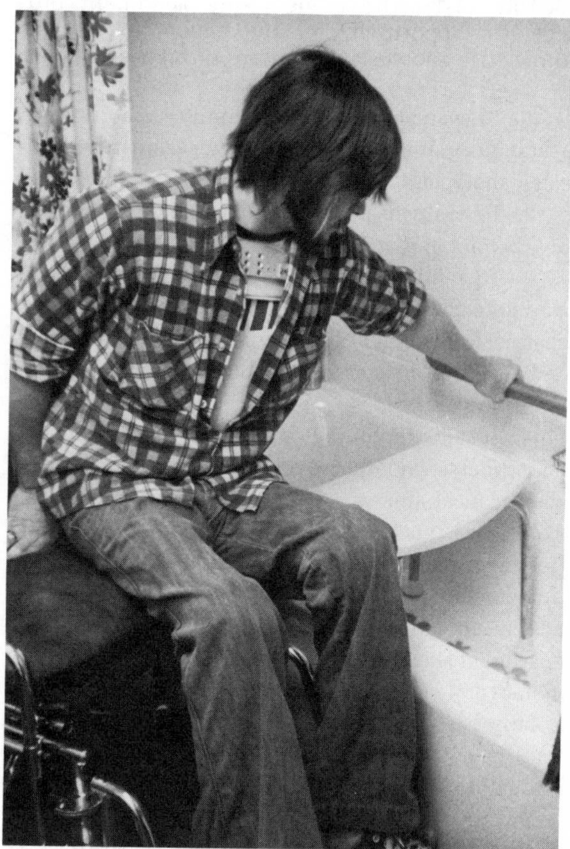

FIGURE 11-10. The homemaking apartment provides an opportunity for the patient to care for himself independently, thus preparing for independent living.

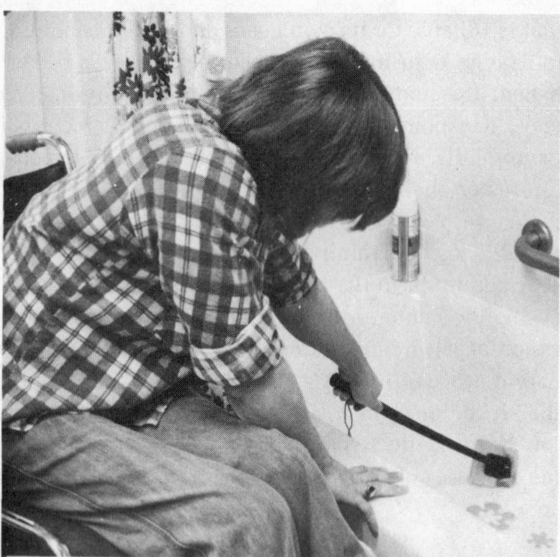

FIGURE 11-11. The homemaking apartment provides an opportunity for the patient to test his knowledge and skills in the care of his own home.

1. To evaluate patient and family capabilities in a homelike situation. Apartment use must be indicated therapeutically.
2. To evaluate physical and/or emotional needs of a patient and/or family.
3. To reinforce and follow through on patient care procedures in preparation for home visit or discharge. To document level of performance of patient and/or family in a protected but independent area.

The staff, including all appropriate treatment departments and therapy services, and the family should meet after an apartment stay to discuss the experience, make possible changes in program or treatment plan, provide for extended family education, and plan for appropriate disposition for the patient. In addition to being an educational tool, an apartment stay can provide a means for boosting the morale and confidence of the patient and family. On a daily basis the apartment lends itself to use as a training area for activities of daily living and for the evaluation of large scale homemaking tasks such as bedmaking and vacuuming.

Home Visits

It is necessary to know the patient's home situation when establishing a treatment plan. Therefore the therapist must first evaluate the living situation so that the initial teaching of skills and information will be pertinent and appropriate. Often the patient or family can provide adequate information but, if problems are indicated in any area, a home visit may be necessary. It may be advantageous to include the patient when making the home visit. Questions can be answered and fears quelled.

The occupational therapist and rehabilitation home economist or other members of the rehabilitation team such as the physical therapist may participate in the evaluation. The following questions should be considered:

1. Is at least one entrance accessible to the patient? Are railings or ramps indicated?
2. Are doorways wide enough for wheelchair traffic?
3. Do doorsills, rugs, or floor coverings hinder safe ambulation?
4. Is furniture placed to provide for a good traffic pattern? Is it sturdy enough for safe transfers?
5. Are the telephone, light switches, television, and radio accessible? Is bathroom adequate for safe transfers? Are grab bars, elevated seats, mats, bathstools, or plumbing modifications indicated?
6. Is the bedroom large enough for independent transfer? Are needed items placed conveniently? Is a commode chair indicated? Are closet spaces enough to accommodate needs? Are storage areas accessible?
7. Is the kitchen of adequate size for safe functioning? Are range, sink, refrigerator, and cupboards accessible for safe use?
8. Are laundry facilities accessible?
9. Is the children's play area available for supervision?

Post-discharge home visits provide a good form of follow-up. The visitor can assess the adjustment to the home situation and the degree of carry-over, make recommendations concerning the problems which might have come to light since discharge, evaluate the effectiveness of the home program and the need for additional services or equipment, and make any necessary referrals to appropriate agencies. Results of the post-discharge evaluation should be shared with all involved departments.

A follow-up questionnaire can be used as an indicator of the necessity of a home visit or it can serve as an indicator of the effectiveness of the homemaker rehabilitation program.

Architectural Design Considerations and Selection

In the Home

It is necessary to evaluate the home circumstances when planning a rehabilitation program and often it is necessary to suggest modifications for making the home environment functional. This initial preparation maximizes the affects of the rehabilitation process.

Timing is important in initiating the subject of home modifications with the patient and family. The patient who has not yet accepted the disability may reject any plans because they seem to be an indication that the disability is indeed permanent. The family also must be ready to accept, cooperate, and be supportive. Both the family and patient must see the need for change and be willing to work with the therapist in assessing the modifications necessary in light of the patient's physical ability. Sometimes it is helpful to have the patient sketch a floor plan and list, if possible, inaccessible areas. A home visit may be necessary to obtain measurements or assess a difficult situation. The family can help by supplying photographs or measurements of the home.

Much has been written concerning home modifications with special emphasis on the kitchen and bathroom. Special requirements have been established for wheelchair functioning, proper work heights, and storage areas (Fig. 11-12). The basic mixing, sink, and range centers have been developed with specifications for equipment and storage techniques. Each of the three types of kitchens—U, L, and aisle—has advantages and disadvantages; these depend on the homemaker, the disability, and the family situation.

Most people are unable to remodel extensively and some, especially apartment dwellers, find it impossible to make any structural changes. Ingenuity and perseverance are needed and can make even the most unlikely places livable. The therapist can merely make recommendations for modifications based on the following guidelines:

1. The dwelling must provide adequate space for entrance and exit. Doorways should be 36 in. wide and ramps 30 to 40 in. wide. Inclines should be of approximately 6 degrees or 1 in. to 1 ft. and should be equipped with railings.
2. Doorsills should be eliminated where possible. The dwelling should enable free movement throughout. Throw rugs should be removed and thick carpets avoided. Nonskid floors are preferred. Furniture should be arranged appropriately to allow a free flowing traffic pattern. Doors may be eliminated or changed to sliding or folding doors or curtains. Bathing and toileting facilities should be provided with grab bars and nonskid flooring. Wall switches should be within easy reach, 36 in. from the floor, and outlets should be 24 in. from the floor. The communication system should be within reach and of a type usable by the patient.
3. The kitchen should be functional and meet needs as determined by the homemaking evaluation.
4. Heating and air conditioning systems may be essential for some disabilities.

Figure 11-13 is a sample of a sketch of bathroom facilities.

In Society

The rehabilitation process cannot be considered totally successful until all disabled individuals are freed from manmade environmental restrictions. Making the home accessible is an important first step, but the individual must not be shut out or shut in by barriers outside the home. In addition to physical barriers there are attitudinal barriers. These are broken each time a disabled individual takes his or her place in society.

Architectural and transportation barriers, however, are not so easily eliminated. Stairs, curbs, heavy doors, inaccessible restrooms and telephones, and public transportation restrict independence of those individuals with mobility limitations. This group includes not only the wheelchair bound but also the blind, deaf, those with assistive walking devices, and those with curtailed mobility as a result of the aging process, arthritis, or other limiting conditions. A barrier free environment would provide freer access for all.

Federal and state governments and public and

(*Text continues on p. 244*)

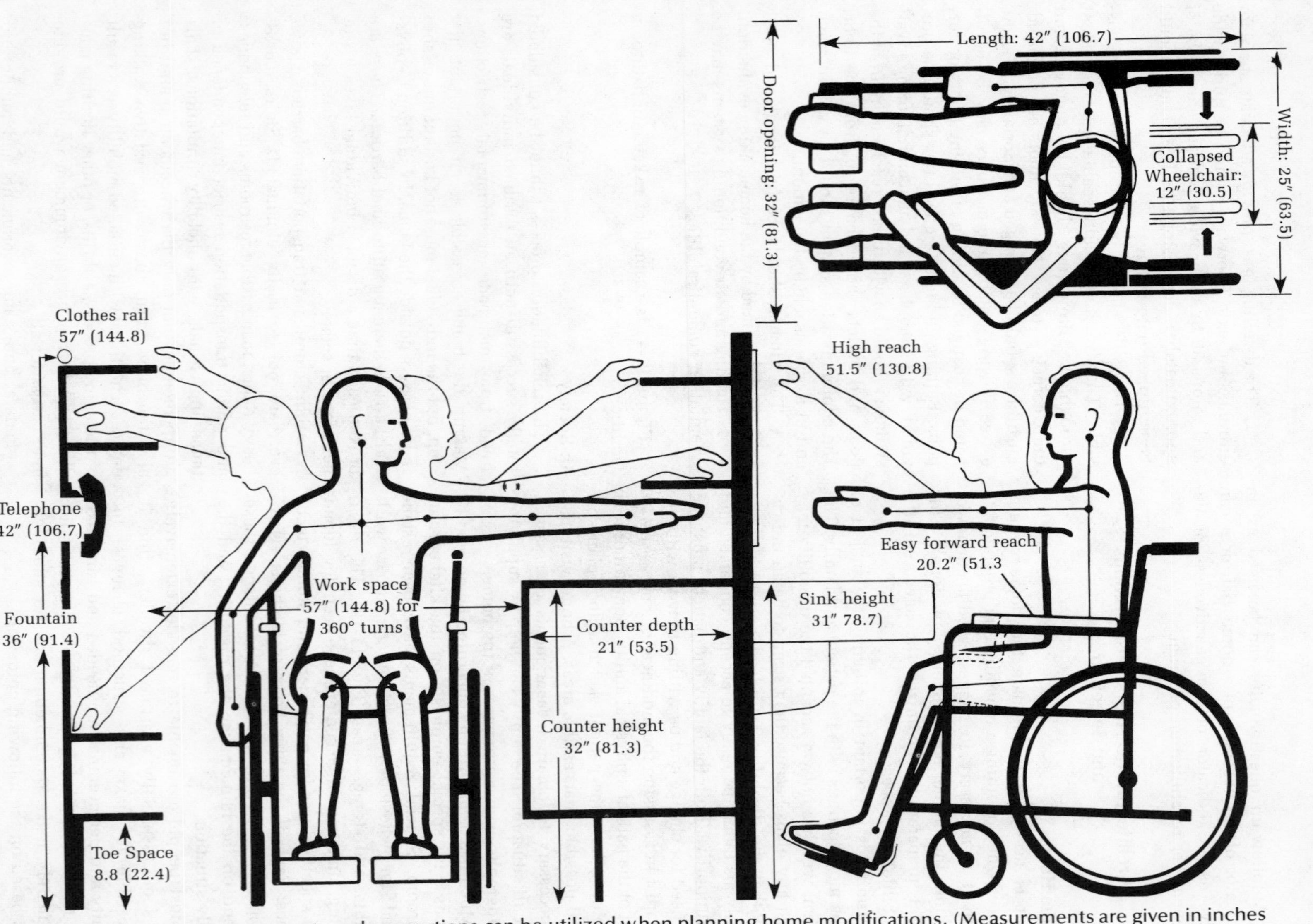

FIGURE 11-12. Basic measurements and proportions can be utilized when planning home modifications. (Measurements are given in inches and centimeters.) Adapted from Humanscale 3.[13]

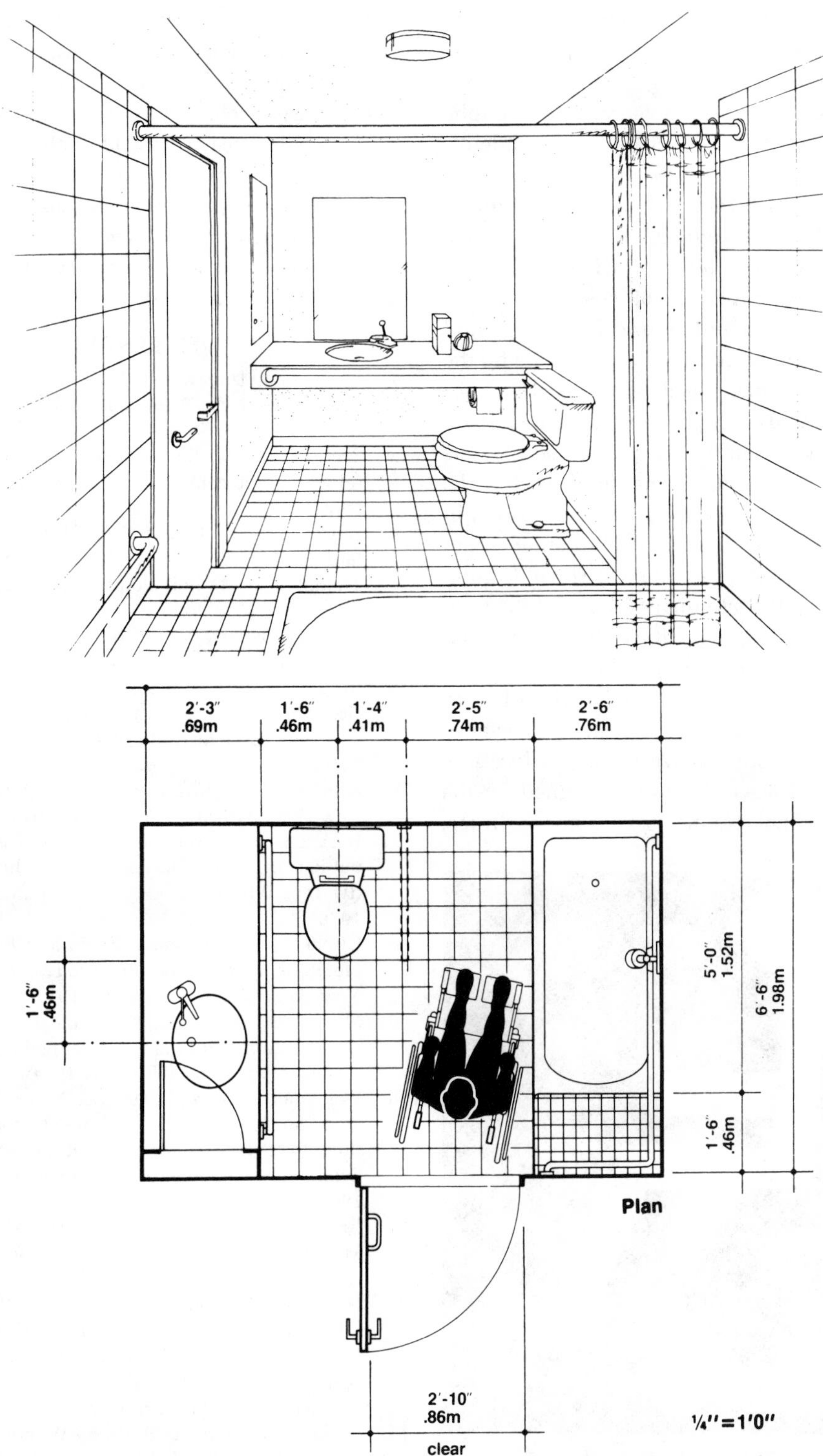

FIGURE 11-13. Two views of a bathroom suitable for the use of most disabled persons. Courtesy of Harkness and Groom.[14]

nonprofit groups are becoming involved in breaking through the barriers that are keeping the disabled from using public buildings, housing, theaters, stores, recreational facilities, restaurants, and public transportation. In the early 1960s the President's Committee on Employment for the Handicapped, with the Easter Seal Society for Crippled Children and Adults, led a compaign that made the public aware of this discrimination. Enactment of the Architectural Barriers Act of 1968 ensured that certain federally funded buildings and facilities would be designed so as to be accessible and usable by the physically handicapped. Federal legislation has established standards, which were revised in 1976, for providing accessibility as prescribed by the American National Standards Institute (ANSI). The Architectural and Transportation Barriers Compliance Board was created by the Rehabilitation Act of 1973. By 1974 every state and the District of Columbia had required the elimination of architectural barriers in public buildings either through legislation, building codes, or executive directives.[15]

The International Symbol of Access (Fig. 11-14), officially in use since 1969, has been of assistance to millions throughout the world in the location, identification, and use of facilities designed for the disabled. The symbol signifies barrier free facilities: ramped entry ways, restrooms with wide stalls and grab bars, 30 inch wide doorways, ground level entry, telephones, drinking fountains, elevator controls within reach, and/or reserved and enlarged parking spaces near accessible entries. The display of this symbol also serves as a means of educating the public to the problems of accessibility faced by the disabled person. The symbol has increased general awareness and acts as a catalyst for the elimination of environmental barriers.

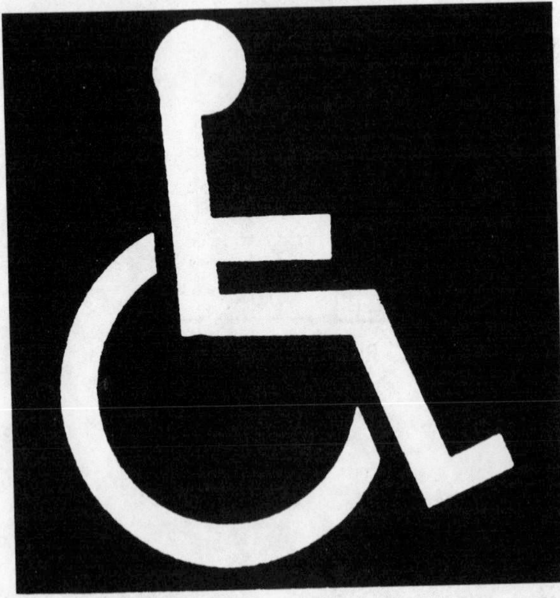

FIGURE 11-14. The International Symbol of Access.

REFERENCES

1. Ford, J., and Duckworth, B.: Physical Management for the Quadriplegic Patient. Philadelphia: F. A. Davis Co., 1974.
2. Zimmerman, M. E.: Homemaking training units for rehabilitation centers. Am. J. Occup. Ther. 20:226, 1966.
3. Zimmerman, M. E.: Activities of daily living. In Willard, H. S., and Spackman, C. S. (eds.): Occupational Therapy, ed. 4. Philadelphia: J. B. Lippincott Co., 1971, pp. 217–256.
4. Ford and Duckworth: Physical Management for Quadriplegic Patient.
5. Rusk, H. A.: A Manual for Training the Disabled Homemaker. Rehabilitation Monograph VIII, pp. 49–50. New York: Institute of Rehabilitation Medicine, 1970.
6. Klinger, J. L.: Self-Help Manual for Arthritic Patients. New York: Arthritis Foundation, 1974.
7. Harkness, S. P., and Groom, J. N., Jr.: Building Without Barriers for the Disabled. The Architect Collaborative Inc., Whitney Library of Design, Cambridge MA, 1976.
8. Klinger, J. L., Friedman, F. H., and Sullivan, R. A.: Mealtime Manual for the Aged and Handicapped. New York: Simon & Schuster, 1970.
9. May, E. E., Waggoner, N. R., and Hotte, E. B.: Independent Living for the Handicapped and the Elderly. Boston: Houghton Mifflin Co., 1974.
10. Waggoner, N. R., and Reedy, G. N.: Child Care Equipment for Physically Handicapped Mothers, Suggestions for Selection and Adaptation. School of Home Economics, University of Connecticut, Storrs CN, 1961.
11. Gross, J. H., and Crandall, E. W.: Management for Modern Families. New York: Appleton Century Crofts, 1963.
12. Handicapped Homemaker Follow-up Study. Harmarville Rehabilitation Center, Pittsburgh PA, 1972.
13. Diffrient, N., Tilley, A. R., and Bardagey, J.: Humanscale 1/2/3. (Designer: Henry Dreyfuss Associates.) Cambridge MA: MIT Press, 1974.
14. Harkness and Groom: Building Without Barriers.
15. Further Action Needed to Make All Public Buildings

Accessible to the Physically Handicapped. Report to Congress by Comptroller General of the United States, July 1975.

BIBLIOGRAPHY

Barrier-Free Site Design. HUD Publication, 1974. (Available from Superintendent of Documents, U.S. Government Printing Office, Washington DC.)

Barton, D. H.: Self-help clothing. Harvest Years, March 1973, pp. 19–23.

Beppler, M. C., and Knoll, M. M.: The disabled homemaker: Organizational activities, family participation, and rehabilitation success. Rehab. Lit. 35:200–206, 1974.

Botwinick, J.: Cognitive Processes in Maturity and Old Age. New York: Springer Publishing Co., 1967.

Bryce, T. E.: A home economist on the rehabilitation team. Am. J. Occup. Ther. 23:258–262, 1969.

Clothes for the Physically Handicapped Homemaker. Agricultural Research Service, U.S. Department of Agriculture, Home Economic Research Report #12, Washington DC, June 1971.

Clothing for the Incontinent Older Child. Disabled Living Foundation, London, March 1972.

Clothing for Wheelchair Users. Disabled Living Foundation, London, September 1971.

Cookman, H., and Zimmerman, M. E.: Functional Fashions for the Physically Handicapped. New York Institute of Physical Medicine and Rehabilitation, New York University Medical Center, 1961.

Friend, S. D., Zaccagnine, J., and Sullivan, M.: Meeting the clothing needs of handicapped children. J. Home Ec. 65:25–27, 1973.

Goldsmith, S.: Designing for the Disabled, ed. 2. New York: McGraw-Hill Book Co., 1967.

Jay, P E.: Help Yourselves—A Handbook for Hemiplegics and Their Families. London: Butterworths, 1966.

Johannsen, W. J., and Thill, J. D.: Effectiveness of homemaking training for hemiplegic patients. Arch. Phys. Med. Rehab. 48:244–249, 1967.

Koch, A. R.: Significance and scope of rehabilitation in homemaking activities. In Rehabilitation of the Physically Handicapped in Homemaking Activities. Vocational Rehabilitation Administration, Washington DC, 1963, pp. 7–16.

Kliment, S. A.: Into the Mainstream: A Syllabus for a Barrier-Free Environment. Prepared under a grant to the American Institute of Architects by the Rehabilitation Services Administration of the Department of Health, Education, and Welfare, June 1975.

Knoll, C. S., and Schwab, L. O.: The outlook for homemaking in rehabilitation. J. Home Ec. January 1974, pp. 39–41.

Krusen, F. H.: Handbook of Physical Medicine and Rehabilitation. Philadelphia: W. B. Saunders Co., 1971.

Kubler-Ross, E.: On Death and Dying. New York: Macmillan Publishing Co., 1969.

Lawton, E. B.: Activities of Daily Living for Physical Rehabilitation. New York: McGraw-Hill Book Co., 1963.

Lowman, E. W., and Klinger, J. L.: Aids to Independent Living: Self Help for the Handicapped. New York: McGraw-Hill Book Co., 1970.

Making Facilities Accessible to the Physically Handicapped. New York State University Construction Fund, Albany, 1974.

Malick, M.: Manual on Dynamic Hand Splinting. Harmarville Rehabilitation Center, Pittsburgh PA, 1974.

Malick, M.: Manual On Static Hand Splinting. Harmarville Rehabilitation Center, Pittsburgh PA, 1973.

May, E. E., and Waggoner, N. R.: Work simplification in child care. In Teaching Materials for the Rehabilitation of Physically Handicapped Homemakers. School of Home Economics, University of Connecticut, Storrs CN, 1962.

McGowan, J. F., and Gust, T.: Preparing Higher Education Facilities for Handicapped Students. Services for the Handicapped, University of Missouri, Columbia, 1968.

McHugh, H. F.: The 1977 family as consumers. J. Home Ec. 69:6–8, 1977.

Mondale, W. F.: Government policy, stress and the family. J. Home Ec. 68:11–15, 1976.

Morgan, M.: Beyond disability: A broader definition of architectural barriers. Am. Inst. Architects J. 65:50–54, 1976.

Nau, L.: Why not family rehabilitation? J. Rehabil. 39: 14–17, 1973.

Newton, A.: Clothing: A rehabilitation tool for the handicapped. J. Home Ec. 65:29–30, 1973.

Olson, S. C., and Meredith, D. K.: Wheelchair Interiors. National Easter Seal Society for Crippled Children and Adults, Chicago, 1973.

Rednick, S. Smith: The physically handicapped student in the regular classroom. In A Guide for Teaching Housing and Home Care. Danville IL: Interstate Printers and Publishers, 1976.

Reference List on Self-Help Devices for the Handicapped. National Easter Seal Society for Crippled Children and Adults, Chicago, 1972.

Rehabilitation of the Physically Handicapped in Homemaking Activities. Proceedings of a Workshop, U.S. Department of Health, Education and Welfare, Washington DC, 1963.

Rusk, H. A.: Rehabilitation Medicine, ed. 3. St. Louis: C. V. Mosby Co., 1971.

Schwab, L. O.: Rehabilitation of physically disabled women in a family oriented program. Rehab. Lit. 36:34–47, 1975.

Schwab, L. O.: Self Perceptions of Physically Disabled Homemakers. Ed.D. Thesis, University of Nebraska, 1966.

Schwab, L. O., and Fadul, R.: Are we prepared for the new rehabilitation legislation? J. Home Ec. 67:33–34, 1975.

Shattel, F. M.: Workshop on Rehabilitation of the Physically Handicapped in the Homemaking Activities. Sponsored by American Home Economics Association, Office of Vocational Rehabilitation, U.S. Department of Health, Education and Welfare, January 1963.

Slater, S. B., Sussman, M. B., and Straud, M. W.: Participation in household activities as a prognostic factor in rehabilitation. Arch. Phys. Med. Rehab. 51:605–610, 1970.

Smith, C. R.: Home planning for the severely disabled. Med. Clin. N. Am. 53:703, 1969.

Steinke, N., and Erickson, P.: Homemaking Aids for the Disabled, 1963. (Available at American Rehabilitation Foundation, 1800 Chicago Avenue, Minneapolis MN 54404.)

Straus, R.: Social change and the rehabilitation concept. In Sussman, M. B. (ed.): Sociology & Rehabilitation. Cleveland OH: American Sociological Association, 1965.

Suchman, E. A.: A model for research and evaluation on rehabilitation. In Sussman, M. B. (ed.): Sociology & Rehabilitation. Cleveland OH: American Sociological Association, 1965.

Switzer, M. E.: Foreword. in Rehabilitation of Physically Handicapped in Homemaking Activities. Proceedings of a Workshop, U.S. Department of Health, Education and Welfare, 1963.

Technical Handbook for Facilities Engineering and Construction Manual. Section 4.12: Design of Barrier-Free Facilities. United States Department of Health, Education, and Welfare, Washington DC, 1974.

Watkins, S. M.: Designing functional clothing. J. Home Ec. 66:33–38, 1974.

Wedin, C. S., and Nygren, L. G. (eds.): Housing Perspectives, Individuals and Families. Minneapolis MN: Burgess Publishing Co., 1976.

Wheeler, V. H.: Planning Kitchens for Handicapped Homemakers. Rehabilitation Monograph 27. New York Institute of Rehabilitation Medicine, New York University Medical Center, 1966.

Yost, Schroeder, Rainey: Home Economics Rehabilitation, A Selected, Annotated Bibliography. 1977. University of Missouri—Columbia, (206 Whitten Hall, Columbia MO 65201, $1.50).

ADDRESSES

American Home Economics Association
2010 Massachusetts Avenue
Washington, D.C. 20036

American Dietetics Association
Publication Department
430 N. Michigan Avenue
Chicago, Illinois 60611

ICTA Information Center
(International Center on Technical Aids)
IACK S-161 03
Bromma 3, Sweden

Schools Offering Homemaker Rehabilitation Programs: Colorado State University, University of Georgia, University of Southern Illinois, University of Missouri-Columbia, University of Nebraska-Lincoln, Ohio State University, Penn State University, and University of West Virginia.

section 3 / Human Sexuality / Marianne Rozycka

Sexuality is becoming increasingly recognized and accepted as a major component of the human personality. This recognition has led to an acute awareness by health professionals of their responsibility to deal directly with the sexuality of their clients.

The subject of human sexuality encompasses a complex and subtle blend of the biological, psychological, social, and interpersonal aspects of being either a man or a woman. Some physiological function and anatomical structure distinguishes male from female (Tables 11-2 and 11-3).

Family responsibilities and other life-roles are influenced by sex. Clothing and the way it is worn reflects sexuality. Even the choice of friends and leisure time activity may be affected by one's sex.

The way we choose to communicate, satisfy, and deal with our sexuality is based upon development of a sexual identity. Freud[1] explored the role and significance of sex in human life. His concept of progression through psychosexual stages was broadened by Erikson[2] in his theories of ego development. Psychosexual theory can be a useful guide in better understanding the subtle interplay of sexuality and personality development. Belmont states "The particular nature and quality of adult sexual behavior

Table 11-2. Female sexual response cycle.

	Able-bodied female	*Disabled female*
Wall of vagina	Moistens	±
Clitoris	Swells	Swells ±
Labia	Swells and opens	Swells ±
Uterus	Contracts	±
Inner 2/3 of vagina	Expands	±
Outer 1/3 of vagina	Contracts	±
Nipples	Erect	Erect
Muscles	Tense, spasms	Tense, spasms
Breasts	Swell	Swell
Breathing	Increases	Increases
Pulse	Increases	Increases
Blood pressure	Increases	Increases
Skin of trunk, neck, face	Sex flush	Sex flush

Adapted from Cole, T., by Glass, D. D.: Sexuality and the spinal cord injured patient. In Oaks, W. W., Melchiode, G. A., and Fisher, I. (eds.): Sex and the Life Cycle. New York: Grune & Stratton, 1976, p. 187. Reprinted with permission.

will be heavily determined by what happens during the child's progression through the psychosexual stages."[3]

The Masters and Johnson[4] studies and those of Kinsey[5,6] highlighted the impact of human feelings on adequacy of sexual expression and communication. Until recently the professional who worked with the disabled person tended to avoid dealing with the client's sexuality because the professional was inhibited by lack of knowledge, by personal uneasiness with his or her own sexuality, or by myths and taboos concerning the sexuality of the disabled.[7] Religious beliefs and socioeconomic and ethnic influences also have an impact on a person's sexual attitudes and knowledge.

Based on work done at the University of Minnesota School of Medicine, Cole has made the following assumptions:[8]

1. Sexual concerns do exist for the disabled person.

2. It may require more than personal experience or opinion to deal with these concerns.

3. A person's ability to solve sexual problems is

(*Text continues on p. 250*)

Table 11-3. Male sexual response cycle.

	Able-bodied male	*Disabled male*
Penis	Erects	Erects ±
Skin of scrotum	Tenses	Tenses ±
Testes	Elevate in scrotum	Elevate in scrotum ±
Emission	Yes	No ±
Ejaculation	Yes	No ±
Nipples	Erect	Erect
Muscles	Tense, spasms	Tense, spasms
Breathing rate	Increases	Increases
Pulse	Increases	Increases
Blood pressure	Increases	Increases
Skin of trunk, neck, face	Sex flush	Sex flush

Adapted from Cole, T., by Glass, D. D.: Sexuality and the spinal cord injured patient. In Oaks, W. W., Melchiode, G. A., and Fisher, I. (eds.): Sex and the Life Cycle. New York: Grune & Stratton, 1976, p. 187. Reprinted with permission.

Table 11-4. Suggested approach in dealing with the patient's sexual problems.

A traditional approach	*because*	*but*	*An approach for the occupational therapist*	*because*
My responsibility is to help people achieve a better state of health. I'll concentrate on that.	Sex is separate from health. If the patient wants to know about sex he/she will find out himself/herself.	Perhaps no one will inform the disabled person about his/her sexual potential.	Initiate discussion and endorse sexuality. Be aware of physiological mechanisms of sex (see Tables 11-2 and 11-3 and Figs. 11-15 and 11-16). Recognize that it is difficult for many people to deal directly with explicit sexuality. Know when to refer a patient to an appropriate team member for specific sexual information.	Healthy sexuality is a part of total rehabilitation and all team members are responsible for helping the patient achieve a better state of health.
Rehabilitation facilities are designed to promote constant interaction sometimes with loss of privacy.	Most learning is done better by interacting with others rather than alone.	Some activities require privacy for learning to occur.	Be sensitive to privacy needs. Don't overreact to human sexual behavior should it occur, e.g., erection during ADL training. When appropriate, recommend opportunity for aloneness, e.g., hospital pass for home visit.	Anxiety-free practice promotes integration.
Sex can be distracting—concentrating a patient's attention on rehabilitation activity will avoid these distractions.	Sexuality is not important to rehabilitation process anyway. If sexuality is recognized it may become unmanageable.	Sex is a natural part of life and awareness of sexuality belongs in the rehabilitation process.	Encourage sexual awareness and responsibility as part of ADL. Teach skills in attractive dressing and grooming techniques including application of cosmetics, after-shave, etc. Teach skills in relating to others as appropriate to patient's need and life-style, e.g., role-playing slow dancing with patient with loss of coordination who plans to attend school dance on weekend with his girlfriend.	Learning of social sexual skill should be expected and encouraged just as people are expected to learn other ADL.

Should a patient demonstrate socially unacceptable sexual behaviors according to hospital standards he/she may be reprimanded or shunned. If it continues he/she may even be discharged.	Hospital personnel should maintain "proper" sex model.	Ignoring or reprimanding a disabled person for testing a self-image of a whole person may communicate that he/she is incompetent and not okay.	Avoid overreacting to behavior with sexual content. Objectively share information with team members so that the behavior can be understood. Deal with the patient as you would like to be dealt with. Encourage the patient to discuss feelings with appropriate team members.	Methods of expressing sexuality can be developed by problem solving rather than punishment.
Many medical, nursing, and therapy procedures must be done no matter how personal they may seem to me.	In a professional relationship objectivity is ensured and I really don't have sexual feelings toward my patients.	Denying our own sexual feelings could inhibit them in our patients.	Deal with personal aspects of therapy openly and sincerely. Be aware of your effect on a patient especially during dressing or bathing training. Acknowledge your patient's effect on you. Realize that nonverbal communication can give the patient input as to his/her own sexuality.	Sexuality is an early concern of many patients. Acknowledging feelings will endorse honesty and responsibility.
When appropriate I answer questions about sexual capacity or sexual attractiveness.	If I initiate an awareness of sexuality the patient may get the wrong idea and will get hurt.	Some people are shy and need "permission" to speak freely about sexuality.	Recognize that we are all sexual beings. Be aware of the possibility of sexual response for the disabled (see Tables 11-2, 11-3, and 11-5). Anticipate sexual concerns and be prepared either to deal directly or to refer to another for help. Take the responsibility to become comfortable with your own sexuality.	The disabled person will appreciate your sensitivity and concern. When sexuality is discussed new disability may be avoided.

Adapted from Cole, T. M.: Mimeographed material from Program in Human Sexuality. University of Minnesota Medical Center, Minneapolis.

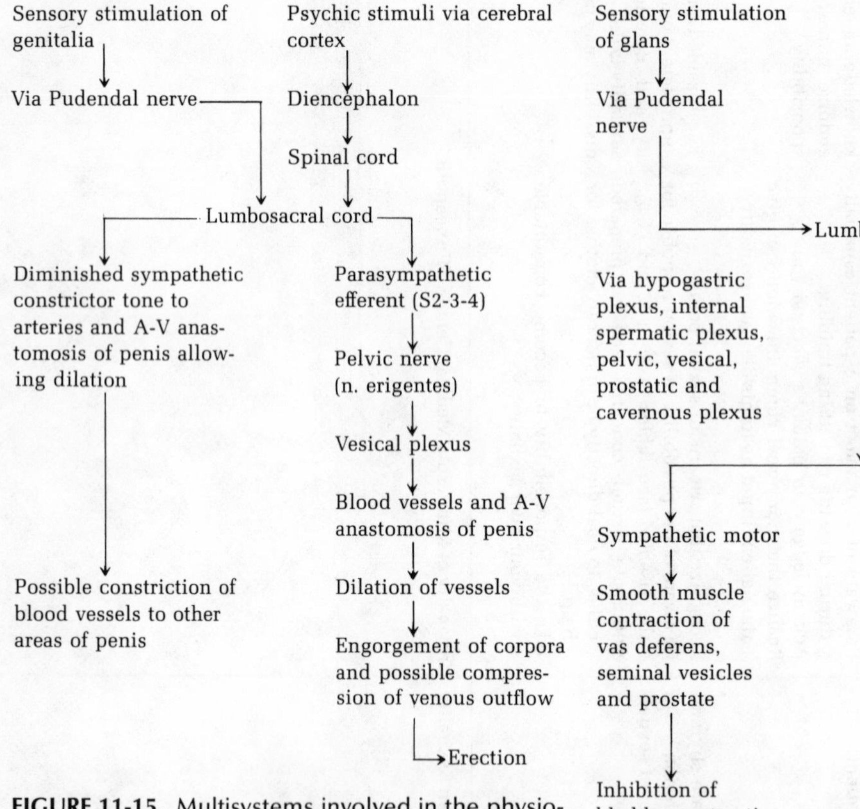

FIGURE 11-15. Multisystems involved in the physiological mechanism of erection. From Glass, D. D.: Sexuality and the spinal cord injured patient. In Oaks, W. W., Melchiode, G. A., and Fisher, I. (eds.): Sex and the Life Cycle. New York: Grune & Stratton, 1976, p. 185. Reprinted with permission.

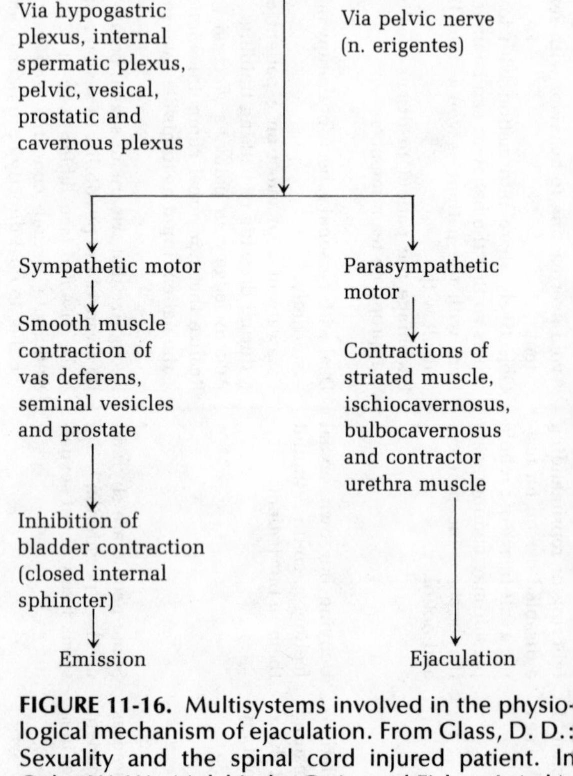

FIGURE 11-16. Multisystems involved in the physiological mechanism of ejaculation. From Glass, D. D.: Sexuality and the spinal cord injured patient. In Oaks, W. W., Melchiode, G. A., and Fisher, I. (ed.): Sex and the Life Cycle. New York: Grune & Stratton, 1976, p. 186. Reprinted with permission.

often hindered by biases, myths, taboos, and overreaction to sexual information or by the same attitudes on the part of the professional.

Many people, including health professionals, find difficulty in dealing directly with explicit sexuality. It is important, however, that the occupational therapist foster a recognition of the fact that all have sexuality and initiate discussion of these aspects of life. By recognizing the sexual components of medical, social, psychological, and vocational aspects of physical disability, the occupational therapist becomes better prepared to assist the disabled with sexual adaptation. Table 11-4 suggests an approach for the occupational therapist in dealing with patients with sexual problems.

There are many resources available to the therapist who wishes to develop an increased understanding of his or her own attitudes and sexuality, thus by accepting one's own sexual self and being able to deal more effectively with the sexual self of the client. The bibliography is designed to be a guide and reference source for those concerned with obtaining more information regarding sexuality.

Table 11-5. Diagnostic significance of sexual functions.

Type of lesion	*Erection*	*Ejaculation*	*Orgasm*
Complete upper motor neuron lesion	Frequent (93%) Always only reflexogenic	Extremely rare (4%) Always following reflexogenic erection	Absent
Incomplete upper motor neuron lesion	Most frequent (99%) Reflexogenic (80%) Combined with psychogenic (19%)	Less infrequent (32%) More often following reflexogenic erections (74%) than psychogenic erections (26%)	Present with ejaculation
Complete lower motor neuron lesion	Infrequent (26%) Always only psychogenic	Infrequent (18%) Always following psychogenic erections	Present with emission
Incomplete lower motor neuron lesion	Frequent (90%) Psychogenic combined with reflexogenic	Frequent (70%) Following psychogenic and reflexogenic erections	Present with ejaculation

Adapted from Bors, E., and Comaar, A. E., by Glass, D. D.: Sexuality and the spinal cord injured patient. In Oaks, W. W., Melchiode, G. A., and Fisher, I. (eds.): Sex and the Life Cycle. New York: Grune & Stratton, 1976, p. 184. Reprinted with permission.

REFERENCES

1. Freud, S.: Three essays on the theory of sexuality, 1905. In Strachey, J. (ed.): The Standard Edition of the Complete Psychological Works of Sigmund Freud. London: Hogarth Press, 1953, Vol. 7, pp. 125–245.
2. Erikson, E.: Childhood and Society, ed. 2. New York: W. W. Norton Co., 1963, p. 445.
3. Belmont, H. S.: Psychodynamic understanding of sexual development in childhood. In Oaks, W. W., Melchiode, G. A., and Fisher, I. (eds.): Sex and the Life Cycle. New York: Grune & Stratton, Inc., 1976, pp. 29–37.
4. Masters, W. H., and Johnson, V. E.: Human Sexual Response. Boston: Little, Brown, Co., 1966, p. 366.
5. Kinsey, A. C., et al.: Sexual Behavior in Human Female. Philadelphia: W. B. Saunders Co., 1953, p. 842.
6. Kinsey, A. C., et al.: Sexual Behavior in Human Male. Philadelphia: W. B. Saunders Co., 1948, p. 804.
7. Cole, T. M., Chilgren, R., and Rosenberg, P.: A new programme of sex education and counselling for spinal cord injured adults and health care professionals. Paraplegia 11:111–124, 1973.
8. Cole, T. M.: Mimeograph outline. Program in Human Sexuality, University of Minnesota Medical School. Sexual Attitude Reassessment Workshop: Moss Rehabilitation Hospital, Philadelphia, 1972.

BIBLIOGRAPHY

Abram, H. S., et al.: Sexual function in patients with chronic renal failure. J. Nerv. Ment. Dis. 160:220–226, 1975.

Andreason, N. J., et al.: Long-term adjustment and adaptation mechanisms in severely burned adults. J. Nerv. Ment. Dis. 154:352–362, 1972.

Birnbaum, M. D., et al.: Psychosexual aspects of endocrine disorders. Med. Aspects Hum. Sexuality 7:134–150, 1973.

Cole, T.: Touching. Sound film available through Multimedia Resource Center, P.O. Box 439, San Francisco CA 94102. 1971.

Cole, T.: Just What Can You Do? Sound film available through Multimedia Center, P.O. Box 439, San Francisco CA 94102. 1971.

Comfort, A.: Sexuality in old age. J. Am. Geriatr. Soc. 22: 440–442, 1974.

De Leon, G., et al.: Heroin addiction—its relation to sexual behavior and sexual experience. J. Abnorm. Psychol. 81:36–38, 1973.

Dlin, D. M., and Pertman, A.: Sex after ileostomy and colostomy. Med. Aspects Hum. Sexuality 6:32, 1972.

Johnson, W.: Sex Education and Counseling of Special Groups: The Mentally and Physically Handicapped, Ill and Elderly. Springfield IL: Charles C Thomas, 1975.

Lemere, F., et al.: Alcohol induced sexual impotence. Am. J. Psychiatry 130:212–213, 1973.

Manson, M. P., et al.: Some psychological findings in the rehabilitation of amputees. J. Clin. Psychol. 9:65–66, 1953.

Meyerowitz, J. H.: Sex and the mentally retarded. Med. Aspects Hum. Sexuality 5:94–118, 1971.

Rosenblum, J. A.: Human sexuality and the cerebral cortex. Fid. Nerv. Sys. 35:268–271, 1974.

Sidman, J. M.: Sexual functioning and the physically disabled adult. Am. J. Occup. Ther. 31:81–85, 1977.
Wagner, N.: Sexual activity and the cardiac patient. In Green, R. (ed.): Human Sexuality: A Healthy Practitioner's Text. Baltimore: Williams & Wilkins, 1975.
Weiss, A. J., et al.: Sexual adjustment, identification and attitudes of patients with myelopathy. Arch. Phys. Med. 47:245–250, 1966.
Wlig, E. H.: Counseling the adult aphasic for sexual readjustment. Rehabil. Counsel. Bull. 17:110–119, 1973.

section 4/Upper Extremity Orthotics/Maude H. Malick

Great strides have been made in the construction of orthotics for the upper extremities using plastic materials as a result of the NASA (National Aeronautics and Space Administration) programs. Reliability in dynamic splinting has increased as a result of the greater sophistication in electronics and external power sources. This is true not only in the United States but also in Europe, South Africa, and Australia. Since low temperature plastic materials are remoldable, splints can be easily constructed or adjusted while the patient waits. Many splints can be custom designed, constructed, fitted, and applied within an hour. Orthoplast, a transpolyisophrene material, allows the therapist to fabricate temporary progressive splinting with minimal effort. Orthotic principles that apply to the low temperature materials are the same as those applying to the metal or high temperature materials. Low temperature materials require more contour or reinforcement when rigidity is required.

A new series of polycaprolactone materials, such as Polyform, Kay-Splint, Aquaplast, and Varioplast, have been introduced recently. These materials can be handled easily if the molding temperature requirements are strictly adhered to. Static and dynamic splints can be constructed readily but should only be considered for three to six months use. Laminated plastic, high temperature materials, and metal are indicated if splint (orthotic) requirements indicate longer wear. Where moving parts such as metal joints, hinges, and telescopic units are needed in the wrist-driven orthosis, they should be constructed and assembled by a qualified orthotist. A good example of this is the Engen telescopic reciprocal wrist orthosis which, in a modular fashion, utilizes laminated plastic, metal, and rods to make an effective orthosis for the quadriplegic patient.

When evaluating the orthotic requirements of the patient, careful analysis should be made of the forearm and hand to evaluate what stability is lacking and what motion is needed in order to perform functional tasks. Range of motion tests and functional motion tests should be used to evaluate strength, range, coordination, and sensory deficiencies, noting whether and where spasticity is present. When orthotic devices are indicated it is important to:

1. fully explain the forearm and hand evaluation to the patient and involve the patient in the design and selection of the orthosis.
2. begin use of the splint early in the treatment program and then discard the splint if it is no longer useful.
3. fabricate the orthosis so that it will be well fitted, designed, and constructed.

The therapist must always consider the psychological aspects of splinting. Patient acceptance may vary but ease of acceptance can be greatly influenced by proper explanation of its necessity to the patient. The orthosis should meet functional requirements and be cosmetically acceptable. Comfort, stability, and value of the orthosis to the patient are probably the greatest factors in patient acceptance.

Initially the splint should be worn only under the therapist's supervision for short periods to be sure no pressure areas exist. Straps must be adequate and secure so that the orthosis retains its correct position. Slipping, with its accompanying misfit, is the greatest cause of pressure areas.

Most ADL activities are performed more usefully when the forearm and hand are in the best functional position. An orthosis provides the proper position, supports weakened muscles, and stabilizes joints. In most cases, the dominant hand, when affected, is splinted but, if both upper extremities are affected, bilateral orthoses may be considered. When shoulder and elbow function are impaired, overhead slings and balanced forearm orthosis (mobile arm supports) should be considered. The patient should be carefully trained with the orthosis and should be given written detailed instructions. The patient should be trained to put on and take off the orthosis and instructed about its proper fit and mechanics. Many simple assistive devices can be quickly constructed with the low temperature plastics on a temporary basis before those of a permanent nature are considered.

ORTHOTICS OF THE HAND

Orthotics and splinting are often used interchangeably, especially in reference to the upper extremity. With the availability of low temperature plastics, the occupational therapist can readily make nearly any splint to meet the splint requirements of patients. Since the number of occupational therapists outnumber the orthotists 15 to 1, the responsibility for hand splinting largely falls to the occupational therapist.

The occupational therapist must assess or evaluate both the patient's affected hand and unaffected hand in order to determine the specific purpose of the splint and the parts to be splinted. The purpose of the splint determines whether the splint should be static or dynamic as well as the regimen in which it is to be used. All splints are a part of an overall patient management program.

Static splints may be protective, supportive, and/or corrective in their design. A static splint may be indicated to protect weak muscles from being stretched by providing the force to counteract a strong muscle group and in this way provide a functional balance while healing is taking place. The splint can support the hand, joint, or arch as a substitute for weak muscles as in the case of arthritis. Corrective splinting can specifically position or force an involved joint or bone into correct or near correct alignment. Static splints have no movable parts and wherever possible should hold the involved forearm and hand in functional position.

All splints must be taken off at intervals and be a part of a maintenance exercise program. The splint and the patient's hand should be washed and dried and the hand carefully replaced in the splint in the correct position. The therapist must always be aware of swelling or edema. Edema can be due to constriction of the splint or its strap. Prolonged static splinting can cause immobility of joints. The patient should be encouraged to use the splinted extremity as much as possible to maintain muscle tone and joint mobility. No splint should immobilize more joints in the hand than is specifically indicated by the evaluations.

All splints should be neat and constructed with careful craftsmanship. They should be light weight, durable, cosmetically acceptable, washable, and carefully designed to avoid loss of the special properties of the thermoplastic material.

Choice of Splinting Materials

There is a wide variety of splinting materials available. Their varying properties must be understood in order to use them properly. They can be classified in four groups:

high temperature materials
moderate temperature materials
low temperature materials
no heat or layered materials

In general, high temperature materials are best cut flat with hand or power tools such as a jigsaw; they should be formed on a plaster positive mold to avoid burning the patient. Low temperature and layered materials may be cut with a scissors; they do not require a mold and can be molded directly on a patient. All materials listed except the layered materials come in sheet form of various thicknesses. Application of the various materials is dependent upon their thickness and rigidity and the design of the splint. The less rigid materials will require more area and contour for support.

High temperature materials include Nyloplex, Royalite, and Kydex. A splint of this type is shown in Fig. 11-17. A moderate temperature material is high impact vinyl. Low temperature materials include Orthoplast, Polyform, San-Splint, Kay-Splint, SOS Plastazote, and Aquaplast. An example of no heat or layered material is Plaster of Paris bandage. In general, low temperature plastic materials are

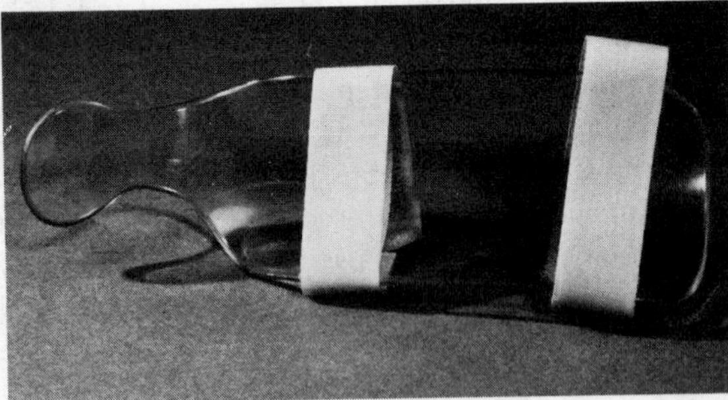

FIGURE 11-17. A simple palmar wrist cock-up splint made out of Nyloplex provides an aesthetically appealing rigid wrist support. Nyloplex is a high temperature plastic which must be formed over a plaster mold.

used for temporary progressive splinting and the high temperature plastic materials for long-term splint requirements.

Construction of the splint requires a thorough knowledge of the properties of the materials and the imagination of the occupational therapist. Patterns and models are guidelines only and should be modified to meet each patient's special requirements. Static splints should never be used longer than is physiologically indicated and should never be used if a dynamic splint would be equally effective. Splints should immobilize only the intended joints, leaving all the adjacent joints free to move. Static splints can:

1. Prevent unwanted motion.
2. Relieve pain.
3. Prevent deformity and contractures.
4. Substitute for weak or lost muscle function.
5. Maintain a functional position for bone, muscle, tendon, or ligaments during a healing process.

Physiological Considerations

It is requisite that each occupational therapist understand the bony skeleton, joint locations, and muscle insertions and functions of the forearm, wrist, and hand. The versatility of motion in the hand depends on the amount of motion in every joint above it. The shoulder, elbow, and wrist must be stable and functional in order to use the hand. Without shoulder motion, the hand is limited to the arc of motion in front of the body allowed by elbow motion. Without elbow motion, the hand is limited to the small arc in which the hand is placed by the wrist.

No matter what splint is used, the hand must be kept in functional position (Fig. 11-18). The functional position of the hand is as follows:

1. Wrist in 30 degree dorsiflexion.
2. Normal transverse arch.
3. Thumb in abduction and opposition and lined up with the pads of the four other fingers.

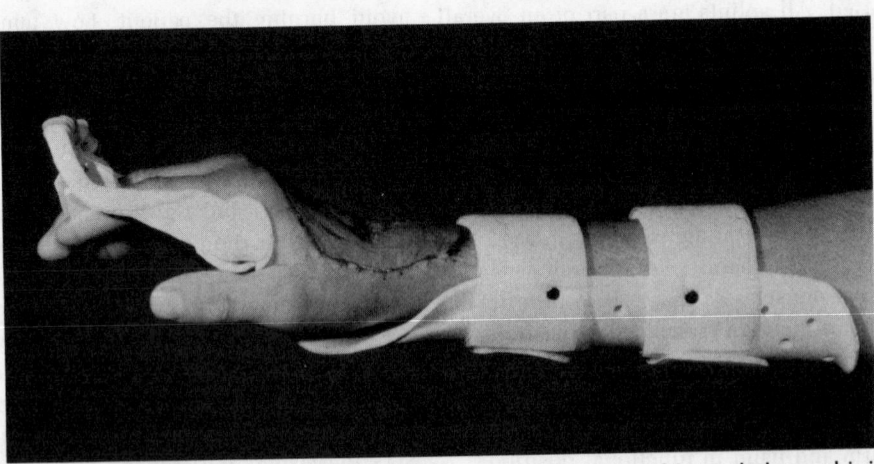

FIGURE 11-18. An orthoplast palmar splint used to maintain the wrist and interphalangeal joints in a functional position. A low profile dynamic outrigger was made to support the fingers. The straps were placed to avoid crossing the dorsum of the metacarpals.

4. Metacarpal and proximal interphalangeal joints in 45 degree flexion.

Palmar Creases

The palmar surface of the hand is covered with thick, tough, and not very pliable skin. This lack of pliability accounts for a system of palmar creases, which allows for flexion and motion. These creases vary slightly on each individual and should act as guidelines for the designing and fitting of each splint. The distal palmar crease must not be impinged upon if full metacarpophalangeal (MCP) flexion is required. Likewise, the thenar crease must not be impinged upon if opposition is required. The wrist creases indicate the best location for a splint strap to stabilize the splint and prevent it from sliding forward.

Arches of the Hand

The palm of the hand is concave from side to side and also in its length. This shape is formed by three arches (Fig. 11-19), which are of prime consideration when constructing a splint.

TRANSVERSE ARCH. The distal transverse arch is also called the metacarpal transverse arch. When the hand is at rest, the arch is slightly oblique. This arch is deepened when the hand is used functionally. The mobility of the fourth and fifth metacarpal within the arch contributes directly to the dexterity of all the fingers. If this metacarpal mobility is constricted, the functional motion of the fingers is directly impaired. Therefore the ability of the arch to deepen should always be considered when designing a splint. There should be freedom and some excursion considered if a palmar bar or support is designed into a splint.

The proper functioning of the thumb depends on the integrity of the transverse arch also. If the arch is depressed, the hand becomes flat and the thumb is unable to oppose the fingers. This opposition is only possible when there is some cupping of the palm and when the curve of this arch is able to be increased voluntarily. Any weakness or damage to this arch will impair the strength, mobility, and precision of the motion of the thumb.

LONGITUDINAL ARCH. The longitudinal arch follows the long lines of the phalanges and metacarpal and carpal bones at a slightly oblique angle and primarily involves the third finger. The mobility of the phalanges (fingers) directly affects the efficiency of the hand grasp.

PROXIMAL TRANSVERSE ARCH. The proximal transverse (or carpal) arch is located at the wrist and is troughlike. It is formed by the annular ligaments and the carpal bones. It is this arch that provides the mechanical advantage to the tendons of the finger flexors by providing the fulcrum.

THE "BALL" AND FUNCTIONAL POSITION. The "ball" is the result of the combination of the three arches.

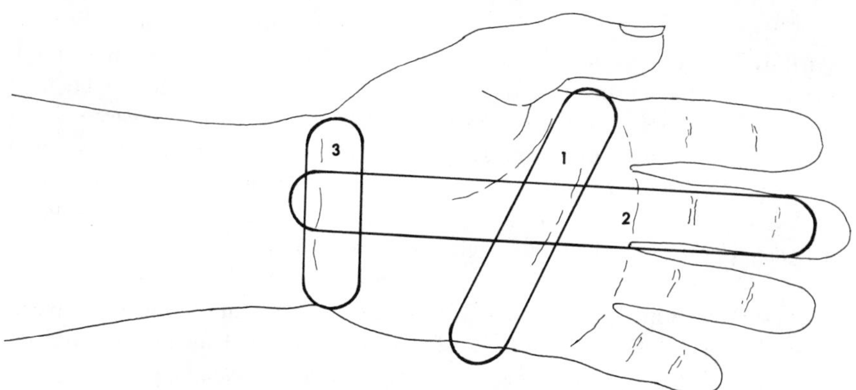

FIGURE 11-19. The three arches of the hand are of primary importance to hand function. *1,* The transverse arch; *2,* the longitudinal arch; and *3,* the proximal transverse arch can be identified easily by the creases of the hand.

It is located directly over the metacarpals which the three arches form. Often the ball is the best pivotal position of support for the hand in a splint. It can be noted when grasping an object. The splint must conform to this ball if it is to fit properly and allow normal function.

When the hand is in the position of function it maintains its arches, slight dorsiflexion of the wrist, and moderate flexion of all the joints of the fingers with the thumb in opposition. This position is maintained primarily by two key sets of joints: the wrist for the hand and the metacarpophalangeal joints for the fingers.

Requirements of a Well Designed Splint

A well-designed and fitted splint should be individually constructed to support, reestablish, or facilitate normal coordinate movement, preserve normal physiological status of muscles, and prevent deformities. The splint should provide the patient with as functional a hand as possible for performing as many activities as possible. This is best done when the splint:

1. Maintains normal arches.
2. Retains normal axis of motion.
3. Permits balanced function of unaffected muscles.
4. Provides most practical prehension pattern.
5. Allows maximal mobility within optimal stability.
6. Frees palmar surface of hand and digits for greatest sensory perception.

Precautions Regarding Pressure Areas

Pressure areas can be created in splinting because force is placed on hand areas for correct positioning. Certain areas are prone to pressure. They are:

1. Dorsum metacarpophalangeal joints with dorsal splints.

2. Palmar (volar) surface of metacarpophalangeal joint of thumb and index finger with C-bar of opponens cuff.

3. Palmar (volar) surface of distal joints of fingers with palmar resting-pan splints, especially with flexion contractures.

4. Dorsal surface of the first phalange of each finger with lumbricales bar.

5. Head of ulna with the wrist strap of the dorsal opponens splint and/or the forearm section bar of the long opponens splint.

6. Metacarpal joint of the thumb just distal to the head of the ulna with the opponens bar.

7. The center of the palm with the palmar (volar) surface of a wrist cock-up, especially when there is wrist flexion contracture.

Pressure areas can be avoided by correct splint designs which include:

1. Following contours of the normal hand and forearm.

2. Placing minimal stretch on joints or muscles in deformed positions over a longer period rather than striving for immediate correction.

3. Increasing surface area to distribute pressure and by using padding.

General precautions include the following:

1. Design and modify splints individually in order to meet the needs and changes in each patient's extremity. The splint should be viewed systematically and reevaluated according to need, fit, and purpose.

2. Wear splints intermittently. The length of time is determined by the physician and/or therapist and usually is not more than ten to twelve hours daily. Splints should be worn only as long as they are performing a function.

3. Avoid tight encircling of the hand to prevent constrictions. There should be no blanched areas where circulation is decreased.

4. Avoid pressure areas over bony prominences.

5. Avoid making too short a forearm section because this will provide inadequate leverage. Conversely, too long a forearm section will impinge on elbow joint (and limit flexion). A good general rule is for the forearm section to be two thirds the length of the forearm. The splint should be checked when the patient is seated.

6. Fit the palmar piece over the metacarpal transverse arch accurately and allow the metacarpal joints to flex at the right angle.

7. Contour sides of finger, thumb, and platform splints to follow the natural curve of the digits. Metacarpal and proximal interphalangeal joints should be flexed to about 15 to 25 degrees. Avoid positions which would lead to hyperextensions of finger joints. The thumb should be held in a functional position of 45 degrees abduction and opposition.

DYNAMIC SPLINTS

Purpose of Dynamic Splinting

Dynamic splinting is the application of a force on a moving part, which remains nearly constant as the part moves. Often it is called active splinting; this refers to the specific and directional mobility that the splint gives the patient's joints by providing forces which substitute for absent muscle power. This joint mobility decreases adhesions, maintains joint function, and prevents ankylosis of the joint.

Dynamic splints must be designed and constructed carefully to provide specific traction with good directional control. Outriggers, which must be placed accurately and secured firmly to the body of the splint, often can be used (Fig. 11-20). The stability and maintenance of splint position on the hand is of prime importance.

A large percentage of patients requiring dynamic splinting are seen in acute care hospitals following surgery or trauma to the forearm and hand and, subsequently, are seen as outpatients and in rehabilitation centers. Dynamic splints frequently are used to substitute for absent muscle power, to prevent contractures or impending contractures, to maintain balance, to promote rest, or to mobilize specific joints.

Dynamic splints may be required for the following:

1. Skeletal substitution
   a. To aid in fracture alignment
   b. To support bones and joints having pathology
2. Muscle balance
   a. For paralyzed muscles
   b. For divided tendons or muscles
3. Joint motion
   a. To preserve joint motion
   b. To increase joint motion
4. Rest
   a. To promote wound healing of newly repaired structures
   b. To treat infection
   c. To relieve pain

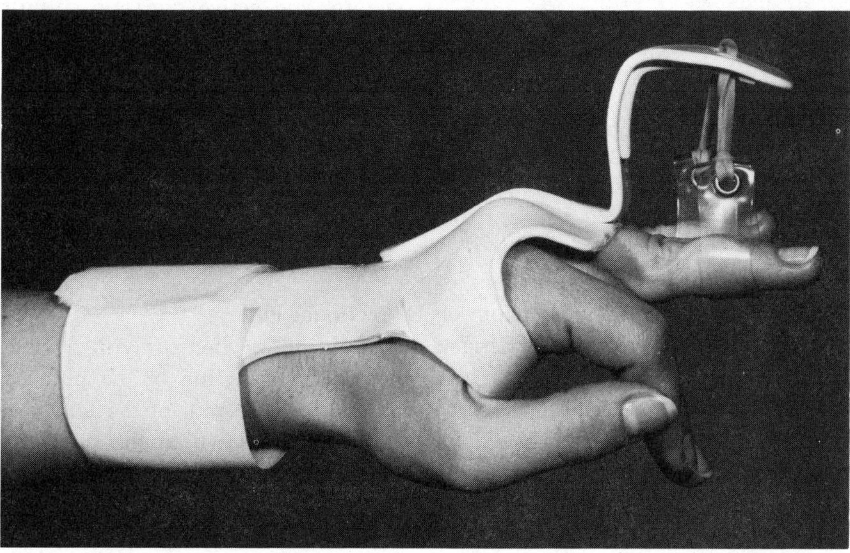

FIGURE 11-20. A dorsal splint with a lumbrical bar incorporating an outrigger. This applies an extension assist to the PIP joints by stabilizing the proximal phalanx.

The patient should be under close supervision of the physician and the occupational therapist. He or she should be encouraged to maintain and restore joint motion, follow the exercise program, and have the splint checked and adjusted regularly. The therapist must maintain an accurate joint measurement progress record.

Medical Principles

Good general medical principles must be considered in dynamic splinting. These principles include:

1. Moving muscles must be given an opposing, balancing force in order to maintain joint mobility and freely gliding tendons. A corrective force, often in the form of a finger cuff and rubber band, is necessary.

2. Movement prevents joint limitation, muscular atrophy, and deformity such as ankylosis.

3. Joints never should be immobilized needlessly.

4. Where there are injuries on the *flexor* surface, the wrist and fingers should be placed in flexion.

5. Where there are injuries in the *extensor* surface, the wrist and fingers should be placed in a neutral (resting) position.

6. Whenever possible, the position of function should be maintained prior to the application of any dynamic unit.

7. The hand should be elevated in the presence of edema since edema causes fibrosis and prevents function. The edema should be reduced as quickly as possible so that early motion can be encouraged and the movement in the uninvolved parts of the hand maintained.

8. Construction of straps which constrict venous return should not be used. Excessive tension of circular straps cause edema and increase the danger of ischemic contractures.

Static Base of the Dynamic Splint

The static base of the dynamic splint is of primary importance in all splinting. This base is the secured (anchored) foundation upon which all the support and moving parts rely. The static base of the splint:

1. provides foundation for proper (functional) alignment of joints.
2. provides a foundation to which the outrigger is attached with its traction components.
3. provides the foundation for a hinge joint.
4. aids in the relaxation of any spastic muscle.
5. allows tissues to adapt to their new position.
6. protects a newly repaired structure.
7. provides the support for proximal parts to allow increased function in distal joints or uninvolved parts.
8. aids in the positioning for edema control.

Immobilization leads to joint stiffness; this must be remembered when constructing the static base of a splint.

Forces

Dynamic splinting provides constant force over a long period of time in contrast to strong, short-term pressure. It operates according to a principle similar to the one an orthodontist uses in straightening teeth. Active motion can be encouraged, for the pumping effect of muscle contraction helps relieve edema and increases joint range of motion. Eight hours of light, steady tension are more successful than vigorous passive exercise for twenty minutes, especially where contractures are present. Progressive alteration to a static splint can draw out a contracture, and active dynamic splinting can aid in maintaining the correction.

Active dynamic splinting has a physiological effect as well, for when the muscles are moving they pump away stagnant fluids that wash out the toxins and the tendons keep gliding and the joints keep moving. Thus, the formation of adhesions is prevented and the good mobility of joints can be maintained.

Directional Pull

In splinting when applying flexion traction to the fingers, the direction of the pull is of paramount importance. The pull of the fingers must not draw them straight down to the palm of the hand but rather obliquely aim them at the scaphoid bone or the base of the third metacarpal. In normal opening of the hands, fingers abduct; in normal closing of the hand, fingers adduct moving in an oblique arc of motion (Fig. 11-21).

All the fingers, except the middle one (which may flex straight down), cross the palm obliquely from 10 to 30 degrees. The same line of pull or of direction should be maintained when finger traction is used. If the splint is incorrectly designed with the finger pulled straight down in flexion, a serious ulnar deviation will appear when the patient tries to extend the fingers. If bone callous has formed, the deformity may need surgical intervention.

Exercise Program

Dynamic splints are used to maintain forces and position as well as to be a part of a graduated exercise and activity program. The combination of good dynamic splinting and an exercise program aids in good hand rehabilitation.

The exercise and activity program aids in the excursion of the joint and is good for maintaining the tone of the skin and improving the circulation to the injured part. A patient also can gain confidence by seeing to what degree the hand can be moved safely. Exercises are best performed by the patient following instructions from the therapist so as not to go beyond the point of pain.

When there is lack of sensation, one must be extremely careful to avoid pressure or increase resistance too rapidly in a traction program. Applying heat prior to the exercise program is often a great help in relaxation and facilitation of movement.

Instructions for the Patient

A patient should understand the purpose of the splint, its accurate positioning, and exactly what motion or movement or range is being sought. The therapist should explain functional anatomy of the hand to the patient. The therapist could demonstrate his or her own hand movement and range of motion so that the patient can understand the regimen more clearly and have confidence in it. The patient can use the unaffected hand to explore normal ranges of motion.

Careful instructions in the use of the dynamic splint are absolutely necessary and written instructions are imperative when a splint is given to the patient on an outpatient basis. The patient should be seen at least once a week to measure range of motion of hand joints. Adjustments must be made as gains are made in the mobilization of joints and as muscle power increases. The regimen is successful when there is improvement, little or no pain, and minimal edema. One must be careful in the follow-up program to make sure that the hand does not begin to shift back into its old or nonfunctional position as soon as the dynamic splint has been removed.

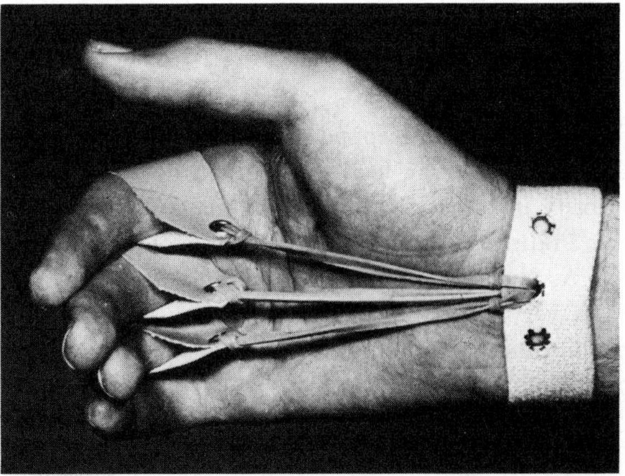

FIGURE 11-21. Dynamic flexion cuff demonstrating the correct line of pull.

BIBLIOGRAPHY

Anderson, M. H.: Functional Bracing of the Upper Extremities. Springfield IL: Charles C Thomas, 1965.

Anderson, M. H.: Upper Extremities Orthotics. Springfield IL: Charles C Thomas, 1965.

Barr, N. R.: The Hand. Principles and Techniques of Simple Splint Making in Rehabilitation. London: Butterworths, 1975.

Cailliet, R.: Hand Pain and Impairment. Philadelphia: F. A. Davis Co., 1974.

Licht, S.: Orthotics, Etc. Springfield IL: Charles C Thomas, 1966.

Malick, M. H.: Manual on Dynamic Hand Splinting. Pittsburgh: Harmarville Rehabilitation Center, 1974.

Malick, M. H.: Manual on Static Hand Splinting. Pittsburgh: Harmarville Rehabilitation Center, 1970.

Wynn-Parry, C. B.: Rehabilitation of the Hand, ed. 2. London: Butterworths, 1974.

section 5/Prevocational Training/Dorothy L. Kester

For many handicapped persons the need to fulfill the self-actualizing feeling of "I can do it too" has priority in the choice of employment. This need is true in direct proportion to the degree of the disability. As the reasons for working and for choice of work vary with individuals so do the reasons and magnitude of the problems that bar people from successful employment.

PROBLEMS

Physical or Medical Problems

It is possible for an apparently minor physical problem to create a complete barrier to returning to work. Consider the house painter trying to paint a ceiling if neck motion were limited, moving the ladder if shoulder motion were limited, or climbing the ladder if hip, knee, or ankle movement were painful. Performance of the same occupation would be hindered by limited tolerance for general physical activity following a cardiovascular accident or respiratory ailment even if ability to perform the specific activities were not affected. Consider the typist with cervical pain, a fractured finger or coccyx, tenosynovitis, or limited visual tolerance.

Some conditions are temporary and do not prevent return to previous employment even before remediation is complete. Other disabilities that are more permanent in nature might not preclude return to work if adaptive devices or environmental changes could compensate for the personal limitation. A third category involves the permanent medical or physical disability that is severe enough to prevent return to previous employment. In this case (or in the case of a person who has never worked), vocational evaluation is available to determine potentials but adjustment programs are also frequently required for mental, emotional, and social problems or other personal reasons.

Mental, Emotional, and Social Problems

In the areas of mental, emotional, and social dysfunction there are problems which may appear to be minor in the home or in many social situations but which are actually major deterrents to employment.

Limited cognitive abilities automatically limit vocational choice possibilities but do not preclude employment. Limited concentration, distractibility, or psychological pressures that limit tolerance for specific activities might preclude employment even though job skills are present. Job skills are meaningless if interpersonal relationships or problem behaviors create friction or reduce productivity.

Life Survival Skills

Skills pertaining to life survival is another problem area which can render job skills meaningless. Grooming, hygiene, and safety skills are as important to the employer and coworkers as to the individual employee. Poor time and money concepts as well as poor social relationships affect employment success, and lack of transportation skills can nullify any possibility of employment.

Job Survival Skills

Factors included under job survival skills overlap some of the other problem areas as well as adding different dimensions. Although it sounds redundant to include life survival skills and interpersonal relationships here, there is a difference between the requirements for social and vocational situations. As one example, in social situations it is possible to choose one's associates but on the job the personalities of one's coworkers are usually more diverse and associates are determined at least in part by the job and the situation.

Sensory Motor Dysfunction

Sensory motor dysfunction does not disappear as the person grows older. The poor motor, tactile, visual, auditory, and/or cognitive skills and tolerances remain; emotional and behavioral problems intensify and ego strength and ability to tolerate stress continue to decrease. Vocational choice is limited or, in many cases, is absent.

Others, who do have the ability to perform higher level occupations, frequently yield to the stresses and end up on lower level jobs. Another group of individuals might have abilities commensurate with employment, but these are negated by emotional or behavioral problems severe enough to prevent success.

Cognitive Dysfunction

Deficiencies in math, reading, reading comprehension, spatial and temporal concepts and relationships and limited ability to deal with abstractions and mental manipulations are problems which may stem from a variety of causes such as retardation, sensory motor dysfunction, or emotional disturbance. Whatever the cause, these problems, in themselves, limit vocational choice and, if combined with other problems, decrease vocational potential even further.

REMEDIATION PROGRAMS

All of the previously mentioned problems may be evaluated and diminished or solved by the occupational therapist, and he or she may design remediation programs. However, some of the occupational therapy skills must be refined or taken into new dimensions and other skills must be learned.

All the adjustment programs involve changing some form of behavior—physical, emotional, social, vocational, and so forth. A variety of techniques should be used to produce these changes but the ones most basic to all of the remediation programs are the evaluative techniques. In many ways these programs could be considered "continuing evaluation" because without a continual evaluation of status there is no foundation on which to determine at any given time what has changed, what needs to be changed, what techniques might work, or when the client reaches the point where he or she has made maximum gains from the program.

Work Tolerance Programs

Work tolerance programs are designed to improve physical abilities or compensate for disabilities, and/or improve poor physical tolerances that interfere with successful employment for a specific job or work in general. Work tolerance programs start with physical and functional evaluations, measurement of joint range of motion, and other pertinent objective measurement techniques. For example, the Minnesota Rate of Manipulation Test is used to measure speed of performance. Frequency of re-testing varies with the length of the program but must be done near or on the day of completion in order to provide meaningful information about the client's accomplishments. The programs are most effective when traditional occupational therapy techniques are combined with job-related tasks that are graded to increase the needed function and/or tolerance for activity.

Clients' individual programs vary considerably depending on the cause and degree of the disability, duration of inactivity, specific difficulties noted the first day, speed of change, and attitude of the client (especially fear of activity). The occupational therapist's knowledge of symptoms and precautions is especially helpful in the early stages of the program for determining whether the client is performing appropriately, underdoing, or possibly pushing too hard. Many clients need to be helped to a more realistic awareness of their capacities through activity combined with counseling. They will not be convinced by purely verbal techniques that they are capable of more activity but must experience it. This experiencing is most meaningful if the tasks are related to the client's work.

These programs follow many of the rules of traditional occupational therapy programs, such as (1) the activities must be within the client's capability but should offer a challenge; (2) the activities must be graded to increase the patient's capability; and (3) in order to create change, the effort required and/or the length of time on a given type of activity must increase.

In reporting to the counselor, whether verbally or in writing, information about present status, expected gains, and potentials must be factual. Motivation, attitudes, behaviors, and emotional status are as important as the physical findings and should, therefore, be included. Check lists or other forms are a concise method for recording these facts but usually cannot provide adequate information. Examples of task performance are more meaningful in many cases but are also inadequate without qualifying narrative or interpretive additions. The narrative section should include specific objective personal and work behavior observations, present status, work readiness, summary, and recommendations. The recommendations are the most important part of a report, in fact the reason for the report; all of the other facts merely provide background information leading to those conclusions.

CASE SUMMARY

Mr. B. was referred for a five-day work tolerance program to determine whether he could return to kitchen installation work following his heart attack.

He was a sturdy-appearing young man whose ability to perform the tests for physical activities was unaffected except for his ability to lift and carry. He was able, after five days, to lift or carry only slightly above half the average load for a man of his age and build. He found, however, that this amount created no problems and was confident that with further work on this at home he would be able to lift the required weights by the time he returned to work.

Activity on the first day consisted of alternate sedentary and active work, with the amount and level of the active work increasing each day. By the fifth day he was working primarily on active tasks such as large wood projects.

He worked accurately and neatly on all assigned tasks, had no difficulty with tasks involving spatial relationships or cognitive functions, and performed well on the basic skill requirements for machine shop work.

Mr. B. gained an understanding of the degree to which he could safely push himself in order to regain further strength and tolerance. He was able to return to kitchen installation work shortly after discharge from the program.

Adjustment Training

There are two major types of adjustment training: personal adjustment training and work adjustment training. They are different in their overall objectives but have some similarities and actual overlapping of individual goals. Methods used for both training programs are similar in that they use work as a major media. The major differences in techniques result primarily from the type and philosophy of the facility and the type and severity of disability in the clients. The techniques vary from learning by experience to well organized behavioral techniques.

Work itself is used as a major catalyst, but many other techniques are also required. Personal, social, and vocational counseling with individuals and groups, role playing, behavior modification, skill training, audiovisuals, guest experts, and field trips are some of the tools that can be helpful with all clients and are usually necessary with those clients who have severe or combinations of dysfunction.

Concurrently with the above techniques, the work and working space can be manipulated to accelerate the rehabilitation process. Depending on the facility, either simulated or actual jobs are utilized to provide a flexible, yet controlled, realistic work environment for the client. At the same time the client is gaining work experience, his or her social, emotional, and vocational behaviors and skills are being evaluated. Long range goals and short range objectives for rehabilitation are determined and procedures planned.

The work assigned might be graded from sedentary to active or the reverse, from gross motor to fine motor, from minimal to high requirements for speed and/or accuracy, from working alone to cooperating with others, or from a task on which speed and attention are externally controlled (as on an assembly line) to self-controlled.

The client might be placed on a specific job primarily for the example peers will set or because they will contribute appropriate peer feedback. This peer feedback is often much more effective than any provided by the supervisors or counselors. Charting or graphing of behaviors, work rhythm, accuracy, and productivity is also an effective means for providing immediate feedback as well as graphically demonstrating progress or regression. Other effective feedback techniques include use of video tape, self-evaluations, tokens, or remuneration.

Group sessions, even when geared for specific learning experiences such as job survival skills, are an economical means of providing other necessary knowledge and skills. These skills include such factors as peer interaction, self-esteem, emotional awareness, amount and appropriateness of verbal and nonverbal responses, and attentiveness.

Generalization and oversimplification is necessary when discussing differing personalities. In actual fact, there is no specific rule for determining what comes next in the learning hierarchy. Each client has his or her own best time when ready to learn a specific thing. Each client differs also as to how much he or she will learn and by which method or combination of methods he or she learns best. The occupational therapist must develop the ability to determine those times, places, and methods for each client.

PERSONAL ADJUSTMENT TRAINING. One of the types of adjustment training is personal adjustment training (P.A.T.). The major goals of P.A.T. are:

1. Decrease behaviors adversely affecting vocational potential.
2. Improve interpersonal relationships.
3. Normalize work-related behaviors.
4. Maximize life survival skills.
5. Improve use of leisure time.
6. Maximize acceptance of the disability.

A major part of this program might require social as well as personal adjustment. Basic math, basic reading or survival words, personal hygiene, health, grooming, dress, manners, appropriate behavioral reaction patterns, social relations, use of leisure time, table manners, relations with peer groups and authority figures, recreation, and dating are areas given attention in personal adjustment training. Persons who need help with these skills usually require assistance with money handling, time concepts and awareness, transportation, appropriate self-expression, human sexuality, desirable character and behavior traits, how to make friends, and building of ego strength and self-confidence combined with acceptance of limitations. In many cases it is also important to assist the family in accepting the client's disability in order to help develop realistic goals for the client.

WORK ADJUSTMENT TRAINING. The second type of adjustment training is in work adjustment. The three major goals of work adjustment training (W.A.T.) are:

1. Maximize vocational potential.
2. Maximize potential for independent living.
3. Maximize potential for emotional and vocational self-support.

A "pure" work adjustment training program involves knowledge of and skill in meeting the requirements of work. It includes such factors as punctuality, attendance, independence and self-support, understanding of the relationships of work to daily living, relationships with co-workers, and acceptance of supervision and authority. However, frequently there is no such thing as pure work adjustment. Poor vocational knowledge or skills usually go hand-in-hand with, or result from, poor personal adjustment. To ignore the developmental hierarchy of these factors can create the additional behavioral and emotional problems of crises, frustrations on the part of the client and work adjustment counselor, and even failure. If the client has not learned what a job is, why people work, or why responsibility, dependability, independence, willingness to accept help, handling of frustrations, personal relationships, health, and hygiene are important, the client has not learned how to keep a job. It is unrealistic, therefore, to teach him how to find a job, fill out applications, or handle a job interview.

New dimensions are added to the value of work itself at this level. In the W.A.T. program the emphasis of the work itself shifts to improving interpersonal relationships, effective use of abilities and acceptance of disabilities, adjustment to work pressures, derivation of work satisfaction, and realism of the client's self-concept as a worker. Many of the skills dealt with in a P.A.T. program are also included in W.A.T. in order to develop the skills to a more mature level.

Once the personal aspects have been developed, the client is ready to continue with the work skills. Learning how to look for and apply for work, how to fill out an application, what is involved in an interview, and what to expect on a new job require a variety of methods and much practice. Guest speakers and field trips should be added at this time, if they have not been used before, to provide more realistic experiences directly related to the world of work.

Vocational-Educational Program

The vocational-educational program is a newer, more complex type of program that was developed for adolescents and young adults with perceptual dysfunction. The goals of this program include:

1. All P.A.T. goals.
2. All W.A.T. goals.
3. Maximize sensory motor integration.
4. Maximize educational skills.

Perceptual dysfunction, in itself, affects vocational potential in many ways: gross motor, fine motor, and tactile problems affect physical skills; apraxia affects visual-motor skills; and visual dysfunction affects visual skills. Each aspect of dysfunction interacts with and compounds the problems created by the others, e.g., tactile dysfunction and poor spatial and temporal skills affect potential for all types of employment. The person's speed of learning; ability to deal with abstractions; emotional, social, and behavioral maturation; and self-concepts and ego strength are also directly affected by the perceptual dysfunction.

The perceptual dysfunction also compounds the difficulties of the rehabilitation process. The following is an example of this situation.

Previous testing may have indicated potential for a specific type of work, such as janitorial, in which the client is interested. In the training program, however, unexpected difficulties arise when the job is broken down into specific tasks. For example, the client stops working after doing only part of the task, ignores obviously dirty areas when cleaning and says he or she can't see anything wrong when told to redo the area, stops to stare into space or have a conversation with a coworker, can't schedule his or her own work, or doesn't start the second task when the first is completed.

When corrected or told to redo a task, the client insists it was done correctly and becomes irate or otherwise behaves inappropriately. The supervisor considers him or her lazy, sloppy, inattentive, and explosive. The supervisor may not realize that the client's time concepts are poor, that the client is unable to conceive of the sequence from task to task or within a task, that poor visual perceptions prevent the client from seeing that the job is not done correctly, and that the client's low self-esteem and poor emotional maturity cause him or her to take the correction as an accusation and one more example of failure.

As a result of behavior problems in combination with unacceptable job performance, the client is discontinued from the training program. The counselor finds another, supposedly easier type of training and the same problems arise; eventually, the case is closed and the client is on his or her own. The person has become increasingly frustrated and, as the frustration increases, self-esteem and willingness to try decreases even further.

A special program is needed for this type of client. Since most multifaceted problems are best remediated through a multifaceted attack, the most effective program for this type of client is one that includes all aspects of the P.A.T. and the W.A.T. programs, placing additional emphasis on educational remediation and adding perceptual remediation and an understanding by the staff of the ramifications of perceptual dysfunction. Adolescents and young adults do accept perceptual remediation and become increasingly motivated as change is realized. Self-esteem, willingness to try new things, speed of learning, accuracy of work, and behaviors all improve as perceptual skills and ego strengths increase. Because of the complexity of these problems and the length of time they have existed, the rehabilitation process is also a lengthy one.

The results that can be attained by the preceding programs are demonstrated by the following case summary.

CASE SUMMARY

F. W. is a nineteen-year-old male who has received special services from a minimum of ten special facilities. Minor surgery was performed at eighteen months, following which he stopped making any attempts to speak. His family was counseled by the crippled children's services; he was diagnosed as aphasic and received speech therapy. Upon reaching school age, he was placed in special education, spent two years at an institute of logopedics, then returned to the public school system for a work experience program. During this time he and his parents were also seen by child guidance services. Many psychological assessments were attempted, each resulting in minimal objective information. However, clinical judgments indicated that F. had much more potential than testing could indicate considering his lack of communication and response, shyness, retiring nature, and extremely immature behaviors.

At sixteen, at the request of the school program director, he became a vocational rehabilitation client and was admitted to the recently developed vocational-education program at the center.

For months after admission, F. insisted on keeping his lunch with him, refused to remove his coat, pulled the coat over his head, and turned his back or actually hid if asked to do anything when other persons were in the area. He hid if any new person appeared and, if talked to firmly, hid for the rest of the day. Communication consisted of grunts and gestures, primarily to indicate that something hurt. Educational skills consisted of counting to three and recognizing most letters of the alphabet. Balance, equilibrium reaction, and perceptual development were poor. Despite these behaviors, it became apparent that he learned physical tasks easily and liked challenges when he worked alone.

He required several months to feel comfortable with persons he saw every day, and six months to be willing to do anything except woodwork in a group situation. Once comfortable, he was willing to attempt new things if he thought he was helping. Following conferences with the staff, his family allowed him to help with increasingly difficult tasks at home.

As self-confidence increased, he began to communicate verbally. A speech evaluation was performed when his speech consisted primarily of nouns strung together with an occasional uninflected verb and a few adjectives. Auditory comprehension for language was at a 6-year level, but auditory memory, fine discrimination, and usage were lower. Therapy was recommended and instituted.

Behaviors, skills, and motivations have improved slowly. He no longer blushes when new people or groups appear and works with new staff members with little hesitation. He does not yet fully understand the productivity aspects of employment, but willingly accepts new challenges. Work quality is very good when he understands what is wanted.

Perceptual development has improved considerably in all areas. He is functioning at approximately the first grade level in reading and math; major gains have been made in his sight knowledge of words, and he is beginning to use phonics to sound out words. He functions semi-independently in simple addition and possesses some skills in money and telling time. Dramatic gains are noted in the amount and variety of verbal output and the use of simple grammatical structures. Speech is not clear, but he willingly repeats if he is not understood. When with his peers, quantity of speech is close to normal, and he talks on the telephone nightly with one coworker.

At a recent conference, his parents requested our assistance with a familial decision. Is F. now ready for an out-of-state move they have been planning for several years but delayed because of his progress? They will investigate possibilities for continuing speech, educational, social, and vocational programs. We concurred with this decision, recommending that social and vocational factors be the primary considerations.

BIBLIOGRAPHY

Brewer, E., Miller, J., and Ray, J.: The effect of vocational evaluation and work adjustment on clients' attitude toward work. Voc. Eval. Work Adjustment Bull. 8:18–25, 1975.

Bottersbusch, K. F., and Sax, A. B.: A Comparison of Seven Vocational Systems, Materials Development Center, Stout Rehabilitation Institute, University of Wisconsin, Menomonie WI, 1976.

Dinneen, T.: Work Evaluation as a technique for improving self-concept. Voc. Eval. Work Adjustment Bull. 8:28–34, 1975.

Granofsky, J.: A Manual for Occupational Therapists on Prevocational Exploration. Dubuque IA: W. C. Brown Book Co., 1959.

Hoffman, P. R.: Work evaluation, an overview. Work Evaluation in Rehabilitation, Reprint Series RS-70-2, 3–18, 1969.

Olshansky, S.: Reply to Kopstein and Lores. Rehabil. Lit. 36:142, 1975.

Raymond, E.: Measuring the interpersonal aspects of work behavior. Voc. Eval. Work Adjustment Bull. 8:19–23, 1975.

Roberts, C. L.: Definitions, objectives and goals in work evaluation. Work Evaluation in Rehabilitation, Reprint Series RS-70-2, 19–30, 1969.

Persons interested in more definitive information on adjustment techniques, will find articles in journals such as:

Journal of Rehabilitation, published by the National Rehabilitation Association.

Vocational Evaluation and Work Adjustment Bulletin, published quarterly by the Vocational Evaluation and Work Adjustment Association, a division of the National Rehabilitation Association.

The American Journal of Occupational Therapy.

Many of the available articles are indexed in Psychological Abstracts and Rehabilitation Literature. The University of Wisconsin-Stout, Menomonie WI, 54751, maintains a Materials Development Center for such materials.

Part Six

General Areas of Occupational Therapy Practice

12

Psychiatry and Mental Health

Elizabeth G. Tiffany

Who are the people with whom the psychiatric occupational therapist works? How do we define the *mentally ill*? Throughout human history mental illness has worn many masks. It has been thought of as demon possession, mystical ecstasy, constitutional inferiority, physiological illness, psychological imbalance, a response to environmental deviations, and an ethical and social problem.

Perhaps the most effective definition today is a functional one. People who, through the centuries, have been called mentally ill, psychiatrically disabled, or maladjusted have been those who have lacked the ability to organize their thoughts, feelings, attitudes, and actions in a way which would permit them to function within society for either a brief or extended period of time. Such a broad definition seems necessary. The phrase "ability to organize" allows for a wide range of etiologies, which include physiological, toxic, psychological, social, and others. Such a definition allows for some consideration of the severe psychological pathologies that sometimes accompany physical illness or trauma and require very special attention if the process of rehabilitation is to be effective. It does not exclude the possibility that the mentally retarded or the neurologically impaired may also have components of psychiatric disability. The phrase "within society" allows for the possibility that the environments and social systems in which people live are varied and that what constitutes healthy behavior in one may be seen as highly undesirable, perverted, or ill in another. We find that, at the outer edges of our definition, the distinctions between "mental" and "physical," "individual" and "societal," tend to become blurred.

Occupational therapy, like medicine, is concerned with the restoration or maintenance of function in people who are ill or otherwise disabled. Like medicine, occupational therapy must always reflect and act upon the base of knowledge of the time. What is known and understood about people and their functioning dictates what is perceived as possible. Like medicine, occupational therapy will always be bound to some degree by the values of the time and the place in which it provides service. Occupational therapy, like medicine, is practiced by people, individuals who bring to their profession their own personal strengths and weaknesses, value systems, needs, and unique ways of perceiving, thinking, feeling, and acting. These factors explain some of the differences one finds in occupational therapy practice, especially in psychiatric settings. They also give urgency to the need to define clearly and in depth the underlying premises of psychiatric occupational therapy practice.

The purpose of this chapter is to examine the principles and practices of occupational therapy as applied to the treatment of mental illness. No examination of this area of occupational therapy is complete, however, without considering the "normal" continuum of human growth (see Chapter 3, Section 1, Human Development). In Section 1 of this chapter, the history of events and trends of psychiatric occupational therapy practice in the United States is traced. The basic elements of the occupational therapy process are considered in Section 2 as they relate to all areas of practice. This is followed in Section 3 and 4 by a discussion of the occupational therapy process itself and the various kinds of settings in which occupational therapists work and the unique approaches to treatment found within these settings. Finally, as a summary, the challenges of psychiatric occupational therapy for the future are considered in Section 5.

section 1 / Historical Roots

On close perusal of the history of psychiatric occupational therapy, it is evident that there are threads of thought which are woven into the fabric of the profession as a whole. These constant strands of thought are what have given the profession its consistent uniqueness throughout the years.

Competence, mastery, self-image, motivation, total function, adaptation, integration, satisfaction—these are some of the key words that appear throughout the literature of occupational therapy. A thoughtful look at their meanings reveals a fundamental belief which has prevailed throughout the history of occupational therapy: the belief that human beings are whole, that mind and body are intricately linked, and that anything that impinges upon or influences one must affect the other. Dunton, one of the founders of occupational therapy, said in 1922, "The primary objects to be obtained by occupational therapy may be divided into two groups, mental and physical, although it is impossible to divorce these functions."[1] To work toward the restoration of function in their physically disabled clients, occupational therapists have relied upon psychological involvement in the *meanings* attached to the *doing* process. To work toward restoration of function in their mentally ill clients, occupational therapists have used movement, doing, touching, sensing, that is, physical factors. In working with all kinds of clients, occupational therapists must be concerned with factors such as stress, anxiety, tension, and learning, all of which have long been demonstrated to have both emotional and physical components.

MORAL TREATMENT—WORK AND PRODUCTIVITY EQUATE WITH DIGNITY

It is generally thought that the principles of "moral treatment" formed the base for modern psychiatric practice and for the specific concern with the uses of activity for treatment as we know it in occupational therapy. What are the tenets of moral treatment which, in the late eighteenth century, were so great a departure from the existing beliefs and practices with regard to the mentally ill? Moral treatment was based on the belief that mental illness occurred as the result of physical and psychological, not mystical, factors. Environmental stresses were recognized as major causes. Therefore, attention to a patient's environment or milieu was a primary concern, and institutions for the mentally ill gave attention to providing pleasant surroundings, kind and consistent treatment, and opportunities for patients to be productive. There was a belief that, no matter how ill or bizarre the patient appeared, there were still healthy parts to his or her personality; therefore treatment should include ways for the patient to develop self-esteem.

The institution to which the mentally ill were sent became their community. At a time when cultural and social systems were homogeneous and communication and transportation methods were limited, the establishment of a fairly uniform institutional community was quite possible. Patients were committed to institutional care for long periods of time and in some instances for life. Moral treatment sought to develop in the institutional community a sense of family living. The milieu was one of daily routines, with chores and responsibilities shared by staff and patients for the good of all. Staff members provided role models for the patients. When staff members and patients both came from the same kinds of cultural and ethnic backgrounds, as they often did during this period, such a milieu could be quite successful.

Because the work ethic was dominant in society, work prevailed as a major means for the individual to experience satisfaction and purpose in life. "The patient is now one of our best workers, and in other respects improves much . . . I had the most rational conversation with him that I had ever had . . . It was truly pleasing to discover such rationality."[2] So wrote Isaac Bonsall, who, in 1817, became the first superintendent of the Friends Asylum in Frankford, located in Philadelphia. Bonsall was describing the effect of occupation on a severely disturbed patient.

THE BEGINNING OF THE PROFESSION OF OCCUPATIONAL THERAPY

Occupational therapy developed into an identified profession during the years after World War I (see Chapter 1). At that time Doctor Adolf Meyer and Eleanor Clarke Slagle developed the use of carefully planned goals and methods for promoting health through the use of activities. It was in the 1920s that Meyer restated the principles of moral treatment and gave a context and philosophy for the development of the profession of occupational therapy.[3] At the same time Slagle began training occupational "therapeutists." She divided their rehabilitation efforts into three distinct groups: those directed towards patients who in all likelihood would continue their lives within the institution, those directed towards return to the community, and those directed towards prevention through the use of a pre-hospital work clinic. The approaches of Meyer and Slagle to the use of activities and relationships, examined in the light of today's knowledge and practice, were remarkably modern—they emphasized developmental needs and had a sense of the importance of preparing the individual patient for functioning within society.[4]

In the 1920s, behaviorism dominated psychology while psychoanalytical theory dominated psychiatry. The pioneers in occupational therapy, however, focused on the patient's outer reality and functional behavior. In the institutional setting, the patient was involved in work assignments. These assignments seemed effective in promoting adjustment.

William Rush Dunton, Jr., the psychiatrist whose commitment and belief in the principles of occupational therapy were at the cornerstone of the profession, wrote several books and articles on the subject. In *Prescribing Occupational Therapy* published in 1928 he systematically categorized activities and kinds of patients. He thoughtfully delineated principles for matching activities with the needs of patients in a way which could be therapeutic. He classified activities in terms of their demands for attention, repetition, physical or intellectual effort, social factors, and criteria for rest, surprise or creativity. He simplified the categories of mental disorders and suggested the kinds of activities that could be most desirable and most therapeutic with each category. He also described the importance of the therapist's approach and attitude for each:

> For the manic—steady, quieting activity to reduce motor restlessness and train concentration; sedative activity, rhythmic and repetitive, with little variety.
>
> For the depressed—stimulating activity, although initially the therapist may need to give a preliminary course of stereotyped activity. The activity should have the potential for replacing the patient's preoccupations with depressive ideation. The therapist must use tact and be sensitive.
>
> For the demented (dementia praecox or schizophrenia)—reeducation activities to train better habits of thought and action. Social activities which would place the individual into simple, structured work with others—activities which demand constant attention to overcome daydreaming, and activities to emphasize reality contact.

> For the paranoid—activities which would create or stimulate interest in concrete things—such as caring for goldfish or canaries, working in hospital industries.
>
> For the psychoneurotic—activities to reduce egocentricity and to allow for the sublimation of repressed conflicts.[5]

In Dunton's work we see a major attempt to analyze activities, to categorize patient needs, and to suggest therapist approaches. He considered the core of the occupational therapy process to be making the correct matches among these elements.

Other proponents of the clear, deliberate application of activities to meet specific patient needs were Louis J. Haas and L. Cody Marsh. Haas' publications, *Practical Occupational Therapy* and *Occupational Therapy for the Mentally and Nervously Ill*, contain interesting, detailed descriptions of crafts projects in addition to theoretical formulations about the use of crafts.[6,7] Haas stated emphatically that "being busy is not necessarily therapeutic."

Marsh, in a speech at the Sixteenth Annual Conference of the American Occupational Therapy Association, defined the uses of carefully matched work assignments as therapy.[8]

1930s AND 1940s—OCCUPATIONAL THERAPISTS AS AIDES TO THE PSYCHIATRIST

In the 1930s and 1940s psychiatric occupational therapists clearly identified themselves as aides to the psychiatrist in providing treatment for the mentally ill. The occupational therapist's activities included music, psychodrama, bibliotherapy, recreation, work, and arts and crafts. In effect, occupational therapy was concerned with the whole person and his or her total life of work and play within the institutional setting.

At the same time that occupational therapy developed as a profession there began a search for theoretical concepts which would provide frames of reference for treatment. Therapists began to be dissatisfied with basing their practice purely on intuitive and empirical success. Occupational therapists saw their roles as closely aligned with the psychiatrist responsible for patients. The situation in which they worked involved a written prescription from the psychiatrist or physician before the occupational therapist could initiate treatment. The prescription gave basic information about the patient, including special precautions, and requested that the occupational therapist provide specified services. The occupational therapist's areas of service to the psychiatrist included (1) diagnostic aid (through the observation of the patient's behavior and performance in occupational therapy), (2) facilitating the patient's adjustment to the hospital environment, (3) supplementing shock therapy, (4) supplementing psychoanalytical therapy, and (5) habit training.[9]

Psychoanalytical Bases and Some Research

The theoretical base for occupational therapy as a true intervention and treatment modality within a psychoanalytical frame of reference was specified by William C. Menninger. His six categories of the functions of activities as treatment are as follows: (1) as an outlet for aggression and hostility, (2) to provide opportunities for advantageous identifications, (3) as atonement for guilt, (4) as a means of obtaining love, (5) to provide opportunities to act out fantasies, and (6) to allow for an experience of creative work.[10] The occupational therapist working within this context needed to have basic knowledge of the principles of psychoanalytical psychiatry and especially of defense mechanisms, as well as a sensitivity to the potentials of given activities for fulfilling the functions described above.

Although intuition, common sense, and empirical success provided the only guidelines in the selection of activities, it is evident from the literature of the time that there were tendencies to seek a more scientific base and to define occupational therapy professionally.

Electric and insulin shock therapies were being employed. These presented special challenges to the occupational therapist. The psychiatric casualties of World War II provided impetus for the development of programs under the Veterans Administration. One is struck by the number of articles written by physicians in collaboration with occupational therapists during this period.

Training Programs for Aides

Obviously, for the number of patients hospitalized, there were never enough trained therapists, especially as training programs grew longer and more academic. The professional occupational therapist, in many instances, became a program planner and a supervisor of aides, particularly in the large hospitals. It became a major concern of professional therapists to find ways to transmit theoretical knowledge to untrained staff members and to facilitate the communication of treatment goals and methods. In the large hospitals, psychiatrically trained physicians were also in short supply. Although the psychiatrist's written prescription could serve an important purpose, effective communication of this kind often was more an ideal than a reality.

1950s—ON THE THRESHOLD OF RADICAL CHANGES

At the beginning of the 1950s, in addition to shock therapies, psychosurgery in the form of the prefrontal lobotomy was added to the list of medical attempts to cure the mentally ill, or, at least to provide symptomatic relief. Occupational therapists had to find ways to work effectively with the lobotomized patient. It was often discouraging. Psychosurgery, although initially considered promising, was to be a short-lived form of treatment.

Psychodynamic principles for treatment and activity analysis were explored in greater depth in the 1950s. The occupational therapist began to look at the patient's behavior and symptoms in terms of "externalized or internalized aggression, projection, withdrawal and regression."[11] Gail Fidler, in an article in the American Journal of Occupational Therapy in 1948, presented an outline of activity analysis through which the materials, tools, actions, and interpersonal relationship potentials of activities could be explored.[12] Professional occupational therapists attempted to match activities with patient needs based on this kind of thinking.

TIME: 1949

PLACE: An Occupational Therapy Shop in a private psychiatric hospital.

The occupational therapist enters her office, a screened off area in the back of the bright, pleasantly decorated large room known as the "O.T. Shop." (A sign, carefully painted in old English script hangs outside the door to designate this fact.) She stops for a moment to smooth her starched white uniform and notes that she will soon have to have her hair cut or fasten it up. On her desk lies a copy of *Discovering Ourselves* by Strecker and Appel,[13] an old book, but one which she finds stimulating and helpful not only in understanding her patients but also in understanding herself.

Her patients have just left and the day is about over. There were ten in this last group, men from the locked ward. An attendant brought them down to her shop and stayed with them for the hour they were there. She thinks, with satisfaction, how much better it is in this bright new area, compared with the dingy basement shop next to the boiler room. It was more than the change that felt good—it was the idea that the hospital superintendent really seemed to appreciate and support occupational therapy. Until the shop was moved two months before she had needed to take supplies to the men on the ward. It seems so much better to get them out of that atmosphere. Here, she could give them so many more things. There are floor looms, where patients can beat out their hostility on rugs. And there is a bicycle jigsaw and a workbench. Good masculine activities. And, of course, the radio, so they could have music. The only drawback is that the men can come only when they're on good behavior. That's a problem she's been thinking a lot abouf. She was planning to get together with the ward personnel to see if there would be some way to put a punching bag up, or something, right on the ward, for the men to use whenever they began to feel upset.

Now, however, her mind was focused on one patient. He was new in the hospital and she had already received a written prescription for occupational therapy from his doctor. She thumbed through a pile of cards on her desk until she found his prescription. The card read:

NAME: John Jones AGE: 31 DIAGNOSIS: Schizophrenia, paranoid type
O.T. PRESCRIPTION: Activities to divert attention from hallucinations, improve reality testing and attention span, increase socialization.
PRECAUTIONS Patient has auditory hallucinations. May become assaultive. Currently being treated with insulin coma therapy. Observe for insulin reactions.
PHYSICIAN: M. Brown, M.D.
WARD: 5B

John Jones had come to O.T. that day. He seemed mild-mannered and polite but a little vague in his thinking, probably because he'd had an insulin treatment earlier. That was the problem with the patients who were getting insulin or electric shock therapy. They sometimes seemed to forget everything or be really out of touch. John Jones had picked copper tooling to do. This had seemed a good choice to the occupational therapist because it would require some planning and attention; its actions involved hard pressure but also controlling, and it was masculine. He already was planning to use it as a gift. He had chosen a picture of two sheep, with a little lamb standing between them. When he started to work on it, he seemed able to follow the directions all right. He said that the little lamb reminded him of himself, in between his mother and his wife. The occupational therapist jots down a little note to mention that to his doctor. She also decides to set aside time to read John Jones' chart before he comes to the shop tomorrow.

The occupational therapist then opens a cabinet and takes down rolls of brightly colored crepe paper, some construction paper, paste, and a box of blunt-pointed scissors. She places these items on a cart, ready to take to the women's locked ward first thing in the morning. They would need an early start to make the decorations for the party that evening.

One more thing, before she could call it a day. She picks up the telephone and calls the lady in charge of the hospital auxiliary. She needs to check out a few more details about the O.T. sale next week.

"Sometimes," she thinks, "I really do feel like a jack-of-all-trades but I like what I'm doing and I feel sure that the activities I give my patients help them. They know I'm interested in them and accept them as human beings." She remembers, in a flash, having seen the movie *The Snake Pit* the week before. "Thank goodness it doesn't have to be like that anymore," she thinks as she locks up the cabinets and desk, puts on her coat, and leaves.

Psychopharmacology—New Possibilities

The mid-1950s saw a major revolution take place in mental hospitals. The introduction of psychopharmacology, the use of tranquilizers and psychic energizers, opened a new world of possibilities. The medicines seemed to reduce most of the gross pathological symptoms and acting out behaviors which previously had interfered with treatment. Social psychiatry and anthropology explored new vistas for handling the problem of mental illness. Maxwell Jones' "therapeutic community" in England received attention.[14] The therapeutic milieu, open-door policies, halfway house, family treatment, aftercare services, and volunteer involvement all became possibilities.

Two major events took place in psychiatric occupational therapy at this time. One was a book; the other was a study which culminated in a book.

In 1954, the book, *Introduction to Psychiatric Occupational Therapy* was written and published by Gail S. Fidler, OTR and Jay W. Fidler, M.D. This book represented professional occupational therapy as the use of productive activities as treatment in a collaborative effort between the occupational therapist and the psychotherapist. It suggested the concept of the occupational therapy area as a laboratory in which the patient could experiment with new ways of handling emotions and developing living skills. It presented a much refined, psychoanalytically-flavored activity analysis process, suggested ways in which groups could be used to facilitate treatment, and encouraged the study of projective techniques. While acknowledging that many occupational therapists were working without psychiatric supervision to the extent described, it encouraged occupational therapists to formulate treatment goals and programs in the most meaningful way on their own and to work toward effective communications with all involved staff. The Fidlers candidly stated, "These views cannot be presented without the realization that occupational therapy is a young field and that there are great potentialities for future development. This is especially emphasized by the fact that the entire field of psychiatry is still in its youth and therefore any of the subsidiary techniques must also be as elementary if not more so."[15]

In 1956, following a two-year study funded by a grant to the American Occupational Therapy Association by the National Institute of Mental Health, a conference of leaders in the field of psychiatric occupational therapy was held at Boiling Springs, Pennsylvania. Under the leadership of Elizabeth P. Ridgway and Gail S. Fidler, the participants explored and questioned many emerging issues of psychiatric occupational therapy practice. These were identified as *use of self, use of group and group techniques, use of activities, creation of the therapeutic milieu, development of special treatment goals as a supplement to psychotherapy,* contributions to psychodynamic formulations through the *use of personality, social, and skills evaluations* and, finally, *bridging the gap between community living and the hospital.*[16] In her introduction to the published proceedings of the conference, Wilma West said, "Several developments and changes in the treatment of psychiatric patients during recent years made this project a timely one. These include an awareness of the reversibility of the process of mental illness, the growth of the team approach and resulting collaboration of all concerned, utilization of group interaction and an increasing emphasis on the total individual and the milieu in which he functions."[17] This is a fair assessment of the state of psychiatric occupational therapy at that time.

TIME: 1957

PLACE: O.T. Shop in a large, progressive state institution.

Barbara and Jack, registered occupational therapists, are seated at the end of a long table near a window in the large, somewhat cluttered O.T. room. They've just come back from lunch and are working together warping a table loom. Two copies of the American Journal of Occupational Therapy lie on the windowsill.

Barbara comments to Jack, "Did you see the article in the September Journal about the study they made—the one that proved that if the occupational therapist is able to work on developing relationships with the patients, the patients become more active?"[18]

Jack replies, "Nope. But it makes sense, doesn't it? I know that sometimes it looks as if I'm goofing off when I just sit and talk with the guys from Ward B but they really do seem to want to come to O.T. and I think I get further with them . . . you know . . . it's like they trust me more."

"Yes," Barbara says, and adds, "By the way, has Dr. Brown started having team meetings for Ward B? He said he wanted to because soon they want to make it an open ward. He wants to start having ward meetings for all the patients too. He really wants to make sure that everybody's involved in the changes."

Jack recalls, "They're supposed to start next week, at eight o'clock Wednesday morning. That's the time when most of the nurses and attendants are around. I wonder how it will work. Incidentally, since you mentioned the Journal, I did look at that article about changes in O.T. due to tranquilizing drugs.[19] Did you see it? I guess because I'm a recently graduated O.T. I'm not so aware of the differences the new drugs are making. I know the things they told us about in school, the kinds of crazy actions we heard about. Well, I just haven't seen them, at least not many of them. What worries me, though, is that half the time I feel as if I'm working with zombies. The article says that a lot of your time and energy used to go into finding ways to channel excess drives, controlling hyperactivity, and so forth. Is that true? I almost think that would make O.T. more interesting!"

Replying to Jack's comments, Barbara says, "Oh, I don't know about that. It got pretty wild sometimes. Now, in some ways it seems easier, but in other ways it seems harder—like working through a mask. And we've got a whole new set of things to watch for, and report. By the way, has Dick complained to you about his eyesight? He was trying to draw the squares on that chessboard he's making and he was having an awful time. Said everything was going blurry on him. Better check it out. Uh-oh, it's one o'clock and the crowd is about to arrive."

They fasten down the pieces of warp with tape, open the supply cabinets, and unlock the O.T. room doors. Jack says, "See you," and retreats through a back door which leads to the men's shop.

A group of twenty women, in hospital dresses, presses through the door. Two nursing aides accompany the group. As if preprogrammed, they go to the supply cabinets, take out boxes neatly labeled with their names, and seat themselves around the table. Some begin to work on embroidery and some on knitting; one goes to an upright loom on which a braided rug has been started. Two of the women, apparently new, stand still until the aides talk them into taking seats at the table. Barbara sits down near them and suggests to them that they draw some pictures. She gives them crayons and construction paper. Barbara is uncomfortable. She has been reading, for the second time, the book, *Introduction to Psychiatric Occupational Therapy*.[20] The scene before her seems so very far removed from the exciting ideas about what O.T. could be. She begins to think about things they could do, especially if the hospital really goes into teams.

She moves about the group of patients, offering help to some, encouraging others, stopping to listen while one complains about a problem in the dining room, occasionally chatting with the whole group about some current event and trying to interest the group in planning an afternoon party to which they would invite their doctors, visitors, or any special friends. The atmosphere is quiet and subdued. It is hard to feel enthusiasm. On another level, Barbara's mind is racing ahead. She's devising a form—one which would list the kinds of information we get about patients when they do activities—the way they use the materials and the way they relate to the O.T. and to each other. And she's planning a new method for reporting to the doctors and nurses. And, remembering that the hospital has just hired a volunteer director, she's thinking about ways volunteers can help them in new kinds of activities. She'll have to talk to Jack about all this.

Government Action Spurs Community Mental Health

The Mental Health Study Act was passed in 1955, establishing the Joint Commission on Mental Illness and Health. The charge of the Commission was to establish priorities and viable methods of services for the mentally ill. *Action for Mental Health*, the report of the commission, was published in 1961.[21] This report proposed a concerted attack on mental illness in the following ways: (1) better distribution and community-oriented philosophical reorientation of psychiatrists; (2) increasing participation of lay people at various levels in programs of prevention, treatment, and rehabilitation; (3) shift of emphasis from institutional to community services; (4) plans for shared federal, state, and local funding of community mental health centers. Thus was launched the community mental health movement.

In 1963, the Community Mental Health Act was passed, mandating the National Institute of Mental Health to establish and fund community mental health centers in local "catchment" areas with populations from 75,000 to 200,000. This gave impetus to the development of new approaches to treatment. Transactional analysis, gestalt therapy, and milieu therapy came to the fore. Family therapy became a treatment of choice for some individuals, with the interesting premise that the mentally ill person in a family may simply be expressing the symptoms for a whole family's pathology.[22] Behavioral approaches to treatment such as desensitization and operant conditioning techniques, developed by Joseph Wolpe and others, grew rapidly.[23] "Token economies" or behaviorally-oriented milieus were developed and seemed promising, particularly in treating the long-term chronically disabled and institutionalized mentally ill, the mentally retarded, and some kinds of childhood psychoses.

Research efforts were intensified in the areas of biochemistry, neurophysiology, metabolic, enzyme, and genetic abnormalities. Psychosomatic illnesses were explored in greater depth. The wholeness of human function and the connections between mind, body, and emotions were proven repeatedly. Each new research finding, it seemed, pointed to new questions and new areas for exploration. Research efforts and techniques were aided by the enormous capabilities introduced by the growth of computer technology.

There was a shift away from emphasis on the long-term, deep methods of treatment by psychoanalysis, and a concerted effort was turned to explore ways in which individuals could be returned to function as rapidly as possible. Partial hospitalization programs opened so that patients could continue to live their lives in the community and attend treatment programs during the day or evening. Mental health professionals, including occupational therapists, began to visit the homes of their patients, and to look into important aspects of work and recreation in the community. Patients, in some settings, began to be called clients, residents, or members. The atmosphere of psychiatry had taken on a new and optimistic perspective.

1960s—SOME CREATIVE CHAOS

The worlds in which psychiatric occupational therapists worked were greatly expanded by these changes. The spirit of experimentation, of questioning, and of unrest which characterized society as a whole during the 1960s permeated occupational therapy as well. Knowledge grew and new techniques were developed for the management of the mentally ill.

The Fidlers published a second book in 1963, *Occupational Therapy: A Communication Process in Psychiatry*.[24] They emphasized the enormous potential of the occupational therapy process as another vital language for communication, especially in view of its use of the nonverbal and its work regarding object relationships. They identified three major emphases for occupational therapy in psychiatry: (1) *treatment*, directly applied intervention in a pathological process to effect change in the patient, with subcategories defined as *psychoanalytic*, *supportive*, and *directive* (repressive); (2) the *mental health process*, by enhancing the milieu and supporting the healthy parts of the individual; and (3) *rehabilitation*, helping the patient to learn to use existing strengths more effectively. This book provided carefully analyzed and synthesized material, especially regarding the meaning of activities and interpersonal transactions in the activity process. Though strongest in its psychoanalytical orientation, it acknowledged as well the changes which were taking place both in psychiatry as a whole and in psychiatric occupational therapy.

The early 1960s were also influenced by the development of instruments for evaluation or assessment of the client. This was a period when there was significant interest in the use of the *Azima Battery*.[25] Gail Fidler also developed a battery, similar to the Azima Battery, through which information about a client's psychodynamics could be obtained.[26] These two batteries, and a number of local modifications of them, used art media and clay. The client's behavior and his or her projections were interpreted to provide meaningful data to aid in treatment planning.

Cognitive-Perceptual-Motor Research

Another very significant development was taking place during the 1960s. A. Jean Ayres was beginning to publish her observations of perceptual motor development and dysfunction in children. Her research, which is still going on, was based on neurophysiology, and seemed to point to some areas of major concern to the occupational therapist working in psychiatry. Lorna Jean King, in Arizona, began a daring experiment with chronic schizophrenics and exhaustive research in the literature on perception, neurophysiology, and mental illness. She adapted and applied the theoretical base and some of the techniques developed by Ayres. The results of her work with severely regressed, institutionalized, chronically ill schizophrenic patients were most encouraging. By the end of the 1960s, it appeared that continued research and application of *sensory motor integrative* techniques for certain groups of patients was indeed indicated and contained heuristic value in terms of other, related psychiatric concerns.

Developmental Theory

In psychological and educational circles during this time there was a growth of interest in the work of Piaget. Developmental theory and especially theories of cognitive development were being explored generally. Psychiatric occupational therapists began to explore the significance of Piaget's work as it might relate to the occupational therapy process in psychiatry.

Activities Therapists

It should be noted that, with the increased attention to direct services for the mentally ill, there were not enough trained occupational therapists to fill the critically needed positions in both institutions and community. New activity specialties grew up: therapeutic recreation, art, music, dance, drama, and horticulture. These specialties grew from at least two roots: (1) independently and in a parallel stream of thought with occupational therapy, based on existing knowledge in education and psychology; (2) as an outgrowth of the training of workers in occupational therapy in the two decades preceding. Each new discipline using activities has sought to develop its own professional identity, its own special areas of practice, and its own research base. Taking as its foundation the same base as occupational therapy, that activity can be used for evaluation and for treatment, the new activity specialties presented a challenge to occupational therapy to refine its own theory and practice and to work toward developing viable ways of communicating and cooperating with them.

American Occupational Therapy Association Funded for Consultant

Under the Social Rehabilitation Services Grant (#123) the American Occupational Therapy Association was funded in 1964 to have a fulltime consultant in psychiatric rehabilitation in the National Office. Through the efforts of this consultant, and with the backing of the American Occupational Therapy Association, a number of regional and national institutes were held across the United States. The main foci of these workshops, which were held between 1964 and 1968, were supervision, group process, object relations, and education. In addition to the effects of deepening the knowledge base and strengthening the skills of practicing therapists, there was a concomitant development of a sense of community among them, as they shared together in the search for greater professional effectiveness.

The project director for this particular grant was June Mazer. Actually, the project RSA#123 had been started in 1958 as a consultancy program in physical dysfunction; at that time Irene Hollis was director. Mary Alice Coombs joined the project in 1961 and it became a joint physical-psychiatric consultancy. In December, 1962, the physical dysfunction phase was concluded. The psychiatric phase continued until 1968. Fourteen regional institutes were held on group process, administration, object relations, and evaluation and twenty-one national institutes were held on education and advanced object relations.

Search for a Comprehensive Theory

The Psychiatric Special Interest Group of the Council on Practice of the American Occupational Therapy Association became especially active on a nationwide basis during the 1960s. There was a surge of interest in exploring ways to incorporate the expanding approaches and the everwidening knowledge base into occupational therapy practice. Local special interest groups flourished in many areas. These groups became forums in which practicing therapists studied together, shared their questions and their ideas, and supported each other as they faced the critical issues which were emerging in psychiatry as a whole. The Psychiatric Special Interest Group, on a national level, participated in a number of special projects.

In 1968 the American Journal of Occupational Therapy invited occupational therapists practicing in psychiatry to submit papers describing the application of concepts to practice. The resulting issue of the American Journal of Occupational Therapy might be considered a landmark as the authors attempted to define theoretical frames of reference and to describe viable approaches to their use. The words of the introduction to the special section describe the situation of occupational therapy in psychiatry at that time: "It is evident that many therapists are involved in the struggle to formulate and/or apply various theories in their practices, even though none of the submitted papers proposed a truly comprehensive theory of occupational therapy. Each article is accompanied by critical discussions and an author's response. We hope that these will stimulate further critical thinking and discussion. Our dream is that this special section may herald the beginning of a period rich in clinical exploration and research."[28] The four articles and the conference report included in this issue focused attention on the difficulties of developing such a comprehensive theory. The authors identified the work still to be done by describing both their thought and their practice.[29,30,31,32,33]

Following the institutes on object relations in 1967, a small group of therapists met in Albion, Michigan, to attempt to relate "a large number of divergent theories and thoughts to a specific framework which would include all aspects of the organism."[34] The object relations institutes and their culminating seminar attempted to explore in some depth the existing knowledge bases in anthropology, sociology, psychology, neurophysiology, and philosophy as well as in psychiatry. There seemed to be little doubt that all of these could be significant in contributing to the knowledge base of occupational therapy. This was a most ambitious task and the problem seemed to be one of providing bridges between all the possibilities. The charge was stated, "A necessary step toward building a body of knowledge specifically related to the kind of experience occupational therapy is able to provide is a frame of reference which utilizes a truly holistic developmental approach."[35]

The climate of optimism, enthusiasm, and investigation characterizing psychiatric occupational therapy at this time was reflected in a number of articles which were published during 1969 and 1970. Mary Reilly and her colleagues and students at the University of Southern California began to make their contributions to the field through the study of the work-play continuum, the patient's real world, and concepts of competence as the keys to the theoretical base of psychiatric occupational therapy.

The "occupational behavior" frame of reference for occupational therapy in psychiatry, as explored and proposed by Reilly, has taken the earliest principles and approaches of occupational therapy as practiced in "moral treatment" and expressed in 1922 by Adolf Meyer and examined them in depth and in the light of current psychological and sociological literature. This group proposed that occupational therapy shift its "initial perspective of patients from diagnostic labels to those of occupational roles of worker, student, housewife, retiree, preschooler and even career patient. . . ."[36] Occupational therapists were urged to look into the influences of the experiences found in childhood play.

In 1970 a symposium, "The Skill Continuum from Play through Work," was conducted in Boston under the sponsorship of the United States Department of Health, Education and Welfare (HEW), Maternal and Child Health Service. The papers presented at this symposium were published in the American Journal of Occupational Therapy in September 1971.[37,38,39,40,41,42,43,44] The important message of this orientation was expressed by Matsutsuyu: "It was found that the perspective based on pathology held few guidelines for working knowledge of healthy function. It is not enough to accept the definition of health as the absence of disease."[45] The framework for this thinking had been expressed earlier by Reilly when she said: "Play, in a chronological or longitudinal sense, we believe, is the antecedent preparation area for work. In a cross-sectional sense, we have found it clinically useful to see an adult social-recreation pattern of behavior as a sublatent support to a work pattern. The entire developmental continuum of play and work we designate as occupational behavior."[46]

TIME: 1969

PLACE: The O.T. office in a day program in a mental hospital of medium size.

Alice W., the occupational therapist, sits at her desk, writing a note. She has just finished working with a group which is planning an issue of the program's newspaper. The clients in the group are Don, a middle-aged man who is just recovering from a depression; Marie, an obese young woman whose obsessive-compulsive tendencies have interfered with her ability to work at her job; and Jim, a nineteen-year-old man who is suffering from an anxiety neurosis.

"How can I express what seemed to be happening when Jim and Don and Marie were starting to plan the next issue of the newspaper?" she thinks, her pen poised above the paper. "It was as if Don and Marie were Jim's mother and father, and he was their little child. And Jim seemed to fit right into that role. Maybe it's because Don and Marie really have had a lot more experience with the paper. On the other hand, we have seen so much of Jim's dependency in just about every aspect of his life. We've seen it in our evaluations too. This is probably just another expression of that. Putting the paper out could be a good way to help him to grow, because he certainly has the basic skills. I'll talk with Don and Marie about letting Jim do the typing first . . . then maybe they'll show him how to do the paste-up, if he's interested."

At this point, there's a knock on the door, and a pleasant-faced woman, the unit's social worker, pokes her head in and says, "They're going to run the videotape of the activity group again, so the group can watch. Maybe you'd better be there for the feedback session."

Alice gets up and goes to the door saying, "You bet. I want to have another look at the way Jim handled the situation. I have a feeling he may want to talk about it. By the way did you want to borrow my Arieti?[47] And sometime could you let me look at your *Freedom to Learn*?"[48]

1970s—SOME REFLECTIONS, THEN A SHIFT OF GEARS: ACCOUNTABILITY

In American society the early 1970s were a time of some disenchantment. Out of the chaotic and creative flux of the late 1960s there emerged a public tiredness. The Vietnam War dragged on, draining off money and manpower that more and more Americans began to feel could be better used. Government spending priorities moved further away from the social and health concerns of the 1960s. The economy seemed doomed to increasing inflation as a worldwide problem. Watergate set off widespread questions about trust and accountability, which had ramifications beyond the political arena, touching business, education, and health care delivery systems. It became increasingly important for all health professionals to justify their services. This meant clearly defining their goals and methods and the populations to be served. Reporting systems needed refinement to be consistent with professional aims and relevant to patients' needs.

Occupational therapy was forced during the late 1960s and early 1970s to look carefully at its uses of work as therapy. For many years, in some of the large public institutions, patients had been assigned to work in the laundry, maintenance shops, farm, and a variety of other areas. Frequently in these assignments patients were able to experience the success of developing real proficiency at given tasks and a sense of being a contributing, productive member of the institutional community. Unfortunately the very positive personal effects which these work assignments had on some patients, also, within the institutional setting, tended to reinforce their need to stay in the hospital. There was not enough attention given the total milieu of the institution and not enough effort put into helping the patients generalize their skills so they could use them in the world outside the institution. From the standpoint of the public it appeared that patient labor was being seriously exploited.

The question of institutional peonage was brought into the courts. (The case, Nelson Eugene Souder vs. Peter J. Brennan, Civil Action 482-73, resulted in a law in April 1974 requiring that patients be paid the statutory minimum wage for performing work within the institutional setting. The date when vigorous enforcement was to proceed was set as December 1, 1974.) Therefore the assignment of patients to work without pay in situations which benefited the institution became illegal. The act resulting from the above-mentioned court action required that institutions provide pay for patients' work. Few institutions could afford either this or the necessary staff and paperwork to justify work as therapy. There were some patients, the seriously institutionalized and chronic, who lost in the process their one successful, however rote, activity. And so, a concomitant, and possibly resultant, movement took place to develop more community, business, and industrial contacts so that patients could be given work assignments in the real world with real remuneration. Occupational therapists needed to examine this concept.

Peer Professionals

At the beginning of the 1970s the psychiatric occupational therapist was plunged into a new and challenging set of perspectives. In many ways the occupational therapist was beginning to accept and identify with a peer professional role along with physicians, social workers, psychologists, and nurses. The search for a unifying theory of occupational therapy had disclosed in sharp relief the unique contributions that could be made by the therapist. The occupational therapist as an "aid to the physician" gave way to the occupational therapist as a co-professional cooperating with a number of other disciplines in the treatment of the mentally ill in at least some of the newer and less traditional settings. The contexts for treatment and the constitution of the treatment teams were considerably extended. By 1970 occupational therapists were working in schools, community programs, and homes in addition to the traditional settings. In some of the more traditional settings, nontraditional staffing patterns and new approaches were being explored.

As popular trends in psychiatry gained momentum and prominence, many occupational therapists working in psychiatry saw the value of learning and gaining skills in their use. Transactional analysis, gestalt therapy, meditation, bioenergetics, assertiveness and effectiveness training, and a variety of humanistic and self-actualization group techniques are just a few of the movements which were beginning to offer new avenues to the development of healthier, more productive and satisfying lives in the general (normal to mildly neurotic) population. Some occupational therapists, as well as psychologists, social workers, and others, saw in these techniques opportunities for enhancing the treatment of their clients. With varying degrees of effectiveness, they incorporated them into existing treatment techniques. This happened most readily and most often in those settings where the occupational therapist's role was blended with the roles of other members of the treatment team.

In 1971 Geraldine Finn presented the Eleanor Clarke Slagle Lecture at the Annual Conference of the American Occupational Therapy Association in Cleveland. Her lecture discussed the societal and technological changes which had taken place during the preceding decades and examined the efforts which had been made at Boston State Hospital to shift occupational therapy services to a prevention model. She identified nine major issues which were part of that process:

1. the function of primary institutions in maintaining the health of the people of a community and the need for occupational therapists to understand the functions, goals and policies of these primary institutions
2. the planning of appropriate programs and services based on man's need to engage in interaction with the objects of his environment in order to maintain his health throughout his life

3. the need to reinterpret the body of knowledge available within the profession of occupational therapy in order to apply it in the service of keeping people healthy rather than in helping people minimize their disabilities
4. the creation of new associations of our available knowledge in order to respond more accurately to the pressing reality needs of today
5. the establishment of an organizational model which will allow translation of abstract plans about activities, human action and the delivery of health services into concrete actions
6. the presence of risk taking and its ramifications on one's ability to function and persevere when faced with an unfamiliar environment
7. the necessity of reexamining communication patterns to ensure real communications among people
8. the need to create a climate of acceptance for a planned program and the development of the skills needed to assist others in seeing the value of these programs
9. the role of supervision in maintaining the performance and professional growth of the staff members.[49]*

The kinds of programs described by Finn included

> early intervention programs for children, consultation services to teachers, inservice programs on developmental screening, and program planning, outreach programs for the elderly, workshops for mothers and preschool children, inservice programs on perceptual-motor development for mental health workers, development of new models of parent education and counseling and the introduction of knowledge about developmental levels of human performance in a community drug program.[50]

The work of Anne C. Mosey, Lela Llorens, and others gave further impetus to occupational therapists in several parts of the country to study and articulate the principles of human development as a basic frame of reference for psychiatric occupational therapy. This approach led to further interest in perceptual and cognitive functioning and the concepts of stress and regression.

The 1970s have also seen the resurgence of interest and attention to the significance of societal attitudes, values, and varying life styles. Community-based programs, partial hospitalization, and home treatment programs have made it essential for occupational therapists to consider the impact of these social changes as well as the impact of their own personal value systems on all aspects of treatment.

Social Change and Definition of Frames of Reference

A new chaos and creative flux developed in society as a whole during the 1970s. The Civil Rights Movement begun in the 1950s extended into concerns which profoundly affect health care professionals. It aroused consciousness and analysis of inequities suffered by many segments of the population. The Women's Movement mobilized many people to think and act to change some of society's most fundamental attitudes and practices. The elderly and the handicapped organized to demand long overdue rights, opportunities, and concern. Homosexuality is no longer considered an illness and people with varying sexual orientations have "come out of the closet." Other taboos have been lifted. Death and dying, as part of the continuum of living, are being talked about and studied. The patient's right to treatment has become a major concern. The nation is experiencing what Alvin Toffler called future shock[51]; we are bombarded with facts, new orientations, and the rapid fabrication and just as rapid decline of materials, ideas, and fads. All of this has enormous significance to occupational therapy, a profession with a commitment to help others to "do for themselves."

In some areas, psychiatric occupational therapists began to experiment and work with behavioral approaches to treatment. Usually working within a team and in a setting where *behavior therapy* was being used, therapists developed methods of treatment based upon schedules of reinforcement, operant conditioning, modeling, shaping, and chaining procedures. For some patients, these techniques

* Reprinted with permission of the American Journal of Occupational Therapy.

proved useful in changing or extinguishing undesirable behavior patterns and in establishing and reinforcing healthy behavior patterns.

At the same time, neurophysiological knowledge and neurophysiological approaches to treatment have been continuing to gain momentum; they promise to make a very significant impact on psychiatric practice. Refinement and development of the work of Ayres and King have continued. There has been increased attention to the effects of the functions of the reticular activating system. In 1975 Josephine Moore, in her Eleanor Clarke Slagle Lecture at the Annual Conference of the American Occupational Therapy Association in Milwaukee, "Behavior, Bias and the Limbic System," spoke eloquently of the need for greater consideration of the influence of basic neurophysiological mechanisms in determining human feelings and actions.[52]

The search for clean conceptual models, clear frames of reference, and a unifying theory of occupational therapy has continued to be a preoccupation of the profession as a whole during the 1970s.

In her book, *Three Frames of Reference for Mental Health*, published in 1970,[53] Mosey discussed three different conceptual approaches to psychiatric occupational therapy: (1) psychoanalytic, (2) acquisitional, and (3) developmental. She suggested that each of these three frames of reference define specific aspects of the occupational therapy process. According to Mosey, each frame of reference has postulates regarding the nature of the individual, the characteristics of health and illness, and viable approaches to evaluation and treatment. Clarity with regard to the frame of reference used in treatment is seen as highly desirable. It permits the therapist to tap into and utilize a specific body of knowledge. It encourages consistency among expectations, goal-setting, and approaches to evaluation and treatment.

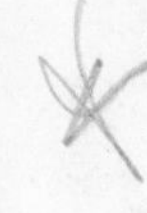

In current practice it seems that the three frames of reference that Mosey identified are indeed viable. For the purposes of this chapter, we shall equate the acquisitional with the behavioral frame of reference. Added to these three frames of reference, there are two others which fulfill the criteria for designation as frames of reference in their own right: the *sensory integrative* and the *occupational behavior* frames of reference.

Mental Health Task Force Makes Recommendations

In 1975 a special task force comprised of psychiatric occupational therapists was appointed by the American Occupational Therapy Association. Their charge was to identify issues of concern in the practice of occupational therapy in mental health and to recommend solutions to identified problems. They surveyed practice in psychiatric occupational therapy and, based on their assessment of the status of occupational therapy in psychiatry, made their recommendations. The recommendations were published in the American Occupational Therapy Association newspaper in September 1976. The task force reported that "mental health practice lacks standardized clinical techniques and therefore is dependent on a conceptualization of the fundamental value of performance which has never been clearly articulated."[54] The task force went on to make recommendations geared to refining the knowledge base and strengthening the technology of occupational therapy practice. Specific recommendations were made regarding research, graduate education, continuing education, and the definition of occupational therapy practice in psychiatry. Although the work of this task force was addressed to psychiatric occupational therapy practice, it had serious implications for the profession as a whole. The recommendations of the task force have been taken very seriously by the membership of the American Occupational Therapy Association, are being widely discussed, and will probably prove influential in affecting the direction of occupational therapy.

TIME: 1977

PLACE: Kitchen area of a Community Mental Health Center.

Bill (a registered occupational therapist with five years of experience in psychiatry) and Rona (an occupational therapy student in the sixth week of her second fieldwork experience) are having a cup of coffee before starting the day. They are in the kitchen, an area partitioned off from a pleasant livingroom, part of the program's small ADL apartment. Bill and Rona have a pile of papers spread out on the table in front of them. They have been discussing the clients.

Rona comments, "I finished checking out Ro-berta yesterday. It didn't work at all to place her in the group on Monday. She just went into her shell and stayed there. So I decided to work with her on a one-to-one basis for a while. She has a lot of rote skills, old familiar schemes, I guess, at a pretty high level—things like making coffee and setting the table—but when she tries something she never did before, or when there's some special emotional strain, she falls apart unless we give her a lot of structure. She seems able to handle only about two steps at a time, so you have to stay near. I think it's really important to give her that support. Don't you?"

Bill comments, "She certainly needs to succeed. Just watch that she doesn't get too dependent."

Rona replies, "I know. That's tricky, and I may need help to recognize it if it's happening. I was thinking—you know, her husband is going to stop by for lunch today. I thought I'd have her make something like grilled cheese sandwiches—which I'm sure she can handle—but use ready-mades like potato chips and tomatoes, and finish it out with ice cream for dessert. She's coming in at ten o'clock to decide the menu and seems to feel okay about going down the street to buy the food. I just think it's important for her to make the meal, but it can't be too complicated. What do you think?"

Bill says, "Sounds good to me. You're using her integrated skills well and that's probably important, because, while it's neat that her husband is coming, it's bound to be somewhat stressful. You know—he's been doing most of the cooking at their house for a couple of years! Good luck."

Bill leaves Rona and goes down a short hall to his office to check his schedule of activities for the day. A 9:30 meeting with the director to review the budget. The meeting would be sticky. Everybody's looking for ways to cut corners and save money. At 10:30, he would work with a small group of clients, men and women, in the workshop next to the kitchen. They would be doing simple repairs to broken pieces of furniture which they had brought in to the center. Most of the work was gluing and clamping, but there were some minor painting and refinishing jobs. He had found that this activity was good, both as evaluation and as treatment.

In the afternoon he would be taking Rona with him to the home of one of their clients. Mrs. Smith, the client, was forty-five years old. An arthritic condition prevented her from getting out of the house. She was depressed and anxious. An occupational therapy program had been started to see if there were ways she could be helped to handle her basic activities of daily living. The situation was difficult because her family were all hard-working, energetic people, who were used to having Mrs. Smith depend on them, but who tended also to resent it silently. And the house was full of architectural barriers.

Somewhere, Bill was going to have to fit in time to read over the AOTA Mental Health Task Force Report again, because there was going to be a local hearing about it that evening. He had read it once and had felt excited about parts, depressed about other parts, and disturbed about some but not all of the recommendations.

"It could matter a lot, how this gets handled!" he thinks.

REFERENCES

1. Dunton, W. R.: Prescribing Occupational Therapy. Springfield IL: Charles C Thomas, Publishers, 1928, p. 9.
2. Bonsall, I. In Van Atta, K.: An Account of the Events Surrounding the Origin of the Friends Hospital. Philadelphia: Williams Brothers Printing Co., 1976, p. 24.
3. Meyer, A.: The philosophy of occupational therapy. Arch. Occup. Ther. 1:5, 1922, pp. 1–10.
4. Slagle, E. C.: Training aides for mental patients. Arch. Occup. Ther. 1:14, 1922.
5. Dunton: Prescribing Occupational Therapy.
6. Haas, L. J.: Practical Occupational Therapy. Milwaukee WI: Bruce Publishing Co., 1944.
7. Haas, L. J.: Occupational Therapy for the Mentally and Nervously Ill. Milwaukee WI: Bruce Publishing Co., 1925.
8. Marsh, L. C.: Shall we apply industrial psychiatry to psychiatry? Occup. Ther. Rehab. 12:1, 1932.
9. Wade, B.: Occupational therapy for patients with mental disease. In Willard, H. S., and Spackman, C. S. (eds.): Principles of Occupational Therapy, ed. 1. Philadelphia: J. B. Lippincott Co., 1947, pp. 99–109.
10. Menninger, W. C.: Psychiatric hospital therapy designed to meet unconscious needs. Amer. J. Psychiat. 93:347, 1936.
11. Wade, B., and Franciscus, M. L.: Occupational therapy for the mentally ill. In Willard, H. S., and Spackman, C. S. (eds.): Occupational Therapy, ed. 2. Philadelphia: J. B. Lippincott Co., 1954, pp. 103–108.
12. Fidler, G. S.: Psychological evaluation of occupational therapy activities. Am. J. Occup. Ther. 2:284, 1948.
13. Strecker, E. A., and Appel, K. E.: Discovering Ourselves, ed. 2. New York: Macmillan Co., 1948.
14. Jones, M.: The Therapeutic Community. New York: Basic Books, 1953.
15. Fidler, G. S., and Fidler, J. W.: Introduction to Psychiatric Occupational Therapy. New York: Harper and Row Publishers, 1954, p. 170.

16. West, W. (ed.): Changing Concepts and Practices in Psychiatric Occupational Therapy. New York: American Occupational Therapy Association, 1959.
17. Ibid, p. xi.
18. Niswander, G. D., Haslerud, G. M., and Dixey, E.: The effect of the professional activity of the occupational therapist on the behavior of acute mental patients. Am. J. Occup. Ther. 11:273, 1957.
19. Elkins, H. K., and Van Vlack, N. M.: Changes in occupational therapy due to the tranquilizing drugs. Am. J. Occup. Ther. 11:269–271, 1957.
20. Fidler and Fidler: Introduction Psychiatric Occupational Therapy.
21. Action for Mental Health. Joint Commission on Mental Illness and Mental Health. New York: John Wiley & Sons, 1961.
22. Nagy, I., and Framo, J.: Intensive Family Therapy. New York: Harper and Row Publishers, 1965.
23. Wolpe, J.: Psychotherapy by Reciprocal Inhibition. Palo Alto: Stanford University Press, 1958.
24. Fidler, G. S. and Fidler, J. W.: Occupational Therapy: A Communication Process in Psychiatry. New York: Macmillan Co., 1963.
25. Azima, F. J.: The Azima Battery. In Mazer, I. (ed.): Materials from the 1968 Regional Institutes sponsored by the American Occupational Therapy Association on the Evaluation Process. Final Report R.S.A.-123-T-68. New York: American Occupational Therapy Association, 1968.
26. Fidler, G. S.: Diagnostic battery, scoring and summary. In Mazer, J. (ed.): Materials from the 1968 Regional Institutes sponsored by the American Occupational Therapy Association on the Evaluation Process. Final Report R.S.-123-T-68. New York: American Occupational Therapy Association, 1968.
28. Mazer, J., and Mosey, A. C.: Introduction to Special Section: Theories of psychiatric occupational therapy. Am. J. Occup. Ther. 22: 398–399, 1968.
29. Diasio, K.: Psychiatric occupational therapy: Search for a conceptual framework in the light of psychoanalytic ego psychology and learning theory. Am. J. Occup. Ther. 22: 400–414, 1968.
30. Tempone, V., and Smith, A.: Psychiatric occupational therapy within a learning theory context. Am. J. Occup. Ther. 22: 415–425, 1968.
31. Mosey, A. C.: Recapitulation of ontogenesis. Am. J. Occup. Ther. 22: 426–438, 1968.
32. Watanabe, S.: Four concepts basic to the occupational therapy process. Am. J. Occup. Ther. 22: 439–450, 1968.
33. Mazer, J.: Toward an integrated theory of occupational therapy. Am. J. Occup. Ther. 22: 451–456, 1968.
34. Mazer, J.: Ibid.
35. Ibid, p. 456.
36. Matsutsuyu, J.: Occupational behavior: A perspective on work and play. Am. J. Occup. Ther. 25:292, 1971.
37. White, R. W.: The urge towards competence. Am. J. Occup. Ther. 25:271–274, 1971.
38. Florey, L.: An approach to play and play development. Am. J. Occup. Ther. 25: 275–280, 1971.
39. Takata, N.: The play milieu. Am. J. Occup. Ther. 25:281–284, 1971.
40. Michelman, S.: The importance of creative play. Am. J. Occup. Ther. 25:285–290, 1971.
41. Maurer, P.: Antecedents of work behavior. Am. J. Occup. Ther. 25:294–297, 1971.
42. Bailey, D.: Vocational theories and work habits related to childhood development. Am. J. Occup. Ther. 25:298–302, 1971.
43. Johnson, J.: Considerations of work as therapy in the rehabilitation process. Am. J. Occup. Ther. 25:303–307, 1971.
44. Matsutsuyu, J.: Occupational behavior: A perspective on work and play. Am. J. Occup. Ther. 25: 291–294, 1971.
45. Ibid, p. 291.
46. Reilly, M.: The educational process. Am. J. Occup. Ther. 23:302, 1969.
47. Arieti, S.: The Intrapsychic Self. New York: Basic Books, 1967.
48. Rogers, C.: Freedom to Learn. Columbus OH: Charles E. Merrill Co., 1969.
49. Finn, G.: The occupational therapist in prevention programs. Am. J. Occup. Ther. 26:65, 1972.
50. Ibid.
51. Toffler, A.: Future Shock. New York: Random House, 1970.
52. Moore, J.: Behavior, bias and the limbic system. Am. J. Occup. Ther. 30:11–19, 1976.
53. Mosey, A. C.: Three Frames of Reference for Mental Health. Thorofare NJ: Charles B. Slack, 1970.
54. A Report of the American Occupational Therapy Association Mental Health Task Force. Occup. Ther. Newspaper 30:1976.

section 2/Elements of the Psychiatric Occupational Therapy Process

Our knowledge base is continually expanding. The momentum for this expansion has been supplied by the growing numbers of therapists involved in graduate study and research. We have committed ourselves, moreover, to the development of conceptual models on which to base our frames of reference for treatment. The issues raised in 1976 by the Mental Health Task Force Report are relevant, reflecting our current states of knowledge and practice in psychiatric occupational therapy.

Conceptual models for psychiatry at the present time are drawn from the knowledge bases of the biological and social sciences. There has been a continuous expansion of knowledge in response to new research findings and in response to the changes in society as a whole. Through the years at least six schools of thought in psychiatry have evolved and these have provided conceptual bases from which the prevailing frames of reference for psychiatric occupational therapy have been derived. These schools of thought may be identified as (1) biophysical, (2) intrapsychic, (3) behavioral, (4) sociocultural, (5) phenomenological, and (6) integrative.[1] The frames of reference which developed in occupational therapy are (1) sensory integrative, (2) psychoanalytic, (3) behavioral, (4) developmental, and (5) occupational behavior.

In the *biophysical* school of thought, research and theoretical formulations focus on problems in the basic anatomical, physiological, and neurophysiological structures of the individual. These include biochemical and metabolic imbalance as well as abnormality or dysfunction as a result of trauma, disease, genetic, and congenital aberrations. In occupational therapy, the *sensory integrative* frame of reference relies heavily upon the conceptual bases and theoretical formulations of the biophysical school of thought.

In the *intrapsychic* school of thought, the concern is with unconscious processes, conflicts based on repressed material, and the health of conflict resolution in each of the successive stages of psychosexual development. The *psychoanalytic* frame of reference takes its conceptual basis and theoretical formulations from the intrapsychic school of thought.

The *behavioral* school of thought is based upon hypotheses and scientifically controlled laboratory research into the ways in which learning is acquired. It is concerned with the specific observable behaviors of individuals and does not acknowledge or attempt to work with unconscious material or thought processes. The *behavior therapy* frame of reference is clearly based on this school of thought.

The *sociocultural* school of thought places major emphasis on the effects of community, cultural, and social forces on the individual. These are seen frequently as defining what constitutes psychiatric illness as well as directly contributing to an individual's ability to function adaptively. The concepts and theories of this school of thought comprise the background for many of the occupational therapy approaches, but are especially influential in the *developmental* and *occupational behavior* frames of reference.

In the *phenomenological* school of thought, major interest is in the individual's perception of self and others, as well as in the effects of societal values on this type of perception. The phenomenological school of thought incorporates knowledge and perspectives from the intrapsychic and sociocultural schools; its concern is highly individualized. The school of thought has lent itself well to preventive and self-actualization approaches. Some of its theoretical premises and conceptual bases may be incorporated into *psychoanalytic, developmental,* and *occupational behavior* frames of reference in occupational therapy.

Another term for the *integrative* school of thought is *biopsychosocial.* This is a comprehensive approach which considers that psychological processes and human behavior are determined by dynamic and complex interrelationships of physical, emotional, social, and cultural processes. The *developmental* and *occupational behavior* frames of reference in occupational therapy rely upon the broad spectrum of knowledge that characterizes this school of thought.

It is evident, in exploring the history of psychiatric occupational therapy, that, in spite of developments and changes in society as a whole and in the theoretical and conceptual bases of psychiatry, the psychiatric occupational therapy process has been consistent in at least one characteristic. It has consciously and deliberately developed methods for using the interactions among four basic elements to promote and maintain function. The four basic elements considered in occupational therapy are: (1) the *client*, or individual who needs help, (2) the *therapist*, or individual who is the helper, (3) the *activity*, and (4) the *context* in which the helping takes place.

The frames of reference which are used in the helping process determine the perspective from which the client's problems are understood, the kind of relationship which is fostered between the therapist and client, the nature of activities used in treatment, and the total context for treatment. Each frame of reference provides its dimensions of understanding about the occupational therapy process; each suggests a way of going about the processes of evaluation, setting objectives, planning and implementing the occupational therapy program.

These factors are the essence of psychiatric occupational therapy. In this part of the chapter, perspectives on these four elements as a foundation for a subsequent consideration of the psychiatric occupational therapy process are explored.

THE CLIENT

When an individual seeks psychiatric treatment the need to do so arises out of problems that are acutely felt. Sometimes it is the client who feels the need and takes the initiative in seeking help, but often, because of the nature of the illness, other people, often family members, friends, work associates, or neighbors, may need to take some responsibility for seeing that the client receives care and treatment. Sometimes, when an individual becomes very ill or severely disturbed, especially if this occurs in a public place, it is the police who are charged with the responsibility for getting the client to a hospital.

What are the problems which make it necessary for an individual to require psychiatric help? They include confusion, disorientation, distortions of perceptions or thoughts, feeling bombarded by stimuli, anxiety, depression, despair, impulsive outbursts, inability to organize, inability to handle feelings, inability to communicate or to relate to others, lack of capacity for pleasure, deficits in judgment in the management of personal or work life, lack of balance in routines of waking and sleeping, tactile defensiveness, poor sense of time, and, frequently, lack of ability to recognize or assess the self or problems. All of these are experienced in some degree by most people at times of stress. It would seem that there are several factors that determine whether experiences may be considered symptomatic of mental illness. These factors are: (1) the severity of the problem, whether it is experienced so acutely that it threatens to cause harm to the individual or to the people around him or her, (2) the length of time the problem is experienced, and (3) the ability of the individual to recognize and undertake measures to change the condition or simply to "bounce back" spontaneously. It is useful to think of mental conditions as degrees of psychiatric function and dysfunction on a continuum that goes from health to illness. In doing so, it is possible to take into account a number of important considerations, such as environmental stress and cultural perspectives, as well as the stress of disease, trauma, or deficit. It also encourages the consideration of preventive as well as treatment, maintenance, and rehabilitation measures.

Underlying the presenting problems of the client, there are at least five major areas that are important: the client's concept of self, ability to test reality, object relationships, ability to cope with feelings, and organization of thoughts and actions.

Concept of self refers to the knowledge and feelings a person has about himself or herself. It includes awareness of one's body and bodily functions, a sense of one's ability to control one's actions, and a sense of competence in doing the tasks of everyday living. Self-esteem and the way a person feels that others see him or her are part of self-concept.

Reality testing refers to the process by which individuals can know that what they perceive, think, and feel is real. It is closely related to self-concept in that one must be able to recognize reality to know one's own strengths, assets, weaknesses, and limits. As in self-concept, reality testing takes place both at a concrete body-experience level and at an abstract social-emotional level. The ability of an individual to process information received from the world is the key to reality testing.

Object relationships refers to the kinds of interactions that take place between an individual and the world which is external to him or her. Objects are both human and nonhuman. Objects meet human needs; through objects we learn about the world; objects are the recipients of our expressions of feelings. The term, object relationships, which springs from psychoanalytic thought, refers to the kinds of perceptions one has of others and the effectiveness with which one gets along with others. It is closely meshed with self-concept and with reality testing.

Coping with feelings refers to the ways in which individuals handle their moods and emotions. All human beings experience some measure of fear, anger, joy, sadness, depression, and elation in the normal course of living. Sometimes strong feelings occur in response to specific events. Sometimes feelings are part of a general mood. They may be felt intensely or mildly. They may debilitate the person who is experiencing them or may be the cause of actions which are destructive to self or others. They may on the other hand energize and enhance one's concept of self and relationships with others. Feelings are powerful motivators to action and bear a direct but complex relationship to thought processes.

Organizing one's thoughts and actions refers to all those cognitive functions which are necessary for an individual to plan a course of action and follow it, to recognize cause-and-effect relationships, to be able to problem solve and to have clear, functional concepts of time and space.

Sensory Integrative Perspectives on the Client

The mentally ill frequently are found to have perceptual difficulties, some of which may be due to the primary disease process and some of which may be due to more transitory factors such as stress or medication. The perceptual process is the core of an individual's ability to organize, integrate, and interpret internal and external or environmental stimuli. Perceptual ability is developed; the earliest experiences of infancy and childhood are critical to the process. Beginning with early tactile and kinesthetic percepts, children develop concepts of their bodies. If this process is interrupted, or if the neurological system is in some way dysfunctional, the resultant perceptual distortions may prevent normal interactions between the individual and the environment and make reality testing and the establishment of healthy, functional cognitive and motor abilities difficult. The resultant distortions in object relationships, both human and nonhuman, may lead to further emotional distress, which may ultimately result in serious forms of maladaptation or mental illness.

The functions of the brain in integrating and screening the sensory stimuli with which human beings are continuously bombarded are of monumental importance in determining human behavior. King, building on the research of Ayres into sensory integration in learning disorders, has developed an exceedingly well documented body of knowledge about sensory integrative dysfunction in patients diagnosed as schizophrenic. Observation of large numbers of institutionalized chronic schizophrenics yielded a common picture: S-shaped posture; shuffling gait; inability to raise arms over head; immobility of the head and shoulder girdle; tendency to hold arms and legs in a flexed, adducted, and internally rotated position; lack of normal hand function; weakness of grip; and lack of motivation. Her hypothesis, based on observation and a search of the literature, is: "Some individuals have defective proprioceptive feedback mechanisms, the vestibular component in particular being first underreactive, and second, underactive in its role in the sensorimotor integration process. This defect, whether genetic, developmental, or the result of trauma, constitutes an important etiological or prodromal factor in process and reactive schizophrenia."[2]

King also indicates that the paranoid schizophrenic syndrome is distinctly different from that of process and reactive schizophrenia. One of the most universal problems of the process and reactive schizophrenic seems to be in the area of perceptual constancy. It is not difficult to understand how this problem would seriously hamper the development of healthy concepts of self, other people, and objects and would interfere with the process of reality testing.

Some of the basic principles underlying the sensory integrative approach to treatment are the following:

1. Early life (probably including prenatal) experiences of vestibular, proprioceptive, and tactile stimulation are important in personality development.
2. Neurological immaturity has a related emotional overlay, which may take the form of full-blown illness.
3. The tactile sense is critical for an individual to learn about the environment and about himself or herself as a differentiated entity.
4. Perceptual constancy is necessary to provide a predictable basis on which to build learning. Lack of visual or auditory perceptual constancy seriously distorts an individual's ability to adapt to both the human and nonhuman environment.
5. When a client's perceptual deficits are identified and understood, a multidimensional remedial approach may be used to help him or her. Movement and sensory activities, carefully selected, have the potential of facilitating or acting as true remediation.

King has experimented and worked with neurophysiological approaches to remediation of sensorimotor integrative dysfunction and has experienced empirical success with these methods. In general, the activities of sensory integration are gross motor ones, selected with two important requirements: (1) that the conscious attention of the patient *must not be centered on the motor process, but on the outcome or object*, and (2) that the *activity must be pleasurable*. The subcorticalization of the experience is most important. It has been Lorna King's observation that when patients make gains in sensory integration, the gains tend to be permanent, and the success of the process usually motivates patients to continue.

The specific kinds of activities are ones which involve vestibular stimulation, heavy work, proprioceptive feedback, sensory input, and awareness of space and form. Both recreational and task-oriented activities may incorporate these elements. Attention may also be directed to the potential of activities in terms of their alerting or stimulating effects and inhibiting or slowing effects. Figure 12-1 gives these general characteristics.

King's work is making a significant impact on the treatment of a heretofore difficult population. She has broken ground for continuing important research.

	ALERTING, STIMULATING		INHIBITING, CALMING
VESTIBULAR	Fast, sudden, jerky, intense		Slow, rhythmic, even
TACTILE	Light touch	Pressure touch	Pressure touch, rhythmic
TEMPERATURE	Cool		Warm—neutral
POSITION	Head up, chest out		Head down

FIGURE 12-1. Effects of activities in terms of neurophysiological mechanisms. Adapted from information obtained at a workshop led by L. S. King.[3]

Behavior Therapy Perspectives on the Client

From the behavior therapy perspective, there are four systems that determine the way learning takes place: positive reinforcement, negative reinforcement, punishment, and extinction. *Positive reinforcement* is a pleasing or need-fulfilling event; *negative reinforcement* is the withdrawal of an unpleasant or aversive stimulus when a change of behavior has taken place; *punishment* refers to the presentation of an unpleasant stimulus; *extinction* is the withdrawal of a pleasing stimulus or the bombardment with the original reinforcer with a resultant decrease in the behavior.

For example, a parent's smiles and praise when the child brings home a good report card are a form of positive reinforcement. The child learns that good grades please his or her parents; if that is important, the child has learned to work for good grades. When a child works very hard to get good grades in order to avoid being nagged and scolded, the child has learned to do so through negative reinforcement. Punishment is the presentation of an unpleasant or aversive stimulus or the withdrawal of a pleasant stimulus following the occurrence of some undesirable behavior. The child might be punished for receiving poor grades by being spanked or scolded or by not being allowed to go out to play. If parents stop praising the child for receiving good grades, the child may stop trying to please them in that way, or, if the parents give too much praise too continuously, the effect will be one of *satiation* and the child will stop trying. These are two examples of extinction.

The behavior therapy perspective is based on scientific laboratory research, originally done with laboratory animals. In terms of treatment procedures, it may permit highly controlled procedures for helping people change their behaviors. Patterns of behavior, even very complex ones, may be altered or reversed, and new ones may be established, if one is able to identify and use effective schedules of reinforcement. The behavioral approaches are concerned with the existing behavior-environment relationships of the individual. The behaviorally oriented therapist, then, would look at the things which an individual *said* or *did* reflecting problems in the areas of self-concept, reality testing, object relationships, coping with feelings, and organizing thinking. The large problems would be seen in terms of the component specific behaviors. Words like "self-concept," "reality testing," and "object relationships" would not be used. One would state instead, for example, something like "the client will initiate a conversation with another client." Certainly, this is a piece of several larger areas of concern, but it is a small, observable, and measurable behavior. Behaviors are identified clearly and specifically and are treated directly. Concern is for the individual's unique and individual patterns of response to feedback.

Sieg[4] has defined behavior therapy in the following way: "the emphasis is on designing conditions which will change the behavior and thus alleviate the problem, rather than delving into psychic or mental reasons for the problem." She describes the process of designing a program to include the following considerations[5]: (1) Identifying the terminal behavior, which means clearly and specifically what behavior needs to be increased, decreased, or shaped. This behavior should be observable and measurable. (2) Counting the behavior which must be done initially, before treatment, to establish the baseline of data upon which treatment will build. Counting or measuring then is done continuously as treatment proceeds. The measured data are recorded, charted, and provided to the client as feedback. (3) Selecting a reinforcer, which involves identifying what supports the behavior, and individualizing the reinforcement so that it will be successful and fair for a given client. (4) Selecting a schedule for reinforcement on the basis of learning theory; the therapist must determine the schedule of reinforcement for the particular client and behavior. (5) If new behavior is to be established, techniques of behavior modification are used. The first is *shaping* in which reinforcement is given for each successive approximation to the desired behavior. The second is *chaining,* in which reinforcement is given for behaviors related to a specific behavior which has been established. (The occurrence of the established behavior is treated as the stimulus for another response which is related. Very complex behavior patterns may be developed through the step by step shaping and chaining of series of responses.) Finally, the therapist (or another person) may *model* the desired behavior and receive reinforcement in the presence of the client. The client may then be reinforced for successful imitation of the behavior.[6]

Behavioral techniques are often unconsciously or automatically applied in life and in many therapeutic circumstances. Behavioral therapy makes the process specifiable and controllable and may be useful to help some clients meet certain desired therapeutic goals.

Psychoanalytic Perspectives on the Client

Psychoanalytic theory has been extensively studied, and many new perspectives based on psychoanalytic theory have developed over the years. The literature is rich in materials that amplify and modify the basic Freudian formulations.

From the psychoanalytic perspective, the client is understood in terms of the powerful interplay between the id or primary drives, the superego or the demands of society, and the ego functions that have developed to mediate their conflict. It is a major function of the ego to maintain contact with reality, and it is the ego that develops ways to help the individual defend against the demands of the id and the superego. Ego functions are clearly and directly related to self-concept, reality testing, object relationships, coping with feelings, and the capacity to organize one's thinking and actions.

The client may also be understood in terms of stages of psychosexual development. Character traits and modes of achieving pleasure or need-satisfaction may be traced to the oral, anal, genital, latency, and phallic stages of development.

In approaching the evaluation and treatment of a client within a psychoanalytic frame of reference, one is concerned with behavior as the overt manifestation of unconscious processes mediated by the ego. All communication and other forms of behavior have both real and symbolic meanings. In therapy, there is a primary concern for the health of the functions of the ego in reality testing, providing effective defense mechanisms and satisfactory interpersonal relationships, and synthesizing all of human experience into logical and adaptive modes of thinking, feeling, and acting. The relationship that develops between the client and therapist is a dynamic one through which the client may be helped to explore, relive, develop insight, and change. The nonhuman objects—the materials, tools, and actions—used in occupational therapy are facilitators to these processes. The ego strength of the therapist is an important factor in the relationship that develops.

It is possible to add the dimension of a psychoanalytic perspective to the basic understanding one has of the client and to focus on providing opportunities for developing and supporting the functions of the ego which will be adaptive. To provide treatment which is purely psychoanalytically based, however, requires that the therapist have thorough self-knowledge as well as a strong theoretical base in psychoanalytic principles.

Developmental Perspectives on the Client

Considered developmentally, the client may be seen to be functioning at any given time at levels which are comparable to those which are experienced in the process of growth and development. The basic principles which relate to the developmental perspective in psychiatry include:

1. The individual grows, matures, and learns in a sequential way. Each gain in structure or function provides the base upon which each new gain is built.
2. The physical, sensory, perceptual, emotional, cognitive, and social aspects of human growth and development are intricately interwoven, and issues, stresses, or gains that take place in any one area will bring about changes in the others.
3. There are special issues and opportunities that present themselves at each period of human development. Through the process of adaptation, the individual explores these issues and opportunities, solves problems, learns, and grows.
4. Under stress of any kind it is a human characteristic to regress to earlier levels of function. Regression may be very brief (seconds or minutes) or may be long-term, depending upon the nature of the stress and the basic health or strength of the individual. Individuals may choose regressive activities deliberately as a method of preserving balance in their lives.
5. In providing experiences to facilitate growth and adaptation, one should consider the developmental issues which present themselves at the client's functional level and the conditions which will make successful achievement possible.

Llorens has been a primary spokesperson for the developmental perspective in occupational therapy. She speaks of occupational therapy as a process of facilitating growth, as well as mastery of self and the environment through a recognition of the needs, abilities, and issues of the growing child.[7] These principles have been translated into a highly successful approach to treatment with adult psychiatric clients.

Mosey, in her "Recapitulation of Ontogenesis," refers to seven adaptive skills on a development continuum and offers suggestions for approaches to treatment to help the client to develop or to regain them.[8] These are listed in Section 1 of Chapter 7 of this book.

Between 1971 and 1973, taking Piagetian formulations of cognitive development, Allen and Lewis[8a] developed an approach to understanding the client whose ability to organize thoughts and actions has regressed to early levels as a result of the stress of the illness. The levels with which occupational therapy may be concerned are characterized in terms of the infant's process of exploring and learning about the world: (1) focus on one's own bodily movements, (2) interest in the effects of one's actions on the environment, (3) use of familiar schemes to achieve an end result, (4) use of trial and error to solve problems, and (5) use of thoughts and images to solve problems. By a thorough knowledge of the Piagetian concepts about the ways the child understands cause and effect, object permanence, and time, and about the conditions that help the child to learn, it is possible to think in terms of structuring occupational therapy experiences through which the client can experience himself or herself as whole and able. Careful identification and use of existing familiar and well integrated "schemes" in an occupational therapy program is an important part of this approach.

An example of the developmental approach to treatment is described by Levy in her careful analysis of a movement approach to the treatment of severely disorganized psychotic patients. Table 12-1 describes the levels of cognition and the behaviors that may be expected at each level. The therapist involves clients in body movement and exercise patterns planned to help in the building of basic cognitive skills. Levy writes: "A significant manifestation of a schizophrenic break is the regression of thought processes to early developmental levels of functioning. Remission from that break hinges on rebuilding the steps toward integrated cognition in developmental order. Movement is the plane on which primal learning must take place, and it is this cognitive level that must be integrated before higher-level thought processes can evolve."[9]

Table 12-1. Piaget's stages and predictable behaviors in the adult psychotic.

	Cognition	*Behaviors*
Stage 1	Functional assimilation	Will perform available schemata
	Generalizing assimilation	Will generalize available schemata to new situations
Stage 2	Able to repeat behavior of models if similar to own behaviors (approximately, at first)	Will imitate if his own body movements are modeled for him
	Beginning to be interested in moderately novel events, actively seeks new stimulation	Will respond to introduction of moderately novel movements
Stage 3	Beginning to perceive effect on environment	Gross-motor activities critical
	Is learning to imitate new behaviors	Is learning direct imitation through progressively more accurate imitation
Stage 4	Is able to imitate directly simple new behaviors	Is able to deal with object-oriented activity

From Levy, L.: Movement therapy for psychiatric patients. Reprinted with permission of the American Occupational Therapy Association, Inc. Copyright 1969, Am. J. Occup. Ther. Vol. 28, No. 6, p. 354.

Table 12-2 gives an analysis of developmental levels that may be found in regressed groups of patients and the related treatment requirements.

Table 12-2. Activity group treatment of regressed schizophrenic patients. Analysis of developmental levels and related treatment requisites.

	Developmental level 6–18 mo.	*Physical/social environment*	*Quality of tasks*
Cognitive Development	1. Undifferentiated self. 2. Cannot conceive end result. 3. Learning via visual imitation if old motor schemes employed. 4. 15 min. attention span. 5. Egocentricity. 6. No covert imagery or abstract sequencing of ideas. 7. Cannot explore properties of objects. 8. Difficulty learning via trial and error.	1. No clutter, noise. 2. Small room. 3. Constant environment in terms of therapist, time, location, etc.	1. Limited number of parts. 2. Limited number of dissimilar parts. 3. Pre-cut projects. 4. Completion within 30 min. 5. Able to be successfully completed by patient. 6. Same project for all patients. 7. Defined as "worthwhile" by patient. 8. Utilize familiar skills, motor schemes. 9. Tasks relate to differentiation of self from others.

(Continued)

Table 12-2. Activity group treatment of regressed schizophrenic patients. Analysis of developmental levels and related treatment requisites. (*Continued*)

	Developmental level 6–18 mo.	*Physical/social environment*	*Quality of tasks*
Social/ Emotional Development	1. Orality/trust. 2. Dependency. 3. Ambivalence. 4. Omnipotence.		1. Allow dependency via structuring task. 2. Promotes development of group cohesiveness. 3. Task allows for "modeling" of therapist. 4. Allows for expression of feeling. 5. Oral gratification in activity.
Group Skills Development	1. Parallel play. 2. Difficulty in sharing. 3. Difficulty in recognizing own and others' feelings and needs.	1. Small group (6 patients). 2. Common table. 3. Male/female group. 4. Area for calisthenics, dancing, cooking.	1. Gradual sharing and cooperation as patient is able. 2. Simple group interaction re task and interpersonal relations in here and now. 3. Same project for all patients.
Perceptual Motor Development	1. Poor shape discrimination. 2. Poor concept of object permanence. 3. Poor figure ground discrimination. 4. Difficulty in fine motor coordination.		1. Simple spatial relationships. 2. Allow for exploration of properties of objects. 3. Deals with object permanence. 4. Use 2 or 3 colors, etc. for discrimination and classification. 5. Familiar motor schemes.
Gross Motor Coordination Development	1. Rigidity. 2. Movements consciously controlled. 3. Loss of smoothness in automatic movements.		

Developmental level 6–18 mo.	*Quality of instruction*	*Quality of therapeutic relationship*
Cognitive Development	1. Visual imitation. 2. Concrete, overt imagery. 3. One direction at a time. 4. Highly structured teaching methods. 5. Repetition of instructions for reinforcement.	1. Firm setting of limits re task and behavior. 2. Acceptance of patient's individuality. 3. Help patient feel safe. 4. Shape desired behavior with smiles/realistic praise. 5. Be specific re expectations of task and behavior.
Social/Emotional Development	1. Praise (reinforcement) for good job. 2. Explicit guidance for correction of mistakes. 3. Clear and consistent instructions.	1. Allow dependency, yet work toward greater autonomy. 2. Provide physical, social support with reassurance. 3. Provide consistent affective response. 4. Continuity of therapists.
Group Skills Development	1. Present task to whole group first. 2. Healthier patient demonstrates steps to other patients. 3. Group comments on individual projects.	1. Promote group belongingness, awareness of others' names, etc. 2. Assist patients in sharing and trusting others in group.

Table 12-2. Activity group treatment of regressed schizophrenic patients. Analysis of developmental levels and related treatment requisites. (*Continued*)

Management problems	*Management techniques*
1. Low frustration level.	1. Therapist openly states problem, shows empathy.
2. Poor impulse control.	2. Restructuring task for greater success.
3. Confusion and short attention span.	3. Limit setting with clear expectations.
4. Demandingness and ambivalence.	4. Tension release via structured gross motor activity.
5. Lability-anger, sadness, joy.	5. Removal of patient from group to another room.
6. Suspicion.	6. Physical contact for reassurance.
7. Passivity.	7. Listens to patient/gives feedback for reality testing.
8. Distractibility.	8. Allow patient participation in decision making.
9. Jealousy among patients re staff.	
10. Massive, overwhelming anxiety.	
11. Blocking, trance behavior.	
12. Delusions, active hallucinations.	

Developed by Diane Maslen for use in the treatment of regressed schizophrenic patients. Sheppard and Enoch Pratt Hospital, Baltimore MD 21204. Reprinted with permission.

In the use of the developmental approach, it is important to note that many normal, healthy, mature adult activities do, in fact, require no more skill than some of the activities of infancy and childhood. For example, hiking, jogging, swimming and many other basic physical activities are at a movement level. Most simple craft activities and some activities of daily living may be broken down and presented in such a way as to meet early levels of integration. The following outline serves as a guideline for group experience that is based on developmental levels.

DEVELOPMENTAL GROUPS*

I. *Aggregate of Individuals*—The individual may interact with one other person, usually the therapist. There is no attempt by an individual to promote interaction outside of the one-to-one relationship.

II. *Parallel Group*—An aggregate of persons who work on individual tasks with minimal requirement for interaction. The leader meets the social-emotional needs of each individual.

   A. Goals:
      1. Increase awareness of self, others, and the environment.
      2. Improve ability to tolerate a nonthreatening group.
      3. Develop beginning sharing behaviors.
      4. Increase attention span.
      5. Reclaim old skills.

   B. Behavioral characteristics:
      1. Attention span—variable (5 min. to 1 hr.).
      2. Verbal but not disruptive.
      3. Nonverbal—(1) quiet (2) withdrawn (3) limited interaction.
      4. Difficulty performing tasks independently.
      5. Requires a structured activity for success to occur.
      6. Ability to attend to individual tasks in the presence of others.

   C. Size and time factors:
      1. 6 to 12 participants.
      2. Length of time variable (20 min. to 1 hr.)

III. *Project Level Group*—Group members interact in a short-term task with others for the length of the task.

   A. Goals:
      To facilitate interaction, verbal and nonverbal, in a short-term task with others. The duration of the relationship is determined by the group activity.

   B. Behavioral characteristics:
      1. Exploration and testing of others, i.e., development of trust.
      2. Difficulty in participating in shared tasks.
      3. Inability to seek assistance of a peer in carrying out a task.
      4. Avoids giving assistance to a peer or provides inadequate assistance.
      5. Fear that others may interfere with task completion.

DEVELOPMENTAL GROUPS* *(Continued)*

6. Tendency to work alone, avoiding contact with others.
7. Lack of understanding that one must help others to receive help from others.
8. Minimal interaction outside of task place.
9. Trial-and-error behavior is observed in the group.

C. Size and time factors:
1. 4 to 10 participants.
2. Length of time variable (30 min. to 1 hr.)

D. Role of therapist:
1. Therapist must meet the social and emotional needs of the individual group members.
2. Provides and/or helps the group to select tasks which require interaction of two or more persons for completion.
3. Therapist usually must provide each group member with specific aspect of the activity to work on and individual instruction when necessary.
4. All materials and tools and equipment must usually be prepared prior to start of each group session.

IV. *Egocentric-Cooperative*—Group members interact cooperatively and competitively in a long-term task (major emphasis of individuals continues to be self-interest).

A. Goals:
1. Group members will be able to select, implement, and execute long-term projects through shared interaction and/or individual response. The therapist provides suggestions and guidelines.
2. Group members will be able to recognize and respect the rights of others.
3. Group members will perceive themselves as belonging to the group both during and after sessions.
4. Group members will be able to engage in cooperative and/or competitive behavior.
5. Group members will be able to assume various group membership roles.

B. Behavioral characteristics:
1. Difficulty engaging in cooperative tasks.
2. Preoccupied with competition or avoids competition.
3. Inability to conform to goals or norms of the group.
4. Disregard for the rights of others.
5. Disrespect for authority.
6. Compulsive, indiscriminate conformity to any authority figure.

C. Size and time factors:
1. 6 to 8 participants.
2. Length of time—1 hr.

D. Role of therapist:
1. Primarily a resource person.
2. Therapist provides minimal assistance (i.e., suggestions, encouragement) so that the group selects plans and executes tasks with much independence.
3. Offers support *and guidance* and continues to satisfy a considerable portion of the individual's social-emotional needs.

V. *Cooperative Group*—Group members satisfy the social-emotional needs of others while interacting in a task, in a same sex peer group.

A. Goals:
1. Increase the individual's ability to express both positive and negative affect in a group.
2. Be able to perceive the needs of others.
3. Be able to meet the needs of others.
4. Become cohesive as a group.

B. Behavioral characteristics:
1. Verbal and aware of other members.
2. Can engage in a shared task.
3. Difficulty in accurately perceiving the needs of others.
4. Difficulty in expressing both positive and negative affect in a group.
5. Difficulty in meeting the needs of others.
6. Attention span adequate to length of task.
7. Task is secondary to need fulfillment.

C. Size and time factors:
1. 10 to 12 participants.
2. Minimum time—1½ hr.

D. Role of therapist:
1. Does not function as an authority.
2. Assists in finding resources (acts as advisor).
3. Offers some support and some need satisfaction.

DEVELOPMENTAL GROUPS* *(Continued)*

VI. *Mature Group*—Group members assume those task and social-emotional roles that promote the general welfare and goal attainment of a heterogeneous group. Leadership is shared.
   A. Goals:
      1. Be able to interact with group members who vary in age, interest, ability, and cultural background.
      2. Be able to assume roles somewhat foreign to the individual's usual pattern of behavior.
      3. Be able to maintain a proper balance between task accomplishment and satisfaction of the social-emotional needs of group members.
      4. Be able to maintain a sense of self-integrity and individuality concomitant with productive participation in a group.
   B. Size and time factors:
      1. 10 to 15 participants.
      2. No time limit.

* Developed by the Occupational Therapy Staff of Norristown State Hospital, Norristown PA. Printed with their permission. Reference: Mosey, A. C.: Occupational Therapy: Theory and Practice.[10]

Occupational Behavior Perspectives on the Client

The infant wakes and makes little vocal sounds. The parent will soon come and feed her. The farmer puts on his overalls and goes out to milk the cows. The school boy finishes his breakfast, picks up his books, and sets off for school. The cashier in the supermarket talks briefly with the manager about the new checkout system, then sets up her counter. The retired teacher looks at her watch, then makes a phone call to ask the plumber to come to fix a leaking pipe. Two college students study together for an exam.

Roles and routines characterize the lives of most human beings. We became psychologically and physically attuned to taking care of our basic needs and to fulfilling the expectations and responsibilities that are part of our lives. In the course of a day and in the course of a lifetime, routines and roles change. Some are normal role changes. The *cashier* in the supermarket may be the *mother* of a school-aged child, the *wife* of an accountant, and the *best bowler* on the church bowling team. Vacation times and weekends permit changes by choice in routines and in roles. But illness and personal crises often cause major disruptions in routines and readjustment of roles.

In the process of development there are factors that enable human beings to establish both the stability and the flexibility needed to support themselves in assuming their roles within society, in carrying out life routines with minimal expenditures of energy, and in coping successfully with changes. Piaget and others have referred to the fact that infants are innately curious and that it is a basic human characteristic to seek stimulation and to value novelty. As children grow and develop they integrate both *knowledge* about the world and the *habits and skills* necessary for living in it. They learn the extent of their abilities to control or to be controlled by other people and events. They learn the "rules" of making things happen. They integrate a sense of time, as it is defined by the culture and society in which they live.

Reilly[11] has described three phases of play through which people learn. The first is a period of *exploration*. When confronted with something new, one is curious and may try to learn about it. New experiences of oneself, new objects, new people, and new procedures bring about a state of arousal. If the novelty is too great, the individual may be afraid and seek to avoid it. If it is too little, there may be no interest evoked. But if the conditions are safe the individual learns rules and develops feelings of hope and trust in the initial exploration of objects and relationships. The second phase is one in which the individual strives to *develop competence*. Through practice and repeated opportunities to experience the effects of one's skills, one develops confidence. The third phase is one in which the individual builds on the trust and self-confidence and works toward *achievement* in terms of externally defined standards as well as those standards which have developed within.

The occupational behavior frame of reference is concerned with clients from the perspective of the roles and the balance of their lives. Play is seen as significant both in childhood and in adulthood to develop and support the knowledge and skills required for carrying out the life roles of society. A strong knowledge base in sociology and psychology as well as in psychiatry is required in order to understand both illness and health in our society. Building upon this base, then, the major concern of the occupational therapist working within this frame of reference is to prevent and reduce the incapacities which result from illness.

Reilly specified six parts of an occupational therapy program based on the occupational behavior frame of reference[12]:

1. The program should incorporate examination of the client's life roles and identification of the skills to support them.
2. The program should reflect developmental stages which help the individual to acquire life skills.
3. The program should provide "natural and legitimate" decision-making opportunities to the client.
4. The milieu must acknowledge competencies, arouse curiosity, deepen appreciation, and demand appropriate behavior across the full spectrum of human abilities.
5. Occupational therapists must recognize and plan for the balance of work, play, and rest in the patient's total life space.
6. The structure of the program should be tailored to the patient and his or her own opportunities to practice life skills.

Medication and the Client

The introduction of psychopharmacology produced a revolution in the treatment of psychiatric problems. While the use of medications has certainly reduced many of the debilitating symptoms of mental illness and has, in many ways, made it possible for clients to function better, it has also produced some new sets of problems. The therapist who works with clients who are receiving medication needs to be aware of the possibility of side effects. In addition to the fact that side effects may be extremely troublesome and upsetting to the client, it is essential that they be monitored closely, so that changes in medication will be made when necessary. Table 12-3 lists some common side effects of medication. Because psychopharmacology is in a continual state of developing new drugs and refining their uses, each mental health professional should check on the medications his or her clients are receiving and their possible side effects and keep this knowledge up to date.

Table 12-3. Medications.

Major medication groups	*Possible side effects*
Amphetamines	Appetite loss, irritability, headaches, insomnia
Anti-anxiety Agents	Drowsiness, incoordination, ataxia
Antidepressants	Excitement, acute hypertensive crises, tremors, ataxia, peripheral neuropathy, impotence, bladder and bowel paralysis, aggravation of glaucoma, jaundice, EKG abnormalities.
Antipsychotic agents	Drowsiness, ataxia, blurred vision, weakness, feelings of unreality, hypotension, parkinsonlike syndrome, akinesia, anergia, dry mouth, facial and tongue hyperkinesias (twitching, blinking, grimacing, sucking, smacking lips), neck and trunk movements, choreoathetoid movements of extremities, tachycardia, constipation, impotence, photosensitivity and allergic skin reactions.

Adapted from DiMascio, A., and Shader, R. (eds.): Clinical Handbook of Psychopharmacology[13]; Physicians' Desk Reference[14]; and Shader, R. I. (ed.): Manual of Psychiatric Therapeutics.[15]

THE THERAPIST

The therapist is only one of many new people to whom the client is exposed when he or she becomes involved in treatment situations. Because psychiatric problems most frequently manifest themselves in chaotic, confused, or destructive interpersonal relationships, the interactions between the therapist and the client may be critical to the desired processes of growth and change.

Although the therapist's role is usually defined by the context, it may not always be entirely clear to the client. It is therefore vital that the therapist be quite clear about his or her role. In the occupational therapy process, the therapist's "use of self" means bringing together knowledge, skills, caring, and basic personality strengths to help the client overcome difficulties and maximize abilities. A therapist is a helper. The kind of helper may vary. The therapist may help by teaching, giving support, aiding in communication, engineering opportunities for growth, confronting problems, clarifying, reinforcing progress, or promoting plans for the future. In the therapeutic context the therapist may be friendly but never the client's "friend," "buddy," or close confidante. This means that the therapist especially must monitor the influence of personal needs and feelings. If, for example, a therapist has a strong need to prove that occupational therapy will cure a client, the therapist risks feeling angry if the client rejects help offered or may feel disappointed if the client fails to respond. Either reaction would be a distortion and ultimately not helpful to the client. Because the maintenance of objectivity within the relationship is important, it is helpful and often necessary for the therapist to have another professional with whom to discuss feelings and events as they arise.

People with psychiatric problems may have great difficulty in developing healthy and health-promoting relationships with other people. Often the relationships that they have experienced either just before becoming ill or throughout longer periods of their lives have been negative. The precedents for human relationships may be fraught with distortions. There may be unrealistic positive or negative expectations of authority figures. Other human beings may be perceived as lacking constancy or predictability or as being threatening or hurtful. On the other hand, the emotional needs of the client may be so powerful as to cloak the reality of the situation in a cloud of wish-fulfillment. Frank[16] has referred to the problems of avoidance, selective inattention, and self-fulfilling prophecy on the part of the client. Fear of being hurt or of an unknown new mode of behavior may function to prevent the client's correction of a pathological self-image. It is the task of the therapist to break through these problems and to develop with the client a new, different set of transactions, ones which will "confirm healthy expectations and disappoint pathological ones."

Initially it is necessary to gain some measure of the client's trust. Trust is a feeling which is based on the perception of the therapist's ability and caring. Trust potentiates motivation. A client who trusts the therapist will be more easily motivated to participate in the occupational therapy process than one who does not feel trust. The issues of trust and motivation are important throughout the entire time the therapist and client are involved with one another.

How are trust and motivation developed? In the therapeutic context there may be many factors. Apart from the direct interpersonal experiences of the therapist and client, there may be the distant uninvolved appraisal the client may make of the therapist based on observations of the transactions between the therapist and other clients or other staff members. There may be the "halo" effect of the encouragement to be involved in occupational therapy from the client's physician, other staff members, or other clients. The client may have made a simple, uncritical judgment based on wish-fulfillment that, if the therapist is on the staff, the therapist must know how to help.

It is, however, in the direct interpersonal transactions between the therapist and the client that true and effective trust is established and reinforced. It is first necessary for the therapist to communicate empathy for the client's feelings and respect for the client as a human being. Such communication may be very simple, like a nod, or asking the client how he or she wishes to be called rather than automatically using a first name, nickname, or a formal name.[17] Communication must be clear and consistent throughout the total process. This is not always easy. The silent, nonverbal client who may be depressed and despairing, for example, may show a strong wish to avoid involvement. The client who may be acting out feelings with hostile language or behavior may seem to be trying to "put the therapist off." The paranoid person who is suspicious or the schizophrenic client who is prompted by hallucinations to behave strangely may make it difficult for the therapist to communicate empathy and respect. Yet, it is these people who most need to feel they are cared for and valued in spite of the strange or threatening behaviors they show. Unless they feel valued it is not really worth the effort for them to invest in making changes. The therapist too must be able to recognize the pain that underlies their behavior in order to wish to invest in making a change process possible. Sometimes this means sitting silently with a client. Sometimes it means confronting behavior or setting clear limits in a way that indicates an expectation that change is possible. It always means maintaining a clear contact with reality and being willing to communicate that reality to the client who needs to know that the therapist can be counted on to point out what is real.

The therapist's own self-confidence and self-knowledge are critical to the development of a truly therapeutic relationship. It is the therapist's knowledge base, combined with the therapist's personal trust in his or her own skills, that make it possible for the therapist to have the confidence necessary to instill confidence in the client. What the therapist knows about the disease or deficit, about the client, and about the kinds of interventions occupational therapy can make will determine the effectiveness of what is communicated about the program. If the client experiences the program as effective, this will promote trust and motivation.

There are a number of fears which often inhibit a client's willingness to participate in occupational therapy. Many of the ordinary things which are part of normal living, such as sometimes expressing anger, or receiving anger expressed by someone else, or making a mistake, may be perceived by the client as extremely risky. In the therapeutic relationship an important contribution may be made when the therapist who is trusted expresses or receives anger without becoming upset, or makes a mistake and is able to admit it.

There are certain other issues that may emerge in the course of a therapeutic relationship in occupational therapy. Among these are dependency, control, and transference. The ultimate goal of the program is to facilitate the client's ability to function as successfully as possible. This means recognizing the issues when they arise, often naming them with the client, and planning strategies for dealing with them. The frame of reference within which the therapist is working will determine the way in which issues are perceived and the kinds of strategies that may be used. For example, dependent behavior will be identified in terms of specific, dependent actions within a *behavioral* frame of reference, and the therapist's role will be to try to develop reinforcement schedules to effect a reduction in the specific behavior. Dependent behavior within a *developmental* frame of reference will be seen in terms of the sequence of developmental needs,[18] and the therapist will try to construct strategies for the client to experience success at the existing level of function so that a sense of competence is fostered, promoting the ability to move toward greater independence.

The *occupational behavior* frame of reference would approach the problem similarly, but with some major considerations being given to the role and functions expected of the client in society. Dependency, viewed *psychoanalytically*, would be regarded as a manifestation of deeper, unconscious needs. As such, it might be dealt with on a symbolic reenactment basis, in which the therapist allows the client to use the activities and the relationship of the occupational therapy process to explore and to relive in a more positive way the events which originally fostered pathological growth. The *sensory integrative* approach would focus primarily on promoting the client's basic perceptual and motor abilities in order to foster a better body image and more effective reality testing. This in turn would lead to a greater sense of or desire for independence in functioning.

At all stages in the course of the therapeutic relationship, initiation, implementation, and termination, it is important to remember that the relationship is a dynamic one involving both therapist and client. Their concepts of themselves and others, as well as their values and biases, will affect the quality and extent of their commitment to a program of change. In this way, an authentic, acting, feeling self on the part of the therapist lends strength to the relationship.

THE ACTIVITY

It has been said that activity is the bridge between one's inner reality and the external world. It is through our activities that we are connected with life and with other human beings. Through the activities in which we engage, we learn about the world, test our knowledge, practice skills, express our feelings, experience pleasure, take care of our needs for survival, develop competence, and achieve mastery over our destinies.

Some element of volition is involved in mental,

physical, and social activities. It is this type of volitional activity that is important in the occupational therapy process. The use of activity which is carefully planned to facilitate change in the client is a unique characteristic of occupational therapy. The activities used in psychiatric occupational therapy are highly influenced by the total treatment context, but also may be significant in *determining* the nature of that context. Limitations on the kinds of activities which may be used are imposed by the environment, materials, or resources available as well as the extent of the therapist's knowledge, skill, interests, and creativity.

Occupational therapists in psychiatry may use activities in a number of ways. General categories into which occupational therapy activities may fall include body movement and exercise, individual and team sports, games, crafts, personal hygiene and grooming, activities of daily living or life skills, prevocational practice, horticulture, work, and creative activity.

Activities may be used as part of the initial assessment process and have, inherently, a function in the ongoing evaluation process. Observation and/or measurement of the client's performance, behavior, and end product in the execution of an activity can yield much valuable information to aid in determining the directions of treatment. The relatively objective nature of data obtained in the activity process is valuable to the therapist and to other members of the treatment team. But most importantly, it is valuable to the client.

A difficult problem which is encountered with a large number of psychiatrically ill clients is their inability to understand their personal assets and limitations. Often activities that involve manipulating objects, tools, and materials and producing something finished at the end provide concrete evidence which can be used to help the client to test reality about himself or herself.

Activities used within a group context or on a dyadic interaction basis, may provide a focus around which the individuals involved can relate to one another. When working together on a task, individuals have an opportunity to explore and practice dimensions of interpersonal relationships in ways that may be either provocative or "safe."

Freely creative or projective activities have long been employed within the psychoanalytic frame of reference, as a communication link with unconscious processes and, as such, have made useful diagnostic contributions.

Occupational therapy is concerned with promoting the ability of clients to function in their own worlds. Activities can provide the ground for exploration and learning, practicing, and achieving mastery. They permit function from the simplest, developmentally earliest, and nonverbal levels to the most complex, most mature levels. It is the task of the occupational therapist to understand the meaning of activity and to know how to determine the potential of each given activity for promoting performance.

Activity Analysis

Activity analysis is essential in making a match between the needs, interests, and abilities of the client and the activities that will help to bring about growth or change. Activities may be analyzed with respect to a number of important dimensions. The frame of reference may determine which dimensions of the activity are to be emphasized and the depth with which some of the dimensions are to be explored and exploited. At this point in the development of psychiatric occupational therapy there is no universally accepted method of activity analysis. In general, it is useful to think of the several aspects of experience and/or functional requirements of the activity, then analyze each of these in terms of its gradability. Time requirements and cultural implications of the activity should also be explored.

One example of an activity analysis based on concepts of human development is given at the end of Chapter 5. Figure 12-2 is another example of a form used to do activity analysis in a long-term hospital setting. Figure 12-3 is an example of the analysis of one specific activity.

Activity analysis based upon a *behavioral* frame of reference will be concerned especially with the specification and seriation of the component parts of the activity, their potential as or need for reinforcement contingencies, and the measurability of data. Activity analysis based upon a *psychoanalytic* frame of reference will pay special attention to the symbolic, expressive, and interpersonal aspects of the activity. Based upon a *sensory integrative*

(*Text continues on* p. 303.)

FIGURE 12-2. Activity analysis in a long-term hospital setting. Developed by the Occupational Therapy Staff of Norristown State Hospital, Norristown PA. Printed with permission.

ACTIVITY ANALYSIS

I. General Information
   A. Name of Activity
   B. Specific Purpose of Activity according to treatment goals

   C. Type of Activity—work related, leisure time, culturally determined, economic implications, role identification, sexual connotation.

II. Materials
   A. Specific Materials
   B. Nature of these materials
      Resistive ____
      Pliable ____
      Controlled ____
      Messy ____
   C. Sensory Input
      Tactile ____
      Auditory ____
      Olfactory ____
      Visual ____
      Taste ____
      Kinesthetic (joint movement) ____
   D. Color
      A. Number and names
      B. Variability (light to dark)

III. Parts of Activity
   A. Number of parts ____
   B. Complexity of part—one step repeated ____, two steps repeated ____, more than two steps repeated ____.

IV. Preparation
   A. Precutting
   B. Provide pattern
   C. Provide sample
   D. Pre-arrangement of supplies (explain)
   E. Re-arrangement of environment (explain)

V. Directions
   A. Demonstration with assistance
   B. Demonstration of each part
   C. Demonstration of whole task
   D. Verbal: part/whole
   E. Written: part/whole

VI. Amount of structure and controls (rules) inherent in activity

VII. Predictability of Results

VIII. Learning Required

	Whole Task	Part One	Part Two	Part Three	Part Four
Old	______	______	______	______	______
Adapted Old	______	______	______	______	______
New	______	______	______	______	______

IX. Decisions required by patient (explain)

X. Attention span (hours, minutes)

XI. Interaction: solitary, parallel play, interaction with one other person, interaction in small group, interaction in large group, competition, cooperation, taking turns.

XII. Communication: little required, nonverbal communication, one word, 10–15 words necessary, common environmental words, reciprocal language, oral directions, reading, writing.

XIII. Motivation: useful, decorative, prestigious, successful, intellectually challenging, effect on others, creative, gratifying.

XIV. Additional Comments:

FIGURE 12-3. Sample of activity analysis form for one specific activity.

ACTIVITY ANALYSIS

Activity: digging and planting a garden plot

Time Requirement (average range for successful completion): one hour.

Average no. of sessions required to complete: one, but may be done in several short sessions, if needed.

Brief Description (including criteria for determining success):

Garden plot 5′ × 5′. Requires digging with spade, raking to remove stones, marking out three rows, planting seeds or small plants.

Success may be determined by the extent to which all the ground is turned over and stone free, and the planting is completed.

Characteristics of Activity	Input	Skills	How can activity be graded?
Physical:			
Gross motor	X	X	The preparation of the 5′ × 5′ plot in advance will determine the amount of physical work required. A new area will require far more effort than a previously dug area.
Fine Motor	X	X	
Strength	X	X	
Rhythm	X	X	
Repetition	X	X	The nature of the seeds or plants will determine how much fine motor skill is required.
Coordination		X	
Passive			
Active		X	

(Continued)

Characteristics of Activity	Input	Skills	How can activity be graded?
Sensory:			
Tactile	X	X	The kinds of tools provided, the kinds of seeds or plants; their relative size, texture, fragility, fragrance. Use of hose or can to water.
Visual	X	X	
Auditory	X		
Olfactory	X		
Gustatory			
Perceptual:			
Tactile	X	X	The kinds of tools, seeds or plants; the amount of lifting, bending, stooping.
Visual space	X	X	
Visual form	X	X	
Vestibular	X	X	
Proprioceptive	X	X	
Kinesthetic	X	X	
Part—Whole		X	
Auditory—Language	possibly		
Auditory figure—Ground	possibly		
Visual figure—Ground	X	X	
Bilateral integration	X	X	
Body scheme	X	X	
Motor planning	X	X	
Cognitive:			Immediate feedback with regard to effects of digging, raking, and changes made in the plot.
Object permanence	X	X	
Causality	X	X	Delayed feedback with regard to growth of plants or harvest crop.
Goal establishment		X	
Goal implementation		X	Therapist may grade means of instruction from use of immediate imitation to verbal or written directions.
Imitation		X	
Trial-and-error problem solving		X	
Seriation		X	Instructions may involve degrees of seriation.
Organize parts into whole		X	Most of the skills involved rely on schemes which are familiar, even if total activity is not.
Interpret signs, symbols		X	

Characteristics of Activity	Input	Skills	How can activity be graded?
Cognitive: (Continued)			
Read			
Use imagination, creativity			
Perceive viewpoint of others			
Test reality		X	
Decenter		X	
Logical thinking			
Hypothetical thinking			
Social-Emotional:			
Control, lead		X	The activity is highly gradable with regard to leadership, dependence, number of interpersonal interactions involved.
Follow, cooperate		X	
Independence		X	The heavy work component may be useful in terms of emotional expression or sublimation.
Dependence		X	
Impulse control		X	
Handle feelings		X	
Work with one other person		X	
Work in a small group		X	
Work in a large group			
Test reality (consensual validation)	X	X	
Play	possibly		

Cultural implications of the activity, with attention to factors which would indicate its relevance to individual life situations:

Activity is familiar to most clients from suburban or rural areas. To city dwellers, the activity may be less relevant, although it tends to be the kind of "new" activity which can be interesting because of its implications for providing a valuable product. The activity is fairly universally understood.

frame of reference, it will be focused primarily on the sensory, perceptual, and physical aspects of the activity, especially in terms of the kinds of input which may be experienced. From a *developmental* perspective, it will be concerned with the parallels between levels of functioning required or expected and developmental levels. In the *occupational behavior* frame of reference, activity analysis will be concerned with developmental levels and the potential of the activity for providing meaningful opportunities for individuals to develop competence and balance within their life roles in society.

There is little doubt that there is a vital need in occupational therapy for in-depth research into the actual meanings of activity as used in occupational therapy and into certain other aspects, such as the transfer of learning.

THE CONTEXT

The settings in which psychiatric occupational therapists currently practice in psychiatry have become varied and complex. Now, in addition to hospitals, one finds therapists working with clients in community centers, satellite clinics, schools, centers for specialized populations, homes, and correctional institutions, to name a few new settings. In terms of space, this means that the occupational therapist does not always work with clients in a well-equipped, well-defined place, such as the Occupational Therapy Shop of a large state hospital. It means that the occupational therapist may often be challenged to plan how to carry out treatment in environments which are not easily controllable but which are close to or part of the realities of the client's life.

The teams with whom occupational therapists work have also become more diversified in the past decade. Instead of, or in addition to, the traditional medical team, occupational therapists in some settings may find themselves working with teachers, business persons, politicians, and members of the clergy as well as the family, friends, and neighbors of the client. Occupational therapists must broaden their knowledge base to include deeper understanding of social, economic, cultural, and political factors and forces. It challenges occupational therapists to become more sensitive to the significance of personal biases and value systems as they affect interpersonal transactions within these contexts.

There is a special need for the occupational therapist to be flexible enough to work in a role which often seems very much blended with the roles of others. This may present either a problem or an opportunity, depending upon how confident the occupational therapist is about the principles of occupational therapy practice and its conceptual bases.

REFERENCES

1. Millon, T.: Theories of Psychopathology and Personality. Philadelphia: W. B. Saunders Co., 1973.
2. King, L. J.: A sensory integrative approach to schizophrenia. Am. J. Occup. Ther. 28:529–536, 1974.
3. King, L. J.: Psychiatric Occupational Therapy Workshop, Temple University, Philadelphia, 1977.
4. Sieg, K.: Applying the behavioral model to the OT model. Am. J. Occup. Ther. 28:422, 1974.
5. Ibid, pp. 421–428.
6. Norman, C. W.: Behavior modification: A perspective. Am. J. Occup. Ther. 30:491–497, 1976.
7. Llorens, L.: Facilitating growth and development: The promise of occupational therapy. Am. J. Occup. Ther. 24:93–101, 1970.
8. Mosey, A. C.: Recapitulation of ontogenesis. Am. J. Occup. Ther. 22:426–438, 1968.

8a. Allen, C., and Lewis, N.: Workshop series notes. Philadelphia PA and Baltimore MD, 1972.

9. Levy, L.: Movement therapy for psychiatric patients. Am. J. Occup. Ther. 28:354–357, 1974.
10. Mosey, A. C.: Occupational Therapy: Theory and Practice. Medford MA: Pothier Bros., 1968.
11. Reilly, M. (ed.): Play as Exploratory Learning. Beverly Hills CA: Sage Publishing Co., 1974.
12. Reilly, M.: A psychiatric occupational therapy program as a teaching model. Am. J. Occup. Ther. 20:66–67, 1966.
13. DiMascio, A., and Shader, R. I. (eds.): Clinical Handbook of Psychopharmacology. New York: Jason Aronson, 1970.
14. Physicians' Desk Reference, ed. 31. Oradell NJ: Medical Economics Co., 1977.
15. Shader, R. I. (ed.): Manual of Psychiatric Therapeutics. New York: Little, Brown & Co., 1975.
16. Frank, J.: The therapeutic use of self. Am. J. Occup. Ther. 12:215, 1958.
17. Purtilo, R.: The Allied Health Professional and the Patient. Philadelphia: W. B. Saunders Co., 1973.
18. Mosey, A. C.: Recapitulation of ontogenesis, p. 427.

section 3/The Occupational Therapy Process: Treatment, Maintenance, Rehabilitation, and Prevention

The process of bringing together the client, the therapist, the activity, and the context for the purpose of providing treatment, maintenance, rehabilitation, or preventive services is the essence of occupational therapy. The context and the status of the client usually determine whether the process is geared to treatment, maintenance of function, rehabilitation, or prevention, although often the therapist may move from treatment to rehabilitation to prevention as the client is helped to achieve increasing autonomy and competence.

The treatment process is one of intervening

directly in the pathology of the client and of effecting changes or interruptions in the illness itself. Behavior therapy techniques and sensory integration techniques in psychiatry are often clearly geared to treatment. So are many of the psychoanalytically-based techniques. Maintenance of function refers to the process which must take place when dealing with clients who have chronic debilitating or deteriorating conditions. Occupational therapy then is based on strengths and geared to the promotion of optimum functioning as long as possible. The developmental and occupational behavior frames of reference place greater emphasis on building upon the strengths and healthy parts of the client; they therefore seem to make their major contributions in the areas of rehabilitation, maintenance, and prevention.

There are five sequential parts to the occupational therapy process: initial assessment, development of objectives, development of plan, implementation of the plan, and termination of the program. Evaluation of the client's progress, keeping records, and making reports are ongoing or periodic processes which keep the program current, relevant, and effective. Table 12–4 and Figure 12–4 are examples of this process.

ASSESSMENT/EVALUATION*

It is essential that the occupational therapist gain a baseline of information about the client before initiating or proceeding with the development of objectives, a plan, and a program. Assessment requires the collection of data and the organization of the data into a meaningful description of the client. In addition to providing an understanding of the client's current illness or problems and their effect on his or her life, it should incorporate information about his or her work, social and cultural worlds, value systems, skills, and interests.

The occupational therapist needs to have the knowledge and judgment to determine what information will be relevant and essential to provide a meaningful occupational therapy program within the chosen frame of reference. There must also be a commitment to an attitude of ongoing evaluation, through which the effectiveness of the program will be determined.

The evaluation process is often helpful in eliciting the interest and cooperation of the client. The establishment of motivation on the part of the client to be involved in occupational therapy is often accomplished through early and continuing collaboration in assessing the problem.

The sections which follow will describe some of the standard ways of doing assessment or evaluation in psychiatric occupational therapy, including observation, getting data from other sources, interviewing, projective techniques, activity evaluation, developmental evaluation, ADL evaluation, prevocational evaluation, perceptual-motor evaluation, inventories, and check lists.

Observation

The skill of the therapist to observe well is critical to all kinds of assessment procedures. The therapist must be able to see, listen to, and pay attention to the intangible feeling tones, which are part of the client's acts and communications, as well as to the more obvious and measurable behaviors. The occupational therapist is in a particularly advantageous position because in the use of carefully planned activities there is a structure for controlled as well as spontaneous observation. Activities provide opportunities for nonverbal and verbal communication to take place.

It is important to think about and know about the kinds of things which may be observed. In a task that involves perceptual motor skill, for example, the therapist must be sensitive to the fact that, if the client consistently changes hands to cross the midline, it may be important; or in a group activity, if a client consistently sits outside of the main circle, it means something. Standardized assessment procedures usually provide guides to observation of relevant behaviors or responses. Before using one of these methods, it is important to review not only the methods to be used but the kinds of general and specific behaviors that might be observed.

Sensitivity to seeing, hearing, and feeling the communications of others is a variable which is subject to a number of factors. Some people are naturally

(Text continues on p. 309.)

* In general, "assessment" is used to mean the initial data-gathering process and "evaluation" refers to subsequent checks on the client's status and effectiveness of the occupational therapy program.

Table 12-4. One example: occupational therapy process in psychiatry.

The client, Ms. S., is a 26-year-old unmarried woman. She lives alone in a small apartment in the downtown area of a small city. She works as a clerk in a supermarket. She became anxious and depressed following transfer to a new location in her job. She has been unable to work or take care of her meals, laundry, and cleaning. After a brief hospitalization during which she received treatment, she was transferred to the day program of a community mental health center. This chart shows the process of treatment and rehabilitation in occupational therapy.

Initial Assessment	*Objectives*	*Plan*	*Implementation*	*Reevaluation*	*Termination*
METHODS USED: Interview, activities configuration, interest inventory, activity battery, records, and team conference.	LONG TERM: Ms. S. will be able to set priorities on her time and energy.	Starting with following a standard schedule of the center, Ms. S. will be encouraged to plan for substitute activities of her own choosing, gradually incorporating activities which are part of her normal life routine.	Ms. S. started working with a task group, attending weekly, joined bowling activity. Followed written schedule of standard activities.	Observation and periodic interviews to review progress.	Treatment on a daily basis was weaned gradually.
INFORMATION GAINED: *Family:* out of touch. *Friends:* a few good friends. *Education:* finished high school, started but did not finish beauty culture course.	SHORT TERM: Ms. S. will be able to plan a schedule of activities for a typical day and follow it with encouragement from therapist.			Ms. S. was initially reluctant but gained interest after a few minor successes.	Evening program is still providing encouragement and support.
Work: present job since high school. Considers work "a drag," but says she was "pretty good at it." *Interests:* television, bowling, paperback mysteries. *Self-care:* used to be "fussy" but in illness unable to cope or care very much. *Self-assessment:* feels "all apart"—but not so hopeless as before hospitalization. Wants to get better.	SHORT TERM: Ms. S. will be able to complete one simple task within reasonable time frame.	Support of therapist, other staff and patient group to be gradually lifted as Ms. S. gains feelings of competence.	Completed individual project of a datebook and calendar for personal use. Began to incorporate personal marketing weekly and to schedule housecleaning in her apartment.	She spent a long time on the datebook, but afterwards began to be interested in filling in plans of her own.	
STRENGTHS: able to work cooperatively and can carry out a task with support. Motivated to improve.			Eventually returned to job—came to center twice a week in the evening for therapy.		
PROBLEMS: decision making, meeting time requirements.					

ACTIVITY THERAPY EVALUATION (Part 1)

I. Collection of data	II. Synthesis and interpretation of data	III. Statement of problems amenable to treatment by activity therapy	IV. Goals	V. Recommendations
1. Interview 2. Observation 3. Reports from A.T. Clinics & other professionals		Work Leisure Self-care 1. Interpersonal skills 2. Cognition 3. Self-expression and awareness 4. Motor 5. Perceptual motor	Short-term Long-term	Level I: O.T., R.T., S.T. Level II: O.T., R.T., S.T. Level III: O.T., R.T., S.T. Basic living skills Physical exercise Art Therapy Dance therapy Assertive training Sex education Vocational rehabilitation Leisure counseling Skill development PAC Social skills Task group Career planning

"Each new patient is interviewed regarding current level of functioning in work, leisure, and self-care. His idea of personal goals, assets, and limitations are evaluated. After this the patient goes through our evaluation clinic which is designed to observe performance in a cognitive task, a small group task, a competitive group, and in an unstructured situation. The data from the interview and the clinic are synthesized into a formal report, the Activity Therapy Initial Summary. This report is fed into the team's assessment for consideration of the total treatment plan. Patients are referred to (1) goal-oriented programs, (2) leisure time skill development programs, or (3) unstructured open activities. Progress notes are fed from the various group leaders to the Activity Therapy Representatives on each hall for summary progress notes which are placed in the medical record. We are also developing guidelines for a discharge summary."

Diane Maslen, M.S., O.T.R.
Director, Activity Therapy

FIGURE 12-4. Sample of activity therapy evaluation. From Activity Therapy Department of Sheppard and Enoch Pratt Hospital, Towson MD. Printed with permission.

ACTIVITY THERAPY EVALUATION (Part 2)

1. Almost never
2. Seldom
3. Occasionally
4. Frequently
5. Most of the time
6. Almost always

Patient's Name ______ Case # ______ Hall ______ Group ______

Date ______ A. T. Staff ______

Dates Attended ______

Reason for not attending ______

	1.	2.	3.	4.	5.	6.
INTERPERSONAL/PSYCHOLOGICAL FUNCTIONING						
A. Demonstrates ability to make own decisions						
B. Absence of nonproductive behaviors (rocking, playing with hands, repetitive movements, preoccupation)						
C. Demonstrates awareness of others' needs/feelings						
D. Cooperation with task, group, staff (verbal/nonverbal)						
E. Expression of affect (spontaneous, clear, appropriate)						
F. Demonstrates ability to initiate, respond, and sustain verbal interaction						
G. Self-direction in unstructured setting and/or task						
H. Demonstrates ability to compromise and negotiate						
I. Demonstrates ability to convincingly state opinions or disagree without aggression						
J. Demonstrates desire to win without hostility						
K. Accepts authority, yet can state own opinions						
L. Accepts body image						
M. Appropriate appearance (clothes, grooming) in relation to role, social group situation, age, and sex						
N. Recognizes and acts on own needs and feelings						
COGNITIVE/TASK SKILLS						
A. Reality orientation (oriented to person, place, time, and situation)						
B. Follows directions (3 oral)						
C. One hour attention span (1=5, 2=10, 3=15, 4=30, 5=45, 6=60 min.)						
D. Demonstrates ability to concentrate despite distraction						
E. Remembers instructions						
F. Can solve problems abstractly (uses covert images)						
G. Demonstrates ability to engage in structured activity without staff encouragement						
H. Neatness in activity						
I. Able to organize fairly complex task (plan, understand, perform)						
J. Tolerates frustration						
K. Appropriate pace in activity						
L. Assumes responsibility for own actions, thoughts, feelings						
MOTOR SKILLS						
A. Adequate posture (shoulders back, head erect)						
B. Endurance (moderate exercise for 60 min.)						
C. Demonstrates spontaneous reactions and reflexes						
D. Demonstrates adequate gross motor, coordination for task (movement patterns, balance, hand-eye coordination, proprioception)						
E. Demonstrates adequate fine motor coordination for task (hand manipulative skills, eye-hand coordination, perceptual motor)						

FIGURE 12-4. *(Continued)*

better observers than others. It is possible, however, for one to develop skills in observation. In addition to basic ability, the perceptual and cognitive "sets" of the observer are important. What will be attended to is directly influenced by what the observer knows about the client and the situation or task in which he or she may be involved and by the expectations which this knowledge may have engendered. One's perceptual and cognitive sets are further influenced by personal biases and value systems and by the level of anxiety or other emotional factors which might enter into the situation. It is important to be aware that this is true and, with that awareness, in the clinical setting, to work toward the achievement of as much objectification as possible. Objectification of the process of observation is helped by planning ahead or by seeking consensual validation from others who may also have been in a position to observe the client.

Interview

An interview is a planned conversation, conducted for a specified purpose. For most clients, the initial interview with the occupational therapist launches the occupational therapy process. It is in the initial interview that the first contact may be made to establish understanding about the purposes of further evaluation and the occupational therapy program itself. It is in the initial interview that the client has an opportunity to share information about his or her problems and situation and to begin to think about making changes.

The therapist needs to plan the interview so that there will be time to explore fully the aspects of the client's history and current status which will be helpful in setting objectives. The types of information gained may depend upon the frame of reference, but there are general areas which provide important information regardless of frame of reference. These might include the client's interests and skills, most recent living situation, existing support systems, what the client thinks about his or her illness, and what the client's hopes for the future are. Other questions that can provide valuable information relate to the client's history. What is the client's educational background? Where and at what kinds of jobs did the client work? How did the client feel about school or work? If he or she left school or work, why? It is in such questions that the therapist gains information about the strengths and weaknesses and the assets and liabilities which have characterized the client's life before illness. The questions the therapist asks the client in the course of the interview will communicate the tone and the interest of the occupational therapist and the nature of the occupational therapy program. The therapist needs to be clear and knowledgeable in the choice of questions, so that they will encourage realistic expectations on the part of the client with regard to occupational therapy.

The environment in which the interview takes place is important. It should be comfortable, quiet, and as distraction-free as possible. This is not always easy to achieve, but it can make a big difference in the success of the interview.

The therapist should clearly state at the outset the purpose of the interview and his or her role in relation to the client. This allows for some further explanation of the purpose of occupational therapy. The therapist's attitudes in the initial interview are the keystone for the rapport and continuing relationship that will be developed. It is essential to feel and to communicate respect, interest, and empathy for the client and confidence that the process will be beneficial.

The information that has been gained in the interview should be available to the client. The notes that the therapist makes during the interview should be made openly. It may be useful for the client to review them. When the interview is reaching its conclusion, the therapist should make this clear to the client. A summary or review of the discussion is often a helpful way to conclude the interview. The therapist will want to let the client know what is to happen next and make an appointment for future contacts and assessment procedures.

There may be other occasions to use the interview technique as an ongoing evaluation procedure. At the termination of the occupational therapy program, especially, an interview may be of great value. It provides an opportunity to review and assess the progress which has been made and to reinforce the learning which has taken place.

The Interest Inventory, Activities Configuration, and Object History described in Chapter 10 provide additional valuable information which may supplement the interview.

Data from Other Sources

There is a wealth of information available from assessment efforts when a team of coprofessionals work together. The pooling of data from all team members may yield a coherent and valid picture of the client. It is essential that the occupational therapist be clear about the pieces of information contributed by team members so that unnecessary duplication of effort (and aggravation to the client) will not occur. For example, a social worker may be able to provide much needed information about the client's home and family.

Psychological tests may give information about certain aspects of the client's intelligence or unconscious motivations. Some tests commonly used by psychologists contain information of special value in developing an occupational therapy plan. The psychiatric occupational therapist may especially wish to check out results in such tests as the Wechsler or Stanford-Binet for intelligence, the Rorschach, Thematic Apperception, and Minnesota Multiphasic Personality Inventory for personality orientation and unconscious material, and the Bender-Gestalt or Draw-a-Person for organic disease. The observations of ward personnel, the charted medications, and comments about transactions between the psychiatrist and client are also significant to understanding the gestalt of the client in the treatment setting.

Activity Evaluation

The careful identification of skills required to carry out activities is the key to treatment in occupational therapy as a whole; the continuing observation of a client's performance is the key to the essential process of ongoing evaluation. Certain specified, uniform tasks, which call upon identified skills for their accomplishment, lend themselves well to the processes of initial and periodic evaluation. The success of the use of activities as evaluation tools relies upon the accuracy and detail of activity analysis. The therapist must be quite clear about the kinds of information that may be gained through the use of a specified task. Almost any task may be used evaluatively, but it is important that the therapist have a clear idea about the skills and time requirements for "normal" performance. It is generally useful to select activities that may be completed in one session, although there may be times when the evaluation of a client's ability to postpone gratification or of a client's frustration tolerance may indicate the use of longer-term projects.

One advantage to the use of activities as evaluation procedures is that the range of traits that can be tested is great and there is wide flexibility in planning. A second advantage is that the use of activities may promote a truly cooperative effort between the client and the therapist in the implementation of treatment. Their heuristic value to the client is in terms of the client's own wishes to feel and to function better. This is easily communicated around activities performance. Establishing the validity and reliability of activity evaluation procedures, however, constitutes one of the major disadvantages of the technique and one of the major challenges to the profession of occupational therapy.

Mosey suggests the use of concepts of present and future levels of functioning as part of the evaluation. "Future" levels of functioning refers to those skills that are related to the client's "anticipated, expected environment."[1] As examples, consider the mother who expects to regain the ability to care for her three children, cook for her family, and keep the house in order; the factory worker who will return to a job requiring attention and manual dexterity, not to mention getting up at five o'clock in the morning; the office manager who will need skills in interpersonal relationships and problem solving. Evaluation of present skills in relation to future demands gives the occupational therapy process a reality and validity which can usually be communicated and mutually understood.

Developmental Assessment

The collection and organization of data in terms of the normal developmental continuum has proven to be useful and empirically successful in the occupational therapy process. Although in psychiatric occupational therapy there has always been some attention to the process of development and to developmental approaches using Freud's concepts of psychosexual development or Erikson's eight crises and the age-specific educational theories, the publication of Mosey's "Recapitulation of Ontogenesis"[2] focused attention on specific ways in which clients could be assessed and treated in terms of adaptive skill development. The organization of adaptive skills may be assessed by a number of different methods and then charted to give a picture of the client. The evaluation of adaptive skills lends itself well to treatment planning. (See Chapter 7.)

Another method, developed by Allen and Lewis, focuses on developmental levels of cognitive skills. The identification of cognitive levels in such a plan is based on the ways in which the client uses imitation and perceives causality, object permanence, and time. Levels of functioning are determined in terms of Piagetian concepts of sensorimotor development and the cognitive gains that are made in normal development during this period. Developmental approaches to evaluation presuppose the importance of identifying the client's current level of functioning as the necessary starting point of treatment. People who are mentally ill regress to earlier stages of development and earlier levels of functioning. The therapist needs to identify not only in what areas and to what levels regression has taken place at a given point in time but also what circumstances or activities tend to make the patient function well and experience success or function poorly and further regress. The Piagetian concept of "familiar schemes" is important and developmental evaluations should include some attention to activities the patient knows well and can perform easily.

Techniques such as interview, activities configuration, and interest and activities evaluations all lend themselves well to contributing to the data used in developmental assessment. In certain settings and with certain kinds of clients, perceptual testing may also be important.

Perceptual-Motor Evaluation

Testing procedures described elsewhere in this book (Chapter 10) have been adapted by therapists for use with psychiatrically disabled clients. These are especially important in pediatric psychiatric problems and with the chronically institutionalized patient. Because most of the standard procedures have been developed and standardized for pediatric populations, their use with adult populations can only indicate trends or possible areas of difficulty. Some therapists have incorporated the Bender-Gestalt, Draw-a-Person, and Purdue tests into their standard testing battery. At the present time, the therapist's ability to observe and identify perceptual-motor performance in a variety of sensory motor activities would seem the basic tool. Walking with a shuffling gait, evidence of auditory or tactile defensiveness, visual or auditory constancy problems, inability to cross the midline in the performance of tasks, rocking behavior, awkwardness, and inaccurate motions are some of the clues indicating the possibility of sensory integrative dysfunction.

Projective Techniques

There is a degree of projection in everything we do and in all things that we produce. As Hammer says, "One's way of walking, whether proudly, boldly, timidly, arrogantly, self-consciously or stridently; one's way of hammering a nail, whether confidently, impatiently, irritatedly, rhythmically or joyfully; even one's way of lacing a shoe, whether one alloplastically places one's foot on a hydrant or fence post thus bringing the shoe up to one's self, or whether one autoplastically brings one's self all the way down to the ground to encounter the shoe lace—all reflect some fact of one's personality."[3]

This element of projection of otherwise often inexpressible parts of the personality is an important part of the total occupational therapy process. Sensitivity to the symbolic as well as the concrete representations in all aspects of doing activities is a primary requirement of good observation. Procedures known as projective tests or techniques are geared specifically to allowing communication of unconscious material in this way.

In settings where the frame of reference for treatment is primarily psychoanalytic, the use of projective techniques may be indicated as a standard form of evaluation. The vast array of unconscious material which a client might present in clay, drawings, or other free-form media has frequently encouraged occupational therapists to work in close collaboration with other therapists, usually psychiatrists. Projective techniques can yield a wide range of diagnostically useful information. The success of the occupational therapist in the use of these techniques is dependent upon a number of factors: (1) the therapist's sophistication about psychodynamics and psychoanalytic theory and practice, (2) the nature of the client population, and (3) the quality and extent of the therapist's own emotional maturity and self-knowledge.

Art, dance, and music therapists rely heavily upon projection as a primary point of entry and ongoing evaluation technique in the therapeutic process. There are a number of projective *testing* procedures, however, which may be used. Standardized tests such as the Thematic Apperception Test and the Rorschach are tools of the clinical psychologist and require specialized training for administering and interpreting. Occupational therapists have developed and adapted some procedures which lend themselves well to the occupational therapy setting.

The prototype of the occupational therapy projective techniques is the Azima Battery.[4] In this, the client is asked to produce something, using first pencil, then fingerpaints, then clay. In this way, the person moves from the simplest two-dimensional, achromatic mode to a more primitive, less controllable, chromatic, two-dimensional mode, and finally to a three-dimensional, regressive mode. In working with the three different materials, the client produces unconscious material. The subtle movement to earlier developmental stages in the sequence is experienced symbolically and often unconsciously through the feeling of the media. This appears to elicit progressively deeper levels of repressed material.

Other projective techniques which have been developed by occupational therapists include the Fidler Diagnostic Battery,[5] the Magazine Picture Collage,[6] and variations of the Draw-a-Person technique. These techniques have proven empirically useful; there have been some attempts to standardize them but there is still much to be done in this area.

Some therapists have sought training and incorporated the use of standardized procedures, such as the House-Tree-Person, or Person-in-the-Rain tests into their evaluation batteries.[7] Group projective techniques, in which the interactional elements of personality are especially communicated, are another interesting variation. Among these would be the production of group drawings, collages, and fingerpaintings.

The sophisticated therapist may learn much about the client's feelings, conflicts, self-image, values, and cognitive processes through the themes and organization created in projective techniques. There are, of course, some important principles which must be understood before undertaking these kinds of evaluation procedures:

1. If the frame of reference for treatment is geared to "sealing over" unconscious material, projective techniques are inappropriate.
2. There must be *consensual validation* regarding the nature of the client's productions. This means that the therapist will discuss with the client the pictures or forms which have been produced. The client may or may not wish to explain their meanings. The therapist should allow the client to take the lead in doing this.
3. There should be no interpretation of unconscious materials or symbols with the client. The therapist and client together should discuss only the material as it is presented.
4. Validation of the information gained in a projective technique should be sought in other observation and evaluation methods. The use of projective materials alone is seldom complete enough for the occupational therapist's purposes.
5. It is important to recognize that these procedures may be fatiguing to the client, and the therapist should plan a time after the testing for him or her to rest with some form of activity which is known to be integrating and nonthreatening.
6. Because projective techniques tend to release more material of a personal nature than some other techniques, the need for the therapist to respect confidentiality is especially important.

Activities of Daily Living, Life Skills

The assessment of activities of daily living in psychiatry must be based on the therapist's knowledge of the demands which may be placed upon the client in his or her daily life. Several therapists have developed lists of the kinds of activities of daily living that should be assessed with most clients. Such activities as basic hygiene and grooming, care for clothing and other possessions, cooking, cleaning, shopping, budgeting, using public transportation, reading a map, understanding and following a timetable, and using the telephone are all part of daily living for most people. Attention to the client's ability to do these things is very important. The client should be assessed in terms of his or her current situation and in terms of his or her future expected situation.[8]

One method of assessing activities of daily living or life skills is to use a questionnaire or interview, and then trying out the various skills. For an outpatient, or the client about to be discharged, a visit to the home may be appropriate. The therapist may learn that life skills for his or her farmer client include getting up at daybreak and tending the chickens and cows or that life skills for an urban secretary include being able to make complicated carpooling arrangements to get to work or that life skills for a mother may mean dealing with the neighborhood children who come to play with her own children.

Prevocational Evaluation

Much of the occupational therapist's work with a client may be directed toward developing skills that may be used in the work world of the client. The kinds of problems which many psychiatrically ill clients encounter with regard to work and which should be assessed and dealt with in occupational therapy generally fit into categories that apply to other areas of their lives, i.e., the ability to organize, to manage time requirements, to get along with other people, to relate to authority figures, to adapt to changes, and to solve problems. It is vital that these kinds of considerations be assessed along with specific skills evaluation procedures. They are probably best assessed through observation of the client in a variety of activities that are structured to provide opportunities for the client to work with other people.

Skills assessments such as have been described in the other chapters may have an important place in the occupational therapist's repertoire in psychiatry. Usually occupational therapists articulate prevocational assessment programs with those provided by other services or agencies, such as Vocational Adjustment Services or the Bureau of Vocational Rehabilitation, and the extent to which the occupational therapist evaluates for specific skills is determined by the kinds of services provided by the other agencies. It is vital that this very important aspect of the client's life should not be overlooked.

DEVELOPMENT OF OBJECTIVES

The tone of the process of assessment is one which should lead directly to the setting of objectives. Objectives are based on the data gained in the process of assessment and, like assessment, should be subject to review and revision as the occupational therapy process is going on. It takes skill to include the client in setting objectives, but it is essential to try to do so. The depressed client, who is caught in a web of static and despairing images about himself or herself, or the psychotic schizophrenic client, who seems to be functioning at a preverbal level, may be difficult to communicate with, but it is nevertheless vital for the therapist to share the objectives which are developed with the client in some way.

The factors that contribute to objectives include information about the client, objectives and frame of reference of the total treatment team, knowledge about the disease process or deficit and the client's prognosis, knowledge about the client's expected future environment, and the realistic possibilities for implementing a plan to achieve the objectives. As objectives are developed it is important to consider the ways in which it will be possible to measure the degrees of success which have been reached in achieving them.

Overall objectives are usually developed by the team. Occupational therapy long-term objectives are designed to promote progress toward the overall objectives. Short-term objectives are developed to provide a series of sequential small steps to bring about progress toward the long-term objective. In the example of the occupational therapy process in Table 12-4, Ms. S's long-term objective was that she should be able to "set priorities on her time and energy." The first short-term objective in accordance with it was that she would be able to "complete one simple task within a reasonable time frame." A subsequent short-term objective was for her to be able to "plan a schedule of activities for a typical day and follow it with encouragement from the therapist." Short-term objectives should represent small increments in the development of healthy patterns of functioning. If it happens that, after assessment, there are no legitimate reasons for developing objectives, occupational therapy probably is not indicated for the client.

DEVELOPMENT OF A PLAN

Initial assessment data about the patient and the objectives for treatment must be translated into a plan of action. A well-designed plan describes for each of the objectives the kinds of activities that will be used, the nature of the therapist's relationship with the client, and the setting in which treatment is to take place. The treatment plan must describe possibilities that can be implemented realistically, taking into consideration any limitations of time, space, and staffing. The treatment plan should be developed in collaboration with the client, or, at least, shared with him or her so that there can be some degree of mutual understanding about the occupational therapy process. In some settings, it is standard practice to have the client sign the treatment plan as a means to achieving this end.

The kinds of considerations which are important in developing the plan are: (1) the meaning of the activities to the client, (2) the suitability of the activities for facilitating progress toward meeting the treatment objectives, (3) the consistency of the plan with the predominant frame of reference for treatment and the methods being used in other services, (4) the accuracy with which the activities are matched to the client's current level of functioning, (5) the gradability of the activities to accommodate to increased function or regression, (6) the adaptability of the activities to meet special needs, and (7) the potential for a successful experience in doing the activities.

Just as the treatment objectives represent an action-oriented summary of the assessment of the client, the treatment plan represents a synthesis of the therapist's knowledge of the potential of activities and relationships as facilitators of growth and performance. A treatment plan is stated in reference to each short-term objective and needs to be flexible enough to permit changes if reevaluation suggests that the plan is not working.

The thoroughness of the therapist's knowledge, the sensitivity with which the therapist has evaluated client's needs, assets, and limitations, and the soundness of the therapist's professional judgment are put to the test as the therapist develops a treatment plan. The plan must be realistic and must relate clearly to the treatment objectives that have been developed.

IMPLEMENTATION OF THE PLAN

The purpose of initial assessment, objective setting, and the development of a plan is to make it possible for clients to be involved in therapeutic programs that are designed as carefully as possible to meet their needs. In one sense the occupational therapy program is a test of the validity of those other measures and of the skill of the therapist in carrying out the plan.

Depending upon the setting and the frame of reference, the therapist may be directly involved with the client or may work in cooperative efforts with other team members in carrying out the program. In some settings the therapist may be only consultative to other services, to community agencies, or to the client, since the program may involve the use of resources away from the primary treatment center. In some instances clients are transferred or discharged before the occupational therapy program can be considered complete. It is a professional responsibility for the occupational therapist to consider and carry out ways of ensuring as much as possible that the client will have continuity in the program.

The issue of trust and confidence is critical to the implementation of the program. The therapist has been able to secure the client's interest in the program and motivation to invest in it. It is therefore vital that the therapist build upon this by maintaining his or her own consistent interest and involvement.

There are three parts of the implementation process. In the orientation phase the therapist reviews the objectives and the plan which have been developed and describes the way the program will be carried out. During the development phase the events of the program should be shown to correlate closely with the objectives that have been set. Formal or informal methods of evaluation of the client's progress should be used. If continuing evaluation indicates that the plan is not working or that the client's needs have changed, it is important to review the objectives and plan as may seem to be indicated. When objectives have been met, or if they become irrelevant, it is time either to terminate the program or to think of new plans to meet new objectives. At the termination of the program, it is a good idea to review with the client the progress that has been made and, perhaps, to work with the client on future plans and future objectives.

Choice of Activities in the Program

The development of the occupational therapy program requires translating the objectives into specific activities. The activities must fulfill the requirements of (1) relevance to the objectives and (2) meaning to the client within his or her normal life space. There are a number of factors which enter into these considerations. Is the activity to be designed so that a success experience may be assured? Are objects and finished products important? Or is the process itself the most important factor? Is body movement important? Are the dynamics of working in a group a factor to be considered? Should the activity be one that involves verbal expression and transactions with others? What about the dimension of time? Is immediate feedback or an immediate result important, or should there be moderate or prolonged delays? These questions can be answered first by looking at the initial assessment of the client. On the basis of that information, and with the knowledge and skills in activity analysis, the therapist should be able to match activities, plans, and objectives.

Figure 12-5 is a schematic representation of the levels on which activities may be experienced and the kinds of activities that promote healthy function at these levels. It is offered as one form of guide to the selection of activities as treatment in occupational therapy.

At the core there is body awareness experience, where movement and sensory input activities are of value. At this level the *process* of the activity is important and automatic and noncortical performance is the measure of success. The focus of the activity is *individual,* although it may be done in a group. It is *nonverbal* but there may be some value in the use of simple naming of the actions or objects presented.[9] It is *immediate,* involving the integration of experiences as they occur.

The second ring is the body effectiveness experience, where one experiences the capability of the body to perform according to some internalized image or standard (exocept). *Individual* sports activities such as swimming, hiking, jogging, climbing or jumping, dancing, and some forms of heavy work may provide for this experience. These activities are primarily *nonverbal* and *process* oriented. They may be accomplished in groups but their focus is *individual.* They involve minimal relationships with external objects apart from the environment in which they take place. They also, like the first experience, involve *immediate* experience.

The third ring refers to the experience of performing actions that have an impact on objects and /or the environment. One experiences the effects of coordination of thoughts and actions, but on a level which is *individual* and personal, not social. It is here that the wide range of crafts activities are especially useful in promoting the ability to see cause-and-effect relationships, object permanence, and problem solving. Some of the basic activities of daily living, such as grooming, hygiene, and simple cooking, also fit this grouping as do individual hobbies, such as collecting stones, birdwatching, and simple horticulture. These activities *may use but do not depend upon verbal activity.* They are primarily *nonverbal.* End *products* as well as *processes* are important. The time frame is short, with *minimal delay* between start and completion.

The fourth ring refers to the coordination of thought, body, and other-relatedness. One experiences the impact of actions and behavior on self and others. At this level we begin to think of using *group* activities by choice as a way of furthering treatment objectives. At this level all kinds of group tasks (including crafts), games, social activities, and more advanced forms of life skills, such as using the telephone and public transportation, shopping or caring for pets may be appropriate. This level is both *verbal* and *nonverbal* and *process* and *product* oriented. There may be *some delay* between start and completion.

The fifth ring refers to the experience of the impact of thought. At this level the individual may be involved in purely intellectual pursuits—reading, learning a language, doing mathematics, art, or music appreciation. These activities may be undertaken as an *individual* or in a *group.* They are more *process* than *product* oriented and tend to be highly *verbal.* The time frame is highly flexible and may involve *considerable delay* between start and completion.

The final, outside ring refers to the creative ex-

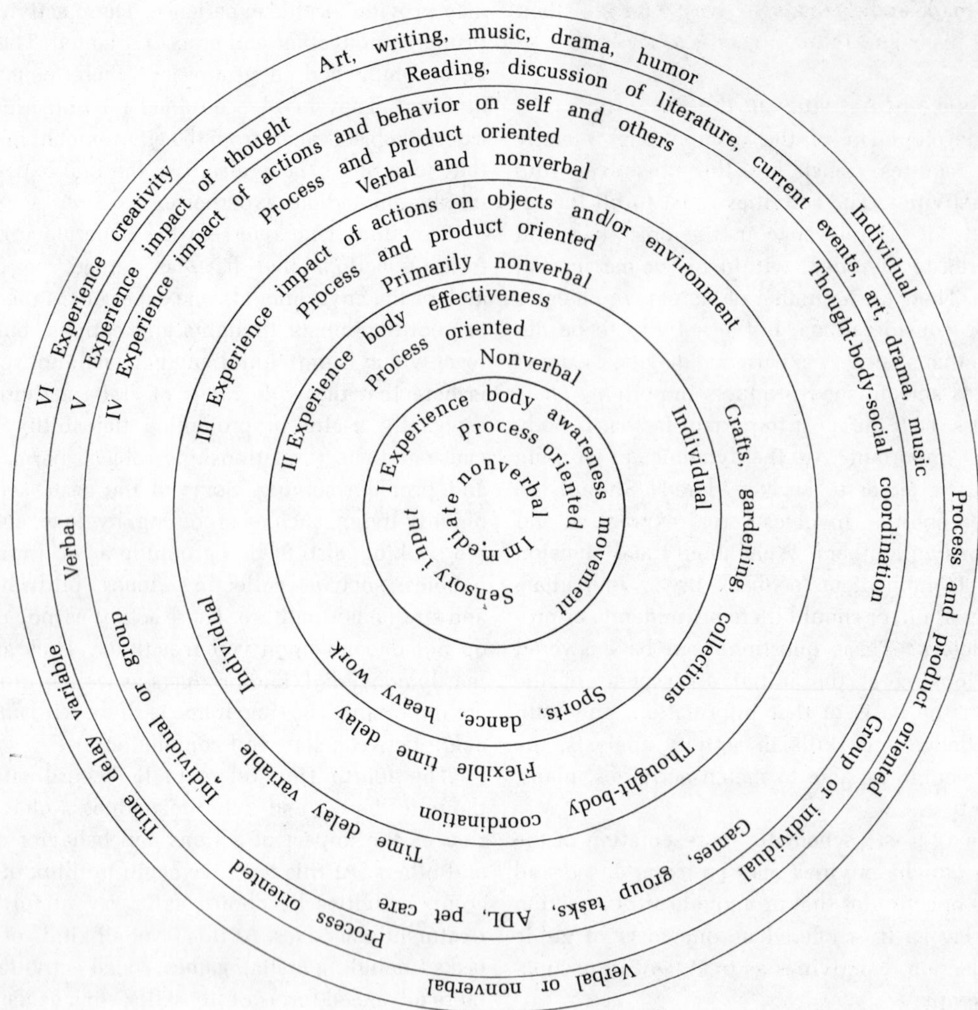

FIGURE 12-5. Representation of experience levels and characteristics of corresponding activities. (See text for explanation.)

perience, that level at which the individual is able to use his or her experiences from all levels and produce something which is new and different and an expression of the self. At this level art, humor, writing, and some forms of planning are used. It is a level which is indicative of high integration and it is one which is seen only occasionally or briefly. It may be either *verbal* or *nonverbal* and is both *process* and *product* oriented.[10] The time frame is *highly flexible.*

The "normal" individual experiences all or most of these levels in the course of living. At each of the levels it is possible to conceptualize movement from issues of survival to the achievement of mastery. A program which will allow the client to experience levels of mastery as a stimulus to exploration of new levels should be planned.

Other issues that must be addressed in the occupational therapy program include the development of autonomy and balance in the client's life. The achievement and maintenance of health may be measured by the degree of control people have over their life activities and the extent to which they have been able to internalize and act upon a sense of balance uniquely suited to themselves. The hospitalized client has very little autonomy in his or her life; concern for balance in rest, activity, and sleep is reflected in the hospital schedule. Even individuals who are not hospitalized but who are seen in outpatient centers seem to have major problems in these two areas. The occupational therapist, in the use of activities as treatment, is in an excellent position to help plan for the development and maintenance of the client's own sense of autonomy and balance.

Finally, a word about the meaning of the activities of the treatment program to the client. In reviewing the data from evaluation procedures, and in targeting the areas for treatment in occupational therapy, one finds important clues as to the level and mode for effective communication. If a client is seen to be functioning at the core area of body awareness, then communication will be nonverbal, and the meaning of the activity will be *in its experience.* King's research has shown that the pleasure derived in activities which effectively meet the patient's level of functioning have a remarkable potentiating effect.[11] Effectively meeting the client's level of functioning means that communication has taken place.

RECORDS AND REPORTS

Because the occupational therapist seldom, if ever, works in isolation, it is essential that accurate records be made and kept current, and that adequate systems of reporting to other members of the treatment team be worked out. Although systems for both record-keeping and reporting vary from setting to setting, their functions remain the same: (1) to provide clear, objective data about the client to aid in guiding future directions of treatment; (2) to permit congruent articulation between occupational therapy and other services; (3) to provide the necessary justification for the cost of treatment, especially where fiscal intermediaries, Professional Standards Review Organization (PSRO), or other forms of utilization review may be concerned.

Four kinds of notes may be written: an *initial note,* giving the results of assessment procedures and the objectives and plan for treatment; *ongoing progress notes,* reporting change or progress toward the specified objectives; *special reports* of incidents, accidents, or especially notable progress; and a *final discharge* summary.

The results of the lengthy initial assessment process may be recorded first in some detail and filed for reference in the occupational therapy office, but it is advisable for the occupational therapist to learn to write a *succinct* report that synthesizes the important factors to be considered and which support the stated treatment objectives and treatment plan. The report, which becomes part of the client's chart, is designed for the purpose of communicating to others; its completeness and clarity are vital.

The written report of the occupational therapy assessment and treatment process has gained greater and greater importance as the public has demanded greater accountability on the part of health care providers. The written note needs to be more than a brief description of what or how treatment has taken place. It should contain a clear statement of the objectives of treatment and of the progress of the client toward achievement of those goals. A note written at the termination of treatment should contain information about the status of the client at discharge compared to his or her status earlier.

The SOAP note, used in some centers, provides a framework for incorporating the important information. SOAP is an acronym for the organization of data as follows: *Subjective:* the client's view of the problem; *Objective:* the clinical findings with regard to the problem; *Assessment:* a listing of important data from the evaluation; *Plan:* a statement of the goals of treatment, the environment and modalities to be used, and the personnel to carry out treatment.

The same principles apply to oral reporting which is done in team meetings or conferences. The dimension that may be added in the conference situation is that it frequently becomes a forum for pooling of information and for problem solving among all members of the treatment team. In this situation, it is especially important for the occupational therapist to be able to articulate clearly the objectives of the program and the baseline of information and knowledge that serve as their foundation.

REFERENCES

1. Mosey, A. C.: Activities Therapy. New York: Raven Press, 1973, pp. 90–93.
2. Mosey, A. C.: Recapitulation of ontogenesis. Am. J. Occup. Ther. 22:426–438, 1968.
3. Hammer, E.: The Clinical Application of Projective

Drawings. Springfield IL: Charles C Thomas, Publishers, 1967, p. 5.
4. Azima, F. J.: The Azima Battery. In Mazer, J. (ed.): Materials from the 1968 Regional Institutes sponsored by the American Occupational Therapy Association on the Evaluation Process. Final Report R.S.A.-123-T-68. American Occupational Therapy Association, New York, 1968.
5. Fidler, G. S.: Diagnostic Battery, scoring and summary. In Mazer, J. (ed.): Materials from the 1968 Regional Institutes sponsored by the American Occupational Therapy Association on the Evaluation Process. Final Report R.S.A.-123-T-68. American Occupational Therapy Association, New York, 1968.
6. Lerner, C., and Ross, G.: The Magazine Picture Collage: Development of an objective scoring system. Am. J. Occup. Ther. 31:156–161, 1977.
7. Hammer: Clinical Application of Projective Drawings.
8. Mosey: Activities Therapy, pp. 90–93.
9. Arieti, S.: The Intrapsychic Self. New York: Basic Books, 1967, pp. 100–101.
10. Ibid., pp. 327–413.
11. King, L. J.: A sensory integrative approach to schizophrenia. Am. J. Occup. Ther. 28:529–536, 1974.

section 4/Contexts or Settings for Treatment

Occupational therapists who work in psychiatry are involved in much innovative programming which is not described here—programming such as providing in-service education to law enforcement officers, working in correctional institutions, and developing community programs for the prevention of drug abuse. The descriptions here are presented not as models but as examples of current occupational therapy practice with references and resources for the reader who wishes to explore them in more detail.

LARGE PUBLIC INSTITUTIONS

Large public institutions include state, county, and federal facilities and institutions run by the Veterans Administration. These hospitals, which evolved during the past 100 years, have provided care for great numbers of people who were unable to function in their homes and communities as a result of emotional problems or actual mental illness. By its nature, because of its being supported by public money, and because there were, until recently, few other kinds of services available, the large public hospital tended to become a catch-all for a wide range of society's problem people, not all of them mentally ill. Many of the large public hospitals were originally built some distance away from population centers. This may have reflected the prevailing attitude of fear which characterized public thinking about mental illness 50 to 100 years ago. The large public hospital usually spread over many acres of ground and incorporated services and functions to make it a fairly self-sufficient community. One may find a farm, stores, post office, laundry, one or more chapels, maintenance services, theater, recreation center, snack bar, medical surgical hospital, and a range of other facilities which make the large institution not unlike a small town.

In a great many of the large institutions, the number of trained professionals has been low. It is not unusual for a physician to have 100 or 200 patients assigned to him or her for care. The use of medications is extensive.

The stable population found today in the large public institution includes a number of chronically ill and geriatric patients or patients with schizophrenia and organic brain syndrome. Many such institutions have, in addition, special units for children, adolescents, drug or alcohol addiction problems, and court-committed cases. The acute care unit or services for newly admitted patients are generally short-term facilities in which screening is done, care is given to individuals during the acute phase of their illnesses, and every effort is made to prevent long-term hospitalization. Whenever possible, individuals are referred to partial hospitalization programs or to community facilities or outpatient departments for continued care. All of these may or may not be on the grounds or part of the institution's programs.

Since the advent of psychopharmacology and the proliferation of outpatient and community services to the mentally ill, there has been a major overhauling of the large public institutions. States have approached their mental hospital systems in a variety of ways, but a central theme has been one of working toward decentralization, returning as many of the inpatients as possible to the community. This has meant, for many patients who had been hospitalized for a significant part of their lives, leaving the security of the institution to live in boarding homes or group living situations in the community. It is obvious that some major efforts have been needed to make adjustment possible. The large public hospitals have been leaders in the development of partial hospitalization programs and such projects as quarter-way or half-way houses and satellite clinics.

Treatment frames of reference in the large public institution are highly variable and, in some cases, would best be termed eclectic. Some sections of an institution may be developed around a behavior therapy frame of reference or "token economy"; others may follow a "reality therapy" model and rely heavily upon the development of a therapeutic community; many institutions have sections that are oriented to modified forms of the psychoanalytic frame of reference.

The occupational therapist has had an important role to play in the large public institution, and it has become increasingly important for the occupational therapist to articulate services with other members of a very complex treatment, maintenance, or rehabilitation team, which includes physicians (who may or may not be psychiatrically trained), nurses, psychiatric aides, social workers, psychologists, dietitians, rehabilitation workers, therapeutic recreators, work adjustment therapists, art, music, dance, and education therapists, and volunteers. Frequently the occupational therapy department is part of a larger "Activities Therapy" or "Adjunctive Therapy" department which includes the other activities oriented workers and professionals. The occupational therapy department may be quite large and may be staffed with a number of on-the-job trained aides or therapeutic workers. Because of the large number of patients to be treated, patients are usually seen in groups, although treatment itself may be individually oriented.

Evaluation and reporting procedures in many large public institutions are specified and standardized in accordance with a government agency. The occupational therapist may, in addition, develop and use a battery of tests and procedures in order to develop viable treatment plans. Any or all of the procedures described earlier in this chapter may be incorporated into the evaluation.

Common problems encountered in the large public hospital include sensory integrative dysfunction; inability to manage self-care, personal hygiene and grooming, time, and activities of daily living; body image distortions; sexual identification problems, and problems with reality testing. One finds in the large public hospital such programs as groups oriented to cooking, grooming, shopping, exercise, gardening, and current events as well as gross motor and sensory integrative activities. Much of the activity of occupational therapy is currently oriented to the preparation of the patient for leaving the institution or for becoming as active as possible if leaving the institution is not feasible. The challenge has been to find ways to develop some degree of autonomy in people who have lived with none for a long time.

PRIVATE HOSPITALS

There are different kinds of private hospitals for psychiatric care and treatment. In general there are hospitals that are staffed with psychiatrists and other professionals and geared to provide team-based services coordinated around clearly defined and shared goals of treatment. There are also hospitals that have been developed to provide a safe, pleasant "rest" for patients who are receiving private, individualized treatment from their psychiatrists who are not, as a rule, part of the regular hospital staff. The role of the occupational therapist in each of these situations is different and these roles will be dealt with separately.

Private hospitals are expensive, so that their patients have tended to be, in general, from a segment of the population that is economically advantaged. Insurance coverage and such programs as Medicaid and Medicare have recently, however, made limited hospitalization in private hospitals possible for all people. Hospitalization periods tend to be short, up to ninety days, as compared with those for the large public hospital. Usually the problems treated are acute. Patients requiring longer hospitalization may be referred to other facilities, such as the large public hospital, or, whenever possible, to partial hospitalization facilities or community mental health centers. In general one sees far less of the long-term chronically institutionalized patient in the private hospital than in the public hospital, but chronic, long-standing problems of adjustment are not uncommon.

The occupational therapist in a team-oriented hospital usually works with at least one psychiatrist, nurses, aides, social workers, psychologists, therapeutic recreation workers, and possibly a number of other activities therapists specializing in art, music, drama, dance, horticulture, and so forth. The size and diversity of the treatment team is dependent upon the size and orientation of the hospital. In smaller hospitals, the occupational therapist working with a staff of aides, therapeutic workers, and volunteers, may be responsible for all activity planning. Figure 12-6 is an example of a department in a private, team-oriented department. (See the Duties of an Activity Therapy Department, which accompanies Fig. 12-6.)

In the second type of hospital, if the occupational therapist is on the staff, the department may be charged with carrying out activities in all areas.

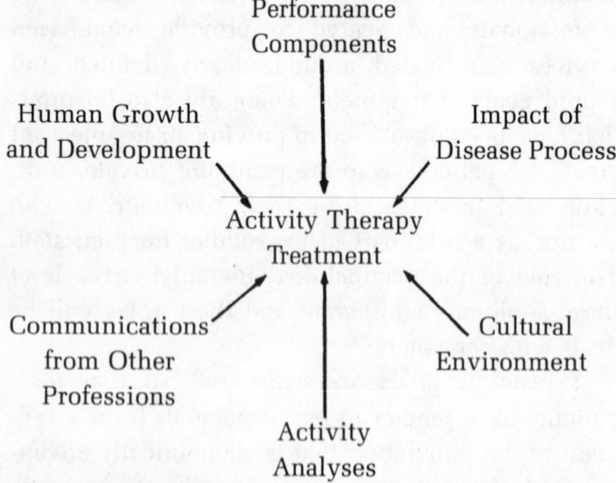

FIGURE 12-6. Input into design of Activity Therapy Department. From Sheppard and Enoch Pratt Hospital, Towson MD. Printed with permission. (See Duties of Activity Therapy Department, which follows.)

COMPONENTS OF ACTIVITY THERAPY*

DEFINITION OF ACTIVITY THERAPY

Activity Therapy is a composite of health professions that utilize activities in the reduction of disease symptoms and the promotion of optimal independent performance in the areas of work, self-care, and the constructive use of leisure time. Individual performance components such as interpersonal skills, communication skills, cognition, motor functioning, self-concept, and perceptual motor abilities are evaluated and treated in order to assist the patient in learning those skills and functions essential to productivity. Examples of activity treatment methods include assertive training, career planning, and work therapy, activities of daily living (cooking, grooming, budgeting, etc.), sex education, social skills and sensory integration activities, exercise groups, movement therapy, and art therapy.

DEFINITION OF MAJOR PERFORMANCE AREAS

Work Skills: Skills essential to securing and maintaining a job, e.g., punctuality, dependability, coordination, problem solving, completion of task, attention to detail, frustration tolerance, awareness of vocational skills and opportunities for placement, comfort with job interview, comfort with authority.

Self-Care Skills: Skills essential to independent functioning in everyday activities, e.g., self-grooming and feeding, use of public transportation, money management, budgeting and cooking, use of community resources.

Leisure Skills: Skills essential to constructive use of leisure time, e.g., knowledge and skills necessary to perform and engage in sports, games, and hobbies.

DEFINITION OF PERFORMANCE COMPONENTS

The learned and developmental patterns of behavior which are the substructure and foundation of the individual's occupational role and ability to function in that role. (Adopted from NIH Report)

1. Cognitive Functioning
   a. Comprehension (level and quality)
   b. Communication skills
   c. Concentration
   d. Problem solving
   e. Time management
   f. Conceptualization and integration of learning (ability to meet new situations)
   g. Time-place-person orientation
2. Psychological Functioning
   a. Coping behaviors, mechanisms, tolerate frustration, control impulses, aware of self-competency and self-limitations
   b. Defense mechanisms
   c. Feelings—awareness of own and others
   d. Self-identity
   e. Self-concept—self-respect, view self as able to influence events

* From Activity Therapy Department, Sheppard and Enoch Pratt Hospital, Towson MD. Printed with permission.

3. Social Functioning (the level, quality, and/or degree of dyadic and group interaction skills)
   a. Dyadic interaction skills: abilities in relationships with peers, subordinates, and authority figures; demonstrating trust, respect, and warmth; perceiving and responding to needs and feelings of others; engaging in and sustaining interdependent relationships; communicating feelings
   b. Group interaction skills: abilities in performing tasks in the presence of others; sharing tasks with others; cooperating and competing with others; fulfilling a variety of group membership roles; exercising leadership skills; perceiving and responding to needs of group members.
4. Motor Functioning
   a. Range of motion
   b. Muscle strength
   c. Endurance
   d. Functional use of body
   e. Gross and fine motor skills
5. Sensory Integrative Functioning
   a. Body schema
   b. Posture
   c. Body integration and awareness
   d. Spatial awareness
   e. Ability to respond motorically to sensory cues
   f. Normal reflex development

Occupational therapy is, on one hand, less guided here because there is no treatment team structure. The range of activities and the extent to which occupational therapy is free to develop therapeutic programs is limited primarily by the occupational therapist's own creativity and/or by administrative policies. Occupational therapy evaluations and reports may or may not be valued, depending upon the orientation of the private psychiatrists. Often, the registered therapist serves as a consultant, not a regular staff member, to such hospitals. The primary goal then is to provide guidance and inservice education.

PSYCHIATRIC WARD OF A GENERAL HOSPITAL

The inpatient ward of a general hospital usually provides emergency or acute care and services to people whose problems have become of such an overwhelming nature that they are unable to continue to function. The patient may be referred from the medical or surgical units of the hospital or by a private physician, often after a precipitous or critical incident such as a suicide attempt. Length of stay in such a facility is usually quite short, often less than two or three weeks.

The inpatient psychiatric ward may be staffed with a dynamic psychiatric team, including psychiatrists, nurses, social workers, psychologists, and occupational therapists. Where this is true the team effort is primarily geared to two major goals: (1) evaluation so that relevant referrals can be made for continued treatment, and (2) provision of a therapeutic climate to provide for optimal rapid reconstitution on the part of the patient.

The kinds of evaluations used by occupational therapy depend upon the treatment frame of reference. Generally, however, occupational therapists use interviews, screening methods to determine organic problems, activity evaluations, and possibly some projective techniques.

Treatment methods are limited to short-term group and individual projects geared to objectives such as increasing reality testing, attention span, and the ability to organize. The understanding and participation of the patient in his or her program is vital, especially if total discharge is imminent.

In such centers, evaluation and reporting techniques used in occupational therapy need to be efficient and accurate as well as rapidly communicated and well coordinated with the efforts of the total staff.

COMMUNITY MENTAL HEALTH CENTERS

Satellite programs, aftercare centers, and community mental health centers have become extensive in terms of the kinds of services offered. Based in "catchment areas" of 75,000 to 200,000 in population, these centers have been developed to care for the mental health and mental retardation needs of the people as close to their homes as possible. The kinds of programs that have been incorporated into community mental health centers include outpatient therapy, crisis intervention, emergency inpatient care, group homes, geriatric programs, therapeutic services to children and adolescents, addiction programs, and a variety of outreach services within the community. Community mental health centers are usually administered and staffed by both professional and lay mental health workers. They have boards of directors composed of community leaders. The community boards may serve as advisory or as governing bodies, and, in most instances, are very active in determining policies and staffing for the centers. Centers are often funded through federal and state sources.

Part of the client population is made up of formerly hospitalized individuals who have been discharged to live at home, in boarding homes, or in group homes. This group of individuals usually attends the center regularly for activities which have been designed primarily to help in adjustment to life outside the hospital.

The occupational therapist may work in several of the programs of the community mental health center. The teams with which he or she works include a psychiatrist, psychologist, social worker, nurse, other activity workers, and, most important, the members of the community. In a community-based service, the objectives of the occupational therapy programs must be geared to helping clients to function optimally in a non-institutional setting and may use community facilities such as neighborhood recreation centers, shopping areas, swimming pools, and ballparks. One innovative approach in community mental health has been to develop programs that are open to the "normal" population as well as to the designated clients. In this way, occupational therapy may get very much involved in preventive programs and health maintenance programs.

Important issues which may be addressed in such a setting include an individual's lack of any sense of autonomy; lack of self-esteem; lack of ability to manage the ordinary demands of daily living including grooming, self-care, sense of time, and organization; lack of assertiveness; need for leisure time interests, habits, and pursuits; need for contact with other people in the community; and fears about jobs and money. See the accompanying example of an evaluation used in a community health center.

INTERCOMMUNITY ACTION, INC.*
Occupational Therapy Functional Evaluation
Activities Program

Name ______________________ BSU # __________

Address ______________________ Tel. # __________

Qualifying Comments   Initial Evaluation __________   Reevaluation __________

A. Concept of Self
1. Activities of daily living:
a. self-care—client performs the following tasks independently
_______ brushes teeth
_______ combs hair
_______ shaves _______ electric _______ safety
_______ washes self _______ body _______ hair
b. clothing and care
_______ wears clothes appropriately
_______ washes clothes by hand
_______ is able to use washer and dryer
_______ is able to fold clothes
_______ is able to perform simple mending
c. food preparation
_______ serves self food
_______ can prepare one dish or part of a meal
_______ can plan for and prepare a simple meal
_______ can plan meals for 1 week
_______ needs supervision when shopping for food
_______ can shop for food independently
d. cares for living area
_______ performs simple chores (list specific responsibilities)
_______ cares for own living area
_______ cares for home and family

* Developed by Christine Hischmann, Mary Goble, and Mary Rogosky, March 1976. Revised by Hischmann, Pollack, Feldsher, and Garvin, December 1976. References: Kolodner, E.: Evaluation Outline, Norristown State Hospital, Norristown PA, December, 1972. Printed with permission.

Qualifying Comments

e. travel—list method of transportation
________ is transported by family
________ is transported by agency or significant other
________ travels with other members of group
________ travels independently

2. Specific skills and interests:

3. Affect (specify):

4. Need satisfaction:
________ feelings of self not being worthy or need satisfaction—unable to respond to therapy
________ relies on therapist to satisfy his/her needs
________ invests energy in another person, but emphasis is on self and what self can get
________ feels satisfied by one-to-one peer give-and-take relationship

5. Dependency:
________ unable to sustain effort despite continued assistance
________ is able to follow through only with continued encouragement
________ needs some encouragement to follow through
________ persists on own with task until completion

6. Ability to organize stimuli:
________ is easily distracted—requires highly structured environment
________ is distracted by external stimuli—can work in structured environment
________ is sometimes distracted by external stimuli—needs some structure
________ is not easily distracted by external stimuli—needs very little structure

7. Maintains focus and attention on program activities:
________ hardly ever
________ occasionally
________ approximately half the time
________ frequently
________ nearly always

8. Responsibility:
________ client rejects all responsibility
________ is unpredictable and hesitant
________ therapist perceives needs; asks client to assume responsibility; client follows through with ________ without ________ assistance
________ client perceives needs but has difficulty accepting responsibility
________ client recognizes and accepts responsibility independently; can be depended on

B. Task Orientation

1. Learning:
________ can imitate several familiar schemes, previously organized into a skill
________ can expand a familiar skill
________ can adapt a familiar skill
________ can imitate new, unfamiliar schemes
________ can imitate new, unfamiliar skills (series of schemes)
________ can expand or adapt new skills

2. Ability to follow directions:
old *new*
______ ______ needs to be physically assisted through motions of activity
______ ______ requires specific step-by-step demonstrations, able to do ________ number of steps at a time

Qualifying Comments

_____ _____ follows simple verbal instructions when accompanied by step-by-step demonstration
_____ _____ follows simple verbal instructions when accompanied by illustrations
_____ _____ follows simple verbal instructions of entire process when accompanied by illustrations
_____ _____ follows simple verbal instructions when accompanied by sample
_____ _____ follows simple verbal instructions
_____ _____ follows complex verbal instructions
_____ _____ follows written instructions

3. Decision making:
_____ unable to make decisions
_____ relies on others for decisions
_____ hesitant—needs to check with others
_____ makes some decisions independently
_____ makes decisions with ease; capable of independent decision making

4. Validation of judgments:
_____ judgments are unrealistic
_____ judgments are usually idiosyncratic and unrealistic—can maintain some control with therapist's guidance
_____ a deterioration of judgment is exhibited with tasks that are personally filled with emotion
_____ seeks help to check judgments on tasks which are difficult
_____ can use cultural norms to assess acts realistically and objectively

5. Adheres to rules and regulations:
_____ hardly ever
_____ occasionally
_____ approximately half the time
_____ frequently
_____ nearly always

6. Critical evaluation:
_____ refuses to listen to critical evaluation or to recognize errors
_____ tends to avoid situations with error risks
_____ has difficulty tolerating error
_____ has difficulty tolerating error, degrading the value of the task
_____ accepts criticism, but withdraws
_____ accepts criticism; profits, but expresses hostility
_____ can tolerate making mistakes and profits from critical evaluation

7. Frustration tolerance and impulse control:
_____ is apt to lose control, easily becomes angry
_____ tends to respond to frustration by withdrawal or anger
_____ with support, can exercise appropriate control
_____ has appropriate emotional control, tolerates frustration without difficulty

C. Concept of Others

1. Communication skills:
_____ mute
_____ cannot communicate in organized, understandable way
_____ has great difficulty communicating thoughts, ideas, feelings
_____ communication is vague but understandable
_____ makes self understood, focusing on essential appropriate factors

2. Is assertive:
_____ hardly ever
_____ occasionally
_____ approximately half the time
_____ frequently
_____ nearly always

Qualifying Comments

3. Group skills:
    ________ isolates self from group
    ________ works on fringes of group; observes members; only therapist-client interaction
    ________ does tasks while associates are present; interaction with associates is limited
    ________ engages in a shared, give-and-take relationship with peers
    ________ can work competitively
4. Relationship to therapist:
    ________ openly defiant of therapist
    ________ questions therapist
    ________ works with therapist inappropriately ____, appropriately ____

D. Motor Skills
1. Motor learning:

	Gross	Fine
________ has difficulty or cannot learn simple motor skills	____	____
________ is able to learn simple motor skills	____	____
________ is able to learn average motor skills	____	____
________ learns complex motor skills	____	____

2. Motor performance:
    Handedness: right ___ left ___
    Performs gross motor tasks within *normal limits:*
    ________ walking
    ________ climbing stairs
    ________ catching medium ball
    ________ running
    ________ sitting
    ________ moving to music (rhythms)
    ________ transfer object from one hand to another
    Performs fine motor tasks within *normal limits:*
    ________ grasp (using a hammer)
    ________ pincer grasp (sewing)
    ________ combination grasp (crocheting)
    ________ finger dexterity (making paper flowers)

E. Summary of Functioning
1. Areas of strength:

2. Areas of weakness:

3. Significant changes:

4. O.T. treatment goals and recommended activities:

By ______________________________

Title ______________________________

The occupational therapist and the community mental health center team is usually involved in preventive services to the public. Often, through counseling and through the use of activities, hospitalization may be avoided. The occupational therapist's concern in the use of activities here may be centered around helping the client to achieve the establishment of healthy patterns and balance in living, especially the ability to both pace himself or herself and to assess the need for help before it is too late.

ADDICTION PROGRAMS*

Centers for the inpatient treatment of those people addicted by drug and alcohol may be located in urban or rural settings, may be private and independent, or may be part of a larger institutional system such as a state hospital or community mental health center. Such centers may be staffed by psychiatrists, psychologists, social workers, nurses, counselors, activities therapists, educational counselors or teachers, and a criminal justice liaison person. An important feature of many addiction programs is that staff positions at different levels are made available to residents (clients) as they recover from their addiction. The incorporation of recovered addicts into staff positions is a valuable addition to the program and provides therapeutic incentives to the ex-addict.

Most inpatient, drug-free addiction programs are developed around a therapeutic community model that is psychologically oriented, promotes shared responsibilities, and gives a fair amount of freedom to the residents. Most of the therapeutic efforts of these programs are group oriented. Reality therapy, behavior modification, and developmental approaches are commonly used.

Usually the client or resident in inpatient drug-free addiction programs is there voluntarily, although he or she may have committed himself or herself to the program as an alternative to going to jail. Many initially enter the program with the intention of "drying out" so that they may return to their lives on the outside. They represent a wide range of population variables with regard to age, sex, intelligence, family background and socioeconomic status. The one outstanding personality characteristic which has been observed by people who have worked closely with addicts is that they seem to have an exceedingly low level of self-esteem. Other characteristics include regression to oral (or earlier) levels of emotional need gratification, underlying depression, limited coping strategies, low frustration tolerance, and a need for intensity of experience. They appear to have some deficit in their ability to process information from the environment. This last deficit, coupled with an apparent need for intensity of experience, raises the question of perceptual or sensory integrative dysfunction. In fact, the apparent need of the addict to avoid responsibility and to flee reality, to lack trust, and to show impulsiveness may be symptomatic of some more basic problems. Motivating the client or resident to stay in treatment beyond the "drying out" period is a major concern for all the staff.

The occupational therapist working in an addiction program may use a number of evaluative techniques. Interviews, activities configurations, observation in activities and in other group settings, and consultation with other staff are the commonly used approaches. The use of sensory integrative methods of assessment may also prove useful.

The need for continual, completely honest and clear communication that is both verbal and nonverbal is essential in the therapist's relationship with the client. The therapist needs to be, in this area especially, aware of personal biases and values, honest about them, and willing to risk anger or embarrassment if in doing so a responsible concern for the client can be communicated.

In order to meet objectives for treatment in occupational therapy, activities should be designed to include provisions for success, developing reality testing, gaining social status, and experiencing clear, strong sensory input. The addict usually needs to develop ways to assess his or her own abilities and problems realistically. He or she also needs to learn ways to incorporate into his or her life styles the advances made. Activities, especially crafts, sports, and games, lend themselves especially well to the kinds of deliberate and tangible confrontations with self needed to make this possible.

* Betty B. Neves, O.T.R., Medical College of Georgia, Augusta, Georgia, 1977, furnished information on this topic.

In the area of drug addiction, efforts are being expended on prevention programs. It has been found that activities are a most viable alternative to the use of drugs. Occupational therapy has an important contribution to make in programs designed to reach the early user or abuser of alcohol or drugs.

PARTIAL HOSPITALIZATION: DAY AND EVENING PROGRAMS

Partial hospitalization programs make it possible for the client to continue to live in the community while receiving treatment on a regular basis. The client who is seen in partial hospitalization programs frequently has been transferred from an inpatient program. The day or evening program may be viewed as a step toward totally independent living. For others, the day or evening program represents an early intervention step, hopefully to prevent more extensive hospitalization.

Many clients who attend partial hospitalization programs are individuals whose adjustment to life has been somewhat marginal for some time. The task of a day program staff is one of providing rehabilitation. Most programs are group and milieu oriented. The team, consisting of psychiatrists, psychologists, social workers, nurses, occupational therapists, and therapeutic recreators usually is closely knit and there may be much blending of roles. The total team, for example, may become trained and responsible for such activities as group therapy and psychodrama.

In settings such as these, the occupational therapist has a special responsibility for providing opportunities for the client to use activities in ways that are relevant to his or her life. Occupational therapy may, for example, develop activity groups built upon problems clients express they have in shopping, using transportation, and balancing their life routines. The occupational therapy model that incorporates the development of skills in managing time and/or balancing work, rest, play, and sleep in their life space is one which is valuable in the partial hospitalization program especially. Planning for the weekend and practicing skills for making friends may be special issues for these clients, as many of them experience great stress from long empty periods during which they have little sense of how to use the time. Having fun in a social setting may also be an important part of the program.

Evaluation procedures in day or evening programs tend to be informal, unless otherwise specified by the hospital or agency. Interview, observation in group activities, and consultation with other staff members are the most commonly used methods. The interest inventory and activities configuration or an adaptation of these methods has proven to be especially useful. Efforts are frequently made to de-emphasize the medical or institutional atmosphere and to develop a sense of community which is normalized in its atmosphere.

CHILDREN'S CENTERS

Children who are hospitalized in inpatient facilities usually are psychotic or so seriously hampered by neurotic or behavior disorders that it is impossible for them to function in a normal setting. Children with less severe problems may be seen in school settings or in outpatient facilities such as those connected with the community mental health center.

Children's inpatient facilities frequently are part of a larger institution but they may be administered and staffed independently. The concept of team is of utmost importance because of the need for sick children to experience consistent treatment. Teams in children's psychiatric facilities consist of psychiatrists, nurses, child care workers, social workers, psychologists, teachers, and a variety of activities therapists. Ideally there is round-the-clock planning for hospitalized children. Parent counseling and family therapy may be an important part of the total program.

Treatment frames of reference in children's centers are usually well defined; psychoanalytic, developmental, occupational behavior, sensory integration, and behavior modification may be used. The occupational therapist and all other workers in a children's setting, regardless of treatment frame of reference, need to have strong, basic knowledge of human development and the ability to work in close collaboration with other members of the team, especially with the child care workers and the teachers. The occupational therapist may or may not be involved in parent counseling or family treatment, but the addition of occupational therapy for these groups is seen as highly desirable.

Occupational therapy evaluation procedures, especially those related to sensory integration, developmental levels, and play, can be of diagnostic value. For purposes of treatment planning in occupational therapy, evaluation may be accomplished in the use of perceptual tests, activities evaluations, observation, and interview. The play inventory techniques described by Takata[1] are especially useful. Occupational therapy may offer play activities to provide sensory motor experience, interactions with others, and the development of basic cognitive skills.

ADOLESCENT PROGRAMS

Special inpatient and outpatient treatment facilities have been developed to provide services to troubled or emotionally disturbed adolescents. Treatment teams in these programs are similar to those of children's facilities and it is equally important for all staff members to have a strong knowledge base in human development.

The kinds of problems presented by adolescents range widely from full-blown psychotic schizophrenic and depressive reactions through neuroses, personality disorders, and mild to severe but transient situational episodes. The normal adolescent world has its special symbols and important objects, different from those of childhood or adulthood, and even the psychotic adolescent needs to have these symbols and objects. The skill of the therapist may well be in knowing how to incorporate the activities that are common to adolescence into projects that meet emotional and cognitive developmental needs of a much earlier period.

GERIATRIC PROGRAMS

Many kinds of programs have been designed to meet the needs of the geriatric population. The occupational therapist with special knowledge and skills in geropsychiatry has an important contribution to make in these programs.

There are community based programs, which serve the function of helping the elderly to maintain and improve their abilities to live productively in society. These programs reach clients who have never been hospitalized or treated for psychiatric disorders but who, as they have grown older, have experienced the debilitating effects of decreasing sensory function and other effects of the aging process and have become less able to cope with the demands of everyday living. The role of a community geriatric center and of an occupational therapist is clearly one of providing preventive services. The occupational therapist who works in one of these centers may be involved cooperatively with many different kinds of people. Centers may be part of an outreach of a church, a settlement house, a special housing project or apartment for the aging, or a school system. The personnel connected with these agencies may be deeply invested in the success of their programs. The range of activities that evolves out of such programs is very wide and may be limited only by financial factors and the ingenuity of the leaders (staff or clients). Musical groups, crafts boutiques, and even small business services are not beyond the possibilities, especially since the major goal is to provide the elderly with opportunities to develop and maintain their fullest sense of productivity and capability.

Inpatient programs for elderly psychotic clients are usually part of a larger institution. Many of these clients are people who have been long hospitalized with chronic psychiatric conditions and have grown old living in the institution. Others have developed psychoses as a result of illness, stress, or organic deterioration in the process of aging.

The staffing for such programs usually includes physicians, nurses, social workers, volunteers, and activity workers, including occupational therapists, with psychological services consulting. Where the clients are infirm or physically ill there is a heavy weighting in favor of nursing services.

Occupational therapy can make a vital contribution in several ways to these clients. The reality orientation which is provided through involvement in activities is much needed. Sensory input activities such as working with fragrant or colorful objects, feeling textures, and tasting good food are the elements of some basic activities designed to help the client to maintain contact with the world. Other kinds of activities, dependent upon the client's physical condition and level of contact, might include discussion groups, cooking groups, preparations for special events like a party or community outing, exercise sessions, and folk dancing.

HOME TREATMENT

Occupational therapists are beginning to provide services to clients in the home setting for psychiatric problems. It has, however, been a practice of some occupational therapists working within a hospital or partial hospitalization program to begin to explore with the client the home and community settings from which he/she comes and to which he/she will return. This has been of great value in helping the occupational therapist know more clearly the demands that may be made upon the client away from the treatment setting. It thus becomes easier for the occupational therapist to help to plan relevant activities for each client.

Watanabe describes four concepts[2] as being critical to consider in the psychiatric home treatment process: (1) life space, (2) mastery, (3) life tasks, and (4) responsibility. These represent long-term targets around which short-term goals and short-term occupational therapy tasks could be developed in the home treatment setting.

When an occupational therapist goes into the home of the client, the occupational therapist is in the client's territory. The occupational therapist's skills in observation and interviewing the client and other significant people, such as family members, close neighbors, or the local grocer, are critical. There is probably no more directly beneficial way to conduct treatment for some clients than in their own homes where their own objects, rituals, and routines can be observed and worked with, provided these things are not so emotionally charged as to contraindicate treatment in that setting at that particular time.

The home treatment team usually consists of nurses, social workers, and physical therapists in addition to the occupational therapist, with the physician as a referral source and consultant. The occupational therapist must be able to provide clear reports that promote coordination of effort.

Frequently the home treatment occupational therapist who is seeing a case for physical dysfunction encounters significant emotional overlays or full-blown mental illness. The occupational therapist then needs to call upon a psychiatric knowledge base to provide the needed services. Home treatment is discussed in detail in Chapter 25.

REFERENCES

1. Takata, N.: The play history. Am. J. Occup. Ther. 23: 314–318, 1969.
2. Watanabe, S.: Four concepts basic to the occupational therapy process. Am. J. Occup. Ther. 22:439–445, 1968.

BIBLIOGRAPHY

Hospital

Allard, I.: A study of the effects of occupational therapy upon perceptual inaccuracies of the schizophrenic. Am. J. Occup. Ther. 23:115, 1969.

Gray, M.: Effects of hospitalization on work-play behavior. Am. J. Occup. Ther. 26:180–185, 1972.

Heine, D. B.: Daily living group. Am. J. Occup. Ther. 29: 628–630, 1975.

King, L. J.: A sensory integrative approach to schizophrenia. Am. J. Occup. Ther. 28:529–536, 1974.

Kolodner, E.: Neighborhood extension of activity therapy. Am. J. Occup. Ther. 27:381–383, 1973.

Levy, L.: Movement therapy for psychiatric patients. Am. J. Occup. Ther. 28:354, 1974.

Mann, W. C.: A quarterway house for adult psychiatric patients. Am. J. Occup. Ther. 30:646–647, 1976.

Psychiatric Ward, General Hospital

Corry, S., Sebastian, V., and Mosey, A. C.: Acute short-term treatment in psychiatry. Am. J. Occup. Ther. 28:401–406, 1974.

Holmes, C., and Bauer, W.: Establishing an occupational therapy department in a community hospital. Am. J. Occup. Ther. 24:219–226, 1970.

Hyman, M., and Metzker, J. R.: Occupational therapy in an emergency psychiatric setting. Am. J. Occup. Ther. 24:280–283, 1970.

McDonald, S. S.: Looking in on Gates-10. Pa. Gazette 75: 32–36, 1977.

Community Mental Health Centers

Auerbach, E.: Community involvement: The Bernal Heights Ladies' Club. Am. J. Occup. Ther. 28:272, 1974.

Becker, R. E., and Page, M.: Psychotherapeutically oriented rehabilitation in chronic mental illness. Am. J. Occup. Ther. 27:34–38, 1973.

Broekema, M. C., Danz, K. H., and Schloemer, C. U.: Occupational therapy in a community aftercare program. Am. J. Occup. Ther. 29:22–27, 1975.

Cromwell, F. S., and Kielhofner, G.: An educational strategy for occupational therapy community service. Am. J. Occup. Ther. 30:629–633, 1976.

Ethridge, D. A.: The management view of the future of occupational therapy in mental health. Am. J. Occup. Ther. 30:623–628, 1976.

Finn, G.: The occupational therapist in preventive programs. Am. J. Occup. Ther. 26:59–66, 1972.

Laukaran, V.: Toward a model of occupational therapy for community health. Am. J. Occup. Ther. 31:71–74, 1977.

Webb, L.: The therapeutic social club. Am. J. Occup. Ther. 27:81–84, 1973.

Addiction Programs

De Angelis, G. G.: Theoretical and clinical approaches to the treatment of adolescent drug addiction. Am. J. Occup. Ther. 30:87–93, 1976.

Dohner, V. A.: Alternatives to drugs—a new approach to drug education. J. Drug Ed. 2:3–22, 1972.

Freudenberger, H. J.: The therapeutic community revisited. Am. J. Drug Alcohol Abuse 3:33–50, 1976.

Jones, K. L., Shainberg, L. W., and Byer, C. O.: Drugs and Alcohol. New York: Harper and Row Publishers, 1969.

Reese, C. C.: Forced treatment of the adolescent drug abuser. Am. J. Occup. Ther. 28:540–545, 1974.

Rinella, V.: Rehabilitation or bust: The impact of criminal justice system referrals on the treatment of drug addicts and alcoholics in a therapeutic community. Am. J. Drug Alcohol Abuse 3:181–184, 1976.

Sendy, E., Shorgz, V., and Alkane, H. (eds.): Developments in the Field of Drug Abuse. Proceedings 1974 of the National Association for the Prevention of Addiction in Narcotics, Cambridge MA: Schenkman Publishing Co., 1975.

Slobetz, F. W.: The role of occupational therapy in heroin detoxification. Am. J. Occup. Ther. 24:340–346, 1970.

Partial Hospitalization

Deacon, S., Dunning, E., and Dease, R.: A job clinic for psychotic clients in remission. Am. J. Occup. Ther. 28: 144–147, 1974.

Kuenstler, G.: A planning group for psychiatric outpatients. Am. J. Occup. Ther. 30:634–639, 1976.

Schechter, L.: Occupational therapy in a psychiatric day hospital. Am. J. Occup. Ther. 28:151–153, 1974.

Solberg, N. A., and Chueh, W.: Performance in occupational therapy as a predictor of successful prevocational training. Am. J. Occup. Ther. 30:481–486, 1976.

Children's Centers

Ayres, A. J., and Heskett, W.: Sensory integrative dysfunction in a young schizophrenic girl. J. Autism Childhood Schizophrenia 2:174–181, 1972.

Barker, P., and Muir, A. M.: The role of occupational therapy in a children's in-patient psychiatric unit. Am. J. Occup. Ther. 23:431–436, 1969.

DiLeo, J. H.: Children's Drawings as Diagnostic Aids. New York: Brunner Mazel, 1973.

Fahl, M. A.: Emotionally disturbed children: Effects of cooperative and competitive activity on peer interaction. Am. J. Occup. Ther. 24:31–33, 1970.

Florey, L.: An approach to play and play development. Am. J. Occup. Ther. 25:275–284, 1971.

Hurff, J.: A play skills inventory. In Reilly, M. (ed.): Play as Exploratory Learning. Beverly Hills: Sage Publications, 1974, pp. 267–283.

Knox, S.: A play scale. In Reilly, M. (ed.): Play as Exploratory Learning. Beverly Hills: Sage Publications, 1974, pp. 247–266.

Llorens, L.: Facilitating growth and development: The promise of occupational therapy. Am. J. Occup. Ther. 24:93–101, 1970.

Llorens, L.: Occupational therapy in community child health. Am. J. Occup. Ther. 25:335–339, 1971.

Llorens, L.: The effects of stress on growth and development. Am. J. Occup. Ther. 28:82–86, 1974.

Llorens, L., et al.: The effects of a CPM training approach on children with behavior maladjustment. Am. J. Occup. Ther. 23:502–512, 1969.

Loveland, C. A., and Little, V. L.: The occupational therapist in the juvenile correctional system. Am. J. Occup. Ther. 28:537–539, 1974.

Masagatani, G.: Hand-gesturing behavior in psychotic children. Am. J. Occup. Ther. 27:24–29, 1973.

Michelman, S.: The importance of creative play. Am. J. Occup. Ther. 25:285–290, 1971.

Shaefer, C. E. (ed.): Therapeutic Uses of Child's Play. New York: Jason Aronson, Inc., 1976.

Takata, N.: Play as prescription. In Reilly, M. (ed.): Play as Exploratory Learning. Beverly Hills: Sage Publishing Co., 1974, pp. 209–246.

Takata, N.: The play milieu. Am. J. Occup. Ther. 25:281–284, 1971.

Adolescent Programs

Caplan, G., and Lebovici, S.: Adolescence: Psychosocial Perspectives. New York: Basic Books, 1969.

Jodrell, R. D., and Sanson-Fisher, R.: An experiment involving disturbed adolescent girls. Am. J. Occup. Ther. 29:620–629, 1975.

Mosey, A. C.: The treatment of pathological distortion of body image. Am. J. Occup. Ther. 23:413–416, 1969.

Shannon, P. D.: Occupational choice: Decision-making play. In Reilly, M. (ed.): Play as Exploratory Learning. Beverly Hills: Sage Publishing Co., 1974, pp. 285–313.

Geriatric Programs

Anderson, E.: A continuity of care plan for long-term patients. Am. J. Public Health 5:2, 1964.

Butler, R., and Lewis, N.: Aging and Mental Health: Positive Psychological Approaches. St. Louis: C. V. Mosby Co., 1975.

Deichman, E., and O'Kane, C.: Working with the Elderly—A Training Manual. Buffalo NY: D.O.K. Publishing, Inc., 1975.

Hasselkus, B. R.: Aging and the human nervous system. Am. J. Occup. Ther. 28:16–21, 1974.

Hasselkus, B. R., and Kiernat, J. M.: Independent living for the elderly. Am. J. Occup. Ther. 27:181–188, 1973.

Leslie, D. K., and McLure, J. W.: Exercises for the Elderly. Iowa City: University of Iowa Graphic Series, 1975.

Lewis, S.: A patient-determined approach within a state hospital. Gerontologist 15:146–149, 1973.

Lewis, S.: Geriatric activity program planning: Occupational therapy community consultancy services, Norristown State Hospital. Paper prepared for Geriatric

Care Symposium, Norristown State Hospital, Norristown PA, April, 1976.
Lewis, S.: Geriatric awareness program: Reclaiming intellectual and social skills among the institutional elderly. Paper prepared for Geriatric Care Symposium, Norristown, Norristown PA, April, 1976.
Lewis, S.: Occupational therapy and geriatrics: Assuming a leadership position. Am. J. Occup. Ther. 29:459, 1975.
Murphy, E. C.: Organic brain syndrome. Paper prepared for Geriatric Care Symposium, Norristown State Hospital, Norristown PA, April, 1976.
Nystrom, E.: The elderly. Am. J. Occup. Ther. 28:337–345, 1974.
Parachek, J. F.: Parachek Geriatric Rating Scale. (Written in cooperation with L. J. King.) Scottsdale AZ: Greenroom Publications, 1976.
Shafer, A. L.: Providing supportive services to the elderly. Am. J. Occup. Ther. 25:423–427, 1971.
Weg, R.: The changing physiology of aging. Am. J. Occup. Ther. 27:213–217, 1973.

Home Treatment

Rozycka, M. F.: The maintenance of community mental health with the family as the unit of treatment. Unpublished manuscript.

section 5/Summary and Challenge of the Future

As theory and practice in psychiatric occupational therapy are traced through the years, a pattern emerges that indicates that the profession has maintained certain consistent awarenesses and concerns. The therapist has sought to promote in clients a sense of wholeness as well as the ability to adapt and function as fully as possible. The therapist has tried to maintain a level of awareness that keeps pace with growing knowledge and advancing technology and with the expanding consciousness that has characterized both health care and society in general. In many ways it seems that the development of the occupational therapy profession in psychiatry and in mental health has been similar to human development. In Piagetian terms, the profession has moved between equilibrium and disequilibrium many times in the past fifty years. New but not greatly discrepant information and knowledge has been assimilated and accommodated to and the practice of occupational therapy has developed and expanded. There have been times when the profession has become curious, ready, and eager to explore new concepts; and there have been times when occupational therapy has needed to practice methods based on a newly acquired conceptual frame. To use White's term,[1] the field of psychiatric occupational therapy has sought to achieve professional "competence."

Allying itself with psychiatry, the profession has been subject to the excitements, dilemmas, and ambiguities that have characterized the development of medical psychiatric practice. As psychiatric practice itself has grown and become diversified, it has had to become more and more responsive to and interested in the changes, diversification, and growth which have taken place in the social sciences. Changes in society have been close to revolutionary. These changes have forced psychiatry and all of its related professions, including occupational therapy, to develop new alliances and new perspectives.

There has been a need to incorporate broader concepts of health and illness and to accommodate to greater demands for preventive services in addition to treatment, maintenance, and rehabilitation. The move has been away from institutional care to diverse community programs. Psychiatric practice as well as occupational therapy practice is in a period of disequilibrium.

Perhaps the psychiatric occupational therapist has only embryonic conceptual models and frames of reference to address some of the issues that currently present themselves. Nevertheless the issues are there to be served. What about the great numbers of chronic institutionalized expatients who have been discharged to live in the obscurity of boarding house rooms and nursing homes? In some instances we have only limited resources even for finding them. What about the runaway adolescent who seems unable to find stability in life? What about the segment of an increasingly aged population which is neither sick nor well but which might be helped to continue to be productive, contributing members of society? What about the effects of more leisure time? What about the increase in computer technology and the devaluation of the work ethic? What about the effects of newly acquired consciousness of racism, sexism, agism, and of the rights of the handicapped? What role do we have in helping our client understand his or her sexuality? Should we accommodate to new approaches or popular fads in mental health? How do we work with other activities therapy professionals whose bases are similar to but not the same as ours? How can we maintain our commitment and work within some of the constraints imposed by standards that often seem to be depersonalizing to the client? How do we deal with increasingly complex concerns for accountability and legality?

These are only a few of the issues that call upon us to explore, study, think, adapt, and grow as a profession. Some of them are critical and some even painful. Some of them are exciting. A profession, which is growing and developing, needs to have two kinds of people: (1) those who stay close to the ordered center, thus maintaining stability and (2) those who dare the outer limits, raising questions, seeking answers, and testing new ideas. The tension which must develop between these two groups is an essential one for it is out of this tension that creativity and vitality are born.[2]

There is no way that a single chapter on occupational therapy practice in psychiatry and mental health can begin to provide the depth or the breadth of the knowledge base that is required to function within even one of its frames of reference or one of its contexts. Rather, I hope this chapter is a challenge to work toward refining the knowledge and defining the practice here presented.

REFERENCES

1. White, R. W.: Motivation reconsidered: The concept of competence. Psycholog. Rev. 66:297–333, 1959.
2. Tiffany, J. S.: The abolition of the threshold: Women and liminality. Unpublished.

GENERAL BIBLIOGRAPHY FOR CHAPTER 12

Alexander, F., and Selesnick, S.: The History of Psychiatry. New York: Harper & Row Publishers, 1966.

Allen, C.: The performance status examination. Paper presented at the Annual Conference of the American Occupational Therapy Association, San Francisco, 1976.

Arieti, S.: The Intrapsychic Self. New York: Basic Books, 1967.

Ayres, A. J.: Sensory Integration and Learning Disorders. Los Angeles: Western Psychological Services, 1972.

Ayres, A. J. and Heskett, W.: Sensory integrative dysfunction in a young schizophrenic girl. J. Autism Childhood Schizophrenia 2:174–181, 1972.

Azima, H., and Azima, F. J.: Outline of a dynamic theory of occupational therapy. Am. J. Occup. Ther. 23:215, 1959.

Barlow, I., and Simkin, S.: The leisure activities and social participation of mental patients prior to hospitalization. Therapeutic Recreation J. 5:161–67, 1971.

Bearison, D. J.: The construct of regression: A Piagetian approach. Merrill-Palmer Quart. 20:21–30, 1974.

Bendroth, S., and Southam, M.: Objective evaluation of projective material. Am. J. Occup. Ther. 27:78–80, 1973.

Benjamin, A.: The Helping Interview. Boston: Houghton Mifflin Co., 1974.

Berlyne, D. E.: Curiosity and exploration. Science 53:25–33, 1966.

Berne, E.: Games People Play. New York: Grove Press, 1967.

Berne, E.: Transactional Analysis in Psychotherapy. New York: Grove Press, 1961.

Bruner, J.: On voluntary action and its hierarchical structure. In Koestler, A., and Smithies, J. R. (eds.): Beyond Reductionism. Boston: Beacon Press, 1969.

Burke, J. P.: A clinical perspective on motivation: Pawn vs. origin. Am. J. Occup. Ther. 31:254–258, 1977.

Coleman, J. C.: Life stress and maladaptive behavior. Am. J. Occup. Ther. 27:129–179, 1973.

Conte, J. R., and Conte, W. R.: The use of conceptual models in occupational therapy. Am. J. Occup. Ther. 31:262–264, 1977.

Cratty, B. J.: Movement Behavior and Motor Learning. Philadelphia: Lea and Febiger, 1967.

Cutting, D.: A review of projective techniques. In Mazer, J. (ed.): Materials from the 1968 Regional Institutes sponsored by the American Occupational Therapy Association on the Evaluation Process. Final Report R.S.A.-123-T-68. New York: American Occupational Therapy Association, 1968.

DuCette, J. and Wolk, S.: Cognitive and motivational correlates of generalized expectancies for control. J. Personality Social Psychol. 26:420–426, 1973.

Ellsworth, P. D., and Colman, A. D.: The application of operant conditioning principles to work group experience. Am. J. Occup. Ther. 23:495–501, 1969.

Erikson, E.: Childhood and Society, New York: W. W. Norton & Co., 1950.

Ethridge, D. A.: The management view of the future of occupational therapy in mental health. Am. J. Occup. Ther. 30:623–628, 1976.

Feldenkrais, M.: Body and Mature Behavior: Anxiety,

Sex, Gravitation and Learning. New York: International Universities Press, 1966.
Fidler, G. S.: The task-oriented group as a context for treatment. Am. J. Occup. Ther. 23:1, 1969.
Florey, L.: An approach to play and play development. Am. J. Occup. Ther. 25:275–284, 1971.
Florey, L.: Intrinsic motivation: The dynamics of occupational therapy theory. Am. J. Occup. Ther. 23:319–322, 1969.
Frank, J.: The therapeutic use of self. Am. J. Occup. Ther. 12:4, 1958.
Freedman, A. M., and Kaplan, H. I. (eds.): The Child—His Psychological and Cultural Development, Vol. II, New York: Atheneum, 1972.
Freedman, A. M., Kaplan, H. I., and Sadock B. J.: Modern Synopsis of Comprehensive Textbook of Pscyhiatry/II. Baltimore: Williams & Wilkins Co., 1976.
Freud, S.: The Ego and Mechanisms of Defense. New York: International Universities Press, 1946.
Gellhorn, E.: Motion and emotion: The role of proprioception in the physiology and pathology of the emotions. Psycholog. Rev. 71:357–372, 1964.
Gillette, N.: Occupational therapy and mental health. In Willard, H. S., and Spackman, C. S. (eds.): Occupational Therapy, ed. 4. Philadelphia: J. B. Lippincott Co., 1971.
Gillette, N., and Mayer, P.: The group method in occupational therapy. In Mazer, J. (ed.): Materials from the 1968 Regional Institutes sponsored by the American Occupational Therapy Association on the Evaluation Process. Final Report R.S.A.-123-T-68. New York: American Occupational Therapy Association, 1968.
Glasser, W.: Reality Therapy. New York: Harper and Row Publishers, 1965.
Goffman, E.: Relations in Public. New York: Basic Books, 1971.
Haas, L. J.: Occupational Therapy for the Mentally and Nervously Ill. Milwaukee WI: Bruce Publishing Co., 1925.
Hall, E. T.: The Hidden Dimension. Garden City: Doubleday and Co., 1966.
Holtzman, P.: Perceptual dysfunction in the schizophrenic syndrome. In The Schizophrenic Reactions. New York: Brunner/Mazel, 1970.
James, M., and Jongeward, D.: Born to Win. Reading MA: Addison-Wesley Publishing Co., 1973.
Jantzen, A. C.: Definitions of mental health and mental illness. Am. J. Occup. Ther. 23:249–253, 1969.
Jones, M.: Beyond the Therapeutic Community. New Haven: Yale University Press, 1968.
Jung, C.: Man and His Symbols. New York: Doubleday and Co., 1964.
Kaplan, B. H., (ed.): Psychiatric Disorder and the Urban Environment. New York: Behavioral Publications, 1971.
Kielhofner, G.: Temporal adaptation. Am. J. Occup. Ther. 31:235–242, 1977.
Kolodner, E.: Neighborhood extension of activity therapy. Am. J. Occup. Ther. 27:381–383, 1973.
Laukaran, V. H.: Toward a model of occupational therapy for community health. Am. J. Occup. Ther. 31:71–72, 1977.
Lawn, E. C., and O'Kane, C. P.: Psychosocial symbols as communication media. Am. J. Occup. Ther. 27:30–33, 1973.
Levy, L.: Movement therapy for psychiatric patients. Am. J. Occup. Ther. 28:354, 1974.
Line, J.: Case method as a scientific form of clinical thinking. Am. J. Occup. Ther. 23:308, 1969.
Llorens, L.: Projective techniques in occupational therapy. Am. J. Occup. Ther. 21:4, 1967.
Matsutsuyu, J.: The interest check list. Am. J. Occup. Ther. 23:323–328, 1969.
Matsutsuyu, J.: Occupational behavior: A perspective on work and play. Am. J. Occup. Ther. 25:291–294, 1971.
Mazer, J., and Mosey, A. C.: Toward an integrated theory of occupational therapy. Am. J. Occup. Ther. 22:451–456, 1968.
McClelland, D. C., Atkinson, J. W., and Lowell, E. L.: The Achievement Motive. New York: Appleton-Century-Crofts, 1953.
Meyer, A.: The philosophy of occupational therapy. Arch. Occup. Ther. 1:5, 1922.
Millon, T.: Theories of Psychopathology and Personality. Philadelphia: W. B. Saunders Co., 1973.
Moore, J.: Behavior, bias and the limbic system. Am. J. Occup. Ther. 30:11–19, 1976.
Moorhead, L.: The occupational history. Am. J. Occup. Ther. 23:331, 1969.
Mosey, A. C.: An alternative: The biopsychosocial model. Am. J. Occup. Ther. 28:137–143, 1974.
Mosey, A. C.: The concept and use of developmental groups. Am. J. Occup. Ther. 24:273–275, 1970.
Opler, M. K.: Culture and Social Psychiatry. New York: Atherton Press, 1967.
Overbaugh, T. E., and Bucher, B.: Use of operant conditioning to improve behavior of a severely deteriorated psychotic. Am. J. Occup. Ther. 24:423–427, 1970.
Piaget, J.: Play, Dreams and Imitation in Children. New York: W. W. Norton & Co., 1962.
Piaget, J.: The Construction of Reality in the Child. New York: Basic Books, 1954.
Piaget, J.: The Origins of Intelligence in Children. New York: International Universities Press, 1952.
Purtilo, R.: The Allied Health Professional and the Patient. Philadelphia: W. B. Saunders Co., 1973.
Reilly, M.: A psychiatric occupational therapy program as a teaching model. Am. J. Occup. Ther. 20:66–67, 1966.
Reilly, M.: Occupational therapy can be one of the greatest ideas of twentieth century medicine. Am. J. Occup. Ther. 16:1, 1962.
Reilly, M. (ed.): Play as Exploratory Learning. Beverly Hills: Sage Publishing Co., 1974.
Reilly, M.: The educational process. Am. J. Occup. Ther. 23:299–307, 1969.
Robinson, A. L.: Play, the arena for acquisition of rules for competent behavior. Am. J. Occup. Ther. 31:248–253, 1977.

Rogers, C.: Freedom to Learn. Columbus: Charles E. Merrill, 1969.

Searles, H.: The Nonhuman Environment. New York: International Universities Press, 1960.

Shannon, P. D.: The derailment of occupational therapy. Am. J. Occup. Ther. 31:229–230, 1977.

Sieg, K.: Applying the behavioral model to the occupational therapy model. Am. J. Occup. Ther. 28:421–428, 1974.

Smith, M. B.: Competence and adaptation: A perspective on therapeutic ends and means. Am. J. Occup. Ther. 28:11, 1974.

Stein, F.: Three facets of psychiatric occupational therapy models for research. Am. J. Occup. Ther. 23:491–494, 1969.

Van Allen, R., and Loeber, R.: Work assessment of psychiatric patients: A critical review of published scales. Can. J. Behavioral Science 4:101–117, 1972.

Watts, F. N.: Modification of employment handicaps of psychiatric patients by behavioral methods. Am. J. Occup. Ther. 30:487–490, 1976.

Watanabe, S.: Four concepts basic to the occupational therapy process. Am. J. Occup. Ther. 22:439–445, 1968.

Watanabe, S.: The activities configuration. In Mazer, J. (ed.): Materials from the 1968 Regional Institutes sponsored by the American Occupational Therapy Association on the Evaluation Process. Final Report. New York: American Occupational Therapy Association, 1968.

White, R. W.: Competence and the growth of personality. In Masserman, J. (ed.): The Ego. New York: Grune & Stratton, 1967.

Wolk, S., and DuCette, J.: The moderating effect of locus of control on achievement motivation. J. Personality 41:59–70, 1973.

White, R. W.: Motivation reconsidered: The concept of competence. Psycholog. Rev. 66:297–333, 1959.

ACKNOWLEDGMENTS

It would be impossible to name all of the patients, colleagues, and students who, over the years, have asked questions, sought answers, and shared knowledge. Appreciation to Christine Hischmann, Diane Maslen, Linda Levy, Ellen Kolodner, Lorna Jean King, Doris Kaplan, and the occupational therapy staffs of the Norristown State Hospital and the Sheppard and Enoch Pratt Hospital for their willingness to share their ideas, charts, and forms, to Betty Neves for sharing her experience and knowledge about occupational therapy in the treatment of addiction, and to Elizabeth Ridgway and Gerald Grant for reading and advice, and to Jennifer S. Tiffany for the many hours in which she shared her editorial skills, objectivity, and moral support.

13

Functional Restoration

Elinor Anne Spencer

section 1 /Theory and Application

The occupational therapist assesses and treats persons who have physical and/or neurological dysfunction. A variety of settings exist, among them the general hospital, rehabilitation center, community health center, nursing homes, public schools, psychiatric settings, outpatient clinics, and the community itself. Consideration of specific programs for persons with physical and/or neurological dysfunction must include recognition of psychological factors. The purpose of this chapter is to present the clinical aspects of physical/neurological dysfunction as they relate to the total picture of the affected person.

LIFE STYLE

The impact of a disease or an injury causing physical and mental disabilities can be devastating. Although the long-term impact may not be recognized in the early stages of disability, which are characterized by psychological denial, it affects the individual in a variety of ways over a period of time. Thus the term *life style* has become important to the occupational therapist and to other professionals working in the rehabilitation field.

Emphasis is on the adult in this chapter; however, when physical disability strikes the young child, there often are effects that he or she will have to contend with in childhood and in adult life. The stage of development and the age of the person when trauma or disease occur can be both advantageous and disadvantageous (Fig. 13-1).

A healthy adolescent who is accidentally shot during a hunting trip, with resulting paraplegia, is fortunate to have reached this stage of physical and social development before the injury. To a degree, the adolescent is prepared to achieve maximum potential in sensory-motor function post-trauma because of being intellectually and experientially aware of what he or she could accomplish pre-trauma.

The child born with cerebral palsy is not so fortunate as to have a guideline to normal functioning. However, having never known this state, it does not act as an unattainable objective, and he or she can experience the joy of learning what he or she can do.

Many of the diseases discussed in this chapter occur in young adulthood. Some occur gradually and are progressive; others occur suddenly and the

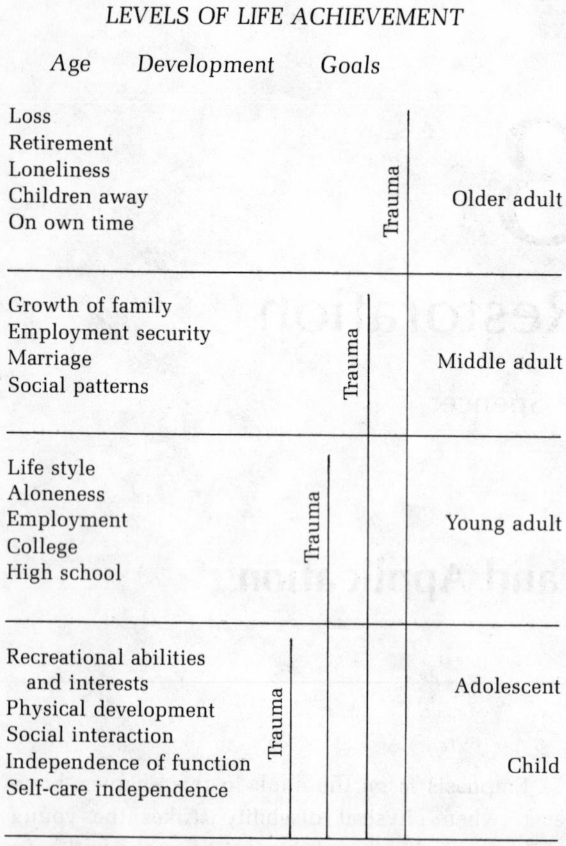

LEVELS OF LIFE ACHIEVEMENT

Age *Development* *Goals*

Goals		Age
Loss Retirement Loneliness Children away On own time	Trauma	Older adult
Growth of family Employment security Marriage Social patterns	Trauma	Middle adult
Life style Aloneness Employment College High school	Trauma	Young adult
Recreational abilities and interests Physical development Social interaction Independence of function Self-care independence	Trauma	Adolescent Child

FIGURE 13-1. Skills and life experiences prior to the occurrence of disease or trauma can be recorded. Rehabilitation goals build on achieved abilities and interests and direct the disabled person toward goals appropriate to his or her level of development.

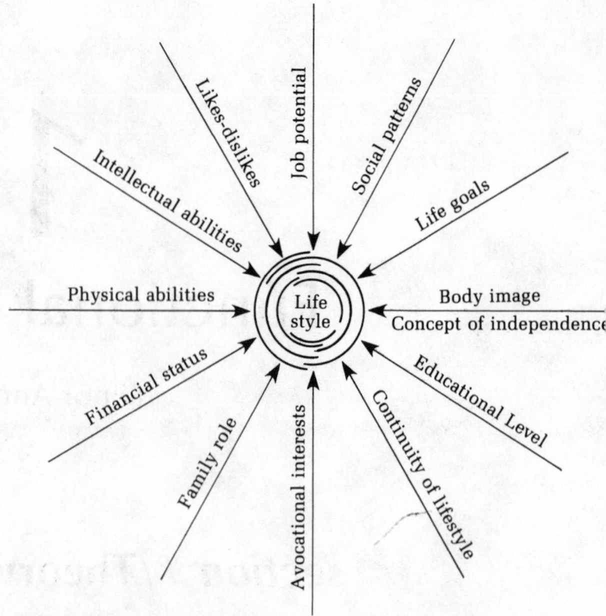

FIGURE 13-2. The impact of sudden trauma or disease affects all aspects of life style, and the severity and duration of the condition taxes the inner resources and assets the person has already achieved.

condition is stable and not progressive. In all of the conditions there is an adjustment to be made on the part of the individual who must contend with what has happened. The individual's life style will be altered. Figure 13-2 illustrates some of the aspects of a person's life style that are affected by disease or trauma; the affected person must adjust to some or all of the changes.

A healthy person naturally finds expression in physical, intellectual, psychological, emotional, sexual, and social abilities and activities. The loss of physical ability can affect all of these. It can hinder the individual's ability in and accessibility to his education, job, friends, and family; it can disrupt his or her pursuit of life goals. Likes and dislikes already established can hinder the setting of new goals. Loss of intellectual abilities can affect learning, achievement of physical potential, and personal relationships. The person's financial status can also interfere with family relationships and pursuit of rehabilitation objectives.

Pre-morbid psychological attitudes can assist the individual in coping with the struggle to regain a continuity of life style and to set new goals to achieve physical and emotional satisfaction. All of these concerns are part of the total rehabilitation program, and the occupational therapist must learn at what point each patient can work through each one most beneficially.

THEORY

One of the basic theories of occupational therapy is the use of performance as feedback to the patient to assist him or her in becoming involved in self-initiated, *purposeful activity* (Fig. 13-3). The use of adaptive techniques to assist in the achievement of independent functions (self-care, social interactions, planning and initiating tasks) is often employed. The occupational therapist's greatest challenge is to motivate a person toward self-direction and achievement for personal satisfaction. To this end the occupational therapist organizes the patient's immediate environment to provide opportunities for successful achievement of independent and productive functions.

If no program were established, some patients would be incapable of self-initiation directed toward changing their life styles and becoming relatively independent. Some create obstacles or, because of denial and depression, refuse to try to improve and to learn necessary skills.

Effective treatment depends on a therapeutic relationship between the occupational therapist and the patient, collaboration of the rehabilitation team regarding the individual patient's treatment plan, a plan relevant to the patient's life style, the setting of realistic goals, and the continual involvement of the patient in the rehabilitation process.

The goals of the occupational therapist are to assist the patient in being more aware of self, abilities, and goals and to aid the patient in adapting to the environment, thereby becoming a viable part of it. The therapist does this by assisting the patient in using his or her body to accomplish desired movements and tasks. The use of activity analysis and adaptation aids the patient in becoming aware of the "new" self and in gaining the ability to function.

The occupational therapist is concerned with the physical, mental, and social health of the person being treated. Different approaches or a combination of techniques are necessary for effective treatment. Major areas which should be considered are:

1. Relationship between the occupational therapist and the patient.
2. Collaboration of the patient in the development and implementation of his treatment plan.
3. Cooperation and communication with the other professionals on the rehabilitation team.
4. Determination of the relevancy of the treatment plan to the patient's life style.
5. Determination of the ultimate goals regarding the patient's reentry into his life style.
6. Consideration of the society, schooling, work, leisure, and family situation which might affect the patient.

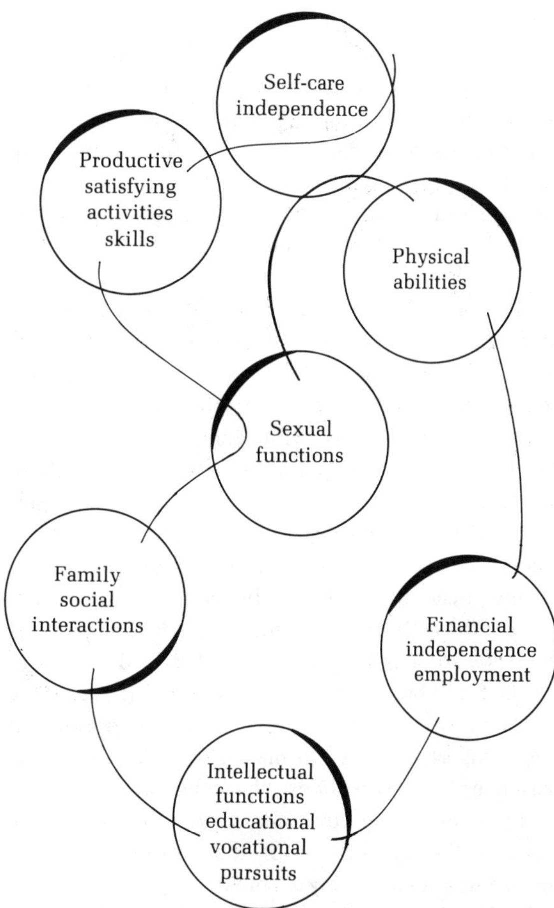

FIGURE 13-3. The use of performance in one area of function to facilitate function in another results from the successful achievement of a given task. The interrelationship of tasks is connected by the thread of achievement.

Unique and essential assets of the occupational therapist are knowledge of normal human development, knowledge of disability, capacity to adapt activities, and skill in activity analysis. With this body of knowledge, the occupational therapist is able to apply therapeutic concepts to activities of daily life.

VALUE OF ACTIVITY

The disabled person may never be able to accept the fact of physical or neurological disability. To work effectively with a person suffering the early stages of permanent disability, the occupational therapist must recognize that the disabled person must make the decisions related to the degree of acceptance and the course to be followed. As in mourning a loss, the disabled person will go through periods of denial, hope, delusion, hate, guilt, complacence, sadness, depression, hostility, adjustment, and, finally, acceptance. The ability to reason aids in passage through these stages, although the person must deal with the disability both emotionally and intellectually.

The patient can do much to make maximum use of remaining physical abilities, adding to them as his or her strength, endurance, and motivation increase. Activity which is specifically and therapeutically directed toward an increase in functional ability can provide important feedback to the patient by showing tangible proof that he or she *can* perform. Although the level of performance may not reach the patient's former physical or intellectual competence, incentive can be derived from small gains if the activity is directed properly. As the gains increase, so does the motivation, the willingness to try, and the beginnings of acceptance. In the early treatment sessions, the patient must be supported in the forms self-expression may take as he or she experiences the feelings described above.

In considering the adjustment to disability through the application of therapeutic activities, the occupational therapist must keep in mind the following factors the patient can learn from the involvement:

1. Getting to know physical abilities and limitations.
2. Learning how to compensate for physical disabilities.
3. Learning the limits of physical tolerance.
4. Learning how to cope with mental and emotional frustrations caused by physical disability.
5. Learning the social, economic, interpersonal, and familial implications of disability, and learning to cope with dependency.
6. Contending with economic problems: the cost of hospitalization, the expense of outpatient treatment and assistive devices, the loss of job opportunities and the necessity to be dependent on someone else (i.e., relatives or society).
7. Adapting to a new functional level of achievement.
8. Learning to compensate for disability by using substitutes for familiar functions.
9. Learning the functional use of leisure time.
10. Learning to organize and to adjust to a new life style.

In the rehabilitation process the patient must be encouraged and allowed to function independently at the level of his or her ability in all areas of activity. This approach begins with self-care and ends with vocational independence. If deprived of the experience of doing independently whatever is possible, the patient will lack the opportunity to work and to struggle through the stages of achieving maximum independence. If a nurse or a therapist does the job, he or she encourages dependency on the part of the patient. When uninvolved in the treatment, the patient loses commitment to the regaining of self-care skills, self-reliance, identity, and individuality. In assisting the patient to regain these functions, the therapist must put aside his or her own needs and comfort to help the patient through the struggle.

Pre-morbid attitudes and associations may work against the patient who suffers debilitating disease or injury (Fig. 13-4). These biases may cause rejection of a deformed limb, scarred face, mechanical hand, brace, or splint. The social implications of wheelchair use may overwhelm the person who will need to adjust to a world that is primarily built for and accessible to the "able-bodied walking." Achievement of the tough tasks of facing the public from a wheelchair, of requesting aid in surmounting a high curb, or of persuading officials to legislate against the construction of architectural barriers is

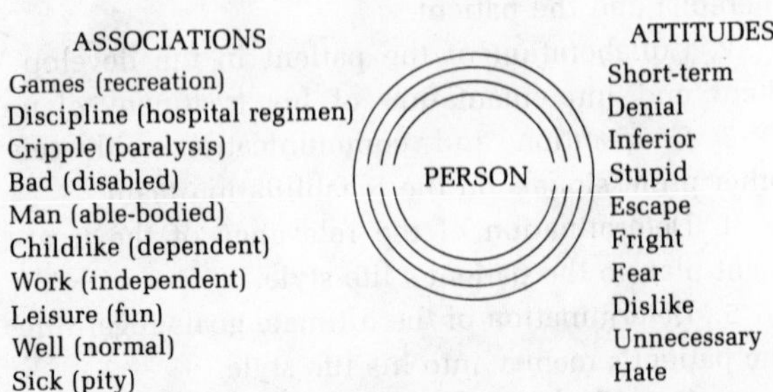

FIGURE 13-4. Personal attitudes, associations, and experiences which can enhance or hinder the patient's concept of his role in the rehabilitation effort.

developed by the enforcement of independent abilities as early and as effectively as possible. Basic dislike of self, lack of acceptance of strengths and weaknesses, lack of ability to deal with others, and vagueness about life goals hinder the achievement of rehabilitation goals.

ENVIRONMENTAL FACTORS

Performance is greatly affected by environmental influences and the way the patient interprets them. The occupational therapy program provides the patient with activities that: (1) create awareness of self in time and space, (2) develop awareness of the environment, and (3) reveal behavior changes and development of abilities. In the effort to assist the patient in these awareness areas, the occupational therapist uses the following objectives in planning the treatment program: active movement and performance by the patient, and active involvement of the patient with those nearby and the environment to provide opportunities, channel abilities, facilitate action, and eliminate barriers to function. Through a program of normal activities in an appropriate environment the therapist assists the patient to establish a new self-image and to accept changes in physiology, feelings, and appearance. The therapist also aids the patient's adjustment in preparation to reenter the home and community and to assume healthy attitudes towards himself or herself and towards the family.

Dunning[1] suggests that occupational therapists are managers of space (to promote stimulation), people (to encourage social interaction), and tasks (to develop skills). In functioning in this role, the therapist analyzes the effects of the patient's surroundings in terms of the patient's response. Deficits, which are revealed in the initial interview and evaluation, lead to appropriate changes in the environment either to stimulate or to inhibit the person. The therapist must assist the patient in gradually adjusting to the challenges of the environment by increasing performance.

Environmental influences can have positive or negative effects on the evaluation and treatment of the patient with physical or neurological disability. The following elements can structure the environment for success:

1. Atmosphere: The occupational therapy room should have adequate and comfortable space, lighting, and temperature. The therapist orients the new patient to the meaning of the room, its contents, and its functions and introduces the patient to the other people in the room. The therapist tries to control the visual and auditory stimuli in order to relieve any anxiety or confusion that the patient may experience.
2. Sensory bombardment: Excessive sensory impulses (visual, auditory, tactile, proprioceptive, and kinesthetic) can cause the patient to become confused, fatigued, and/or negative. Therefore, the therapist controls *all* of the stimuli surrounding the patient.
3. By using voice and body in a supportive, nonthreatening way, the therapist becomes a therapeutic tool.
4. An acceptable level of achievement, commensurate with the patient's interests, is necessary to provide positive feedback.
5. In some situations familiar objects may be threatening to the patient during the early stages of treatment. Therefore, unfamiliar activities and exercises may be better for initial evaluation and treatment.

The occupational therapist assists in providing an optimum environment for the patient. The arrangement of furniture in the patient's room, bed location in relation to the door and/or to other patients, accessibility of personal items, proximity to the call button, and accessibility and ease of use of the bathroom all contribute to the patient's mental and emotional well-being. Regardless of where the patient eats and socializes (own room, cafeteria, or dining room) the facilities should be accessible and should encourage independent functioning; the patient should be with compatible persons during meal times and for social functions.

In the occupational therapy room, depending on the goals of the treatment program at a given time, the patient should be allowed to work in a secluded area if desired or to work in proximity to other patients who could have a therapeutic effect on his or her functioning.

The family can be therapeutically involved in the treatment. When appropriate, the family is invited to participate in the patient's exercises and activities.

However, visits from family and friends can have a variety of effects on the patient; while some people may be encouraging and may stimulate functional recovery, others may be patronizing or pitying and thus may retard progress. The objective of stressing environment interaction is assisting the patient to adjust to returning home and to use his or her skills to arrange the environment for maximum function and minimum stress.

REFERRAL OF THE PATIENT

Theoretically the person may be referred to occupational therapy by anyone recommending evaluation, treatment, or consultation regarding various problem areas. This is permitted by the American Occupational Therapy Association (AOTA); however, it does not apply in all cases. For example, in the hospital, nursing home, and other medically-oriented settings, a patient must have a written, signed referral from a physician in order to be eligible for third party payment. Lack of third party reimbursement can prohibit occupational therapy service to the patient and can cause him or her to lose valuable assistance in regaining independent function.

Although each patient must always be considered individually in evaluation and treatment procedures, there are general principles that should be applied in recording pertinent evaluation information.

The *referral form* is the means by which the occupational therapist receives the formal request for treatment. Whether or not the referral is from a physician, there are some essential points of information that should be included. Figure 13-5 is a sample form. Note the inclusion of:

1. Patient identification (name, address, phone number, name of next-of-kin, birthdate, admission date, and insurance information).
2. Name of facility or department.
3. Identification of the form ("Request for evaluation and treatment").
4. Diagnosis.
5. Precautions or pertinent data.
6. Request.
7. Signature of physician.
8. Date of request.

On the form illustrated in Figure 13-5 the therapist writes the evaluation report directly below the referral information. In some cases the referral may appear on a physician's order form in the patient's chart, which includes such orders as medications, consultations to other physicians, and requests for services.

Treatment recommendations and progress notes are added consecutively on the form. This is quite different from the problem-oriented system commonly used in many medical settings. In the latter, all persons reporting on a patient use the same form consecutively and refer to a problem list in reporting information rather than each discipline using separate forms. (See Chapter 26.)

GENERAL EVALUATION PRINCIPLES: CHRONOLOGY AND CONTENT

Although it is helpful to have an organized routine for the evaluation of a new patient, it is frequently necessary to adjust the routine to meet the needs of the patient. For example, if a patient is physically fatigued, the therapist can evaluate an aspect of his or her condition that will not cause additional fatigue. Similarly, if the patient is anxious because of emotional stress and mental fatigue, the therapist should choose an evaluation area and method that will be acceptable, comfortable, and tolerable. For the most accurate results of the evaluation procedures, it is essential to adjust the chronology of the assessment according to the individual's needs. The evaluation should be done as quickly and as thoroughly as possible.

Before beginning the evaluation, the therapist determines the duration of the patient's stay in the hospital and how much time will be spent in occupational therapy. This will be helpful in determining the extent of evaluation appropriate to the treatment to be provided. The patient should not go through hours of evaluation which, while giving the therapist much information, may not be appropriate to the treatment program. Unfortunately, this imbalance may occur when there is a lack of team effort in setting initial goals, when the evaluation is more extensive than necessary, or when the evaluation is poorly organized and overly time consuming. It is important to remember that the patient does become mentally and physically fatigued during the evaluation;

NAME OF FACILITY
OCCUPATIONAL THERAPY REFERRAL

Patient Identification

REQUEST FOR EVALUATION AND TREATMENT

Diagnosis:

Precautions or Pertinent Data:

Request:

_______________M.D. _______________

Signature Date

REPORT OF EVALUATION AND TREATMENT

Date Signature

FIGURE 13-5. Sample occupational therapy referral form.

it should include an equal balance of positive feedback and information to the patient and should be accomplished in a realistic amount of time.

Clinical Evaluation Techniques

The occupational therapist uses four basic clinical evaluation techniques: (1) observation, (2) interview, (3) formal and standardized testing procedures, and (4) informal performance testing. Each technique provides a different approach to gathering information and is used to achieve and maintain optimum therapeutic contact with the patient. Usually, in the course of the total evaluation and treatment programs, all are used, either separately or in combination.

Observation

The most important technique is that of observation. The therapist must continually be aware of how he or she, the environment, and the tests are affecting the patient. Signs and symptoms of the patient's physical and mental condition should be observed closely. Observation requires no previous contact with either the patient's chart or other people. It can thus be used effectively in the absence of external information from written or personal sources.

By observing the patient's facial expression the therapist can detect paralysis, drooling, spasticity, confusion, expressions of alertness, fatigue, happiness, sadness, or pain. The position of the patient's arms and legs can indicate spasticity, flaccidity, deformity, or pain. The patient's sitting position can tell the therapist of muscle imbalance, discomfort, or lack of voluntary control. The patient may wear splints or slings, indicating some deficit in normal function. If the patient can walk into the room, he or she may display a gait produced by the use of braces, crutches, a prosthetic limb, a cane or walker as well as revealing a degree of paralysis not necessitating these aids. The patient's skin may exhibit the effects of exertion or anxiety by appearing sweaty or red or becoming pale and clammy. Undue pressure from a splint or brace can be detected by red or ulcerated marks or sores. If the therapist asks the patient to perform a task, the response can reveal hearing loss, muscle weakness, and/or incoordination.

Interview

The points already mentioned in regard to observation can be used in the interview. Again, little might be known about the patient and his or her condition. The interview (combined with observation) is the opportunity to find out information helpful to the therapist in planning the therapeutic program. Informal discussion with the patient can set him or her at ease with the therapist and the environment.

Most persons do not tolerate persistent questions about themselves at this point in their rehabilitation, but they may wish to share information regarding their problems in order to try to deal with them. The sincere therapist who observes the patient's reactions during the interview can often pick up valuable information about the patient's interests and concerns and can regulate the interview according to the reactions and attitudes of the patient.

The attitude of the therapist must be acceptable to the patient if he or she is to trust and confide in him or her. The interview need not be rigidly formal nor need it be completed in a single session. The initial contact marks the beginning of the relationship between patient and therapist. The relationship may last a long time (depending on the rehabilitation needs of the patient) so this beginning is crucial for the setting of the therapeutic relationship. Atmosphere, environment, privacy, duration, and comfort are important during the interview.

Formal and Standardized Testing Procedures

These tests provide objective results by comparison of the test results with standardized norms for functional abilities. The tests consist of specific procedures and equipment used in a standardized way. Included are measurement of passive and active joint range of motion using a goniometer, manual muscle testing procedures, grip strength using a dynamometer, prehension strength using a pinch gauge, and sensory testing including two-point sensory discrimination, light touch, and stereognosis.

Objective testing of coordination can be accomplished with dexterity tests such as the Crawford Small Parts Dexterity Test (Fig. 13-6), the Pennsylvania Bimanual Work Sample, the Minnesota Rate of Manipulation Tests (Fig. 13-7), the Bennett Hand Tool Test, and the Nine-Hole Peg Test.

Tests of perceptual-motor function include the Ayres Battery, the Frostig Battery, and the Minnesota Spatial Relations Test (Fig. 13-8). Treatment centers use a variety of specific tests to measure performance according to norms; these are but a few of those commonly used.

Informal Performance Testing

There are instances in which it is necessary to modify evaluation techniques to the individual patient according to his or her disability, perceptual dysfunction, and mental attitude. Although objective tests provide a measurement of abilities as compared to standard norms, further evaluations are done to determine the patient's specific abilities and limitations in function in order to establish treatment approaches.

The therapist evaluates the patient's abilities

by assessing how well he or she accomplishes specific tasks. What are limitations of strength, coordination, or range of motion as indicated by ability shown in reaching for, grasping, or placing objects? (Fig. 13-9) How well is the patient adjusting to limitations? This can be assessed by the character of his or her social interactions with other patients, mental tolerance of the social context and activity of the occupational therapy room, and ability to work with his or her spouse and/or the therapist in reviewing self-care abilities in light of eventually going home, where the assistance of a family member may be needed.

Performance testing also involves the assessment of the patient's problem-solving ability in accomplishing a task involving several steps. For example, a woodworking project may be used to test the perceptual-motor abilities of the patient with brain damage. The therapist observes the way the patient plans the project, his or her visual perception, eye-hand coordination, concept of verticality, and proper use of tools.

In performance testing it is essential to set up the task so that, even though difficult for the patient,

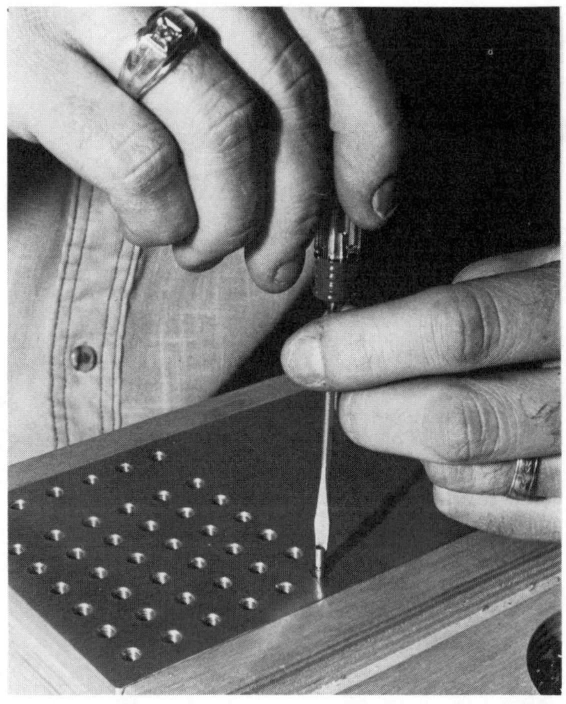

FIGURE 13-6. Crawford Small Parts Dexterity Test, a bimanual small tool coordination test.

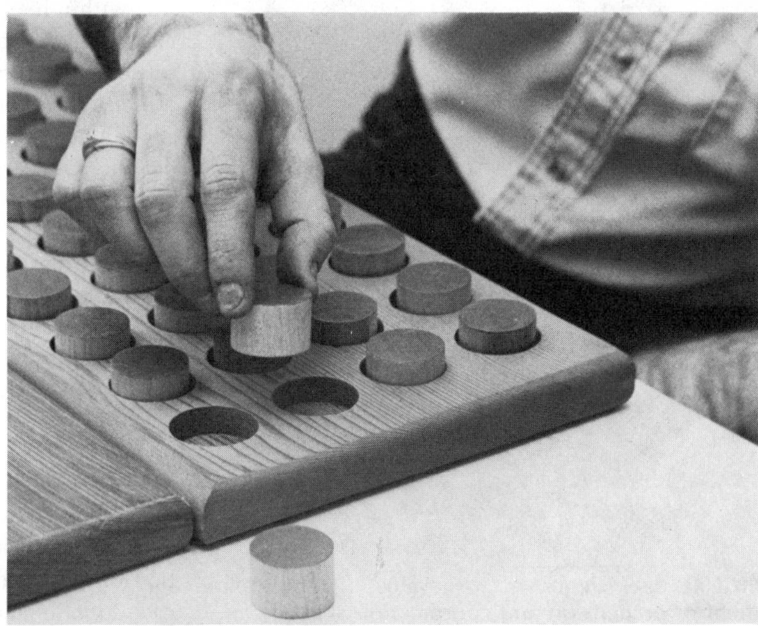

FIGURE 13-7. Minnesota Rate of Manipulation Tests, a manipulation test for unilateral and bimanual dexterity and coordination through repetition of set patterns.

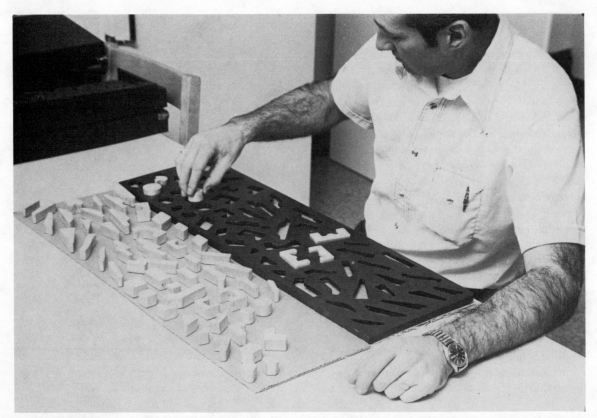

FIGURE 13-8. Minnesota Spatial Relations Test, a standardized test to evaluate visual-motor perception and organization.

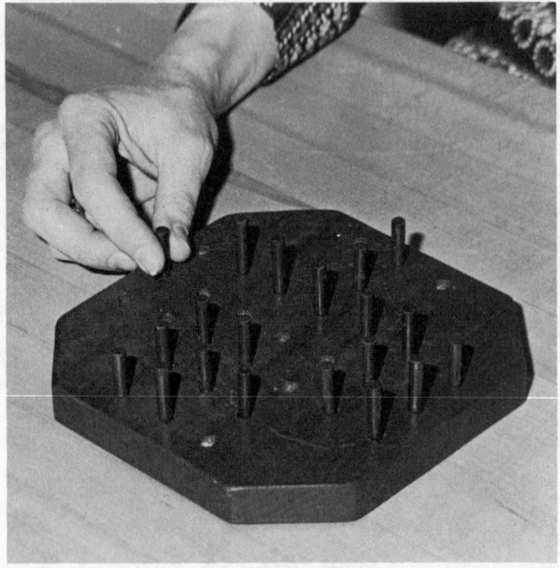

FIGURE 13-9. Pegboard for evaluation and treatment of prehension and coordination skills.

it is within his or her abilities. The use of a familiar task in evaluation may be threatening because it causes the patient to become acutely aware of the loss of ability. Performance testing must include a balance of success along with evaluation of functional deficits. Otherwise the patient may become overly discouraged or negative toward the occupational therapist, and such an attitude can hinder achievement and progress.

Occupational Therapy Worksheet

The occupational therapy worksheet presented here is commonly used to record information derived from the evaluation of the patient. It is referred to as a "worksheet" because it is *not* included in the chart; rather, it assists the therapist in noting information which will be included later in the formal summarized chart report. In addition to the documentation of the basic information regarding the patient, each functional area is delineated for ease in record-

Discharge Date: ____________

OCCUPATIONAL THERAPY WORKSHEET

Name: ______________________
Address: ______________________
Age: ______ Education: ______________
Occupation: ______________________
____
Marital Status: ______ Children: ______________
Other: ______________________

Admission Date: ______________ Ward: __________
Diagnosis: ______________________
Pertinent History: ______________________
O.T. Referral: ______________________
____
Dr. ______________ Date: ______________
Precautions: ______________________

House: Location: ______________ Entrance: ______________ #Floors: ______________
Bathroom: ______________ Architectural Barriers: ______________________
____

EVALUATION: (ROM, strength, coordination, balance, sensation, spasticity, endurance, psychological and perceptual dysfunction)

Upper Extremities: Hand Dominance:
____

RUE: ______________________
____
LUE: ______________________
Bilateral: ______________________
____

Trunk and Lower Extremities:
____
____

Perceptual Functioning: (visual, auditory, motor planning, stereognosis, proprioception)
____
____

Mental Functioning: (attention, awareness, behavior, retention, reception, abstract reasoning, problem solving)
____
____

ADL: (position, balance, mobility, assistive devices used, motivation, perceptual deficits)

Hygiene/Grooming: ______________________
____
Dressing: ______________________
____
____
Self-Feeding: ______________________
____
Writing/Reading: (signature, tracing, copying, spontaneous writing and reading, dominance, field cut, neglect, sight)
____
____

HOMEMAKING: (food preparation, clean-up, safety, home modifications, assistive devices, positioning)
____
____
____

INTERESTS: (vocational, avocational, skills and abilites)
____

SPLINTS AND ASSISTIVE DEVICES: (type, date given, recommendations)
____
____

TREATMENT PLAN
(goal, procedure, positioning, assistive device, activity)

DATE: ____________

Signature

ing information. Additional sheets are sometimes used to supplement this form with detailed information regarding range of motion, perceptual functions, manual muscle testing, activities of daily living, and/or homemaking. This depends on the needs of the individual patient.

At the end of the worksheet there is space for inclusion of the treatment plan. Ideally, following the evaluation, the therapist and the patient design the treatment plan. If the therapist uses the evaluation information creatively, he or she should be able to formulate the goals of treatment and the methods to be used with the patient to achieve these goals.

These methods include the positioning of the patient for treatment, adaptations to the equipment used or types of assistive devices provided the patient, use of splints and other assistive equipment (for example, arm supports). The goals may include unilateral or bilateral improvement in self-care and/or homemaking skills, prevocational readiness, resocialization, functional achievement, and regaining of motivation.

A helpful addition to the worksheet would be to note both the patient's progress and any conference notes regarding the patient. These sheets not only provide a guideline to the therapist but also can aid a substitute therapist if necessary.

Checklist

The use of a checklist format is an efficient method of recording objective information. The inclusion of the date on which the measurement was made is essential in order to maintain an accurate record of progress. This is also important in determining at what point a change in the treatment program is necessary.

This type of format can be used efficiently for the following types of evaluations:

1. Range of motion
2. Manual muscle testing
3. Sensory testing
4. Perceptual testing
5. Dynamometer and pinch-gauge testing
6. Activities of daily living
7. Homemaking
8. Splint check-out
9. Assistive device check-out

It is helpful to have a variety of these forms which can be used when needed. Once gained, the information can then be summarized on the worksheet and on the chart. The checklists are usually considered worksheets; however, they are sometimes included in the chart as primary data. Sometimes a stringent procedure must be followed for approval of the placement of additional sheets in the chart. Also, a short, succinct summary is preferable to lengthy, overly-detailed information; it is more likely to be read. Notes should always be dated and signed, and updated when necessary.

TREATMENT

General Principles

The objectives of occupational therapy in the treatment of the patient with physical and neurological conditions include five major areas: (1) awareness of self, (2) maximum level of self-care independence, (3) restoration of functional ability, (4) exploration of vocational and avocational potential, and (5) socialization and adjustment to new life patterns.

AWARENESS OF SELF. Frequently the patient seeks a defense from the misery of accepting a disabling condition or a long-term progressive illness by denying its existence. Although physical or intellectual deficits may be an obvious result of the illness, the patient may still either consciously or subconsciously deny the occurrence or the implications of his or her condition. The occupational therapy program emphasizes the patient's major objective and, in doing so, provides the patient with the opportunity to see him or herself as a thinking, doing being. Through the performances of tasks directed toward achievable accomplishments, the patient is encouraged to become aware of abilities and problems on a daily basis. The task is directed toward self-accomplishment and self-awareness. In treatment, it is therapeutic for the patient not only to succeed but also to fail occasionally. Failure can be tangible proof to the patient that he or she is denying inability. Although he or she may become depressed, hostile, or discouraged in knowing, it is only in knowing both strengths and weaknesses that the patient is able to see what abilities he or she has and what abilities he or she must try to regain. The denial of limitations prevents the patient from seeing himself or herself as he or she is.

MAXIMUM LEVEL OF SELF-CARE INDEPENDENCE. The responsibility for assisting the patient in independent self-care techniques falls generally to the occupational therapist in collaboration with the nurse. The occupational therapist assesses the problems that the patient has in self-care. For example, if the patient is unable to distinguish between objects of different shapes or colors or is unable to relate to vertical or horizontal positions, the patient may be unable to determine the front, back, or sleeve of a shirt. A person with a flaccid arm cannot handle eating utensils in the usual manner and thus may have to learn how to cut meat one-handed, switch the fork to the non-dominant extremity, or use a plate guard for control.

The occupational therapist analyzes these problems, determines the approach to be used in dealing with them, and teaches the patient the techniques to be used. The nurses then follow through to see that the techniques are used in the patient's daily activities.

In some instances the patient can accomplish self-care and eating by performing the tasks in a different way rather than by using special devices or equipment. However, when various devices are necessary (examples: elastic shoe laces, Velcro closures, or elastic thread), or when the patient must master a new skill (one-handed shoe-tying or one-handed meat cutting), all possibilities should be explored to ensure minimum reliance upon but maximum effectiveness of the special equipment or the acquired skill. Effectiveness in self-care provides the patient with independence rather than dependence upon others; this aids not only the patient, but also helps in family relationships. The accomplishment of self-care tasks leads to further successes and motivation.

RESTORATION OF FUNCTIONAL ABILITY. The restoration of functional ability may precede or follow the emphasis on self-care activity. The exercise of the body and the sensory awareness that the patient uses and develops in the accomplishment of self-care tasks are correlated to specific activities directed toward the restoration of functional ability. These activities include specific exercises to improve strength, range of motion, coordination, and function.

The emphasis of the occupational therapy program is on active rather than passive exercises and on utilizing the abilities of the patient. Although assistive equipment (suspension slings, wheelchairs, lapboards, and splints) may assist the patient passively, the objective of their use is to assist the patient in achieving the maximum level of independent and active functioning. For example, the suspension sling may facilitate arm movement of the quadriplegic, enabling him or her to bring both hands together; with the use of tenodesis function, the patient can eat independently, practice buttoning clothes on a board, write, or type. A variety of assistive equipment may be needed to encourage function and to prevent fatigue during exercise activities.

The occupational therapy room should provide an atmosphere of activity, an emphasis on productive achievement, and an encouragement to try. Activity should be geared toward that which is acceptable and interesting to the patient so that he can see its relation to the total rehabilitation objectives. Often the patient rejects a treatment situation because he cannot face not being able to do things he has done in the past; he resents doing things in an inferior way, doing "child's play," or not being able to function at his expected standard. He may become belligerent and refuse to participate in the therapy program. The occupational therapist must make every effort to devise appropriate treatment programs to prevent negative reactions by the patient.

EXPLORATION OF VOCATIONAL AND AVOCATIONAL POTENTIAL. The occupational therapist should discuss future vocational plans with the patient and concentrate training in the areas related to the vocational goal. For example, the patient who is attending school might wish to spend time improving hand writing and note taking skills. Job tasks may be simulated in occupational therapy for the patient who can return to work. If new vocational goals are set, such as bookkeeping or mechanical drawing, the patient may become proficient in performing these tasks using hand splints.

Avocational interests should be explored, especially when vocational goals are not feasible, in order to give the patient an interest in life. Hobbies such as reading, writing, painting, and drawing can be pursued even though physical limitations require use of adapted equipment to perform many activities.

SOCIALIZATION AND ADJUSTMENT TO NEW LIFE PATTERNS. The occupational therapist can assist the patient in making satisfactory adjustment to a disability and restore self-confidence by concentrating on accomplishments and capabilities and also by providing opportunities for social interaction. The patient should be encouraged to participate in recreational programs and in the patient-governing bodies that are active in many rehabilitation facilities. To ease the fear of taking part in outside social activities because of "looking different," the patient should be encouraged to go on outings such as bowling, baseball games, and movies while still in the hospital. These activities make the patient begin to function as a member of a community in preparation for discharge into the community. Upon discharge, each person should be encouraged to participate in social and community affairs and to attend functions that were part of his or her life before the injury.

Summary

In summarizing treatment, the principles of approach are the following:

1. Set the environment for success by creating a therapeutic milieu.
2. Orient the individual treatment program to the patient's interests and abilities.
3. Use passive range of motion to encourage active patterns of movement.
4. Demonstrate adaptation techniques in the way the patient is expected to perform.
5. Establish long-term goals with regard for the implications of the disability and potential achievement.
6. Establish short-term goals to achieve positive feedback and satisfaction for the patient for accomplishment of long-term goals.
7. Work on the short-term goals one at a time to establish the patient's acceptance of the disability and the rehabilitation program.
8. Include the patient in setting the long- and short-term goals as he or she is receptive to them.

9. Engage the patient in productive, purposeful activity.

10. Encourage resocialization for motivation, acceptance, and adaptation.

Approaches and Correlation with Other Disciplines

The ideal treatment approach to a patient is the *team approach* in which formal and informal interaction are encouraged among all persons working with a patient for the purpose of developing and implementing a unified treatment program. This team includes the patient and his or her family as well as health care workers.

In the rehabilitation approach there are overlaps in evaluation and treatment among the physicians, nurses, physical therapists, occupational therapists, speech therapists, social workers, and vocational rehabilitation counsellors. Overlaps can be useful in carryover of activities and in the continual monitoring of the patient's progress. Communication among the disciplines is necessary to encourage coordination rather than antagonism over "who does what" with the patient. For example, the occupational therapist works with the physician regarding the medical precautions related to body positioning, mental and physical tolerance of activity, and progression of pathological symptoms. A coordinated self-care program involves the cooperation of the nurses in the inclusion of the methods of the occupational therapist in the patient's daily hygiene, grooming, dressing, and eating. The occupational therapist coordinates the morning dressing program and general exercise activities with the physical therapy program so that the patient's physical gains are used throughout the treatment day and he or she does not become overly fatigued. The speech therapist aids team members in effective communication with patients with speech deficits. As the social worker deals with the patient and family, he or she needs to know the patient's treatment programs and progress in order to interpret "what and how" the patient is doing, to convey this information to the family, and to assist the patient in understanding the daily program. The vocational rehabilitation counsellor relies on the occupational therapist's evaluation of functional ability to determine the patient's role in education, job return, placement, or relocation.

A functional definition of roles among the team members is essential for communication and effective rehabilitation of the patient. The specific roles of each member of the team may vary in different treatment centers.

Team members are important sources of information and support to one another. For example, a patient may come into the occupational therapy room and develop signs of extreme fatigue, such as sweating and difficulty in breathing. The occupational therapist contacts the physician or the nurse for assistance in determining the cause and seriousness of the patient's symptoms. The occupational therapist contacts the physical therapist to determine techniques for the patient's safe and successful transfer from one chair to another, for information about whether he or she will be safe standing to perform a woodworking project or whether a patient can safely stand and walk in the kitchen for assessment of homemaking skills. Both occupational and physical therapists should coordinate muscle testing, range of motion, sensory testing, and assessment of physical tolerance and balance. The speech therapist and occupational therapist work together in designing the treatment approaches for the aphasic patient. Realistic vocational planning by the counsellor is aided by the occupational therapist, who assesses the functional abilities of the upper extremities, the intellectual level of functioning in applied tasks, and the patient's general physical tolerance. The physician aids in developing realistic planning in terms of the prognosis and the patient's mental approach to rehabilitation.

Discharge Planning

The end result of a well-coordinated team approach is effective discharge planning, with all team members contributing to the plan for the patient's reentry into the community. Discharge planning had long been considered the province of the social worker. However, with the development of the team approach and the growth of rehabilitation, discharge planning has broadened from the concept of placement of a person following discharge to actual preparation for discharge.

This preparation includes medical considerations (continuation of medication, follow-up visits, plans for future treatment procedures); provision of assistive equipment for home exercise functions and activity or independence in daily living; counselling of the family regarding the patient's self-care and general activity; and a home visit to determine the presence of architectural barriers and to evaluate the patient's potential for functioning in the home.

These concerns are best met by beginning discharge planning upon admission and at the time of first contact with and evaluation of the patient. By first finding out the patient's home environment, life style, educational level, and occupation, the team can create a treatment plan that will assist the patient in preparing to go home while he or she is still in the hospital. If the total treatment plan is geared toward meeting the needs of the patient upon discharge, he or she is encouraged to see the importance of therapy for realistic discharge planning rather than as a program which has no relationship to what the patient regards as the most crucial problems at home. Discharge planning by the occupational therapist is a realistic approach to treatment, geared to the eventual return home of the patient.

REFERENCES

1. Dunning, H.: Environmental occupational therapy. Am. J. Occup. Ther. 26:292, 1972.

section 2 / Major Disabilities

A "disability approach" to evaluation and treatment is presented in this second section. The approach to specific evaluation, adaptations, and treatment will be discussed through the symptom complexes of the major disabilities seen by occupational therapists in the rehabilitation setting. The purpose of this structure is to correlate techniques with specific conditions; it does not imply that approaches discussed in one section cannot be used, where appropriate, with another disability.

The occupational therapist working in a rehabilitation program must evaluate and treat persons suffering disabilities resulting from a variety of diagnoses. Those discussed in this chapter are:

1. Neurological conditions: cerebrovascular accident (CVA), head injury, multiple sclerosis (MS), Parkinson's disease, spinal cord lesions, polio, the Guillain-Barré syndrome, amyotrophic lateral sclerosis (ALS), myasthenia gravis, muscular dystrophy (MD), carpal tunnel syndrome, and Volkmann's ischemic contracture.
2. Orthopedic conditions of the upper and lower extremities.
3. Arthritis (osteoarthritis and rheumatoid arthritis).

NEUROLOGICAL CONDITIONS

Neurological conditions include a large variety of diagnoses and clinical manifestations that occur according to the location of the lesion within the nervous system. Diagnoses discussed in this section include cerebrovascular accident (CVA, stroke, hemiplegia), traumatic head injury, multiple sclerosis (MS), Parkinson's disease, spinal cord lesions, polio, the Guillain-Barré syndrome, amyotrophic lateral sclerosis (ALS), myasthenia gravis, muscular dystrophy (MD), and peripheral nerve injuries.

Lesions in the brain are caused by cerebrovascular accident, head injury, multiple sclerosis, and Parkinson's disease and result in intellectual, personality, physical, and emotional changes. Lesions in the spinal cord and nerve roots include spinal cord injury, polio, and the Guillain-Barré syndrome and result in paralysis of the extremities with respiratory, bowel, and bladder involvement. Myasthenia gravis and muscular dystrophy are primarily diseases of the muscles resulting in dysfunction. Multiple sclerosis, Parkinson's disease, myasthenia gravis, amyotrophic lateral sclerosis, and muscular dystrophy are progressively debilitating conditions. Depending on the severity of the trauma, there may be significant recovery potential for the person suffering from cerebrovascular accident, head injury, spinal cord injury, the Guillain-Barré syndrome, and peripheral nerve injuries. Although spinal cord injury, polio, and the Guillain-Barré syndrome may show a similar clinical picture in hospitalization, they vary in prognosis.

One way of distinguishing clinical manifestations of neurological conditions is by distinguishing upper motor neuron from lower motor neuron lesions. The upper motor neuron lesion (UMN) occurs in the corticospinal or pyramidal tract, located in the brain or spinal cord. Resultant conditions are hemiplegia, paraplegia, or quadriplegia. The location and extent of the lesion determines the extent of the paralysis. The clinical signs include loss of voluntary movement, increased muscle tone (spasticity), pathological reflexes in the limbs, and sensory loss.[1] The principle causes of UMN lesions are cerebrovascular accident, brain tumor or trauma, amyotrophic lateral sclerosis, multiple sclerosis, and spinal cord transection or compression.

UMN conditions resulting in impairment of cerebral functions are cerebrovascular accident (internal brain trauma), head injury (external brain trauma), and multiple sclerosis (disease). UMN conditions *not* resulting in impairment of cerebral functions are spinal cord injury (external trauma) and amyotrophic lateral sclerosis (disease).

Lesions in the extrapyramidal system result in disorders of muscle tone and involuntary movements, e.g., Parkinson's disease. Conditions of ataxia resulting from proprioceptive disorders can be caused by lesions in the spinal nerve roots (spinal ataxia) or in the cerebellum and its pathways (cerebellar ataxia).[1] Common causes of ataxia are head injury, brain tumor, and multiple sclerosis.

The lower motor neuron lesion (LMN) occurs in the anterior horn cells, nerve roots, and the peripheral nerve system, causing flaccid conditions of monoplegia, paraplegia, triplegia, and quadriplegia. Diseases contributing to LMN lesions usually are systemic and have symmetrical involvement; an exception to this is polio, which can have widely scattered effects in the limbs. The presence of lesions results in loss of voluntary function, flaccid paralysis, sensory loss, and atrophy. The principle causes are polio, the Guillain-Barré syndrome, ischemia, peripheral nerve injuries (see chapter 22) and brachial plexus injury.

Neurological impairment depends on the location of the lesion rather than on the nature of the lesion (Table 13-1). Therefore there is some similarity in the treatment of neurological disorders according to the site of the lesion. Impairment can involve intellectual functions (perception, problem solving), mental processes (personality, behavior, motivation), motor functions (muscle power, bladder and bowel control), sensory functions (proprioception, sensation, stereognosis, hearing, and sight), coordination (ataxia), and involuntary motions (tremor).

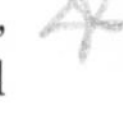

General

Evaluation

The evaluation of the brain-damaged patient with neurologic impairment includes techniques to assess motor, sensory, integrative, expressive, receptive, passive, active, intellectual, perceptual,

Table 13-1. Correlation of location of lesion with resultant pathology, organic manifestations, and course of disease.

Location of lesion	*Pathology*	*Organic Manifestation*	*Course of disease*
Brain	Cerebrovascular accident Head injury Multiple sclerosis Parkinson's disease	Intellectual Personality Physical Emotional Communication	Nonprogressive Nonprogressive Progressive Progressive
Spinal cord	Spinal cord injury Polio Guillain-Barré syndrome	Physical	Nonprogressive
Muscle or myoneural junction	Myasthenia gravis Amyotrophic lateral sclerosis Muscular dystrophy	Physical Communication (motor)	Progressive
Extremity	Peripheral nerve injury	Physical (local)	Nonprogressive

and attitudinal responses. A practical approach to assessment includes the setting of the environment and the therapist's eliciting maximum response from the patient. Frequently, treatment approaches must be used in evaluation to make accurate assessments. The length, progress, and type of evaluation technique used depends on the patient's physical and mental tolerance and comprehension, because all areas of function are interrelated and influence each other.[2] At the beginning of evaluation a means of communication must be established since the patient may lack speech and/or comprehension of instructions.

PRAXIA: MOTOR ABILITY. The therapist compares the two sides of the patient's body during evaluation. Except in cases of bilateral hemiplegia or accompanying factors such as previous fractures, arthritis, or other neurological problems affecting the sound extremity, bilateral evaluation gives an indication of the impairment on the opposite side. For the confused patient, checking the passive range of motion of both extremities before requesting active movement may help to give him or her a clearer idea of what is required. Most patients do not understand complicated technical terms, and demonstrations using passive range of motion help. This technique will also help the apraxic patient, who cannot initiate the voluntary motor act although he or she may have the motor ability to perform.

The therapist checks both passive and active range of motion, strength, reflex activity, coordination, proprioceptive and kinesthetic sense, postural reactions, and bilateral integration. These techniques will need to be modified depending on whether the patient is in bed, in a wheelchair, or ambulatory.

Safety precautions during motor evaluations are essential and, although the patient may verbally indicate no deficits, the therapist must evaluate to make certain of the patient's condition. In the assessment of the patient's motor ability, activities can be provided to stimulate strength and coordination and to detect apraxia. The patient's vision should be occluded to evaluate proprioceptive and kinesthetic sense.

The ability of the patient to perform the motor act may be more functional when he or she is asked to perform a task such as reaching for an object in the therapist's hand or touching a part of his or her own body. Return of muscle function in the hemiplegic patient follows the developmental patterns of synergies; therefore the therapist should observe the patient's active movements for signs of synergistic patterns. The therapist should also observe the position of the patient's limbs at rest for signs of spasticity, edema, muscle weakness, or neglect. These can be noted in the posture of the patient lying in bed or in a sitting position.

SENSORY FUNCTIONS. The therapist touches the patient lightly to determine the patient's perception of the location of tactile stimulus. This can be done either from distal to proximal or vice versa; however, sensory and motor deficits are usually increasingly impaired from proximal to distal. The patient is asked to occlude vision by looking the other way or by closing the eyes. Although a blindfold may be necessary for the patient who is unable to look the other way or does not comprehend the reason for closing the eyes, this may be a frightening technique. The therapist can perform the test by covering the testing area or by placing the patient's arms under a table while sitting opposite the patient.

The patient's fingers are touched with rough and smooth objects to determine texture discrimination; familiar objects of varying sizes, shapes, and weights are presented to determine stereognosis. In the case of hemiplegia the uninvolved extremity should be checked first so that the patient understands what is being asked; then the affected hand and arm should be checked. This provides some positive input and feedback and encourages the patient regarding intact functions.

VISUAL PERCEPTION. The therapist should first determine whether the patient wears glasses or has a visual acuity deficiency. The patient should be asked to identify familiar objects or words; this can be done either verbally (if the patient can speak) or by a process of elimination (pointing or selecting). The therapist should determine the patient's accuracy in color, size, and shape discrimination. Tests standardized on a child population can be used to make observations in the area of figure ground, spatial relations, and form constancy. The patient should be asked to read a sentence written in large letters or an advertisement from a magazine and to write his or her name. This determines the ability to form letters and to interpret them; reading, writing, and block designs can be used to detect the presence of field cut or neglect of the visual field.

BODY SCHEME. The use of the body and neglect of intact functions can be determined in the evaluation of sensory and motor functions already discussed. The use of the draw-a-person test, figure assembling tests, identification of body parts, and self-care assessment assist in determination of the function of the total body awareness. The patient's left-right discrimination and directionality may be affected.

INTELLECTUAL FUNCTIONS. Ability to write is tested by asking the patient to write his or her name. If the patient is unable to do this, the therapist gives assistance by forming the letters, asking the patient first to trace and then to copy them. Close observation reveals perceptual disorders in spatial relations, directionality, and concepts of form. If the patient is able to write spontaneously, the following activities should be checked: ability to copy letters and numbers, to do simple arithmetical problems, and to answer questions related to a written paragraph. Problem solving and construction abilities can be evaluated later by assessing the patient's ability to plan such activities as a simple woodworking project or a weaving project and to learn to follow step-by-step procedures.

GENERAL APPLIED MENTAL FUNCTIONS. In the course of the specific evaluations, consideration should be given to the patient's attention span, distractibility, comprehension of verbal and demonstrated instructions, remote and recent memory, and sequential memory. Since mental and physical tolerance may be limited, particularly in the early stages of rehabilitation, attention should be focused on positive performance with termination of the evaluation or treatment before the patient becomes fatigued or discouraged. The therapist should make sure that every assessment period has positive aspects and should verbally encourage the patient regarding intact functions and progress.

APPLIED FUNCTIONS. The assessment of applied functions includes combinations of the specific evaluations mentioned previously. It is essential to pinpoint areas of deficit so that they are considered in the assessment of the more complicated and threatening daily functions such as self-care. If the therapist has accurately and carefully evaluated physical, sensory, intellectual, and integrative abilities, he or she uses this information in evaluating the specific deficits in applied functions.

SELF-CARE. The self-care evaluation should be done in the situation in which the patient feels most comfortable. Evaluation of grooming and dressing should be done in privacy to prevent the patient's discouragement at not being independent in a task which he or she previously could perform. Evaluation of self-feeding skills can be done either in the occupational therapy room or in the patient's room, depending upon the patient's desires and mental state. The use of the nondominant, sound extremity may be embarrassingly incoordinated, and the patient may need practice to accomplish one-handed self-feeding. It is often desirable for the patient to gain skill in self-feeding before eating in a public place. Evaluation to determine the need for splints, assistive devices, and changes in methods of performing an activity accompanies the assessment of self-care skills; the therapist should observe the patient's work in self-care activities.

The careful evaluation of all self-care areas is essential to the patient's regaining self-esteem and respect through the retrieval of independent functional ability. Attention to these areas assists the patient in regaining a sense of reality and of his or her individual role in the family.

SPLINTING AND ASSISTIVE DEVICES. As the functional deficits are determined by the therapist, consideration is given to the use of splinting to provide positioning against spasticity and resultant deformity, to stimulate muscle functions, to increase the patient's awareness of desensitized extremities, and to protect nonfunctioning extremities for future functions. Using assistive devices in early treatment can support the use of functioning muscles and can provide functions to increase the patient's independence.

Occupational Therapy Program

The occupational therapy program incorporates three major areas: (1) identification of function through evaluation procedures, (2) development of function through use of specific activities to increase function, and (3) integration of function into the patient's routine tasks. The program is determined by consideration of the patient's deficits and abilities discovered in the formal evaluation and identification of treatment priorities. When the program is established it is explained to the patient. When feasible the therapist and the patient work out the program together.

POSITIONING. The appropriateness of the patient's position for function is essential, whether in bed, in a wheelchair or a regular chair, standing, or walking. The therapist should evaluate the patient's balance and awareness of position and should show the patient different positions that may be used comfortably and safely. If necessary, extremities should be placed in the optimum position for motion. Among devices and concepts which aid the patient are a mirror for visual feedback, gravity for ease of movement, repetition of movement for sensory awareness, sensory contact for reinforcement, bilateral use of the extremities for midline crossing and integration of two sides of the body, and supportive devices to minimize fatigue and maximize function.

VESTIBULAR STIMULATION. Activities involving movement which changes the plane of the patient's head in space should be used. Among these are games involving spatial concepts: shuffleboard (from the wheelchair or while standing), table shuffleboard, catching a ball or beanbag, hitting a ball, dancing, or marching.

CORRELATION OF SENSORY INPUT. Gradual controlled increase in stimuli in all activity should be provided. In all task-oriented activity there is a variety of sensory input: visual, auditory, tactile, proprioceptive, and vestibular. Reinforcement of sensory cues assists memory development and orientation through repetition and familiarity; this increases awareness. Associations should be made between and among activities, i.e., the correlation between vertical-bilateral sanding and pulling up one's pants.

TECHNIQUES OF SENSORIMOTOR STIMULATION AND INHIBITION. Techniques providing fast irregular rhythms characterizing stimulation include vibration, pressure, tapping, stretching, joint compression, brushing, icing, resistance, and visual and auditory stimuli.

Techniques of inhibition include warmth, slow stroking, gentle shaking or rocking, pressure on the insertion of a muscle, and joint compression. In addition, cool colors, soft regular rhythms, and soft even-speaking tones can be used.

SPLINTING AND SLINGS. The provision of splints and slings for the brain-damaged patient remains a controversial subject among physicians, physical therapists, and occupational therapists. This controversy is caused by the variety of treatment approaches and settings available. Those using sensorimotor facilitation techniques tend to discourage splinting because it counteracts the use of neurophysiological techniques, but those in settings where these techniques have not been and generally are not used tend toward the traditional concepts of splinting and the use of arm slings. The provision of assistive devices should be carefully assessed and should correlate with other treatments, thereby providing the patient with the maximum advantage of all treatments.

In the early stage of hemiplegia, when the extremity is flaccid and concern is for positioning to prevent deformity, contractures from spasticity, and edema, a static hand-forearm splint can be used to maintain the extremity in a functional position. As the patient begins to regain function, the need for a splint should be reassessed to determine whether it can be used as a night splint, allowing the hand freedom during the day for functional activities.

With the restoration of the upper extremity musculature, a static cock-up splint to support the wrist both at rest and during activity is often recommended. This may have a C bar at the thumb web space to prevent contracture. Dynamic splinting (the long opponens with an outrigger and finger cuffs, for example) to encourage active use of the fingers during resistive functional exercises may be appropriate.

Orthokinetic splinting providing mobilization and support can be used for (1) relief of pain, (2) increase of muscle strength, (3) increase of range of motion, (4) muscle reeducation, and (5) improvement of coordination. This type of splint uses a minimum of static coverage where inhibition is desired and acts as a facilitator of paralyzed extensor muscles through the use of wide elastic straps over the muscle bellies and tendons. The orthokinetic concept is a dynamic one; its purpose is function rather than immobilization.

The arm sling is commonly used to support the flaccid arm and to prevent subluxation of the shoulder. If shoulder musculature is functioning and the articulation is not subluxed, the sling is used only during ambulation to offset the pull of gravity and to prevent edema of the hand. While the patient is seated in a wheelchair, other devices should be used to support and position the arm; an overhead suspension sling, a lapboard, arm trough, or padded wedge placed on a lapboard can prevent edema of the hand. Positioning is important—*every effort must be made, both in bed and chair positioning, to prevent edema* in the hand. Although the arm sling is an easily recognizable means of support for the paralyzed arm, care must be taken *not* to use a sling that will cause shoulder pain, increase in spasticity, and subluxation as a result of poor design, application, and/or use. A balanced forearm orthosis or suspension sling with an overhead bar can be attached to the wheelchair to both support the arm and facilitate movement.

AUDITORY STIMULATION. Keeping in mind the environmental effects on the neurologically impaired patient, the therapist can use auditory stimulation therapeutically. Verbal cues can be used supportively, as reinforcement, and for orientation. In the same manner, socialization can be used for auditory discrimination and localization as well as for providing verbal feedback. Music can be used for relaxation during or after effort or as a rhythmic accompaniment to gross motor activity during the use of the spring suspension sling.

TACTILE STIMULATION. Application of stimuli to the skin of the involved extremity over flaccid muscles, using touch and moderate pressure, can result in improved sensory response and increased motor function. Passive cutaneous stimulation by the therapist, using stroking, pressure, brushing, and object pressure, stimulates sensation. Manipulation of shapes in both the affected and nonaffected hand encourages feedback from the normal extremity. Pressure over the muscle belly, joint, or tendon stimulates individual muscle response. Cutaneous stimulation from tools adapted with surface textures encourages security of grip and sensory stimulation. Rolling in bed during dressing and bathing stimulates the patient's body awareness. Self-stimulation and location of the affected extremity during self-care activities encourages range of motion, bilateral awareness and integration, and increases function.

VISUAL STIMULATION. When the patient comes for treatment, he or she should be oriented to the occupational therapy room, with furniture, people, and activities being pointed out and identified. The furniture can be used to relate form constancy and color and shape discrimination.

When denial or neglect of a visual field or extremity is shown, the patient should be encouraged to look at his or her body during exercises and activities. Cutaneous and verbal stimulation can draw attention to the extremity, and the patient should be encouraged to place the arm on the table even though not using it actively in a task. Visual tasks such as object assembly, puzzles (Fig. 13-10), reading the newspaper, writing, or copying encourage visual organization.

FUNCTIONAL ACTIVITIES. The patient focuses on the activity instead of the goal of specific muscle or extremity function. The goals should be inherent in the activity; thus doing the activity should accomplish the goal.

Sensory stimulus is developed through adapted cutaneous contact with tools, the beater of a loom, or the handle of a sander. Sensory discrimination is stimulated through the adapted tools as well as by the use of materials such as clay, sand, or theraplast. Gross motor reaching and throwing activities to stimulate proprioception and kinesthetic awareness such as shuffleboard and beanbag, ball, and dart throwing are useful. Use of the skateboard attached

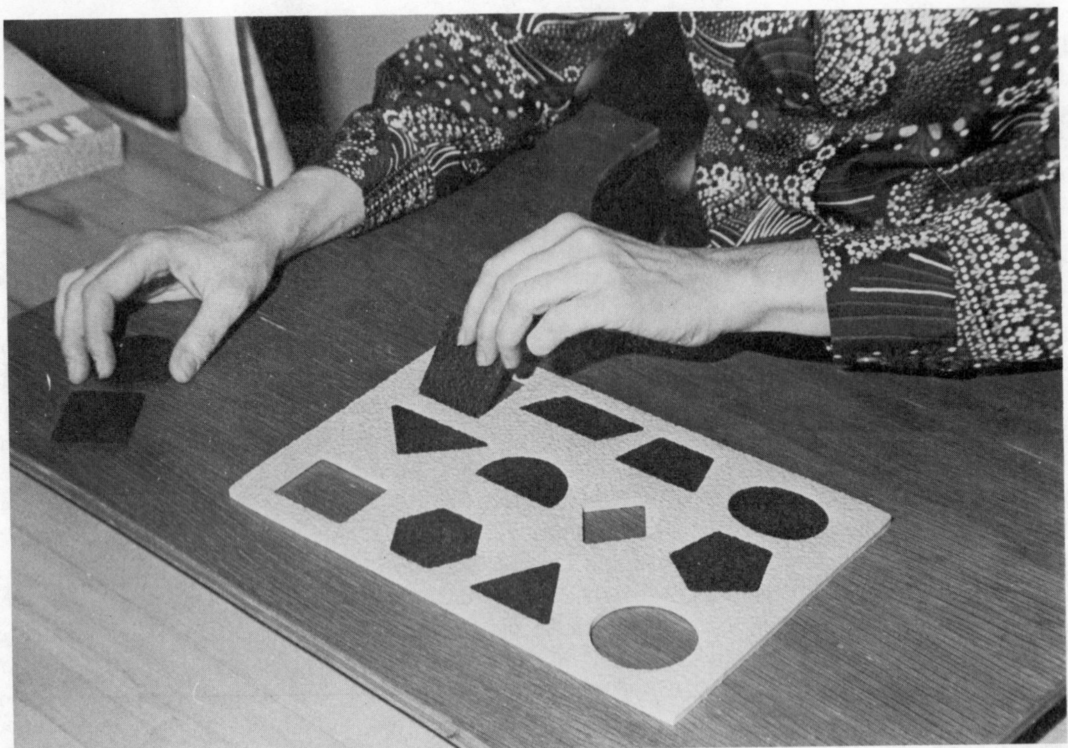

FIGURE 13-10. Puzzles assist the patient in visual-spatial perception and discrimination tasks, tactile sensation, coordination, prehension, and placement skills.

to the forearm for directed range of motion activities stimulates upper arm active movements. Adaptations can be made for holding a pencil and drawing patterns on paper or on a horizontal blackboard during directed skateboard movement.

Suspension slings and pulley systems incorporating weighted or counterbalanced resistance are both supportive of weak extremities and facilitative to movement. They may be used in conjunction with activities to increase shoulder and elbow function. The addition of a functional hand splint may be used to encourage positioning and grasp. Activities such as weaving, woodworking, and especially sanding, planing, and filing can be adapted to incorporate movements with gravity assisting for diagonal patterns and to encourage midline crossing.

Trunk stability and correct positioning are encouraged during all activities. Stability of trunk and joints proximal to those being used are necessary for self-directed, goal-oriented, coordinated acitivty.

Cerebrovascular Accident

The cerebrovascular accident (CVA) is a lesion in the brain commonly referred to as a stroke or a shock because of its sudden onset; it results in paralysis of one side of the body (hemiplegia). The lesion is characterized by an interruption of the blood supply to the brain tissues caused by thrombus, embolus, anoxia, hemorrhage, or aneurysm. Precipitating factors may include a history of hypertension, arteriosclerosis, or congenital artery wall weakness. Although hypertension and arteriosclerosis contribute to the vessel breakdown or occlusion in the older adult, congenital vascular weakness can result in an aneurysm, a common cause of hemiplegia in the young adult.

Vascular disease can cause a complete CVA with a full picture of hemiplegia or a transient ischemic attack (TIA) because of vascular insufficiency. The TIA may result in brief and spotty impairment of neurological function; it is frequently a warning of the probability of CVA in the future. The treatment of the patient with either a complete CVA or TIA not only should be geared toward rehabilitation of the present problem but also should include prophylactic techniques to prevent further occurrence of TIA or CVA.

Other causes of hemiplegia include external trauma (a blow on the head or a fall striking the head), heart attack, and brain and spinal tumors. In these cases the character of the condition may vary slightly from the cardiovascular lesion but, because many of the symptoms are similar, evaluation techniques and treatment procedures used in CVA can be applied.

In this section the evaluation and treatment of the person suffering a CVA is emphasized and the role of the occupational therapist in the intensive rehabilitation regimen of a team-oriented approach is discussed. Because of the number and complexity of the manifestations facing the patient and the impact of these conditions on daily life and family, all team members must work together in the rehabilitation process.

Definition

The lesion in the brain that causes hemiplegia usually occurs in one hemisphere and affects the contralateral limbs and face. The result is commonly referred to as right or left hemiplegia, depending on the side of the body involved. However, in discussing CVA and hemiplegia, it is essential to distinguish between the location of the CVA (right hemisphere) and the location of the hemiplegia (left side of the body). Should the CVA occur in the left hemisphere, the hemiplegia will be located on the right side of the body.

Depending upon which side of the brain is involved, there can be, in addition to motor and sensory deficits, impairment of perceptual and cognitive functions, of premorbid personality, of motor planning and problem-solving abilities, and of judgment (Table 13-2). Urinary continence, motivation, and a sense of social awareness and responsibility may be lost.

A lesion can affect both hemispheres of the brain, thus causing bilateral clinical signs.

Impact of Hemiplegia

Whether the person is affected by the sudden onset of CVA or by the shock of external trauma causing hemiplegia, the results of the condition can have a devastating impact on his or her life. The adult patient may be going to school, completing vocational or academic training in preparation for employment, secure in employment, nearing the peak of vocational goals, nearing retirement, or retired. In all of these situations, the patient may suffer the threat of not returning to his or her previous life style and/or occupation. The severity of the brain damage, the pre-morbid health conditions, the patient's attitude toward the condition and rehabilitation, the support of family, and the restoration of various functions are all factors in rehabilitation.

While the patient's developmental level prior to the CVA was that of an adult, the effect of the CVA may reduce the patient's physical and mental levels to those of a child. The patient may be unable to accept the arduous recuperation of lost functions through specific "childlike" activities such as strengthening of limbs and development of coordination; learning again to read, write, and speak; or developing independence in self-care and toilet functions. Frequently the patient denies the full implications of self-involvement in the recovery of these functions; he or she may be unable to cope with the multitude of problems facing him or her and the family, or the patient may be suffering actual damage to brain tissues which control motivation and adjustment. The adult hemiplegic patient tends to look back to normal functioning and imposes pre-morbid standards on present abilities.

Sensorimotor losses are accompanied by changes in body image and personality which affect both the patient and family and can strain their relationship. Confusion resulting from brain trauma can leave the patient unable to establish self-direction and purposeful motivation or to understand simple conversations. The effects on the patient's personality may result in a change in values, having an effect on level of performance. Because the older adult suffering a CVA has "all that has been gained to lose," one of the most difficult problems for both the patient and the therapist is the patient's belief

Table 13-2. Cerebrovascular accident.

Artery	*Areas of Brain affected*	*Manifestation*
Internal carotid	Frontal lobe Parietal lobe Temporal lobe Internal capsule Optic nerve	Aphasia (dominant hemisphere) Contralateral hemiplegia Homonomous hemianopsia
Anterior cerebral	Anterior part of internal capsule Tip of frontal lobe Surface of cerebral hemisphere to parietal-occipital junction	Contralateral monoplegia (leg) Sensory loss Mental confusion Apraxia Aphasia (dominant hemisphere)
Middle cerebral	Convolutions of cerebral hemisphere Lateral orbital-frontal region Internal capsule Anterior thalamus	Contralateral hemiplegia (primarily arm) Contralateral facial weakness Aphasia (dominant hemisphere) Homonomous hemianopsia Sensory loss
Posterior cerebral	Midbrain $^{2}/_{3}$ Temporal lobe Middle occipital lobe Posterior internal capsule	Contralateral hemiplegia Hemi-anesthesia Homonomous hemianopsia Ataxia Tremor
Basilar	Pons Medulla Cerebellum	Symptoms from 3rd to 12th cranial nerves Loss of proprioception Cerebellar dysfunction
Cerebellar	Midbrain Pons Cerebellum	Cerebellar ataxia Contralateral loss of pain and temperature

that he "has lived his life" and there is nothing left.

The following factors contribute to disorientation, confusion, malfunction, and lack of progress:

1. Auditory deficit: receptive and/or expressive aphasia.
2. Impairment of verbal expression.
3. Deficits in learning ability which affect performance.
4. Impairment of previously independent function.
5. Denial and neglect of affected extremities.
6. Distortion of time and place which affects the ability to plan the future.
7. Loss of tactile sensation and function which impedes motor function.
8. Loss of proprioceptive and kinesthetic awareness which hinders bilateral integration.
9. Apraxia or loss of voluntary motor activity which hinders functional ability.
10. Visual-perceptual deficits such as field cut or visual field neglect.

These deficits, although common, may not be present in all hemiplegics.

PHYSICAL MANIFESTATIONS. A lesion in the brain, usually localized in one hemisphere, results in motor impairment in the contralateral side of the body. Complete (-plegia) or partial (paresis) flaccid paralysis of the upper and lower musculature and facial muscles is manifested in the loss of active mobility of the involved extremities. While passive range of motion is complete initially, gradual onset of spasticity presents the threat of increased muscle tone impeding active range of motion and causing contractures and deformity. The severity of involvement depends on location and extent of the lesion. Some patients may begin to gain voluntary muscle power a few days following the CVA. Others may experience no return for months or years. For some the ability may never be regained. Impairment of the dominant extremity necessitates a change of dominance, and loss of bilateral coordination with a possibility of partial loss of strength and coordination in the sound extremity.

SENSORY DEFICITS IN EXTREMITIES. Sensory impairment is manifested in peripheral reception of stimuli, tactile functions in the affected hand, and general sensory awareness. Manifestations of peripheral impairment include lack of sensation of cutaneous stimuli (temperature, touch, pain); inability to locate the area of stimulus; inability to identify the position of the extremity (proprioception); inability to identify a familiar object through tactile sensation (stereognosis); inability to effect the motor act (apraxia); inability to correlate purpose and accomplishment of tasks (ideational apraxia); and inability to carry out new purposeful activities while retaining ability to perform routine activities (ideomotor apraxia). Lack of sensory functions and impairment of sensory receptors in the extremities affect motor functions by causing lack of feedback. Bilateral integrative functions are also affected by sensory deficits.

VISUAL DEFICITS. Double vision (diplopia), loss of half of the visual field (hemianopsia), and neglect are three common manifestations of visual impairment. Loss of part of the visual field prevents the patient from seeing objects on the right or left side. The patient is unaware of this "cut" in the visual field until he or she realizes that a paragraph makes little sense because he or she can read only half of it or when he or she drives the wheelchair into the side of a doorway or only half dresses thinking the task has been completed.

Visual field neglect occurs when the patient ignores visual stimuli on the side of hemiplegia when confronted with simultaneous stimuli from both visual fields. This occurs when visual fields are intact.[3] Distortions in the perception of spatial relations (vertical, horizontal, oblique) result in impairment in deriving meaning from visual stimuli and in using this information in intellectual functions.

COMMUNICATION DISORDERS. Both left and right hemiplegic patients show communication disorders in the early stages following CVA; however the right hemiplegic tends to retain more severe deficits in speech, verbal reception, and language because a lesion in the dominant hemisphere (usually the left) affects all language areas to some degree. Specific problems that occur are impairment in interpretation of the meaning of spoken and written words (receptive aphasia), impairment of the ability to use speech and to write communicatively (expressive aphasia), and impairment of motor function of speech (dysarthria). Distorted auditory reception, loss of hearing, and inability to locate auditory stimuli or to make meaning of them can affect the speech response. Apraxia is the impairment of the voluntary ability to use the speech mechanisms; the patient may possess these functions but is unable to use them. Despite apraxia, the patient may be able to use the tongue, lips, or speech mechanisms for automatic and reflexive actions such as chewing or blowing.

INTELLECTUAL AND PERCEPTUAL DYSFUNCTIONS. With the disturbance in sensorimotor reception and expression, the hemiplegic patient frequently demonstrates impairment in abstract reasoning. The severity of this condition depends on the auditory, visual, and tactile abilities which remain intact. Learning is affected by sensory deficits that impede learning through the use of auditory instructions, reading, imitation, and demonstration. The prognosis for restoration of independent function depends on the patient's ability to receive and to organize information for learning and implementation.

FUNCTIONAL IMPLICATIONS. With sensory and motor loss in the arm and leg on the affected side of the body, the hemiplegic person functionally becomes one sided. Activities such as rolling over in bed, eating, dressing, bathing, grooming, and two-handed activities are now limited by the paralysis of an arm and a leg. Not only are the specific peripheral functions impaired, but the sense of integration of the body is also affected by the cerebral lesion. The patient may find it difficult to adjust to a necessary change in hand dominance. Activities requiring total sensorimotor awareness are affected. The patient may deny or neglect the functional implications of this condition and may grow to depend on others for assistance in daily functions and responsibilities. The rehabilitation program is geared both toward achievement of maximum independence and toward family awareness and acceptance of the patient's level of function.

Self-Care Skills and Activities of Daily Living

The level of accomplishment in self-care skills and activities of daily living by the hemiplegic patient is largely dependent on *motivational, perceptual, judgmental,* and *sensory-integrative* factors. While both right and left hemiplegic patients suffer motor paralysis or limitations, there are distinctions in the effects of the locations of the lesions.

Functional areas largely affected by a lesion in the right hemisphere of the brain are those involving motivation, perception, judgment, and sensory integration. Therefore the left hemiplegic patient may deny the affected extremities, have visual or sensory neglect or denial, have distortions in concepts of movement and spatial relations, have lost the concept of the motor act, or lack motivation for self-improvement. These deficits may be more of a hindrance to function than are motor paralysis and physical limitation.

The left hemiplegic patient is more likely to suffer difficulties in tasks such as seeing all the food on the plate or finding eating utensils, grooming the left side of the body, dressing the whole body, or walking than the right hemiplegic patient.

With the left hemiplegic patient, daily exercises and activities are directed toward increasing sensory awareness and carrying over this awareness into self-care functions. Exercises and activities should include developing visual and proprioceptive awareness of the patient's involved extremity, encouraging the patient to turn the head to the affected side to include the part missing from sight because of field cut or neglect, and increasing the patient's proprioceptive awareness of the involved extremity through developing bilateral functions. Although distortion in body image concepts may hinder the patient's self-care independence, the practice of self-care techniques and activities can aid awareness and integration of bilateral functions.

The right hemiplegic person, while also suffering motor paralysis and/or impairment, usually does not incur the problems with judgment encountered by the left hemiplegic person. However, the right hemiplegic person shows varying degrees of communication disability.

The patient whose limitations in function are primarily in the motor areas (i.e., a person with flaccid or moderately spastic extremities) can learn techniques of self-care fairly easily by using sound extremities to assist affected ones.

The occupational therapist assists both right and left hemiplegics in self-care feeding, dressing, bathing, and grooming tasks as soon as medically possible and incorporates these skills into the patient's daily program. The patient is also encouraged to use one-handed techniques and assistive devices, such as a rocker knife for cutting meat one-handed, Velcro attachments on clothes for ease of fastening, and elastic shoe laces. Bathing and grooming are assisted by long-handled sponges, bath mitts, and adapted nail clippers for one-handed use.

Psychological and Social Implications

Mention has been made of the devastating effect of hemiplegia on the person. Not all persons, of course, react in the same way to catastrophic illnesses or disabilities. Often the reactions will reflect pre-morbid taboos and fears. The patient's gains from rehabilitation are, to some degree, dependent upon attitudes developed prior to the CVA.

The patient who is lacking in motivation and is depressed is difficult to rehabilitate, and may become a burden to him or herself and to the family. Often the patient is the breadwinner or the homemaker. The loss of ability to carry out these family responsibilities affects both the patient and the family. The family may undergo financial hardships because of the hospitalization, and this may be a further worry to the patient. At times the family finds it difficult to function without the hospitalized member and needs counselling to understand the course of rehabilitation and to solve the seemingly insurmountable problems of daily living.

Social implications for reentry into the home and community include adjustment to permanent functional deficits, dependence on assistive equipment (braces, slings, and/or a wheelchair), and financial insecurity. The person may no longer be able to drive or to work because of visual and intellectual deficits. Developing a new life style may be necessary.

Vocational Implications

For the young or middle-aged adult suffering hemiplegia, the effect on vocational potential can be serious, depending on skills previously attained and the impairment of intellectual functions. Return to a previous vocation depends in large measure on the type of job the patient was doing, the patient's status in the company, the understanding of the employer, and the patient's ability to regain employable skills.

Frequently job competition is too great for reentry of the worker with permanent hemiplegia. The worker who is no longer able to pursue a vocation suffers a loss in self-esteem, self-image, status in the family, and status in society. Prevocational evaluation for alternate job possibilities and training programs to learn new skills are part of the rehabilitation program.

Head Injury

Head injuries are caused by direct trauma to the skull. Common causes are automobile accidents, industrial accidents, blows or wounds, and falls. Head injury occurs in 70 percent of the persons injured in traffic accidents and falls.[4] Resulting trauma is concussion, contusion, laceration, or compression. Although both skull fracture and brain damage can occur, one may occur without the other. The significance of injury to the head is the resultant state of the brain rather than the state of the skull.[5] A variety of neurological symptoms and manifestations can result from head injury.

Depending on the location and extent of the lesion, the patient's symptoms may be of short duration, latent, or extended over a long period of time. Post-trauma manifestations can be marked. They can include loss of consciousness, dizziness, headache, vertigo provoked by sudden change in position, confusion, emotional reactions which may result in convulsions or combativeness, and disorientation in time and place. Personality disorders, amnesia, and delirium may also occur.

These may be accompanied by intellectual deficits, blindness, diplopia, hemianopsia, olfactory dysfunction, and auditory deficits. Physical symptoms include quadriparesis, unilateral or bilateral hemiparesis, initial decerebrate rigidity, and speech deficits. Restoration of functional, intellectual, social, psychological, and physical manifestations may require a period of years if the patient's injury is severe.

The patient may demonstrate physical and mental deficits similar to those of a person who has suffered cerebrovascular accident (CVA). However, patients with traumatic head injuries are usually in their teens or twenties. Also, mental manifestations and personality changes are often more blatant than those seen in CVA. These prevent the head-injured patient from interacting with the environment. The patient may seem to have actually lost contact with his or her surroundings.

Occupational Therapy

The initial task of the occupational therapist is to determine a means of communicating with the patient. When lack of spontaneous speech exists, the patient may not respond verbally to questions, comments, or simple requests from the therapist. A code system of communication may have to be worked out between the therapist and the patient. For example, the therapist may ask the patient to indicate "yes" by closing the eyes or lifting an arm. Disorientation and confusion may also result in the patient's being unable to communicate.

Memory deficits may prevent the patient from remembering or recognizing people or events from day to day; therefore continual repetition of tasks and symbols might be necessary until the patient's memory is extended. Personality changes, loss of inhibitions, distortions of judgment, and lack of abstract reasoning combine with the patient's memory loss to hinder problem solving and learning ability. The patient may also display a short attention span, distractibility, and fear of insanity, particularly when blindness, disorientation, amnesia, or a combination of physical, psychological, and intellectual manifestations are present.

Physically, the patient may initially be tactually defensive or hypersensitive, may be apraxic, may demonstrate incoordination (tremor or ataxia), and may develop spasticity later in the recuperation period.

Treatment begins with assessment of a method of communication, of sensorimotor deficits, orientation, and functional abilities. The patient is then treated symptomatically with the treatment program directed toward self-awareness and awareness of objects and toward initiation and accomplishment of purposeful activity. Development of the patient's motor strength and coordination is combined with activities to encourage his social awareness and interaction with others. Graded intellectual and problem-solving tasks (reading, arithmetic, and writing) aid the patient in regaining function.

Treatment may begin with basic visual and tactile discrimination and sensorimotor activities such as self-care skills, exercise activities, and games. Initially the occupational therapist works with the patient in quiet surroundings, gradually increasing auditory and visual stimuli. The patient is provided with activity simple enough to assure success but complicated enough to hold interest. As physical and mental tolerance increase, the therapist can expand the complexity of the patient's environment.

The patient's educational and employment goals depend upon the overcoming of intellectual and judgmental deficits and development of integrative abilities.

Multiple Sclerosis

Multiple sclerosis (MS) or disseminated sclerosis is a progressive disease of the nervous system. It begins with the destruction or dissemination of the myelin sheath of the nerve fibers and progresses to the eventual formation of multiple sclerotic plaques or patches which affect the white matter of the brain and spinal cord. These plaques may also be found in the gray matter of the cerebral cortex and in the cranial and spinal cord roots.[6]

Characterized by exacerbations and remissions, the disease may pursue its course for many years. It usually affects young adults (ages twenty to forty) during their period of greatest productivity. Although the cause of the disease is unknown, influenza, respiratory infections, pregnancy, surgery, and trauma may be precipitating factors; change in climate, fatigue from overwork, and poor dietary habits have also been implicated as possible factors. Nervous tension and irritability may precede the onset of physical symptoms.

The clinical picture may be hemiplegia, paraplegia, or quadriplegia, and the patient's prognosis and life span are variable. While the average life span of a person with MS may be twenty years, it can vary from three months to forty years; some remissions can last as long as twenty-five years.[7] There may be long and almost complete remissions in the early stages of the disease. However, after middle age, the course of the disease often progresses.

Symptoms appear in two general modes. The first is characterized by a single lesion or several isolated lesions which result in neuritis, double vision, weakness in a limb, or numbness in a part of the patient's body. The second is insidious and is manifested in a slowly progressive weakness of one or all limbs. Accompanying spinal symptoms include spastic paraplegia, superficial sensory loss in the lower limbs and trunk, impairment of postural sensibility and sense of vibration, and spastic/ataxic gait.[8]

Common early signs of MS include nystagmus (lateral oscillating movement of an eye to one or both sides), slight intention tremor in one or both upper limbs, and exaggeration of tendon reflexes. These initial symptoms may disappear over a period of weeks or months, leaving only slight residual physical signs; however, the cumulative effects of multiple lesions later cause permanent changes in the patient's nervous system.[9]

Symptoms of the advanced case of MS include scanning or staccato speech and slurring of syllables, nystagmus, dissociation of conjugate lateral movement of the eyes, weak and grossly ataxic upper limbs, severe paraplegia, sensory loss, incontinence, episodes of euphoria, depression, and irritability, impairment of postural sensibility, and astereognosis.

Although muscular wasting or atrophy are rare, motor weakness may appear in the patient's extremities, trunk, and face. The patient may experience a feeling of heaviness in the spastic extremities and may lose postural sensibility in limbs and trunk.

Incoordination is a frequent problem for the patient with MS. Intention tremor is accompanied by muscle imbalance in hands and arms, and the tremor may develop in head movements during the later stages of the disease. When the patient must perform tasks requiring accurate movement, the tremor may increase. Ataxia is evident in the gross movements of both the upper and the lower extremities.

The patient suffers sensory deficits manifested by numbness, impairment of positional and joint sense, fine tactile discrimination, hypersensitivity to contact, postural sensibility and vibration sense, and astereognosis.

The patient's ability to communicate verbally may be hindered by dysarthria caused by spastic weakness or ataxia in muscles of articulation. In some instances the speech impairment may become so severe as to render the patient unintelligible.

In some cases the patient with MS may display only ocular symptoms for many years. Although the patient's vision usually improves within a few weeks of the initial onset of symptoms, residual damage to the optic nerve is manifested in optic atrophy.

The patient may exhibit some reduction in intellectual efficiency and some emotional changes; he or she may suffer wildly contrasting moods, going from euphoria to depression very quickly. These fluctuations in mental and physical ability are characteristic of the patient with MS and must be considered during evaluation and treatment. The patient is a victim of gradual and intermittent loss of physical and mental control, resulting in emotional reactions and irritability.

Occupational Therapy

General rehabilitation goals include passive and active range of motion, stretching exercises to reduce spasms and spasticity, reeducation of muscles to control coordination and maximize general strength and function, and encouragement and support of the patient regarding his or her capabilities. Because the patient is prone to anxiety and tension, the occupational therapist emphasizes maintenance of functional abilities and stresses avoidance of becoming chilled or fatigued and of avoiding situations where injury may occur. Decreased sensation, incoordination, transient blindness, and judgment impairment can create life-threatening conditions for the patient with MS.

When evaluating the patient with MS, the occupational therapist considers the following areas:

1. Using passive range of motion to determine spasticity or inconsistent muscle response.
2. Employing active range of motion exercises to determine the patient's strength and to detect the presence of intention tremor, incoordination, and lack of sensation or body balance.
3. Testing the patient's eyesight and functional use of extremities in ADL.
4. Evaluating the patient's intellectual functions and emotional stability.

Treatment consists of providing the patient with exercises and activities that present graded resistance to weak muscles, prevent substitution patterns from developing, and employ repetition to encourage the patient's physical endurance. The occupational therapist must pay close attention to the patient's fatigue factor because the patient may not recognize or admit fatigue.

The patient should be encouraged to engage in exercises and activities that employ all extremities, but he or she may become discouraged with hand activities if sensation and coordination are poor and if intention tremor is prevalent. If the patient has the muscle power and endurance, activities should be performed from both a seated and a standing position.

The patient may need assistive devices and reeducation in ADL; he or she should be encouraged to participate in social functions to maintain the ability to relate to family and friends.

In all activities the patient must be assisted in adjustment to the progression of disability. The patient may deny the gradually worsening condition and become euphoric in an attempt to hide the lack of acceptance and to ward off depression. Euphoria may prevent acceptance of assistive devices and may cause establishment of unrealistic goals. The occupational therapist can aid the patient in the establishment of realistic long- and short-term goals, maintenance of self-care, and avoidance of anxiety.

Parkinson's Disease

Parkinson's disease is a slowly progressive disease of the brain which may be produced by a number of different pathological states. This chronic condition is caused by the degeneration of neurons in the substantia nigra and globus pallidus causing damage to the basal ganglia. This may be precipitated by carbon monoxide and manganese poisoning, encephalitis, senile brain changes, and arteriosclerosis. Disturbance of motor function is characterized by slowing of emotional responses and voluntary movement, muscular rigidity and weakness, slowly spreading tremor, and a shuffling gait.

Symptoms may appear over a period varying from months to years. Gradually the person takes on an attitude of immobility evidenced by a masklike face and staring eyes. Limbs and trunk assume a flexion attitude, and there is little rotary movement of the cervical spine and little free swinging of the arms. The person's arms tend toward adduction; wrists tend to extend and fingers to flex at the metacarpophalangeal joints and extend at the phalangeal joints with loss of tenodesis action.

Movements are characteristically slow with some weakness in voluntary movements and loss of associated movements. Intrinsic movements are awkward and incoordinated. Reduction in range of motion which limits articulation causes slurred, low volume, and monotone speech. There is a tendency to drool. Chest excursion may be decreased because of muscular rigidity, thus decreasing the vital capacity.

Involuntary movements of extremities are generally described as having a "cogwheel" or "leadpipe" rigidity; the former shows jerky tremor while the latter is smoothly rigid. Although these patterns of movement are common, the manifestations may be unequal on both sides of the body. The tremor may be seen as a rhythmic, alternating movement of the opposing muscle groups, often described as a "pill-rolling" movement, effected by the thumb and fingers at the metacarpophalangeal joints. The tremor may shift from one muscle group to another. It usually is present when the patient is at rest and often is diminished when the patient voluntarily moves the affected limb; the tremor increases with emotional excitement, although it can be inhibited temporarily by conscious effort.

Full passive range of motion is usually maintained, although contractures can occur in the patient's hands and feet because of his or her rigid posture; this rigidity can also cause muscular pain, but it does not result in sensory loss. Therefore, the patient may exhibit restlessness, frequently changing position for comfort.

The gait typical of Parkinson's disease is easily recognizable as slow and shuffling with small steps and a tendency toward lurching. The patient appears propelled by momentum and he is unable to stop quickly. He or she is described as having a festinating gait, hurrying with small steps in a bent attitude as if trying to catch up to the center of gravity.[10]

Occupational Therapy

Treatment is directed toward graded resistive exercises to increase strength and coordination, gross motor activities to encourage general mobility and increase chest excursion, fine patterns of movement for maintenance of productive abilities, maximum independence in ADL, and encouragement of motivation, self-esteem, and socialization.

Because the gradual development of rigidity and immobility in patients are characteristic of Parkinson's disease, auditory stimulation such as music can be used to encourage body mobility through rhythmic marching, dancing, clapping, and singing, either individually or in groups. Sports can be used for motivation, socialization, and movement; ball-throwing, ping pong, darts, and shuffleboard also increase strength and speed of movement in all extremities. In gross motor activities, balance, coordination, and breathing patterns are emphasized.

Craft activities can be used to maintain gross and fine coordination, strength, and concentration as these are required for general self-care functions. Activities should be designed so as to encourage good posture, increase mobility, and stimulate successful accomplishment.

Spinal Cord Injury

The rehabilitative process for the person with spinal cord injury requires adjustment to a lifelong disability. The work done in the general hospital or the rehabilitation center provides the initial medical care, protects the patient for future life involvement, works toward achievement of maximum levels of bodily movement and function, and supports psychological preparation for self-motivation in daily activities and goals. It is a mere beginning to the life the person will have to lead as a paraplegic or quadriplegic.

The initial program with the person with spinal cord injury is crucial to his or her total well-being. Rehabilitation is the preparation for making achievable, satisfactory goals for the future. It is a gradual move from total dependence to maximum independence, from the shock of functional loss to acceptance of achievable abilities. It is to these ends that the occupational therapist designs the treatment program.

The occupational therapist has important contact with the patient at various stages in the rehabilitation process. The goals change as the patient moves from one stage to another.

Injury to the spinal cord results in temporary or permanent paralysis of the muscles of the limbs. Temporary manifestations are caused by compression of the cord without transection or puncture, while permanent paralysis is caused by fractures and dislocations which puncture or transect the spinal cord.

Injuries are caused by trauma including gunshot wounds, stab wounds, falls, automobile accidents, and sports accidents. The most common of these is the automobile accident resulting in forced flexion and hyperextension of the trunk causing fracture and dislocation of the vertebrae. Initial symptoms include flaccid paralysis of the affected extremities with spasticity occurring after the spinal shock stages, loss of all sensation and increased reflex activity below the level of the lesion, and incontinence of bowel and bladder. In many cases secondary injury results from improper handling at the scene of the accident.

It is essential in the early care of the spinal cord injured to prevent the patient from becoming either overly discouraged or overly hopeful. Some doctors advocate telling the patient his or her chances of walking and the degree of permanent paralysis immediately to avoid false hopes. All too often the patient is initially told that he or she will recover full functions and, when the full implications of the injury are finally discussed, the patient finds it difficult to accept permanent paralysis. In the early stages of hospitalization the patient tends to deny the extent of the injury. At this stage, however, denial is a protection from the realities that must be faced and may actually help the patient through the devastating effects of the initial trauma.

Level of Lesion

Disability, treatment, and function of the spinal cord injured person depend on the level and extent of the lesion. The condition referred to as *quadriplegia* occurs from injury in the cervical and possibly high thoracic areas of the cord and results in muscular deficiencies of the upper extremities, trunk, and lower extremities. *Paraplegia* occurs from injury to the thoracic and lumbar cord areas and results in muscular paralysis in the trunk and lower extremities. The terms *quadriplegia* and *paraplegia* refer to paralysis of the limbs, while *quadriparesis* and *paraparesis* refer to weakness of the limbs.

The level of segmental innervation determines the effect of the trauma incurred (Fig. 13-11). The extent of the injury determines the functional outcome.[11] Muscles innervated by segments at and below the level of injury are affected. Although a functional estimate and expectation can be approximated given the diagnostic level of injury, other factors may retard or change the expected rehabilitative prognosis. Among these factors are accompanying injury, respiratory complications, head injury, decubiti, lack of motivation, damage to the vertebral column, urinary infection, spasms, and sensory loss.

FUNCTIONAL IMPLICATIONS FOR SPECIFIC LESION LEVELS. Table 13-3 describes some of the functional differences among patients with cervical lesions.

The initial treatment of the *quadriplegic* patient (paralysis of all four limbs) is skeletal traction through the use of head tongs. Traction is applied for approximately six weeks, after which the patient

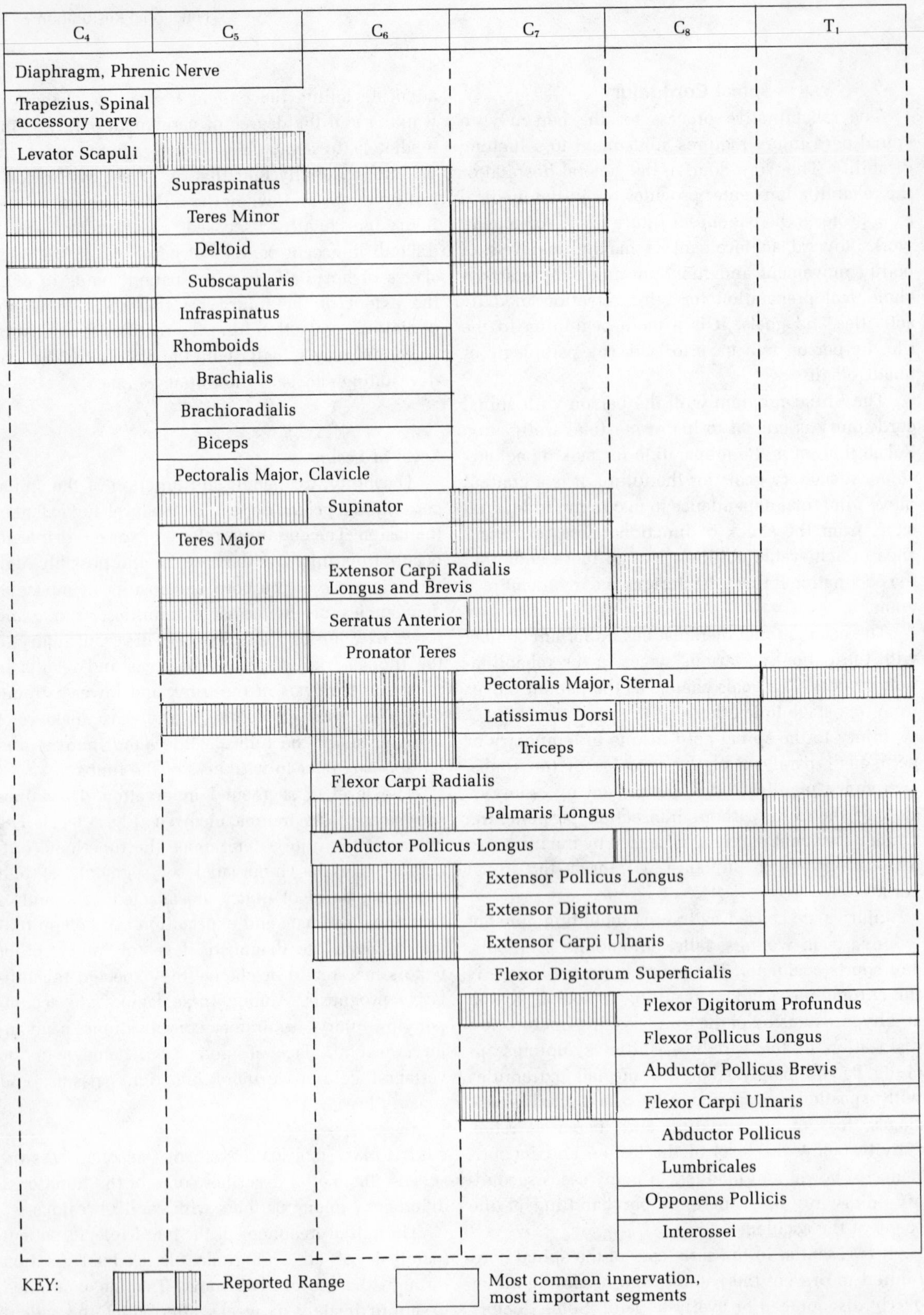

C_4 C_5 C_6 C_7 C_8 T_1

Diaphragm, Phrenic Nerve

Trapezius, Spinal accessory nerve

Levator Scapuli

Supraspinatus

Teres Minor

Deltoid

Subscapularis

Infraspinatus

Rhomboids

Brachialis

Brachioradialis

Biceps

Pectoralis Major, Clavicle

Supinator

Teres Major

Extensor Carpi Radialis Longus and Brevis

Serratus Anterior

Pronator Teres

Pectoralis Major, Sternal

Latissimus Dorsi

Triceps

Flexor Carpi Radialis

Palmaris Longus

Abductor Pollicus Longus

Extensor Pollicus Longus

Extensor Digitorum

Extensor Carpi Ulnaris

Flexor Digitorum Superficialis

Flexor Digitorum Profundus

Flexor Pollicus Longus

Abductor Pollicus Brevis

Flexor Carpi Ulnaris

Abductor Pollicus

Lumbricales

Opponens Pollicis

Interossei

KEY: —Reported Range; Most common innervation, most important segments

FIGURE 13-11. Innervation level of muscles of the upper extremity.

Table 13-3. Functional implications of cervical cord lesions.

Level of cervical lesion	*Remaining musculature*	*Active mobility*	*Functional loss*	*Functional implications*	*Occupational therapy implications*
C_4	Sternocleidomastoid Upper trapezius	Neck movements Shoulder elevation	Respiratory endurance Upper extremity functions Trunk sensation and control Lower extremity sensation and control General endurance General independent mobility	Total dependency in self-care Dependency on external devices for upper extremity movement and productive activity Confined to wheelchair Can propel electric wheelchair	Requires assistance in communication skills: tape recorder, electric typewriter (using hand typing sticks, headstick, mouthpiece, electronic communication board), electric page turner for reading, talking books (records) Uses external powered (electric or CO_2) functional hand splints and arm supports for upper extremity activity in the wheelchair Can engage in light recreational and avocational activities for ROM, strength, interest, and motivation
C_5	Sternocleidomastoid Trapezius Rhomboids Partial rotator cuff Partial deltoids Partial biceps	Neck movements Shoulder elevation Scapular rotation, adduction Partial elbow flexion Weak or no sensory function	Ability to change from supine to prone position in bed Ability to achieve sitting position in bed Independent trunk control and sensation Lower extremity sensation and control Wrist and hand functions	Use of externally powered devices for arm and hand functions Assistive devices for self-feeding Dependency in self-care and transfers Can propel electric wheelchair	Devices described above may be necessary Dynamic tenodesis splints for writing, grasping, and other hand functions Mobile arm support, balanced forearm orthosis, or suspension slings for general upper extremity support and mobility Special equipment or devices for telephone, TV operation, eating, drinking Recreational and avocational activities for ROM, strength, interest, motivation
C_6	All muscles of C_4 and C_5 level Partial serratus anterior Partial pectoralis Partial latissimus dorsi Deltoid Biceps Partial extensor carpi radialis	All movements of C_4 and C_5 Scapular adduction, flexion, extension Weak trunk control Shoulder flexion Elbow flexion Wrist extension (tenodesis function for grasp) Weak sensory function in hand	Weakness in trunk control, affecting balance Lower extremity functions Weakness in grasp, release, and prehension	Can achieve sitting position in bed by using trapeze bar (above bed) or rope attached to foot of bed Can assist in wheelchair transfer Can propel regular wheelchair Can use assistive devices for self-care Fairly mobile arm control Weak tenodesis function	Dynamic tenodesis splints for hand functions Assistive devices for independence in self-care: razor holders, utensil holders, pencil holders, extended handles for reaching, dressing loops for pants, sliding board for transfers, devices for toilet needs (catheter and leg bag, suppository management) Friction adaptations to wheelrims or knobs for pushing wheelchair using thenar eminence of hand Typing sticks Push-ups in wheelchair for arm strengthening and prevention of decubiti Independent living skills Driving with hand controls and wheel knobs Vocational goals
C_7	All muscles of C_4, C_5, C_6 level Finger flexors Finger extensors	All movements of C_4, C_5, C_6 Moderate trunk control Functional grasp and release Sensory function of hand	Weakness in trunk control Weakness in intrinsic muscles of the hand and isolated finger functions Limited dexterity and general hand strength	Independent bed and wheelchair mobility Independent bed/wheelchair transfers Strong arm control Has grasp functions and coordination without splints Nonfunctional ambulation for standing and short distances	Assistive devices for toilet activities and lower extremity dressing Upper extremity activities for physical restoration without splinting Can drive with hand controls and do car transfer Independence in daily living and community involvement Vocational and avocational goals

is immobilized in a neck support from two to four months.[12]

The position of the patient in traction is supine or prone in a completely extended position for protection of the spinal cord. The patient may be placed either on a Stryker frame bed which rotates horizontally or on a Circo-electric bed which can be turned by changing the angle from horizontal to vertical on a 180-degree axis. These special beds are used to aid in the important change of position for skin and limb protection; the change must be made by the nurses every two hours. The tilt-table commonly used in physical therapy assists in positioning the patient in the vertical position. If he or she is not gradually acclimated the patient tends to become dizzy when his or her head is brought to a vertical position after weeks spent in traction.

The early treatment of the quadriplegic patient consists of turning, massage, and passive range of motion to maintain freedom of movement and to prevent contractures. Following the traction period, general conditioning exercises are provided, including proper breathing and training in rolling. Self-care is begun as soon as possible to relieve anxieties regarding bodily functions and to prevent dependency on others. Following the bed stage, the patient is encouraged to adjust to the vertical position by being put on the tilt-table. When tolerance increases sufficiently the patient begins sitting in a wheelchair.

Skin and Limb Care

Protection of the skin and prevention of contractures are essential in the care of both the quadriplegic and the paraplegic patient. Because sensation is lost below the level of the lesion, the patient is unable to detect pressure from external objects and is unable to change position because of muscle paralysis. Thus position changes must be made by nurses or attendants. The skin is susceptible to injury from the shearing force of sheets, pressure from footboards used for positioning, and the gravitational effect of the limbs immobile on the mattress. Decubitus ulcers (pressure sores) develop from local anemia caused by this pressure and appear over bony prominences. Even though air mattresses and water mattresses are used and routine position changes are followed, decubitus ulcers can still occur.

The patient must be instructed in the importance of turning in bed or shifting weight when in the wheelchair. As a patient becomes more mobile, instruction should be given as to how to check all areas of the body; this can be done by the patient's using a long-handled mirror to check the back, buttocks, and lower extremities.

Because the flaccid extremities yield to the pull of gravity, they are properly positioned using sand bags, pillows, or footboards to prevent the stretching of the weak muscles and the development of contractures which will limit future function of the limbs. Pressure from bed clothes must be avoided, and the patient's limbs should be visible. Prism glasses can be used so that the patient can see his or her extremities and inform the nurse when position should be changed.

Rehabilitation

The goals of rehabilitation for the quadriplegic and paraplegic patient are maximum level of self-care from a wheelchair, recognition of physical and intellectual abilities and potential, resumption of family life, education, and/or employment, and acceptance of the condition.

Common problems incurred by both the quadriplegic and the paraplegic are depression, dependency, decubiti, contractures, spasticity, atrophy, weakness, urinary tract infection, boredom, hostility, and lack of motivation.

Use of adaptive equipment may be required for substitution of motion, problems of decreased trunk balance, compensation for reduced reach from the wheelchair, and for limitation in locomotion. Assistive devices may be needed to perform the self-care activities of personal hygiene, grooming, and dressing.

Discharge planning must begin immediately with protection of the flaccid extremities for future functioning, establishment of long-term and short-term goals, gradual conditioning to enable the patient to tolerate an upright position, establishment of maximum use of the upper extremities in self-care and productive activities, and acceptance of permanent paralysis and wheelchair living (Fig. 13-12). The patient must be encouraged to develop physical and intellectual resources with which to combat the difficulties of living.

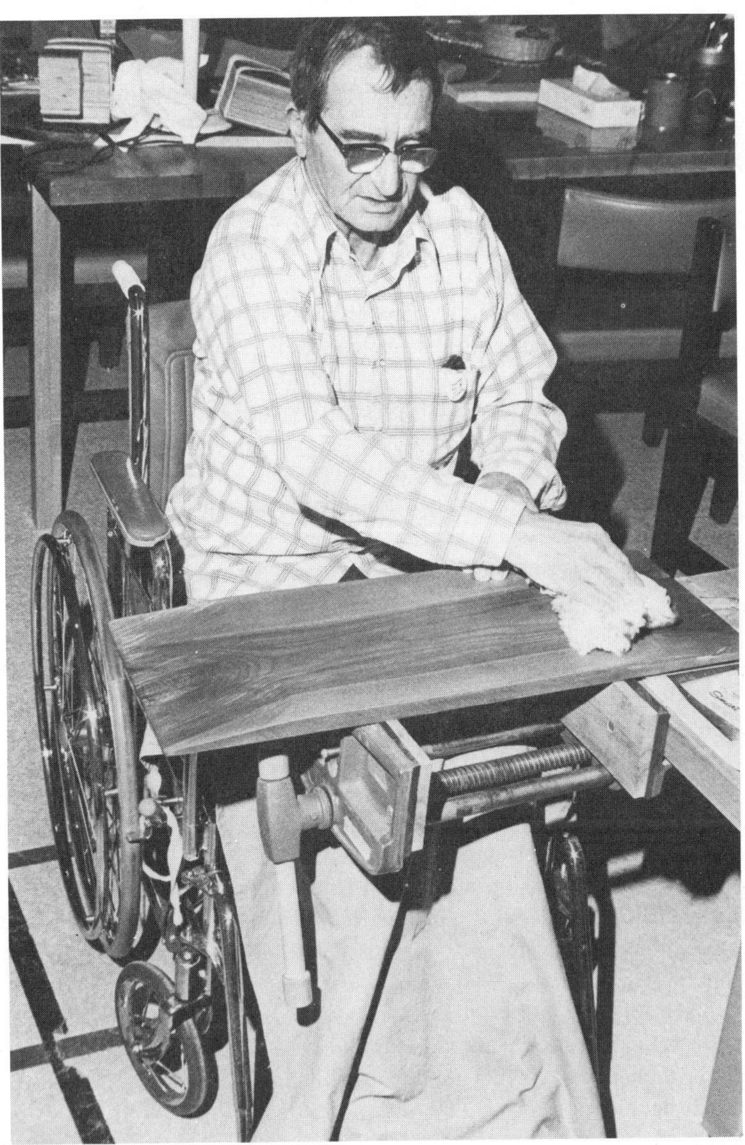

FIGURE 13-12. A paraplegic patient works on his transfer board for upper extremity strengthening and adjustment to wheelchair living.

Occupational Therapy and Quadriplegia

BED PHASE. Evaluation while the patient is confined to the bed consists of the following steps:

1. Read the chart for restrictions of bed position because of fracture or dislocation of the spinal column.

2. Check for proper alignment of the extremities and trunk for prevention of stretching of paralyzed muscles.

3. Check all extremities for the presence of reddened areas indicating pressure.

4. Determine need for hand splints to maintain functional positioning or for functional use.

5. Check the level of sensation of the patient's trunk, arm, and hand by asking the patient to identify the location of touch. Passive position of extremities and tactile sensation of an object placed in the hand must also be checked.

6. Gently move the extremities to determine pas-

sive range of motion when the patient does not have restrictions in arm movements and check limitations caused by pain, fractures, spasticity, hypersensitivity, or contractures.

7. Request that the patient move the extremity in active range of motion. Use gravitational assist by holding the paralyzed extremity to aid movement.

8. Encourage the patient regarding functional and sensory abilities.

9. Talk with the patient regarding interests, the hospital stay, feelings, and primary concerns.

Treatment during the bed phase requires the following:

1. Check daily on proper positioning for prevention of decubiti and contractures.

2. Gently massage and stimulate sensory receptors over upper extremities.

3. Move the patient's upper extremity joints in gentle, full, passive range of motion daily, telling the patient when you are moving the extremity and how.

4. Provide splinting to prevent tightening of muscles and deformity. Provide functional splinting to encourage tenodesis function and to stimulate sensory function.

5. Attach suspension slings to the traction bar above the bed; these slings stimulate and facilitate active movements of the patient's shoulder and elbow by spring action of the sling (Fig. 13-13).

6. Use a hand cuff or mitt on the sling to stimulate wrist extension during shoulder adduction and elbow flexion movements for the establishment of tenodesis function of wrist and fingers (see Fig. 13-13).

7. Use arm slings with elbow and wrist straps to support arms for maximum active movement and hand functions; use a palmar cuff with a pocket for insertion of a spoon or a pencil so the patient can use arm movements in productive activity.

8. Encourage active range of motion of all joints of the upper extremities by using gravitational assist.

9. Encourage active range of motion by providing gentle resistance to joints and muscle groups in hands and arms.

10. Use assistive devices such as bath mitts to encourage active arm range of motion for bathing. This increases body awareness.

11. Set up an electric page turner over the bed on the bedtable so that the patient can operate it with palm contact (Fig. 13-14) or with movement of the chin or shoulder if he or she lacks lower arm function.

12. Provide prism glasses to prevent the patient's developing eyestrain in viewing television or seeing visitors from a supine position (Fig. 13-15).

13. During all treatment in this phase, encourage the patient to use all active movement possible to increase power and functional ability. By doing this the patient becomes involved and assumes responsibility for the rehabilitation process.

14. Provide activities in which the patient is interested.

15. Provide psychological support throughout the treatment regime.

16. Coordinate occupational therapy techniques with nursing and physical therapy personnel and other members of the rehabilitation team. This aids the patient in gaining maximum function and minimizes fatigue and frustration.

WHEELCHAIR PHASE. When the patient has progressed to sitting in a wheelchair, the following evaluation procedures are used:

1. Range of motion: Move the limbs through complete passive range of motion at all joints, one at a time, being careful not to cause pain in sensitive joints, particularly in the shoulders and elbows. Give support to the flaccid or weak limbs by holding them carefully during range of motion. Check for both spasticity and deformity in the upper extremity joints.

2. Muscle strength: Provide gravitational assist to determine if the patient can resist gravity and give gentle resistance as tolerated to determine muscle strength.

3. Sensation: Note the presence of pain in passive movement. Occlude the patient's vision; touch the skin lightly with your finger and determine if the patient responds to the stimulus. Progress from distal to proximal areas. To evaluate two-point discrimination, sharp touch, and localization of stimuli, touch the skin with a sharp object such as a sharpened dowel stick or two-point pressure gauge. Determine first whether the patient responds to the stimulus, can localize the stimulus, and can distinguish if

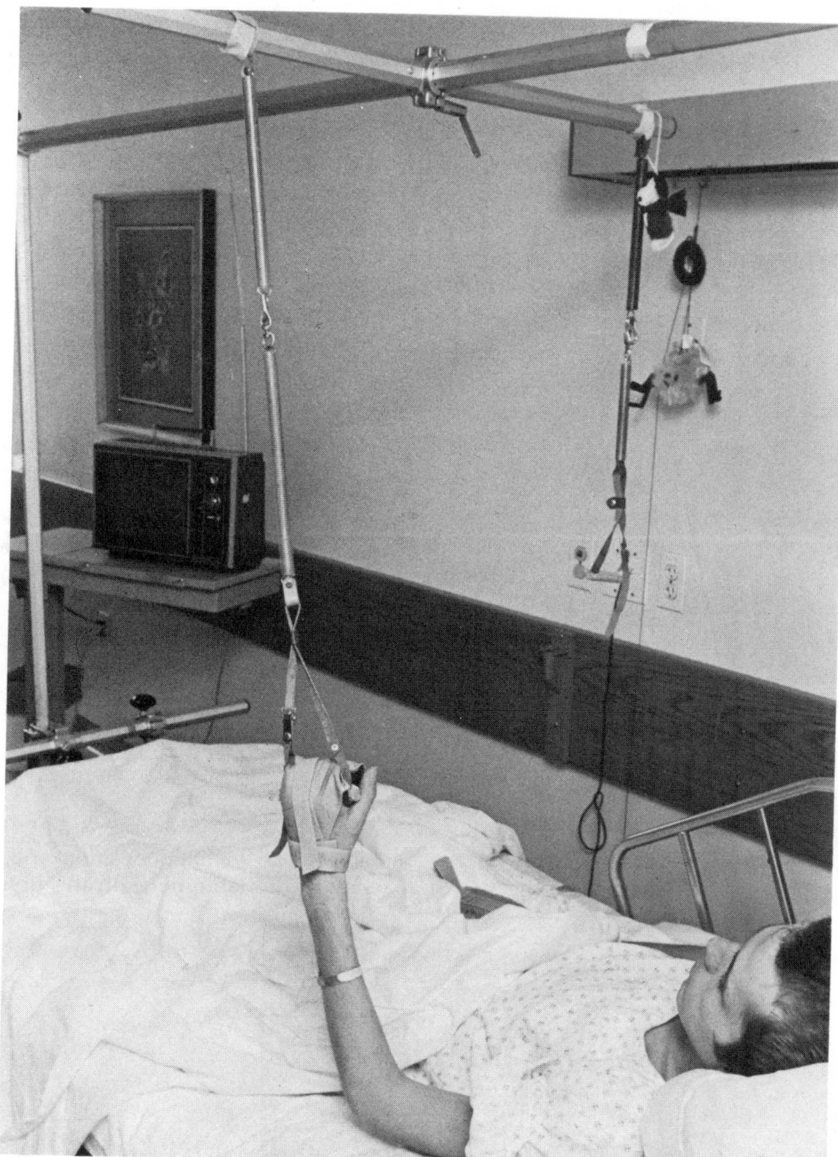

FIGURE 13-13. Overhead bed traction frame used for attachment of a spring suspension sling and positioning mitt to facilitate upper arm active exercise against resistance. A pulley system can also be attached to vary and to increase resistance.

there were one or two stimuli. Place an object between the patient's thumb and fingers, move it around in the palmar area, and then ask for recognition of the object by its size, shape, and texture to determine stereognostic function.

4. Position sense (proprioception): Move the body part to be tested gently in reciprocal movements and then ask the patient to identify the position of the limb when stopped. The patient may feel the movement but may not be able to identify the position without seeing it.

5. Patterns of movement: Provide the patient with a reaching or grasping task to perform, i.e., picking up a 2″ x 2″ foam block, reaching to the shoulder, or reaching for an object held in the air. Observe the pattern of movement to determine functioning muscles and the presence of spasticity. Observe any substitution patterns the patient may use

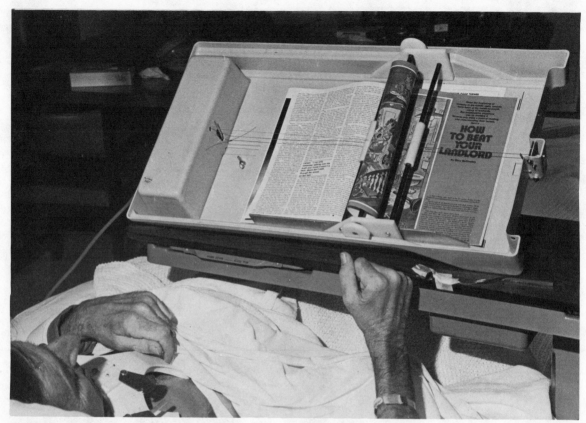

FIGURE 13-14. Electric page turner placed on the bedtable in an inclined position and operated by a quadriplegic patient by palm contact on the switch attached to the table beneath the right corner of the machine.

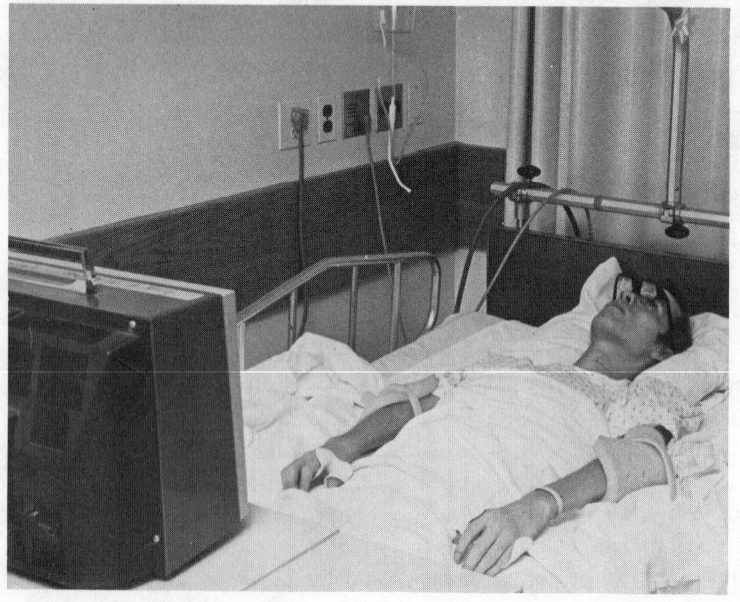

FIGURE 13-15. Prism glasses prevent eyestrain in viewing television while the quadriplegic patient is in a supine position. Note use of foam elbow protection against skin breakdown from pressure on the bony parts. Note thumb splints for passive positioning in opposition.

to the detriment of others which should be strengthened.

6. Functional activities: Determine actual gross grasp, prehension, coordination, strength, and tenodesis function. Determine the patient's ability to perform functional activities such as picking up an object and placing it, reaching for an object, using two hands constructively, writing, pushing and pulling objects, turning pages of a book. Use objects of varied weights, sizes, and texture. Present tasks within the patient's functional ability as determined by range of motion, muscle power, sensation, position sense, and patterns of movement already observed and evaluated. Do not ask a patient to do impossible tasks.

7. During all evaluation procedures, assist the patient in movements when necessary. Do not allow fatigue or discouragement. Emphasize what *can* be done and encourage the patient to do it. Be explicit in instructions and demonstrate when necessary. Terminate the evaluation before the patient becomes fatigued and try to end with accomplishment.

8. Talk with the patient regarding his interests so that the treatment program can include activities that are related to these interests and aid the patient in setting realistic long- and short-term goals.

9. Determine the patient's trunk control for free movement of the upper extremities in isolated asymmetrical use and use in ADL functions.

10. Evaluate the need for assistive devices and/or splints for restorative exercises and activities in addition to those needed for positioning and self-care activities.

11. Evaluate self-care and all activities of daily living including self-feeding, grooming, toileting, bathing, dressing, writing, clerical skills, and homemaking skills. The physical plan of the home must also be evaluated.

12. Prevocational evaluation: Evaluate functions for job skills and employment potential when the patient has mastered upper extremity functional activities and activities of daily living within his or her limits.

General Treatment Procedures and Techniques

POSITIONING. Exercises and activities can be done in almost any position if both the patient and the equipment are properly situated. In preparation for exercise or productive activity, the patient should be positioned with concern for optimum biomechanical advantage in function.

Bed: Upper extremity activities can be assisted by the use of an inclined lapboard in the supine and sitting positions with suspension slings attached to traction frames.

Prone position on a Circo-electric bed: When the patient is prone (face down) on the Circo-electric bed, he or she can use gravity for shoulder flexion and elbow extension. A table is necessary to provide support in elbow flexion if the patient lacks lower arm functions. If the patient is in a prone position, independent feeding should be encouraged using slings and a palmar cuff and having the tray, with a nonskid mat, placed under the bed. Plates that have plateguards allow the patient to pick up the food independently.

Wheelchair position: Good position is necessary. The patient is generally seated on a cutout seatboard with a gel, water, or air cushion for hip positioning and prevention of decubiti. The chair should have an extended back, arm, and foot support. A lapboard, suspension slings, or a balanced forearm orthosis can be attached to the wheelchair.

Standing table: This device is often used by the patient wearing braces. It aids in trunk strengthening, standing tolerance, and upright positioning. Activities done at the standing table may also be accomplished by some patients using a belt support at a work table.

ACTIVITIES FOR FUNCTIONAL RESTORATION. All activities should increase upper extremity joint range of motion, strength, physical tolerance, grasp, and psychological adaptation. These activities should also include the use of assistive equipment, which will increase the patient's capacity to function independently and result in the realization of maximum capacities.

Manipulation of pegs and of other objects of varying sizes, weights, and textures improves the patient's grasp, reach, and ability to place objects. The activity teaches isolated arm and hand functions and provides the patient with experience in using assistive equipment.

Constructive activities (e.g., woodworking) can be adapted to provide range of motion and strengthening of the upper arms and trunk muscles. If the patient has poor grasp, a palmar cuff, bilateral handles, or holding mitts can be used with tools for such tasks as sanding, sawing, planing, or drilling.

Diversional activities are provided for the pure fun of engaging in a game with another person. These activities such as checkers, chess, or Scrabble can be done in bed or in a wheelchair. Arm supports may be needed and the patient may require hand splints; however he or she is able to engage in competitive activity.

Some adapted activities provided for the spinal cord injured patient are:

1. Use of table-based power tools such as a small jigsaw, drill press, and/or a printing press. These can have extended handles for easy reach and control.
2. Use of handpower equipment, secured if necessary to substitute for lack of control.
3. Vertical and adjustable angled chalkboards for gross arm and writing exercises.
4. Use of ropes attached to loom harnesses to change the shed using the arms when lower extremities are paralyzed.
5. Special handles on the loom beater to provide supination or pronation exercises.
6. Use of a pulley and weight system attached to the loom beater for strengthening upper extremities by providing resistance.

All activities offer possibilities for adaptation. Some of the activities mentioned are helpful to the paraplegic patient as well as the quadriplegic patient because they provide a means to increase strength, endurance, and balance for the trunk and upper extremities. The quadriplegic patient needs these functions for wheelchair manipulation and activities, but the paraplegic patient needs upper arm strengthening for wheelchair maneuvering over long distances, transferring, standing in braces, and walking with crutches. The build-up of maximum upper extremity strength is essential to the paraplegic. Engagement in an upper extremity activity program is crucial to the beginning of productivity from a wheelchair and leads to independence in daily living tasks, increased responsibility, and, eventually, employment. The paraplegic patient should experience all aspects of functioning from a wheelchair before leaving the rehabilitation setting.

ADAPTATIONS TO ACTIVITIES. When the patient is confined to bed or to the reclining wheelchair, it is often difficult to set up activities that the patient will be able to see and reach. Both the position and the patient's lack of upper extremity mobility place limitations on activity. However, the following are examples of adaptations which can be provided for the quadriplegic patient in bed or in a wheelchair.

In the bed position the following adaptations are possible:

1. Use of the bedtable to position activities (books or visual puzzles) which can be performed by using prism glasses.
2. A table lapboard with a bottom edge can be placed over the patient's chest; this can be inclined and stabilized (using projecting legs) to hold reading materials or other items.
3. Commercial bookholders are useful.
4. Suspension slings can be attached to the traction frames on the bed.
5. Slings, mirrors, and activities can be attached to the Circo-electric bed frame.
6. Activities can be placed on a chair or low table for the patient who is prone on the Circo-electric bed. Feeding trays can also be placed on a chair.

The following adaptations will provide wheelchair activities:

1. An inclined treatment table aids the patient during early treatment when still in a reclining wheelchair.
2. Vises and clamps are used to position and stabilize activities.
3. A lapboard on the wheelchair aids arm positioning and provides an accessible work surface.
4. Controls normally operated by the feet (e.g., a sewing machine control) can be extended and placed on the table so that they can be manipulated by the arms.

FUNCTIONAL SPLINTS: TENODESIS. The quadriplegic patient is provided with a tenodesis or flexor-hinge hand splint when he or she has achieved active dorsiflexion (hyperextension) of the wrist. It is with active motion against resistance that the patient is able to channel movement through the splint into a strong and functional prehension grip. The tenodesis splint uses the natural function of the finger tendons to tighten in wrist hyperextension and to relax in wrist flexion. Although the patient is able to effect this function voluntarily with sufficient active wrist extension without the splint, strong grip may be lacking in thumb-finger contact. The splint is applied to give the patient power for the functional needs of prehension.

There are various forms of splints that are commonly provided; some are for trial and training while others are permanent. Trial tenodesis splints may be made by the occupational therapist from thermoplastic materials. The patient is taught how to use the splint in active grasping and releasing and in coordination activities. The flexor-hinge hand splint is made by the occupational therapist or the orthotist for permanent use and is usually made of metal or high temperature plastic. The patient may continue to use the splints if they aid in daily activities or eventually may discard them as muscle power and substitute functions are gained.

If the patient does not have active wrist extension against gravity and resistance, other types of hand-wrist tenodesis splints may be needed to provide the function of grasp. These may be electronically or carbon dioxide (CO_2) controlled to effect an independent grasp. The use of these devices depends on the motivation of the patient, as they require tolerance of noise and the pressure of harnesses and special rigging as well as the acceptance of complicated assistive equipment to substitute for natural functions.

Occupational Therapy and Paraplegia

BED PHASE. Evaluation during the bed phase of paraplegia consists of the following:

1. Check restrictions of movement as noted in the chart with regard to the status of the spinal cord injury and other possible injuries.
2. Check the position of the patient for proper alignment of the paralyzed trunk and lower extremities.
3. Check the passive and active range of motion of the upper extremities (which should be normal, but may be weak).
4. Interview the patient in regard to general interests, goals, and expectations.

During treatment, the following procedures are followed:

1. Provide the patient with upper extremity activities for gentle, active exercise of his or her arms while supine: reading, book games, craft activities.
2. Provide the patient with an inclined table lapboard and prism glasses for ease in performing upper extremity activity.
3. Provide activities that offer resistance in hand functions to increase strength and to decrease mental frustration: theraplast, leatherwork, making models, copper tooling, macrame, weaving, and woodcarving.

MOBILE BED AND WHEELCHAIR PHASE. When the restrictions of mobility are removed, the paraplegic patient can begin self-care activities such as bathing in bed or in the wheelchair. A long-handled sponge will help in reaching the feet. Self-care activity increases self-awareness, responsibility, and self-esteem.

At this time, if the patient is able to turn in bed and to reach a sitting position, upper extremity dressing can be done in bed as tolerance of the sitting position increases. When the patient can sit for longer periods, lower extremity dressing in bed may be begun. For this, a long-handled reacher may be needed.

Some adjustment time may be required to regain a sense of balance and body use when the patient first moves from the bed into a wheelchair. When this is accomplished, all bathing and grooming can be done before a mirror and upper extremity dressing can be done in the wheelchair. Unless the paraplegic patient is hindered by severe spasticity in the legs, all self-care activities should be able to be accomplished independently. It is crucial to the rehabilitation of the paraplegic that the patient be encouraged to assume these responsibilities as functional ability is regained. Self-care activities not only provide independent functions but also provide important daily exercise in balance, strength, and coordination. Since fatigue may be experienced in the early accomplishment of these tasks, the treatment program must be coordinated with other therapies. All rehabilitation team members must be informed of the patient's level of accomplishment, so that all efforts are coordinated toward the patient's achieving maximum independence.

The continuation of productive upper extremity activity is also essential because the paraplegic person will eventually need to adjust to *life* in a wheelchair. In many cases the paraplegic patient will want to have the opportunity to learn to use braces and crutches to walk; however, the braces are heavy and walking requires much strength. Because the cost in energy is very high, the patient often resorts to the wheelchair for ease of travel; this occurs after a trial time which may last for months or years.

Life in a wheelchair, however, requires that all activities be done in a sitting position. The patient will be dependent on his or her arms for mobility, vocation, and avocations (Fig. 13-16). The resourceful paraplegic individual can do virtually anything from a wheelchair—except climb steps or pass through narrow doorways and reach appliances and counters that are too high.

The occupational therapy program consists of developing upper extremity productivity which will lead to prevocational and vocational planning. Skills begun in occupational therapy during hospitalization can greatly assist the paraplegic person in accepting limitations and using abilities for developing employable skills and healthy attitudes.

Regular chair: The patient who is able to transfer with or without a sliding board, can practice this skill in occupational therapy by transferring to a regular chair. The chair should have both a firm back and firm seat. Working from a regular chair increases the patient's trunk and upper extremity strength and mobility.

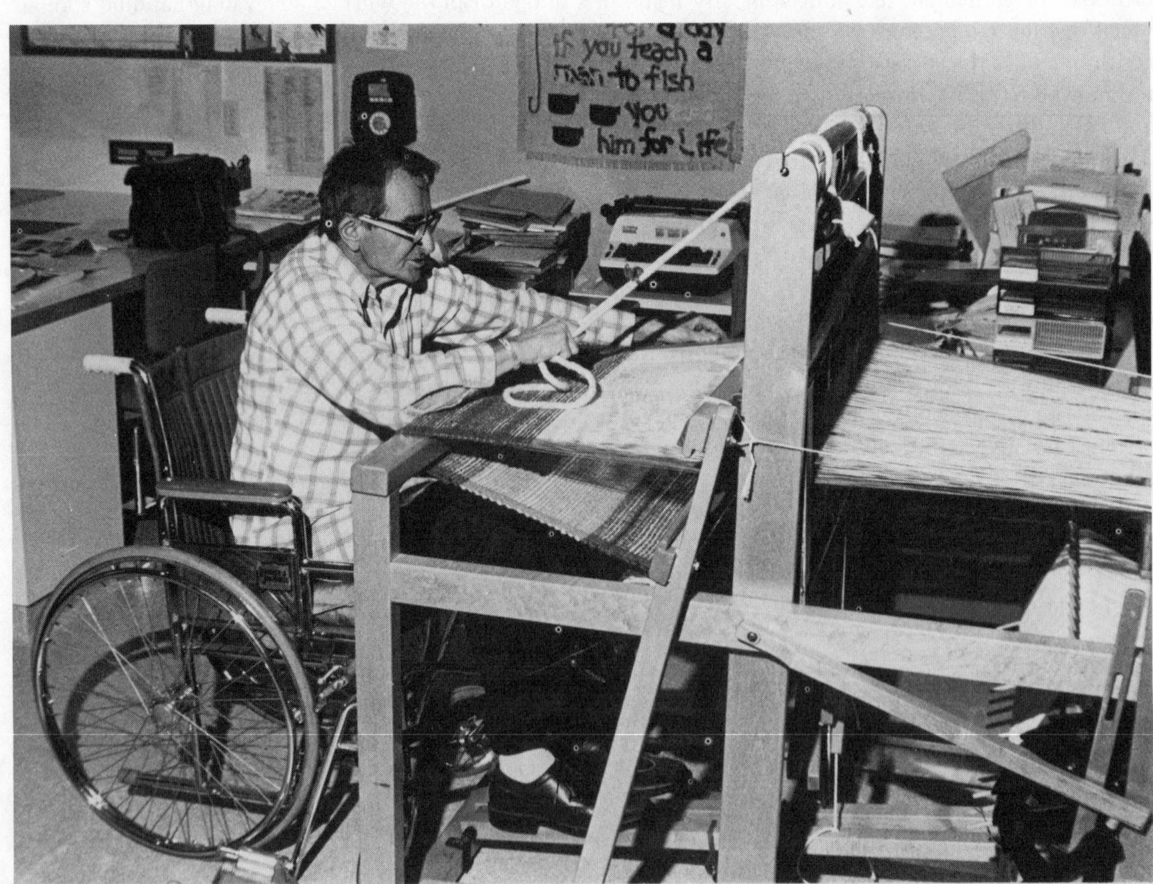

FIGURE 13-16. Ropes are attached to harnesses of the floor loom to enable the paraplegic individual to change the shed with his arms instead of his paralyzed legs. The addition of weights to the beater and the harnesses provides resistance for arm and trunk strengthening.

ACTIVITIES OF DAILY LIVING. Barring the complications of decubiti and excessive spasticity, the paraplegic person is able to learn to be essentially independent in self-care. The high-level paraplegic may have some problems with lower extremity dressing because of trunk instability and loss of muscle strength for balance; however, various assistive devices can help a person overcome these problems. With training the paraplegic person can function independently in self-care from bed and wheelchair, can perform household activities from a wheelchair, and can transfer, drive with hand controls, and perform vocational skills. Major problems will be those caused by architectural barriers outside of and within buildings, problems which impair mobility and make job-seeking extremely difficult.

The daily accomplishment of self-care and other independent or assisted activities can provide the spinal cord injured person with maintenance of range of motion, strength, and both physical and psychological endurance. The patient's abilities in these areas should be discussed with the family so that they will encourage as much independence as possible.

ASSISTIVE DEVICES. The paraplegic individual needs fewer assistive devices than does the quadriplegic person. The former generally uses a seatboard and special cushion for the wheelchair, a transfer board, a long-handled reacher for dressing or retrieving objects from high places or the floor, and wheelchair accessories (drink holder, ashtray, and carrying bag).

General Considerations for the Spinal Cord Injured

WHEELCHAIR PRESCRIPTION. The wheelchair will become a way of life for the spinal cord injured person in most cases. Therefore it must be prescribed for individual comfort, safety, maneuverability, and independence. A poorly fitted wheelchair can contribute to deformity, muscle disuse, decubiti, and decreased motivation for function and socialization. The wheelchair needs of the paraplegic and quadriplegic patients are different.

In most cases the paraplegic person will be able to propel a wheelchair inside with ease and outside on smooth ground (less easily on rough ground). The paraplegic person is independent in self-care activities and virtually all aspects of daily living. The wheelchair should be heavy duty but lightweight for ease of lifting in and out of a car; should be as narrow as possible for easy passage through doorways and maneuvering in bathrooms; should have swing-away removable footrests for transfer and proximity to cabinets and work areas; and should have removable desk arms at a comfortable height for arm positioning, transfer, and proximity to tables and counters. A seatboard with a special cushion to prevent decubiti is sometimes used to maintain good positioning of trunk and hips. The foot pedals should clear two inches from the ground for safety over bumps and rough ground, the depth of the seat should extend to two inches proximal to the knee bend; and the back height should extend no farther than three inches below the axilla to allow free movement of the arms but to provide needed trunk support. Pneumatic tires are often recommended for ease and safety over rough ground and for a comfortable ride. However, because these tires need to be checked for sufficient air pressure and do go flat, they are contraindicated when the patient is unable to attend to these functions or does not have access to someone who can help. Hard rubber tires may be more practical in this case.

While the wheelchair for the quadriplegic individual has the same requirements, there are some additional needs. For ease of maneuvering, the quadriplegic person may require knobs or plastic friction sheaths on the wheel rims for easier propulsion or a motorized chair with touch controls. The back should be higher than that of the paraplegic's chair since the quadriplegic has loss of trunk control and needs extra support. A brake extension may be necessary for independence in locking brakes. Heel loops and leg rests are needed for foot and leg positioning, and a safety belt may be needed for balance. Although a wheelchair with a reclining back may be used in early treatment to compensate for the quadriplegic patient's tendency to get dizzy, it is not recommended during later periods. It can increase the patient's dependency on the reclined position, which limits upper extremity function.

The wheelchair should be ordered as soon as possible in the rehabilitation program to encourage the patient's early association with functioning in a wheelchair.

DISCHARGE PLANNING. The patient and family are included in the rehabilitation program as soon after admission as possible and are fully informed of all of the stages of the rehabilitation process. The process begun in the hospital continues at home and in the community. The patient maintains a relationship with the rehabilitation team to achieve planned goals upon discharge.

During hospitalization the rehabilitation team may encourage the patient to go home on weekends so that he or she can begin to face the adjustments he or she will have to face upon discharge and can use acquired skills in the home environment. These visits alert the family as to the patient's capabilities, progress, and general program. It is from these visits that the patient, family, and therapist can work together on home planning and architectural renovations.

RETURN TO SCHOOL. The patient's vocational goal and discharge plan may include returning to school. The social worker or occupational therapist checks the school for the presence of architectural barriers that would prevent the easy entrance into the building and access to rooms, bathrooms, cafeteria, and other areas. A system of carrying books, obtaining optimum work surfaces and heights, and note-taking may be needed by the quadriplegic patient. The school personnel should be informed of the importance of full involvement of the wheelchair-confined person in all aspects of the educational environment and should be encouraged to aid in his or her acceptance by peers.

AVOCATIONAL ACTIVITIES. Activities that are provided the patient for restoration of function can become outlets for avocational needs. As the spinal cord injured person works through adjustment to wheelchair living, avocational outlets are needed for venting feelings as well as for providing a sense of accomplishment. As new patterns of movement develop, the patient can apply these in hobbies and leisure activity at home. Many spinal cord injured people have benefitted greatly from participation in organized sports such as basketball, swimming, ping pong, and weightlifting and, by competing on a national level, have achieved resocialization, achievement, and an increased sense of self-worth.

DRIVING. One of the most common social problems facing the wheelchair-confined person is the lack of adequate public transportation. Therefore it is essential that the paraplegic person become independent in driving skills using hand controls, in independent car transfers, and in placing the wheelchair in the car.

Many quadriplegic individuals can also drive with hand controls and steering knob, but they may need assistance getting in and out of the car, and most will need help in getting the wheelchair into the car.

Many automobile manufacturers now can outfit a van with hand controls and a hydraulic lift, making it much easier for the spinal cord injured person to travel. However, these vehicles are expensive to buy, to insure, and to operate.

PREVOCATIONAL CONSIDERATIONS. The employment potential of the spinal cord injured person is not necessarily correlated with the injury and its manifestations. A person with a debilitating injury is able to return to work if he or she is motivated, possesses employable knowledge and skills, is offered necessary reassurance from family and friends, and is able to find a job.

Although the patient may have to change former vocational goals, the functional occupational therapy program should provide the spinal cord injured person with knowledge and the desire to achieve.

Poliomyelitis and Guillain-Barré Syndrome

Poliomyelitis and Guillain-Barré syndrome, both lower motor neuron (LMN) lesions, result in flaccid paralysis and atrophy of the extremities. Polio results in an immediate and long-term paralysis of muscles, necessitating the eventual use of substitutions for function. In extreme cases the patient may require extensive functional devices and mechanisms for respiration; more commonly the patient may need splints, arm supports, braces, and/or assistive devices for self-care and other upper extremity functions.

The patient with Guillain-Barré syndrome, unlike the polio patient, has a good prognosis for recovery. Factors affecting recovery are premorbid physical condition, motivation, return of muscle function, and the character of the rehabilitation program.

For both the patient with polio and the one with Guillain-Barré syndrome, a common precaution in the rehabilitation program is the avoidance of fatigue in order to protect future functions. Psychological support, practical use of returning musculature in productive activity, and social stimulation are essential for the patients with each disease if they are to become involved in the rehabilitation objectives.

Poliomyelitis

Because of the extensive and effective use of vaccines, poliomyelitis is no longer prevalent in children's hospitals or in adult rehabilitation centers. The occupational therapist occasionally encounters a patient who has had a history of polio which complicates the current admission for treatment. There are times in a pre-vocational or vocational program when the therapist may need to evaluate the functional ability of the post-polio client.

Polio is an acute infectious disease caused by a virus which affects the anterior horn cells of the gray matter of the spinal cord and the motor nuclei of the brain stem.[13] The result is widespread or localized muscular paralysis with subsequent atrophy. The effect of the paralysis may be asymmetrical and patchy in character, resulting in paralysis in some muscles of one limb and none in others, causing an imbalance. Although the lower limbs are more often affected than the upper limbs, clinical conditions may demonstrate complete or partial monoplegia, hemiplegia, paraplegia, or quadriplegia. Sensation, however, is intact.

Symptoms include loss of cutaneous and tendon reflexes in the affected muscles, flaccid paralysis of the muscles affected, atrophy, subluxation of adjacent joints, general body weakness, respiratory and circulatory effects, and imbalance of muscle power. Contractures can occur in stronger muscles because of weakness of antagonist muscles. Asymmetrical paralysis of spinal muscles can result in scoliosis. Retarded bone growth can occur in the affected limbs.

TREATMENT. Early medical treatment begins with immediate and complete bedrest; physical activity increases the risk of further paralysis. Hot packs are provided to relieve muscle pain, and the patient is positioned to protect limbs from contracture and deformity. A tracheotomy may be necessary to provide an airway, and there may be a need for assistance in ventilation for the patient unable to breathe independently because muscles of respiration are weak. Various types of respirators and ventilators are used and might be required throughout the patient's life. During the phase in which the patient is receiving assistance in respiration, a *gentle* program of maintenance of passive and active functions is used.

Massage, passive and active range of motion with graded resistance, provision of splinting for prevention of contractures, and functional training follow as the patient regains physical tolerance. Surgical considerations include tendon transfers and arthrodesis to improve function and correct deformities.

The prime precaution in treating the patient with polio is to avoid muscle and body fatigue. Fatigue can result in further weakness and, if the muscles are overworked, loss of function can occur. Aside from this serious problem, it can cause the patient to miss hours of necessary treatment because of the debilitating effects of fatigue in one treatment session. Respiratory and cardiac stress must also be avoided. Signs of labored breathing should be looked for and, if necessary, the treatment should be terminated. The patient's muscle function should be continually evaluated for signs of imbalance.

Treatment sessions should be timed within the span of the patient's physical tolerance in order to avoid general body fatigue. In order to maintain and increase the patient's range of motion, endurance, and coordination, exercises and activities should be progressive and resistive and should be done symmetrically. Prevention of substitution patterns is important in the initial treatment program to encourage strengthening of weak muscles; however, when optimum muscle power has been reached, the patient may have to learn to use substitution patterns to assist in independent functions.

Arm supports and splints can be used both to minimize fatigue and to aid the patient in positioning weak extremities, particularly if there is shoulder girdle involvement. The balanced forearm orthosis (ball bearing feeder) can be used successfully for self-feeding, hygiene, upper extremity dexterity tasks, and other activities. Gravity can be used to assist weak musculature. For the severely involved polio patient, provision of special equipment becomes essential for continuation of upper extremity functions. Devices such as an electric wheelchair, electric page turner, tape recorder, prism glasses, talking books, and special splinting can be helpful. With the proper equipment the severely involved but well-motivated patient can adjust to adaptive functioning for daily activities and employment.

One of the most significant contributions the occupational therapist makes is providing assistance through adaptive and supportive activities for maximum productivity and social involvement. Because the effect of the disease is permanent, the patient with severe upper extremity involvement must adjust to being assisted by using complicated mechanical and electronic systems to substitute for or assist with arm positioning and hand activities.

Guillain-Barré Syndrome

Guillain-Barré syndrome is an acute disease of the nervous system that involves the spinal nerve roots, peripheral nerves, and, occasionally, the cranial nerves.[14] It is characterized by a hypersensitive response of the peripheral nervous system resulting in polyneuritis or inflammation of the nerves following a viral infection. The disease can affect either sex at any age. The acute phase involves rapid onset of paralysis of the limbs with accompanying sensory loss and muscle atrophy.

The initial illness, followed by flaccid paralysis, may affect all four limbs at once or may begin in the legs and spread upward to the arms. It may involve muscles of respiration. Proximal and distal muscles of the limbs are usually affected symmetrically. Reflexes are diminished or lost, sensation is impaired in the extremities and the muscles are tender, but all sensory modalities are not impaired.

Prognosis is varied and improvement may be sporatic. Almost complete recovery may be gained within three to six months or more, or the recovery may be incomplete with slight remissions, serious relapses, or the occurrence of a plateau. The patient may regain independent ambulation but retain some residual weakness and incoordination in all extremities with some atrophy in the intrinsic muscles of the hands. The patient who makes slow progress may develop atrophy which, if unattended, can hinder the effective use of the hands in manipulative tasks. The patient with weakness and incoordination may require lower extremity braces to substitute for the lack of strong leg muscles.

OCCUPATIONAL THERAPY. The patient with Guillain-Barré syndrome generally benefits from an intensive rehabilitation program. With the initiation of rehabilitation techniques as soon as the patient has reached medical stability, activities are introduced to encourage active muscle use in order to prevent atrophy or the wasting of muscles.

General rehabilitation goals include maintenance of nutrition, prevention of contractures, gradual diminution of the initial rest program, passive and active range of motion exercises for affected extremities, activity for muscle strengthening and coordination, restoration of sensation, increase in activity according to the patient's tolerance, splinting to prevent deformity from atrophy and disuse, a self-care program to encourage independent functions, assistive devices to encourage functional use of extremities, and development of work tolerance for prevocational preparation.

The occupational therapist designs a program geared to the *gradual* improvement of active functions. Because the patient may be totally paralyzed when first referred to occupational therapy, the first consideration may be to provide splints to maintain the functional position of fingers, thumbs, and wrists to prevent contractures from poor positioning. While on bedrest, the patient can benefit from the stimulation and encouragement of light social activities such as visits from family and friends, watching television, and supportive visits from the therapist, who engages the patient in positive conversation regarding interests while performing passive range of motion exercises. It is important to maintain free joint motions of the wrist and fingers for grasping activities which use tenodesis function.

Early treatment is similar to that of the spinal cord injured quadriplegic. The therapist must consider maintaining the patient's full passive joint range and encouraging active range against gravity. In addition, the therapist provides psychological support and therapeutic social stimulation and encourages the patient to use special devices such as an electric page turner, which can provide the satisfaction of reading independently but requires a minimum of movement to operate.

As the patient improves medically and begins to regain motor power, the occupational therapist provides activities which require increasing ranges of motion, coordination, and strength. The development of strength in specific muscles encourages the strengthening of other muscles.

However, as has been stressed, *care must be taken not to fatigue the patient.* Fatigue can be prevented by the therapist's providing the patient with suspension slings or arm supports for positioning and for facilitation of movement for hand functions. As the patient's motor power begins to return and coordination improves, care should be taken to vary activities between gross and fine, resistive and nonresistive, so that maximum gain can be derived without undue fatigue to the patient.

Specific activities of the upper extremities should encourage coordinated movements maintaining good body alignment to minimize the development of substitution patterns. The patient whose recovery is steadily progressive needs assistive devices *only* to prevent fatigue and substitution; usually these are not needed permanently. However, the patient whose progress is slower should be encouraged to use assistive equipment to gain strength and function.

From the beginning of treatment, self-care activities can encourage sensory and motor stimulation. Self-feeding and grooming can be started when necessary arm functions begin to return, even if a palmar cuff is used to substitute for grasp. Dressing can be started when physical tolerance increases and the patient has sufficient active range of motion.

As the patient regains functions, the program should be upgraded to challenge strength and coordination. The patient should be encouraged to function independently whenever possible and to ask for assistance only when needed. Along with the physical therapist, the occupational therapist monitors the patient's regaining of individual muscle control and checks for muscle atrophy.

Because the prognosis for the return of the patient's ambulation and functional upper extremity ability is generally good, the recovering patient is encouraged to participate in an activity program in which abilities for maximum independence can be developed. Recreational activities such as sports serve to improve physical endurance and coordination. (For specific adaptation of activities, assistive devices, and self-care techniques, see the section on spinal cord lesions earlier in this chapter.)

Amyotrophic Lateral Sclerosis

Amyotrophic lateral sclerosis (ALS) is a chronic systemic disease of unknown cause that affects the corticospinal system from the cortex to the periphery. It is characterized by degenerative changes which are most evident in the anterior horn cells of the spinal cord, motor nuclei of the medulla, and corticospinal tracts. The loss of nerve cells causes progressive wasting of the muscles, particularly evident in the upper extremities and in those muscles innervated by the medulla.[15]

The onset of ALS is gradual and steadily progressive, and the disease is generally fatal within one to six years.[16] It is nonhereditary.

Symptoms may first occur in muscles most used by the patient in his occupation or at the site of an injury.[17] Muscular atrophy usually begins in the intrinsic muscles of the hands and arm musculature; the patient complains of weakness, stiffness, and clumsiness of the fingers. Although the onset usually is centered symmetrically in the upper extremities, it can vary in location and severity. Thenar and finger flexor atrophy generally occur prior to atrophy of the extensors.

Weakness extends proximally from the hands to the shoulders. From the shoulders, the weakness moves to the tongue, where atrophy and paresis of the lips, tongue, and palate cause slurred speech which eventually becomes unintelligible. The patient's ability to swallow is also affected. As the patient's extensors become involved, weakness in the trunk, loss of head control, and lower extremity paralysis occur; eventually all reflexes are lost.

Treatment

ALS is treated symptomatically to provide maintenance of nutrition, to prevent fatigue, to prevent respiratory infections, and to avoid exposure to cold. Drugs can be used to control problems in swallowing, spasticity, and respiratory and urinary infections.

The rehabilitation program includes moderate

activity to maintain strength through muscle re-education and passive exercises to prevent contractures. The exercise program provides relaxation and alleviation of spasticity. Self-care techniques require the use of assistive devices to substitute for the patient's gradual loss of motor function. Gait training, with braces, is used when the patient can tolerate standing.

The occupational therapist provides both physical and psychological assistance to the patient with ALS. Therapeutic techniques and activities should be used with care to maximize functional benefit and minimize fatigue. Passive range of motion by the occupational therapist can provide relaxation in addition to maintaining maximum range of motion in the joints. The passive range of motion exercises should be followed by a short, active exercise period determined by the patient's muscle power.

The use of assistive equipment can aid the patient in retaining as much function as possible. A wheelchair, suspension slings, arm supports, and positioning aids can stimulate the patient to socialize, to care for him or herself, and to engage in activities which provide a day-to-day enjoyment of life.

Myasthenia Gravis

Myasthenia gravis is a progressive, degenerative disease that affects the myoneural junction. Impairment of conduction of nerve impulses to muscles occurs because of a presynaptic or post-synaptic block at the receptors on the motor endplates caused by a lack of release of the enzyme acetylcholine necessary for conduction.[18]

Beginning with a gradual onset, this chronic disease is characterized by intermittent, abnormal fatigue of isolated muscle groups. In later stages it results in permanent weakness of some muscles and muscle atrophy in others. The disease usually affects young adults, with females being more commonly affected than males.

The most common symptom of myasthenia gravis is abnormal muscular fatigue, most frequently observed in the eye muscles; this symptom is accompanied by ptosis (drooping of both upper lids) and diplopia (double vision). In addition the patient may present weakness of the facial muscles; total eye closure; retraction of the angles of the mouth; weakness of the bulbar musculature necessary for chewing, swallowing, and articulation; dyspnea (shortness of breath); weakness in the trunk and limbs; and general fatigue. Initially these symptoms are exacerbated when the patient is fatigued but they may disappear following rest.

In the later stages of the disease the patient experiences difficulty in swallowing and speaking. Eventually the patient becomes bedridden and immobile with severe permanent paralysis and contractures.

Remissions (decrease in symptoms) and improvement in general muscle strength and function may be marked and can last for years. However, sudden attacks of weakness caused by physical exertion, infection, or childbirth occur.

Occupational Therapy

The therapist's prime concern in working with the patient with myasthenia gravis is to aid the person in regaining muscle power and endurance; the therapist must take care not to cause debilitating fatigue. Because this disease is characterized by remissions, the recuperating patient may be able to regain functional abilities in upper extremities and independence in self-care and, in some instances, may be able to walk. If physical tolerance can be maintained during rehabilitation, the patient might be able to return to a nonexertive form of work. Overexertion must be avoided and respiratory problems must be prevented. He or she should be encouraged to employ work simplification techniques, therapeutic breathing, and energy conservation during activities.

The therapist should provide gentle, nonresistive activities that are interesting to the patient. These activities should be creative and productive and should provide the patient with psychological and intellectual stimulation to maintain a concept of self-worth.

In the later stages of the disease the bedridden patient may lack the ability to use the arms. Should this occur, the patient can benefit from electronically-controlled devices which substitute for nonfunction, thereby enabling the patient to operate a tape recorder, record player, television set, or radio. Such devices have been produced in the United States and England; although they are now expensive to manufacture and to repair, they enable the severely disabled person with intact intellectual abilities to communicate with the outside world and to have control over the immediate environment. For example, electronic activation of heating systems, windows, doors, telephones, lights, recording systems, and typewriters can be included in the installation. A discussion of the social and intellectual stimulation that can be provided to the patient severely disabled with myasthenia gravis appears in Dorothy Clark Wilson's book, *Hilary*.[19]

Muscular Dystrophy

Muscular dystrophy (MD) is a disease of the muscle cell which causes progressive degeneration of specific muscle groups. This disease is of unknown origin and is characterized by variation in the size of individual muscle fibers caused by initial swelling of muscle groups; the result is a pseudohypertrophic (enlarged) appearance of muscles. Although this false enlargement gives the appearance of a very strong extremity, it is caused by an excess of fat in the tissue and is eventually followed by atrophy.

The disease affects children, adolescents, or young adults. The most common type of MD is pseudohypertrophic muscular dystrophy, which normally affects males and is inherited as a sex-linked recessive genetic defect. It may occur sporadically or may affect several siblings.[20]

Symptoms appear during the middle of the first decade of life: a previously normal child begins to walk clumsily, tends to fall, and has difficulty getting up after a fall. The characteristic pseudohypertrophy of the muscles manifests itself in the calves, glutei, quadriceps, and deltoids. These muscles are enlarged and firm to the touch but they usually are weak. In some cases this manifestation may appear in the triceps and forearm muscles. The accompanying atrophy usually affects the proximal more than the distal muscles. Muscle impairment can cause weakness of the extensors of the spine, resulting in lordosis, weakness in the knees, and diminished tendon reflexes. While sensation and intelligence are unimpaired, the child with MD may be limited by the rapid onset of severe physical limitations and confinement to a wheelchair. Schooling may be interrupted and capacity to progress with peers may be diminished.

Early signs of MD are manifested in the sloping appearance of the patient's shoulders; this is caused by weakness in the shoulder girdle. Contractures are common in the later stages of the disease, caused by weakness in muscle groups whose antagonists remain comparatively powerful. An example of the developing contracture is seen in the patient who walks on his or her toes because of progressive weakness of the anterior tibial muscle and the tendency of the biceps and hamstrings to shorten. When the patient becomes confined to a wheelchair, contractures occur in the trunk, causing postural changes.

Occupational Therapy

Because MD results in a gradual loss of muscle power and control, the rehabilitation program is directed toward the maintenance of range of motion and strength through the continuation of self-care and functional skills. Contractures can be prevented through passive range of motion exercises, proper positioning of the patient in the wheelchair for arm function, active exercises and activities for the arms, and assistive devices.

As the weakness increases, assistive equipment such as arm supports are used to assist the patient in reaching, self-feeding, and other arm and hand activities. Special devices may be needed for bathing and dressing and for diversional and productive activities. The therapist should also provide the patient with a home exercise program which can maintain the existing muscle power and allow the patient to participate in various pursuits. Although the life span of the patient with MD is shortened, he or she can continue a relatively normal life with the use of adaptive equipment and assistive techniques.

Peripheral Nerve Injuries

Peripheral nerve injuries result from direct trauma to the extremity and affect all muscles innervated below the point of injury. Common causes include fractures, dislocations, crush injuries, compression, and lacerations. Primary impairments include sensory and motor dysfunction, contractures, deformity, and swelling. Continuing malfunction of the nerves can cause long-term or permanent muscle dysfunction, deformities of the hand, sensory loss, and trophic changes.

Occupational Therapy

The general rehabilitation goal is to return the patient to a maximum level of function and independence. The injury may have caused serious damage to the patient's sensorimotor system, resulting in the loss of extremity function caused by the blockage of conduction of impulses. Depending upon the location and severity of the injury, the patient may suffer a long-term disability. The rehabilitation program focuses on return of the patient's capacity to use the extremity and on development of sensory and motor function. Physical and cosmetic changes in the extremity may cause difficulties in the patient's psychological adjustment to disability.

From the initial immobilization in a cast to later dynamic splinting by the occupational therapist, treatment must be carefully monitored. Specific forms of splinting are used protectively and as a forerunner and stimulus to function. The design of the dynamic splint provides minimal coverage of the patient's extremity but allows flexible, controlled use of the hand. Elastic or spring finger cuffs facilitate movement. The affected extremity needs exercise to prevent disuse atrophy. Because there may be muscle imbalance following nerve injury, the splint prevents overstretching of the strong, unaffected muscles. Correct alignment is essential to provide the patient with mechanical advantage and to preserve functional potential.

Skin changes and sensory deficits may be caused by poor circulation. Therefore, a concern of the occupational therapist is maintaining the integrity of the patient's skin.[21] The therapist checks the effect of splinting and other devices on the affected extremity, uses cutaneous stimulation to encourage functional return of sensation, and helps the patient develop an awareness of pain, temperature, and tactile discrimination. With these supportive concepts, the patient can avoid further injury to the desensitized limb.

Passive and assisted movements of the limb restore the flexibility of the joints. Gentle passive range of motion, accompanied by heat and warm water, facilitates movement. As the patient's strength increases, the occupational therapist increases the resistance provided by various exercises or activities. However, care must be taken not to fatigue the patient or overstretch weakened muscles. The therapist's observation should include checking to make sure that the patient is not using substitution patterns that impair the development of function. Sensory stimulation includes manipulation of objects of different sizes, textures, weights, and shapes.

Contractures impede rehabilitation. Once they occur, it is difficult to release them by passive stretching which may cause joint damage if done improperly. Splints can be useful in preventing contractures in the early phase of treatment.

The therapist may use static or dynamic positioning to support the patient's joints in maximum normal alignment and muscle balance. Specific designs for splints will depend on the patient's functional capacity.

The occupational therapist encourages the patient to develop maximum functional use of the impaired extremity. Total body use is important in reintegrating the disabled extremity with the rest of the patient's body; activities which are gradually upgraded in resistance encourage the patient's coordination, increase function, and augment general physical and mental tolerance of the condition. However, the occupational therapist must be careful not to overwork the patient because excessive exercise can cause edema in the affected extremity, creating stiffness in the joints, thus hindering his or her range of motion. (For additional information see Chapter 22 on Hand Rehabilitation.)

Carpal Tunnel Syndrome

The carpal tunnel syndrome results from compression of the median nerve at the wrist's transverse carpal ligament, resulting in paresthesia and pain involving the first three fingers of the hand, the forearm, and the wrist. Usually the symptoms are worse at night than during the day. Forced and sustained positions of the wrist can cause pain. Driving for long periods, knitting, typing, and/or carrying packages can exacerbate the symptoms.

The syndrome is characterized by joint swelling, sensitivity on joint flexion and extension, and pain caused by maintenance of a fixed position. There is a sensory loss in the median nerve distribution and the thenar eminence may display atrophy.

Carpal tunnel syndrome is caused by rheumatoid arthritis, malunion of a wrist fracture, tumors, diabetes mellitus, and occupational stress.

Steroid injections may be used for local treatment; however, these can cause additional trauma to the joint and surgical intervention for release of pressure may be required. Immobilization of the patient's wrist in a neutral position may provide relief at night and allow performance of heavy activities during the day. It is important to advise the patient to avoid activities that cause stress.

Volkmann's Ischemic Contracture

This debilitating condition of the upper extremity can occur directly after trauma or can result from swelling within restricting bandages or casts. Two thirds of the patients with Volkmann's ischemic contracture are under thirty years of age and most are between the ages of two and sixteen.[22] The condition usually results from fractures of the humerus. Other causes include damage to the brachial or the axillary artery from gunshot wounds or from embolus, rupture, trauma, or pressure involving the forearm.

Ischemia is caused by swelling in the arm. Interference with circulation in the lower arm deprives all involved tissues of their blood supply. The rapid onset results in initial necrosis of tissue and progresses to fibrosis and contracture. The intrinsic muscles of the hand are affected by "glove anesthesia," and there is impaired nutrition of the patient's hand and forearm.[23]

The clinical picture reveals an edematous, cold, numb forearm; the patient's hand is blanched and has a smooth, glossy appearance. The patient has difficulty moving the hand and has paralysis of the flexor, extensor, and intrinsic muscles of the hand along with loss of sensation. The patient's arm muscles are tender, swollen, and hard over the forearm. Contractures may be present with flexion in the distal joints and extension in the proximal joints of the fingers. Extensors of the fingers may be functional; however, the patient may be limited to extending the fingers with wrist flexion because of tight flexor tendons. Median, ulnar, and radial nerves are involved with the median nerve being most affected. Muscle atrophy occurs and the bones become osteoporotic. In children, bone growth is retarded and deformity is increased.

Medical treatment involves immediate removal of the restricting cast or bandages, reduction of the fracture, and release of the pressure causing the ischemia. Release of the nerves, nerve repair, and tendon and nerve transfers may be done along with excision of the necrotic areas and skin grafting. Because of the continuous initial progressive contracture, a splint is provided to maintain extension of the wrist and fingers.

Occupational Therapy

The role of the occupational therapist is to provide specific passive and active range of motion and strengthening exercises to aid the patient in regaining maximum use of the extremity. The therapist uses techniques to provide positioning to prevent deformity, to support maximum use of the hand and arm, and to encourage use of both extremities in assisted bimanual activity, and offers counselling regarding acceptance of appearance of the arm. The prognosis for restoration of function of the patient's hand depends on the severity of the condition, the availability and feasibility of surgical procedures, and the motivation of the patient. The patient may be required to change hand dominance and to adapt to the functional and cosmetic aspects of the disability.

The activity program stresses maximum use of the involved extremity with specific grasping exercises to utilize the functional gains of surgery. In providing splints for finger traction, the therapist must pay attention to preventing cutaneous pressure areas because of decreased sensation.

The occupational therapist assists the patient in adapting to one-handed activities, giving instructions in using the involved extremity as an assist in holding or carrying items and in using gross arm motions in bilateral movements. The patient is also trained in coordination and use of the unaffected arm.

If surgical repair has been done to the tendons or nerves, the patient may require reeducation in functional movements and splinting may be necessary to maintain the capacity to use the injured extremity. The occupational therapist must also encourage the patient to accept the condition and to deal with both the limited function and the appearance of the arm.

ORTHOPEDIC CONDITIONS

Among those patients with orthopedic conditions who are referred to occupational therapy are those with hand injuries and persons with hip, back, upper and/or lower extremity fractures which confine them to bed or cause them to be placed in traction. For persons with upper extremity injuries, the surgeon may request functional training for increasing range of motion, strength, and coordination; provision of assistive devices for self-care; static and dynamic splinting for upper extremity injuries; and diversional activities for those in traction. The number of patients with orthopedic conditions seen and treated by the occupational therapist depends on the recognition of the value of occupational therapy by the orthopedic surgeon.

Evaluation

The evaluation varies depending on the type of injury and the extent of the patient's immobilization. For example, a patient with a neck injury may be seen initially while in neck traction. If the spinal cord has not been injured, there may be weakness but not paralysis in the extremities. The patient with a lower back injury may have full upper extremity function but be confined to supine positions in bed and may have restrictions on back movements with or without lower extremity dysfunction. The patient with a lower extremity fracture may have full use of the arms but be confined to bed in leg traction, or there may be precautions against hip flexion. A person with an upper extremity orthopedic injury may be in bed, in a wheelchair, or ambulatory.

In preparing to evaluate the patient, the occupational therapist should review the medical factors pertinent to the patient's injury and the present medical condition. These factors include the type of fracture, length of time and type of immobilization, alignment and progress of bony union, presence and extent of nerve involvement, presence of infection, precautions of mobility, safe joint movement and muscle stretching, and consideration of removal of supporting casts, braces, or splints during activity or exercise.

Evaluation should include passive and active range of motion of the joints proximal and distal to the immobilized joint(s); general mobility of all extremities; positioning alternatives for the patient; feasibility of the patient's using a wheelchair or walking; and the existence of accompanying factors such as paralysis, trophic changes, edema, pain, fatigue, contractures, scar tissue, and psychological problems. The occupational therapist evaluates the patient's level of functional ability and independence in activities of daily living.

General principles of treatment of the affected limb include the following:

1. Support of the injured part to relieve trauma, to prevent further destruction of tissue, to ensure proper alignment of the extremity, and to prevent pain from joint limitation.
2. Prevention of disuse atrophy in the musculature surrounding the traumatized area. The patient should be encouraged to maintain strength, range of motion, and function.
3. A therapeutic exercise program for reeducation of muscles and joints.
4. Encouragement of normal functional return following immobilization and gradual use of the extremity in unilateral and bilateral coordination activities.
5. Assistance in the patient's adjustment to cosmetic and functional changes caused by trauma.

A patient may have pain in the extremity caused by the trauma itself or by immobilization; such a patient may not be motivated to participate in a full program of exercise and activity. The therapist must encourage the patient to become involved in rehabilitation in order to prevent deformities, substitution of motor patterns, and pain in the weakened limb.

The orthopedic patient with an upper extremity trauma may remain in the acute care setting for a relatively short period of time but long enough for adequate setting of the fracture, healing of surgical sites, and stabilization of medical complications. Initial casting is usually done by the physician, but the occupational therapist may be requested to assist in preparing for future adjustment of splinting in coordination with a functional exercise and activity program.

Occupational Therapy

Shoulder disabilities may occur postoperatively in cases involving tumor, traction, immobilization, fracture, or periarthritis. Clinical signs include pain, muscle atrophy, shoulder weakness, contracture of the adductors with the inability to rotate externally, fear of movement, and stiffness. Following heat, massage, and whirlpool activity in physical therapy, the occupational therapy program should include graded activities to increase strength, range of motion, and function by using such activities as the floor loom, printing press, woodworking, macrame, and basketry. The patient should be encouraged to participate in recreational activities such as shuffleboard, darts, bowling, and ball games to develop full use and integration of the injured extremity. The patient's physical tolerance and fatigue level should be the gauge used for gradation of the patient's program. Prevocational evaluation becomes part of the treatment program for the patient who will be able to return to work. The occupational therapist works closely with the vocational rehabilitation counsellor in identifying specific job-related abilities. The industrially oriented program is basically one of regaining work tolerance in a graded conditioning program.

For upper extremity injuries, activities such as using hand tools and power machinery, painting, and shoveling are used. The conditioning program should utilize productive work tasks and activity time should be increased as the patient's endurance develops. However, the patient should be monitored for signs of pain, swelling, or fatigue.

Home activity programs should be developed to encourage the patient to maintain a general conditioning program.

Patients who have a fractured forearm or hand may require a splint as a supportive device for strenuous activity. Unless there is peripheral nerve involvement from the injury, the orthopedic surgeon usually provides the initial splint. However, the occupational therapist may be asked later to provide a dynamic splint to encourage finger function. The most useful treatment is functional training in the use of the injured extremity. Productive activity is essential to the achievement of this goal. Graded manual activity and specific dexterity training in the affected hand are essential for the regaining of functional abilities. If the patient cannot regain adequate use of the hand through functional activity, counselling for alternative job training and placement may be required.

Patients who suffer residual effects from surgery (scarring or amputation) may need cosmetic adjustments. The occupational therapist can counsel the patient, pointing out assets and helping the patient accept the additional trauma of cosmetic disfigurement.

When a patient has suffered a fracture of a lower extremity, the occupational therapy program begins with activities to provide diversion while the patient is confined to bed. When the patient is able to stand and bear weight on the injured extremity, he or she can begin a program of standing tolerance and general reconditioning. Lower extremity active exercises include graded, resistive exercises of the extremity, coordination exercises, and use of the extremity involving the entire body.

Adaptations to the floor loom, printing press, bicycle, and woodworking equipment can aid the patient in gradual increase in strength and coordination. Work-simulated tasks designed for the injured worker offer preparation for the demands of the job (Fig. 13-17).

For the patient who has had a back or leg injury, work activities include weight bearing, lifting, carrying, climbing, and bending. Activities such as lifting, carrying weights, climbing ladders, shoveling, chopping wood, pushing a wheelbarrow, and pulling heavy objects are given and upgraded according to the patient's tolerance. Specific activities for strengthening a limb and increasing tolerance which are used for the patient having a lower extremity injury include balancing and exercising using adapted equipment such as a bicycle saw, or treadle sander, lathe, or printing press.

Fractured Hip—Hip Replacement

The patient with a fractured hip or with a hip replacement is commonly referred to the occupational therapist by the orthopedic surgeon, rheumatologist, or physiatrist. The patient benefits from diversional activities, self-care training, assistive devices, home evaluation, and home adaptation.

During the bedrest stage following surgery the patient may benefit from diversional activities that

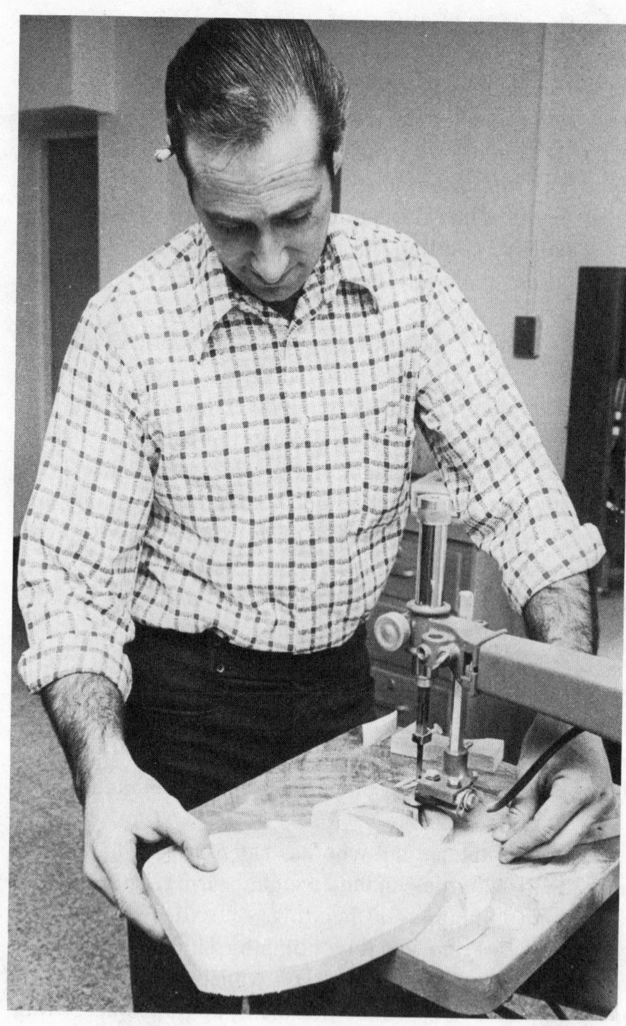

FIGURE 13-17. A patient recovering from an industrial injury to his back uses the power saw. The occupational therapist can evaluate standing tolerance and prevocational performance during performance of this activity.

assist in psychological adjustment and divert attention from pain. When there is medical clearance for the patient to move around in bed, he or she should be encouraged to participate in morning hygiene and self-care. Because the patient may be restricted in the use of the hip joint in flexion and resistive movements, long-handled reachers and special hooks can provide assistance in dressing. When the physician concurs, range of motion of the hip should be encouraged during activity. However, the rehabilitation process must be gradual.

The patient may be discharged from the hospital before he or she has fully recovered from the injury or surgery; therefore, a home program should be established for him or her in protecting the hip from further injury and to encourage him or her to exercise and participate in self-care activities. The occupational therapist instructs the patient in both protective precautions and the use of various devices that can assist in self-care. The patient should avoid bending the hip more than ninety degrees and crossing the legs at the knees or ankles. A firm, knee height, straight-backed chair with arm rests should be used. Reclining chairs are very difficult for the patient to get into or out of, can cause the patient to fall, and should be avoided. Toilet seat extensions and firm pillows in low chairs can insure proper height for adequate transfer and comfort.

The patient should be advised to sleep in a supine position, to promote good alignment of the hip joints. If the patient is accustomed to turning in bed, a pillow should be placed between the legs to inhibit movement.

Other aspects of the patient's home program include instruction and advice in the use of assistive devices for bathing (long-handled sponges, soap on a rope, and nonskid safety strips in the shower), for dressing (long-handled shoehorn, stocking aids, elastic shoe laces, and reachers), and for other activities of daily living. A "walker bag" attached to the crutch may be used to carry small objects. Cars with low reclining seats should be avoided when possible, but a cushion may be used to raise the seat to a comfortable height.

ARTHRITIS

Arthritis can affect a person of any age, has a variety of causes and effects, and can be of short duration or a lifelong condition. It can be the effect of local trauma or the aging process (osteoarthritis) or that of systemic infection (rheumatoid arthritis). Although it is commonly thought that arthritis is an affliction of the elderly, it may also be a handicap of the young. Persons with arthritis may be referred to occupational therapy on either an inpatient or an outpatient basis.

Degenerative joint disease (DJD) or osteoarthritis, is the less feared type of the disease. The occupational therapist usually sees the person with degenerative joint disease during an outpatient visit. Although DJD most commonly affects fingers at the proximal interphalangeal and distal interphalangeal joints with minimal or no pain, other frequently traumatized joints are the ankles, knees, hips, and elbows. DJD often occurs in people who have been active in sports or whose jobs have caused strain on their joints, or it accompanies the aging process. The swelling associated with DJD is in the bony structure, not in the soft tissue as is the case with rheumatoid arthritis.

Treatment of DJD primarily is local, consisting of rest, relief of pain, and protection of the affected joints. Heat and therapeutic exercises should be provided on a gradual, upgraded basis.

Rheumatoid arthritis is a progressive systemic disease resulting in inflammation, pain, and structural changes in the affected joints. Characterized by remissions and exacerbations, rheumatoid arthritis results in progressive limitation and deformity. Many persons suffering rheumatoid arthritis referred to occupational therapy are between the ages of twenty and forty. They exhibit swollen, reddened, and painful joints with or without deformities and complain of pain during and after excessive use of the affected joints. Because of the limitations imposed by the disease, the person's functional ability, physical appearance, and mental tolerance are affected. Treatment must be geared toward assisting the patient in combating the debilitating effects of the disease and in maintaining maximum independent functions. The occupational therapist is concerned with aiding the person in a self-directed program of home treatment following hospitalization.

The clinical picture of rheumatoid arthritis is mainly centered on the joints, where there may be subluxation, dislocation, pain, swelling, stiffness, and deformity. Muscle atrophy may occur because of limitations in joint movement and decreased activity. Contractures may occur from both decreased muscle activity and prolonged immobilization. Skin changes and loss of weight are characteristic. The patient may eventually need braces, crutches, or a wheelchair for locomotion; splints to prevent deformity and provide function; and a variety of assistive devices for self-care.

Functional problems caused by arthritis arise from limitations in active and passive movement. Among the causes are joint limitations; fear of pain; actual pain; and decreased strength affecting reach, grasp, and coordination.

Before discussing evaluation techniques and treatment programs, it is essential to review precautions.

1. *Dislocation and subluxation:* Avoid overactivity of the affected joints. Avoid resistive exercises.

2. *Pain and swelling:* Do not exercise the extremity of a patient who is in the acute stage of rheumatoid arthritis. Encourage active range of motion without resistance. Keep the patient warm and comfortable.

3. *Fatigue:* Use suspension slings for support against strain and fatigue. Do not exceed the patient's endurances and do not allow fear to develop.

Minimize strenuous activity and alternate activity with rest.

4. *Over-exercise:* Work within the patient's limits of pain, swelling, and/or tolerance.

5. *Muscle atrophy:* Exercise should be limited to the patient's maximum active range of motion. If the patient can work against resistance, use it in an activity to encourage strengthening of muscles.

One of the surgical procedures to combat the symptoms of rheumatoid arthritis is synovectomy. It is performed early in the course of the disease to relieve pain and swelling, release contractures, and prevent arthrodesis of joints. Other surgical procedures include arthroplasty and replacement of the hip, knee, elbow, or metacarpophalangeal joints. These surgical procedures may be successful in relieving pain, aligning joints, establishing function, and increasing range of motion. When a surgical procedure is considered, the occupational therapist should inform the surgeon of the patient's functional ability so that function may be retained after surgery. The patient's attitude and expectations regarding surgery are crucial to rehabilitation.

Evaluation

The referral of the patient with arthritis might specify splinting and/or maintenance of functional abilities. Participation in diversional or productive activities; provision of assistive devices; techniques for self-care, joint protection, and work simplification; home evaluation; and removal of architectural barriers may or may not appear on the formal referral, but they must be considered by the occupational therapist.

Following the referral, the therapist considers the medical information in the patient's chart and specific recommendations from the referring physician. Determination of the duration of the disease, previous treatment, and the current phase of the arthritis are important in the therapist's evaluation. During the evaluation the therapist carries out the following:

1. Observe the patient's extremities for signs of redness, swelling, atrophy, discoloration, surgical scars, malalignment, joint deformities such as boutonnière or swan neck, or deviations from normal alignment (hyperflexion, hyperextension, abduction, adduction, or ulnar deviation).

2. Observe the relaxed limbs for signs of atrophy, joint limitation, pain, or discomfort.

3. Check for splints, braces, or other special equipment. Determine the patient's ability to use and care for the devices provided.

4. Gently move the extremities through the passive range of motion, noting the presence of subluxation, joint limitation, muscle tightness, and/or pain.

5. Ask the patient to move extremities through all ranges of motion. Insist that the patient indicate if there is pain.

6. Check the patient's muscle strength by providing some resistance.

7. Provide activities that evaluate the functional use of hands and arms:
   a. *Grasping:* Small objects such as nuts and bolts or jigsaw puzzle pieces.
   b. *Handling heavy objects:*
      1. A hammer, using one hand.
      2. A can of sugar, using two hands.
   c. *Reaching:* Ask the patient to place a book on a shelf, turn on a faucet, or open a drawer.

8. Ask the patient to use hands in activities such as writing, removing a letter from an envelope, counting money (either change or bills), and finding a page in a book.

9. Determine whether or not the patient is independent in self-care: bathing, grooming, eating, transferring from one position to another, walking, and carrying needed items.

10. During the entire evaluation, observe the patient's performance. Look for signs of mental and physical fatigue. Vary the evaluation activities so that the patient can complete them without unnecessary pain, frustration, and joint stress.

11. Encourage the patient, listen to his or her needs, interests, and concerns. Emphasize abilities. A positive approach can aid the patient by improving both physical function and mental outlook.

12. Do not prolong evaluation sessions beyond the patient's mental or physical tolerance. Correlate the occupational therapy program with other aspects of the patient's rehabilitation.

Treatment

Specific Approaches

The approaches to treatment must be individualized to meet the needs of various patients. The outpatient may be seen for the first time at the request of a physician for the construction of resting splints and/or splints to protect joints and to provide improvement of function, for energy conservation orientation, and for the provision of assistive devices. The outpatient often has a family to care for, a job to perform, or school to attend. With the implementation of various aids and programs, the patient can perform different tasks with greater ease and comfort, and can gain the satisfaction of accomplishing chosen activities with less pain and stress. Following the remission of painful symptoms requiring medical treatment, the patient may need only a few treatment sessions. The homemaker can be assisted in organizing time and tasks to minimize tension. The employed arthritic client can be assisted in self-evaluation of job activities and can learn how to adapt equipment or arrange the work schedule. The student can learn ways to ease the strain of note-taking in class and of carrying books and equipment. The student should also be encouraged to participate in social activities and engage in recreation.

The inpatient is likely to be on bedrest during the acute stage of arthritis. Evaluation and initial treatment may be accomplished during this time. During the period of inflammation, there should be little stress on joints, and daily activities of bathing and feeding should be assisted. Bathing can be simplified with the use of a bath mitt or a long-handled sponge. For meals the patient can be provided with a fork with a built-up handle, a serrated knife, a large-handled plastic mug, easily managed food containers, and a rubber mat upon which to place plates.

Bed positioning is extremely important to prevent deformities and to encourage the most beneficial, comfortable, and successful means of functioning. The patient should use a firm mattress: he or she should lie flat in the supine position with arms and hands straight at the sides. A small pillow may be used if necessary. Light covers should be used to minimize weight on sensitive limbs.

Prism glasses for television viewing or seeing visitors can minimize fatigue and strain during this period. A book holder which can be angled for bed use, and a lapboard placed in a comfortable position, can be used for reading and writing. All items should be placed within easy reach.

During the period of bedrest the patient often suffers pain from inflammation of the joints and requires encouragement and diversion more than active exercise. Exercise when used should *not* include resistance at this time.

Poor positioning of the extremities may cause pain, poor alignment, stiff joints, deformity, and general discomfort. Thus, splints may be indicated during the acute inflammatory stage of rheumatoid arthritis.

The importance of positioning continues when the patient is sitting in a chair, uses a wheelchair, and/or walks. When the patient is able to sit in a chair for activity, attention should be given to proper alignment of the body. A high-backed chair should be used for trunk and head support. Feet should be placed firmly on the floor and firm cushions should be used to raise the patient to a comfortable position. Good positioning minimizes strain, encourages mechanical advantage in functions, and prevents deformities.

When the patient is in a wheelchair or is ambulatory, the occupational therapy program becomes more intensive. As soon as medically feasible, the patient can engage in light activities which employ maximum active range of motion. Needlework, Turkish knotting, light weaving, and painting can be used to strengthen the patient's upper arm and hand and increase range of motion and coordination.

The occupational therapist is responsible for teaching the patient the use of assistive devices and techniques which can aid in self-care and homemaking activities. For example, built-up handles can be used for toothbrushes, combs, hairbrushes, eating utensils, and cleaning implements. Built-up handles, mitts, and rubber mats for cooking utensils aid the homemaker. Dressing can be assisted by the use of long-handled implements, and reachers can be used to grasp objects from the floor or from high places.

The arthritic patient's home can be made safe by the addition of railings at stairways, removal of heavy doors and scatter rugs, provision of easily managed latches on doors and cabinets, and arrangement of furniture and work areas for ease of movement and function. The occupational therapist can advise the patient in these labor-saving and safety factors.

Principles of Treatment

The following principles are important for the occupational therapist to know:

1. *Control of the rheumatoid process.* Physicians who treat the person with rheumatoid arthritis attempt to control the disease with anti-inflammatory and analgesic drugs; they also encourage bedrest during the acute phases of the disease and following surgery in instances of severe destruction of the joints. Although one or a combination of these procedures may succeed in retarding the rheumatoid process for a period of time, the patient may continue to have exacerbations of the disease leading to periods when rest and therapeutic exercise are necessary. When the patient's joints show a reduction of swelling and inflammation, the rehabilitation program can begin.

2. *Joint mobility through range of motion* (Figs. 13-18 and 13-19). Passive and active range of motion of all extremities are essential for good functional restoration. Passive and active range of motion should be employed to determine the presence of pain and joint limitation. Active range of motion with resistance should be encouraged only after the therapist has determined that pain, swelling, and inflammation have been reduced.

3. *Functional training.* The occupational therapist uses functional training to make the patient aware of both his limitations and his abilities. Analyzing the patient's daily activities can lead the therapist to provide specific self-care techniques, diversional activities, productive activities, and joint protection aids.

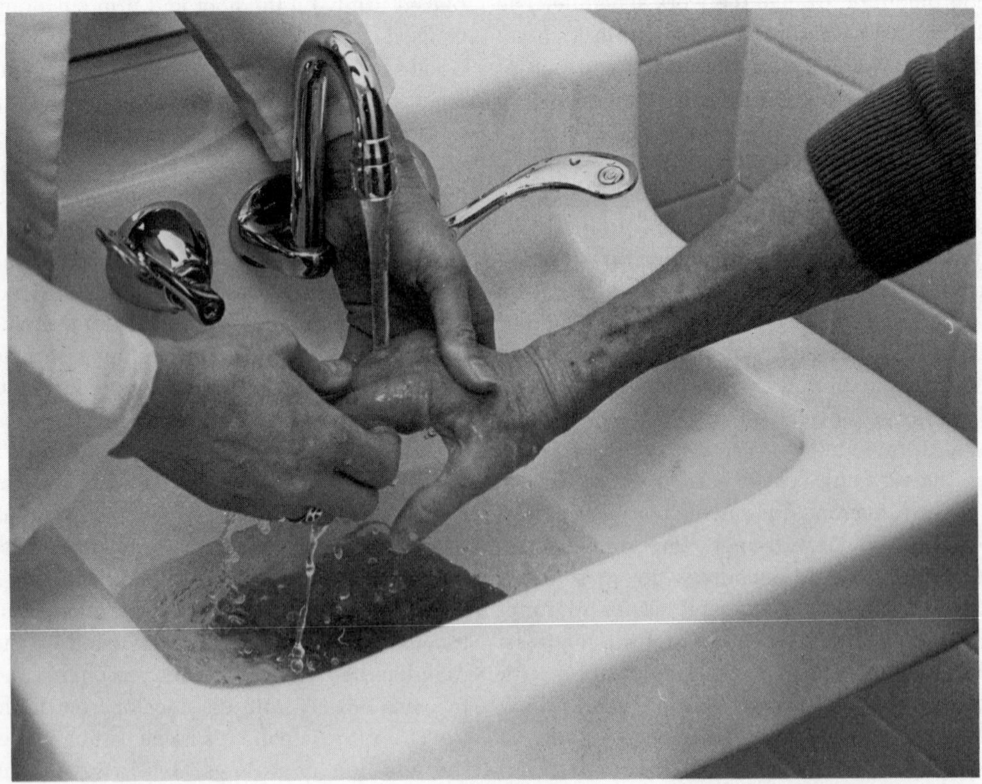

FIGURE 13-18. Warm water and percussion are used to stimulate and soothe painful arthritic joints during passive exercise done in preparation for activity.

4. *Maintenance of muscle power.* The patient with rheumatoid arthritis may exhibit weakness. Deformities may prevent functional use of muscles and joint alignment may be continually challenged. Without adequate joint function, muscle power is reduced, but the use of a functional hand splint can properly align muscles, joints, and tendons. Activities requiring strength must be used carefully in the arthritic patient's therapeutic program (Fig. 13-20). Too much resistance can cause joint pain. The occupational therapist must avoid activity which will cause fatigue to the patient, and must make the patient aware of limitations on his or her strength.

5. *Independence in self-care.* Because of the existence of pain and joint limitations characteristic of arthritis, the patient may suffer deficiencies in self-care, may avoid dressing, or may request assistance in basic activities of daily living. The therapist should encourage the patient to use self-care techniques as therapeutic exercises, employing assistive devices and special equipment to conserve energy and avoid further joint destruction.

6. *Increase physical and mental endurance.* The person with rheumatoid arthritis is subjected to frequent hospitalizations. Exacerbations and remissions are common, and the patient displays frustration caused by the inability to cope with family or job responsibilities.

The therapist should encourage the patient to develop a regime of alternate rest and work which will protect joints and conserve energy. The patient should also be instructed in the principles and use of joint protection techniques. The development of awareness of the disease's nature can help both the patient and his or her family cope with physical limitations that result from tension, overwork, or pain.

7. *Assistive devices.* These devices should be used only to increase function or to protect impaired joints. They should be lightweight, simple to operate, and acceptable to the patient. They should encourage independent function. If the patient cannot use the device easily, the patient will discard it.

8. *Home program.* The occupational therapist must stress the need for the patient with arthritis to continue the therapeutic program at home. Among the elements of discharge planning are a home visit to determine architectural barriers, necessary rearrangement of furniture and toilet facilities, assistance with work space and appliances, and development of specific devices.

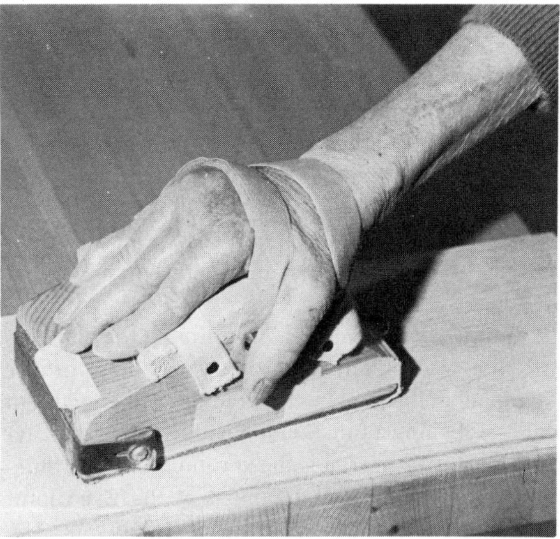

FIGURE 13-19. This patient has rheumatoid arthritis and has had surgical replacement of the metacarpophalangeal joints. She is using the sanding block for resistive activity to achieve active range of motion and muscle function of the arm. The patient's hand is positioned in maximum passive extension of the metacarpophalangeal joints.

Splinting

The provision of splinting for the patient with rheumatoid arthritis is both crucial and controver-

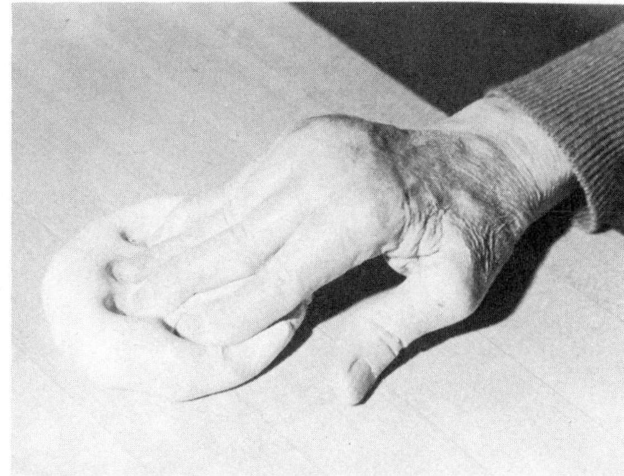

FIGURE 13-20. Soft resistive theraplast material provides specific finger exercises for the patient with rheumatoid arthritis.

sial. As Hollander wrote, "It is usually much easier to prevent a deformity in arthritis than to correct one."[24] Some experts believe that no splint at all is preferable to a splint that causes decreased function or deformity in the patient with arthritis.

The purposes of splinting the arthritic are provision of support to diseased joints, alleviation of pain, prevention of deformity, maintenance and promotion of function, and establishment of functional alignment.

Splints are used at night to maintain the patient's extremity in a static position, providing proper alignment of the joints without undue stress on them and establishing a functional position for daily activities. Because the wrist is the key joint for hand function, stabilization and alignment of the wrist joint must be done prior to splinting of the fingers. The splint used at night can be a volar splint extending from the distal third of the forearm to the fingertips, with abduction and extension of the thumb. In some cases the thumb may be left free and the splint may terminate at the distal portion of the metacarpophalangeal joints. This construction may be necessary to prevent stiffening of the phalangeal joints in extension since they should be slightly flexed.

Daytime splints also maintain functional alignment of the arthritic patient's wrist and fingers; however, the splints must be of different types from those used at night. If the patient's pain is at the wrist, static positioning can stiffen the joints and thus the splint must be removed and the joints allowed full range of motion several times during the day. Dynamic splinting must be controlled to prevent both pain from movement and deformity from poor positioning. The palmar aspect of the splint can terminate at the palm. Finger cuffs and rubberbands can be used to provide finger mobility with an outrigger for positioning and resistive activity. With this type of positioning, it is essential that the wrist be stabilized to minimize trauma to the finger joints.

After the occupational therapist has constructed the splint(s), they should be inspected to ensure that they provide proper support and comfort to the patient. Splints should be lightweight, cover a minimum amount of skin, and be easily applied or removed (Fig. 13-21). The patient must be advised to

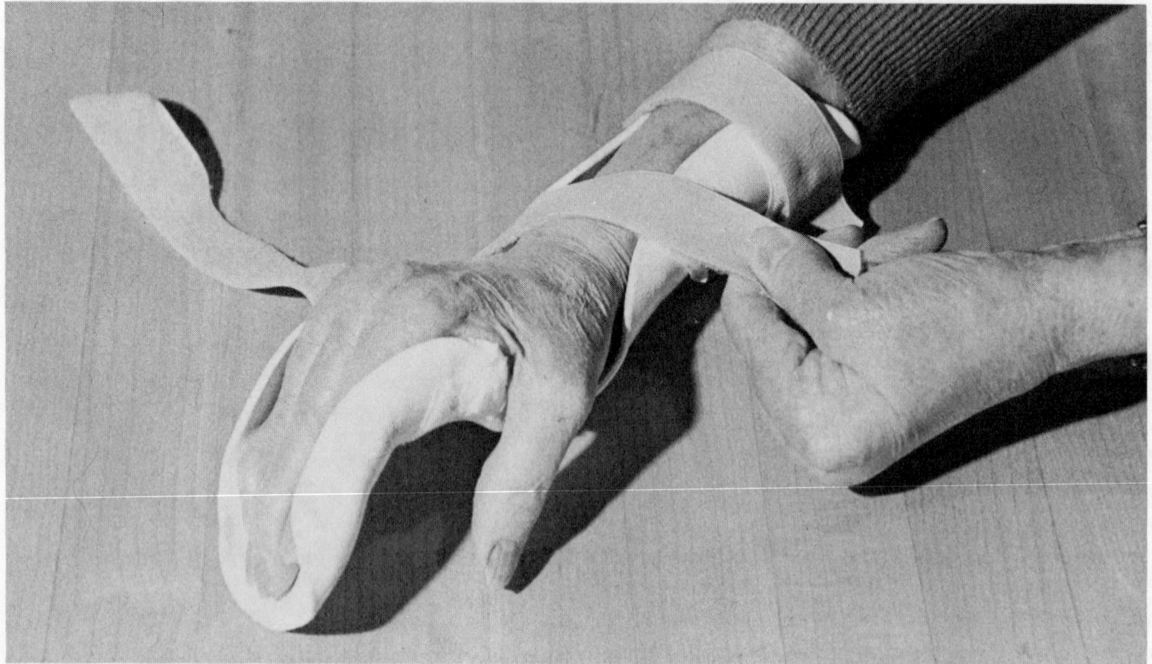

FIGURE 13-21. A patient with rheumatoid arthritis puts on her volar splint, which is used for night resting and proper positioning.

inform the therapist of areas of irritation and to use both passive and active range of motion exercises in conjunction with the use of the splint.

Principles of Joint Protection

Education in joint protection is an essential part of the occupational therapist's work in rehabilitation. Because of pain and instability, some arthritic patients fear further damage to the joints and therefore avoid using them. On the other hand, an arthritic patient may deny the disability, avoid preventive precautions, and actually cause destruction and deformity.

The patient must become involved in the rehabilitation process, carrying over program principles learned during hospitalization. Among these principles of joint protection are the following.

1. Avoid positions that cause deformity. The therapist should encourage the patient to look carefully at the affected extremities to determine whether or not natural positions are resulting in redness, swelling, or pain. Tests for both passive and active range of motion should be discussed with the patient so that he or she recognizes how to avoid excessive strain during daily activities.

2. Avoid sustained positions. The occupational therapist should teach the patient that maintaining a fixed position places stress on specific joints. For example, the longer a person grasps an object, the greater the likelihood of pain and stiffness upon release of the object. The arthritic must be encouraged to change position or activities frequently, encouraging the reciprocal muscle movement to stretch tightened muscles and to relieve pressure on the joints.

3. Use the strongest joints for heavy work. Patients with arthritis must be taught to compensate for weakened joints and to try to develop bilateral capacity.

4. Do not start what you cannot stop. Arthritic patients are characterized by ambition and an involvement with the work ethic. These traits impair the patient's ability to create a pace compatible with the disease. The occupational therapist must instruct the patient in energy conservation, organization of tasks, and awareness of fatigue.

5. Use joints to the greatest mechanical advantage. Certain activities can be done more easily in a standing position; among them are mopping a floor, mixing a cake, or washing one's hair. Among activities which are more easily done while seated are reading a book, working on a puzzle, doing needlework, or sewing. The crucial element here is not only putting the body in the most advantageous position of function but also preventing stress on other joints. If the mechanical aspects of different positioning for different activities are analyzed thoroughly by the therapist, the findings can be valuable in assisting the therapist in adapting positions and activities to increase function. Not using the body in a position that utilizes strong muscles and joints effectively may cause strain and even present a safety hazard.

6. The patient must be taught to respect pain. Although one can sometimes detect the signs of pain on someone's face or can learn of pain through the patient's complaint, pain itself is highly subjective. Tolerance levels of pain vary and, when there is a sensory deficit, the perception of pain may be entirely lacking. In periods when the arthritis is active the patient may complain of severe pain, and there may be visible inflammation of joints. In the stages following acute attacks of arthritis, the pain must be considered when planning activity programs. It must be conveyed to the patient that joint protection is for the purpose of improving and maintaining function rather than restricting function. This is often misinterpreted and the patient ignores the suggestions for optimal bodily functions in the presence of arthritis. Improper use of joints can increase pain. Lack of attention to position change and activity change can cause pain. Mental denial, frustration, or tension can cause improper use of joints and put undue strain on them. The patient must plan activities to maximize function and range of motion.

REFERENCES

1. Rusk, H. A.: Rehabilitation Medicine, ed. 3. St. Louis: C. V. Mosby Co., 1971, p. 449.
2. Willard, H. S., and Spackman, C. S. (eds.): Occupational Therapy, ed. 4. Philadelphia: J. B. Lippincott Co., 1971.
3. Mossman, P. L.: A Problem-Oriented Approach to Stroke. Springfield IL: Charles C Thomas, Publishers, 1976, p. 188.
4. Cave, E. F., Burke, J. F., and Boyd, R. J.: Trauma Management. Chicago: Year Book Medical Publishers, 1974, p. 269.

5. Bannister, R.: Brain's Clinical Neurology, ed. 4. London: Oxford, 1973, p. 207.
6. Brain, B., and Walton, J. N.: Brain's Diseases of the Nervous System. London: Oxford, 1969, p. 494.
7. Bannister: Brain's Clinical Neurology, p. 394.
8. Ibid., p. 392, 393.
9. Ibid., p. 392.
10. Brain: Brain's Disease, p. 525.
11. Long, C., and Lawton, E. B.: Functional significance of spinal cord lesion level. Arch. Phys. Med. Rehabil. 36:249, 1955.
12. Rusk: Rehabilitation Medicine, p. 321.
13. Bannister: Brain's Clinical Neurology, p. 347.
14. Brain: Brain's Disease, p. 814.
15. Ibid., p. 595.
16. Alpers, B. J., and Mancall, E. L.: Clinical Neurology, ed. 6. Philadelphia: F. A. Davis Co., 1971, p. 598.
17. Brain: Brain's Disease, p. 598.
18. Bannister: Brain's Clinical Neurology, p. 329.
19. Wilson, D. C.: Hilary. New York: McGraw-Hill Book Co., 1963.
20. Bannister: Brain's Clinical Neurology, p. 323.
21. Licht, S. (ed.): Rehabilitation and Medicine. Baltimore: Waverly Press, 1968.
22. Boyes, J. H.: Bunnell's Surgery of the Hand, ed. 5. Philadelphia: J. B. Lippincott Co., 1970, p. 240.
23. Ibid.
24. Hollander, J. L., and McCarthy, D. J., Jr.: Arthritis and Allied Conditions. Philadelphia: Lea & Febiger, 1972, p. 603.

BIBLIOGRAPHY

Blakiston's Gould Medical Dictionary, ed. 3. New York: McGraw-Hill Book Co., 1972.

Bobath, B.: Adult Hemiplegia: Evaluation and Treatment. London: Heinemann, 1971.

Brunnstrom, S.: Movement Therapy in Hemiplegia. New York: Harper & Row Publishers, 1970.

Buckwald, E.: Physical Rehabilitation for Daily Living. New York: McGraw-Hill Book Co., 1952.

DePalma, A. F.: The Management of Fractures and Dislocations, Vol. 1, ed. 2. Philadelphia: W. B. Saunders Co., 1970.

Dorland's Illustrated Medical Dictionary, ed. 25. Philadelphia: W. B. Saunders Co., 1974.

Dunning, H.: Environmental occupational therapy. Am. J. Occup. Ther. 26:292, 1972.

Erlich, G. E. (ed.): Total Management of the Arthritis Patient. Philadelphia: J. B. Lippincott Co., 1975.

Farber, S. D., and Huss, J. A.: Sensorimotor Evaluation and Treatment Procedures, ed. 2. Indianapolis: Indiana University–Purdue University, 1974.

Ford, J. R., and Duckworth, B.: Physical Management for the Quadriplegic Patient. Philadelphia: F. A. Davis Co., 1974.

Galbreaith, P.: What You Can Do for Yourself. New York: Drake, 1974.

Garrett, J. F., and Levine, E. S.: Psychological Practices with the Physically Disabled. New York: Columbia, 1962.

Gilbert, A. E.: You Can Do It From a Wheelchair. New Rochelle NY: Arlington House Publishers, 1973.

Gruen, H.: A postoperative dynamic splint for the rheumatoid hand. Am. J. Occup. Ther. 24:284, 1970.

Gutmann, J. (ed.): Rehabilitation of the Injured Workman. Dubuque IA: W. C. Brown Co., 1962.

Haymaker, W., and Woodhall, B.: Peripheral Nerve Injuries. Philadelphia: W. B. Saunders Co., 1953.

Hirschberg, G. G.: Rehabilitation. Philadelphia: J. B. Lippincott Co., 1964.

Jones, M. (ed.): Work Adjustment as a Function of Occupational Therapy. Dubuque IA: Brown, 1962.

Krusen, F. H., Kottke, F., and Ellwood, P. M.: Handbook of Physical Medicine and Rehabilitation, ed. 2. Philadelphia: W. B. Saunders Co., 1971.

Kulkulka, G. G., and Basmajian, J. V.: A preliminary report: Biofeedback training for early finger joint mobilization. Am. J. Occup. Ther. 29:469, 1975.

Licht, S. (ed.): Stroke and its Rehabilitation. Baltimore: Waverly Press, 1975.

MacDonald, E. M.: Occupational Therapy in Rehabilitation, ed. 2. London: Bailliere, Tindall, and Cox, 1964.

MacDonald, E. M. (ed.): Occupational Therapy in Rehabilitation, ed. 4. Baltimore: Williams & Wilkins, 1976.

Malick, M. H.: A preliminary prosthesis for the partially amputated hand. Am. J. Occup. Ther. 29:479, 1975.

Marmo, N. A.: A new look at the brain-damaged adult. Am. J. Occup. Ther. 28:199, 1974.

Marmo, N. A.: Discovering the lifestyle of the physically disabled. Am. J. Occup. Ther. 29:475, 1975.

May, E. E., Waggoner, N. R., and Hotte, E. B.: Independent Living for the Handicapped and the Elderly. Boston: Houghton Mifflin Co., 1974.

McCombs, R. P.: Fundamentals of Internal Medicine. Chicago: Year Book Medical Publishers, 1971.

McKenzie, M. W.: The role of occupational therapy in rehabilitating spinal cord injured patients. Am. J. Occup. Ther. 24:257, 1970.

Morris, A. F., and Brown, M.: Electronic training devices for hand rehabilitation. Am. J. Occup. Ther. 30:376, 1976.

Moskowitz, R. W.: Clinical Rheumatology. Philadelphia: Lea & Febiger, 1975.

Newsom, M. J., et al.: An occupational therapy training program for the $C_{5\text{-}6}$ quadriplegic. Am. J. Occup. Ther. 23:126, 1969.

Pearson, P. H., and Williams, C. E.: Physical Therapy Services in the Developmental Disabilities. Springfield IL: Charles C Thomas, 1976.

Rider, B.: Effects of neuromuscular facilitation on cross transfer. Am. J. Occup. Ther. 25:84, 1971.

Sattely, C.: Approaches to the Treatment of Patients with Neuromuscular Dysfunction. Dubuque IA: W. C. Brown Co., 1962.

Shafer, R.: Occupational therapy for lower extremity problems. Am. J. Occup. Ther. 28:99, 1974.

Silverstein, F., French, J., and Siebens, A.: A myoelectric hand splint. Am. J. Occup. Ther. 28:99, 1974.

Taylor, D. P.: Treatment goals for quadriplegic and paraplegic patients. Am. J. Occup. Ther. 28:22, 1974.

Wagner, E., and Zimmerman, M.: Approaches to Independent Living. Dubuque IA: W. C. Brown Co., 1962.

Wasserman, P., and Giesecke, J. (eds.): Health Organizations of the United States, Canada, and Internationally, ed. 3. Washington DC: McGrath, 1974.

Wilson, D. C.: Handicap Race. New York: McGraw-Hill Book Co., 1967.

Wilson, D. C.: Take My Hands. New York, McGraw-Hill Book Co., 1963.

Wilson, D. J., McKenzie, M. W., and Barber, L. M.: Spinal Cord Injury: A Treatment Guide for Occupational Therapists. Thorofare N.J.: Charles B. Slack, 1974.

Wright, B. A.: Physical Disability—A Psychological Approach. New York: Harper & Row, 1960.

PUBLICATIONS AND PAMPHLETS FOR HANDICAPPED PERSONS

A Source Book: Rehabilitating the Person with Spinal Cord Injury (Superintendent of Documents, United States Printing Office, Washington DC 20402)

Accent on Living (Accent on Living, Inc., P.O. Box 726, Gillum Road and High Drive, Bloomington IL 61701)

Active Handicapped (The Active Handicapped, Inc., 526 Aurora Avenue, Metairie LA 70005)

Do It Yourself Again. Self-help Devices for the Stroke Patient (American Heart Association, New York NY 10010)

Home Care Programs in Arthritis: A Manual for Patients (Allied Health Professions of The Arthritis Foundation, 1212 Avenue of the Americas, New York NY 10036)

Rehabilitation Gazette (Rehabilitation Gazette, 4502 Maryland Avenue, St. Louis MO 63108)

Rehabilitation World (U.S. J. International Rehab. Information, 20 West 40th Street, New York NY 10018)

Self-Help Manual for Arthritis Patients (Allied Health Professions of The Arthritis Foundation, 1212 Avenue of the Americas, New York NY 10036)

The Squeaky Wheel (National Paraplegia Foundation, 333 North Michigan Avenue, Chicago IL 60601)

You and Your New Hip (Occupational Therapy Department, University Hospitals of Cleveland, Cleveland OH)

RESOURCES

American Academy of Physical Medicine and Rehabilitation
30 North Michigan Avenue
Suite 922
Chicago, Illinois 60602

American Congress of Rehabilitation Medicine
30 North Michigan Avenue
Chicago, Illinois 60602

American Heart Association
44 East 23rd Street
New York, New York 10010

American Speech and Hearing Association
9030 Old Georgetown Road
Washington, D.C. 20014

Arthritis Foundation
1212 Avenue of the Americas
New York, New York 10036

Georgia Warm Springs Foundation
330 Madison Avenue
New York, New York 10017

Goodwill Industries of America, Inc.
9200 Wisconsin Avenue
Washington, D.C. 20014

International Society for Rehabilitation of the Disabled
219 East 44th Street
New York, New York 10017

Muscular Dystrophy Association of America, Inc.
810 Seventh Avenue
New York, New York 10019

Myasthenia Gravis Foundation, Inc.
230 Park Avenue
New York, New York 10017

National Amputation Foundation
12–45 150th Street
Whitestone, New York 11357

National Easter Seal Society for Crippled Children and Adults
2023 West Ogden Avenue
Chicago, Illinois 60612

National Multiple Sclerosis Society
257 Park Avenue, South
New York, New York 10010

National Paraplegia Foundation
333 North Michigan Avenue
Chicago, Illinois 60601

National Parkinson Foundation, Inc.
1501 Northwest 9th Avenue
Miami, Florida 33136

National Recreation and Park Association
1601 North Kent Street
Arlington, Virginia 22209

National Rehabilitation Association
1522 K Street, N.W.
Washington, D.C. 20005

ACKNOWLEDGMENTS

Sincere appreciation to the administration and staff of Eastern Maine Medical Center, Bangor, Maine. Particular thanks to the occupational therapists for their patience, encouragement, and assistance and to Ron Gregory for taking photographs and to the patients who were willing to be photographed. Thanks also to Patricia A. Curran for editorial and typing assistance.

14

Minimal Brain Dysfunction

Elnora M. Gilfoyle and Ann P. Grady

"Meet my son Johnny. He can't read. Oh he's bright enough; he sure can learn lots of other things. Why he's a whiz at math. When it comes to reading and spelling, sometimes I think he is just lazy or maybe his teacher doesn't know how to teach him. Johnny's a big, handsome boy, isn't he? He's got a lot of friends to play with but they never seem to stay around too long. Guess he is so strong they are afraid of him. He does strike out and starts to hit frequently. He doesn't mean to hurt; he likes his friends. He doesn't look like a sensitive boy but he surely is. He cries a lot and gets his feelings hurt. His friends tease him—call him Gork, Clumsy-duck, Dum-dum, and Retard. Oh, I understand why they tease him. Sometimes he is clumsy. Once he tripped and fell over the printed design in the carpet at school. And he is in a special reading class but that doesn't seem to help as he still can't learn to read.

"He has always been different from my other children. Even as a baby he was more fussy and never liked to be held. He was slow to sit and walk, but since he learned he never stops. He is in constant motion, never sits still. At least we don't have to worry about too much TV. Can you believe it, he wouldn't watch 'Sesame Street.' Couldn't pay attention or sit still long enough. Johnny was always so active we tried to give him extra activities out-of-doors. He has trouble handling sports and playground equipment. He was five before he could ride his tricycle and we still have training wheels on his bicycle. John's dad is a very patient man and doesn't expect him to be a super star but even he got frustrated trying to teach him to catch a ball. He just gave up.

"We enrolled John in a preschool program when he was three, but he was disruptive and cried a lot. The teacher recommended that we wait for a year to try preschool again. She suggested that we have our doctor examine him to be sure John was well. We took him to our doctor and he told us that John was okay and that he would outgrow his problems. Well he is eight now and he isn't growing out of his problems. They seem to get worse, and it is harder and harder for his Dad and me to handle him.

"What's wrong with us as parents? What have we done to our boy? What's wrong with our boy? Can someone help me?"

INTRODUCTION

Such terms as learning disability, educational handicap, central processing dysfunction, sensory-integrative dysfunction, perceptual-motor handicap, dyslexia, developmental deviations, and minimal brain dysfunction are currently being used to describe a population of children similar to Johnny.[1] Children like Johnny have neural impairments which interfere with the normal process of maturation and development. These children have difficulty in organizing information from the environment for use.[2]

The purpose of this chapter is to define and discuss the problems of these children, to present some aspects of evaluation and treatment, and to explore the roles and functions of occupational therapy with these children. Although the term *minimal brain dysfunction* (MBD) is used here, many other terms are synonymous.

Definition

Minimal brain dysfunction (MBD) is a diagnostic and descriptive category of neurodevelopmental lags.[3] The child with MBD looks normal and rates average or above on tests of intelligence, but learning, behavior, and functional performance problems persist. The deviations in the neural functions of this child interferes with and delays the process of sensorimotor-sensory integration (SMS), thus affecting ability to adapt. (See Chapter 3, Section 2.)

MBD is the result of maldevelopment of the brain, occurring in utero or in early childhood. The diagnosis of MBD comprises a varied group of symptoms that describe the neurodevelopmental performances in relation to sensorimotor, language, cognitive, and social-emotional skills. The diagnosis of MDB is based on findings that are considered abnormal or pathological with reference to the child's age. The findings indicate a delay or lag in certain aspects of the child's development and maturation. A younger child with the same findings may be regarded as normal.[4]

Symptoms

Kinsbourne[5] describes MBD as a neurodevelopmental lag. The lag or delay in the neural development may affect any part of the nervous system; consequently MBD may manifest itself with varied symptomatology. In addition there may be a lag in some areas of performance and not in others. The more common problems noted in children with MBD follow. The list is not all-inclusive but gives a general "feel" for the problems of a child with MBD. A child may not have all the symptoms, and the presence of the symptoms does not in itself mean that MBD is present.

CLUMSINESS OR SENSORIMOTOR PROBLEMS. Children with MBD are frequently described as being clumsy and awkward. Their development, as related to sensorimotor skills, may be retarded. When they do achieve a skill, the quality of performance seems inefficient, uncoordinated, and clumsy. The patterns of posture and movement are influenced by primitive lower level reactions. These children have difficulty learning and performing such complicated tasks as dressing, tying shoes, riding tricycles, jumping rope, and catching a ball.

HYPERACTIVITY/HYPERKINETIC. Children with MBD may appear to be tense. The muscles may feel tight as if the child were in constant preparation for quick movement. The children who are described as being hyperactive have difficulty sitting still; they shuffle their feet and wiggle in their chairs. They get up from their sitting position and frequently run around aimlessly. They impulsively strike out at their environment. These children are much more active than other children of the same age. They appear to be driven into constant motion, although their activity is without purpose. Hyperactive children are frequently described as wild, undisciplined, and behavior problems.

HYPOACTIVITY/HYPOKINETIC. There are a few children with MBD who are inactive. These children are very slow. They avoid moving around and give the impression of being lazy and not interested in the environment. They may appear to be floppy, as if they were a rag doll. Frequently they appear to be weak and overly relaxed. They may have poor joint stability as if they were double-jointed. Because they are not disruptive, they are described as being good children.

DISTRACTIBILITY. Children with MBD who are distractible switch their attention and frequently change their interest and thoughts quickly from one thing to another. They cannot focus their thoughts or control their attention to do the tasks at hand. Any activity in their environment may attract them and consequently distract them from their task. These children may appear to be daydreaming or not listening and paying attention to others within their environment. They become disruptive in a group such as a classroom.

IRRITABILITY. Some children with MBD are highly irritable. They cry frequently, have frequent mood changes, and get their feelings hurt easily. These children become irritated and frightened by events that do not bother other children, such as being touched, held, or bumped. They may have accented fears of animals, other people, and loud noises. They may explode into tantrums frequently.

LANGUAGE DIFFICULTIES. Children with MBD have a variety of speech and language problems. Frequently they are slow to learn to talk and may display some articulation problems. They have difficulty discriminating between sounds or words. Some of the children have problems sequencing sounds or blending sounds into words and words into sentences or retaining the spoken words of a conversation. They cannot distinguish or focus on the pertinent sounds from those less important to the task at hand because all sounds within the environment may be perceived with the same intensity.

COGNITIVE-LEARNING DIFFICULTIES. Although these children have the intellectual capacity to learn and may be considered quite intelligent, they may have special problems with learning to read, print, write, spell, or do math. The children may have difficulty distinguishing differences and similarities of visual forms and shapes. Therefore the written symbols of language cannot be perceived for use in reading and math. They frequently reverse letters, numbers and words, and even entire sentences beyond the time when other children have ceased reversing. Sequencing a series of letters into words or words into sentences presents problems. The children frequently have memory difficulties and seem to forget how to accomplish the simple daily living tasks. Their learning problems are directly related to disorders of perception.

DIRECTIONALITY PROBLEMS. The child with MBD may have problems perceiving "right," "left," "up," "down," "after," and "before." These children have difficulty mastering their own position in relation to space. They lack a sense of direction. Directing their own movements through space toward some goal or position becomes a complicated task that may not be achieved.

LATERALITY-HANDEDNESS. Children with MBD are frequently very slow to establish a hand preference or dominance. They may use the left and the right hand interchangeably. Although the age and the importance of establishing laterality and/or handedness has not been clearly established, it has been noted that children with MBD are slower to develop this preference than other children.

Etiological Factors

There are a variety of etiological factors which may result in MBD, but specific causes are not presently known. The problems of MBD are influenced by prenatal and perinatal factors, length of gestation, the degrees of environmental enrichment or deprivation, and the demands of the environment upon the maturing organism.[6,7,8,9] It is generally accepted that the presence of disease, trauma, and nervous system pathology affects the course of maturation. Recent research and reports in the literature are also being directed to the effects of food additives, allergies (food, chemical, and inhalants), and abuse upon the neurodevelopment of children. The more accepted etiologic factors do not differ greatly from those associated with the profound central nervous system disorders such as cerebral palsy or mental retardation.[10]

There is no one etiological factor but a varied group of suspected antecedents. Although the factors may vary there is an underlying neural processing condition that effects maturation and development which results in MBD. The current literature proposes that the neurodevelopmental lags of many of the children with MBD may be due to an impairment with the processing or integrating functions of the nervous system.[11] During the maturational-developmental periods of infancy and childhood the maturing nervous system cannot organize and integrate the experiences from the environment for use.

There is a correlation between the nervous system's maturation, purposeful environmental stimuli, and the adaptive response.[12] When the nervous system is deprived of meaningful stimuli and when the nervous system cannot make a meaningful response to the stimuli, effective maturation cannot take place.

Harris[13] portrays the nervous system as "a series of interacting functional units" which have a continual interplay at different structural levels. The units carry a variety of information and, if one unit works ineffectively, the other units are affected in some manner. Maturation and the resulting developmental behaviors become disorganized in proportion to the degree of involvement or impairment of the neural connections or the interaction between the units and nuclei and between integrative structures.[14] Maldevelopment results from the inadequate maturation of the nervous pathways.

Myelination of these pathways and synaptic connections do not develop fully nor at their proper time. Factors contributing to a deficit in maturation include:

1. abnormal input (sensory deprivation, incorrect assimilation)
2. abnormal output or function (meaningless, purposeless accommodation)
3. abnormal feedback (inadequate, faulty association/differentiation).[15]

The abnormal system evokes purposeless, generalized, nonrepetitive activity which provides inadequate blending of the neuromusculoskeletal functions (Chapter 3, Section 2). The nervous system does not make use of the environmental experiences and cannot be conditioned to establish appropriate nervous pathways and connections for the development of posture and movement patterns. The child continues to adapt with lower level behaviors which are described as neurodevelopmental lags.

To emphasize the concept of neurodevelopmental lags, compare the expected normal prehension pattern of the three-year old in Figure 14-1 with the total grasp pattern of the four-year-old child with MBD in Figure 14-2. The immature adaptation of the pattern observed in Figure 14-2 is indicative of the lower level behaviors of the adaptation process of the eighteen-month old in Figure 14-3. Although the grasp pattern of the child with MBD (Fig. 14-2) is not identical to the grasp pattern of the eighteen-month old (Fig. 14-3), influences of the primitive pattern can be noted.

Another example of neurodevelopmental lag is presented in Figures 14-4, 14-5, and 14-6. Manipulative prehension is the mature adaptation process for handling a crayon as illustrated with the child in Figure 14-4. The child with MBD (Fig. 14-5) adapts

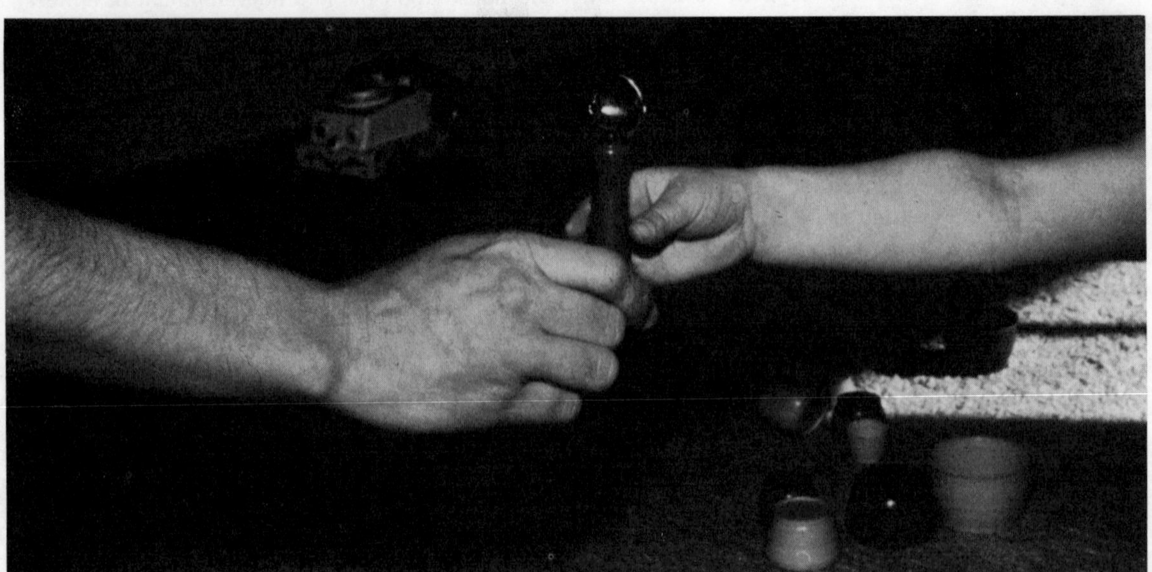

FIGURE 14-1. Normal prehension pattern of the four-year old.

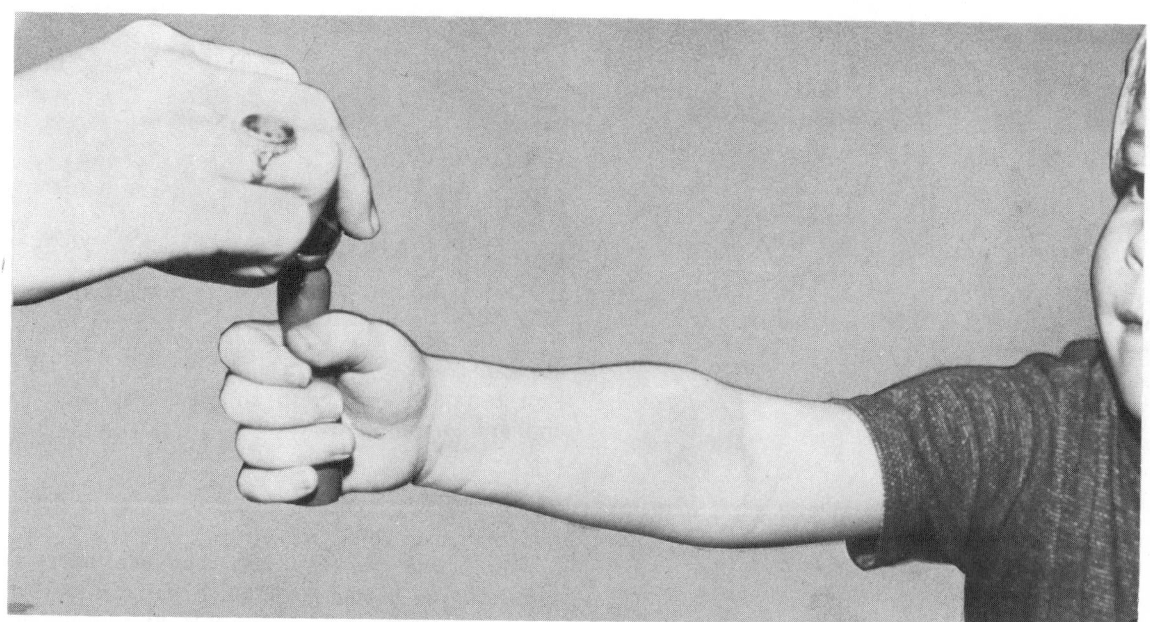

FIGURE 14-2. Total grasp, the immature prehension pattern of a four-year old with minimal brain dysfunction.

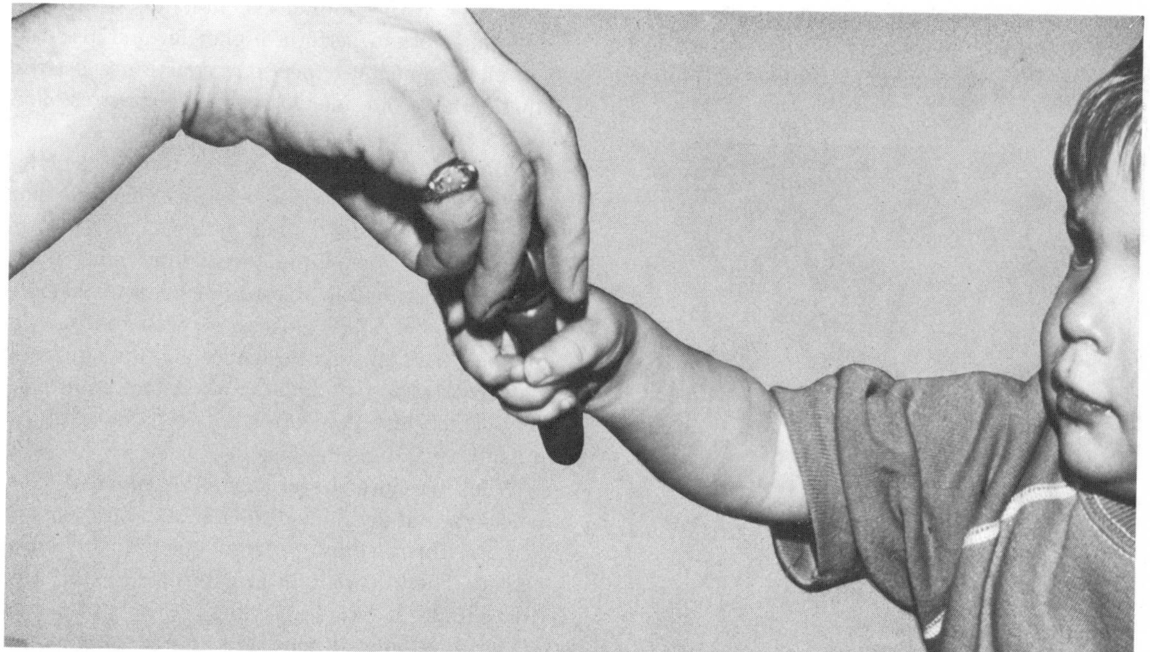

FIGURE 14-3. Total grasp, the normal prehension pattern for an eighteen-month-old child.

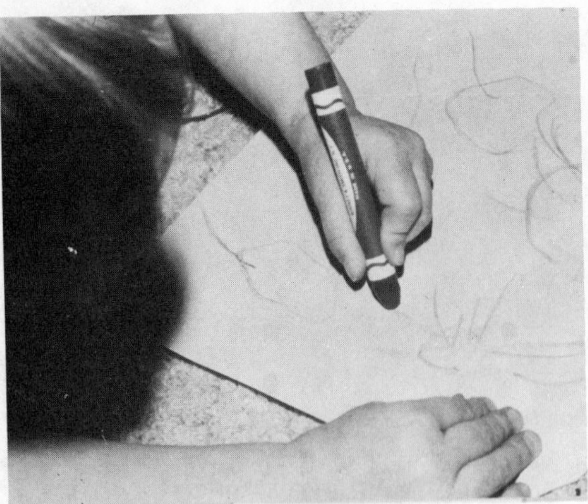

FIGURE 14-4. Manipulative prehension, a mature adaptation.

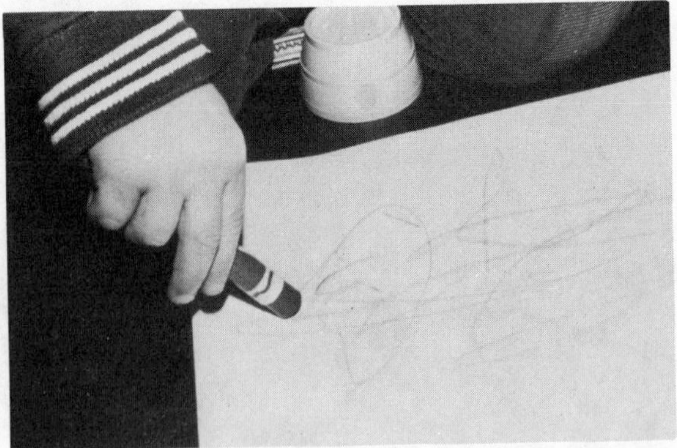

FIGURE 14-6. Palmar grasp, a mature adaptation for an eighteen-month-old child.

with a lower level behavior of palmar grasp, which is likened to the pattern used by the eighteen-month old in Figure 14-6.

During the developmental course of the child with MBD environmental experiences do not facilitate higher level adaptations and the self-system does not process and integrate stimuli for effective interaction, and, thus, neurodevelopmental lags result. When a child cannot make use of the information from the environment to facilitate development, he or she will continually adapt with a spatiotemporal stress reaction.[15]

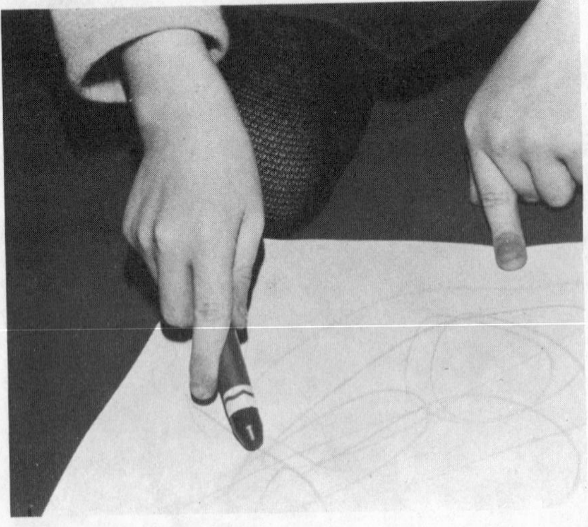

FIGURE 14-5. Palmar grasp, an immature adaptation.

The normal process of spatiotemporal stress as discussed in Chapter 3, Section 2 can be applied to the dysfunction patterns of a child with MBD. In the normal process, higher level behaviors are enhanced by the repetition of activities as the nervous system integrates the experiences into its repertoire. The child with MBD cannot benefit from repetition or mere activity because the experiences are purposeless or meaningless for the nervous system's use. The child with MBD continues to function with lower level behaviors to perform higher level skills. Each new environmental experience constitutes a stress situation and continues to constitute stress as experiences are repeated.

Prior adaptations have not become integrated into the self-system for use in the association/differentiation component of adaptation. Therefore the essential elements of the lower level adaptations cannot be modified to adapt higher level behaviors. Spatiotemporal stress reactions will continue to influence the child's performance and the child will adapt with primitive patterns of posture and movement. Thus, repetition of primitive patterns results in neurodevelopmental lags.

When the normal everyday environmental experiences cannot be utilized to facilitate development, then an intervention program should be implemented. The intervention program for a child with MBD should be based upon the concepts of normal human development and have a neurodevelopmental approach.

NEURODEVELOPMENTAL INTERVENTION

A neurodevelopmental approach for the treatment of MBD is one that intervenes in such a manner as to effect change upon the maturational process. Neurodevelopmental intervention is based upon the following premises:

1. Development is a function of the maturation of the nervous system.

2. Maturation occurs as a result of the modification of the nervous system by the integration of experiences through a spatiotemporal adaptation process.

3. Development occurs through a spiraling sequence with lower level behaviors becoming modified by repeated experiences. The acquisition of higher level behaviors is dependent upon a certain degree of adaptation of the previous behaviors.

4. The developmental process of a child with MBD represents neurodevelopmental lags. Immature spatiotemporal adaptation with disorganized SMS integration accounts for some aspects of this impairment.

5. The developing nervous system has the capacity to compensate for impairments by forming new connections during the early periods of maturation. The plasticity or flexibility of the formative nervous system enhances the capacity for the adaptation process to modify the interconnections of the functional system of the brain.[16,17]

6. An intervention program that therapeutically structures the environment and employs sensory input, motor output, and sensory feedback is believed to lower the threshold of previously unresponsive brain cells through the process of summation and convergence.[18] These processes appear to influence neural organization and ultimately establish new engrams, thus facilitating maturation.[19]

We have utilized these premises in constructing a model for an occupational therapy intervention program. The model has as its basis the theory of the spatiotemporal adaptation process of assimilation, accommodation, association, and differentiation and the inherent sensorimotor-sensory (SMS) integration. The spiraling continuum, as discussed in Chapter 3, Section 2, is utilized to illustrate the concepts of the development of adaptation and thus provides a basic "road map" for facilitating spatiotemporal adaptation.

Within the spatiotemporal adaptation model, the theoretical framework of the spiraling development of neuromusculoskeletal functions, as described in Chapter 3, Section 2, provides the necessary reference point from which the occupational therapist can:

1. assess the presence and degree of dysfunction
2. establish the treatment goals
3. plan and select the specific treatment methods and media to be utilized
4. implement the selected program to achieve the treatment goals

The therapist utilizes the knowledge of the spiraling process of reflex/reaction maturation and the development of mobility/stability muscle patterns as the guide for sequencing the program. A neurodevelopmental program will make use of certain aspects of the process to facilitate the desired response; it will not mirror the spiraling steps of development.

To further explain this concept, consider the case of Johnny presented at the beginning of this chapter. An occupational therapy assessment identified that Johnny's postural patterns were influenced by the more primitive righting reactions. For example, when Johnny would sit in a chair and turn his head, his trunk would turn also. The head/trunk turning pattern disrupted his sitting balance and affected his performance with desk activities. The head/trunk rotation pattern was also noted with rolling, standing, and walking activities. Utilizing the spiraling process as the framework, the therapist could identify the need for Johnny's self-system to differentiate head and trunk rotation components and adapt them to higher level equilibrium reactions. In a neurodevelopmental program, it is not necessary to have Johnny return to an identified specific developmental level and bring him along the course of development. A neurodevelopmental program utilizes the principles of the process of development and applies methods and media that facilitate a desired response.[20]

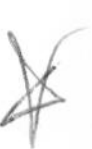

Within the neurodevelopmental program, a

variety of media and methods may be employed by the therapist to facilitate the process desired. The methods and media chosen are dependent on the identified capabilities and needs of the child, the immediate goals to be accomplished, the therapist's knowledge and skills with the media and methods, the age of the child, and the physical setting where the program will be implemented. The reader is referred to Chapter 7, Section 2, regarding the treatment process for an orientation to the variety of treatment methods which can be applied to a neurodevelopmental approach.

Although the media and methods chosen may vary, there is an underlying commonality of the use of purposeful activity that is unique to the occupational therapy program. Purposeful activities include the complete continuum of self-care, work, play, exercise, and recreational and leisure time activities. The activity is the media used to facilitate the child's purposeful response.

A purposeful response is defined as that which is appropriate for the task and useful to the nervous system through meaningful sensory feedback. An activity becomes purposeful when the nature of the activity requires the participant to function in a manner that facilitates the desired response. For an activity to be purposeful it must provide direction and an effort that is more mature or at a higher level than that experienced with past behaviors.[21] For example, a child's sitting on a large ball and bouncing up and down can be purposeful activity. The nature of the activity directs the sitting and movement patterns of the child in such a manner that equilibrium reactions can be facilitated. It is the therapist that identifies and directs the activity so that the nature of the activity can facilitate a higher level performance.

Inherent within purposeful activity is the therapeutic purpose or goal that is achieved by the child's doing the activity. Purposeful activity is utilized as a media to elicit the child's own discovery of the environment. On a conscious or cortical level, the child's participation may be directed to the joy of doing and completing the activity. On the unconscious or subcortical level, the child's participation elicits a meaningful response that results in the enhancement of neurodevelopment.

Purposeful activity is used to facilitate maturation and not to develop a sensorimotor skill. The child's output or motor response is the therapeutic means of reaching the objective of therapy through the sensory feedback. The child's self-system integrates a process that can then be used to adapt new experiences as well as being applied to a variety of activities. Purposeful activity becomes occupational therapy treatment only when it directs a higher level response that enhances neural integration.[22]

In summary, a neurodevelopmental program for the child with MBD is based upon the theory of spatiotemporal adaptation. The spiraling framework of neuromusculoskeletal functions is the therapeutic reference point for evaluation, planning, and implementation. The principles of the reflex/reaction maturation and mobility/stability development are utilized by the therapist to sequence the occupational therapy program. The therapist and the program are concerned with the *process* employed to achieve an activity and not the achievement of the activity. Inherent within the occupational therapy neurodevelopmental program is the use of purposeful activity to facilitate a meaningful response for the child's self-system. Purposeful activity is treatment when it directs a response that enhances neural integration.

ROLE AND FUNCTIONS OF THE OCCUPATIONAL THERAPIST*

The goal of an occupational therapy program for a child with MBD is to facilitate maturation so that the child can achieve his or her highest level of functioning. In order to achieve the goal, the therapist structures the environment and provides appropriate purposeful activities that facilitate SMS integration by directing a higher level response from the child. Through the child's performance with the therapeutic milieu, the child can adapt the environmental experiences in an organized manner, thus facilitating higher level behaviors.

To carry out the goal of therapy, the occupational therapist has three basic and interrelated roles:

* The material presented in this section was developed for the American Occupational Therapy Association Continuing Competency Project, Contract #NO1-AH-44116, Department of Health, Education and Welfare, Appendix V. "The Roles and Functions of the Occupational Therapist in the treatment of the Developmentally Disabled Client." E. Gilfoyle, O.T.R.

1. an evaluator of the child's adaptation process
2. a planner of the neurodevelopmental program
3. an implementer of the program

The evaluating, planning, and program implementation roles of the occupational therapist can be delivered in a variety of settings, including the hospital/clinic, home, school, day care centers, residential facilities, and public and private agencies. To carry out the roles, the therapist may work in cooperation and collaboration with the child and his or her family and with other persons interested in the child (teacher, physician, nurse, psychologist, etc.). The program may be carried out on a one-to-one basis (child-therapist), with the child and family, or with small or large groups. The physical setting for the therapy program and the persons involved, either directly or indirectly, in the program is determined through the evaluation process.

Evaluation Process

A neurodevelopmental treatment program begins with a thorough evaluation of the child's functioning process. A child may be referred for occupational therapy services by a physician, psychologist, teacher, social worker, or the child's family. After receiving the referral, the occupational therapist evaluates the child's performance in order to identify the developmental level of occupational performance skills and the components needed to achieve those skills. Occupational performance skills are the behaviors and practical abilities of an individual used to perform self-care, school/work, and play/leisure time activities. The components of occupational performance skills are those biological and psychological processes utilized in order to accomplish skilled behaviors. Included are sensorimotor-sensory, psychosocial, cognitive-language and cultural components (Fig. 14-7). In addition to the consideration of the affects of the components upon the performance, the evaluation must consider the relationship of the components to each other as to how they influence behavior.[23]

Self-help tasks include *feeding* (i.e., the child's ability to suck, chew, swallow and handle eating utensils, motivation and interest in feeding, ability to understand directions); *dressing* (i.e., putting on and taking off garments, fastening garments such as buttons, zippers, and tying shoes, obtaining and putting garments in storage areas such as drawers and closets); *hygiene/grooming* (i.e., brushing teeth, combing and washing hair, washing and caring for body and bodily needs); *object manipulation* (i.e., use of telephone, keys, money, and watch); *communication* (i.e., verbal abilities and breath control as related to speaking and task performance, written communication).

Play/leisure time tasks include *stability and mobility* to move within the environment (i.e., rolling, sitting, creeping, standing, walking, running, jumping, and climbing); *object manipulation* (i.e., toys, games, reading materials, pencils, crayons, scissors, paper, recreational equipment such as balls, gloves, racquets, and bicycles); *psychosocial aspects* (i.e., motivation, interest, ability to get along with others, frustration tolerance, and social competence).

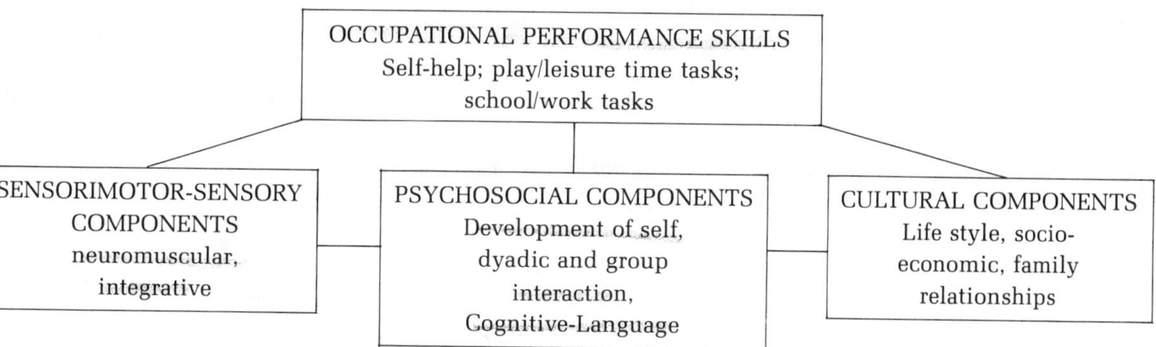

FIGURE 14-7. Functional performance behaviors.

School/work tasks include *perceptual-motor* (i.e., paper pencil/desk activities, ability to plan movements (praxis), visuospatial relationships for perceiving and copying forms and symbols for math, language, and reading, body schema and image, rhythmic activities, hand-eye and body-eye coordination, and ability to plan gross movements in space); *homemaking* (i.e., kitchen activities such as handling utensils, washing dishes, sewing, washing and ironing clothes, cleaning and dusting, making beds, and cleaning up room).

These examples of occupational performance skills can be used to observe the child's functioning abilities and needs. By observing the child's functional performance the therapist considers the underlying components necessary in order for the child to achieve skilled performance with self-help, play/leisure time, and school/work tasks. Identifying the developmental level of the components is the essential element for program planning and implementation.

The ability to achieve occupational performance skills may be the goal for the child; however it is the facilitation of the components that provides the child with the abilities needed to achieve the performance skills. Therefore the occupational therapy evaluation must identify the developmental needs regarding the components. The components are grouped into three main categories—sensorimotor-sensory, psychosocial, and cultural.

1. Sensorimotor-sensory components: *neuromuscular* (i.e., range of motion, muscle strength, muscle tone, endurance, functional use of body with patterns and postures of movements, volitional, spontaneous movement and control, and general physical fitness); *integrative* (i.e., presence and influence of primitive patterns of reflex/reactions, presence and influence of mobility and stability patterns of posture and movement, reception and perception of sensory stimuli and the adaptive response to the stimuli, body schema and body language used).

2. Psychosocial components: *knowledge and use of self* (i.e., ability to perceive self-needs, feelings, conflicts, defenses, coping behaviors, sexuality of self, self-respect, feelings of competence, acceptance of successes and failures, self-awareness and identity); *motivation and need drives* (i.e., anxiety/frustration tolerance, impulse control, expression of feelings, interest and concerns with self, activities, and others, and defensive, submissive, and aggressive behaviors to incoming stimuli); *dyadic interaction* (i.e., peer relationships, demonstrating trust, respect of another, relationships with subordinates and authority figures, perceiving and responding to another's needs and feelings, ability to cope with stress, level of interaction with objects and persons such as eye contact, touching, withdrawal, and repetitive movements); *group interaction* (i.e., sharing, cooperation, respect of others, competition, exercising group membership roles, social competence, dependency/independency, gratification, ability to perceive social feedback); *cognitive and communicative* (i.e., ability to follow verbal and written instructions, comprehension and expression, concentration, problem solving, time management, and reality orientation).

3. Cultural components: cultural and ethnic background, value orientation, family relationships and activity patterns, socioeconomic status, architectural barriers, attitudes of family toward dysfunction and disability, and family motivation and expectations.

Although the occupational therapist's program for the child with MBD may focus on the SMS components to modify performance, the therapist must take a holistic approach by considering all aspects of the child's behavior as it relates to the development of occupational performance skills. Knowledge and understanding of how the psychosocial and/or cultural components have an effect on SMS behaviors is vital to treatment planning and implementation.

In order to gain the needed information regarding the components related to the child's functional abilities and needs, five basic procedures of an evaluation process must be considered. The procedures are:

1. Interviewing the child and the family regarding the developmental history, the presenting problem(s), the child's family's objective for the program, and the life-style.

2. Observation of the child's occupational performance skills and components.

3. Use of testing procedures such as standardized and / or nonstandardized tests to identify the child's abilities and needs with occupational performance skills and components.

4. Consultation with the other persons that are directly involved with the care of the child (i.e., teacher, physician, psychologist) regarding the child's needs and progress.

5. Analysis, recording and sharing of the findings of the occupational therapy evaluation with the child / family and the other persons directly involved.

These procedures are carried out throughout the evaluation process of initial screening, formative evaluation, and the reevaluation. Initial screening is a process utilized to determine the child's general abilities and needs and to determine the suitability of occupational therapy services. Upon receiving a referral, the therapist collects and compiles information from the referring source, the child / family, and other persons involved. The information is reviewed and analyzed in order to decide the suitability for service, to select those behaviors which should be further evaluated, and to select those evaluation procedures to be used. The initial screening procedures may include personal or telephone interviews, observation of the child's performance with a few selected skills, and screening tests to establish the need for more in-depth evaluation.

The data obtained from the initial screening process are summarized and the therapist formulates recommendations regarding further evaluation and types of services which will meet the child's needs. During the initial screening process, the therapist may establish that the child would benefit from the service of another specialist. The therapist takes the responsibility to contact the family and refer them to another more appropriate source.

When the child is accepted for further occupational therapy evaluation, the therapist establishes the amount of time and cost for conducting the evaluation and contacts the family to schedule appointments. In addition, the therapist must explain the formative evaluation to the family, what will be done and why, what information will be obtained, the time and cost, and so forth. Should financial assistance or transportation be needed, the therapist refers the family to the appropriate source.

Contact with the initial referring source is made in order to inform and share the plans for further evaluation. Records of the initial evaluation findings must be maintained.

The purpose of the formative evaluation is to provide the in-depth understanding of the child's capabilities and needs so that a program can be planned and implemented. In addition, an evaluation establishes a baseline of developmental performance which can be used in the measurement of progress and the effects of the program.

The formative evaluation can be grouped into three categories: (1) that dependent upon special tests, (2) that dependent upon observing behavior, and (3) that dependent upon the interview and developmental history.

Special Tests

Standardized tests aid in determining what tasks a child can accomplish as compared to the expected performance for children of a given age. The tests yield a performance score. However, the score does not reveal the method or approach the child used to accomplish the tasks, nor does it describe the basis for failure. The information regarding the process must be gained through clinical observations and by the therapist's interpretation of what the test items may reveal. The scores of tests give a skeletal overview while the observations provide the "flesh," and enable the child to be seen as a true human being.[24]

A test is an extension of the examiner. The test provides a systemized and standardized method of observing behavior. One important value of a test is the opportunity it gives the examiner to observe the process of a child's functioning.[25]

Any examiner must be trained and supervised in the use of standardized test materials. Without proper training and supervision an examiner might administer the test in an improper manner, misinterpret test items, score the test improperly, and fail to observe pertinent behavior. Table 14-1 includes a listing of some of the testing materials that are

Table 14-1. Evaluation instruments.

Author	Reference number	Test
Ayres	25	Southern California Sensory Integration Tests
Bayley	26	Bayley Scales of Infant Development
Beery	27	Developmental Test of Visual-Motor Integration
Berges	28	The Imitation of Gestures
Denhoff	29	Meeting Street School Screening Test
Egan	30	Developmental Screening 0–5 Years
Fiorentino	31	Reflex Testing Methods for Evaluating CNS
Frostig	32	Developmental Test of Visual Perception
Gesell	33	Developmental Diagnosis
Kephart	34	Purdue Perceptual-Motor Survey
Kirk	35	Illinois Test of Psycholinguistic Abilities
Milani-Comparetti	36	Developmental Examination in Normal and Retarded Children

available and appropriate to use for the evaluation of the performance of a child with MBD. The list is not complete and the reader is referred to reference books on testing in the libraries.

In addition to standardized tests, a therapist may utilize nonstandardized materials such as checklists, inventories, or test items. A nonstandardized test may be used as an organized means to observe behavior and can be valuable for perceiving and interpreting the child's process of development. The score of a nonstandardized test may serve as a baseline by which the child's progress can be measured; however the score cannot be used to compare the child's performance to that of other children's performance of a given age.

Observations

A child comes to an evaluation with varied symptomatology. The examiner's goal is to learn as much as possible about the behavior of the child. The therapist needs to know what the behavioral process is and how the behavior is accomplished or why the behavior cannot be accomplished. In the evaluation process there is no substitute for observations gained during the examination.

The observations begin the moment the examiner first sees the child. Does the child show anxiety? Does he speak softly, slowly, or is he explosive? Is he neatly dressed? Does he follow the conversation? How does he approach a test item? How does he handle material? Is he rigid? Does he recover from failure? The list of questions and observations is endless. The skilled and experienced examiner makes use of the observations.

Interview and History

An important part of a comprehensive evaluation is gained by the interview and history of the child / family. The interview can give information about the family's reaction to the child, clues about the nature of the involvement, and reaction of the child to his or her problem(s). The interview provides insight into the child's feelings about the evaluation and feelings about his / her life-style. The history indicates the types of experiences and stimulation the child may have encountered. History reveals likes and dislikes such as what toys, games, and entertainment the child may prefer. Interview and history reveal what the child is allowed to do at home, what constitutes a typical day, how the child plays with toys, games, his friends, and so forth. The history provides an insight into the child's behavior by considering the outstanding developmental landmarks such as when the child rolled over, sat, stood, creeped, walked, spoke words, rode a tricycle, handled scissors, and printed his name. In addition it is important to know if anything occurred prior to the evaluation that may affect the performance of the child such as a spanking, threat, and, more importantly, the cultural, emotional, or socioeconomic deprivation that may have a relevance to the child's performance.[37]

The examiner analyzes, interprets, and synthesizes all the material gained from tests, observations, interviews, and history. These sources provide the comprehensive information upon which the neurodevelopmental program will be implemented.

The findings of the evaluation are recorded and discussed with the child / family. The written report of the formative evaluation includes the referral information, evaluation procedures used, standardized test scores, findings from interviews and observations, interpretation of test / evaluation results, and recommendations for occupational therapy services. The report is a permanent part of the child's record and must be shared with all persons concerned with the child. The report must be in intelligible and meaningful language for the reader or listener. It must be as concise as possible, yet the significant and essential findings must not be left out.[38] The method of reporting is determined by the situation and the people with whom the therapist communicates.

Should the report be given verbally during a conference, the therapist must record the dates, discussion, and interpretation of the conference. The reporting conference may add new or different information that is vital to the evaluation findings. The reporting conference with the child / family is an ideal time to establish the immediate and long-range goals with the child / family for the occupational therapy program.

Reevaluation

The reevaluation process may be ongoing or may include another formative evaluation sitting. The purpose of the reevaluation process is to provide a means to measure change and the effectiveness of the neurodevelopmental program. The reevaluation process may include the informal review of written progress notes and observations made during the treatment program. In addition, the therapist may assess the child's progress and the appropriateness of the methods and media being used by periodically repeating the formative evaluation process. When the reevaluation process includes testing materials that were also used during the initial formative evaluation, the therapist must be certain that the appropriate length of time between testing situations has occurred and that the program has not included practice with test items nor activities that are very similar to those used for test items.

The results of the reevaluation process are recorded and shared with the persons concerned. The therapist recommends discontinuation of the program when the services are no longer needed, feasible, or beneficial. When appropriate, the occupational therapist is responsible for developing a follow-up plan which includes referral to other agencies, programs, or personnel as needed.

Planning Process

The purpose of the program planning process is to establish the immediate and long-range goals for the occupational therapy program and to determine the methods and media most appropriate for accomplishing the determined goals. Goals are established collaboratively with the child / family and with other persons working with the child. Goals to maximize functioning may include maintenance of the current level, prevention of dysfunction, restoration of functioning, and facilitation of higher level performance. Goals are based on the child's current and potential level of occupational performance skills; the assessment of the components needed to achieve performance skills; the motivations, interests, and needs of the child / family; the accessibility of treatment programs; and the previous and predicted life-style of the child / family. The program goals are shared with the child / family and with other persons concerned with the child's care. The goals are recorded in appropriate records and may be modified as the need arises or as results from the reevaluation process indicate revision.

The planning process includes the therapist's selection of the methods and media to be used in order to accurately and appropriately accomplish the established goals. The selection of the methods and media is dependent upon:

1. therapist's knowledge and competence level with the specific method / media
2. availability of supervision / consultation for therapist when needed
3. child's interest, motivation, age, and developmental level
4. child's developmental occupational role tasks (infant, preschooler, student, etc.)
5. physical setting for the program
6. availability of equipment / supplies

The methods / media that are used in the program should be recorded in the appropriate records. During the treatment process the methods / media may be modified according to the determined changes in the child's performance and according to the effectiveness of the methods / media.

Implementation Process

The neurodevelopmental program of the occupational therapy service is the process of utilizing intervention methods and media to achieve the established goals for the child. The program includes a variety of purposeful activities and therapeutic methods to maximize development, maturation, and independence of occupational performance skills and the components to achieve the skills. The major emphasis of the neurodevelopmental program is the development and maturation of the components of the skill so that the child can attain the occupational performance skill as a result of the development of components. Aspects of the implementation process were discussed earlier in this chapter.

The uniqueness of the occupational therapy program is the utilization of purposeful activities to enhance neural integration and facilitate higher level performance skills. Although the major emphasis of the occupational therapy program for children with MBD is the facilitation of SMS development, the aspects of the psychosocial and cultural components are vital considerations in the program. The therapists must take a holistic approach to the evaluation and treatment for the child with MBD.

REFERENCES

1. Chalfant, J., and Schefflin, M. A.: Central Processing Dysfunction in Children: A Review of Research. N.I.N.D.S. Monograph, No. 9, 1969.
2. Ayres, J.: Sensory Integration and Learning Disorders. Los Angeles: Western Psychological Services, 1972.
3. Kinsbourne, M.: Minimal brain dysfunction as a neurodevelopmental lag. Ann. N. Y. Acad. Science 205:268–273, 1973.
4. Gilfoyle, E., Grady, A., and Moore, J.: Children Adapt. Thorofare NJ: Charles B. Slack. In press.
5. Ibid.
6. Ibid.
7. Apgar, V.: Perinatal problems and the central nervous system. In The Child with Central Nervous System Deficit. Children's Bureau Publication, No. 432, 1965, pp. 75–77.
8. Chalfant and Schefflin: Central Processing Dysfunction.
9. Goldman, A. S.: Predisposing genetic and metabolic factors. In The Child with Central Nervous System Deficit. Children's Bureau Publication, No. 432, 1965, p. 8.
10. Gilfoyle, Grady, and Moore: Children Adapt.
11. Ayres: Sensory Integration.
12. Moore, J. C.: Concepts from the Neurobehavioral Sciences. Dubuque IA: Kendall Hunt, 1973.
13. Harris, F. A.: Multiple-loop modulation of motor outflow: A physiological basis for facilitation techniques. Phys. Ther. 51:391–396, 1971.
14. Harris, F. A.: The brain is a distributed information processor. Am. J. Occup. Ther. 24:264–268, 1970.
15. Gilfoyle, Grady, and Moore: Children Adapt.
16. Harris: The brain distributed information processor.
17. Norton, Y.: Neurodevelopment and sensory integration for the profoundly retarded multiply handicapped child. In Price, A., Gilfoyle, E., and Myers, C. (eds.): Research in Sensory-Integrative Development. Rockville: American Occupational Therapy Association, 1976, pp. 64–71.
18. Harris: Multiple-loop modulation.
19. Norton: Neurodevelopment and sensory integration.
20. Gilfoyle, Grady, and Moore: Children Adapt.
21. Ayres: Sensory Integration, p. 36.
22. Ibid., p. 126.
23. Gilfoyle, Grady, and Moore: Children Adapt.
24. Gilfoyle, E.: The three faces of Ev. In Perceptual-Motor Dysfunction Evaluation and Training. Proceedings of Occupational Therapy Seminar. University of Wisconsin, Madison, 1966, pp. 55–70.
25. Ayres, A. J.: Southern California Sensory Integration Tests, Los Angeles: Western Psychological Services, 1972.
26. Bayley, N.: Bayley Scales of Infant Development. New York: Psychological Corporation, 1969.
27. Beery, K., and Buktenica, N.: Developmental Test of Visual-Motor Integration. Chicago: Follett Publishing Co., 1967.
28. Berges, J., and Lezine, I.: The imitations of gestures. In Clinics in Developmental Medicine, No. 18. London: Heinemann, 1965.
29. Denhoff, E, et al.: Developmental and predictive characteristics of items from the Meeting House School screening test. Develop. Med. Child Neurol. 10:220, 1969.
30. Egan, D., et al.: Developing screening, 0–5 years. In Clinics in Developmental Medicine, No. 30. London: Heinemann, 1969.
31. Fiorentino, M.: Reflex Testing Methods for Evaluating C.N.S. Development, ed. 2. Springfield IL: Charles C Thomas, 1965.

32. Frostig, M.: Developmental Test of Visual perception, ed. 3. Palo Alto: Consulting Psychologists Press, 1964.
33. Gesell, A., and Armatruda, C. S.: Developmental Diagnosis. New York: Halber, 1947.
34. Kephart, N., and Roach, E.: Purdue Perceptual-Motor Survey. Columbus: Merrill, 1966.
35. Kirk, S. and McCarthy, J.: Illinois Test of Psycholinguistic Abilities. Urban IL: Institute for Research and Exceptional Children, 1968.
36. Milani-Comparetti, A., and Gidoni, E.: Routine developmental examination in normal and retarded children. Develop. Med. Child Neurol. 9:631–638, 1967.
37. Gilfoyle: Three faces of Ev.
38. Ibid.

Peds 414-418

15

Pediatrics

Celestine Hamant

A multitude of factors affect the practice of occupational therapy; in no area is this more true than in pediatrics. A little over a generation ago children with chronic conditions such as polio, juvenile rheumatoid arthritis, and tuberculosis often spent months, sometimes years, in hospitals. A tonsillectomy kept a child in the hospital for a week or more. Few children with myelomeningocele survived; leukemia and other childhood cancers were rapidly fatal. Non-educable mentally retarded children were placed in institutions or kept at home and child abuse was hardly discussed.

Our society has changed with time: medical advances of great magnitude have been made; various groups have formed for mutual support and have pressured for their legal rights; federal legislation has attempted to make health care more accessible to all children. More severely damaged babies are surviving, and disabled children, like the general population, are living longer. Some disabling diseases have been controlled (e.g., polio and tuberculosis). Even children with illnesses still considered terminal (such as cystic fibrosis and some forms of cancer) are enjoying many more years of life. Outpatient and overnight surgery are commonplace and the average length of hospital stay is five to seven days. All of these factors, plus occupational therapy research into child development, have caused the practice of pediatric occupational therapy to change markedly.

Having enumerated so many changes, can we assume that anything has remained the same? Yes, of course. Children still develop in a relatively orderly fashion with certain milestones preceding others and certain skills building on others. Play is still the primary occupation of children, through which they learn, develop, and grow. Children still have caretakers, parents or others, on whom they depend for the necessities of life, including love and security. Children's basic needs have not changed. Unfortunately, even temporary hospitalization can interrupt the developmental continuum, halt play activities, and interfere with the normal parent-child relationship.

According to Llorens:

> An additional premise stated that physical or psychological trauma related to disease, injury,

environmental insufficiencies, or intrapersonal vulnerability can interrupt the growth process.

The effect of an adverse physical, social, or emotional condition, one which inhibits or stresses rather than facilitates optimal growth and development, can be considered interruptive.

Hospitalization which unfortunately is often a necessary component of many diseases and injuries can also be considered disruptive to optimal growth and development as well as the condition necessitating it. Intervention to facilitate continued growth and development in such cases would minimize the negative effects.[1]

This chapter considers the relationship of occupational therapy and general pediatrics in the acute medical care facility.

THE INPATIENT WITH AN ACUTE PROBLEM

Referral

Referrals come to the occupational therapy program from a variety of sources. Usually the physician completes the referral or includes occupational therapy in the orders section of the chart. Referrals can also be requested by the occupational therapist's screening new admissions, by another health care professional, or by a parent recognizing the need for occupational therapy service. In an acute medical facility, all referrals are signed by a physician.

The referral may contain a great deal of, or very little, information. Minimal information includes the diagnosis and precautions in addition to patient identification information. The checklist type referral is used as an educational tool for physician and others (Fig. 15-1).

Evaluation

After the referral is received, thorough evaluation is carried out. Occupational therapists have many evaluation tools to choose from and it is important that appropriate ones be selected. Accurate use of standardized tests is imperative for the documentation of valid, reliable results. Some examples of evaluations used in the pediatric occupational therapy department at James W. Riley Hospital for Children, Indiana University Medical Center, are:

Alpern-Boll Developmental Profile
Bayley Scales of Infant Development
Denver Development Screening Test
Evaluation of Daily Living Skills
The Gesell Developmental Evaluation
Joint Range of Motion Test
Marianne Frostig Developmental Test of Visual Perception
The Purdue Perceptual-Motor Survey
Reflex Testing Methods for Evaluation of Central Nervous System Development
Southern California Sensory Integration Tests

Much evaluation of the young child can be done through observation of behavior (type of grasp, strength, and so forth) and through questioning the parents, if they are reliable.

Evaluation results are recorded so that they are easy and meaningful for others to read and understand as well as useful for the occupational therapists.

Treatment Planning

Once the evaluation has been completed, treatment planning is done. Treatment planning is based on the results of evaluations, but many other factors are also considered: prognosis, precautions (isolation, attached apparatus), length of hospitalization, accessibility of patient for treatment, projected occupation of the patient (school, play, ADL). Even more important in treatment planning is involvement of the patient and his/her parents (or caretakers). A home visit may be indicated in order to plan for the patient's return to the home situation. The physician and other health care team members should be consulted as appropriate. To plan a treatment program without involving the patient, family, and health team is to invite failure.

Some patients who are acutely sick will have only short-term goals; others will have both long- and short-term goals as well as numbers of treatment objectives. In the latter case, it is important to carefully prioritize the objectives, so as not to overwhelm the patient or occupational therapist by trying to accomplish everything at once.

OCCUPATIONAL THERAPY REFERRAL—PEDIATRICS

Diagnosis:

Precautions:

Activity:	Limited ☐	To clinic:	On stretcher ☐			
	Unlimited ☐		In wagon or wheelchair ☐			
	Bedrest ☐		Ambulatory ☐	☐ Inpatient	☐ Outpatient	

☐ Developmental evaluation and treatment

☐ Observation of performance

Increase or maintain

- ☐ 1. Muscle strength
- ☐ 2. Physical tolerance
- ☐ 3. Range of motion
- ☐ 4. Coordination
- ☐ 5. Upper extremity use

Develop

- ☐ 1. Awareness of self, others and environment
- ☐ 2. Improved self-concept

Meet psychological and emotional needs arising from

- ☐ 1. Separation from home
- ☐ 2. Physical restraint
- ☐ 3. Reaction to hospitalization, surgery and/or procedures
- ☐ 4. Environmental deprivation
- ☐ 5. Behavioral regression
- ☐ 6. Other

☐ Splinting (describe below)

☐ Adapted positioning equipment (describe below)

Training in special skills related to

- ☐ 1. Self-care
- ☐ 2. Use of upper extremity prosthesis
- ☐ 3. Eating and feeding
- ☐ 4. Blindness and severe visual limitations
- ☐ 5. Perceptual-motor functions

☐ Behavior modification program

☐ Home program

Remarks:

Date Signed M.D.

FIGURE 15-1. From Occupational Therapy Department, James Whitcomb Riley Hospital for Children, Indiana University Medical Center, Indianapolis. Printed with permission.

Treatment Implementation

After treatment has been carefully planned, it is carried out either at the bedside, in the occupational therapy department, or in some other area, depending on the condition of the patient and the goals of treatment.

The three major types of treatment approaches used are: functional, developmental, and supportive. It is difficult to define specifically where one approach stops and another begins, and it is not unusual to employ all three approaches at once with the same patient. For purposes of clarification, general definitions of treatment types follow:

Functional: relates to a specific function which either has been lost and is being relearned or is being learned for the first time. A specific skill (dressing, feeding, play) is involved, or an activity leading to that skill (splinting, positioning, ROM) is carried out.

Developmental: relates to the achievement of developmental milestones. It is used more often with children with delayed development, mental retardation, or both, who have never possessed the abilities being developed.

Supportive: relates to psychological and emotional needs and problems. It is dependent more upon the relationship between the therapist and patient than on the activity used.

Documentation

The importance of clear, accurate documentation cannot be overstressed. Reevaluation, using the same tools as the initial evaluation, is an effective method to validate progress. It is equally important to document lack of progress or regression. Various formats for the recording of information are in use (see Chapter 26). In most places the entire facility uses the same format (e.g., Problem Oriented Medical Record, POMR). The Medical Records Department can be helpful in planning documentation methodology.

Follow-Up

Because of the short hospitalization of most pediatric inpatients with acute conditions, the occupational therapists in such centers must be knowledgeable of state-wide facilities to which the children can be referred upon discharge. Actual contacts and referral arrangements with occupational therapists around the state are often made by phone since there is rarely time for letterwriting except to confirm and document discharge plans.

If there is no pediatric occupational therapy service in the area where the patient lives, the patient may have to return to the acute care facility for periodic outpatient follow-up care with an ongoing home program.

Home programs are prepared in collaboration with the patient, if possible, the family and, if indicated, the health care team. The therapist presents the final program to the patient and appropriate family members (e.g., mother, father, and babysitter) both verbally and in writing and asks them to demonstrate treatment procedures to be sure that the instructions have been clearly understood.

Many patients, who are seen initially as acutely sick inpatients, are assigned to a specialty outpatient clinic upon discharge for periodic (e.g., quarterly) follow-up by the health care team. In this situation, the occupational therapist often serves as a consultant, responding to specific questions or concerns communicated by the patient's school, local treatment center, or home care agency. All occupational therapists should familiarize themselves with facility policies regarding communication of patient information, authorizations required, and so forth (see Chapter 26).

Summary

Although many pediatric patients who are admitted for short-term inpatient stays in acute medical facilities do not require occupational therapy, there are many who do.

Treatment objectives depend upon diagnosis, length of stay, precautions, funding sources, availability (and ability) of family members, and outside occupational therapy referral sources. The occupational therapist may be called upon to participate in the diagnostic process through evaluation and / or observation. He or she may provide supportive treatment for the patient who has regressed emotionally during a hospitalization requiring painful, frightening, and often unexplainable procedures as well as separation from family. Developmental treatment may be provided for the younger child whose extended acute episode requires physical restraint, so that the developmental level can be maintained. Functional treatment is indicated, for example, for the patient suffering from acute trauma, who may require ADL training, splinting, and adaptive equipment.

CASE STUDY 1

An occupational therapy referral was received on May 5, 1974, for developmental evaluation and treatment for Tommy R. The diagnosis was "failure to thrive" secondary to frequent vomiting.

Tommy was seen in the occupational therapy department when aged eleven months. A Gesell Developmental Evaluation was performed. It was noted that his highest area of performance was motor, which was normal. His adaptive skills were about one to two months low: personal-social skills were very low and language was nonexistent. Tommy was visually alert, but his affect was blunted and he seemed to give the tester only vague recognition. Since the child had not vomited during the testing period, the therapist decided to try leaving him alone, left the observation room, and walked into an adjoining viewing room. At her departure the child did not cry or attempt to follow her but crept to the middle of the room, sat up, and vomited.

In subsequent treatment sessions it was noted that, as long as the therapist engaged the child in active play and participated with him, no vomiting occurred but, when left alone, even with many toys, he vomited frequently. With this information and after extensive consultation with the physician and the family, the child was given a diagnosis of "maternal deprivation."

Tommy's mother had never been able to develop an appropriate relationship with him. Indicative of this problem was a question asked of the therapist in a session in which the therapist was showing Mrs. R. how to interact with her child: "You don't expect me to *play* with him do you?" However, Mrs. R. indicated interest in learning to work with Tommy and was referred for guidance counseling in the local area. It was decided that the child needed more attention than Mrs. R. could provide at that time so a full time babysitter was arranged and the home program was explained to her as well as to the parents. The family was referred back to the local physician for follow-up.

An outpatient visit six months later showed marked improvement. Tommy had stopped vomiting, had begun to gain weight, and was making rapid gains in all areas of development. Speech had developed to within two months of normal.

In a one year follow-up, Tommy's development was normal for age. The babysitter had been decreased to part-time and Mrs. R. was interested in discontinuing the babysitter and placing the child in a day care program for young children. This was encouraged and occupational therapy was discontinued in June 1975.

The original referring physician recently wrote to one of the hospital staff physicians to state that Tommy is now in nursery school, doing very well, and performing at a normal level in all areas.

CASE STUDY 2

Barbara G. was referred to occupational therapy on June 14, 1976, at age three years and ten months for feeding training. She had been injured in an automobile accident on May 5, 1976, in which she sustained a fracture of the right clavicle and a depressed skull fracture. At the time of admission she was comatose; by the date of referral she was semicomatose.

The therapist observed Mrs. G.'s feeding of Barbara in the hospital, since Mrs. G. was staying around the clock with her. It was noted that the child chewed and swallowed without choking, her jaw was stable, and she was able to move food around in her mouth with her tongue, using protraction, lateralization, and retraction effectively.

The therapist contacted the physician indicating that feeding training was not needed but that a program to increase environmental awareness and muscle strength was in order. The appropriate referral was sent and the program was begun on June 16, 1976. Initially Barbara responded to auditory and tactile but not visual stimuli; she was able to grasp objects with her left hand. A program was given to the mother to carry out in the hospital including talking to the child and providing various olfactory, auditory, tactile, and visual stimuli. The occupational therapist followed the child daily while in the hospital. By June 24, 1976, it was noted that Barbara moved her right arm voluntarily during bilateral activity play and smiled to express enjoyment of activities. At the end of the occupational therapy sessions she would moan as if protesting leaving and refused to indicate good-bye.

Mrs. G. was very enthusiastic about the program and her ability to participate in it. Treatment goals included developing and encouraging:

1. environmental awareness by continuing visual, auditory, and tactile stimuli
2. bilateral upper extremity activities
3. fine hand usage bilaterally
4. verbalization

The patient was discharged in July 1976 with an extensive home program (see accompanying program) to provide the mother with a variety of therapeutic activities from which to choose. Mrs. G. has consistently been able to work effectively with Barbara.

HOME PROGRAM FOR BARBARA G.
JULY 9, 1976

Occupational Therapy

1. *Body Parts.* Can use a puppet or doll of Barbara's. Talk about the puppet or doll's eyes, nose, etc. Have the puppet or doll point to Barbara's body parts. Have Barbara point to her own body parts. Pick out two to three to specifically work on, then increase them as she learns them.

2. *Books.* Use books that have simple, fairly-large pictures in them. Best if picture only has one to two things in it. Talk about the things you see, point to them. If you don't have a book like this, you can take magazine pictures and mount them on cardboard to make your own book.

3. *Imitation of Words and Sounds.* Encourage Barbara to make sounds. Make a point to call objects by name. Talk about things you are doing to her, for her, or with her.

4. *Ball Play or Bean Bags.* Encourage Barbara to throw a ball or bean bag to someone. Depending on how large the ball is, she may need to use one hand or both hands. With the bean bags encourage her to throw with both hands, first with one and then the other.

5. *Water Play.* Use a pan of water and have several things Barbara can put in and take out. Play with her, talk about what you're doing. Encourage her to find the things in the water. Use things that feel different when they're wet such as a cup, plastic toy, sponge, etc.

6. *Cardboard Box.* Take a cardboard box such as a shoebox. Cut three holes in the top. Make them different

shapes and sizes. Take three or more objects that will fit easily through the holes such as a block, pop bead, clothespin, etc. Encourage Barbara to find a hole to fit them in. After all the blocks are through the holes, encourage her to remove the lid to find them. Can also do this with a coffee can, oatmeal box, etc.

7. *Cookie Sheet.* Take a cookie sheet and put sand, sugar, oatmeal, or other similar substance on it. Encourage Barbara to spread it around with her fingers. Make designs in it. Can also use a small basin. With a cup, spoon, and other such items encourage pouring, scooping, etc.

8. *Play Doh.* Encourage Barbara to squeeze Play Doh using both hands. Roll it, pound it, etc.

9. *Singing Games.* Play see saw, sing Nursery Rhymes, etc. Any kind of singing game would be good for Barbara.

10. *Puzzles.* Simple one piece puzzles. Encourage Barbara to remove the puzzle parts. Work on getting her to try to replace them.

11. *Balloons.* Tie a balloon to a string. Encourage Barbara to bat the balloon in the air. Encourage her to use two hands.

12. *Stacking.* Take four to five empty shoe boxes. Tape the lids so they won't open. Encourage Barbara to stack them on top of each other. See if she will follow your verbal commands and not need demonstration.

13. *Dressing.* Encourage Barbara to assist you with dressing her. Try to get her to lift her arm and put it through a sleeve. Take off a top, but leave her arms through one sleeve, see if you can get her to pull it the rest of the way off.

14. *Discourage Flinging.* Since Barbara likes to throw toys, encourage her to do something more purposeful with the toys she plays with. Have everyone in the family work on this. Be consistent; if she starts to throw a toy redirect her to something else.

If you have any questions or problems, please feel free to contact me at 264-8211.

Supervisor
Occupational Therapy Dept.
Riley Hospital for Children.

Barbara was reevaluated in August 1976. Testing showed normal activity in all areas; the therapist reported this to the parents and told them that if her performance remained normal at her next return visit, occupational therapy would be discontinued. She was seen in November 1976, where all skills on the Gesell Developmental Evaluation were within normal limits. Barbara was discharged; her parents have the phone number of the occupational therapy department and are free to call for an appointment if any new problems arise.

CASE STUDY 3

Terry F. is a normally intelligent, very sensitive five-year-old boy who is an only child. He has a diagnosis of bilateral hydroureter nephrosis and, at the time of admission, had bilateral nephrostomies, a suprapubic catheter and an indwelling catheter. His symptoms began one year ago and since that time he has had numerous hospitalizations and surgical procedures. This was his second admission within four months. He was referred to occupational therapy on May 14, 1976, for supportive treatment as a result of increased depression and recent suicidal statements. When initially seen, Terry was hyperactive and his mother, who was with him, was obviously very tense.

Terry demonstrated a very short attention span and a refusal to try anything new. When he asked to perform an activity that was too strenuous for him and was told that this was not possible at this time, he shouted with great hostility, "You're mean to me, you hate me," and began to cry. Terry's mood swings were very rapid but he did respond to direct, simple explanations and directions. Occupational therapy goals at the time were to:

1. Establish a supportive consistent relationship.
2. Provide appropriate outlets for hostility and aggression.
3. Promote successful experience through one-step activities leading to goal achievement in order to increase self-confidence and esteem.
4. Provide an atmosphere for exploration of feelings related to the many medical and surgical procedures and the unusual number of tubes and stomas in and on his body.
5. Provide age appropriate activities and maintain an active interest in the environment.

Terry was seen daily by a certified occupational therapy assistant for the remainder of his hospitalization. Following the death of a friend of his on the unit, Terry's depression got worse; he began to have fantasies and refused to eat. This proved to be a short-term relapse and by June 2, 1976, it was reported that Terry was actively participating in activities and taking pride in various finished projects. He related stories of his home life and seemed anxious to return home. He was discharged on June 4, 1976.

On July 26, 1976, Terry was readmitted for urinary tract infection and was referred to occupational therapy for continued supportive therapy during hospitalization. At this hospitalization he exhibited no depressions or fantasy behaviors but was once again quite active initially and was very conscious of his scars, wanting to cover them up with BandAids. Treatment goals included providing age-appropriate activities during his hospitalization and providing opportunities for him to explore his feelings regarding his physical appearance.

Terry was treated by a male occupational therapy affilitate with whom he was able to relate well. There was much discussion about body scars and the affiliate happened to have had an appendectomy. Terry responded well to his activity sessions and talked about what he planned to do when he returned home. One day he removed the BandAids from his scars and stated that he "no longer needed them." Terry has not been readmitted to date.

CASE STUDY 4

Steven T. was referred to occupational therapy in May 1976 for developmental evaluation and treatment. His diagnosis was ventricular septal defect with pulmonary stenosis. The Bayley Scales of Infant Development were administered and the results indicated that the child was functioning within normal limits in all areas except motor development which was attributed to weakness secondary to cardiac problems. He was given a home program and arrangements were made for homebound therapy in the local community.

Steven returned in September 1976 at age ten months for admission resulting from the development of glaucoma; his cardiac condition had stabilized. The new referral to occupational therapy was primarily for evaluation in activity and development, since Mrs. T. had noted a decrease in the child's general response during the past few months. The physician's evaluation had elicited very little response from the child and because of the previous near normal occupational therapy evaluation results, the physician questioned whether some sort of degenerative disease was involved in addition to the visual and cardiac problems.

The therapist noted that when Steven was tested in normal light conditions, he generally kept one or both eyes closed because of light intensity, so his reactions to the presentation of materials were extremely limited. She decided to administer the same evaluation in dim light to see whether he would be able to respond more appropriately. The results of the evaluation in dim light demonstrated a motor development of seven-and-a-half months and all other areas at the nine-month level. After consultation with the physician, it was determined that the child's general one-month delay could be related to the visual problem and the motor development was further delayed because of energy limitations. An appropriate home program involving the use of dim light was developed for the parents and the information was transmitted to the homebound therapist in the local area. It is anticipated that this child should have potential for relatively normal development, if the glaucoma is able to be stabilized. The family, however, is having many problems; Mr. T. is unemployed and is an alcoholic, and there are other children in the family, so that Steven's follow-up care is primarily dependent on the homebound therapist. Steven will be placed in a day care program as soon as he is old enough and his condition has stabilized. He will continue to be followed in occupational therapy in conjunction with Cardiac Clinic.

CASE STUDY 5

Bethann D. was referred to occupational therapy on April 22, 1975, at the age of ten years with a diagnosis of second and third degree burns over 40 percent of her body, concentrated on her thorax and arms. Bethann was evaluated and found to be depressed and quiet but receptive to some suggestions for activity. Her mother was staying with her and was cooperative in participating in the occupational therapy program. Goals included:

1. bilateral upper extremity activities to encourage active range of elbows and shoulders
2. supportive therapy for fear and depression
3. bilateral axillary splinting when appropriate

On April 25, 1975, orders for axillary splinting were received and the patient was fitted that day with bilateral airplane splints to hold both arms in ninety degree abduction, full elbow extension, and fifteen degrees of wrist extension. The splints were constructed of orthoplast and reinforced for stability. Both the nursing staff and Mrs. D. were instructed on care and application of the splints.

As Bethann improved, the upper extremity activity program was increased. During activity sessions she talked to her therapist about her fears that she might die; the therapist was able to assure her that she was getting better but communicated Bethann's fears to her physician and the nursing staff so that they might also reinforce her improvement.

In June 1975 she was started on an activities of daily living program including dressing and self-care. Being very well aware of her body and how it looked, she began to discuss with her therapist the concerns she had about her scars. The occupational therapist worked with the Social Service Department to arrange for an older girl who had had similar burns and who was healed to come in so that Bethann could see how her scars might look in the future. Releases for growth and breast development were discussed with her and her mother. On July 10, 1975, Bethann was discharged from the hospital.

In December 1975 Bethann returned to the hospital for release of burn scar contractures of both axillas. Her mother admitted that she had not been following the splint-wearing protocol that had been prescribed. New splints were made and have been worn appropriately since that date. Bethann returned to the occupational therapy department in March 1976 for some adjustment in the splints needed because of growth and weight gain. She was readmitted to the hospital in July 1976 for release of burn scar contractures resulting from growth. New bilateral axillary splints were made at this time. Bethann will continue to be followed until her growth years are over.

THE INPATIENT WITH A CHRONIC CARE PROBLEM

Those children with disabling conditions (amputee, cerebral palsy, myelomeningocele) or with long-term degenerative diseases (muscular dystrophy, central nervous system disease) often have repeated hospitalizations and are followed on a long-term basis in outpatient clinics.

Referral

In order to maintain continuity of care, patients of this type are followed consistently by the same occupational therapist whether they have inpatient or outpatient status. This therapist initiates a referral for physician signature whenever necessary, depending on the purpose of admission and length of projected stay.

Evaluation

Since the patient and family are known to the therapist, the evaluation process may differ from that for the inpatient with an acute condition. Evaluation may involve working out with the family the best way to manage a normally ambulatory child who has been placed in a spica cast or body cast. The period of hospitalization may not be the appropriate time to attempt a thorough reevaluation of a patient with a chronic illness. On the other hand, however, a child whose condition is degenerating may require total reevaluation to see how much ability has been lost.

Treatment Planning

As indicated previously for the acute problem, treatment planning should involve the patient, family, and health care team. For the chronic care patient who is temporarily hospitalized the plan may involve maintenance of learned skills, especially if the child is mentally retarded and loses skills easily. After discharge, the patient may return to the previous home program.

Planning for the child with a degenerating condition includes grading activities down to accommodate decreasing strength, coordination, mentation, attention span, and energy. It may also include the provision of adaptive equipment to be used by the family in the care and management process if the child is to remain at home.

Treatment Implementation—Approach to the Older Child

The patient is treated in the occupational therapy department, at bedside, or in an alternate location, if indicated. For the older child or the teenager who has repeated admissions, it is important to encourage as much continued independence and decision making as is possible. The teenage repeater may be able to be responsible for procuring his or her own referral from the doctor and making arrangements with the therapist for treatment time. He or she can be given great latitude in the type of activity selected, relating to the treatment goals that he or she has helped to develop. Cooperation and a feeling of self-worth are greatly enhanced by such an approach.

The older child who does not wish to participate in occupational therapy may be encouraged and positively reinforced for cooperation but is not forced to participate unless he or she is performing well below the normal mental level for chronological age. All children must be able to find meaning in therapeutic activity:

> "Here I sit at
> A great big loom
> Making God knows what,
> For God knows whom."[2]

Documentation

It is equally important to thoroughly document information on patients, particularly those with degenerative conditions, who have repeated admissions to maintain an up-to-date record of their performance level, status of adaptive equipment, and so forth. The importance of accurate and thorough documentation for third party and/or welfare coverage, chart audit, and court subpoena is covered in Chapter 26.

Follow-Up

Chronic and/or degenerative patients are often seen in outpatient clinics at the same facility where they are hospitalized. The occupational therapist must keep track of return appointments, coordinating his or her own follow-up of the patient with the clinic visits if the family lives a long distance from the hospital.

The home program is a critical part of follow-up care. It must be kept in mind that the priorities of the therapist may not be those of the family. If the family is to carry out the program, it must be viable and meaningful for them.

Summary

The inpatient with a chronic care problem and his or her family are often known to the therapist. Because of the rapid turnover of resident physicians and others in a large hospital, the occupational therapist is often one of the few familiar faces to the patient and family over a period of time. This continuity of care is of great importance and should be provided whenever possible.

Since many of these patients are medically active over periods of years, consistent and thorough communication is essential—with the family, school, local welfare and home care agencies, and local treatment centers.

CASE STUDY 6

Harry M. was referred to the myelomeningocele (MM) treatment team in April 1968 at the age of one year with a diagnosis of myelomeningocele at the L_1 level with hydrocephalus and a functioning Holter valve. His level of development at that time, with the exception of the motor level which was at two to four months, was at the seven to ten month level. Harry has been on a developmental program in occupational therapy since that time.

Although Harry has had consistent follow-up by the treatment team, extensive and varied family problems have hindered his progress.

Mr. M. deserted the family of four children, and Mrs. M.'s skills limit her to only very menial, low-paying jobs. She is an obese woman whose own health problems and family problems are overwhelming to her. She also has been unable to utilize the limited resources in the rural community where they live. In addition, Mrs. M. is overprotective of Harry, taking care of him rather than encouraging independence.

Although he had learned to walk at age seven, he was nonambulatory by age nine because of weight gain. In November 1976, Mrs. M. inquired whether Harry could be taught to walk again. The physician explained that it would require several surgeries to relieve contractures as well as extensive weight reduction and a lengthy training program.

Mrs. M. was asked to consider this for one month and return to clinic with a decision. At that time she decided not to pursue walking but rather to have Harry accommodate to a wheelchair life-style. Mrs. M. has become more interested in having Harry "take care of himself" and so arrangements were made for another home visit and for a reevaluation of ADL skills. The evaluation indicated that Harry is wearing diapers which leak when he is in school and odor is a problem. He is in the second grade of public school and his teacher is planning to recommend special education next year. He is dependent in dressing, bathing, and self-care. He can transfer, but cannot get out of the bathtub or into the family's truck.

The long-term occupational therapy goal is ADL independence. Short-term goals have been simplified to attempt to ensure success for Mrs. M. and Harry so that positive reinforcement might stimulate greater effort. A bathtub seat has been ordered and some clothing adaptations are being tried.

The treatment team is following this family once a month. Unfortunately there are no local resources available for frequent follow-up and support.

CASE STUDY 7

Judy H. was referred to occupational therapy on February 11, 1976, for developmental evaluation and treatment, adapted equipment positioning, and feeding evaluation and training. Judy is a two-year-old child with central nervous system degenerative disease of unknown etiological factors. She was reportedly normal until one year of age when she began to develop seizures and to deteriorate. At the present time she has several seizures per day, has no head control, and is spastic in all four extremities.

Judy was fitted with an adapted wheelchair with a head rest (See Chapter 20 for details of adaptive positioning equipment). The evaluation showed weak suck and swallow patterns. A facilitation program for lip closure, sucking, and swallowing was developed and taught to her mother. The patient was followed daily throughout hospitalization and was discharged on February 25, 1976, with her equipment and feeding program.

She was readmitted on April 15, 1976; at this point her physical status had degenerated slightly and she was no longer able to hold her head up even for a few seconds at a time. Crossed chest straps had to be used continually in order to keep her upright in her wheelchair. Mrs. H. had noticed increased lethargy. Her feeding facilitation program was altered and a "preemie" nipple with an enlarged hole was used. As Judy's care was becoming more complicated and time-consuming, the family was urged to consider residential placement.

The patient was readmitted in August 1976; she no longer responded to visual stimuli, responded to auditory stimuli only on occasion, was no longer able to suck or swallow voluntarily, and was placed on nasogastric tube feedings with plans for a gastrostomy. Mrs. H. reported that, at this point, she was alone in caring for Judy because her husband and relatives panic when they are asked to perform any of her care. She was, however, adamant in keeping Judy at home. It was stressed to the mother that some effort should be made to get away for short periods of time and do things that she enjoys, such as bowling. She seemed realistic about the child's prognosis and was coping adequately. Elbow restraints were made because Judy chewed on her fingers and caused them to bleed.

The patient was seen in outpatient clinic in November 1976; she was tolerating her gastrostomy feedings and weighed sixteen pounds. She no longer cried, was less responsive, and was developing increasing hypertonicity. The elbow restraints no longer needed to be used continually as Judy had less interest in chewing her hands. Mrs. H.'s only break at this time from Judy's full-time care was for grocery shopping and going to the Laundromat; however, her emotional status seemed to be adequate and she was being followed by social service.

Judy was seen again in outpatient clinic on January 26, 1977. Her wheelchair continued to fit well and was helpful in changing her position and enabled Mrs. H. to keep Judy in sight while she did housework. Judy had become opisthotonic when awake, requiring flexion bed positioning to break up the extensor thrust which was demonstrated. Use of the wheelchair was reemphasized. The patient and her mother were to be seen in March during her next outpatient clinic appointment.

CASE STUDY 8

John W. was referred to occupational therapy in March 1972 with a diagnosis of acute lymphocytic leukemia and osteoporosis. He was fourteen years old and was referred for needs arising from separation from home and restrictions including bedrest. During that admission he had to spend much of his time in a total extension body cast and, when out of the cast, he was on bedrest. This, in addition to his reaction to his diagnosis, caused depression. He became involved in structured projects which he was allowed to select and he enjoyed treatment sessions with his therapist. He began to talk more and initiated conversation about his health and family, displaying a good sense of humor.

His next admission was in July 1974. By this time he was sixteen-years old and obviously more serious and solemn. He complained that he should be out working instead of being in the hospital. John was from a large, relatively-poor family. Goals during his second admission included:

1. constructive use of time during hospitalization
2. activities and experiences to provide a stimulating environment
3. outlet for expression of feelings

John again became involved in occupational therapy, enjoying more complicated activities and conversing with therapists.

His third admission was in August 1974. His parents continued to be supportive and he once again was able to become involved in activities. By this time he was able to procure his own referral from his physician and to contact his therapist to set up his own treatment program.

His last and most lengthy admission was in November 1974. By this time he was quite weak but, although he showed apathy at first, he did involve himself in occupational therapy again. On his previous admission he had done some leather work which he enjoyed; on this admission he discussed with the therapist the fact that he knew this was going to be his last Christmas and he felt he was too old to ask his father for money to purchase presents for his parents and siblings. Because he had not been able to work during the summers, he had no money of his own, so he asked to make some projects to give to his family for Christmas. The therapist encouraged his plan and he selected leather projects. Although he was too weak to do any carving or stamping, he was able to tool and used leather dyes very effectively to create interesting designs in his projects. John worked diligently, often asking to take the projects to his room in the evening and on weekends so that he could complete them in time for Christmas. He did complete all of his gifts and was discharged just before Christmas.

John died in January 1975 and, when Mrs. W. contacted his occupational therapist to tell her of John's death, she stated that the leather Christmas gifts had made Christmas even more meaningful for the entire family since he was able to give them something that he had done himself. She indicated that everyone in the family was using gifts that John had given them except his father, who keeps his wallet in a drawer and looks at it periodically as a reminder of his oldest son.

CASE STUDY 9

Jennifer A. was first seen in March 1974 at the age of eleven months for developmental evaluation; diagnosis was "delayed development." The Gesell

Developmental Evaluation showed that Jennifer was at least one to two months behind in all areas of development. Another problem area was feeding; Mrs. A. stated that the patient used a baby bottle and ate strained foods and that when junior food was introduced the patient either choked or vomited. A feeding evaluation was done which showed no physical abnormality in the feeding process, but that her feeding problems were due only to not being accustomed to anything but strained foods. All testing results were explained to Mr. and Mrs. A. who were told that there were delays in all areas of the patient's behavior. A home program stressing developmental activities was given.

Mrs. A. brought Jennifer in for occupational therapy reevaluation on April 23, 1974. Some gains were noted including increased active sitting balance and increased bilateral upper extremity use. On this visit the child was accompanied to the department by her brother as well. Mrs. A. had obvious difficulty in controlling the brother's behavior. After the evaluation was over, the mother became upset and cried; she expressed guilt feelings about both children, stating that if she could be different the children would be better. Mrs. A. said that she had little support from her husband in the childrearing process and that she was unable to find a babysitter because both of her children were such problems. The boy, aged three, appeared to be a behavior problem; Mrs. A. said that "someone evaluated him and said that he was 'emotional'." The occupational therapist referred the brother to the Child Guidance Clinic for evaluation and treatment. Because Jennifer was making developmental gains very slowly, occupational therapy visits were indicated only every two or three months; however, because Mrs. A. seemed to need a great deal of support, the therapist continued to see the patient monthly and gave the mother positive reinforcement for appropriate parenting.

In May 1974 Jennifer was eating junior foods but was still not doing any finger feeding. Mrs. A. brought with her on this visit a female friend who seemed very supportive and was able to reinforce the gains that the child had made. The patient's brother was being seen in the Child Guidance Clinic. Jennifer's home program was upgraded each time to reinforce with Mrs. A. the progress that the child was making. (See home programs for Jennifer A.) By June 1974 the patient was able to chew and swallow a regular diet and was beginning to finger feed. By November 1974, at age nineteen months, Jennifer was functioning between the ten and fifteen month level; she was beginning to cooperate in dressing and remove simple clothing. The need for consistent discipline was stressed as Mrs. A. reported the child was beginning to have temper tantrums and was showing more manipulative behavior. Mrs. A. was urged to enroll Jennifer in a preschool program at the local center for retarded children, which she did in September 1975.

In November 1975 Mrs. A. was pleased with the preschool program which Jennifer attended two half days a week. The occupational therapist observed that Mrs. A. was using more effective and appropriate discipline with her child. Communication with her teacher in May 1976 indicated that the child was walking and running, using single words to express her desires, and could name simple pictures. She fed herself independently with utensils and assisted with dressing. She began full day preschool classes in the fall of 1976. In November 1976 Jennifer was three years and seven months old. Her performance level ranged from two to three years; she was able to ride a tricycle, match four basic colors, join two words, and begin to dress herself. She was much more interested in her environment. Mrs. A. was recently given the option of discontinuing from the active occupational therapy program and going on a P.R.N. (as needed) basis, since Jennifer is involved in the preschool program and doing well, but Mrs. A. preferred to continue with occupational therapy at scheduled periodic intervals. Her next appointment was arranged for March 1977, when dressing skills were to be evaluated and toilet training to be initiated.

Home Program for
Jennifer A.
4/23/74

1. Try to feed all junior foods and/or table foods. You can continue to use a bottle, but try to offer a cup at least for one meal.
2. When Jennifer plays on her stomach, put toys in front of her so she has to go after them. Don't let her roll over.
3. Encourage Jennifer to take toys out of a small box. You might have to move her through the motions.
4. Continue the other activities on the first program.

Home Program
for Jennifer A.
5/10/76

1. Work on the concept of "one" and "many." Tell her to take one cookie or give you one block.
2. Try working on "same" and "different" or "like." Ask Jennifer to find one toy just like another one. You can use magazines to look at pictures.
3. Work on "big" and "little." Find the big toy or block, etc.
4. Work on "on" and "under." For example, tell Jennifer to put something on a chair or under the chair.
5. Make a "word box." Put 3 to 5 familiar objects into a box. Ask Jennifer to find an object. Ask her to tell you what is inside.

ADDITIONAL PEDIATRIC SITUATIONS

There are some special situations which occur in pediatrics that cannot be adequately addressed either under acute or chronic care. Brief discussions and case summaries about these follow:

Neonate

The sick newborn or "at risk" premature infant is often treated in the large, acute care pediatric center. These children, because of their tenuous states, are often in isolettes for weeks or months with oxygen and mist, IVs, and gavage feeding. They may require physical restraint to prevent accidental dislodging of tubes. As a result, while their occupation should consist of eating, sleeping, and sensorimotor investigation, they frequently lack normal tactile, visual, auditory, gustatory, proprioceptive and even olfactory stimulation, as well as missing the primary time for mother-child "bonding." Much more research needs to be done into the ramifications of this deprivation relative to future psychological and emotional development.

CASE STUDY 10

Bonnie C. was referred to occupational therapy at age three weeks with a diagnosis of prematurity, gastroschisis, and bowel atresia. She was referred to occupational therapy for developmental evaluation, treatment, and home program. At this time she was in an isolette with an ileostomy bag, a hyperalimentation (HA) line, a gavage tube, and an IV. A reflex test was administered on July 24, 1975; results indicated that Bonnie had a strong sucking reflex and was an active baby who tested in the normal prenatal range. Some lag was identified in grasp reflex, primitive righting, extensor thrust, and crossed extension reflexes. The occupational therapy plan was to see Bonnie twice daily for short periods of time for developmental stimulation. Program goals were to increase tactile awareness, develop postural adjustments to position change, and encourage attention to visual and auditory stimuli with retesting in one month to determine rate of progress and define further treatment goals. It was noted that Bonnie's arms were restrained at her sides in order to keep her from dislodging the various tubes she had in place.

A one-month reevaluation indicated that Bonnie had become very irritable when awake and slept most of the time. At this point her treatment program was continued with the exception that small toys were introduced because she had been moved to an "open air" crib. Bonnie's periods of wakefulness were brief; she seemed to require constant position change to keep her awake. She did, however, passively regard the therapist. Her arms were still restricted to prevent pulling out her tubes. Goals at this time included increase in head control and eye contact and social response to interaction.

In December 1975 treatment goals were increased to include gross motor activities with emphasis on reaching, head control, sitting balance, and visual tracking. Neuromuscular facilitation techniques to oral musculature to increase strength of suck was included in her program. By the end of December Bonnie was able to suck strongly enough to take her bottle and had begun to reach, grasp, and respond more consistently to her therapist.

Further surgical procedures were indicated in early January 1976, and Bonnie's condition deteriorated markedly. She was returned to her isolette. Occupational therapy goals had to be reduced to supportive treatment with only tactile and verbal stimuli being presented. By the end of January 1976 Bonnie was six and one half months old, had had numerous surgical procedures, and still had an HA line, a gravity fat emulsion IV, and a gastrostomy. She had developed head control but had no sitting balance, continued to be seen twice a day for fifteen to twenty minute periods, was irritable, cried frequently, and tired easily but did respond to her therapist. Goals were upgraded to include:

1. Reach and grasp objects with free (non-IV) hand.
2. Visual regard and tracking of objects with head participating.
3. Auditory responses such as head and eye turning toward sound.
4. Increase suck strength by neuromuscular facilitation to oral musculature followed by pacifier use.
5. Tactile stimulation to increase awareness and response to a variety of textures.

Upright bed positioning was provided in an effort to get Bonnie into a sitting position to increase her head control and expand her visual field.

During Bonnie's hospitalization her parents visited often, worked with the therapist, and were able to carry out the treatment program but had never had their child at home or been responsible for her care. She continued to improve and, following a two-week stay in the Parent Care Unit where parents practice caring for children with special needs, she was discharged at age ten months in May 1976. At that time her developmental age varied from sixteen to thirty-six weeks. She was given a home program and a return date of July 1976. Unfortunately no local resources could be identified to help this young family. A reevaluation with the Gesell Developmental in July 1976 indicated that Bonnie's level of development had not increased since discharge. In discussion with the parents, it became evident that Mrs. C. had not been able to carry out the home program because of the amount of adjustment she had to make in having the child home and because of the lengthy feeding sessions. A total review of the mother's day helped both parents see how their time was utilized. Mr. C. agreed to take over some of the housekeeping chores and to work with Bonnie in the evening, thus giving his wife more time with the child during the day.

The next appointment was in November 1976, at which time Bonnie was sitting independently indefinitely, and was able to move from sitting to prone. All other skills were at the forty-week level and the parents were positively reinforced for their successful carrying out of the program and for the child's progress. They were very pleased when they were given an upgraded home program and Mrs. C. stated that it was like "passing to the next grade in school." Bonnie continues to be followed and is doing well.

Long-Term Patient

Occasionally, in an unusual circumstance, a child will spend a long time (more than a year) in a setting designed for acute care. When this occurs, the occupational therapist should be involved in the development of a plan related to the occupation and development of the child on a long-term basis.

CASE STUDY 11

Sarah J. was hospitalized immediately following birth with a diagnosis of hyaline membrane disease and microthorax. Most children with a diagnosis of microthorax do not live past the age of six months. Sarah was referred to occupational therapy in March 1970 at age one month for developmental evaluation and treatment. Her initial treatment was very similar to that in the study of Bonnie C. As Sarah J. grew up, however, she remained in the Intensive Care Unit (ICU) of the hospital since she was on a ventilator and could not breathe on her own at all. Her development was particularly hindered by the fact that her arms had to be restrained to keep her from dislodging her oxygen tubing and the fact that she never had an opportunity to see other children play. At the age of six months, a developmental reevaluation was done by the occupational therapist which showed that Sarah was two months behind in adaptive, motor, and personal-social skills. Since Sarah seemed to be holding her own physically, a case conference was called to determine whether the ICU staff felt that they could provide any kind of normalization of life-style for this child in such an abnormal situation.

The nursing staff on the unit were challenged by the possibility of having this child on a long-term basis and procedures were established whereby the home program would be carried out by the nursing staff on ICU with the occupational therapist treating the child and serving as a consultant to the unit for the child's development. With the encouragement of a very understanding and involved physician, activities such as mirror play and finger painting were introduced to the Intensive Care Unit.

As the child grew older, tubing, which attached her to her ventilator, was increased in length to allow for more excursion and to increase her gross motor activity ability. By this time a corner of the intensive care unit was assigned to her, and she became the proud owner of a small sandbox and a "large pan" swimming pool in which she splashed, wearing a bikini that the nurses had purchased for her second birthday. Shortly thereafter a potty chair was installed and toilet training was in progress; she had learned to feed herself in the usual messy manner.

In her third year, she accomplished toilet training and began dressing and undressing skills despite the tubes, which now were attached to a helmet that she wore in order to keep them from getting dislodged during her very active play periods. Once the helmet had proved successful, she was given permission to move about the hospital when accompanied by a nurse and a respiratory therapist. Her oxygen tanks and ventilator were put on wheels and she enjoyed having tea parties with some of the other hospitalized children and often ate lunch on other units. Her development was normal, except for language and, though she could not speak, she developed quite an intricate pantomime system. She was started on lessons in sign language.

Sarah delighted in coming to occupational therapy and thought it was one of the best rooms in the hospital. During the summer she was able to go outside where she enjoyed swinging and playing ball. For her third birthday she received a tricycle and the vision of her riding down the hall as fast as possible with the respiratory therapist running behind with the oxygen tanks was a delight to all. Throughout her hospitalization her parents and older brothers visited almost daily, since they lived in the immediate area. At age three years and four months it was decided to try to wean her off the ventilator and see if she could breathe on her own to determine whether there was any chance of her living outside the hospital environment. This was a very slow process but eventually it was successful. In anticipation of her eventual discharge her occupational therapist began to make recommendations for some normalizing activities (e.g., she had never ridden in a car).

She was not quite four years old when she was discharged from the hospital and was able to go home for the first time. She had spent several weekends there previously so that she was acclimated to the situation. Her family was outstanding and was able to care for her very well and to promote her general development. Her outpatient hospital visits were joyous occasions when she visited all of her old friends.

Early in her fifth year she was hospitalized twice for pneumonia and it became apparent that her body was outgrowing her lung capacity. Her parents made the decision that they did not want her life sustained artificially and this decision was respected by her physician. In October 1974 she developed a serious case of pneumonia and was rehospitalized. At age four years and eight months she died in the same Intensive Care Unit in which she had spent the majority of her life.

Isolation

The child who has to remain in isolation for long periods of time (more than a week), especially if he or she feels relatively well, becomes a special challenge for the occupational therapist. The feelings of rejection, of "being bad—or else they wouldn't put me in here by myself," of loneliness and boredom, and of frustration combine to cause depression and despair. Children thus confined cannot make physical contact with adults as the mood strikes them and often suffer from "touch hunger."

The needs of such a child for a treatment program that includes long-term, self-motivating, clean activities as well as some control on the part of the child over his or her environment is critical for maintaining psychological and emotional equilibrium.

CASE STUDY 12

George D. was admitted to the hospital in May 1974 at age ten with a diagnosis of infection associated with hemophilia. This child was known to have behavior problems and, although he had been hospitalized before, this was the first time he had been isolated. His behavior became an increasing problem; the situation became really serious when he became self-abusive and began to strike his arms and legs against the bed rails, eventually causing a serious hemorrhage in his knee. George was referred to occupational therapy and it was determined that a behavior modification program would be developed for him. The occupational therapist worked with George to determine what kinds of activities he enjoyed and then collected a number of projects and games that could be self-initiated and done independently.

It was determined that if any of the nursing personnel noticed George doing any of the activities that the therapist provided for him, or if he was quietly watching television, reading a book, resting in his bed, or some other nondestructive behavior, he would be given a "point." The point tally was kept on a board in the window of his door. Every ten points earned a star and stars added up to one of several kinds of rewards.

A reward could be either a specific treat, e.g., ice cream before bedtime, or he could contract for a certain amount of someone's time, e.g., a half hour of one of the nurse's time to read him a story or a certain amount of the therapist's time to play a board game with him. In addition to the earned time, he also was seen twice a day by a certified occupational therapist assistant who introduced new activities and games that he could learn to do by himself. Within a week George's destructive behavior had been eliminated; his positive behavior, reinforced with rewards, had replaced it.

George received visitors only very rarely since his family lived out of town and included a number of children, two of whom, in addition to George, were hemophiliacs.

There were no further behavior problems during the hospitalization and George was discharged in August 1974.

THE IMPORTANCE OF PLAY—PREVENTIVE TREATMENT

The importance of play in the life of a child cannot be overestimated. George Bernard Shaw summarizes thus, "all children should be tirelessly noisy, playful, grubby-handed except at mealtimes, soiling and tearing such clothes as they need to wear, bringing not only the joy of childhood into the house but the dust and mud as well; in short, everything that make the quiet and order of sickness and nursing impossible."[3]

It is not unusual for an occupational therapy referral to read "adjustment to hospitalization," and this probably is a realistic goal for the older child and the teenager. For the younger child, preschool and below, a number of considerations need to be made. In *Young Children in the Hospital*,[4] Robertson describes three stages that the young child goes through when separated from his mother—protest, despair, denial.

In the protest stage the young child needs his or her mother and is used to her response to his or her cries. This child's reaction is to cry and shout. In the despair stage he or she still needs mother but feels hopeless and gives up. If the mother should visit at this time, he or she will rage at her. Unfortunately, the mother may then be asked not to return, since her presence "upsets the child." In the denial stage the child represses feelings for the mother who has "failed," forgets the mother, and becomes interested in the immediate surroundings. Hospital personnel are likely to rejoice, thinking that the child has finally "settled in." However, such a child often has difficulty in adjustment when returned home, suffering from insecurities and night fears.

The obvious answer is not to separate young children from their families, especially from the mother, if at all possible, and many pediatric hospitals now have live-in arrangements. Even with this system, however, a play program is essential to maintain the developmental level of the hospitalized child and help him/her learn from experiences.

The hospital play program is often but not always provided by the occupational therapy department. In some hospitals this program is run by recreation therapy; at the James W. Riley Hospital for Children in Indianapolis, Indiana, Child Life Services is in charge of this type of program. An activity or play program is a necessity for any inpatient acute care pediatric hospital. Provisions should also be made for evening and weekend coverage as well as weekday programming.

CONCLUSION

The occupational therapist who chooses to work in the acute pediatric setting will find that he or she spends 50 percent of the time working with adults under stress—the patients' families. The child belongs to the family and not to the therapist nor the hospital. The therapist must be able to work with and care about children who are sick, children who are irritable, children who are mentally retarded, children who are disabled, children who are disfigured and deformed, children who have degenerating conditions, children who are dying—and the families of all of these children.

The therapist must be able to accept each child at the point where he or she is, physically, mentally, emotionally, socially, and help the child take the next step toward being able to achieve his or her occupation at the highest possible level, for only then will the child have the chance to live life with satisfaction.

REFERENCES

1. Llorens, L. A.: The effects of stress on growth and development. Am. J. Occup. Ther. 28:82–83, 1974.
2. Dimock, H. G.: The Child in the Hospital. Philadelphia: F. A. Davis Co., 1960, p. 106.
3. Lindheim, R., Glaser, H. H., and Coffin, C.: Changing Hospital Environments for Children. Cambridge: Harvard University Press, 1972, p. 1.
4. Robertson, J.: Young Children in Hospital. London: Tavistock Publications, 1970, pp. 12–14.

BIBLIOGRAPHY

Burton, L.: Care of the Child Facing Death. Boston: Routledge & Kegan Paul, 1974.

Florey, L.: An approach to play and play development. Am. J. Occup. Ther. 25:275–280, 1971.

Geist, H.: A Child Goes to the Hospital. Springfield IL: Charles C Thomas, Publishers, 1965.

Gray, M.: Effects of hospitalization on work-play behavior. Am. J. Occup. Ther. 26:180, 1972.

Hamovitch, M. B.: The Parent and the Fatally Ill Child. Los Angeles: Delmar Publishing Co., 1964.

Hardgrove, C. B., and Dawson, R. B.: Parents and Children in the Hospital. Boston: Little, Brown & Co., 1972.

Huss, A. J.: Touch With Care or a Caring Touch? 1976 Eleanor Clarke Slagle Lecture. Am. J. Occup. Ther. 31:11–18, 1977.

Matsutsuyu, J.: Occupational behavior: A perspective on work and play. Am. J. Occup. Ther. 25:291–94, 1971.

Noble, E.: Play and the Sick Child. London: Faber and Faber, 1967.

Plank, E.: Working with Children in Hospitals. Cleveland OH: Western Reserve Press, 1971.

Robertson, J.: Hospitals and Children: A Parent's Eye View. London: Tavistock Publications, 1962.

ACKNOWLEDGMENTS

To the occupational therapy staff at the James W. Riley Hospital for Children, Indiana University Medical Center, for their assistance in the preparation of this chapter.

16

General Medicine and Surgery

Carole Hays

Occupational therapists in a general hospital have a unique opportunity to contribute to the total health care of individuals. The individuals in this setting are acutely ill, many have more than one problem, their diagnoses are in the process of being identified, and their adjustment to problems is just beginning. Many of the medical and surgical diagnoses that an occupational therapist must deal with in a general hospital are those that have been covered in other sections of this book, that is, cerebral vascular accident, spinal cord injuries, and arthritis. In a general hospital the occupational therapist's approach towards individuals with such diagnoses and others that will be covered in this chapter is somewhat different because they are treated in the acute stage of the disease. The therapist must see each patient as a human being with a unique set of problems which must be viewed with sensitivity and creativity.

There are many facilities, agencies, and institutions where an individual may receive health care, but in the United States the general hospital is second only to the private doctor's office in the delivery of health care services. General hospitals serve all ages from birth to death. They are most frequently the entry point for all types of diagnostic, medical, and surgical problems ranging from birth defects to traumatic quadriplegia. In some areas of the country, general hospitals provide all of the acute rehabilitation and chronic care programs for both physical and mental disorders; in other areas they serve as a primary care provider for acute problems and as a referring agent to rehabilitation centers, home care programs, mental health facilities, chronic care institutions, and other health care systems.

One first needs to consider the very nature of a general hospital. It is important to recognize that a general hospital exists for acute care problems or for episodic care. With this philosophy and the new enforcement of it by hospital utilization review committees, the patients have very short-term hospitalizations which nationally range anywhere from 5.4 days to 11 days. Therefore it is essential that occupational therapists assess the potential benefit of treatment to referred patients so that recommendations can be made regarding whether the patient should be discharged, kept in the hospital for a longer period of time, or sent to another facility. Because of the short-term hospitalization, many times the therapist only has time to complete the assessments and program planning and the implementation is done by a therapist in another center, in the patient's home, or through home health care agencies. Discharge planning is vital in assuring that all patients receive quality care.

The procedure that the occupational therapist utilizes in a general medical and surgical setting is based upon problem solving. The process of providing occupational therapy services to patients includes data gathering, analysis of available information and evaluations, program planning, program implementation, documentation on the medical record of all the services rendered, continual reassessment and reevaluation of the patients and their goals, modification of the original plan based upon reassessment, home visits, discharge planning, aftercare programs as appropriate, and follow-up by the occupational therapist until the patient has reached a maximum level of functioning.

The process of initiating an occupational therapy program is essentially the same in general medicine and surgery facilities regardless of the specific diagnostic categories. With this in mind the next section will be an overview of occupational therapy assessment and will be followed by examples of specific approaches to selected diagnoses and problems.

ASSESSMENT

The assessment of the patient should include a maximum amount of information gathered in a short period of time; an interview form is often helpful.

REFERRAL INFORMATION. This section should include the date of admission to the facility, who referred the patient to occupational therapy (whether that be a physician or another health care professional), and the age and birthdate of the patient. It should also include the diagnoses that are being addressed in occupational therapy treatment and other additional diagnoses that are affecting the patient's life. The reason for the referral should be documented.

PHYSICAL STATUS. The current physical status of the patient is the next area to be assessed. Initially this should include the reason for admission, the onset of the problems, progression of the symptoms, previous hospitalizations, medications, other complaints, past medical history if applicable, mobility, mental status, sitting balance, visual deficit, range of motion, strength, sensation, coordination, and physical tolerance. In many instances it is not practical to do a complete and specific evaluation of the patient's physical status at the time of initial interview. However, whether the individual functions within normal limits and where deficits exist should be recorded and then a complete evaluation can be accomplished as part of the overall treatment plan.

ENVIRONMENT. The family situation, including the patient's marital status, family members at or near the home, people who are with the patient during the day and night, and which family members are employed needs documentation. There should be a brief description of the home accessibility including whether it is in an urban or rural setting; type of structure; whether it is a house, apartment, upstairs flat, etc.; number of levels; number of steps between levels; number of stairs the patient utilizes in daily living; and the number of rooms. The patient's mode of transportation outside of the home also needs to be assessed. Is he or she a licensed driver? Does he or she use a bus or other forms of public transportation? Does he or she assist with driving, or do others have to drive?

SELF-CARE. During the initial assessment the present self-care status should be documented. Independence requires that the patient perform every aspect of that task without assistance. The occupational therapist should ask and record if the patient does or does not use adaptive equipment. The areas of self-care that should be considered are eating, dressing, toileting, washing, bathing, mouth care, shaving, hair care, make-up, and nail care.

COMMUNICATION. The interviewer should listen carefully to the patient's speech and determine whether impairment is present. If possible, a sample of the individual's writing should be obtained. The patient should be asked about past and present typing skills and the availability of a typewriter. Accessibility of and ability to use a phone at home and in the hospital should be determined as well as the type of phone used by the patient.

OCCUPATION/EDUCATION. Data should be gathered regarding former, present, and proposed occupations. Periods of employment, education or training, and job requirements and responsibilities should also be documented.

DAILY RESPONSIBILITIES AND ACTIVITIES. This should include home and/or job responsibilities, leisure time activities, amount of time the patient is active, daily routine, who is presently carrying out the patient's responsibilities, and if these people can be depended on to continue during the recovery of the individual.

PATIENT'S GOALS. The individual's long- and short-term goals need to be documented. Included should be the patient's understanding of the disability or disease, response to a brief description of the occupational therapy program, and attitude towards the occupational therapy program.

THERAPIST'S IMPRESSION. The potential benefit of treatment, presumed reliability of patient responses and interpretation of patient responses, should be recorded.

OCCUPATIONAL THERAPY PROGRAM PLAN. This section should state plans for specific evaluations, treatment objectives, treatment modalities, follow-up or referral considerations, and estimated duration of occupational therapy treatment.

EXAMPLES OF TREATMENT PROGRAMS

The assessment process is essentially the same for each referral received, but individual treatment plans are developed for each patient based on the information gathered. Certain aspects, however, are common within specific diagnostic categories.

A complete example of a treatment program is presented for myocardial infarction. Cardiac disease is the most common cause of death in the United States, and patients with this diagnosis are frequently treated in general hospitals. Some other examples of treatment plans and special services for patients with other problems are presented in less detail.

Myocardial Infarction

Myocardial infarction (M.I.) is an event that causes permanent heart damage. Tissue anoxia from occlusion of the arterial blood supply results in necrosis of muscle fibers in an area of myocardium. Eventually this shrinks and scars. The extent of functional impairment varies with the amount of damage, area of damage, length of time since the event, and patient cooperation during the acute and convalescent stages. Arrhythmia, valvular damage, thromboembolism, shock, pump failure, and anxiety states may contribute to prolonged recovery times.

The primary goal of the rehabilitation program for individuals with the diagnosis of recent acute myocardial infarction is to return the patient to maximum functional abilities by creating a therapeutic environment that not only promotes a healing of the damaged myocardium but also helps prevent any further insult to the heart. The objectives to be achieved in helping the patient reach this goal are (1) provision of a systematic approach to the advancement of activities throughout the patient's convalescence, (2) active participation by the patient and family in the cardiac rehabilitation program, (3) provision of an explanation to the patient of the disease process and its consequence for life style, and (4) provision of emotional and psychological support for the patient and family by all members of the team.

When dealing with an acute medical problem such as myocardial infarction, it is essential that the occupational therapist consult with the nursing staff and review the medical records daily to keep current on the patient's status. The occupational therapist must also consult with the physician to determine from a medical standpoint when the patient's activity level should be reduced, sustained, or upgraded.

After receiving a referral from a physician, reviewing the medical records and consulting with the nursing staff on the patient's condition that day, the occupational therapist should initiate the program by completing an initial assessment. With the data gathered from the physician, the nurse, the medical record and the interview form, the therapist will be ready to begin planning a treatment program.

Stages of the Treatment Process

Each stage of the treatment process involves four basic areas of daily living—self-care, mobility/ambulation, exercise, and other activities of daily living or recreation. The occupational therapist usually does not see the patient during the time of complete bedrest, which is considered stage one. Stages two, three, and four are defined by energy expenditure and the patient is progressed from one stage to the next after consultation with the primary physician.

STAGE ONE. An activity chart should be given to the individual during the first contact (see accompanying activity chart). The purpose and stages of the program are explained and appropriate initial activities are filled in by the therapist. The purpose of an activity chart is to demonstrate visually to the patient, family, and other staff the level of physical activity permitted. The activity program serves to maintain and increase physical tolerance, to prevent loss of muscle tone, to promote means of relaxation, to develop interests to replace previous more strenuous activities, and to aid in long-term rehabilitation and adjustment to convalescence.

STAGE TWO. At stage two, some of the self-care activities allowed are washing hands and face, feeding self in bed, fingernail care, brushing teeth, and feeding self in a chair with feet elevated. In the mobility/ambulation area the patient should be able to utilize a bedside commode with the cardiac method of transfer and start sitting with feet elevated in a chair twice a day for 20 minutes. After the therapist's observation to ascertain that the condition is stable, sitting can gradually be progressed to 60 minutes three times a day. Other activities allowed include listening to the radio, reading a book that is in a bookstand or otherwise supported, reading a newspaper or magazine, using the telephone for 3 to 5 minutes at a time with two or three calls a day, doing crossword puzzles, or writing short letters. When the patient tolerates this level of activity the therapist consults with the physician about advancing the patient to stage three.

STAGE THREE. During stage three, in the area of self-care, the individual should be able to bathe (except for the back and legs) in bed or seated near a sink, to shave with an electric razor, to comb short hair, and to dress and undress in bedclothes. Regarding mobility/ambulation, a patient should first be able to walk to the bathroom for toileting, progress to walking in the room three times a day, and then progress to walking in the room as desired. Other activities which can be incorporated during stage three are watching television while in bed and reading a newspaper. Light activities such as yarnwork, table games, or light crafts can also be initiated. When able to tolerate all stage three activities, the patient can progress to stage four, in consultation with the physician.

STAGE FOUR. During stage four, in the area of self-care, the individual should be independent in eating if seated in a chair and in dressing and undressing in street clothes. The patient may take a shower. The individual should be able to do some activities such as going to an occupational therapy clinic, a hospital beauty parlor or barber shop, or coffee shop. At this stage, ambulation includes walking in the hall at a slow pace of approximately two miles per hour or 44 feet in 15 seconds. This should be progressed until the patient is able to walk in the hall at three miles per hour or 66 feet in 15 seconds. Other acceptable activities would include getting items out of drawers and the closet, observing and participating in activity programs such as talking, singing, and light crafts, and sitting outside in warm weather. The individual should also be able to begin some stair climbing.

Criteria for stopping any activity or failure to progress an activity during patient monitoring include signs and symptoms of ischemia and/or undue fatigue, chest pain, shortness of breath, dizziness, diaphoresis, pallor, cyanosis, and nausea. Another sign of caution is incomplete recovery with symptoms of fatigue one hour after an activity has been completed. All changes need to be analyzed within the context of the situation or activity. In all cases of distress, consultation with the attending physician

CARDIAC REHABILITATION PROGRAM ACTIVITY CHART

Name: ____________________ Room: ____________________

Admission: ____________________ Date program started: ____________

Doctor: ____________________

Occupational Therapist: ____________________

○ Supervision needed ○ Can do without supervision ○ Activity no longer applies	1–1.5 Mets. Stage II	1.6–2.0 Mets. + U.E. Tension (Static) Stage III	2.1–3.0 Mets. Stage IV
Self-care	Wash hands and face ○ Feed self in bed ○ Fingernail care ○ Brush teeth ○ Feed self in chair with feet elevated ○	Bathe body in bed except back and legs ○ Shave self (seated, electric razor) ○ Comb hair (short) ○ Bathe body except back, seated at sink ○ Dress/undress in bedclothes ○	Eat in dining room in w/c. ○ Dress/undress in street clothes ○ Go to beauty parlor in w/c. ○ May take shower ○
Mobility	Bedside commode with assisted transfer ○ Chair rest with feet elevated: bid. 20 min. ○ bid. 30 min. tid. 20 min. *As tolerated . . . tid. 30 min. ○ tid. 45 min. ○ tid. 60 min. ○	Walk to bathroom for toileting ○ Progress to walking in room tid ○ Walk in room ad lib ○ Sit in chair ad lib ○	Walk in hall—slow pace 44 ft. ○ Walk in hall 44 ft. in 15 secs. (2 mph.) ○ Walk in hall 55 ft. in 15 sec. (2.5 mets.) (2.5 mph.) Walk in hall 66 ft. in 15 secs. (3.0 mets.) (3 mph.) ○
Exercise	Deep breathing every hour—5 deep breaths ○ Shoulders—1 arm at a time ○ Quad. setting—1 leg at a time ○ Hips and knees—1 leg at a time ○ Ankles and toes—1 leg at a time ○	Quad setting ○ Hips and knees ○ Straight leg raising—1 leg at a time ○	Straight leg raising ○ Trunk side bending ○ Trunk twisting ○
Other activities	Listen to radio ○ Read light weight book with bookstand or otherwise supported ○ Use of telephone 3–5 mins., 2–3 calls/day ○ Crossword puzzles ○ Write short letters ○	Watch T.V. in bed sitting ○ Read newspaper ○ Yarn activities ○ Table games and activities ○ Light craft activities ○	Get items out of drawers, closet. . . . ○ Observe, participate in recreation programs in w/c talking, singing, table games ○ Sit outside in warm weather, not in hot sun ○ Stair climbing ○

is required before either initiating or resuming activities. Observations and actions taken are to be noted on the medical record.

It is not in the purview of this section to go into detail in the field of telemetry and electrocardiogram monitoring. Therapists who work in facilities that now have telemetry as a part of cardiac monitoring during the treatment program have further guidelines and methods of evaluating when to stop an activity. Comparisons between a resting, baseline tracing and the most recent electrocardiogram strip on the medical chart may reveal significant differences, such as recently developed arrhythmias. A therapist who is employed in a work situation that has these tools available will need further in-service training and continuing education in the use of the telemetry, treadmill, electrocardiogram monitoring, and physical exercise programs. They are now being provided across the country by occupational therapists, physical therapists, physical educators, and others.

Environmental Evaluation

In addition to the activity program, the therapist and the cardiac patient will need to evaluate the patient's environment. If the patient is to be discharged some of the information needed is the physical structure of the home including accessibility of rooms and utilities, home accessibility from the outdoors, levels and locations of bathrooms and the patient's bedroom, and kitchen and work area locations and structures. The individual's primary home management responsibilities, the family members' responsibilities, child care responsibilities, and availability of outside help should also be assessed.

Further information on job requirements and duties needs to be obtained including the hours of work required; the physical demands of the job including sitting, walking, climbing, lifting; the individual's view of the mental demands or stress of the job; production rate and output on the job; and the patient's responsibility for others. Free time available from work also needs to be determined. This would include lunch time, coffee breaks, and if the patient can take extra time if needed during the day. The therapist should discuss what kinds of facilities are available at the place of employment such as elevators, restrooms, health facilities, and areas available for resting. The usual method of getting to and from work, the distance and travel time spent from home to work, and the distance and availability of a bus from the parking lot to the building entrance are additional considerations.

The other aspects of the patient's returning to work that need to be evaluated include the company's attitude towards part-time employment increments until an employee is able to resume full-time employment, the feasibility of a change of job within the company, and the policies of the company regarding sick leave, vacation, and retirement. All possible income such as sick pay, disability insurance, social security, other family members' salaries, and public assistance should be considered. Planning must take into account the attitude of the patient about returning to the same job, consideration of a job change, and willingness to work. Based on the information gathered, the therapist supplies the physician and the patient with recommendations about return to work, vocational (work) evaluation, retirement, employment opportunities that may be open to the individual, or referral to a vocational rehabilitation service. Many people are able to resume employment, but they usually are not ready until two to three months after the myocardial infarction. It is usually recommended that they begin work on a part-time basis.

Another treatment objective is a review of work simplification. This should relate to the individual's situation including home and vocational responsibilities and avocational interests.

Psychosocial Aspects

Consideration of the psychosocial problems is essential when dealing with a patient with myocardial infarction. The individual with myocardial infarction goes through the common stages of coping with illness, including disbelief, shock, denial, anxiety, anger, depression, and, finally acceptance and adaptation. The patient's mood may reflect boredom, restlessness, anger, depression, anxiety, and/or loneliness. Some of the goals of the cardiac rehabilitation program should be to decrease the patient's and family's fears through the process of education and to facilitate understanding of the disease/injury and what it is realistic to expect. The therapist should encourage the view that successful recovery from injury leads to a relatively normal and productive life. The patient and the family are able to observe concrete evidence of progress through the use of the activity chart which documents increased activity levels and increased strength and endurance without discomfort. It is important that the therapist maintain daily contacts to establish rapport and allow maximum opportunity for discussion of the myocardial infarction risk factors, the roles of activity, stress, limitation of activities, relationships, return to work, signs and symptoms of fatigue, and ischemia. By the time of discharge the patient and family should have a clear understanding of these factors and should be reassured about a safe return home.

Prior to the patient's discharge, a home program should be developed in conjunction with the physician and the other team members. Included here is an example of a basic home program that was developed by the occupational therapist and the clinical nurse specialist in cardiology and reviewed by the physician. In some facilities a dietician, social worker, and other professionals may be part of the home care team. Even though there are some basic premises for preparing home programs, each program must be developed for an individual patient on a personal basis and must be reviewed with the patient and family before discharge. Telephone contact with the patient one to two weeks after discharge to check on his or her functional status and answer any questions that have arisen is also helpful.

AN INTERVIEW

Ronald, a forty-nine-year-old male, was admitted through the emergency room with sudden onset of gripping chest pain radiating to the medial aspect of his left arm and the left side of his jaw. The pain lasted for forty-five minutes. He had no history of angina, shortness of breath, or diaphoresis. His diagnosis was an anterior myocardial infarction (M.I.). This is a brief interview with him one month later.

"What can you tell me about yourself?" "Well, I'm an automotive engineer with a large automobile company. My wife and I have four children—two are married, one is away at college, and my fourteen-year-old son, Joe, is living at home. As you know, I've recently had a heart attack and have had to be at home on a limited activity program."

"How do you feel about your activity program?" "I was very upset at the beginning. I didn't believe I had had a heart attack and really could see no purpose for a cardiac rehabilitation program. The doctor, nurse, and therapist took the time to explain what had happened to me and what was necessary for me and my family to do to get me back to work and really live again. The therapist started by putting an activity chart on my bedside stand so I could see what I was allowed to do while I was in the hospital. Before I went home I was given a home program by the occupational therapist and the nurse."

"How is the home program going?" "Well, it does help me set limits on myself and at the same time keep working on the things I'm allowed to do. I believe I'm beginning to understand that if I want to return to my job I have to follow the program to give my heart a chance to heal."

RONALD'S HOME PROGRAM

I. First week at home (approximately fourth week after M.I.)
   A. Self-care
      1. Eating—May eat three meals at the kitchen table, with family members present.
      2. Bathing—May use shower or bathtub. Use lukewarm water and have all necessary articles nearby.
      3. Dressing—May dress self; wear comfortable, loose-fitting clothes.
      4. Grooming—All activities allowed.
      5. Hair care—Have wife or son wash your hair while you are seated in a chair.
   B. Ambulation
      1. Walking—Walk inside for the first week at home. May walk on main level and between rooms as desired. In addition, you should walk 75 ft. to 100 ft. this week.
      2. Sitting in chair—As tolerated.
         a. Never sit for more than one hour without getting up for a short walk.
         b. When possible elevate your legs while sitting and do not cross legs.
   C. Rest
      1. Rest at least one hour after each meal. This may be done in a chair with your legs elevated.
      2. Rest quietly or nap for at least one hour in the late afternoon.
   D. Activities
      1. Visiting—Limit visitors to family and close friends. Do not allow visitors to interfere with scheduled rest periods.
      2. Car rides—Do not take trips in the car for the first week.
      3. Meal preparation—Once cooking utensils are placed on stove, counter, or table you can prepare one meal a day. Do not move, lift, or carry pots and pans or food to the table.
      4. Housework—Do not participate in general household tasks or yardwork for this week.
      5. Sexual activity—Not generally permitted until the sixth week.

6. Other activities
   a. May continue any projects begun in the hospital.
   b. May do table top activities for one hour three times a day, such as cards, puzzles, models, drafting, or painting.

II. Second week at home (fifth week after M.I.)
   A. Self-care—unrestricted
   B. Ambulation
      1. Walking
         a. May walk 100 ft. to 200 ft. daily, gradually increasing amount over the week. If symptoms of fatigue, chest pain, shortness of breath, or dizziness occur, cut back to first week's level.
         b. Avoid stairs and any steep inclines in walking.
         c. May sit on porch if outside temperature is 40°F. (near 5°C.) or warmer.
   C. Rest
      1. Continue resting after meals for one hour.
   D. Other activities
      1. Rides in car—May go for rides in car as a passenger three times this week. Rides cannot exceed one hour.
      2. Visiting—Same as first week.
      3. Meal preparation—May prepare two meals a day this week. Must not lift or carry food, pots, or pans. Sit at table to work when possible.
      4. Household—May wash dishes, if already placed in sink. Do not wash pots and pans. This should not be done until after resting one hour after eating. May put dishes and silverware away if not more than two plates are lifted at a time. May dust. May assist in cutting and preparing vegetables if seated. May assist in household plant care if seated.
      5. Other activities—Can work a total of 4 hr. daily, spread throughout the day. Continue previous activities. May also begin assembling light wood projects (no sawing). Allowed essential business conferences, provided they are not too numerous (one per day), protracted, or associated with tension.

After completion of these two weeks a routine visit to your physician is indicated. Based on the physician's findings concerning your general progress additions to your rehabilitation program will be made.

Swallowing Program for Dysphagic Adults

A swallowing program is done in close cooperation with the medical, nursing, and dietary staffs, the patient, and the patient's family. The occupational therapist, prior to involvement in a dysphagia program, must review the anatomy and physiology of the complex swallowing mechanism, including the specific volitional and reflexive components. The occupational therapist must understand the nerves that affect swallowing, musculature action, and what signs and symptoms may be present.

Swallowing impairment often results from acoustic neuroma, brain stem tumors, radical neck surgery, laryngectomy, long-term tracheostomy, multiple sclerosis, myasthenia gravis or other progressive neurological diseases, cerebral vascular accidents, and Guillain-Barré syndrome. In developing a program for persons with swallowing problems, the therapist should complete an initial assessment as presented earlier, obtaining a general history of the patient, including specific facts related to the swallowing problems. There needs to be an evaluation of the peripheral speech and swallowing mechanisms, including resistance to mouth opening, jaw deviation, tongue deviation, strength of the tongue on protrusion and retraction, soft palate function, and laryngeal closure.

Prerequisites for Treatment

Before implementing a swallowing program, there are several prerequisites. The first is that the patient must be mentally alert and able to follow instructions, carry them over from day to day, and concentrate on the task well enough to support a reflex behavior. Secondly, the physiological potential to swallow must be ascertained from the evaluation. Lastly, a gag reflex must be present.

If a patient has little or no gag reflex unilaterally or bilaterally, a stimulation program needs to be attempted before food is introduced. In addition, tongue mobility and good laryngeal closure should then be established through tongue exercises and stimulation to ensure propulsion of food through the mouth to the esophageal opening.

Treatment Program

Exercises to strengthen the mechanical swallowing abilities of the patient include exercises for tongue lateralization, tongue elevation, tongue retraction, strengthening the cheeks and lips, chewing, swallowing, and gag reflex. Facilitation with pressure, vibration, and ice might be used along with the exercises.

The precautions in implementing a swallowing program for a patient include awareness of aspiration, including choking and gagging on foods and liquids; observation for food coming out of the mouth, tracheostomy, or nose; and daily checking of the patient's weight, hydration, and intake and output to make sure the patient is receiving enough nourishment.

When the patient is ready to attempt oral feeding several things are important to consider in the diet selection. Select the diet keeping in mind the other methods by which the patient may be receiving nutrition or hydration (I.V., nasogastric, or other tube feedings), the therapist's evaluation results, and the patient's food preference. Specific foods are selected to provide the patient the most sensory feedback possible to enhance the volitional and reflexive components. Considerations are (1) food with low specific gravity such as liquids or purees does not excite pressor receptors in the mouth or, more importantly, the soft palate and has the tendency to leak into the trachea; (2) casein in milk products thickens mucous secretions thereby decreasing sensation; (3) pureed food may not have an aroma and often tastes bitter; (4) sweet food decreases saliva and, (5) sour food facilitates swallowing.

The patient must trust the therapist in order to comply with the program. There are numerous emotional ramifications resulting from the inability to eat and the necessity for relearning the process. It is usually an unpleasant experience; it is uncomfortable and can be painful. The patient is often embarrassed because he or she may be sloppy. The emotional support provided by having a confident therapist present during meals can be the most important treatment offered.

When oral food swallowing is initiated the nasogastric tube should be removed, if possible, since it depresses the gag reflex, irritates the mucous membranes, and increases secretions. It also prevents tight closure of the nasopharynx passages. Intravenous fluids are usually continued since this prevents dehydration in the patient. The patient should sit in a chair at ninety degrees; the neck should be slightly flexed and the body tilted forward during the meal and for one hour afterwards. The food should be placed in the mouth at the point where the patient will get the most sensory feedback for the taste, pressure, and temperature of the food. The patient should be started slowly with small amounts of food.

Preferably the patient is fed small portions five times a day rather than large portions three times a day. The patient needs to be supervised by the occupational therapist initially with each meal and can then be followed by the nursing staff, if instructed properly by the therapist. The ultimate goal is for the therapist to instruct the patient and family in the swallowing program well enough to allow them to continue the program until independence is reached.

By following a program of evaluation, therapeutic exercises, and treatment, the majority of patients do note improvement and some have complete resolution of their swallowing problem.

Role of the Occupational Therapist in Death and Dying

The occupational therapist has a unique background in physical, psychosocial, and occupational performance needs. Integration of this knowledge gives the therapist the ability to see a person as a human being rather than a disease process. Therefore, an occupational therapy service program for individuals who are dying can provide psychological support and active participation within the patient's capabilities. The activity provided should be in concert with the patient's goals and physical and mental capabilities and should provide a feeling of self-worth and productivity.

The therapist must be secure in his or her own attitude towards death and dying. The therapist must be able to listen, hear, understand, be sensitive to, and be able to respond verbally or nonverbally to spoken and unspoken requests. The ability to recognize when a patient needs you and being willing to take the time regardless of personal or professional schedules is essential. It is usually recognized that the sicker and closer to death the patient is the less personal attention he or she receives from the hospital staff. The patient continues to receive good medical and nursing care but less love. It is an occupational therapist's responsibility to be sensitive, to be aware, to provide meaningful activities, and to care.

Death and Dying

CASE SUMMARY

Ada was a thirty-six-year-old mother of eight children with a diagnosis of acute leukemia. Her family could only visit on weekends because she lived 100 miles from the hospital. She was referred to occupational therapy with the problem of reduced energy level and was instructed in work simplification and home management techniques. The therapist also worked with Ada and her family to set up a household routine that provided built-in rest periods so she could continue to be independent and function as a wife and mother. Because of her husband's request Ada was not told her diagnosis.

Two weeks after discharge the therapist called Ada to find out if the home management plan was functioning. Ada and her husband were satisfied with the program and the household was running smoothly. Follow-up contacts after six months and one year were made and the family was still managing well.

At the age of thirty eight, Ada was readmitted to the hospital since the disease process had progressed rapidly. It was then determined that she only had a few weeks to live. She was again referred to occupational therapy for supportive care. One of Ada's goals was to make individual items of similar quality for each of her eight children, which would last as a remembrance and a reminder that she loved them. The therapist helped Ada select items within her capabilities and which Ada enjoyed doing. They were graded from the first project, which was the most difficult, to the last item which required less strength and was less complicated. The grading of the activities was necessary because she was expected to decline in awareness and physical capability.

The last item that Ada was making was a ceramic piggy bank which required several coats of one-color glaze. On the final day she was in bed with intravenous fluids running and was alert for only one or two minutes at a time. During these intervals she still wanted to complete the project. The therapist had to help hold the brush in Ada's hand in order to finish. She and the therapist completed the glazing at 2 p.m. The therapist returned at 4:30 the same afternoon and told Ada that the piggy bank would be fired and ready the next day. No one else was in Ada's room. Her family had been notified of the severity of her condition and were on the way to see her.

Ada asked the therapist to stay with her and hold her hand. During the remaining few hours Ada was awake and alert only a few minutes at a time. She talked about her family and was told by the therapist that they were coming. She was concerned and was reassured by the therapist that she had completed all the projects and that each child would receive the presents she had made. What Ada wanted most was contact with a caring human being who would be with her at the end. Ada's respirations ceased at 6:30.

Cancer

The term "cancer" is used by the public to refer to a myriad of separate diseases with a common bond. They all begin with a disorderly growth of cells in a malignant neoplasm. The autonomous growth of abnormal tissue invades or replaces normal tissue. It can also spread to distant sites, and this is termed "metastasis."

The location, rate of growth, spread of growth, and amount of interference with function determine the pathological effects of the disease. It often strikes in middle age although no extreme of age is unaffected. Causative factors have been identified but the process remains incompletely understood. The means of slowing, arresting, or curing the disease include surgery, chemotherapy, and radiation. These can result in amputation, seriously altered ways of functioning, change in self-image, adjustment of lifestyle, and varying states of well being.

Occupational Therapy for Patients with Radical Mastectomy

A referral to occupational therapy should be obtained from the physician as soon as possible after admission or after surgery. Occupational therapy services for the woman having a radical mastectomy are designed to help prevent problems of decreased shoulder range of motion and edema, to provide education through discussion, to demonstrate available adaptive equipment such as bras, prostheses, clothing including bathing suits, and cosmetics to obscure scars. The therapist should provide activities that are therapeutic, explain which activities are contraindicated postoperatively and facilitate the patient's psychological acceptance of her amputation and her return to the family. Physical activity usually does not begin until four to ten days postsurgery on consultation with the patient's physician. The specific objectives are based on the problems the patient presents with due consideration of any other complicating problems such as decreased strength, obesity, and hemiplegia. There should be a review of household work simplification, work simplification, and activities beneficial to the patient.

In coordination with the social service department, psychological support for the individual and the family should be offered. There are some community agencies that can be very helpful to the woman with a mastectomy, such as the Reach for Recovery Program of the American Cancer Society. The patient should be referred if appropriate. Following discharge from the hospital there should be a review and reinforcement of material presented during hospitalization and outpatient treatment if necessary.

Diabetes Mellitus

In diabetes mellitus, blood sugar becomes elevated as a result of a deficiency of insulin. There are other associated metabolic variations and vascular changes. The disease is controlled by stimulation of insulin production with oral medication, lessening insulin requirements by diet or weight loss or with the administration of insulin. Balance must be achieved between available insulin, intake of food, and consumtion of energy in activities. Long-standing diabetes may lead to decreased vision from retinal vessel disease, kidney lesions with failure, neuropathies, arteriosclerosis, and peripheral vascular disease causing gangrene and perhaps damage severe enough to require amputation.

There are four primary objectives for occupational therapists when working with a patient admitted to the hospital with diabetes. They are (1) providing regulated activity to assist in insulin regulation, coordinating normal home activity with hospital routines, (2) providing an environment to allow the individual to demonstrate knowledge of diet regulation, (3) evaluating and teaching compensatory skills when the patient has lost function as a result of associated complications resulting in visual loss, sensory loss, or amputation, and (4) providing psychological support.

Following the initial interview of the patient, the therapist needs to evaluate the home and work routine and to calculate the calories expended by the individual on a normal day. The treatment program then focuses on providing activities to simulate home calorie expenditure during the hospitalization. Specifically these may include self-care, activities of daily living, recreation, avocational interests, walking, climbing stairs, exercises, or real work experiences such as collating, typing, filing, or woodworking. By providing the regulated activity program, the physician and dietician will have a better basis for insulin and diet regulation.

The role of the occupational therapist in diet regulation is to evaluate the previous dietary regime and the patient's level of responsibility for it by talking to the dietician, patient, and patient's family. The therapist would then provide the patient with an opportunity to apply dietary knowledge by planning and preparing a snack and/or a meal. The treatment plan may provide for therapeutic trips to stores and/or restaurants which will help determine the individual's ability to maintain the diet independently.

The patient also needs a supportive milieu in which to express feelings about diabetes mellitus and achieve realistic acceptance of it. The therapist should be able to help minimize malingering by provision of an activity program and simulated home management responsibilities. Close coordination and a team approach with the physician, nurse, dietician, patient, family, and occupational therapist is essential.

A program for an individual with complications or decreased function focuses on necessary compensatory skills. The program could include additional goals in ADL skills, communication, amputee training, or work simplification. Referral to appropriate community agencies, rehabilitation centers, or other health care systems may be needed.

Chronic Obstructive Pulmonary Disease

Patients with chronic obstructive pulmonary disease (C.O.P.D.) have difficulty moving air in and out of their lungs because airways are narrowed by spasms, secretions, or loss of elasticity of lung tissue, which allows air to be trapped in the lungs. Chronic obstructive pulmonary disease results from emphysema, chronic bronchitis, bronchiectasis, diseases that cause pulmonary fibrosis or cardiac disease. Symptoms include decreased physical tolerance, shortness of breath, cough with production of sputum, chest pain, hemoptysis, and noisy respirations.

Four primary objectives for occupational therapists when treating patients admitted to the hospital for chronic obstructive pulmonary disease are

(1) evaluating and teaching compensatory skills for loss of physical tolerance including work simplification and energy conservation, (2) exploration of job responsibilities and vocational (work) evaluation to decrease occupational exposure to dust and toxins, (3) provision of graded activity programs, and (4) psychological support.

The initial interview should provide the occupational therapist with information for development of treatment plans. The plans must be individualized to facilitate as normal function as is physically possible. By providing a regulated activity program the occupational therapist provides the physician with a better baseline for the regulation of medicines. The occupational therapist may work in conjunction with the physical therapist and the respiratory therapist in the development of a breathing exercise program.

SPECIAL TREATMENT PROCEDURES

Therapeutic Trip

The therapeutic trip is a community outing in which the occupational therapist and patient go outside the confines of the hospital. The purpose of a therapeutic trip is to provide the patient with practical experience while the therapist evaluates and instructs the individual in regards to the following:

1. Architectural barriers.
2. Application of previously learned skills such as transfers or handling of money.
3. Ability to assume responsibility such as obtaining from the physician a "leave on pass" order, gathering any necessary equipment, and donning appropriate clothing.
4. Ability to organize and plan, such as allowing adequate time for the event, making transportation arrangements, and obtaining equipment needed.
5. Ability to problem solve and be flexible.
6. Ability to interact practically and comfortably with the public.
7. Ability to manage a wheelchair, crutches, walker, or cane.
8. Judgment about safety factors and when to seek help.
9. Dependence/independence of patient in all areas including the initiation and carrying through of plans.

Prior to a therapeutic trip the above objectives and methods of achieving them are discussed with the patient. Prior to, during, and following the trip the patient is expected to assume as much responsibility as possible. Following the trip the patient and staff member should assess the patient's functioning and problem areas. Follow-up treatment programs and services are based on the outcomes of the therapeutic trip as assessed by the therapist and patient.

Home Assessment

If the patient or therapist foresees problems in the patient's return to home from the general hospital, the therapist should arrange to do a home assessment before the planned discharge. Ideally, the therapist should arrange for the patient and the other members of the household to be present in the home during the assessment.

If possible, treatment and evaluation of performance should be completed prior to the home visit. The purpose of the home assessment is to see if barriers in the home environment will conflict with performance. By doing the home assessment before discharge the therapist can make realistic recommendations to the patient and implement further treatment goals to ease the transition from the hospital to the home. The therapist can also determine whether further services are needed on an inpatient or outpatient basis, whether a referral to a home care program is necessary, or whether discharge to another type of facility is indicated.

The home assessment can be fairly standardized and often a form or questionnarie is helpful. All rooms and hallways that the patient will utilize need to be evaluated for maneuverability regarding carpeting, mobility on surfaces, adequate turning radius, furniture placement, and presence of throw rugs. The location, height, and ease of operation of plugs and switches needs to be noted as well as the presence of adequate lighting. Threshold, direction of door's opening, ability to operate knobs and locks, and door width need to be considered. The location, heights, and capability of moving of furniture must be recorded. In regard to stairs, the height, number of flights, presence of rails (including sturdiness and whether they are on one side or both), and frequency of their use need to be documented. Specific observations necessary for various areas of the home are listed in the accompanying home assessment report.

OCCUPATIONAL THERAPY HOME ASSESSMENT REPORT

Patient's Name
Address
Telephone Number

Date:

People who participated:
Number of levels:
Which rooms on each level:

	ACCESSIBLE ADEQUATE	NON-ACCESSIBLE INADEQUATE	RECOMMENDATIONS AND/OR CORRECTIONS NEEDED
OUTDOORS			
1. Terrain			inclines, mobility on varying surfaces
2. Porch/Patio/Balcony			
a. Stairs			railing; size; number; height
b. Doors/Doorways			threshold; direction of opening; operate knobs and locks; width
c. Maneuverability			furniture; carpeting; mobility on surfaces; adequate turning radius; throw rugs
d. Furniture			location; height; transfers
e. Plugs/Switches			location; height; ease of operation
3. Parking/Garage			distance to entrance; incline
4. Compliance with City Ordinances			ramping; exits; fire codes; building permits
5. Entrances—Front Side/Back			steps; railings; surfaces; direction of opening threshold; operate knobs and locks; width
HALLWAYS			
1. Maneuverability			as above
2. Plugs/Switches			as above
LIVING ROOM/DINING ROOM			
1. Doors/Doorways			as above
2. Maneuverability			as above
3. Furniture			as above
4. Plugs/Switches			as above
5. Lighting			amount location
KITCHEN			
1. Doors/Doorways			as above
2. Maneuverability			as above
3. Stove/Burners			operation and visibility of controls; location; gas/electric
4. Oven			operation and visibility of controls; open/close door; operate broiler; height; pull out/in oven rack
5. Refrigerator/Freezer			height of handle and shelves; depth; open/close doors
6. Dishwasher			loading/unloading; operate controls; portable/built in; detergent
7. Sink			garbage disposal; direction of approach; manage faucets; height; depth; countertop space; stopper
8. Plugs/Switches			as above
9. Storage			ability to reach; handles; organization; adequate amount
10. Working Surfaces			countertop heights; depth; direction of approach
11. Transportation of Items			distances; continuous surfaces for sliding objects; wheeled cart; lapboard; walker apron
12. Small Appliances			location; operation; work saving
13. Furniture			as above

(Continued)

OCCUPATIONAL THERAPY HOME ASSESSMENT REPORT (*Continued*)

	ACCESSIBLE ADEQUATE	NON-ACCESSIBLE INADEQUATE	RECOMMENDATIONS AND/OR CORRECTIONS NEEDED
BATHROOM			
1. Doors/Doorways			as above
2. Stairs			as above
3. Maneuverability			as above
4. Sink/Countertop Space			as above
5. Tub/Shower			manage faucets; nonskid surfaces; height; transfer; need for grab bar and/or chair
6. Toilet			need for grab bars; location of toilet paper; height; operate lever; direction of approach; transfers
7. Plugs/Switches			as above
8. Mirror			height; location
9. Medicine Cabinet			height; location; open/close door
BEDROOM			
1. Stairs			as above
2. Doors/Doorways			as above
3. Maneuverability			as above
4. Closets			direction of approach; height of rod and shelves; open/close door
5. Dresser			height; location; open/close drawers
6. Furniture (Bed/Chair)			location; heights, transfers
7. Plugs/Switches			as above
8. Lighting			as above
BASEMENT/REC. ROOM			(evaluate if use is necessary or desired)
1. Stairs/Lighting/Railing			as above
2. Doors/Doorways			as above
3. Maneuverability			as above
4. Plugs/Switches			as above
5. Furniture			as above
COMMUNICATION SYSTEMS			
1. To contact others outside home			telephone (emergency numbers easily visible, location, type, operation); signal in window; warning light
2. To contact those within home			intercom; buzzer system; bell
CLEANING			
1. Laundry Facilities			washer/dryer; location; load/unload; operate controls; detergent
2. Supply Storage			ability to reach; handles; organization; adequate amount
3. Use of Equipment			open/close containers of cleaning equipment; vacuum; mop; dustpan; broom
4. Garbage Removal			location; city ordinances; secure and tie bag; transport; use of other person
USE OF COMMUNITY RESOURCES			
1. Transportation			public (cab, bus, train); personal
2. Shopping Facilities			distance; type (mall, street); restroom facilities; use of other persons; phoning orders; architectural barriers
3. Social and Recreational Facilities			distance; architectural barriers; restroom facilities (church, parks, clubs, theaters)
4. Medical Facilities			distance; architectural barriers; restroom facilities; emergency arrangements; transportation

OCCUPATIONAL THERAPY HOME ASSESSMENT REPORT (*Continued*)

	ACCESSIBLE ADEQUATE	NON-ACCESSIBLE INADEQUATE	RECOMMENDATIONS AND/OR CORRECTIONS NEEDED
ADDITIONAL CONSIDERATIONS			
1. Other Rooms			frequency of use; accessibility; need for cleaning
2. Windows			height; location; open/close; lock; shades/curtains
3. Thermostat			location; height; operation and visibility of controls
4. Precautions when patient is alone			communication system; adequate food, water, medication bowel/bladder care
5. Pursuit of Avocational interests			location of supplies; adequate space
6. Yardwork and Repairs			use of other persons; storage; use of equipment

SUMMARY AND RECOMMENDATIONS: Briefly summarize; include persons responsible for carrying out recommendations, if possible; suggested follow-up

Date of Visit: ______________

Length of Visit: ______________

Signature: ______________

SUMMARY

The variety of problems that an occupational therapist encounters through referrals, evaluation, and treatment in a general hospital is limited only by the therapist's skills, knowledge, and ability to problem solve. Some additional diagnoses that might be encountered and guidelines for approaching patients suffering from them are listed in Table 16-1. The functional goal for each patient is to be as independent as possible.

The patient's problems can be as simple as an inability to open jars or as complex as adjusting to life in a wheelchair, learning about adaptive equipment, and discovering new methods of accomplishing daily life tasks. This chapter is just a beginning. To be a good occupational therapist one must con-

Table 16-1. Problems encountered with guidelines for solving.

Diagnosis	*Common problems encountered*	*Occupational therapy services rendered*
Parkinson's disease	Muscular weakness Tremors Extreme rigidity	Activities of daily living Therapeutic activities to increase coordination, range of motion, and muscle strength Work simplification
Rheumatic heart disease	Decreased physical tolerance Poor cardiac reserve	Work simplification Energy conservation Graded activity program

(*Continued*)

Table 16-1. Problems encountered with guidelines for solving. (*Continued*)

Diagnosis	*Common problems encountered*	*Occupational therapy services rendered*
Scleroderma and other collagen diseases	Excessive fatigue Limited range of motion Decreased muscle strength	Therapeutic activities to maintain and/or increase range of motion and muscle strength Physical tolerance programs Activities of daily living Splinting Psychological support
Blood dyscrasias	Excessive fatigue	Work simplification Energy conservation Graded physical tolerance program
Renal insufficiency	Dependency on artificial dialysis Limited energy Variety of neurological manifestations Limited work potential	Hospital and home program to help maintain a balance of fluids and body chemistry by medication, activity, and diet Graded physical tolerance program Vocational (work) evaluation Avocational pursuits Activities of daily living
Hip fracture	Self-care problems, especially reaching, transfers, and lower extremity dressing Household management Nonoperative fracture treated by bed-rest and/or traction	Self-care evaluation and treatment Avocational program Work simplification Physical tolerance program
Hemophilia	Hemorrhage into joints causing limited range of motion	Activities to maintain and/or increase range of motion Vocational (work) evaluation Static splinting to prevent contracture or deformity Self-care evaluation and treatment
Obesity	Limited reach Poor cardiac reserve Poor self-concept Lack of appropriate work skills	Graded physical activity program Self-care evaluation and treatment Activity assimilation program Vocational (work) evaluation Behavior modification
Low back pain	Pain-medication cycle Inability to carry out life tasks	Work simplification with emphasis on proper methods for lifting and carrying Activity assimilation program Psychological support Behavior modification Vocational (work) evaluation
Thoracic surgery—cardiac	Decreased physical tolerance Unable to carry out home management tasks Employment concerns Fear of surgery	Work simplification Energy conservation Graded activity program Psychological support Vocational (work) evaluation
Psychosomatic illness	Inability to function in daily life tasks	Behavior modification program Psychological intervention Avocational pursuits Energy expenditure programs

tinue to acquire and apply new knowledge and skills throughout one's career.

ACKNOWLEDGMENTS

With special acknowledgments to Barbara Bly, O.T.R., Betty Cox, C.O.T.A., and Carolyn Creighton, M.D., and thanks to Ann Fish, O.T.R., Anne Hull, O.T.R., Leslie Kamil-Miller, O.T.R., Julie Smith, O.T.R., Ann Woodman, O.T.R., and the entire occupational therapy staff at the University of Michigan Hospital.

BIBLIOGRAPHY

Banus, B. S.: The Developmental Therapist. Thorofare NJ: Charles C. Slack, 1971.

Beeson, P. B., and McDermott, W. (eds.): Textbook of Medicine, ed. 14. Philadelphia: W. B. Saunders Co., 1975.

Berzins, G. F.: Occupational therapy program for the chronic obstructive pulmonary disease patient. Am. J. Occup. Ther. 24:181, 1970.

Bockus, H. L.: Dysphagia. In Gastroenterology, ed. 2. Philadelphia: W. B. Saunders Co., 1963, Volume I, Chapter 3, pp. 54–59.

Burnside, I. M.: Touching is talking. Am. J. Nurs. 73:2060–2063, 1973.

Creighton, C. A., et al.: Who helps the diabetic? New Physician, April 1973.

Doty, R. W.: Neural organization of deglutition. In Code, C. F. (ed.): Handbook of Physiology. American Physiological Society, Washington DC, 1968, Section 6, Volume IV, pp. 1861–1902.

Dysphagia and Heartburn. In Harvey, A. M. (ed.): The Principles and Practice of Medicine, ed. 18. New York: Appleton-Century-Crofts, 1972, Section IX, Chapter 65, pp. 687–694.

Ellis, H.: Dysphagia. In Hart, F. D. (ed.): French's Index of Differential Diagnosis, ed. 10. Baltimore: Williams & Wilkins, 1973, pp. 217–221.

Exercise Testing and Training of Apparently Healthy Individuals: A Handbook for Physicians. New York: American Heart Association, 1972.

Farber, S. D.: Sensorimotor Evaluation and Treatment Procedures for Allied Health Personnel, ed. 2. Indianapolis: Indiana University Press, 1974, Chapter IV, pp. 53–67.

Gambescia, R. A., and Rogers, A. I.: Gastroenterology, dysphagia, diagnosis by history. Postgrad. Med. 59:211–216, 1976.

Griffin, K. M.: Swallowing training for dysphagic patients. Arch. Phys. Med. Rehabil. 55:467–470, 1974.

Handbook on Third-Party Reimbursement for Occupational Therapy Services. American Occupational Therapy Association, Inc., Rockville MD, October 1976.

Hays, et al.: Guidelines for Interpretation of Occupational Therapy in General Practice and Rehabilitation. Michigan Occupational Therapy Association, January 1970.

Huss, A. J.: Touch with care or a caring touch? 1976 Eleanor Clarke Slagle Lecture. Am. J. Occup. Ther. 31:1977.

Krusen, F. H., et al.: Handbook of Physical Medicine and Rehabilitation, ed. 2. Philadelphia: W. B. Saunders Co., 1971.

Kubler-Ross, E.: On Death and Dying. New York: Macmillan, 1971.

Larsen, G. L.: Conservative management for incomplete dysphagia paralytica. Arch. Phys. Med. Rehabil. 54: 180–185, 1973.

Larsen, G. L.: Rehabilitating dysphagia mechanica, paralytica, pseudobulbar. J. Neurosurg. Nurs. 8:14–17, 1976.

McCorkle, R.: Effects of touch on seriously ill patients. Nurs. Research 23:125–132, 1974.

Morse, R. L.: Exercise and the Heart. Springfield IL: Charles C Thomas, 1972.

Phillips, M. M., and Hendrix, T. R.: Dysphagia. Postgrad. Med. 50:81–86, 1971.

Pomerantz, et al.: Occupational therapy for chronic obstructive lung disease. Am. J. Occup. Ther. 29:1975.

Preston, T.: When words fail. Am. J. Nurs. 73:2064, 1973.

Semple, T., et al. (eds.): Myocardial Infarction, How to Prevent, How To Rehabilitate. International Society of Cardiology, 1973.

The American Heart Association Cookbook. New York: David McKay Co., 1973.

Wenger, N. K.: Coronary Care: Rehabilitation after Myocardial Infarction. New York: American Heart Association, 1973.

Wright, I. S., and Fredrickson, D. T.: Cardiovascular Diseases—Guidelines for Prevention and Care. The Inter-Society Commission for Heart Resources, Bethesda MD, 1973.

17

Gerontology

Linda A. Johnson

Although awareness of aging and the special needs of the elderly has been a vital part of the concern of cultures for many centuries, the scientific investigation of the aging process and study of the social consequences of aging populations are to a great extent post World War II phenomena. The definition of "gerontology" is literally the study of later maturity and old age in its biological, psychological, and sociological aspects. The term "gerontologist" is applied to those educators and researchers who study problems of aging as they are currently manifested.

Individuals in professions such as occupational therapy who deal primarily with the elderly in their practice are usually only called "gerontologists" when they also deal in research on problems of aging which they encounter among their clients. Occupational therapists have traditionally used the term "geriatrics" to describe this phase of practice; however, geriatrics refers specifically to the physiology and pathology of old age. There is considerable evidence, with the broader concept of this field, to support the use of gerontology as the descriptive word for this practice area rather than geriatrics.

Occupational therapists operate using the medical model but go beyond the classic model in stressing the normalization process. Within this process, accepting necessary limitations of chronic disability, the therapist's role is that of a facilitator who enables the individual to make decisions on goals, assures awareness of realistic alternatives, and assists in achievement of goals. Each old person has his or her own readiness to capitulate to disability. Given the same degree of disability, some would choose independence to whatever degree it is possible, and others would prefer the security of a protective environment.

Insofar as therapists are able with their clients to achieve realization of this concept basic to occupational therapy theory, they must work within current gerontological theory and public policy. Occupational therapists, by seeking individualized solutions to problems encountered, can make a unique contribution to the field of gerontology. Contrary to other disciplines which develop theories describing what they see going on in society,[1] occupational therapists deal with individuals, enabling them to make choices. There is a real question as to whether the former approach does not, by its very nature, deal in self-fulfilling prophecy, predetermining the results of intervention, whereas the latter approach allows intervention to be flexible based on individual needs, choices, and possible solutions to problems.

THEORIES OF AGING

Sociologists, psychologists, and biologists have produced theories to explain what they see as phenomena of later adulthood and old age. An understanding of these theories is helpful in understanding both the basis of public policy and the rationale behind much research in gerontology. Some of the major theories are touched on in this section.

Sociology

The *disengagement theory of aging* was one of the first theories developed by sociologists and has been a center of controversy ever since.[2] It states that there is a gradual, mutual withdrawal or disengagement of the individual and society from each other, and that this is a natural and inevitable process which continues until the final withdrawal into death. This theory has been repeatedly questioned and challenged by gerontologists.

The *continuity theory*[3] is based on the assumption that identity is a function of relations and interactions with other people. Individuals who are most successful continue to maintain interaction with society after retirement, involving themselves in appropriate community, family, and interpersonal relationships. They continue to maintain both identity and ego strength.

The *activity theory*[4] is closely related to the continuity theory, and, with that theory, is accepted increasingly as research supplies more supporting evidence. It suggests that the majority of aging persons maintain fairly constant levels of activity and engagement with society and that the amount of engagement or disengagement is more influenced by past life-style and socioeconomic forces than by any inevitable biological or psychological force within either society or the individual. It proposes that maintaining or developing substantial levels of physical, mental, and social activity contributes to successful aging.

Psychology

The *psychoanalytic view*[5] states that the sense of identity established in early life produces consistent behavior throughout life, that character structure becomes relatively fixed in early adulthood, and that, even though the ego becomes an increasingly strong change agent, the essential nature of the personality remains stable. Jung and Erikson took exception to this theory. Jung described the increase in introversion in middle and late life, and the reorganization of value systems. Erikson outlined eight stages of ego development, each representing a crisis or choice for ego development. Erikson's eight stages of development[6] are:

1. Development in the infant of a sense of trust versus distrust.
2. Development in later infancy of a growing sense of autonomy versus a sense of shame and doubt.
3. Development in early childhood of a sense of initiative versus a sense of guilt.
4. Development in middle childhood of a sense of industry versus a sense of inferiority.
5. Development in adolescence of a sense of ego identity versus role confusion.
6. Development in early adulthood of intimacy versus ego isolation.
7. Development in middle adulthood of generativity (expanding ego interests and a sense of contributing to the future) versus ego stagnation.
8. Development in late adulthood of a sense of ego integrity (a basic acceptance of one's life as having been inevitable, appropriate, and meaningful) versus a sense of despair, equated with a fear of death.

Peck felt that Erikson's eight stages should be expanded, that his sixth and seventh stages cannot successfully be deferred beyond the age of thirty, leaving the eighth stage to represent in a "global, non-specific way all the psychological crises and crisis-solutions of the last forty or fifty years of life."[7] He suggests four stages that occur in middle age and three in old age. Peck's stages in middle age[8] are:

1. Valuing wisdom versus valuing physical powers, utilizing the wisdom gained through the lifetime's experience to accomplish a good deal more than younger people in a different way to compensate for waning physical powers.

2. Socializing versus sexualizing in human relationships, redefining men and women as individuals and companions, the sexual element becoming decreasingly significant.

3. Cathectic flexibility versus cathectic impoverishment or the ability to shift emotional investments from one person to another or from one activity to another.

4. Mental flexibility versus mental rigidity. This critical issue may arise in middle age when individuals have reached peak status, have worked out the answers to life, and may be tempted to avoid further effort to devise new or different solutions.

In old age, he continues[9] with:

5. Ego differentiation versus work role preoccupation, frequently precipitated by retirement, necessitating development of alternatives that can produce a sense of satisfaction and worth.

6. Body transcendence versus body preoccupation or the ability to create satisfying relationships and develop creative activity of an intellectual nature to combat the tendency to preoccupation with bodily ills.

7. Ego transcendence versus ego preoccupation, the development of an awareness of the enduring significance of one's achievements as contributions to the future to overcome an inward preoccupation and withdrawal.

Social psychologists have other theories such as that of Brim[10] who argued that there are no personality dispositions that are persistent across situations, that personality can be defined as the sum of social experiences and social roles. Another approach represented by Schaie[11] is that of concern for cohort differences. He suggests that we should look to social and historical contexts more than to developmental processes for explaining differences between age groups.

Biology

Biological theories of aging[12] deal largely with attempts to discover causes for cellular deterioration resulting in the various aspects of biological aging. Scientific knowledge has become so extensive that simple explanations no longer suffice. One theory considers the question of whether the aging process constitutes deliberate biological programming or if the present life span of an individual is all that can be expected, considering the chemical complexities of the human being. Another is that of the accumulation of copying errors, which holds that the individual eventually dies because cells develop copying errors and those errors in copying, in turn, reduce metabolic efficiency and interfere with the capacity for repair.

PRESENT SOCIAL CONDITIONS OF THE AGED

Recent Legislation

Public awareness, since World War II, of the growing number of individuals over the age of sixty-five and the appalling conditions under which a great many were living culminated in the federal Older Americans Act of 1965 and the Comprehensive Services Amendments of 1973. This latter strengthening legislation provides a variety of services and resources:

Title II	Establishment of the federal Administration on Aging.
Title III	Grants for state and community programs on aging to develop a system of coordinated and comprehensive services to provide alternatives to institutionalization.
Title IV	Personnel training and research in aging.
Title V	Acquisition and staffing of multipurpose centers.
Title VI	Volunteer programs for senior citizens (Foster Grandparents Program, R.S.V.P., etc.).
Title VII	Nutrition programs (communal dining, meals on wheels).
Title VIII	Library services for the aged, grants to universities for utilizing their resources

	on problems of the aged, especially housing and transportation.
Title IX	Community service employment for older Americans.

State and federal programs are providing homemaker services for the elderly, and an increasing number of home health services are now available under Medicare legislation. Federally funded day care and day health care centers are being developed in several parts of the country. The Supplemental Security Income program was established in 1972 to provide direct cash benefits to aged, blind, and disabled individuals in need of the basic necessities such as food, clothing, and shelter. Increasing numbers of senior citizens are becoming active in groups promoting legislation to their advantage at both state and national levels. Recent major legislation has laid the groundwork which can result in a marked improvement of the quality of life for our aging population.

Health Care

Medical research and health programs have contributed to a lengthening life span for Americans. In the period since 1930, life expectancy for a woman has increased by fifteen years and for a man, eight years. Eighty-six percent of the noninstitutionalized population over sixty-five have one or more chronic conditions. Of these individuals, approximately 81 percent have no limitation of mobility. Older people do have more and longer hospital stays, more doctor visits, more days of disability, and more drug expense, usually for chronic conditions, than those under sixty-five. In a report for the Gerontological Society in 1975, Weg[13] observes that the cost of purchasing health care for the older population is complicated. Their need for medical care increases at the same time as their income is reduced by retirement. Needs develop for long-term care with the prevalence of chronic conditions, diseases, and impairments. In 1973, the per capita health care expenditures of older persons were three-and-a-half times higher than for those under sixty-five. Medicare paid 40.3 percent of the cost out of a total of 64.5 percent paid for by public programs. Weg further reports that there are too few health care facilities, with a shortage of personnel and insufficient funds to meet the need. Communities lack training programs for caretaking personnel and education programs for the public. Coordination of services and agencies involved with programs for the older population is poor.

Status of the Aged

Our society has not defined effective or satisfactory roles for old people. They do not even have a definitive group name as do children, adolescents, young adults, and the middle aged. Schmerl,[14] in *The Gerontologist*, argues that the term "elders" should be used to refer to individuals of advanced age, in order to avoid negative connotations. In the same journal, an official publication of the Gerontological Society, "they" are referred to as older adults, senior citizens, the elderly, older Americans, the aging, the aged, and old people. With many occupations lowering retirement age, the designation of retired persons joins that of grandparents in referring to individuals who are younger, often by as much as twenty years, than the generally accepted age of 65. Neugarten[15] refers to three categories of age: the young old, middle old, and old old. Cain,[16] using a different context, has retitled these categories "frisky, frail, and fragile," thus indicating, among other implications, an appropriate level of care that should be provided. Millions of individuals between the ages of sixty and one hundred, with their infinite variety, defy categorizing. Still, researchers and providers of service routinely categorize them to facilitate the planning of service programs and the development of theoretical foundations for those programs.

Needs of the Aged

Personal adjustment for the aged requires finding self-fulfillment through socially accepted means. Tibbitts[17] lists the needs of the aged as follows:

1. to render some socially useful service
2. to be considered a part of the community
3. to occupy increased leisure time in satisfying ways
4. to enjoy normal companionships
5. to achieve recognition as an individual

6. to have opportunities for self-expression and a sense of achievement
7. to receive health protection and care
8. to experience suitable mental stimulation
9. to have suitable living arrangements and family relationships
10. to find spiritual satisfaction

To achieve these goals, which he describes also as rights, Tibbitts[18] suggests certain obligations which must be fullfilled earlier in life:

1. to become and resolve to remain active, alert, capable, self-supporting, and useful as long as circumstances permit, and to plan for retirement.
2. to learn and apply sound principles of physical and mental health.
3. to develop potential avenues of service after retirement.
4. to share with others the benefits of one's experience and knowledge.
5. to adapt to changes which age will bring.
6. to maintain constructive and pleasant relationships with family, neighbors, and friends.

Attitudes Toward Aging

Our youth-oriented, technological society has, by its very nature, created some of the problems of aging. Rapid technological advance has made obsolete many of the skills accumulated by our elders in their lifetime. The young tend to ignore or disregard their counsel. A transient population has been destructive to the three-generation family concept. Many young people have no intimate contacts with old people.

The mass media projection of the "young is beautiful" concept implies, when it is not stated overtly, that "old is ugly." We are told to get rid of that gray in our hair, prevent wrinkles in our skin, use the toothpaste, deodorant, or soap that will keep us sexually attractive. Even Geritol is advertised by the young and beautiful. Old people are often pictured as cranky, demanding, incompetent, and ill.

Current attitudes toward the elderly still closely resemble those reflected in the 1952 study done by Tuckman and Lorge.[19] They asked a group of young people and another of old people to describe old age. Both groups characterized old people as economically insecure, in poor health, lonely, resistant to change, and failing in physical and mental powers. Add to these stereotypes the concrete facts of our current inflationary economy with high unemployment, and it is not surprising to note some antagonism in the controversy over retirement age or opposition to increased benefits for the aged. Attitudes change slowly, and the responsibility for growth of more positive concepts of aging becomes the responsibility of those individuals who work in the field of gerontology.

THE OCCUPATIONAL THERAPIST IN GERONTOLOGY

The Clients

The young or "frisky" old who have a comfortable income, satisfactory family and community relationships, and good health might be seen in the hospital for an acute illness or a fracture but not usually by agencies and institutions dealing with chronic conditions requiring long-term intervention. The population described as the "frail" and "fragile" or high risk elderly are those most often seen by health care personnel. The physiological processes of aging have taken their toll and feelings of independence, dignity, and self-worth have likewise deteriorated. The process of aging varies with individuals, subject to hereditary, socioeconomic, and environmental factors. This is known as differential aging. For some people, the body deteriorates, leaving the intellectual functioning more or less intact; for others, intellectual functions deteriorate, while the body remains healthy; and for some, both systems seem to deteriorate at much the same rate.

Physiological Deficits

The physiological process of aging results in diminution of reflexes, sensory losses, an increase in chronic disabling conditions, increased fragility of bones as a result of calcium loss, and decreased efficiency of central nervous system integrative functions. Diminution of righting reflexes results in an increased tendency to fall, since the individual is less able to catch himself or herself in time when tripping. Physical self-confidence is lost and the individual becomes increasingly cautious. Also, being more prone to suffer broken bones, the old person becomes more and more timid about venturing out into unfamiliar territory.

A gradual loss of hearing contributes both physical and psychological dangers. Physical dangers arise with failure to hear sirens, oncoming cars, people approaching from behind, and other warning signals. As familiar background noises, such as birds singing and footsteps passing, diminish, the person feels increasingly isolated. Paranoid feelings may develop with failure to distinguish conversations, as the individual wonders if people are talking or laughing about him or her. There is increasing withdrawal as communication becomes more difficult, and both the individual and those nearby gradually cease making the effort to communicate.

The gradual dimming of sight causes a great many problems. Glaring light may be temporarily blinding. Loss of depth perception makes it difficult to see steps and to differentiate the bottom step from the floor. Difficulty in reading labels could cause confusion in taking medications. Combined with other reflex and sensory losses, failing sight adds to the fear of falling.

There are also more subtle sensory losses such as touch, smell, and taste, which reduce pleasure in one's environment, from the lovely feel of soft fabrics to the sensory pleasure of food. A reduced energy level resulting from both physiological and psychological factors affects ability in all of the above faculties to whatever degree they remain intact.

Finally cerebral integration mechanisms are reduced, which affect the speed of learning, the ability to store information, and appropriate integration of sensory input and motor output.[20,21]

Mental Deficits

Goldfarb[22] has been prominent in the struggle to differentiate the diagnosis of chronic brain syndrome or senile dementia from a variety of diagnoses ranging from malnutrition to acute drug reaction, most of the latter being capable of producing permanent damage if not diagnosed properly. He divides the mental disorders of geriatric patients into two categories. The first, functional disorders of mood and thought, can occur at any age; these are unaccompanied by any evidence of brain damage. The second, organic disorders, is related to the physical status of the brain tissue. These two types may appear together. Organic disorders refer to the psychiatric syndromes resulting from diffuse brain damage. The term "acute" is used when the dysfunction is reversible; "chronic" is the term used when it is irreversible. Goldfarb defines acute brain syndrome as the "transient, reversible, mental impairment related to disorders such as infection, pain, malnutrition, heart failure or coronary thrombosis, malignancy, drug intoxication, or cerebrovascular accident."[23]

Studies in northern Europe and England, quoted by Juel-Nielsen,[24] show that the prevalence of all forms of psychoses among the aged, including severe senile and arteriosclerotic psychoses, other organic syndromes, and functional disorders, varied from 6 to 8 percent. This seems to represent a consistent and reliable measurement of the core of severe mental disorders in old age. Opler[25] notes the increase of psychosomatic disorders in modern societies. He states that psychosomatic illness in all ages is symptomatic of masked depression, for which the peak occurs statistically in the group past middle age. Psychiatric nomenclature for depression runs the gamut from normal grief and reactive depression because of deprivations to such psychotic categories as manic depression and involutional melancholia or agitated depression. Opler feels that the "psychodynamics of the aging process depend upon cultural attitudes towards elderly persons as a category of human beings, which can, in turn, influence their treatment as well as their self-assessments."[26]

By far the greatest single mental health problem of the aged, and the most pervasive in its consequences, is depression. Lewinsohn and coauthors[27] discuss the difficulties of defining depression, and begin by analyzing the behaviors commonly exhibited by persons diagnosed as depressed. They then report being impressed with the similarities between the behavior of depressed individuals and that of many elderly persons. Low self-esteem, loss of interest, feelings of emptiness and hopelessness, depressed libido and appetite, feelings of rejection, psychosomatic symptoms and complaints, and a progressive reduction in rate of activity are common to both.[28]

Old people in our society tend to wait for a crisis before seeking medical help for a variety of reasons.

Cost and difficulty in access to the services needed are major factors. Public education regarding availability of services as well as preventive measures and home safety information is a responsibility of all health professionals, including occupational therapists.

The Institutionalized Elderly

Five percent of the population over sixty-five described as institutionalized are found primarily in nursing homes. A few are chronic schizophrenics who have grown old in state mental hospitals. Currently most of the elderly with psychiatric illnesses are found in nursing homes. The average age upon admission is rising slightly, and almost all residents have three or more chronic conditions. Many new residents suffer a period of mild to severe confusion which abates once adjustment has been made to the new surroundings. This process of adjustment requires the skillful support offered by staff members. Without it, and sometimes even with it, many old people die rather quickly after such a radical change. Moving to the nursing home may be the most radical change of the individual's lifetime, and occurs when he or she is both physically and mentally least able to cope with such a transition. For most individuals, this move is viewed as "the beginning of the end." They must part with most of their personal possessions; few are fortunate enough to have the privacy of their own room. Ability to continue making personal decisions may vary with the degree of physical or mental infirmity but is, at best, considerably restricted. There is a heightened awareness of impending death. Institutional management, in spite of recent improvements in many areas, is still geared more toward the convenience of staff than toward the individual needs of residents and tends to be dehumanizing.

The Therapist's Role

The skills of the occupational therapist are put to a real test, especially the ability to evaluate the individual's capacity "to relate to and master his environment and provide a program design which speaks to his task mastery needs."[29] Personal relationships are particularly important to these people who usually have few contacts with others. The therapist should like and feel comfortable with the elderly. It is important to remember that individuals tend to see themselves as others see them.[30] For those isolated in a nursing home, each personal contact assumes enormous importance either in building or in destroying the client's self-image. One must be especially careful to avoid a judgmental approach regarding a resident's values and life-style.

It may be necessary to visit with an individual several times in order to discover the information necessary for a good evaluation. Factors of age, class, ethnic and national origin, sex, and educational level may have to be dealt with before a level of mutual trust has developed which will permit the resident to discuss his or her concerns with the therapist and which will enable the therapist to hear those elements which are important to that individual. Above all, the unique qualities of each person must be recognized and respected.

Activity Programming

Activity programming in a nursing home has received a great deal of attention recently with the Medicare regulations requiring a full-time activity director. Many states have followed Medicare requirements for nursing home certification. Many states also require a consultant for the activity director; this in many cases is an occupational therapist.

Activity for activity's sake is no longer acceptable. Each patient should be interviewed, goals established *with* that patient, and activity plans established which contribute to those goals. Activity goals should correlate with those of the nursing department. The American Nursing Home Association's publication "Winds of Change" states that "an activity program in long term care facilities means the conscious management of daily living through creating, supporting, developing, and restoring the appropriate life style of the residents in the direction of personal and social autonomy."[31] The California State Department of Health in its licensing regulations for nursing homes defines an activity program as "a program which is staffed and equipped to meet the needs and interests of each patient to encourage self-care and resumption of normal activities."[32] The patient is encouraged to participate in activities suited to his or her individual needs. Scheduled group and independent activities are designed to make life more meaningful, to stimulate and support the desire to use physical and mental capabilities to their fullest extent, and to enable each individual to maintain his or her highest attainable social, physical and emotional function, sense of usefulness and self-respect.

It is exciting to see many of the basic premises of occupational therapy incorporated so specifically in legislation designed to improve the quality of life for those old people who live in nursing homes and other long-term care facilities. In many states occupational therapists have influenced the development of such legislation.

Reality Orientation

Reality orientation (RO) is a program that was developed in the Veterans' Hospital at Tuscaloosa, Alabama, by Folsom for a population of severely withdrawn mental patients.[33] It is designed to be used twenty-four hours a day by the entire staff to orient the patients, reminding them of their names, the date, where they are, what time it is, what they ate at their last meal, and what the next holiday is. It includes a half-hour session five days a week for drill on these items. It also involves utilizing a consistent attitude in approaching a given patient, determined by the patient's diagnosis. It was a remarkably effective program with that patient population and has been recommended for use in nursing homes with severely withdrawn patients.

In many nursing homes reality orientation has changed its focus over a period of time. Gubrium and Ksander[34] raised serious questions regarding the purpose and the methodology of reality orientation, particularly the more structured classroomlike session. Materials for the session include an RO board with the requisite information and a clock with movable hands to indicate the time. During sessions the patients read the information on the board in response to questions and are asked what happens at indicated times. The authors observed little correlation between the answers expected and actual timing of events in that setting. They raise questions about the relevance of RO as a therapeutic program for institutionalized elders. They suggest that behavior therapy in general is imperialistic in that it imposes one group's definition of living on another in the name of allegedly objective rehabilitation.

The routine question and answer format has largely been abandoned in favor of such things as a reminiscence group which permits the exchange of early experiences of many sorts such as holiday celebrations and cooking favorite foods. These can be done at any intellectual level, promote interpersonal relationships and a sense of belonging, stimulate thought processes, and bring back pleasant memories. Remotivation groups is the title used to describe a discussion group that utilizes a familiar object such as a pinecone, a seashell, or a milkweed pod to provide sensory stimulation and to stimulate the association process with poems, songs, personal experiences, or occupations associated with the object. Variations are endless. Underlying these group processes is the belief that every individual approaching the close of life needs to have a sense of having contributed a significant spot in history.[35] Establishing a person's contribution to humanity builds a sense of dignity and integrity. Behavior and mental activity characteristic of a specific phase of life are very likely specifically suited to resolving the problems of that phase. The prevalence of reminiscing in the later stages of life suggests that it has adaptational significance in the process of closure.[36]

Elders in the Community

More than 60 percent of the elderly population live in metropolitan areas, mostly in the central city. Forty percent live in non-metropolitan areas but in towns rather than on farms. The three most populous states—California, New York, and Pennsylvania—account for just over a fourth of the older population. Add Florida, Illinois, Ohio, Texas, and Michigan, and the eight states account for over half of the older population. In an inner city section of Portland, Oregon, a 1975 survey reports that 50 percent of the elderly live alone, 25 percent are below the poverty level, 38 percent are isolated, and 11 percent of those report no contact with friends. A projected 20 percent suffer to some degree from mental or emotional problems. Problems encountered by this population include transportation, housing, shopping, access to medical facilities, isolation, and fear for their safety. Remembering that, of the current old age population, 12 percent have completed less than five years of school and only 32 percent have finished high school, it becomes clear that these individuals have a great deal of difficulty coping with a highly bureaucratic service delivery system.[37] Case finding itself is a difficult problem for service providers. Many individuals are isolated in their rooms, only leaving their rooms for essentials such as buying food, and are suspicious of anyone seeking to invade their privacy. Educating these individuals to understand the use of available services, to say nothing of the principles of good nutrition and home safety standards, is exceedingly difficult. Future generations of elders who are better educated and more aware of available services will be less of a problem in this respect.[38]

Intervention Techniques

It is important that all providers of services to these elders remember that, while they share common problems of poverty, increasing disability, poor nutrition, poor housing conditions, and isolation and loneliness, these people are individuals with strengths as well as weaknesses and abilities as well as disabilities. Strengths and abilities must be recognized in order to reinforce waning self-esteem, desire for independence, and ability to improve the quality of life within the range available to them.

Professionals, volunteers, and others who intervene in the lives of this population must avoid several pitfalls if the results of their intervention are to be productive for the individual. One cannot overemphasize the importance of recognizing the dignity, integrity, and worth of every individual no matter how deplorable the conditions under which the person lives, or how poor his or her self-esteem. It is almost inevitable that the individual who is poor and old and in need of a variety of services will also be the product of a different social class, a different cultural and environmental background from that of the person making contact to provide assistance. That chasm must be bridged primarily by the provider of services.

Lady Bountiful who goes into a home, pats the old person on the head, saying how terrible the living conditions are, how awful the person looks, and how the therapist is going to take the old person in hand and take care of him or her can only make a bad situation worse. Under these circumstances, especially when the elderly person has lost confidence and fears not only what he or she views as a hostile society but also his/her own potential inability to cope with life and approaching death, it is far easier to foster an increasing dependence on the service provider than it is to encourage a growing self-confidence and sense of independence. In addition, human beings have a frightening desire to play God, with all the ego reinforcement that role offers. Building a desire for independence in the elderly person requires a nonjudgmental acceptance of the person, which can enable the person to see himself/herself as a worthwhile person. Attempts to make the individual over according to an image which may be more acceptable to the intervener are counterproductive. It is necessary to know the individual sufficiently well to encourage him or her to recognize the variety of real options and to set his or her own goals. Finally comes the difficult task of enabling the individual to attain those goals. Rapport, trust, and a mutual respect for each other's integrity are the bases for successful intervention.

Opportunities for Occupational Therapists

The occupational therapist is concerned with three aspects of health care for the aged: preventive care, acute care, and chronic or long-term care. There are an increasing number of job opportunities for therapists in all three areas, although not all are specifically designated as occupational therapy positions and some require additional training.

Preventive Care

Multiservice centers offer social and recreational opportunities for elders and are usually housed with a variety of other services such as legal aid, nursing clinics, Housing and Urban Development offices, income tax consultants, and other appropriate services. They serve as a community center for senior citizens. Directors of these centers could appropriately be occupational therapists. The centers provide an excellent opportunity for community education on health, nutrition, and safety measures to aid in prevention of illness and accidents as well as promote physical and mental health.

Hospital discharge planners act as liaison with the community when a patient is discharged from the hospital, contacting community agencies that provide appropriate follow-up care in the patient's community. Such agencies as senior citizens' centers, hot lunch programs, Meals on Wheels, Visiting

Nurse Association, home health agencies, and homemaker services can assist in completing the patient's rehabilitation and aid in maintenance of independence. Planners frequently make home visits to determine the adequacy of the home environment. An occupational therapist is well qualified for this role.

Home health aide training is done in Oregon for the State Department of Health by occupational therapists. The therapists provide the same type of training given to restorative aides in nursing homes: range of motion, ADL techniques, transfer and gait training techniques, basic nutritional principles, and safety measures.

Preretirement planning is another area occupational therapists are entering. In increasing numbers, corporations, unions, businesses, and continuing education centers are offering courses for individuals to begin planning for the economic, social, and leisure changes after retirement.

Planning housing for older people is an area with great potential for occupational therapists. Elimination of architectural barriers, planning work areas suitable for the disabled (particularly kitchen and laundry areas), providing protective devices such as appropriate doorknobs for the arthritic or feeble, and compensating for poor eyesight with well-lighted stairs, handrails, and well-marked top and bottom steps are considerations unknown or overlooked by most architects and builders. While initially these devices are no more expensive than ordinary construction, they can be quite costly later. There is a desperate need for appropriate housing for the partially disabled within the community.

Public education opportunities are exemplified by the Seattle therapist who is working with a video tape expert from a local public broadcasting station. They are investigating the possibility of utilizing video tapes to involve tenants of a high rise residence for the elderly in discussion of the change of pace and life-style which benefit the arthritic and to demonstrate protective devices to prevent deformities.

Acute Care

Hospitals and stroke care units are a familiar site in which occupational therapists treat the aged patient. These roles are discussed elsewhere in this text.

Home health agencies, having come into effect since the enactment of the Medicare law, may be less familiar. They are established under Medicare to meet federal guidelines, though they are not limited to Medicare patients. They provide at least two services, nursing plus one or more of the following: occupational therapy, physical therapy, speech therapy, and social work. Some are associated with county or state health departments or local hospitals. They are limited to the treatment of the homebound patient, providing essentially the same services as those available in rehabilitation centers, and can also provide any special equipment needed for the patient. In addition to filling a therapist's regular role, the occupational therapist with some administrative training could initiate and direct a home health agency.

Arthritis treatment centers, found in hospitals, clinics, outpatient centers, or doctors' offices, should include occupational therapy. The therapist's interpretation, in concrete terms in a living situation, of the doctor's prescription for a balanced regime of rest and exercise is often critical to success for the patient. Ability to teach energy saving methods of performing everyday living and housekeeping tasks and to point out simple adaptations that can be made in the household and new ways of performing familiar tasks can be the means of preventing otherwise inevitable deformities.

State receiving hospitals and crisis care units for the treatment of acute psychiatric problems are also familiar to occupational therapists. Their role in these settings is discussed elsewhere and is virtually the same as for other age groups.

Detoxification centers are growing in number in urban areas to treat the acute stages of alcoholism. Many of their patients are aged. There is an increasing recognition of the role occupational therapists can play in the evaluation and treatment of the alcoholic.

Chronic Care

Rehabilitation institutes and skilled care facilities, formerly called extended care facilities, actually fall between the areas of acute and chronic care. Occupational therapists are well recognized as part of the rehabilitation team. The aged form a large part of their patient population. Therapists should assume responsibility for ensuring good follow-up care for these patients when they are discharged.

Nursing homes providing skilled care are required to have a full-time activity director. Few nursing homes have occupational therapists on their staff, although many have recognized the advantages of hiring certified occupational therapy assistants as activity directors. Occupational therapists often act as consultants to the activity director, provide inservice training for staff members, and sometimes also provide direct service for individual patients. The consultant's objective is to integrate concepts of restorative care into the overall plan of patient care in the skilled nursing facility. To accomplish these goals, the consultant works with the administrator, the director of nurses, and the activity director.

Day care centers and day health care centers are being developed in many urban areas. They are designed to provide an additional alternative to institutional care for individuals with varying degrees of physical and/or mental disability. Ideally, they provide structured activity within a therapeutic environment, offering group process to the outpatient as well as one-to-one therapy when needed. A private facility in Beverly Hills is an example of a psychiatrically oriented adult day treatment center.[39] The On Lok Senior Day Health Center in San Francisco has been established as one link in a planned chain of services and programs needed to maintain the frail elderly in the community.[40] The focuses are on health care, physical and occupational therapy for rehabilitation and maintenance, social services, and nutrition. The Levindale Adult Treatment Center in Baltimore offers a wide variety of social, maintenance, and rehabilitation services to fragile persons whose major functional limitations place them at risk of institutionalization.[40a] Occupational therapists usually are participants in the treatment team but too seldom assume administrative and developmental responsibilities for the programs.

State mental hospitals are familiar sites for occupational therapists and have many aged patients. Notable among contributions by occupational therapists in evaluation and treatment of chronic schizophrenics is that of Lorna Jean King, reported in the *American Journal of Occupational Therapy*, October 1974.[41]

Homes for the aged, boarding homes for the aged, retirement homes, retirement villages, and public housing units for the aged must be mentioned separately for, at present, there is little or no involvement by occupational therapists in most of these sites. The contributions that could be made at administrative as well as planning and evaluation levels are as numerous as in the other areas mentioned. They require a combination of the requisite skills and the ability to prove the need for their qualifications to those who are financially accountable for the operation of such facilities.

Occupational Therapy's Contribution

The unique contribution of occupational therapy to the field of gerontology was mentioned in the introduction to this chapter and has been implied throughout. Other disciplines operate from theories derived from observations of group manifestations in society. From these theories, they serve and advise their clients, anticipating results predicted by statistical data. There is always the possibility that the client's reactions may be the result of the professional's expectations. Public policy is determined by the existing norms as interpreted by researchers and theoreticians and, hence, reinforces those norms. The occupational therapist, with the basic premises from which he or she operates, can provide a new dimension to this process. Consider the emphasis upon the individualization of treatment planning; goal setting, and of implementation of the normalization process for the patient or client. With this philosophy, if results are documented and published, a whole new range of options could be introduced into the services provided. These basic premises are described in the 1974 report of the Task Force on Target Populations:[42]

1. The human being has a capacity for intrinsic self-directedness and decision making. The occupational therapy laboratory can help persons exercise those capacities, become aware of options for life style, and develop competence in areas of living important to the individual.

2. The occupational therapist uses an integrative approach to the patient or client on two levels: a) the part of the individual which is

dysfunctional or in which there is a deficit which is seen as being an integral part of a larger whole which the program for maintenance, treatment, or remediation must consider; and b) the human body is an integrated system, and the therapist must consider the impact of programming upon the area in which there is a deficit or dysfunction and upon the mind and body of the individual as a whole.

3. The occupational therapist has a unique way of looking at and evaluating problems and situations that is goal-oriented versus diagnostic.

4. The occupational therapist is concerned with demonstrated change in occupational behavior, that is, the person's use of time, energy, and attention to rest, play, and work. As persons engage in occupations and decision making, the goal-oriented actions become a catalyst for the development and strengthening of new behaviros.

5. The occupational therapy laboratory, wherever located, should be a resource which helps persons become aware of options for their life styles; become self-directive; and become competent in whatever activities are undertaken. As such, occupational therapy is reality oriented.

6. The active use of mind and body in learning and performing occupational tasks affects the central nervous system and produces a level of internal integration which is not achieved through either physical or mental activity undertaken independently or passively performed, such as passive exercise or passive range of motion. Furthermore, the results of performing such occupational tasks provide immediate and concrete feedback to each individual which facilitates self-judgment and decision-making based on internal concepts rather than on external controls or demands. This is an important stage in helping persons toward independence.*

* Reprinted with permission of the American Occupational Therapy Association, Inc. Copyright 1974, Am. J. Occup. Ther. Vol. 28, No. 3, pp. 160–161.

Implied in these premises are critical factors too often forgotten or ignored by professionals from many disciplines in working with elderly clients. The inherent decision-making ability of human beings does not magically disappear at age sixty-five, as our youth oriented society often implies. Options for life-style should refer to the individual's choices within the limits of real possibility, not those of a professional plan of what would be good for that individual. *There is no formula for "understanding old people"*—old people are as different and as complex as human beings at any age.

The therapist must see himself or herself as a facilitator whose professional qualifications can enable a client to make the best possible use of remaining capabilities to achieve his or her own goals. It is in the realm of goal setting that particular care must be exercised to listen to the individual, to identify sufficiently with that person, to help the person realize what he or she can realistically achieve, and to assist the individual in setting goals that are not only possible but important and affirming.

There is a great temptation to assume that old people are sick people and assign them what Parsons calls a sick role[43]: The assumption is made that the sick person is unable to fulfill social responsibilities and, furthermore, should not do so; the sick person cannot make himself/herself well and therefore, must be cared for; being ill is undesirable, so the individual has an obligation to cooperate with those who care for him or her in order to become well. With this concept as an almost subliminal assumption, it is easy to see how providers of services to the aged might fall into a caretaker role rather than that of a facilitator towards independence. A very human tendency to exercise power over fellow human beings can lead to an even more insidious leaning toward the role of benevolent dictator. The therapist must be both objective and concerned—objective enough to make a realistic evaluation and concerned enough to discern patient oriented goals.

Need for Research

Occupational therapy's unique frame of reference can be applied to many research areas. Critical research, utilizing a survey of current literature and applying it to specific provision of services, is practically non-existent in the field at present. Neugarten[44] points out the need to delineate processes that underlie adult change and especially to find operational definitions. She also complains that the phenomena that preoccupy the experimentalist are seldom those that concern the professional dealing with real life problems of clients. There is need to point out factors of environment, experience, and social roles that are primary in understanding stability and change in adult personality. Establishment of objective measures to define the categories of "frisky, frail, and fragile" would enable more appropriate assistance to be offered to those individuals involved than does the present use of actuarial tables of probability.

Care must be taken to pose initial questions in research projects so as to ensure valid results.[45] In developing the methodology, the researcher must remain objective and should carefully review related studies, assessing their validity in the context of the current study. The final step, which must not be overlooked, is ensuring availability of the research to those professionals who may profit from it. Occupational therapists often fail to publish their studies in appropriate journals outside their own field and, hence, are scarcely recognized in the broad field of gerontology.

DEATH AND DYING

As long ago as 1948 a satire was written about American funeral and burial practices.[46] A critical analysis of these practices was written fifteen years later by Mitford.[47] In the past few years the topic of death and dying has achieved widespread attention in classrooms; newspaper, magazine, and journal articles; books; seminars; television documentaries; and talk shows.[48] The more scholarly work has come primarily from psychologists and psychiatrists, concerned mainly with suicide, grief, and the dying patient.

The earliest popular book on the care of the terminally ill patient is *Care of the Dying* by Saunders.[49] Her philosophy of normalizing the lives of patients and their families is of special interest to occupational therapists.

Perhaps the most famous book on the subject is one by Kubler-Ross, *On Death and Dying*.[50] Her humane and realistic approach and her ability not only to listen herself to the dying patient but also to teach others to do so has done much to reduce the fear and anxiety formerly aroused by proximity to a dying person. She describes five stages of adjustment or coping mechanisms necessary for most people to achieve an acceptance of death. The first is denial, a buffer against the shock, and an attempt to postpone the inevitable. The second is anger. During this stage, the patient may become hostile and difficult to cope with. Bargaining is the third, during which time the patient seeks a variety of means to alter or postpone facing the fatal diagnosis. Depression, the fourth phase, has two different aspects: a reactive depression, when it is helpful for the patient to discuss fears and anxiety with a good listener, and a preparatory grief, which requires a more silent presence, supportive of the patient's emotional preparation for death. The final stage, acceptance, will occur if the patient has time and has had sufficient support to work through the other phases. Some of these stages may recur, often several times, before the final stage has been reached. Acceptance is characterized by the absence of anger and depression, almost an absence of feeling, a sense of quiet expectation.

Kastenbaum[51] suggests that there are some things we do not want to know about old men and women. We may resist the prospect of becoming intimately involved in the old person's world, vulnerability, anxieties about death. "Why let ourselves in for vicarious suffering? Why borrow misery from the future? Aversion from intimate contact with the aged is common." Kastenbaum feels that a self-discovery component should be added to the training of those preparing for a career with the aged.

The aged person must either make some type of adjustment to the thought of impending death or build up defenses as shields against the prospect.[52] A realistic acceptance of death is a part of emotional maturity.

It is commonly held that one's life passes in review when facing death. The theory of the life review, developed by Butler, suggests one such mechanism.[53] Life review is defined as a process of looking backward that has been set in motion by the imminent prospect of death. Butler feels that it accounts for the increase of reminiscence in the elderly, that it contributes to the occurrence of certain disorders in later life, particularly depression, and that from it also evolve such characteristics as candor, serenity, and wisdom among certain old people. It occurs not only in old people but in younger people who expect death, such as those who are fatally ill or condemned to death.

Contemplation of early experiences from the perspective of age often results in expanded understanding and may give new and significant meaning to life. It is tragic when the insight leads to a sense of total waste. One group who seems prone to depression and despair are those who avoided living in the present, expecting the future to bring the rewards they sought. This philosophy brings great disillusionment in old age. Those who have consciously injured others, whose guilt is all too real, suffer terribly in this process. Butler feels that, possibly as a result of the life review, personality can change in old age. He has noticed positive, affirmative changes reported by the aged themselves.

Feifel,[54] as well as other investigators, confirmed that, for many old people, a belief in a life after death is a great comfort, going a long way to reduce the element of fear. For a few individuals, a strong belief in retribution for sins in the afterlife is very threatening. It is a great comfort for many to have children and grandchildren in whom they see a continuity of their own life.

The therapist who works with old people must first examine carefully his or her own attitudes toward dying and death. What causes the fear and anxiety which often prompts hospital or nursing home staff, from the aide to the doctor, to avoid unnecessary contact with dying patients? As Kastenbaum[55] suggests, there should be a conscious analysis of one's attitudes and training to prepare one to assume a constructive role with individuals who are anticipating death. A therapist can let the old person know in an appropriate manner, that it is all right to talk about death, if he or she wishes to do so, now or at some future time. The patient who is threatened by impending death often has a great need to discuss it. Family members often are too emotionally involved to be able to listen comfortably. Even the doctor, committed to the saving of lives, may be unable to respond appropriately. Health care personnel who have come to terms with their own anxieties may provide the necessary empathy and support.

Patients in nursing homes, for the most part, see death as preferable to continuing illness or chronic disability. According to Kalish's concept,[56] these persons may already have become "socially dead" in their own eyes as well as in the eyes of others, and thus view their impending death as timely and welcome. The occupational therapist may be able to stimulate interest in enabling the staff members to become more aware of the needs of dying patients. The staff should be alert to the need of some patients to discuss and resolve old conflicts and to assure themselves that their lives have indeed had some meaning. Above all, the dying patient should not be ignored and neglected. The dying patient should be enabled to put his or her affairs in order, to make a will, to discuss funeral arrangements, and to ascertain any other matters that should be resolved. These procedures, appropriate to occupational therapy, are important to the patient to achieve "closure," enabling him or her to be at peace with self and family, create a feeling of fulfillment, and a sense of worth as an individual.[57]

REFERENCES

1. Butler, R. N.: The life review: An interpretation of reminiscence in the aged. In Neugarten, B. (ed.): Middle Age and Aging. Chicago: University of Chicago Press, 1968, pp. 18–30.
2. Palmore, E.: Sociological aspects of aging. In Busse, E. W., and Pfeiffer, E. (eds.): Behavior and Adaptation in Late Life. Boston: Little, Brown & Co., 1969, pp. 58–59.
3. Neugarten, B.: Personality change in late life: A developmental perspective. In Eisdorfer, C., and Lawton, P. (eds.): Psychology of Adult Development and Aging. Washington DC: American Psychological Association, 1973, p. 324.
4. Palmore: Sociological aspects, pp. 57–59.
5. Neugarten: Personality change, pp. 314–316.
6. Erikson, E. H.: Childhood and Society, ed. 2. New York: W. W. Norton Co., 1950, p. 85.
7. Peck, R. C.: Psychological developments in the second half of life. In Neugarten, B. (ed.): Middle Age and Aging. Chicago: University of Chicago Press, 1968, p. 88.
8. Ibid., pp. 88–92.
9. Ibid., pp. 90–92.
10. Brim, O. G.: Socialization through the life cycle. In Brim, O. G., and Wheeler, S. (eds.): Socialization after Childhood. New York: John Wiley & Sons, 1966, p. 316.

11. Ibid., p. 317.
12. Busse, E. W.: Theories of aging. In Busse, E. W., and Pfeiffer, E. (eds.): Behavior and Adaptation in Late Life. Boston: Little, Brown & Co., 1969, pp. 18–27.
13. Weg, R. B.: The Aged: Who, Where, How Well, 1974–1975. Mimeographed paper. Report for the Gerontological Society Convention, Portland OR, 1975.
14. Schmerl, E. F.: In the name of the elder: An essay. Gerontologist 15:5, Part I, 386, 1975.
15. Neugarten, B.: Aging in the year 2000: A look at the future. Gerontologist 15:1–40, 1975.
16. Cain, L. D.: Age Status and Social Structure. New York: Rinehart & Winston, 1963, p. 193.
17. Tibbitts, C.: The evolving work-life pattern. In Tibbitts, C. (ed.): Handbook of Social Gerontology. Chicago: University of Chicago Press, 1960, pp. 123–125.
18. Ibid.
19. Tuckman, J., and Lorge, I.: The best years of life: A study in ranking. J. Psychol. 34:137–149, 1952.
20. Hasselkus, B. R.: Aging and the human nervous system. Am. J. Occup. Ther. 28:16–21, 1974.
21. Eisdorfer, C., Nowlin, J., and Wilkie, F.: Improvement of learning in the aged by modification of the autonomic nervous system activity. Science 170:1327–1329, 1970.
22. Goldfarb, A. I.: Aging and Organic Brain Syndrome. Pamphlet from McNeil Laboratories. Produced by Health-Learning Systems, Inc., Bloomfield NJ, 1974.
23. Ibid.
24. Juel-Nielson, N.: Epidemiology. In Howells, J. G. (ed.): Modern Perspective in the Psychiatry of Old Age, Vol. 6. New York: Brunner-Mazel, 1976, p. 354.
25. Opler, M. K.: Anthropological aspects. In Howells, J. G. (ed.): Modern Perspective in the Psychiatry of Old Age, Vol. 6. New York: Brunner-Mazel, 1975, p. 192.
26. Ibid., p. 187.
27. Lewisohn, P. M., Biglan, A., and Zeiss, A. M.: Behavioral treatment of depression. In Davidson, P. O. (ed.): The Behavioral Management of Anxiety, Depression, and Pain. New York: Brunner-Mazel, 1976.
28. Ibid., p. 140.
29. Johnson, J.: Report of 1974 Task Force on Target Populations, Part I. Am. J. Occup. Ther. 28:160–161, 1974.
30. Palmore: Sociological aspects.
31. Winds of Change. Pamphlet from American Nursing Home Association, Chicago, 1971.
32. Livingston, F. M., and O'Sullivan, N. B.: Occupational Therapy Consultancy in the Skilled Nursing Facility —An Overview. Southern California Occupational Therapy Consultants Group, Los Angeles, 1976.
33. Folsom, J. C.: Reality orientation for the elderly mental patient. J. Geriatric Psychiatry 1:291–307, 1968.
34. Gubrium, J. F., and Ksander, M.: On multiple realities and reality orientation. Gerontologist 15:142–145, 1975.
35. Peck: Psychological developments, p. 91.
36. Butler: The life review, pp. 486–496.
37. Weg: The Aged: Who, Where, How Well.
38. Neugarten: Aging in the year 2000.
39. Turbow, S.: Geriatric group day care and its effect on independent living. Gerontologist 15:508–515, 1975.
40. Lurie, E., et al.: On Lok Senior Day Health Center: A case study. Gerontologist 15:1–50, 1975.
40a. Rathbone-McCuan, E., and Levenson, J.: Impact of Socialization Therapy in a Geriatric Day Care Setting. Gerontologist 15:338–342, 1975.
41. King, L. J.: A sensory-integrative approach to schizophrenia. Am. J. Occup. Ther. 28:529–536, 1974.
42. Johnson: Report of 1974 Task Force.
43. Parsons, T.: The Social System. Glencoe IL: Free Press, 1951, p. 436.
44. Neugarten: Personality change, p. 318.
45. Birren, J.: Principles of research on aging. In Neugarten, B. (ed.): Middle Age and Aging. Chicago: University of Chicago Press, 1968.
46. Waugh, E.: The Loved One. London: Chapman and Hall, 1948, pp. 549–551.
47. Mitford, J.: The American Way of Death. London: Hutchinson, 1963.
48. Lofland, L. H. (ed.): Toward a Sociology of Death and Dying. Beverly Hills: Sage Publications, 1976.
49. Saunders, C.: Care of the Dying. New York: Macmillan Publishing Co., 1959.
50. Kubler-Ross, E.: On Death and Dying. New York: Macmillan Publishing Co., 1969.
51. Kastenbarm, R. J.: Epilogue: Loving and dying and other gerontological addenda. In Eisdorfer, C., and Lawton, P. (eds.): The Psychology of Adult Development and Aging. Washington DC: American Psychological Association, 1973, p. 701.
52. Jeffers, E., and Verwoerdt, A.: How the old face death. In Busse, E. W., and Pfeiffer, E. (eds.): Behavior and Adaptation in Late Life. Boston: Little, Brown & Co., 1969, p. 163.
53. Butler: The life review, pp. 486–496.
54. Feifel, H.: Attitudes toward death. In Feifel, H. (ed.): The Meaning of Death. New York: McGraw-Hill Book Co., 1965, p. 172.
55. Kastenbarm: Epilogue: Loving and dying, pp. 700–702.
56. Kalish, R. A.: A continuum of subjectively perceived death. Gerontologist 6:73–76, 1966.
57. Gammage, P. S., McMahon, P., and Shanahan, P.: The occupational therapist and terminal illness: Learning to cope with death. Am. J. Occup. Ther. 30:5, 1976.

BIBLIOGRAPHY

Adams, J. E., and Lindeman, E.: Coping with long term disability. In Goelho, G., Hamburg, D., and Adams, J.: Coping and Adaptation. New York: Basic Books, 1974.

Arenberg, A.: Cognition and aging: Verbal learning, memory, and problem solving. In Eisdorfer, C., and Lawton, P. (eds.): Psychology of Adult Development and Aging. Washington DC: American Psychological Association, 1973.

Blackman, D. K., Howe, M., and Pinkston, E. M.: Increasing participation in social interaction of the institutionalized elderly. Gerontologist 16:1, Part I, 69–76, 1976.

Graney, M. J.: Happiness and social participation in aging. J. Gerontology 30:701–706, 1975.

Havinghurst, R. J.: The future aged: Use of time and money. Gerontologist 15:1, Part II, 10–15, 1975.

Kahn, R. L.: The mental health system and the future aged. Gerontologist 15:1, Part II, 24–31, 1975.

Kaplan, J., and Ford, C. S.: Rehabilitation for the elderly: An eleven year assessment. Gerontologist 15:393–403, 1975.

Kline, C.: The socialization process of women: Implications for a theory of successful aging. Gerontologist 15:486–492, 1975.

Lewis, S.: A patient determined approach to geriatric activity programming within a state hospital. Gerontologist 15:146–149, 1975.

Neugarten, B., et al.: Kansas City studies of adult life. In Neugarten, B., et al.: Personality in Middle and Late Life. New York: Atherton, 1964.

Oelrich, M.: The patient with a fatal illness. Am. J. Occup. Ther. 28:429–432, 1974.

Payne, E. C.: Depression and suicide. In Howells, J. G. (ed.): Modern Perspective in the Psychiatry of Old Age, Vol. 6. New York: Brunner-Mazel, 1975.

Sheppard, H. L.: Work and retirement. In Binstock, R., and Shanas, E. (eds.): Handbook of Aging and the Social Sciences. New York: Van Nostrand Reinhold, 1976.

Veterans Administration Hospital: Guide for Reality Orientation. Nursing Service, Tuscaloosa AL, 1970 (revised, mimeographed)

Ward, R.: Review of research related to work activities for aged residents of long term care facilities. Am. J. Occup. Ther. 25:348–351, 1971.

Part Seven

Special Areas of Practice

18

Occupational Therapy for Problems with Special Senses: Blindness and Deafness

Ann Starnes Wade

Sighted, hearing individuals occasionally discuss and try to imagine what it would be like to be blind or deaf. Events enjoyed largely through visual or auditory channels are mentioned. Therapists and teachers may simulate a disability by wearing blindfolds or special ear plugs before beginning work with blind or deaf persons. These temporary situations offer some insight into the experiences of persons who lose vision or hearing after they have learned their way about in the world and have developed the ability to communicate with others. They offer much less understanding of the plight of the person who loses sight or hearing in infancy or early childhood or who is born blind or deaf. There is no adequate way for sighted, hearing people to think without using mental visual images or an inner verbal language. It is difficult to imagine how one's own early physical, emotional, and social development and learning would have occurred in the absence of one or both of these significant special senses.

The purposes to be served by this chapter are to review briefly the functions of vision and audition; to consider the problems of blindness, deafness, and a combination of both, whether congenital or acquired; and to describe, examine, and explore special considerations and responsibilities of occupational therapists who work with persons whose vision and/or hearing is absent or impaired.

SIGNIFICANCE OF VISUAL AND AUDITORY SENSES

Interdependence with Other Senses

Both vision and hearing are *distant* senses. These are primary channels by which most individuals gather information and receive pleasure from the environment without making physical contact with it. *Near* senses of touch, movement, taste, and smell are also important; information transmitted via touch-tactile, kinesthetic-proprioceptive, gustatory, and olfactory channels requires direct contact or, in the case of olfaction, closer range.

Use of all available significant sensory information permits the organism to perceive or give meaning to an object, phenomenon, or event most efficiently and accurately. Particularly during infancy and early childhood the individual seeks to touch, manipulate, taste, and smell him or herself and the surroundings, as well as to look and to listen. All senses function in the neonate, although function and effective stimuli are *relatively* unsophisticated. The individual can seek and find gratification through near sensory channels throughout life; however, as the individual matures, it is generally true in many societies that one will gradually reserve touch, manipulation, and smell for intimate relationships, personal experiences, self-care, and safety. Vision and hearing become increasingly sophisticated and reliable in the course of normal development. The match between near and distant sensory data gathered and integrated during early exploration and manipulation of the world gradually enables the child to identify human and nonhuman sounds, objects, scenes, and events through visual and auditory information. The child's perceptions and responses are influenced by past experience, emotions, current physiological state, and data in subcortical and cortical association areas.

Contributions of Vision and Hearing

Contributions of the visual and acoustic senses are understandably great in the development and continuation of *communication skills*, *perceptual-motor ability*, *psychosocial function*, and *cognitive capability*. This should not imply that a blind or deaf person cannot develop and use all intact sensory systems to their full extent.

Communication in ordinary society includes spoken and written words and symbols sent, received, and understood. Both the verbal and the nonverbal content of the message are important. Much information is conveyed via the visual sense through facial expression, gesture, handwriting, demonstration, and diagram. The auditory sense allows a person to hear his or her own sounds and language and culture's sounds and spoken language, which the individual gradually learns through imitation, reinforcement, repetition, association, and experience. It detects messages from vocal tone, telephone, doorbell, radio, alarm clock, and the like.

Such *perceptual-motor abilities* as object recognition, visualization and use of space, localization of sound and objects, sequencing of directions, and timing of actions depend heavily on sight and hearing. In the *psychosocial area* vision and audition are used in conjunction with the tactile and kinesthetic senses to enable one to identify the self as separate from the environment. The distant senses also permit reinforcement of the early spontaneous smiling response which facilitates interpersonal relationships between caretakers and infant. Communication skills obviously play another major role in intra- and interpersonal relationships as well as in *cognitive or intellectual development*. Ability to see, hear, and use language plus all the other aforementioned abilities enable a person to learn from experience and books, to classify, to plan and organize, to solve problems, and to evaluate one's own performance.

Deficits in Vision

The legal definition of blindness in the United States refers to visual acuity that cannot be corrected to better than 20/200 feet or 6/60 meters. That is, the legally blind person, even with maximum correction, cannot see the Snellen or similar chart with the stronger eye from a distance of 20 feet or 6 meters any better than a person with normal visual acuity can see it from 200 feet or 60 meters. An individual may also be considered legally blind if he or she has no peripheral vision, that is, the visual field is restricted to less than that of a 20-degree angle so that he or she sees no more than what a fully sighted person might see through a tube or tunnel.[1,2]

Legal definitions of blindness allow a wide range of visual problems and abilities to be classified as blind. Total blindness, the complete inability to see, accounts for about 20 percent of these.[3] A person may be legally blind yet have some *near visual acuity*, corrected or uncorrected, sufficient to read ordinary newsprint, large print, or something in between the two. Normal near visual acuity can be described as 14/14, achieved by accurately reading the fourteenth, or smallest print line on a Jaeger test type reading card at a distance of 14 inches.[4] Unless there is an eye disease that contraindicates, there is apparently no damage to the visual system even if the individual must hold a book or object only a few inches from the eyes. Each individual will vary in the manner and effectiveness with which he or she uses his or her visual acuity.

A blind person may have *no* awareness of environmental light, may have *light perception*, which is awareness of light versus dark, or may have *light projection*, which is the ability to indicate the light source.[5] The capacity of a legally blind person to perceive enough visual information to permit safe independent movement in the environment is called *travel vision*. So far this is the only major functional definition which emphasizes visual ability rather than disability.[6]

About half a million persons in the United States have been classified as legally blind, but many visually impaired persons do not meet the criteria for legal blindness. One functional definition of visual impairment refers to those who cannot read ordinary newsprint, which requires a corrected visual acuity of 20/50.[7] There are about one million of these functionally blind persons in the United States.[8] A person blind in one eye may not be classified as legally blind if acuity in the functional eye is greater than 20/200. These individuals, as well as those with scotomas, amblyopia, color blindness, and central nervous system disorders of visual perception, warrant special attention for their problems.

Causes of childhood blindness include hereditary problems such as Tay-Sachs disease, retinitis pigmentosa, congenital cataracts, albinism, and glaucoma. Even subclinical cases of maternal rubella, especially during the first trimester of pregnancy, may result in damage to either the visual, auditory, circulatory, or central nervous system or to combinations of these. Thus maternal or congenital rubella is one cause of congenital blindness. Retrolental fibroplasia, once a leading cause of early blindness, has declined with attention to the amount of oxygen that can safely be administered to the premature or distressed infant. Accidents, diseases such as encephalitis, and malignancies can produce visual impairment or blindness at any age. Lowenfeld[9] stated in 1971 that there were more than 25,000 school-aged blind children in the United States.

One study revealed that of the blind population in California, 85 percent had lost their vision after age forty-five; half of the total group had become blind after age sixty-five.[10] The major causes of adult blindness are diabetes, cataracts, and glaucoma. Pain is usually associated with the more rapidly progressing type of glaucoma and with other conditions that include increased intraorbital or intracranial pressure. Vascular disease and multiple sclerosis can lead to visual problems in the adult population.

Some visual field deficits are of psychogenic origin. One way to differentiate these from deficits resulting from other causes is to ascertain what the person sees at varying distances from the visual display. Ordinarily, as a person steps back from an item he or she has been viewing, the visual array expands accordingly. Similarly, the person with organic tunnel vision, as though looking through the viewfinder of a camera, can see more as he or she moves farther from the subject or scene. Persons with psychogenic field deficits characteristically do not perceive an expanded visual array at a greater distance; they continue to identify only the original subject matter.[11]

Deficits in Hearing

Deafness has been defined as the inability to hear and understand speech. This definition has been used for the National Census of the Deaf Population and in the Model State Plan for Vocational Rehabilitation of the Deaf.[12] In a 1969 report the deaf population was estimated at 250,000.[13] Schein stated that of chronic physical disabilities in this country, impaired hearing occurs most often, to the extent that in 1976 there were approximately 13.6 million hearing-impaired persons, of whom 1.7 million were deaf.[14] The nondeaf hearing-impaired persons might be called hard-of-hearing; by definition this indicates that, although impaired, the sense of hearing is functional, with or without a hearing aid.[15]

The person who cannot hear and understand speech may be described according to the phase of life at which deafness occurred. An individual is said to be *congenitally deaf* if he or she was born that way, *prelingually deaf* if he or she lost his hearing prior to the development of speech, or *prevocationally deaf* if he or she became deaf before reaching nineteen years of age.[16]

Intensity or loudness, the amplitude of sound waves, is measured in decibels or dB. Ordinary conversation registers approximately 60 dB. The frequency of sound waves, known as pitch, is usually measured in cycles per second or hertz. The lower-pitched speech sounds are those such as *o* in *go*, *d* and *g* in *dog;* higher tones include *f* in *puff*, *s* in *say*, *school*, and *this*. Adequate auditory perception of speech requires hearing between 500 and 2000 hertz (low to high respectively) but frequencies from 16 to 16,000 hertz are audible to persons with normal hearing. Early hearing impairment may first be detected when testing for sounds at 4000 hertz. Loss is usually gradual and may go unnoticed or undiagnosed for some time. If audiometric tests reveal an average auditory loss of 16 dB for frequencies of 500, 1000, and 2000, the individual is considered to have a *beginning hearing impairment.* A person is classified as *deaf* when the average auditory loss is 82 dB or more for those frequencies.[17]

There are two major categories of deafness. In *middle ear* or *conduction deafness,* when sounds are conducted by air rather than bone, there tends to be greater difficulty in hearing lower frequencies. The greater problem in *perception* or *nerve deafness* is for the higher frequencies, whether sound is conducted by air or bone. If the hearing impairment involves the cochlea, slight increases in sound intensity may, through recruitment, be perceived as much louder, even to the point of pain.[18]

Deafness that occurs in children may be attributed to hereditary nerve deafness, brain defects, birth trauma, and infections. Congenital rubella, maternal ingestion of certain medications during pregnancy, and early infections such as cerebrospinal meningitis and encephalitis may cause deafness.[19, 20] Premature infants and those whose blood type is incompatible with their mother's Rh negative type have a higher incidence of deafness than other infants.[21] Ten of the fifty-seven identified forms of genetic deafness also involve visual problems at some time of life. Genetic counseling has been advised.[22,23]

Otosclerosis, which may first be identified during adolescence, is the primary cause of deafness among active adults.[24] Continuous loud noise can damage the inner ear, but there are no conclusions regarding intermittent intense noise. Incidence of deafness increases with the age of the population. Although more women than men have otosclerosis, after age fifty-five there are more men than women with hearing loss.[25,26]

Deaf-Blindness or Blind-Deafness

Both combinations of this term are included in the title because some libraries catalog according to the second term, even though most use the first. As suggested in the preceding sections on visual and hearing deficits, the combined loss of both distant senses may be due to hereditary or congenital causes, to infections, or to central nervous system trauma and may be complicated by the aging process. The rubella epidemic of the mid-sixties resulted in a relatively large population of deaf-blind children, now 11 to 14 years of age, as well as those with single sensory losses. Because of the other organs affected by the rubella virus, some of the deaf-blind children suffer cardiac problems, motor and/or mental retardation, hyperactivity, and, in some cases, autistic-like behaviors.[27] Just as the individual terms, deafness and blindness, are broad, including a wide range of abilities and limitations, so is the deaf-blind category. Persons may be totally deaf and blind, partially sighted and totally deaf, hearing impaired and completely blind, or mildly to moderately impaired in both vision and hearing. Educational programs for deaf-blind children have accepted, under the guideline established by the National Study Committee on Education of Deaf-Blind Children in 1954,[28] any child whose disabilities prevent his or her benefitting from programs offered the blind or the deaf child. Generally speaking, the most progress has been made by children who became adventitiously disabled, rather than congenitally deaf-blind.

Deaf-blindness in adulthood is discussed near the end of this chapter.

OCCUPATIONAL THERAPY FOR THE DEVELOPING INDIVIDUAL WITH IMPAIRED DISTANT SENSES

Basic human needs, such as those for physical and psychological warmth, safety, and security are universal. Certain tasks, including the development of the abilities to distinguish self from environment and to trust, are required of each individual for successful progression through and contribution to life. The occupational therapist must use knowledge of these in any treatment setting.

Although human needs and developmental tasks are essentially the same for sighted and blind, hearing and deaf individuals, the methods, timing, and evidences of attainment and accomplishment of these may vary. To illustrate the similarities and differences of needs and tasks among developing individuals, I have chosen to discuss the sensory aspects of the development of object recognition and, less extensively, the more sophisticated, interdependent accomplishments of object permanence, establishment of trust, interpersonal relationships, and language. These are all aspects of object relations. The intent of the discussion is to encourage the reader to use knowledge of normal human development and needs, to recognize when variations in methods and results are necessary and relatively normal, and to apply that general and specific knowledge to plan and provide effective intervention for each patient.

Object Recognition

Object recognition, the ability to identify a human or nonhuman object in some personally meaningful way, is fundamental to the development of object permanence and thus also is a significant aspect of the establishment of trust. Consider how an infant recognizes a very important object, his or her mother. Sensory information is available from the mother regarding the visual display of two eyes, mouth, hair color, size, and movements; the tone and rhythm of her voice, heartbeat, and footsteps; the ways she touches and handles the child; the "feel" of her skin, hair, lips, and ring; the vibration of her heartbeat, steps, and voice; the scent of her cologne, breath, and body; and the taste of her fingers, flesh, and, if breastfeeding, milk. The list is not exhaustive but deliberately includes information available through all sensory channels: visual, auditory, kinesthetic, proprioceptive, touch-tactile, temperature, olfactory, and gustatory. From such an array or certain aspects of it the infant develops the concept of mother, into which many women could fit for a short time; however, the infant can usually distinguish his or her mother from another woman at an early age.[29] (Discrimination of strangers begins at approximately 24 weeks.)

Object Recognition and the Blind Child

If the infant described in the preceding paragraph is blind he or she will come to associate all but the visual stimuli, which he or she cannot receive, with his or her mother. So long as he or she can hear, smell, or feel her in some meaningful way, he or she can then recognize his or her mother. If these stimuli are absent, even though the little one is within the mother's vision, to the infant she is absent; in fact, until the infant develops object permanence, she ceases to exist. Ordinarily vision plays a significant role in object recognition, but if the blind infant has sufficient opportunity and encouragement to use and refine the other senses while manipulating and responding to human and nonhuman objects, the milestone will be reached. The blind child's ability to hear and to begin to associate words with objects and events becomes particularly important to the development of object recognition and permanence, relationship-building, and concept formation.

Fraiberg[30] and her fellow psychiatrists have studied the development of blind and sighted children. They have found that otherwise normal, totally blind infants (1) tended to lie passively in their cribs with their arms abducted to either side, elbows flexed to 90 degrees, hands at head level; (2) could distinguish parents from a stranger by the age of six to eight months even when all were silent and the stranger attempted to hold the infant just as his parents did; (3) did not spontaneously reach for objects unless shown by auditory input, from tapping the toy on table or floor, that the object they had just been holding or touching was within reach; (4) could localize sound at about ten months of age; and (5) began to creep only after they could both localize sound and reach. Finally the blind children developed the apparently innate smiling response as do sighted infants but did not further develop or maintain true smiling in infancy, except occasionally for the mother, probably because imitation and reinforcement of the smile were hardly possible. Interpersonal relationships between parents and infant can be affected by this apparent lack of facial responsiveness on the part of the infant.

Object Recognition and the Deaf Child

If all other senses are intact and appropriately stimulated, the nonhearing child will develop object recognition, object permanence, and interpersonal relationships based on visual, manual, and physical exploration and the internal and external results of these experiences. Nonverbal communication through smiling, other lip and facial expressions, body language, gestures, and demonstration will be the basis for the young deaf child's "labeling" of objects, events, and feelings. Later more formal manual signs, finger spelling, lip or speech reading, printed words and symbols will supplement the infant language. If the nonhearing child's back is turned or the child is not visually attending in the parent's direction, the child's inability to respond to his or her parent's words or footsteps as one or the other approaches may affect their relationship. However, when the child does see them, their appearance may be acknowledged with a genuine smile and animation.

Particularly before a definite diagnosis of deafness, the young child may be perceived to be stubborn, withdrawn, peculiar, or retarded as a result of apparently fluctuating attention. Actually this behavior depends in part on the availability of meaningful sensory input in the given situation, a significant factor for every individual. The fact that early babbling can occur in deaf as well as in hearing infants may lead to the false assumption that the child hears. It appears that this is a phenomenon of normal oral motor development. Since the child cannot hear the parents' reinforcement of the babbling, he or she is unable by auditory-imitative means to continue development of the sounds of his or her culture.

Mindel and Vernon,[31] a psychiatrist and a psychologist who have worked and lived with deaf persons and their families, have suggested that many deaf persons tend to use a mannerism reminiscent of the age at which it is natural and acceptable to communicate without words. The mannerism is the smile, which for the sighted but deaf infant is reinforceable and one of the foundations for a warm relationship with mother, father, and others. Rather than conveying a true feeling of pleasure, a deaf person of any age may smile at the speaking, hearing person both to conceal the fact that he or she did not understand all of the spoken message and to avoid embarrassing the speaker.

Language development can and will occur in deaf, blind, hearing, and sighted persons, but its achievement must be judged in terms of one's ability to express, receive, interpret, and respond to immediate and recorded communication rather than with specific reference to the spoken word and the printed page.

Object Recognition and the Deaf-Blind Child

The world of the infant who is both deaf and blind consists only of those human and nonhuman objects that can be felt, smelled, tasted, and manipulated. Fortunately many deaf-blind individuals have some vestige of one or the other distant sense, so that residual vision or hearing, however small, can be used to aid in motivation, orientation, exploration, and satisfaction of many such children. Recalling the tendencies toward passivity of blind infants, and the attentional problems of deaf infants, one has some notion of the probable need to *bring* the world *to* the deaf-blind infant and vice versa, *and* in a manner appropriate, acceptable, and meaningful to the child. Until touched, this infant may receive no stimuli that say someone or something is near. Medical staff and parents may not initially have been aware of the profound sensory loss and thus may have found no reason to handle the newborn differently from any other full-term or premature infant.

Mouchka,[32] the knowing parent of a deaf-blind child, who has also had experience with other similarly handicapped youngsters, noted that these infants behave differently, within three categories: (1) they do not respond to any apparent stimuli but remain passive; (2) they consistently respond vigorously, protectively, and hypersensitively to any attempt to handle them; or (3) they cry most of the time whether they are being handled or left alone. These findings correlate with reports from parents and caretakers of other deaf-blind children and with those of Chess and associates,[33] psychiatrists who have studied children handicapped as a result of the rubella syndrome. Additional cardiac and neurological problems can compound the sensory deficits and make homeostasis even more precarious, which may explain the extreme sympathetic nervous system responses of some multihandicapped children as well as the apparent vegetative state of others. Before object recognition can be attained there must be homeostasis and sufficient meaningful sensory information to permit the infant to sense and respond to the mother or another object. A trusting relationship is based at least in part on sufficient appropriate stimuli which the infant can somehow perceive as satisfying, predictable, and dependable. The demanding and frustrating roles of parents of such handicapped children require ongoing acknowledgment, support, and guidance by empathetic, creative, and competent health care professionals.

Object recognition and permanence, relationships, and communication can be developed slowly if the infant is neurologically and motorically able to tactually and kinesthetically experience and explore self, mother, father, crib, food, toys, and larger environment, augmented by relevant sensory information through all possible channels. Consistent tactual symbols and signs, tactile-kinesthetic rhythms, motions, and vibrations will gradually become representative of objects and events experienced, contributing to crude language development and the establishment of trusting relationships with others who can use the language.

Special Considerations in Occupational Therapy for Developmental Sensory Loss

The pediatric or developmental occupational therapist selects from a comprehensive set of developmental evaluation instruments based on observation of the individual child with parent and nonhuman objects, interview with parents, and information gained through referral and available records. Realistic treatment is planned according to findings and to child and family needs and abilities. There are some factors that merit special attention when the patient is deaf, blind, or both, with or without additional problems. This is equally true when diagnosis is tentative and when the referral to the facility is for complete evaluation, diagnosis, and recommendations.

Need for Meaningful Activity and Interaction

In view of the tendency of blind infants and many deaf-blind infants to lie passively wherever they are placed, movement of arms, legs, head, and entire body must be encouraged through verbal, other auditory, and tactile stimulation. Position changes such as being rolled in both directions to prone or gently bounced or rocked on parent's knees should help stimulate appropriate reflexes, muscle tone, and interaction with the environment. Whether or not the infant sees and hears, those handling the infant should speak and sing to him or her, use natural facial expression and body language, and provide and encourage tactile and kinesthetic experiences. Use of natural speech, facial, and body expression also helps the sighted, hearing person be at ease and facilitates more relaxed interaction. The infant, child, or adult who can perceive some of the visual or auditory input receives that much more information about the experience.

The therapist as well as family members must be alert to what forms and methods of interaction and movement appear to have meaning and to offer satisfaction to the infant or child. From this angle, the therapist can determine how to use and supplement those methods to increase the child's purposeful exploration of self and environment. If the individual prods, bites, or spins, alternative acceptable methods of equivalent stimulation should be planned and provided. Sensory integrative treatment strategies may well be indicated for many or all blind and/or deaf children.

Whether deaf, blind, or both, the developing individual needs assistance or guidance in exploring. The deaf child's experiences require accompanying consistent and appropriate visual symbols such as gestures, manual signs, facial expressions, lip movements, and printed words to establish internal and external communicable terms for attributes and names of persons, objects, daily activities, events, emotions, and eventually ideas, problem solving, and abstract thinking. If blind, the child needs auditory and tactile input for the same reasons, as well as to provide perspective. Tactile-kinesthetic guidance and demonstration are needed by the deaf-blind child. All need time with responsive individuals to use the terms or symbols they learn, to receive corrective and positive feedback, to feel valued, and to be encouraged to continue to reflect and to build on the purposeful exploration.

Use of Residual Distant Senses

Infants, children, and adults who have the ability to distinguish light from dark, to see shadows, to actually see items upon very close inspection or with great magnification can safely be permitted and encouraged to do so. Such use of the eyes will not jeopardize vision.[34] In fact, this residual vision may greatly enhance motivation, orientation, mobility, exploration, and learning. The mother of a blind infant with a pin-point type vision for light encouraged the little one to reach, creep, and eventually walk toward her by holding a tiny flashlight just beyond the infant's reach.[35] In so doing, the infant's mobility, physical fitness, and exploratory learning were greatly facilitated. The rewards of light and mother's warmth and praise made the accomplishments particularly satisfying steps to further feats. Eye glasses, monocular magnifying lenses, and other magnification devices can be used to enhance residual vision.

The deaf child who cannot hear conversational speech well enough to distinguish meaning but responds to the telephone, his or her name shouted from another room, or a loudly ticking clock held near the ear may benefit from a hearing aid. Ability to hear loud sounds or certain frequencies can be used at least for safety and emergency measures, but only if approved by the child's physician and audiologist should it be employed as an aid to motivation and attention.

Use of residual vision will not improve acuity but does appear to improve visual perception. The more one uses what sight remains the more the individual becomes proficient and adaptive in the ways one seeks and uses visual information. The same seems true for hearing. Certainly the use of any residual is of special importance in the development of the deaf-blind child.

The occupational therapist and others working with blind or deaf infants and children must be alert to any evidences that the little one has some residual vision or hearing. Performance in more natural play and interactive settings may differ significantly from behavior in formal or standardized testing situations.

Use of Intact Senses

Objects and interchanges that require ultimate use of each sensory modality allow both evaluation and enhancement of the child's sensory abilities. The occupational therapist must observe all available clues in a situation when evaluating the child's method(s) of identifying or approaching objects and tasks.

Toys and situations should provide for some separate and many combinations of visual, auditory, tactile, kinesthetic, olfactory, and gustatory experiences. To be most meaningful, experiences should be centered around a particular activity or place. For example, bathtime offers feel of water, water and air temperatures, sides of tub, washcloth, soap, and shampoo; of being dry and wet; of acting upon the water, soap, washcloth, own body, and tub toys; of feeling body parts, undressed, scrubbed, wiped, rinsed, patted, and dressed or not dressed. Smells of clothing, soap, shampoo, and bodies offer olfactory stimulation. Stimuli abound; so do opportunities for healthy interaction, evaluation, teaching, and learning in a real world context. Appropriate orientation to the activity, such as introducing the bath water to fingers and hands first while holding the infant comfortably, securely, encouraging the infant to swish the water about, should make the experience more acceptable and pleasurable. As the child develops, he or she can be assisted to note the water faucet and handles, similarities in structure and function to those of the lavatory and sink, and to use them with supervision and independently as he is ready to do so safely. Meaningful communication about the what, how, when, and why of the task, about how well the child does it, how it feels, and with whom he or she does it—repeated with slight variations each time the child engages in the activity—add to concepts of the child's own body, performance and worth, the task, and environment.

Family Involvement and Counseling

The blind and/or deaf infant does not know, early in life, that he or she lacks certain sensory abilities. Parents and other family members will be acutely aware of the lack by the time a diagnosis is made and acknowledged, if not before then. Some parents may have been seeking diagnosis and help for months. Reactions of various family members are very likely to be those experienced to any loss, from shock, disbelief, and denial to grief, helplessness, guilt, and anger, to possible over-identification and empathy, but hopefully, with help, to a coming to terms with the reality of ability as well as disability and to a suitable plan of action.[36] It is apparent to those who work with severely developmentally handicapped children that the emotional needs of the family must be met in order for the child to achieve maximum benefit from a carefully planned habilitation program. Because of the nature of the child's handicap and impact on the family, needs are changing but continuous.

In the early weeks and months support and counseling may be provided through parent groups, individual counseling, reinforcement of everything families are doing correctly for the child, and instruction with demonstration of additional helpful ways to handle, care for, and stimulate the child with emphasis on those which best fit the family's life style and child's needs. Parents, grandparents, and siblings need objective explanations of the disability, reasonable expectations and limitations, type of treatment, and so forth.

If the child is extremely passive or obviously hyperreactive, families, physicians, and therapists need to explore the reasons and experiment with possible solutions. They must understand that the behavior is not directed personally at them but is symptomatic of the child's physiological state and should support each other while treating the child to the best of their knowledge and ability.

Among those things that all families of blind, deaf, or deaf-blind infants and children can do are to place the child in the midst of family activity during most of the child's waking hours, including him or her as much as possible by touch, voice, sight, smell, and movement without overstimulation; to communicate clearly and consistently with the child and each other; and to watch for and find pleasure together in step-by-step progress toward realistic goals. Activities include trips by auto, foot, tricycle, or bicycle to the grocery store, neighbor's house, church, school, and park as well as meals, story time, free play, games, chores, and company at home. Established hours, places, and equipment for meals, sleep, and self-care may add to the child's security and sense of time. Parents also need some time away from the handicapped child for their own mental health; health care personnel may need to assist them to find and use qualified babysitters, as well as resources such as preschools, play groups, reading material, and instruction in special communication methods so they and their children may learn a common language.

School Readiness[37,38,39]

The occupational therapist can be of significant assistance as consultant or provider of direct services in the areas of human development, activities of daily living in the broad and specific senses, play, and school readiness for the child and family. Many accomplishments which constitute school readiness are common to all children: satisfactory emotional development, ability to follow directions, many concrete experiences, and adequate peer and peer group relationships. Readiness for school for the totally blind child should especially include language development to the extent that by the time the child enters school he or she can speak clearly enough to be understood, ask and answer questions with more than a single word, provide name and address; tactual and auditory discrimination which enable the child to discern meaning and purpose from what is felt or heard; mobility and good relaxed posture; good use of both hands; and an awareness that words and ideas may be communicated in tactual form (braille). The last may be accomplished by putting braille labels on familiar objects and possessions and by reading stories from preschool books printed in both type and braille, the reader showing the child how to move fingers along the line of braille as the words are read but not attempting to teach braille.

The deaf child's readiness should especially include the common accomplishments with emphasis on emotional development, interpersonal relationships, many concrete experiences and language development through sign, gestures, facial expression, and possibly some printed words. There are obviously more examples of words in our environment for the deaf child to see but the child must also know that they have meaning. Also necessary are some acceptable effective ways to gain attention as by touch or visual signal; the child needs to be able to seek appropriately the attention of others to understand and follow simple directions such as "come here," "put this there," "sit down."

Schools and Other Training Facilities

Residential and day schools for the deaf and for the blind are available in at least one metropolitan area in most states. Some blind schools now have units for deaf-blind or multiply handicapped persons. An increasing number of visually or hearing impaired students are attending public school classes with sighted and hearing peers. Self-worth, self-care, communication, relationships with adults, and other social skills may become more difficult and even more important as the individual reaches adolescence. Counseling and guidance, indoor and outdoor athletic pursuits, drama, creative writing, other artistic endeavors, and school clubs may facilitate these.

Some secondary schools for blind and deaf students offer shop, homemaking, typing, bookkeeping, and physical education as well as college preparatory courses; they may include classes for personal development, sex education, marriage and family living, leisure and additional vocational preparation. Junior high or high school blind students usually receive orientation and mobility training for independent travel, but preschool blind children have also benefited from the services of orientation and mobility specialists.[40]

Post-secondary education is available to qualified deaf and blind graduates, who can apply for comprehensive services through state divisions or bureaus of vocational rehabilitation. Some programs have been specifically planned to serve deaf students exclusively or in conjunction with hearing students.* They offer skilled counseling in basic academic areas and also in social, vocational, and coping skills, which have been found to be less than adequate in many deaf secondary school drop-outs.[41] For this and other reasons, many deaf students are encouraged or required to enter preparatory or vestibule programs before beginning a formal vocational, technical, or professional program.[42,43]

If the preceding educational opportunities are not feasible for them, persons who have a developmental sensory loss along with other serious physical or intellectual limitations may be served through special classes in public or private day and residential facilities or by educational and health care personnel who come to the child's home.

Future Planning

In the event that a person lacks the physical, psychosocial, or intellectual ability to join the work force, run a home, and generally be an independent member of society, several possibilities exist. These include living at home or in a group home, sharing in household management, chores, and recreation with possible participation in community endeavors, and a sheltered workshop program. Those with serious multiple problems may be independent or semi-independent in ADL within a supervised setting; others may require custodial care. To be appropriate, the environment must provide sufficient meaningful sensory stimuli and experiences, encourage maximum possible use of resident's abilities, and include knowledgeable, sensible, caring personnel, who can and will communicate with each individual in a manner he or she understands.[44,45]

Periodic reevaluation is as necessary for correct treatment and placement as the comprehensive evaluation on which immediate and future planning are initially based. This seems particularly true for the person with multiple developmental disabilities in view of sometimes lengthy plateaus before progress is made and the interaction of the individual, the several disabilities, and the environment.

* Post-secondary educational programs include Gallaudet College, Washington DC; National Technical Institute for the Deaf, Rochester NY; Rochester Institute of Technology, Rochester NY; and three regional programs: Delgado Junior College, New Orleans, Seattle Community College, and St. Paul Technical Vocational Institute.

Resources

For the comprehensive and long-term habilitation required by many persons with visual and/or auditory developmental disabilities, many persons and agencies, methods, and materials are required. These are discussed much more thoroughly in a number of publications, some of which are listed in the bibliography for this chapter.

Whether or not they function formally as a team, a number of professional persons will work with the deaf and/or blind child and his family in the course of treatment. These may include the physician(s) (pediatrician, neurologist, ophthalmologist, otolaryngologist, otologist, psychiatrist), nurse, social caseworker, psychologist, audiologist, optometrist, hearing and speech clinician, occupational therapist, physical therapist, parent, special educator, braille or sign teacher, classroom teacher, recreation specialist, rehabilitation teacher, orientation and mobility specialist,* and vocational counselor. The need to coordinate information and habilitation efforts is obvious.

Regional centers for the deaf-blind as well as local, state, regional, national, and overseas associations for the blind and for the deaf provide general and specific information and assistance to their spe-

* *Peripatologist* is the technical term for orientation and mobility specialist used in Eastern United States.

cial populations, their families, and professional workers; some also are actively involved in education of the general public. Personalized correspondence courses to guide parents in promoting optimum development of their deaf and deaf-blind children under five are available at little or no charge.[46]

Methods and Materials

In addition to the developmental evaluations and tasks available in the pediatric occupational therapy department, the therapist may wish to obtain the Callier-Azuza Scale[47] for evaluation of the deaf-blind or multiply handicapped infant or young child. It is advisable to assemble or check for freshness the containers, droppers, and substances used for testing olfactory and gustatory senses and to add to the collection of manipulable objects and surfaces so that many same, similar, and contrasting textures, weights, shapes, temperatures, actions, sounds, colors, and functions are included. Careful observation and reporting of how the child uses and/or responds to these as well as to the persons present is essential for treatment, continuous evaluation, and program revision.

Activity or task analysis will be invaluable for assessment, for teaching and treating the child and family, and for the setting of goals and objectives in small enough increments for the gratification and morale of child, family, and professionals. The needs for developmentally and individually appropriate, realistic objectives and for minute steps cannot be overemphasized.

The daily schedules or patterns of living of the child and family are important data. They contribute to overall assessment of actual and potential emotional, social, physical, and cognitive-perceptual-motor development of the child. In addition, such information may be indicative of family values and certainly serves as a guide to the type home program and support most appropriate for the individual family.

Equipment and many methods used with the blind, deaf, or deaf-blind child will be similar to those used with other children. Some of these are presented in chapters on sensory integration, pediatric occupational therapy, cerebral palsy, and mental retardation. Toys should include crib toys, pull toys, cash registers, cars, trucks, dolls, puppets, balls, wagons, tricycles, and so forth. The blind child should be given three dimensional objects and puzzles unless the two dimensional item has meaningful form such as circle, square, heart, and triangle. The blind child and the deaf child should have some toys with and some without deliberate auditory qualities like bells, chimes, clicks, and vibrations. The same is true of toys with lights and movement. Some dolls are now manufactured with more realistic genitalia. Natural inclusion of these dolls* in the young child's possession could help in acceptance and naming of the whole body, if parents, teachers, and others are willing and able to assist the child appropriately. Books, games, music, scissors, crayons, and paint should be introduced by persons prepared to help the child use, understand, and enjoy them. Eating and cooking utensils are more appropriately used for their intended purposes rather than as potentially confusing toys for blind or deaf-blind youngsters. Pets are fine when any child is old enough to be gentle with them.

Most early teaching-learning will occur through imitation and modeling of significant others. The demonstration and behavior should correspond to all the child's senses.

Identification of clothing and understanding of top, bottom, inside, outside, on, and off are important to deaf and blind children. Even though the deaf child can see the garment, the child also needs help in learning the words, methods, and acceptable combinations. The blind child should also be helped to learn where and how clothing is stored, what goes together, and what to do with it when undressing. Discussion of colors and patterns and sewing and care of garments is pertinent for older blind children.[48]

The therapist who plans to work with any of these children is encouraged to study further, beginning with agencies and references given in this chapter. Some of the material on adventitiously blind and deaf persons may also apply, and vice versa.

* Dolls include but are not limited to black and white Baby Brother Tender Love by Mattel; Little Siblings—baby boy and girl dolls carried by Constructive Playthings; and others by Ideal and Horseman.

OCCUPATIONAL THERAPY FOR ADVENTITIOUS LOSS OF VISION AND HEARING

Previously sighted persons who lose their vision are frequently referred to as the adventitiously or newly blind. Adventitious deafness, in parallel fashion, denotes a substantial or total loss of hearing after one has had functional use of the auditory sense. The loss may be sudden or gradual. It may occur superimposed upon or secondary to another disabling condition, as the only disability, or as one of multiple disabilities incurred through accident or illness. The occupational therapist may also encounter adventitiously and developmentally blind and/or deaf persons referred to general or psychiatric hospitals or to rehabilitation, day center, or geriatric facilities for problems other than their sensory losses.

Problems of physical and emotional health may or may not be complicated or precipitated by blindness or deafness. If the patient is hard-of-hearing or has low vision rather than being totally deaf or blind, treatment of another condition may be complicated because the vision or hearing impairment may not be immediately apparent. Two important responsibilities of health care professionals are to establish effective two-way communication with the patient and to determine the full extent of particular problems and capabilities, including vision and hearing, in preparation for appropriate treatment and follow-up. One of the greatest needs of mentally ill deaf persons frequently is that of a means of communicating.

Newly Blind or Visually Impaired Adult

A person who has suddenly or gradually lost all sight has lost a major source of information, pleasure, communication, and mobility. How quickly and adequately the person passes through the stages of responses to loss depends upon premorbid personality and abilities, attitudes toward blindness and blind persons, and the attitudes and services of family, friends, and health care personnel. Any visually impaired person should be oriented to the surroundings, his or her condition, and to persons visiting and working with him or her.

As soon as medically stable the newly blind person can assume responsibility for personal care and for much personal business. This can be both psychologically and physically rehabilitating. To make it possible, items needed must be within reach and must be identifiable. The bedside stand, table, chairs, and room should be organized and unchanged, unless the patient is verbally and physically oriented to any necessary alteration. Doors should be completely open or completely closed to prevent collision with a partially open door. In approaching the patient, the occupational therapist should speak directly to him or her in a natural tone of voice, introducing him or herself by name, profession, and function, addressing the patient by name, and avoiding speaking loudly unless it is known that there is also a hearing loss. It is almost always appropriate to shake hands but initially the therapist should be prepared to give some verbal indication of the intent. Hand-to-hand contact gives the patient somewhat more control and information than touching him or her on arm or shoulder.

The newly blind person, whether in hospital, home, or rehabilitation facility, may be experiencing shock, denial, hostility, depression, resignation, or some combination of these. The occupational therapist should check the patient's records to learn the cause and circumstances of his blindness, the date of onset, prognosis, concomitant conditions, occupation, response to blindness, and other pertinent information. Such data, combined with the referral and the therapist's professional knowledge and healthy, realistic attitudes toward blindness and people, provide the right base for initial and future encounters. The therapist and the blind client will discuss what the client is able to do in the immediate environment, current problems, and what the client expects to be able to do when discharged. Immediate tasks include personal care, communication, and some mobility. Problem solving with the client about any difficulties in these areas helps him or her succeed and also sets the tone for rehabilitation. While the client demonstrates how he or she places, locates, and uses such things as comb, brush, water glass, radio, the therapist can observe apparent tactile, kinesthetic, and auditory abilities, approach to the task, degree of organization, control, and emotional tone. It is important that the client be successful at some aspect of self-care or other tasks and that both the client and the therapist recognize the success. The therapist must therefore be prepared to teach or provide an appropriate and successful experience if the client cannot. Some blind persons may need little or no rehabilitation beyond understandable explanation of the condition, acceptance as an individual of worth, accurate responses to questions, presentation of safety, organization, and management principles, and names, telephone numbers, and addresses of agencies and resources for the blind. Others may require individual and/or group treatment and short- or long-term follow-up for psychological as much as physical reasons.

Organization of life space is important for each person with little or no vision. When items have a particular location in a room, closet, or drawer, they are more readily and appropriately used. Work simplification principles apply and may be taught to the client. Systems for hanging clothes by style and color and/or by outfit, folding and identifying money, and arranging study and other work space will help maximize potentials of all blind or partially sighted persons.[49] Personal care is particularly important because it is comprised of familiar and repeatable skills, it influences and reflects the self-concept of the person, and it influences others' attitudes toward the individual and toward blindness. The person must be encouraged to use good posture, to look or turn directly toward the one to whom he or she speaks, and to interact with sighted, blind, and partially-sighted individuals. He or she may wish to extend the right hand when meeting others or invite a firm handshake. Personal care including bathing, hygiene, dressing, and care of teeth and hair are more likely to be routine, automatic, and quickly resumed. Tactile symbols can be sewn (French knots), glued, or tacked to clothing and containers to designate colors, names, and so forth.

The newly-blind older child, adolescent, or adult should be evaluated, trained, and reevaluated for efficient effective use of other senses: auditory, kinesthetic, tactual, olfactory, and gustatory. Refinement of other sensory abilities does not automatically occur when one loses vision.[50,51] The person should be assisted in learning to localize and discriminate sounds. Until the individual can do this, even ordinary conversation may be difficult since it is no longer possible to use visual cues to enhance understanding and gather nonverbal feedback. If the person has residual vision, he or she should be assisted to augment and use it. Some environmental sounds could be recorded to expedite training, but actual situations are preferred. Ability to detect temperatures as well as to feel and manipulate objects is important for safety as well as function. Consider, for example, pouring hot coffee into a cup. The client's pouring hand should find and grasp the wood or plastic handle safely. Accurate pouring can be practiced by placing the other palm and fingers around the cup, pouring directly in the center of the cup, and hearing and feeling the heat as the hot liquid rises to desired level. Prerequisites for this task include the ability to pour cold liquids successfully.

Other skills requiring stereognosis and kinesthesis are eating and all related activities such as buttering bread, cutting meat, and managing salt, pepper, and sugar. Although these skills were likely automatic for the newly blind, and can again be mastered, the client may be particularly sensitive regarding eating in the presence of others. Early meals could be more comfortable with relatively easily managed foods and reasonable privacy; the occupational therapist can assist the patient with some skills before or after mealtimes so that conversation and only essential questions and problems receive attention during the meal. Visualizing the plate as a clock face assists communication about the location of food and other items, such as meat at six o'clock and water glass in line with one o'clock.

It is possible for some previously-sighted blind persons to continue writing by hand with the use of writing guides and check writing guides available through the American Foundation for the Blind. Touch typewriting is another very feasible means of communicating with sighted persons. Tape recorders may permit private correspondence between the blind person and others, eliminating the need for a sighted individual to read the contents of personal mail. Talking books are available in a variety of subjects. If the individual desires and has the tactile perception to do so, he or she may seek instruction in braille reading and writing. There are braille typewriters and braillewriters which the client may wish to use later. The therapist should assist in finding a braille teacher. In preparation, the patient should develop the tactile and manipulative abilities of both hands and might enjoy games using braille playing cards, Scrabble, bingo, and conventional dominos or chess and checkers.

Use of the telephone also maintains communication. The dial and pushbuttons of the phone can be memorized as can numerous telephone numbers. Braille or tactile symbols of some kind could be introduced for recording and recognition of some little used or new numbers. Blind and physically disabled persons may also identify themselves and request a number from the information operator.

Mobility is of great importance. Independent travel skills should be taught by specially trained teachers called orientation and mobility specialists. A full course in orientation and mobility requires approximately 180 hours for the adventitiously blind person.[52] Prior to or along with the course, family, friends, workers, and the blind person should quickly be taught the correct way for the blind to use a sighted guide. The guide walks about half a step ahead of the blind partner, who grasps the elbow of the guide by hand. It becomes less necessary for the guide to alert the partner to curbs, stairways, turns, and stops since the blind person can detect these through the guide's movements. Obstacles such as doorsills, sidewalk cracks, or ice should still be identified and located for the blind person; sights and landmarks along the way can be described for enjoyment and enlightenment. The client should also practice detecting changes in surfaces underfoot, e.g., grass, gravel, carpet, wood, cement. Some blind persons may eventually use guide dogs. Special training courses are available for this.[53]

Corrective and positive feedback should be given the blind person regarding posture, appearance, and performance so that he or she may become as proficient and attractive as possible. Dark glasses may be worn if the cosmetic appearance of the eyes is not or cannot surgically be made acceptable. A variety of attractive styles, shapes, and tints are available.

The intended or current vocation of a newly blind person should be carefully considered for creative problem solving and/or related alternative career choices. The occupation should offer sufficient remuneration and employment opportunities and be compatible with the interest, abilities, attitudes, aptitudes, and qualifications of the blind client.[54] Adequate mental health and motivation of the client are vital prerequisites and thus may become treatment objectives for some persons.

Rehabilitation of those who lose much but not all of their vision should include evaluation of all sensory, manipulative, and travel abilities and problems. Safety, organization, eye-hand coordination, problem solving, and available resources should be introduced or reviewed. Magnifying glasses and monocular lenses, adequate indoor and outdoor lighting, and large print books and magazines can be of great help. Light, bright colors on oven controls and step edges may be useful. Studies[55] of the reduced visual perception of the elderly have shown that signs consisting of white or bright yellow letters and symbols against a dark ground are more easily read than the reverse. Because of the yellowing of the lens, colors in the blue, green, or violet range become more difficult to distinguish, making it advisable to use brighter colors of red, orange, and yellow.

In rehabilitation of the older partially- or totally-blind person it is particularly important to consider the preferences, lifestyle, and personality of the client and to recognize that the client has credible ideas, routines, and needs. (See also Chapter 17, Gerontology.) Possible reduced physical movement and/or tactile perception may require more ingenuity of all concerned to make the human and nonhuman environment accessible and satisfying. The diabetic blind person may lack sufficient tactile perception for braille reading but may be able to use a special syringe (available from the American Foundation for the Blind) for injection of insulin.

Deaf or Hard-of-Hearing Adolescent and Adult

If deafness occurred prior to adolescence it may have adversely affected language development and use. Considering spoken language as a tool for thinking, questioning, interacting, and working through problems, one can understand that reduced communication ability can complicate adolescence. Mindel and Vernon[56] have mentioned that the verbal testing and aggression which hearing adolescent males use as an outlet is less or unavailable to deaf males. Its replacement by physical aggression or other acting out further hinders the deaf adolescent's relationships with others and consequently his perception of himself. The occupational therapist and others who work with these young men can assist in healthy emotional and social development by providing experiences allowing male identification, active expression of feelings and energy, understandable feedback, and success. They may wish to integrate hearing and hearing-impaired adolescents of same and opposite sexes in comfortably structured situations.

Regardless of age, if a hard-of-hearing or deaf person has difficulty in attending to or acceptably attracting attention from others, the therapist may need to assist the person in developing this ability. It may be through brief objective explanation of the hearing impairment to new acquaintances with a polite request that they touch the client in a certain manner, move into his visual field, or give him or her a note. If the deaf person has impaired or no speech, he or she will have to make the request through gestures or the written word. The deaf person may also need to sit or stand where it is possible to receive maximum visual input. If he or she does not speak at all, he or she must use some acceptable audible signal or touch the person whose attention is wanted, approaching from the front to minimize surprises.

The adventitiously deaf or hard-of-hearing person will likely have and use speech, although its inflection may become somewhat flat. The person can be reminded to speak with expression, feeling it as he or she did when he/she could also hear it, just as the blind person continues to use familiar facial expressions. Sign language, finger spelling, speech-reading, facial expression, and written communication will enable complete communication. The combination is referred to as *total communication*. If only speech and speech-reading (lipreading) are permitted or possible, the deaf person will receive only part of the message, and less as the number of persons involved increases. If this is the case, seating and lighting must be sufficiently close and bright for the facial and lip movements to be seen. As speakers change in a discussion group, an additional cue through larger movement like standing or raising an arm can be used.

Fortunately most dormitories and playgrounds, if not all classrooms, of deaf schools and the colleges and technical schools serving deaf persons permit and offer total communication.[57] Some schools are integrated with deaf and hearing students so that social development can be richer; in some instances hearing students take notes in carbon copy type notebooks so that a deaf or hard-of-hearing classmate can also have a written record of the lecture or discussion which he or she watches.[58] The more complete the communication the more likely the deaf person is to understand shades of meaning.

The person who gradually or suddenly loses the ability to hear conversational speech suffers a very real sense of isolation. It is possible for him or her to feel that others have excluded, are talking about, or do not care about him or her. If the hearing loss is amenable to a correctly prescribed and fit hearing aid the deaf person must adjust to and learn to use the hearing aid. Monaural aids can increase the hearing in one ear to match the better ear. Binaural aids can enhance audition in both ears. If the person participates in group activities and travels about the community and beyond, hearing in both ears is particularly useful and safer. Binaural or stereophonic hearing enables most persons to localize sound and therefore is very important for partially-sighted and blind persons.[59]

Not all persons can adjust to hearing appliances. Some magnify all sounds; others magnify the higher frequency sounds which may be diminished in elderly persons. Some speech and hearing personnel have found it worthwhile to train the person in the use of a hearing aid, keeping the appliance in the clinic until the person has adjusted to it.[60] Considerable time may be required for training and follow-up, depending upon the individual, but these measures reduce rejection of the hearing aid and accompanying isolation. Occupational therapists working with persons who are still adjusting to hearing aids can structure the environment so that the hearing-impaired person initially communicates on a one-to-one basis with little or no background noise, gradually adding other persons or background sounds until these can be tolerated and managed in combination. It is also necessary that personnel as well as the owner of the hearing aid know how to put on and care for the appliance, test and replace the battery, and adjust the volume. Activity may cause the volume control of some aids to slip so volume should be checked; this could be made easier by marking the control and surrounding area with a line to indicate the usual position.

Smaller-size group activities might be more pleasant and beneficial for deaf and hard-of-hearing persons, whether the task of the group is to learn manual signs and finger spelling, to discuss problems and alternatives, to review a book, to prepare a meal, or to play cards. As individuals become more experienced in communicating by new methods, the group size and amount of communication required can be increased. Some individuals may tend to interrupt unless they can see all members' faces. Whether newly or congenitally deaf, these persons and their hearing friends can enjoy drama, art, church, dancing, sports, and television together as participants or spectators.

Deaf persons need to use their vision, vibratory, and olfactory senses for safety on the street and at home. Some deaf persons are very safe drivers, using bilateral exterior mirrors as well as the interior rearview mirror. As with any driver, emotional maturity and stability are important behind the wheel.

Doorbell, telephone, and alarm clock signals can be augmented or replaced with lights. Some persons may be able to hear telephone conversation by adjusting the volume control or asking the telephone company to do so. Technology is such that some cities have telephones which convert auditory messages into readable ones, but these are expensive and not yet in widespread use. There are also telecommunicators which utilize typed messages from one unit to another.

It has been noted in several situations that the person who lacks adequate hearing has tended to assume a servant role, whether it be washing the dishes, watching the children, carrying firewood or groceries, pushing a wheelchair, or polishing the car. The person's visual sense has shown him a task to be accomplished, he or she derives satisfaction through successful performance, and he or she contributes in this manner to others in the family or group who may be conversing so rapidly amidst much confusion that the deaf member is unable to follow the thoughts. Reduction of confusion and background music, careful seating or placement of persons in the group and purposeful inclusion of the deaf individual through questions, signs, gestures, and attentive listening to whatever language he or she uses should help ensure that the deaf individual becomes and remains more than just a servant. It should also help to prevent or reduce any paranoid feelings. It is to the occupational therapist's and the patient's advantage that the therapist be able to communicate by signing (sign language). If the caseload includes many deaf persons, I believe it is imperative that the occupational therapist learn sign language.

Marriage and family living can be as challenging and satisfying to the mentally-healthy deaf person as to blind or sighted hearing persons. The deaf person can fulfill his or her parental responsibilities equally well as long as there is some way to communicate with school and other personnel. Some deaf persons have hearing ear dogs that alert their owners to such things as doorbells and baby's cry. If both parents lack both hearing and speech, however, it is important for the language development of their hearing children that the children receive language stimulation regularly during their early years. The children would also develop sign language under their parents' influence so that, in effect, they become bilingual. The need for early language stimulation can be met only by coordinating casefinding through prenatal and maternity care with prompt follow-up and enough competent paid or volunteer personnel to provide consistent stimulation until the children can attend preschool.

Combined Visual and Hearing Losses in Adulthood

The loss of both hearing and vision in adulthood will likely necessitate psychological and physical rehabilitation, including compensation through equipment and methods that use the full extent of tactile, kinesthetic, and olfactory senses, cognitive abilities, and previously learned skills. Although the person can continue to speak with or without loss of inflection and possibly write and type, he or she will need to receive communication by means of a hearing aid if that is possible, by manual signs on hands and arms, by printing letters on palm, by lip reading with fingers, by braille or magnified written messages, and/or by physical demonstration such as being moved through a particular activity.

The American Foundation for the Blind offers at cost a machine called a Tellatouch which makes it possible for a deaf-blind person who knows braille to communicate with someone unfamiliar with the manual alphabet. They also manage a travel concession plan which permits the blind or deaf-blind person to travel with a sighted guide for a single fare on most buses and trains in the United States.

Evaluation of the variety, completeness, and satisfaction of tactile, kinesthetic, olfactory, and gustatory information available to deaf-blind persons may reveal problems. This applies in the home, the retirement center, nursing home, and in the larger environment for work, shopping, worship, or recreation. To promote safety and to structure space it may be important to change flooring and guide rail textures to indicate a stairway is nearby or to define an area, to continue guide rails across doorways with some signal that one has reached a doorway and not a corner, and to teach family and personnel guiding and communication methods whether or not the person uses a long cane. The totally deaf person can sense substances and vibration through the cane but can no longer gain auditory information with it. Gardening with scented and unscented plants, baking or cooking, woodworking, sculpting, hiking, swimming, boating, dancing, visiting, and many other endeavors are possible for the person who wishes to continue or to revise his or her lifestyle. It may be more difficult to communicate but that may make it just that much more important. Occupational therapy can play a significant role in helping these persons return to or continue to live productive, satisfying lives.

REQUIREMENTS OF THE OCCUPATIONAL THERAPIST WORKING WITH BLIND AND DEAF PERSONS

The basic personal and professional knowledge, skills, and attributes required by occupational therapists are good preparation for work with persons who are blind, deaf, or deaf-blind. This work also requires (1) healthy, informed attitudes toward blindness and deafness; (2) a balance of patience, objectivity, and empathy; (3) ability to evaluate thoroughly, discriminatingly but efficiently; and (4) ability to solve problems and organize creatively and practically. Interpersonal skills must extend to families, other personnel, and agencies as well as to patients. Quality of voice and body language may make more difference to blind or deaf persons. Natural use of the words "see," "look," "watch," "listen," and "hear" is acceptable and desirable. It may be necessary to pitch the voice lower and to speak relatively slowly when working with those who have high frequency or other partial hearing losses. Body language may need to be modified so the intended messages can be conveyed.

For maximum effectiveness the therapist should learn to communicate in all or most modes used by clients. Until the therapist can learn the mode used by a particular client, he or she should find and use a qualified interpreter. In some instances the patient or family might like to teach the therapist the most important words. Correspondence courses in braille[61,62] and books[63,64] and community courses on manual alphabet and sign are available to most interested persons. The therapist should have at least basic knowledge of magnifying lenses, eye glasses, hearing aids, audio and visual equipment, and special devices and methods. Although no one can completely understand what it means to be deaf or blind, each is encouraged to experience occlusion of hearing and/or vision in supervised situations including self-care, travel, conversation, shopping, and whatever problem situation the therapist and client are attacking. Fuller appreciation of problems will contribute to their solutions. Insight and understanding can also be gained by reading several biographies or autobiographies that present the ideas, experiences, and recommendations of persons who live with a sensory loss.

REFERENCES

1. Chusid, J. G.: Correlative Neuroanatomy and Functional Neurology, ed. 15. Los Altos CA: Lange Medical Publications, 1973, p. 85.
2. Lowenfeld, B.: Our Blind Children: Growing and Learning with Them, ed. 3. Springfield IL: Charles C Thomas, Publishers, 1971, pp. 9–10.
3. Hutchinson, E., and Wagner, E.: Occupational therapy for the blind and partially sighted. In Willard, H. S., and Spackman, C. S.: Occupational Therapy, ed. 4. Philadelphia: J. B. Lippincott Co., 1971, p. 491.
4. Chusid: Correlative Neuroanatomy, p. 261.
5. Lowenfeld: Our Blind Children, p. 10.
6. Bourgeault, S. E.: Blindness—a label. Ed. Visually Handicapped 6:1–5, 1974.
7. Hutchinson and Wagner: Occupational therapy for blind and partially sighted, p. 490.
8. Services for the Blind Person, the Public and the

Professional. American Foundation for the Blind, New York, p. 1.
9. Lowenfeld: Our Blind Children, p. 8.
10. Atchley, R. C.: The Social Forces in Later Life: An Introduction to Social Gerontology. Belmont CA: Wadsworth Publishing Co., 1972, p. 54.
11. Chusid: Correlative Neuroanatomy, p. 85.
12. Schein, J. D.: Model state plan for vocational rehabilitation of deaf clients. In Proceedings of the Congress on Deafness Rehabilitation. J. Rehabil. Deaf 10: 13–17, 1976.
13. Adler, E. P. (ed.): Deafness: Research and professional training programs on deafness. Sponsored by the Department of Health, Education and Welfare. J. Rehabil. Deaf, March 1969, Monograph 1, pp. 6–7.
14. Schein: Model state plan.
15. Stevenson, E. A.: report of the conference on nomenclature. Am. Ann. Deaf, January 1938. Cited by Bender, R. E.: The Conquest of Deafness. Cleveland: Press of Western Reserve University, 1970.
16. Schein: Model state plan.
17. Chusid: Correlative Neuroanatomy, p. 267.
18. Ibid., p. 268.
19. Sereni, F., and Principi, N.: Clinically harmful consequences of drug administration to the pregnant woman and the infant. In Ziai, M. (ed.): Pediatrics, ed. 2. Boston: Little, Brown & Co., 1975, pp. 55–58.
20. Mindel, E. D., and Vernon, M.: They Grow in Silence: The Deaf Child and His Family. National Association of the Deaf, Silver Spring MD, 1971, pp. 25–30.
21. Ibid., p. 27.
22. Ibid., p. 26.
23. Altshuler, K. Z.: Sexual patterns and family relationships. In Rainer, J. D., Altshuler, K. Z., and Kallman, F. J. (eds.): Family and Mental Health Problems in a Deaf Population. Department of Medical Genetics, New York State Psychiatric Institute, Columbia University, 1963, pp. 107–108. (See also pp. 232–233 in which Rainer identifies "Recommendations for future research," and pp. 234–248 in which Kallman discusses "Main findings and some projections.")
24. Chusid: Correlative Neuroanatomy, p. 267.
25. Atchley: Social Forces in Later Life.
26. Chusid: Correlative Neuroanatomy.
27. Chess, S., Korn, S., and Fernandez, P.: Psychiatric Disorders of Children with Congenital Rubella. New York: Brunner-Mazel, 1971, pp. 82–87; 120–130.
28. Report of the National Study Committee on education of deaf-blind children, 1953, 1954, p. 28. Quoted in Robbins, N.: Auditory Training in the Perkins Deaf-Blind Department. Perkins School for the Blind, Watertown MA, 1964, p. 1.
29. Gesell, A., and Armatruda, C.: Developmental Diagnosis: Normal and Abnormal Child Development, ed. 2. New York: Harper & Row Publishers, 1969, p. 435.
30. Fraiberg, S.: Parallel and divergent patterns in blind and sighted infants. Psychoan. Study Child 23:264–300, 1968.
31. Mindel and Vernon: They Grow in Silence.
32. Mouchka, S.: The deaf-blind infant: A rationale for and an approach to early intervention. In Proceedings from the Fourth International Conference on Deaf-Blind Children, August 1971, at Perkins School for the Blind, Watertown MA, pp. 212–225.
33. Chess, Korn, and Fernandez: Psychiatric Disorders of Children.
34. Cohen, W. J.: The role of the service agency. New Outlook for Blind 55:275–281, 1961.
35. Personal communication with Joseph Parnicky, Professor of Social Work, Ohio State University, Columbus, November 1975.
36. Mindel and Vernon: They Grow in Silence.
37. Lowenfeld, B., Abel, G. L., and Hatlen, P. H.: Blind Children Learn to Read. Springfield IL: Charles C Thomas, Publishers, 1969.
38. Mindel and Vernon: They Grow in Silence.
39. Dale, D. M. C.: Deaf Children at Home and at School. Springfield IL: Charles C Thomas, Publishers, 1967.
40. Personal communication with Robert S. Hall, Orientation and Mobility Specialist, Michigan Rehabilitation Center for the Blind, Kalamazoo, April 1977.
41. Improved Vocational, Technical and Academic Opportunities for Deaf Persons. Final Report, August 1974. (Robert R. Lauritsen, Project Director, St. Paul Technical Vocational Institute, 235 Marshall Avenue, St. Paul MN 55102)
42. Ibid.
43. National Technical Institute for the Deaf. Official Bulletin, October 1975. Rochester Institute of Technology. (Admissions Office, One Lomb Memorial Drive, Rochester NY 14623)
44. 1975 and 1976 presentations by Joseph A. Koncelik, Associate Professor of Industrial Design, Ohio State University, and Leon A. Pastalan, Institute of Gerontology, and Architecture Department, University of Michigan.
45. Pamphlet describing The Elderly Deaf Center of Ohio. (6971 Sunbury Road, Westerville OH 43081)
46. Teacher's Guide: John Tracy Clinic Correspondence Course Learning Program for Parents of Preschool Deaf-Blind Children. (John Tracy Clinic, 806 West Adams Boulevard, Los Angeles CA 90007)
47. Stillman, R., et al.: The Callier-Azuza Scale. Callier Center for Communication Disorders, University of Texas/Dallas. (1966 Inwood Road, Dallas TX 75235)
48. Personal communication with Lynne V. Hall, Registered Occupational Therapist, Western Michigan University, April 1977.
49. If Blindness Occurs: Practical Suggestions for Those Who Live or Work with Newly Blinded Persons. (Booklet) The Seeing Eye, Inc., Morristown NJ.
50. Hutchinson and Wagner: Occupational therapy for the blind and partially sighted, p. 492.
51. Yeadon, A.: Toward Independence: The Use of Instructional Objectives in Teaching Daily Living Skills

to the Blind. American Foundation for the Blind, New York, 1974, pp. xiv–xvi; xxiii–xxv.

52. Koestler, F. A. (ed.): The Comstac Report: Standards for Strengthened Services. New York: National Accreditation Council for Agencies Serving the Blind and Visually Handicapped, 1966, p. 231. Cited in Lydon and McGraw: Concept Development for Visually Handicapped Children, revised ed. New York: American Foundation for the Blind, 1973, p. 5.
53. If Blindness Occurs.
54. Routh, T. A.: Rehabilitation Counseling of the Blind. Springfield IL: Charles C Thomas, Publishers, 1970, pp. 56–75.
55. Pastalan, L. A.: Lecture and demonstration at Ohio State University, Columbus, 1970.
56. Mindel and Vernon: They Grow in Silence, p. 10.
57. Ibid., pp. 3–6.
58. National Technical Institute for the Deaf, Official Bulletin.
59. Bergman, R., et al.: Auditory Rehabilitation for Hearing Impaired Blind Persons. American Speech and Hearing Association Monographs, March 1965, No. 12, pp. 23–26.
60. Ibid., pp. 27–29.
61. United States Library of Congress, Division for the Blind and Physically Handicapped, Washington DC.
62. Hadley Correspondence School, 620 Lincoln Avenue, Winnetka IL.
63. A Basic Course in Manual Communication. Communicative Skills Program, National Association of the Deaf, Silver Spring MD, 1973.
64. Riekehof, L. L.: Talk to the Deaf: A Manual of Approximately 1000 Signs Used by the Deaf of North America. Springfield MO: Gospel Publishing House, 1963.

BIBLIOGRAPHY

Ayres, A. J.: Sensory Integration and Learning Disorders. Los Angeles: Western Psychological Services, 1972.

Asenjo, A.: A Step-by-Step Guide to Personal Management for Blind Persons. American Foundation for the Blind, New York, 1970.

Bauman, M. K.: A Manual of Norms for Tests Used Counseling Blind Persons. American Association of Workers for the Blind, Inc. (1511 K Street, N.W., Washington DC 20005), undated. (The report deals with a 1966–1967 study of testing practices. A Manual of Norms was published separately by the American Foundation for the Blind in 1958 and with their permission was reprinted in this single booklet.)

Bauman, M. K.: A Report and a Reprint: Tests Used in the Psychological Evaluation of Blind and Visually Handicapped Persons. American Association of Workers for the Blind, Inc.

Bauman, M. K.: Guided vocational choice. New Outlook for Blind 69:354–360, 1975.

Bauman, M. K., and Yoder, N. M.: Adjustment to Blindness—Reviewed. Springfield IL: Charles C Thomas, Publishers, 1966.

Bernstein, H. W.: Special approaches in learning processes for the deaf. Volta Review 76:42–51, 1974.

Bolton, B. (ed.): Psychology of Deafness for Rehabilitation Counselors. Baltimore: University Park Press, 1976.

Carroll, T. J.: Blindness: What It Is, What It Does, and How to Live With It. Boston: Little, Brown & Co., 1961.

Chase, J. B.: Developmental assessment of handicapped infants and young children: With special attention to the visually impaired. New Outlook for Blind 69:341–349, 1975.

Contents of proceedings: Congress on Deafness Rehabilitation. J. Profess. Rehabil. Workers with Adult Deaf, July 1976 Vol. 10 (entire issue).

Cristarella, M. C.: Visual functions of the elderly. Am. J. Occup. Ther. 31:432–440, 1977.

Detecting infants' hearing loss. (and) On hearing loss. (News and Reports section) Children Today 3:30–31, 1974.

Fox, J. V.: Improving tactile discrimination of the blind: A neurological approach. Am. J. Occup. Ther. 19:5–7, 1965.

Garfield, J. B.: Follow My Leader. New York: Scholastic Book Services, 1957. (Paperbound: TX 561) (Written for school age children, this story about a newly blinded boy clearly presents many aspects of rehabilitation for blind persons, including use of guide dog.)

Gibson, J. J.: The Senses Considered as Perceptual Systems. Boston: Houghton Mifflin Co., 1966.

Godfrey, B. (ed.): Orientation of Social Workers to the Problems of Deaf Persons. Proceedings of the Workshop of the same title, sponsored by the Vocational Rehabilitation Administration, U.S. Department of Health, Education and Welfare, and the School of Social Welfare, University of California, held at Berkeley, November 1963.

Gregory, S.: The Deaf Child and His Family. New York: John Wiley & Sons, 1976.

Guldager, V.: Body Image and the Severely Handicapped Rubella Child. Perkins School for the Blind, Watertown MA, 1970.

Hill, L.: Nationally speaking: Working with blind preschoolers. Am. J. Occup. Ther. 31:417–419, 1977.

Miller, E., and Bentley, E. I.: Listen to the Sounds of Deafness. Supplementary Educational Center, Metropolitan Atlanta Region, 1655 Peachtree Street, N.E., Atlanta, GA 30309. Reprinted by National Association of the Deaf, May 1970.

Moersch, M. S.: Training the deaf-blind child. Am. J. Occup. Ther. 31:425–431, 1977.

Monbeck, M. E.: The Meaning of Blindness: Attitudes Toward Blindness and Blind People. Bloomington: Indiana University Press, 1973.

Moor, P. M.: Comprehensive care services for the young child who is visually impaired. New Outlook for Blind 69:193–200, 1975.

Morse, J. L.: Answering the questions of the psychologist assessing the visually handicapped child. New Outlook for Blind 69:350, 1975.

O'Brien, R.: Early childhood services for visually impaired children: A model program. New Outlook for Blind 69:201–206, 1975.

Schreiber, F. C.: State of deafness. Proceedings of the Congress on Deafness Rehabilitation. J. Rehabil. Deaf 10:7–12, 1976.

Sevel, D., and Hart, J. A.: Occupational therapy for the hospitalized eye patient. Am. J. Occup. Ther. 23:339, 1969.

Sullivan, T., and Gill, D.: If You Could See What I Hear. Hardcover by Harper & Row Publishers, New York; paperbound by Signet Books, New American Library, Bergenfield, NJ, 1975.

Tactile sex ed. Human Behavior 6:54, 1977.

Thompson, D. S.: Language. New York: Time-Life Books, 1975. (See especially A life without sound, pp. 30–41.)

RESOURCES

Alexander Graham Bell Association for the Deaf
3417 Volta Place, N.W.
Washington, D.C. 20007

American Association to Promote the Teaching of Speech to the Deaf
7342 Rural Lane, Mt. Airy
Philadelphia, Pennsylvania 19119

American Foundation for the Blind
Information Department, Publications Division
15 West 16th Street
New York, New York 10011

American Printing House for the Blind
1839 Frankfort Avenue
Louisville, Kentucky 40206

Association for the Education of the Visually Handicapped
919 Walnut Street
Philadelphia, Pennsylvania 19107

Centers and Services for Deaf-Blind Children
Bureau of Education for the Handicapped
Project Center Branch—Room 2036
Division of Educational Services
7th and D Streets, S.W.
Washington, D.C. 20202

Howe Memorial Press
549 East Fourth Street
South Boston, Massachusetts 01227

International Association of Parents of the Deaf
814 Thayer Avenue
Silver Spring, Maryland 20910

Industrial Home for the Blind
57 Willoughby Street
Brooklyn, New York 11205

John Tracy Clinic
806 West Adams Boulevard
Los Angeles, California 90007

National Association of the Deaf
905 Bonifant Street
Silver Spring, Maryland 20910

Perkins School for the Blind
Publications Department
Perkins Research Library and Evaluation Service
Department for Deaf-Blind Children
Watertown, Massachusetts 02172

Professional Rehabilitation Workers with the Adult Deaf, Inc.
814 Thayer Avenue
Silver Spring, Maryland 20910

ACKNOWLEDGMENTS

The author appreciates the assistance of the following persons who read and made suggestions and contributions to large portions of this chapter: Yvette Gardner, Family Interventionist, and Mary L. Smith, Teacher, Deaf-Blind Unit, Ohio State School for the Blind, Columbus; Lynne V. Hall, O.T.R., Western Michigan University, formerly with the Michigan Rehabilitation Center for the Blind; Robert S. Hall, Orientation and Mobility Specialist, Michigan Rehabilitation Center for the Blind, Kalamazoo; and Patrice E. Moore, O.T.R., Ohio School for the Deaf, Columbus.

H. Kay Grant, O.T.R., Director of the Division of Occupational Therapy, School of Allied Medical Professions, The Ohio State University, read the entire chapter. I appreciate her editorial suggestions, her encouragement, and her role in my work with deaf-blind children.

19
Mental Retardation

Reba M. Sebelist

Sam is a seventeen-year-old male who demonstrates symptoms of mental retardation.[1] His parents were told by social service agencies' staff members, physicians, and well-meaning friends to care for his physical needs but not to expect much mental progress. Not being really sure what the term "mentally retarded" meant, Sam's parents decided to keep him at home rather than to institutionalize him as recommended. Siblings were expected to help care for him and to give in to all his whims—a truly one-sided arrangement.

The lack of guidance, assistance, and respite care have produced a family filled with confusion and guilt because of both their lack of ability to meet Sam's obvious needs and their concern for his future care.

Being nonverbal and incontinent, Sam evidences his frustrations by kicking out and biting himself when thwarted in both physical and mental actions, refusing to attempt new or unfamiliar activities, and meeting his ego needs through voluntarily eating only a few favored foods. Lack of educational opportunities has limited his world a great deal, with most of his learning coming from general television viewing. Contacts with persons other than his family are rare because of his unpredictable behavior. This results in a small confined world for Sam and a restriction of human contact and opportunity for the whole family.

This is a composite case history with mostly negative connotations, yet one which could probably be matched in reality anywhere in the country. Although this is a nation of skills and opportunities with so-called rights for all, this is not true for all citizens. The physically and mentally handicapped have been the recipients of much physical and verbal abuse. Mentally retarded individuals have been locked in bedrooms by families who were confused about what to do, full of guilt regarding "why did this happen to us," upset by their inability to cope, and ashamed. They feared that relatives, neighbors, or friends might discover their so-called disgrace.

As demeaning as this physical abuse might be to the mentally retarded, verbal abuse is much more destructive of human worth. Terms such as "dummy," "moron," "low-grade," and "kids" have a much more dehumanizing effect. After hearing this designation over the years, individuals begin to refer to themselves and their peers in the same manner—a self-perpetuating process of breaking down their sense of worth.

Well meaning groups have attempted to change labels from early ones like "idiot" or "imbecile" to "trainable" or "educable." These new, supposedly complimentary, terms are now being fought by organizations such as the National Association for Retarded Citizens (NARC), which changed its name from the National Association for Retarded Children. Throughout this chapter, the retarded are referred to as individuals who have feelings, rights, obligations, and ego needs.

Changing of designation is a long and slow but positive experience. Society is being forced to observe the change evidenced by retarded individuals when positive acceptance is given to them upon completion of success experiences. Accomplishing this goal is not a matter of simply "watering down" everyday procedures but rather constructing ones that are at the correct levels of development and skill for the individuals concerned. Nothing succeeds like success, as the cliché states—the retarded are people who respond to success experiences.

DEFINITION

What is mental retardation? The *Random House Dictionary of the English Language* refers one to the term "mental deficiency" which it defines as "lack of some mental power or powers associated with normal intellectual development resulting in an inability of the individual to function fully or adequately in everyday life."[2] This definition does not differ significantly from the one developed in 1973 by the American Association on Mental Deficiency (AAMD): "Mental retardation refers to significantly subaverage general intellectual functioning existing concurrently with deficits in adaptive behavior and manifested during the developmental period."[3]

It is apparent from the definitions that the mentally retarded do not demonstrate only one area of difficulty but do, indeed, manifest an interaction of multiple factors among which are sociocultural, psychological, and physical influences. A more extensive discussion of the AAMD definition with emphasis on the effect of the various factors is available in *Occupational Therapy for Mentally Retarded Children.*[4]

Therapy for Mentally Retarded Children—Mental Retardation versus Mental Illness

Frequently the public does not comprehend the difference between mental retardation and mental illness. Some very basic differences are indicated in Table 19-1.

Table 19-1. Differences between mental retardation and mental illness.

Mental retardation	*Mental illness*
Primary defect in intellect.	Intellect relatively unimpaired.
Usually oriented in time and place.	Difficulty with time and place orientation.
Not curable, long term.	Often significant cure possible.
May not differ in aptitude, interests, and feelings.	Cluster of behaviors differing from normal.

Incidence

The people known as mentally retarded comprise approximately 3 percent of any given population. The greatest number of these individuals demonstrate symptoms at birth or shortly thereafter. The remaining, acquired retardates, are mentally retarded as a result of problems occurring after the neonatal period.

Within this 3 percent there is a further percentile breakdown based on the individual functioning level. Those considered to be profoundly retarded comprise 1 5/10 percent, severely retarded 3 5/10 percent, moderately retarded 6 percent, and mildly retarded 89 percent.[5]

Using 3 percent of a *given* population as a point of reference it would be simple to deny need for individualized special programming. However, when it is placed into perspective as 3 percent of the *total* population, a very large number of individuals emerge who require aid in meeting particular needs.

HISTORICAL PERSPECTIVE

An historical review provides an understanding of the specialty area of mental retardation as well as the motivating forces of those currently involved with planning and demanding accountability.

History tells us that in early times the mentally retarded were ignored, received little or no care, or were placed in the woods to fend for themselves or die. Life for the average person was short and living arduous; hence it was extremely difficult to support those who were different and required extra care.

Another reason for the desertion and persecution of these individuals is that they were thought to be possessed by demons.

During the Middle Ages the role of the court jester was usually filled by a retarded individual. Observations of art of the time shows individuals now diagnosed as having Down's syndrome filling the role. Frequently, when these individuals lived with their families, they filled the role of "village idiot." Those who fill the role today run errands, carry messages, and so forth for a small tip but, more importantly, for gaining social acceptance and a sense of self-worth.

Various religious orders became so distressed with the lack of physical care, the ridicule, and abuse given the retarded that they built sheltered communities. Unfortunately, along with the kindly intended isolation, a sense of hopelessness grew. No change was envisioned. Good care and shelter were provided but there was little mental stimulation; this in turn caused more regression and deterioration.

In the 1800s, Jean Itard, a physician who worked with the deaf, became involved with a boy about twelve years of age who had been captured in the forest of Aveyron, France.[6] The lad had been diagnosed as severely retarded by Pinel, an associate of Itard. Feeling that intellectual performance and potential could be affected by environmental stimulation and opportunity, Itard began working with sensorimotor techniques to achieve this goal. Initially he began working with Victor (his name for the young man) through the sense of hearing. After occluding visual stimuli he bombarded Victor with auditory stimuli and required from him an acceptable response. Next he required discrimination of types of noises, proceeding afterwards to verbal clues. As soon as possible the blindfold was removed, but Victor would frequently request its use to rule out extraneous visual distractions. Itard concluded this probably was an attempt by Victor to reduce visual stimuli, his most frequently used, and highly sophisticated sense. When Victor was able to respond to emotions such as anger, sadness, and happiness in vocalizations, Itard proceeded to the sense of touch. Following a similar procedure he then proceeded to the senses of smell and taste. This was a very promising sequence of training but one which was soon to be discarded only to be resumed in the latter part of the 1900s. Itard worked with Victor for five years and, although gains were made by this previously animalistic "Wild Boy of Aveyron," they were not sufficient for him to fit into the "dandified" Paris society; Itard felt he had failed. He did indeed fail if we use the goal of fitting into that society as a criterion; nonetheless, his greatest contribution was to effect attitudinal change regarding the mentally retarded.

Seguin, a student of Itard, elaborated upon Itard's work and developed what he called the "physiological method" of training. After coming to the United States, Seguin became a prime mover in the opening of residential facilities such as Fernald in Massachusetts and Germantown (now Elwyn) in Pennsylvania. His involvement led to the establishment of an organization, now the American Association on Mental Deficiency (AAMD).

As with most specialty areas, unqualified persons promised cures which they could not effect since mental retardation is not a curable illness but a condition. Many felt that, if the condition could not be cured, time, money, and energy expended were wasted. As a result, these unqualified persons caused a reversal in feelings regarding the potential of the mentally retarded and negated the work of Itard and Seguin with a resultant return to the sense of hopelessness.

This attitude of futility continued with the development of larger residential facilities mostly in isolated areas. Society was convincing itself that it was meeting the needs of the mentally retarded by assuring them care for their basic physical needs.

By the end of World War II emphasis shifted and came to include programming by the National Association for Retarded Citizens (NARC), an organization formed for parents of retarded children and interested lay persons. For the first time, professionals were being held accountable for both resultant behavioral change and utilization of funds.

Following lengthy litigation between the Commonwealth of Pennsylvania and parents regarding the availability of educational opportunities for mentally retarded, a Right to Education Consent Agreement was implemented in 1973.[7] This guarantees educational opportunities for all mentally and physically handicapped to an age of twenty-one years. This was indeed a major accomplishment for the parents who were supported in the action by the Pennsylvania Association for Retarded Citizens (PARC), an affiliate of NARC. Many other states are studying the agreement for possible implementation in their educational programs.

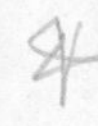

Public Law 94-142, The Education For All Handicapped Children Act, was passed by the federal government in 1975. The major effect of this act on occupational therapy is that all special education programs were to have physical or occupational therapists available either on their staffs or as consultants by September 1977.

A positive change has now been seen in the role of training centers. Funds had not always been available to provide personnel to effect change. Society had been content to have the retarded isolated or institutionalized to receive mostly custodial care. Professionals had not assumed responsibility for preparation to work with the mentally retarded. Pressure from organizations such as NARC along with federal and state regulations have forced accountability by staff. They, in turn, have demanded and are receiving more efficient and appropriate training from colleges, universities, and professional schools which are producing staff members less hesitant to assume responsibility for education and training.

METHODS OF CLASSIFICATION

Intelligence Quotient

For many years the only method used to designate the functioning level of the retarded was the measurement of intellectual skills. The evaluator would utilize instruments and issue an IQ score. These scores have both positive and negative aspects. The skilled evaluator is a valued program team member. Conversely, an inexperienced evaluator can do irreparable damage.

The IQ score with a descriptive statement frequently would influence the amount of effort expended on the individual. It would then remain on the record permanently. Staff members with large case loads would have to set priorities. An individual who scored 40 to 45 would most often be chosen for participation in a program before one who scored 20 to 25. Little thought was given to motivation, previous program exposure, or plateauing. The individual with the low score might be motivated and ready for change. It is not only unfair but also unrealistic and weak programming to base decisions on IQ evaluations only.

A skilled evaluator, who looks at the total person, the physical abilities and limitations, verbal or nonverbal communicative state, and so forth and then chooses an evaluation instrument that is appropriate, can do invaluable work. This type of evaluator elicits responses that produce a higher functioning level and aids the treatment team in developmentally designed programming.

Many states require that a numerical IQ score be given. This information is useful for record keeping, statistics, and research but is not in itself meaningful for the goal directed team.

Medical Diagnosis or Causation

The World Health Organization (WHO) has been concerned with obtaining uniform information for international sharing. WHO feels this process would clarify communication in addition to encouraging sharing for improvement of international health concerns.

In the United States, to implement the request of WHO, the International Classification of Diseases has been utilized by the medical team in an attempt to classify mental retardation according to etiology or causation.

Initially a number from 310 to 315, based on intellectual functioning according to the Revised Stanford-Binet Tests of Intelligence Forms L and M, is assigned: 310 for borderline, 311 for mild, 312 for moderate, 313 for severely, and 314 for profoundly retarded. The 315 designation is for those who have not been assigned a specific functioning level but who demonstrate behaviors associated with retardation.

Following this number is a fourth digit signifying a clinical subcategory based on etiology: .0 following infection and intoxication, .1 following trauma or physical agent, .2 with disorders of metabolism, growth, or nutrition, .3 associated with gross brain disease (postnatal), .4 associated with diseases and conditions resulting from unknown prenatal influence, .5 with chromosomal abnormality, .6 associated with prematurity, .7 following major psychiatric disorder, .8 with psychosocial (environmental) deprivation, .9 with other (and unspecified) conditions. There may come to be a fifth and sixth digit listed as a means of further pinpointing causation.

Hence, for one example, the numerical designation 314.5 indicates that an individual is profoundly retarded as a result of chromosomal abnormality. The greatest value of this type of classification is the ease of comprehension and research usage. This system does, however, remove the human element while social agencies and families are attempting through legal maneuverings to give human dignity to the mentally retarded.

Information including numerical designations desired by the mental retardation section of the International Classification of Diseases is available in the *Diagnostic and Statistical Manual of Mental Disorders* (DSM-II).[8]

It is desirable to know the etiological factors but this information is not essential for program planning. Combining of the two classifications provides information regarding the IQ and the etiological factors but does not indicate what the individual is capable of doing and thus should not be used in isolation as a determinant for training.

Education

A frequently used classification method is one that was designed for use by educators. Terms such as life support, dependent, trainable, and educable are assigned. These terms are meaningful to those who use them daily but are relatively useless to the general population.

The use of case histories for providing relevant information has been frustrating because the focus in the past has been one of describing what has been done and does not include either past or present performance levels of the individual. The use of the educational terms also reinforces in most instances the same lack of information.

Adaptive Behavior Level

The AAMD definition refers to impairment in adaptive behavior as being demonstrable in the mentally retarded. As early as 1955, Sloan and Birch[9] began defining these behaviors. A Monograph Supplement to the *American Journal of Mental Deficiency* prepared by Heber[10] gives four levels of behavior with the following three appropriate age groupings. Descriptive paragraphs are given for Levels 1, 2, 3, and 4 with Level 4 referring to maximal ability and vocational adequacy. Useful as this information was, it still was not an adequate system of classification. Thus, it was updated in 1973 with age level delineation of skills in areas such as activities of daily living, communication, physical, social, self-motivation, and occupation.[11] This method now offers quick reference with information indicating at what level on the developmental continuum the individual is functioning. It also provides a possible recommendation for setting achievable goals.

Composite Classification

Finally, a compilation of information that is meaningful is evolving. From the generic term of mental retardation it is possible to progress through the use of demonstrable IQ score, etiological factors with indications of possible progressive deteriorating conditions, educators' designation, and conclude with adaptive behavioral levels. A combination of all these factors is not only desirable but essential for designing a program to meet the needs of the individual.

ASSESSMENT

As with all aspects of programming for the mentally retarded, assessment must be a combined effort. Some well-staffed centers are implementing a decentralized system of management, which can be an asset for evaluating abilities and limitations. A group of experienced professionals is charged with the responsibility of devising composite evaluative measures affecting the full range of activities existing at the center. This composite evaluation device is administered by either the professional services staff or by other qualified evaluators working in the unit. The results of the testing are shared with the combined staff working with the involved individual.

Not only is the more structured and formal assessment utilized but also the professional services staff meets with the direct care staff to learn the individual's level of response in the residential unit, and, with representatives of other program staff, to ascertain behaviors, gains, regressions, or plateauing.

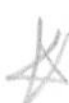

In addition, the professional service staff observes each individual in a variety of program experiences for on-site evaluation and completion of an all inclusive assessment.

This sophisticated level of assessment will not be possible in all centers because of size of staff and assigned multiple responsibilities. However, a complete goal-oriented training program cannot exist without evaluative measurements, for, if no initial or reevaluative information is available, change cannot be measured. However there continue to be programs where change is recorded only through periodic subjective progress notes without an initial assessment having been performed.

Regardless of the sophistication of the assessment team or the materials used, the most important factor is the relevance of the instruments used for measuring the desired results. As the use of a standardized test written in English is unfair to a Spanish speaking person so, also, is one for the mentally retarded that is not level appropriate. After defining the purpose of a specific assessment and the goals to be achieved, the instrument with the greatest potential for determining the functional level of the individual is chosen and administered.

There is a controversy regarding where assessments should be done. Valid arguments can be presented to substantiate various points of view. Concerns include questions of where the activity is usually done, the discomfort of the individual being evaluated in a strange setting, the distractibility of the individual, and so on. Just as it is true that most people function better in a familiar environment, it also follows that the distractions of that same area might affect performance. The professional doing the assessment must make the decision regarding the location, time of day, and family members present when choosing the optimal setting.

A representative listing of some instruments having demonstrated their potential usefulness with the mentally retarded follows. Although the list is incomplete, it is presented to illustrate the scope of available formal instruments. With most mentally retarded individuals, the number of areas to be assessed is such that one or more program areas may be involved in doing the evaluations that are peculiar to the contribution of their disciplines. A more comprehensive description of each of these instruments with validity and reliability can be found in the *Seventh Mental Measurement Yearbook* edited by Buros.[12] With all screening devices it is essential to remember that they are only as useful as the skill of the evaluator in comprehending the behaviors of very young children.

Many occupational therapy departments devise evaluation forms to meet the requirements of their service. The tool can be as simple or as complex as desired but should elicit such information as physical status, mental functioning level, and adaptive behavioral level. Other information contained is dependent on the age level served, the type of program, and the relationship of the department to other program services. It is suggested that an instrument based on the type described by Currie[13] is most useful. This type of instrument evaluates neuromuscular status, perceptual-motor abilities, activities of daily living, and performance abilities.

Intelligence and Developmental Scales

BAYLEY SCALES OF INFANT DEVELOPMENT. Devised for use with infants from two to thirty months of age, this instrument has a mental scale, motor scale, and an infant behavior record. It does not predict potential abilities but does establish an infant's current status in relation to others of the same age. The instrument aids in recognition and diagnosis of sensory and neurological defects as well as emotional distress or disturbance. It is standardized and has good reliability.

DENVER DEVELOPMENTAL SCREENING TEST. This is a screening device for children from two weeks to six years of age. Four sections evaluate gross motor, fine motor-adaptive, communication, and personal-social development. The score sheet with its key gives the average age by which each skill should be attained. In addition, the score sheet provides columns for reevaluation, thus producing a quick composite reference. This is a practical, efficient evaluative tool.

PEABODY PICTURE VOCABULARY TEST. This instrument was devised for use with persons aged two and a half to eighteen years. The individual responds to verbal clues by indicating the correct picture from a choice of four. Negative features of this instrument are that directions are given in English, thus making it invalid for persons who speak other languages. It does not take colloquialisms into account. A very useful instrument for nonverbal individuals, it only requires pointing to the correct picture. The motorically involved can also be evaluated as the test pictures are of a good size and are well separated on the page. The positive aspects of this test outweigh its negative features.

STANFORD-BINET INTELLIGENCE SCALE (IQ). This very old instrument was devised for use with individuals aged two years or older. The current third revision was published in 1960 and combines items from Forms L and M to become the Revised Version Form L-M. This utilization of the better items is felt to produce a more valid instrument. The instrument relies heavily on verbal ability. It requires the use of six different items from a possible seven for each age level. Although this tool has good validity, it does not adequately evaluate older severely-retarded individuals.

WECHSLER INTELLIGENCE SCALE FOR CHILDREN. A stable general purpose scale, this instrument was devised for use with individuals from five to fifteen years of age. From the composite of twelve subtests, information is accumulated for verbal, performance, and full scale scores. The division of items in this scale is based on content rather than level of difficulty. Some evaluators consider this the reason why the scale is easy to administer as well as successful in gaining responses from children. Individually administered, this instrument is valid in measuring immediate mental functioning.

ILLINOIS TEST OF PSYCHOLINGUISTIC ABILITIES. The recommended age range for use of this instrument is two to ten years. In the development of this tool, the original purpose was to produce a device to be used as a diagnostic tool for analyzing intellectual deficits in the learning disabled and mentally retarded. Nine subtests evaluate communication performance in decoding, association, and encoding; levels of language organization; and channels of input and output of language. Although there are areas needing some revision, this instrument has served the purpose of diagnosing learning difficulties. A practical, valid test, it can be a valuable tool.

GOODENOUGH-HARRIS DRAWING TEST. The age range of this test is three to fifteen years. This updating of the Draw-a-Man test presents an opportunity to use a quick, nonthreatening instrument that frequently evokes useful verbal comments while the individual is completing the task. Of vital importance in the use of this instrument is the *purpose* for the use. As a result of motoric difficulties and impaired mental functioning the retarded individual responds not only as a definite individual but also as one who has obvious aberrance. Recognizing these limitations the evaluator must know how to administer the test and be skilled in the use of the information it evokes.

Adaptive Behavior

VINELAND SOCIAL MATURITY SCALE. This instrument has been widely used although no true standardization has been done. Results are based on the experience of the developer. An important feature of this instrument is that the information comes from a general population sample. Because of the subjective nature of this test, the relationship between the evaluator and the individual being tested may have either a "halo" or negative effect on scoring. It is a useful broad evaluation of adaptive behaviors.

ADAPTIVE BEHAVIOR SCALE. This instrument was published by the American Association on Mental Deficiency in 1969 and is composed of two scales, one for ages three to twelve and the other for ages thirteen and older. The tool was developed for use with the mentally retarded and emotionally maladjusted.

The scale devised for adults, thirteen years and older, measures behaviors in the areas of independent functioning, physical development, economic activity, language development, number and time concept, occupation-domestic, occupation-general, self-direction, responsibilities, and socialization in Part One. Part Two evaluates factors such as violent and destructive behavior, antisocial behavior, rebellious behavior, untrustworthy behavior, withdrawal, stereotyped behavior, and odd mannerisms, inappropriate interpersonal manners, unacceptable vocal habits, self-abusive behavior, hyperactive tendencies, sexually aberrant behavior, and psychological disturbances. Since many of the behaviors listed have more than one item to be evaluated, the final score totals the assigned point values from each item.

This is a broad scale and when utilized presents a global view of the individual. The scale is a well-constructed and easily administered tool which has much to offer in assessment of easily discernible areas for habilitation training.

Perceptual Motor

MARIANNE FROSTIG DEVELOPMENTAL TEST OF VISUAL PERCEPTION, THIRD EDITION. The age range recommended for this test is three to eight years. Measuring visual perceptual skills in five areas, the instrument contributes valuable data to the clinical team. The global scores have reasonable reliability.

Although this tool is a good instrument, the value of its use with the mentally retarded is limited to individuals with higher levels of functioning. Low scores are not necessarily an indication to start perceptual training but might rather indicate that the instrument was not the most appropriate one for testing the individual.

THE PURDUE PERCEPTUAL MOTOR SURVEY. This tool was designed for use with children six to ten years of age and aids in identification of children lacking in perceptual motor abilities necessary for acquiring academic skills. As such, it has potential for use with the so-called borderline and mildly retarded but is not useful with the severely or profoundly retarded. It is an action or performance survey. Thus, it is easily administered to the individual who cannot read.

HABILITATION TRAINING

The training of a mentally retarded individual requires the cooperation of many persons filling a variety of roles. The mentally retarded individual, dependent upon his or her functioning level and comprehension, must be a team member. Lack of desire and motivation or a high degree of resistance could interfere with the success of a well-planned developmentally-appropriate training sequence.

The family must be involved in a positive manner and must be given much encouragement and reinforcement in an attempt to allay unwarranted guilt feelings. It must be aided in adjusting to the facts that progress will be slow, gains small and in some cases minimal, and yet they must be demanding and supportive of the retarded individual so that the greatest level of achievement possible is obtained.

The individual may require drugs to aid in control of seizures or aberrant behavior or may use dietary supplements. For example, an individual having causative phenylketonuria (PKU) requires a dietary supplement for maintenance or prevention of further changes. Although physicians and nurses are busy, most will respond to questioning about the individual's medication record. In turn, the medical representatives have the responsibility of informing other team members of changes in the medicinal regimen, especially if consequences or side effects, which could influence the program, are anticipated. Physicians are becoming more aware of the type of contribution the occupational therapist may make, but it is the responsibility of the occupational therapists to make their skills and contributions clear.

The psychologist and social case worker are vital team members. They frequently can elicit from the individual or the family information that is important to program development. The skill of these people can be helpful in the evaluation and compilation of program goals and can forge another link in the development of a total program team.

The staff members considered to be giving direct service vary with almost every center; they are the persons who have daily contact with the individual. They are known by a variety of names: mental retardation aides, child care workers, resident living aides, and so forth. This group provides a vital source of information because they see retarded individuals for extended periods of time; they can report on specific needs, the carry-over of learning from therapies, the reaction of the individual to peers and activity, the individual's tolerance of frustrations and response to daily living situations.

The interaction of physical therapy, occupational therapy, speech therapy, education therapy, recreation therapy, and other concerned persons should occur not only at unit staff meetings but whenever a concern arises. The staff should feel free to discuss problems without having to follow a rigid bureaucratic process; however the staff does have the responsibility to share information with supervisors so they can be aware and able to contribute to the program.

Each and every staff member must have a concern for the retarded individual. The dietary staff will cooperate if time is taken to explain why a special food or preparation is needed. The carpenter might help by making large pieces of equipment such as relaxation chairs, standing tables, and prone boards. These support staff members can be involved in the program; they are able to give much worthwhile help.

The occupational therapist is not working in an isolated area but must offer aid and solicit the same from the total staff. Specifically, occupational therapists are working with a team to develop level appropriate training to aid each individual. The team must set realistic goals, be able to accept slow progress in achieving them, be content to accept temporary plateauing when it occurs, and be prepared to increase training emphasis when the individual evidences readiness for progression in the program.

ROLES OF OCCUPATIONAL THERAPY WITH THE MENTALLY RETARDED

Occupational therapy assists in improving the individual's ability to meet the demands of his or her culture with satisfaction and in a manner that is acceptable to and compatible with that environment. It is essential that the occupational therapist have a knowledge not only of normal growth and development but also of the cultural and social requirements the particular individual must fulfill. Those from a ghetto in a large urban area have different demands to meet than do those from the farming heartlands. In addition, there must be an awareness of the differences resulting from their social, cultural, and value systems as these too affect program implementation and cooperation of both the individual and the family.

The diversity of skills possessed by occupational therapists makes it possible for them to fill a variety of roles both in administration and in providing direct service. In a small understaffed center, the occupational therapist may be expected to be the one providing recreational activities in addition to occupational therapy. In other settings the implementation of an approved work training program may be the occupational therapist's responsibility. As staff is acquired in other disciplines, the occupational therapist is able to relinquish some of these extra duties.

Larger, more completely staffed centers for the mentally retarded present different types of roles. Here, the occupational therapist is delegated responsibilities traditionally assigned to him or her. The therapist is, in addition, able to have frequent contact with members of other disciplines. Each discipline can be an able extension of the others. The occupational therapist might prepare an individual for physical therapy treatment and yet accomplish an occupational therapy goal—that of teaching self-dressing, for example. The teacher reinforces physical and occupational therapy by using adapted equipment or proper positioning. The era of each discipline working as an isolated entity is past and occupational therapy must become a working member of the team.

Occasionally the occupational therapist is placed in an administrative role. One difficulty here might be keeping occupational therapy in its proper perspective as a part of the team. All disciplines must become contributing members of the team coordinated by an administrator whose major responsibility is to utilize the skills of each as required by the mentally retarded individual at a given time.

In centers for habilitation training of the mentally retarded, occupational therapy methods have followed the traditional use of arts and crafts with increased use of appropriate neurodevelopmental activities to aid each individual's sequential development. Both of these approaches are valid. The major decision is which form of treatment should be used to meet the needs of the individual being served.

Traditional

Initially there were few available trained staff who understood the needs of the retarded for participation in gainful activity. Little activity was available beyond occasional entertainment. This lack of activity produced fertile ground for regression (even in those with a higher functioning level), self-abuse, public masturbation, fights, broken windows, destroyed furniture, and torn clothing. These negative behaviors reinforced society's attitude that the retarded person could not be taught or benefit from positive experiences.

A few determined staff would not accept this attitude and began implementing arts and crafts activities based on the premise that busy work is better than idle hands. This was a positive step for some individuals, as was evidenced by improved ego strength. Much fine work was produced but usually little thought was given to the individual's symptoms, interests, or desired goals. A negative feature of the arts and crafts programs was that most were self-funded: individuals had to produce in order to buy supplies, making production the primary function of the activity.

The low institutional housekeeping budgets produced another type of traditional programming—that of the individual's doing much of the work around the institution that was not done by paid help. Properly assigned and supervised work within the institution is a useful therapeutic tool. However, the mentally retarded person was often put to work in areas of need (laundry, grounds, kitchen) for long hours with little or no compensation beyond a pinch of tobacco, a cigar, or a cup of coffee. Days off were unheard of, with the retarded individual frequently doing more physically demanding labor than the paid staff.

This type of abuse led to involvement by labor unions. After much discussion, numerous law suits, and negotiations, the pendulum has swung to the other extreme. Individuals may work only if they agree, sign a voluntary consent form, and receive the minimum wage or prevailing wage, whichever is higher, pro rated to the level of performance. This federal regulation affects the use of therapeutic work as a part of habilitation since many refuse to participate in it voluntarily. Also, most live-in centers have not been given increased funds either to hire the retarded individual or to employ additional staff.[14]

Both types of activities described had much to offer but were abused. Occupational therapists were involved in both types of programs, were distressed by what was happening, and joined other team members in designing program goals indicating availability and quality of program which would produce the potential for change in individuals served.

Current

As an example of current practice, the system developed in one state is described. In Pennsylvania, the directors of occupational therapy departments serving the Commonwealth Department of Public Welfare Office of Mental Retardation institutions for the mentally retarded defined major program areas where occupational therapy has a valid contribution to make toward eliciting behavioral change. The list is not to be considered a complete, all-inclusive one but instead is one that is subject to revision and updating. Each of the areas are discussed more fully later in the chapter but are recorded here for a global view of their thinking. Some areas are evaluation, maintenance, research, resource, and consultancy. The areas listed cannot be considered as separate entities as there are many situations in which their functions overlap. They were difficult to define and are impossible to separate; therefore staff must be prepared to see needs in one or more program areas, set priorities, and plan the program accordingly.

There also appears to be a variety of function and program types to meet specific needs. The group of directors of occupational therapy had difficulty in separating the role responsibilities but have listed them for more clarity of comprehension.

Although these program areas were defined for institutional training, they are also relevant to community centers that provide day care, special education, preschool, and infant stimulation programs.

THE OCCUPATIONAL THERAPY PROGRAM

Assessment Evaluation

The intent of evaluation is to appraise and assess functioning levels of the individual. This may be done for program placement within the occupational therapy service or upon the request of a member of another discipline. A physician, psychologist, or community agency may ask that evaluation be done in order to determine the readiness of the individual for program or to determine the individual's current functioning level.

Instruments for screening, aid in determining the need for further evaluation in specific areas. However, if it has been determined previously that the individual presents symptoms of physical or mental retardation, then further screening is repetitious and unnecessary. Assessment should then be used to determine the level of function of the individual.

Most therapists use a selected battery of instruments. One caution is that the chosen battery must be appropriate and produce meaningful results. A department may assemble a collection of standardized tests with good reliability and validity that produce results to meet their needs. Others may devise a composite battery of their own, combining appropriate materials for their needs. No one instrument or battery will fill all needs. How extensive the battery should be is dependent upon the function of the center, the age of individuals served, and the basic goals of the service. It would be meaningless for a preschool program to compile a prevocational interest and skill battery or for an infant stimulation program to develop a battery on cognitive tasks or refinements of self-care. The type of battery promulgated by Currie[15] is broad enough in scope to cover many age and involvement levels but can be limited to meet specific needs.

Evaluation is not a one-time experience. It is an ongoing process to provide current and updated information on level of ability. Within the training process one must be careful, however, not to teach items used in the test. It is easy to elicit good scores on evaluation yet have poor results in performance if an individual has become test-wise. Evaluation is necessary but must be utilized with care and much skill.

A major responsibility of the occupational therapist is the preparation of clear, concise, and comprehensive reports. If occupational therapists are to function usefully as evaluators they must produce reports which are understandable, meaningful, and useful. Long reports are meaningless because they may not be read thoroughly.

Neurodevelopment

All individuals follow an essentially similar sequential pattern of development. Some, the gifted, progress more rapidly; some, the retarded, progress more slowly. But for each there is a sequential pattern to be followed. The mentally retarded persons have had their sequence interrupted in some manner —physical, mental, emotional, or as a result of multiple factors. They will therefore require special training in order to progress along the developmental sequence.

For years, well-meaning and skilled therapists were using adaptive support devices such as braces and splints in order to get individuals into the upright position and ambulating. When the individuals did not progress it was determined that they were too handicapped, too retarded, or too uncooperative. Little thought was given to developmental sequence.

Frustration on the part of the staff and lack of progress on the part of the individual caused a review of programs of different types and goals. Staff began to question whether the goals were appropriate for the skill level of the individual. Finally various techniques aimed at developmentally-realistic goals evolved with therapists providing sensory stimuli to the individual in order to aid the integration process and permit performance of a motor act. Of vital importance is the awareness of normal growth patterns, the proper level, and type of sensory input needed to achieve the desired result. A person, for example, must have head control before sitting and be able to knee-stand before standing in the upright position.

As in many other areas of dysfunction there is no one technique to meet all the needs. The occupational therapist must evaluate and, after determining the technique most appropriate, proceed with program implementation. There must be constant contact with the other disciplines to utilize their skills and achieve the greatest potential function for the individual in this highly specialized treatment process.

Multiply Handicapped

Many individuals who are designated as mentally retarded are also multiply handicapped. Some are blind, deaf, nonverbal, cerebral palsied, or have missing or incomplete body parts. Many of these involvements alone would demand much adjustment in life style and learning process. When coupled with mental retardation, these problems are severely compounded. A sensory disturbance may be the only manifestation but more often it is accompanied by a motor disturbance which indeed produces a complex training need.

There is much overlapping in this program area. The primary need may be in the neurodevelopmental level or in the area of activities of daily living. The role of the occupational therapist must be to determine the need, set the priority for the service, and proceed to implement the indicated program.

Emotionally Disturbed

This program area encompasses a wide scope of problems ranging from the difficulties of mildly and moderately involved individuals to the persons who demonstrate autistic type behaviors.

The multiple problems faced by the mildly and moderately retarded do not preclude emotional disturbances. Frequently they are alert enough to recognize their difference, feeling society's rejection acutely, and yet strongly wanting to be a part of that society. Many internalize their feelings and develop physical malfunctions such as ulcers and colitis. Occupational therapy can aid these individuals by providing an outlet for and encouraging the release of feelings. The release felt while using the beater on a floor loom or wedging clay is immeasurable and it also is a positive, acceptable behavior. The results derived from the use of various activities are shared with the program team for utilization of all those working with the individual.

Programming for those who demonstrate autistic type behavior must first determine whether the individual is profoundly retarded or is demonstrating such symptoms as a result of extreme emotional distress. The assistance of the total program team is vital in making this decision before goals can be set and programming instituted.

This is an expensive type of programming initially because it requires a one-to-one relationship, but the results are gratifying to the total team. The occupational therapist may be the original worker in the process or may be called upon as a consultant or resource person.

Activities of Daily Living

The majority of mentally retarded individuals appear unable to meet daily self-care needs because of their functioning level. For years, the staff and families of the mentally retarded, in the interest of saving time, have met these needs. On rare occasions inability to learn is the main cause for the individual's not performing self-care activities. More frequently the mentally retarded person has not been required or permitted to undertake his or her own self-care. The behaviors demonstrated by the retarded in this area are often related to the demands made upon them.

It is unfair if the individual is given an unpressed buttonless shirt or blouse and then criticized for sloppy appearance. Likewise, if open zippers are permitted, the therapist is negligent in training for community living. Similarly there should not be one dress code for the retarded persons and another for the staff. There must be consistency in what is expected or accepted.

Use of cosmetics and hair styling should be realistic and meet reasonable current standards. Proper use of cosmetics is a useful tool in teaching body scheme and image.

Self-feeding for some individuals is a slow process and often staff have done the feeding. Frequently, small inexpensive dishwasher-safe adapted utensils can be made and utilized for more independent self-feeding.[16] More involved adaptations may require greater on-site assistance from the occupational therapist and demand the training of other staff members in their use and purpose. Adapted equipment should be kept as simple as possible in both construction and complexity in order to encourage use by all staff.

Self-care in personal hygiene is frequently avoided by most disciplines. The use of the toilet and toilet tissue and handwashing must be encouraged. Teaching of self-care for menstrual needs is increasing. Unfortunately little is being done to instruct individuals about or to discuss these bodily functions.

Sex education must be faced realistically, and the occupational therapist must be prepared to explain or answer questions in a manner comprehensible to the individual. The use of proper names for body parts is encouraged. One should not expect that a lesson explained once is learned. As with all individuals, the retarded have normal urges and are concerned about them. The therapist should answer questions factually and truly in a manner that can be understood.[17]

A successful method of teaching self-care in feeding, dressing, and personal hygiene appears to be using the process known as *chaining. Forward chaining* means building upon a series of simple steps, to develop a more complex series, and finally to complete the task. For example, the donning of slacks would progress from having the individual insert his feet into the leg openings, to pulling up the trousers, and finally to fastening them. For some individuals, *backward chaining* is an easier learning process. This involves having the individual first complete the task—buttoning, fastening the clamp, pulling up the zipper—and then expanding to include the pulling up process, and finally the insertion of feet into the leg openings. Each procedure ends with the same result, but the manner used is dependent upon the individual's perceptions and physical status. Chaining can be utilized for teaching most activities of self-care through individualized occupational therapy training as well as through sharing the process with the direct care staff for reinforcement and implementation.

Vocational Exploration

The extent of the role of occupational therapy in this area varies according to the roles taken by other disciplines. It may be that, in one setting, a registered occupational therapist has the responsibility for evaluating potential, planning, and implementing the total program. In a larger, more completely staffed center, the occupational therapist's role could be that of evaluation through offering work experiences for exploration and determination of readiness for progression to workshop assignment.

It is imperative that the therapist be aware of the individual's feelings toward work and those of his or her culture. To many, the ability to work is a sign of health and usefulness. Unfortunately many mentally retarded persons feel they do not have any responsibility in this area. The occupational therapist can be of value to the team by attempting to motivate the individual to become involved in a work training experience.

Maintenance

For the want of a better term, the descriptive word "maintenance" is assigned to this program area. The term is used to designate programming for those who have reached what is probably their maximum level of functioning. The goal is to prevent regression.

The individual with a progressive disorder needs assistance in retaining ability in range of motion, activities of daily living, and cognition for as long as possible. The aid that the therapist can give the individual and the family is important. There are few progressive disorders causing mental deterioration among those diagnosed as mentally retarded. However, those that do exist require additional skill and effort from the program team.

The normal aging process and the acquisition of additional physical or neurological involvements compounds the care and responsibility of the program teams. A senile eighty-year-old mentally retarded individual may demonstrate behaviors similar to those seen throughout his or her lifetime but he or she will probably demonstrate less skill than other eighty-year-old senile individuals. This individual requires an evaluation and adjustment of goals by the program team to assist in functioning at his or her highest level.

Although the term maintenance can be interpreted negatively, in this aspect of programming it is given a positive connotation and is meant to be an area where therapy is not only desired but strongly indicated.

Research

Unfortunately few occupational therapists have been involved in the area of research and those working with the mentally retarded have been just as remiss. A wise man once said something to the effect that, "It is not the so-called retarded who are retarded. It is those who work with them who are lacking in skill to provide aid." Occupational therapists are involved in providing facilitation of change and are attempting to meet current needs but understaffing, heavy case loads, and required paperwork have frequently been used as excuses for avoiding involvement in research.

Many times a therapist may say a patient has reached his or her maximum level of function when this may be an evasive statement for not knowing what to do next. The frustration felt by an individual who apparently cannot control drooling is an excellent example of an aspect of training where joining with the speech therapist in research might produce results for improvement in chewing, swallowing, cosmetic appearance, and ego strength for the involved individual.

Research does demand time, but the occupational therapist has the responsibility to become more involved in sharing findings with others. Research projects also improve level of skill.

Resource and Consultancy

The increase in numbers of small facilities providing interim care, extended care, and community living arrangements, and the requirement that such centers have a registered occupational therapist as a consultant in order to meet government regulations for funding provides another potential role for the therapist working with the mentally retarded.

Agencies such as AAMD and NARC have encouraged the return of those who can profit from living in such settings to community centers. Being closer to the family has been desired by many but the level of functioning requires more care than the family can provide. In addition, many mentally retarded persons with no families can be placed in a center where they might go to a workshop and return to minimal supervision at nighttime. Others who require more skilled care may be placed closer to their families so family members may visit them more easily.

The role of occupational therapy can be that of assisting the staff in providing needed adaptations for self-care, in developing an activity program that is therapeutic, and in aiding the staff to meet the particular needs of the mentally retarded individuals so that they may adjust more easily to a new and different life style.

CASE STUDY

Carol, at the time of admission to occupational therapy, was a twelve-year old diagnosed as profoundly mentally retarded with autistic-like behavior.

An illegitimate daughter of a borderline intelligent mother, Carol was rejected at birth. The infant was placed in a foster home but was transferred many times because she was unable to adjust. She was a difficult feeder and poor sleeper, essentially a silent child and apparently fearful of human contact. Rimland, in his work *Infantile Autism*,[18] advances the theory that this type of behavior may evolve as a result of maternal rejection in utero. If one agrees with this theory then the behavior can be explained. However, for occupational therapists in a training center, the main concern was how to evoke behavioral change in Carol.

Admission behavior was that of a nonverbal, incontinent, pretty, fairly-well-nourished adolescent who spent her waking time pacing or moving in a whirling pattern. Sleep habits were poor. Carol had difficulty relating to humans but did have an attachment to a rolled bib which she used to slap herself. The palm of her right hand was used to slap her face with enough intensity to cause bleeding on occasions.

In an attempt to restrict self-abusive behavior, Carol was dressed in a jumpsuit with hand pockets which was laced up the back. This protective procedure was deemed necessary by medical service but further compounded Carol's withdrawal by limiting her sporadic positive hand movements.

It was impossible to utilize formal evaluative procedures, so goals were determined as a result of extended observation of Carol in her residential area. These goals were determined after discussion with the program team involved: (1) obtain eye contact and pleasurable human contact, (2) negate self-abusive behavior, and (3) develop self-feeding since this was her one area of voluntary human contact.

It was decided that liquids were an acceptable primary reward so they were given with secondary verbal praise and physical contact when possible.

Much time was spent in aiding Carol to react to her human environment: walking with her, waiting for her to walk by (when she stopped she was given a drink), and reaching to touch her. Finally the big day came when she voluntarily reached to touch the therapist. Concurrently, reduction in self-abusive behavior occurred, permitting removal of the jumpsuit and the use of dresses and other normal attire.

The decision was made to progress to self-feeding because food is an oral reinforcer and fulfills a very basic survival need. First, Carol was fed while standing in her living unit. Next, the therapist sat making it necessary for Carol to come to the spoon, while being encouraged to sit beside the worker. Finally she was able to sit at a table while being fed. The next step was to aid her in grasping, filling, and inserting the spoon into her mouth. Physical assistance was reduced to pressure on the ulnar border of her hand, then discontinued. Other residents who also were beginning self-feeders were added to the table with Carol who was able at the end of about eighteen months to self-feed with acceptable behaviors for her developmental stage.

The improved contact with her environment and demonstrated reactions aided in determining the next goal—that of toilet training and self-care in this area.

Small but meaningful gains were made, giving Carol an increased sense of self-worth through actions that meet physical and psychosocial requirements.

THE FUTURE AND THE MENTALLY RETARDED

What does the future hold for the mentally retarded? One outstanding advancement is the demand for accountability. Families, community agencies, funding sources, and professional organizations are demanding proof of the results of time, energy, and funds expended. Staff no longer can report impressive looking statistics for attendance at mass activities, numbers of pounds of food served, tons of laundry washed, or gallons of water used. They are expected to produce behavioral change in individuals, with some exhibiting extreme change which will permit independent living, apart from the family unit. In others, seemingly minimal change in self-care is seen; these changes permit more active participation within an institutional community. These extremes on the continuum are based on degrees of change which are obtainable based on the individual's skill level. If an individual can sit in a chair rather than lie down, self-feed rather than be fed, or be continent rather than wear diapers, the time and energy spent in training are justified.

Involvement of families must continue to increase. Initially families were encouraged to institutionalize and forget a retarded family member. For those who conformed to this counsel, there was development of increased guilt and shame. This was compounded, on the rare occasions that they were permitted to visit, by the lack of recognition on the part of the mentally retarded individual and in some instances by lack of interest on the part of the staff. For those who kept the family member at home, stress was placed on the total family by a society that did not understand, gaped, and commented on aberrant behaviors. Fortunately these types of abuse have lessened, and families are being involved as a total unit in a variety of treatment community activities.

The increased involvement of the family unit is only one product of family counseling. The family is being given help in adjusting to the needs of any member who is mentally retarded; it is aided in deciding where and when to go for assistance and in comprehending how to obtain and ask the maximum level of function of the retarded individual. The family is helped in planning for the care of the individual when the primary family can no longer meet his or her needs.

Advances have been made medically which will make the prevention of mental retardation caused by some factors a reality. Genetic counseling will be of immeasurable importance. Individuals who have potential for conceiving an involved child will be so informed and counseled.

Those known as high-risk mothers because of age, exposure to infection, and possible genetic complications have access to the amniocentesis procedure. This involves the removal of about 10 cubic centimeters of amniotic fluid which contains fetal cells. The fluid is analyzed relative to a number of metabolic disorders and chromosomal content with the recommended remediation being given by the physician.

Much progress has been made with an even greater prospect for the future as a result of prenatal care. Early care during pregnancy will aid in improving the nutrition of both the mother and the baby. Various medical and dietary supplements providing a well-balanced diet will aid in the reduction of premature births as well as in the prevention of disorders such as hyperthyroidism that result from endocrine imbalances.

Some geographical areas are now developing a high-risk registry. Individuals considered to be potential candidates for extended care are listed in the registry and observed closely.

Increased use of tests at birth, such as those for phenylketonuria, will determine if there will be a need for dietary supplements for the baby. The use of the supplement may not totally eliminate the effect of these causative factors but will surely reduce the potentially severe level of retardation.

Expansion of programs such as infant stimulation, Head Start, and others will affect the numbers of those who are considered to be retarded as a result of insufficient stimulation during early and formative years.

When a study is made of all potential causative factors of mental retardation, it is apparent that the current advances will not eliminate retardation. Many causes, such as unknown prenatal influences or trauma, are not yet preventable but the gains made recently do present a positive indication for future reduction of the incidence of mental retardation and for more efficient care for those affected.

REFERENCES

1. Smith, D. W., and Marshall, R. E. (eds.): Introduction to Clinical Pediatrics. Philadelphia: W. B. Saunders Co., 1972, p. 181.
2. Stein, J. (ed.): The Random House Dictionary of the English Language. New York: Random House, 1967.
3. Grossman, H. J. (ed.): Manual on Terminology and Classification in Mental Retardation. Baltimore: Garamond/Pridemark, 1973.
4. Copeland, M., Ford, L., and Solon, S.: Occupational Therapy for Mentally Retarded Children. Baltimore: University Park Press, 1976, p. 27.
5. Ibid.
6. Itard, J.: The Wild Boy of Aveyron. Century Psychology Series. Englewood Cliffs NJ: Prentice-Hall, 1962.
7. Goldberg, I., and Lippman, L.: Right to Education. New York: Teachers College, Columbia University, 1973.
8. Diagnostic and Statistical Manual of Mental Disorders (DSM—II), ed. 2 American Psychiatric Association, Washington DC, 1968.
9. Heber, R. (ed.): A Manual on Terminology and Classification in Mental Retardation. Monograph Supplement to Am. J. Mental Deficiency, ed. 2. American Association on Mental Deficiency, Springfield IL, 1961, p. 64.
10. Ibid., p. 63.
11. Grossman: Manual on Terminology and Classification, p. 23.
12. Buros, O. K. (ed.): The Seventh Mental Measurement Yearbook. Highland Park IL: Gryphon Press, 1972.
13. Currie, C.: Evaluating function of mentally retarded children through use of toys and play activities. Am. J. Occup. Ther. 23:1, 1969.
14. Employment of Patient Workers in Hospitals and Institutions at Subminimum Wages. U.S. Department of Labor, Washington DC. U.S. Government Printing Office, 1975.
15. Currie: Evaluating function of mentally retarded children.
16. Nathan, C.: Please Help Us Help Ourselves. Occupational Therapy Department, Indiana University Medical Center, Indianapolis, 1970.
17. De la Cruz, F. F., and LaVeck, G. D.: Human Sexuality and the Mentally Retarded. New York: Brunner-Mazel, 1973.
18. Rimland, B.: Infantile Autism. New York: Appleton-Century-Crofts, 1964.

BIBLIOGRAPHY

Anderson, F.: Fay's First Fifty: Activities for the Young and the Severely Handicapped. Augusta GA: Strothers Printing, 1974.

Banus, B. S.: The Developmental Therapist. Thorofare NJ: Charles Slack, 1971.

Baumeister, A. A.: Mental Retardation. Chicago: Aldine Publishing Co., 1967.

Ellis, N.: Handbook of Mental Deficiency. New York: McGraw-Hill Book Co., 1963.

Fiorentino, M. R.: Reflex Testing Methods For Evaluating CNS Development. Springfield IL: Charles C Thomas, Publishers, 1972.

Gellis, S. S., and Feingold, M.: Atlas of Mental Retardation Syndromes. Washington DC: U.S. Government Printing Office, 1968.

Haynes, U.: A Developmental Approach to Case Finding. Washington DC: U.S. Government Printing Office, 1967.

Houts, P., Scott, R., and Leaser, J.: Goal Planning with the Mentally Retarded. Milton S. Hershey Medical Center of the Pennsylvania State University, Hershey, 1973.

Koch, R., and Dobson, J. (eds.): The Mentally Retarded Child and His Family. New York: Brunner-Mazel, 1971.

Koestler, F. A. (ed.): Reference Handbook for Continuing Education in Occupational Therapy. Dubuque: Kendall/Hunt, 1970.

Krajicek, M. J., and Tearney, A. I. (eds.): Detection of Developmental Problems in Children. Baltimore: University Park Press, 1977.

Moore, J. C.: Neuroanatomy Simplified. Dubuque: Kendall/Hunt, 1969.

Mysak, E. D.: Principles of a Reflex Therapy Approach to Cerebral Palsy. New York: Teachers College Columbia University, 1963.

Price, A., Gilfoyle, E., and Myers, C. (eds.): Research in Sensory Integrative Development. American Occupational Therapy Association, Rockville MD, 1976.

Robinson, H. B., and Robinson, N. M.: The Mentally Retarded Child. New York: McGraw-Hill Book Co., 1965.

Rothstein, J.: Mental Retardation. New York: Holt, Rinehart & Winston, 1961.

Seguin, E.: Idiocy and Its Treatment. (reprinted) New York: Teachers College Columbia University, 1907.

Smith, D. W.: Recognizable Patterns of Human Malformation. Philadelphia: W. B. Saunders Co., 1970.

The Child with Central Nervous System Deficit. Children's Bureau Publication Number 432-1965, Washington DC. U.S. Government Printing Office, 1965.

West, W. (ed.): Occupational Therapy for the Mentally Handicapped Child. Chicago: University of Illinois, 1965.

Wolfensberger, W.: Normalization. National Institute on Mental Retardation, Toronto, 1972.

20
Cerebral Palsy

Margaret V. Howison, Joyce A. Perella, and Doris Gordon

In the area of cerebral palsy the occupational therapist is effectively able to focus attention on the integration of the many aspects of a child's development including the physical, sensory, perceptual, emotional, cognitive, cultural, and social aspects. It is necessary for the occupational therapist to know the normal developmental sequences before appropriately evaluating and treating the individual with cerebral palsy.

Normal development is presented in Chapter 3. This chapter attempts to reinforce those concepts and develop a rationale of occupational therapy intervention for individuals with cerebral palsy.

HISTORICAL PERSPECTIVE

Although not documented initially by name, cerebral palsy has been identified from earliest times. Perhaps this describes the one who was "a cripple from his mother's womb, who never had walked," (Acts 14:8) or "the man who was sick of the palsy." (Matthew 9:2)

It was not until 1843 that William John Little of England (1810-1894) first discussed "infantile spastic paralysis" which became known as "Little's disease." In 1862 Little presented an accurate paper on the etiologic factors of cerebral palsy. This described the problem as one resulting from prenatal, natal, and immediate postnatal influences.[1]

For many years cerebral palsy treatment was approached from a surgical perspective. The early enthusiasm for surgical intervention to correct deformities, provide stability, and improve motor control soon waned as assessment showed that deformities reoccurred or new ones developed. Much of the basis for treatment came from the success in treating poliomyelitis.[2]

In 1932, Winfield M. Phelps (1894-1971) became more aware of the necessity for exercises, muscle training, and bracing. Prior to 1932 he had completed his orthopedic training in Boston, where Bronson Crothers was developing the new field of pediatric neurology. As a result a beginning program for treatment of cerebral palsy evolved.[3] Phelps, who coined the term cerebral palsy (C.P.) to dissociate it from mental retardation, gradually did less surgical intervention except for bone deformities on older children.

From Phelps' era there gradually evolved various

approaches of nonsurgical therapy which emphasized neuromuscular training. These approaches include Fay and Doman-Delacato with the neuromuscular reflex therapy; Bobath with the neurodevelopmental treatment approach; Rood with the neurophysiological approach; and Kabat, Knott, and Voss with proprioceptive neuromuscular facilitation. (See Chapter 7, Section 2.)

Recently there has been an increasing interest in cerebral palsy. Persons involved in the fields of neurology and psychology have studied early disorders more carefully; this has led to a closer study of the early stages of development. At the same time those persons working in the area of pediatrics have advanced the knowledge regarding the newborn and the newborn's neurological status. These changes and increased interest have led to both earlier diagnosis and more successful treatment.[4]

The application of modern sophisticated obstetrical and neonatal care, together with the treatment of infants under one year of age (before disordered postures and movements are established), suggest that, in many cases, disorders may be prevented.[5] Consequently fewer severely involved children are now being referred for treatment, and those who are are younger than those referred ten years ago. It is exciting to speculate what the situation will be in ten more years. Hopefully there will be many less severely involved children who will be able to lead relatively normal and productive lives.

DEFINITION, INCIDENCE, AND ETIOLOGY

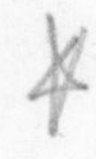

Cerebral palsy is defined as a nonprogressive lesion of the brain occurring before, at, or soon after birth and which interferes with the normal development of the immature brain. The resulting impairment of the coordination of muscle action with an inability to maintain postures and balance and to perform normal movements and skills is common to all cases.[7] Because the parts of the brain are interrelated, there may be many associated neurological abnormalities such as sensory deficits, speech problems, sensory integration deficits, intellectual impairment, seizure disorders, and emotional problems.

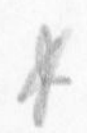

The incidence of cerebral palsy has been estimated at approximately two per one thousand live births.[8]

Cerebral palsy seems to be caused by complications prenatally in 30 percent of the cases, perinatally in 60 percent of the cases, and postnatally in 10 percent of the cases.[9]

Prenatally cerebral palsy may be inherited or acquired. Acquired causes are infection such as toxoplasmosis, rubella, and cytomegalic inclusion disease; prenatal anoxia (lack of oxygen) such as umbilical cord around the neck; prenatal cerebral hemorrhage (abnormal bleeding) such as maternal toxemia or direct trauma; Rh factor such as kernicterus resulting from Rh complications; metabolic disturbances such as diabetes; harmful exposure to roentgen ray; bleeding in the first trimester; drug toxicity such as vitamins A and D; or multiple births.[10]

Perinatal causes are anoxia from respiratory obstruction, placental abnormalities, maternal anoxia, hypotension, or breech delivery; trauma or hemorrhage from disproportions and malpositions, forceps application, holding head back, induced labor, sudden pressure changes in a precipitate delivery, prolonged labor, or cesarean delivery; or prematurity.[11]

Postnatal causes are trauma from skull fractures, wounds, and contusions of the brain or subdural hematomas; infections from meningitis, encephalitis, or brain abscesses; toxicity from lead, arsenic, and coal tar derivatives; vascular accidents such as congenital aneurysms or hypertensive disorders; anoxia from CO_2 poisoning, strangulation, or hypoglycemia; or neoplasms or the developmental effects of tumors, cysts, or hydrocephalus.[12,13]

CORRELATION OF NORMAL DEVELOPMENT AND DEVELOPMENT IN CEREBRAL PALSY

The correlation study presented should facilitate a preliminary understanding of the influence of all abnormal tonic reflex activity on normal motor developmental sequence as it relates to cerebral palsy. The study is not complete, and the reader is encouraged to refer to the References and Bibliography for more information.

Normal Postural Reflex Mechanism

In review, normal motor development is dependent upon normal postural tone. The tone must be high enough to provide mobility and stability but not so high as to prevent both movement and stability. The normal postural reflex mechanism provides the foundation upon which all purposeful movements and skills are performed.[14] Righting, equilibrium, and protective extension reactions are defined as the normal postural reflex mechanism. These reactions are subcortical, automatic responses which develop in a definite sequence.

RIGHTING REACTIONS.[15-17] Righting reactions are the first to develop and function. They perform the following:

1. Provide normal alignment of the head with the trunk and the trunk with the limbs. This function is demonstrated by the neck righting response present at birth until six months of age. Turning of the infant's head to the side is followed by log rolling of the trunk as the trunk strives to maintain alignment with the head.

2. Provide normal position of the head in space with the mouth horizontal and the face vertical. For instance, the labyrinthine righting reaction, a vestibular response, facilitates head extension against gravity in prone position. The response is present from one month of age throughout life. It is considered the key to normal development since head extension increases normal extensor tone throughout the body. The labyrinthine righting response develops in supine position at six months of age and laterally at eight months of age. These responses also remain throughout life.

3. Provide postural orientation and adjustment by vision. This function is accomplished by the optical righting reactions which develop simultaneously with the labyrinthine righting reactions in prone, supine, and lateral positions. Optical righting reactions remain throughout life.

4. Provide rotation within the body axis as influenced by the body on body righting reaction. This reaction overrides the neck righting response, begins at six months of age, and remains until five years. The rotation is essential and enables the child to roll segmentally from supine to prone and to return roll from prone to supine. Rotation also enables the individual to assume sitting and quadruped positions.

EQUILIBRIUM REACTIONS.[18-20] Equilibrium reactions are automatic responses that enable the individual to maintain or regain his balance when the center of gravity has been displaced. These are vestibular responses that develop in a definite sequence. The mature response consists of the head and the trunk righting toward the high body side; extension, abduction, and external rotation of extremities toward the high body side; and extension, abduction, and internal rotation of extremities on the low body side. Equilibrium reactions develop in prone and supine positions at six months, four-foot kneeling at eight months, sitting at ten to twelve months, kneeling at fifteen months, and standing at fifteen to eighteen months. These reactions remain throughout life.

The righting and equilibrium reactions interact.

PROTECTIVE EXTENSION REACTIONS.[21] These reactions function to protect the head and body when falling. These automatic reactions consist of extension of extremities. Protective reactions begin at six months in prone suspension. In sitting they develop forward at six months, laterally at eight months and backwards at ten to twelve months. Reactions also develop in kneeling and standing and remain throughout life. (See Chapter 10, Section 3, for developmental reflexes and reactions.)

Progression Through Eight Months

By eight months of age the infant has progressed through the following stages of gross motor development:[22]

Stage I (3 to 4 months). Characterized by symmetrical and midline orientation of extremities, head control, and forearm support in prone position. This is demonstrated by the infant's extending the head in midline and bearing weight on forearms when lying prone. When supine, the infant is able to bring hands together in midline orientation.

Stage II (4 to 5 months). Highlights the beginning of symmetrical extension/abduction of limbs. The infant begins to stretch (extend) arms and legs when lying on abdomen. In supported standing, the infant bears almost all weight on extended legs.

Stage III (6 months). Emphasized by strong extension/abduction patterns of the limbs. This is exemplified by the infant's bearing weight on a fully extended arm while reaching forward with the other extended arm for a toy while in prone position. In back lying, the infant will reach forward with fully extended arms to be picked up and will take feet to mouth with legs extended and abducted.

Stage IV (8 months). Characterized by the beginning of spontaneous rotation within the body axis as well as trunk control and balance. The infant moves from prone position to sitting and then from sitting to prone position. Ability to sit unsupported for one minute is present.

Progressing through these stages of normal development enables the eight-month-old child to roll segmentally from prone to supine position and vice versa, as influenced by the body on body righting reaction. This acquired rotation also enables the child to go from a prone position to a sitting position and vice versa, using the support of protective reactions to do so. Independent sitting is developing and protective extension reactions forward and sideward are used for support and balance while in the sitting position. Crawling on the abdomen backward and forward is accomplished by pushing and pulling with the arms. The child pulls to a standing position using a half kneel while holding on to furniture and putting full weight on lower extremities.

Equilibrium reactions are established in prone and supine positions, are developing in sitting but are absent in standing. Righting reactions are present. A combination of optical and labyrinthine righting reactions enable the child to right the head in prone, supine, and lateral positions. Neck righting has been overridden by body righting on the body since six months of age. This provides the necessary rotation to enable the child to segmentally roll and assume the sitting position. Protective extension reactions are present from forward suspension and in sitting to the front and sides. They are absent in the back.[23] The transfer of objects from hand to hand is common. Radial palmar grasp and voluntary release of objects held in hands are developing.

It becomes evident that the normal eight-month-old child has developed mobility and begins to explore and interact with the environment. However, the individual with cerebral palsy at eight months of age or older may or may not be able to accomplish these tasks. Brain damage may interfere with the maturational process of the central nervous system and this results in a pathological release of abnormal tonic reflex activity. This influence can interrupt the normal motor developmental sequence at any stage.

TONIC LABYRINTHINE REFLEX. The tonic labyrinthine reflex (TLR) is normally observed from birth to approximately four months of age. It is a vestibular response characterized by increased extensor tone in supine and flexor tone in prone positions. In individuals with cerebral palsy, an abnormally strong TLR response in supine may dominate the individual (Fig. 20-1). This increased extensor tone in supine may be characterized by severe hyperextension of head and trunk. The shoulder girdle is retracted with the arms externally rotated, abducted, and elbows flexed with fisted hands. The lower extremities are strongly extended at hips and knees with the legs internally rotated and adducted. The ankles are plantar flexed.

The individual when strongly dominated by this abnormal pattern, will not be able to right or flex the head forward in the supine position. Increased abnormal tone inhibits rotation and the individual will not be able to roll from supine to prone or assume sitting or any higher developmental position. Most likely the arms cannot be brought forward and oriented in midline, nor can the hands be brought to the mouth. In addition, the normal postural reflex mechanism will be absent. Respiration and feeding will also be abnormally affected.

Presence of severely abnormal increased flexor tone in the prone position is a result of the tonic labyrinthine reflex. The head is flexed and the shoulder girdle is protracted with arms tightly flexed and adducted against the chest. The hands are frequently fisted with the thumb adducted across the palm of the hand. Lower extremities are also adducted, flexed at the hips and knees, and positioned under the abdomen. Sometimes increased extensor tone versus flexor tone can dominate in the lower extrem-

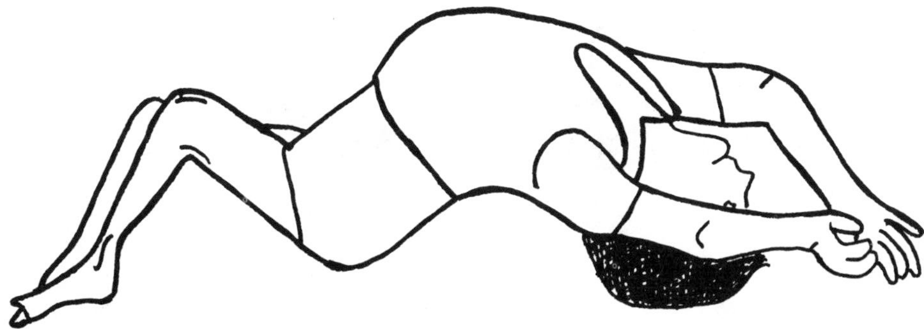

FIGURE 20-1. Tonic labyrinthine reflex (TLR) in the supine position. The illustration shows severe extensor tone of the TLR called opisthotonos.

ities (Fig. 20-2). When dominated by abnormal severe flexor tone, the individual with cerebral palsy will have difficulty turning his head from side to side or righting his head against gravity in prone. The increased flexor tone will also inhibit the progression in the developmental prone sequence, i.e., weight bearing on forearms (prone prop), to weight bearing on extended elbows with hands open, to quadruped position, to kneeling position, to half kneeling, to stand. Rotation within the body axis will also be inhibited by the increased flexor tone and will prevent rolling segmentally from prone to supine positions or assuming prone to sitting. Prehension patterns will be impossible as a result of fisted hands. The normal postural reflex mechanism will not develop because postural tone is abnormal or hypertonic.

ASYMMETRICAL TONIC NECK REFLEX. The asymmetrical tonic neck reflex (ATNR) can be observed in normal development from one to six months of age. It is a primitive response elicited by the stimulation of proprioceptors in the neck muscles. This response is characterized by increased extensor tone in the extremities of the face side; increased flexor tone in extremities on the skull side. Normally the infant is not dominated by the primitive response and can move out of it with little effort. The ATNR reaction seems to assist the normal infant in developing unilateral swiping (reaching) as he visually regards his outstretched (extended) arm and hand.[24] The response (ATNR) also appears to serve as a preparatory response for rolling over with the extremities on the lower body side extended and the extremities on the upper body side flexed while the head is turned.

Persistence of the ATNR beyond six months of age may indicate pathological factors and central nervous system dysfunction (Fig. 20-3). Domination of a strong abnormal ATNR response in the individual with cerebral palsy will result in the lack of the development of body symmetry (normally established by four months of age). The head will lack midline orientation as the abnormal increased tone will result in the head deviating to the side. Increased tone will also prevent the ability to orient the hands together in midline and to bring the hands to the mouth. Asymmetry may also be noted in the trunk and, if it persists, can lead to scoliosis of the

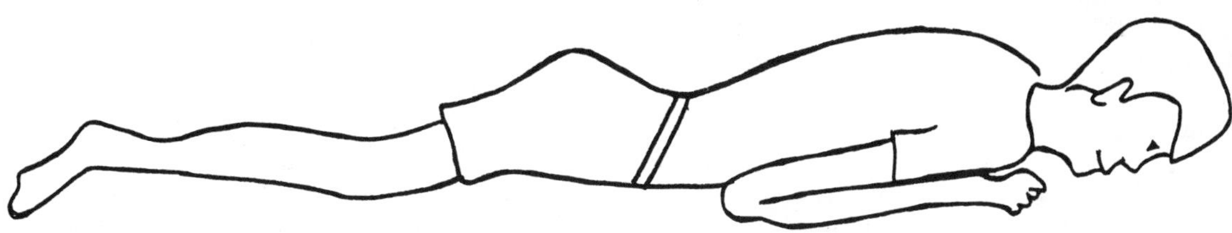

FIGURE 20-2. Tonic labyrinthine reflex in the prone position.

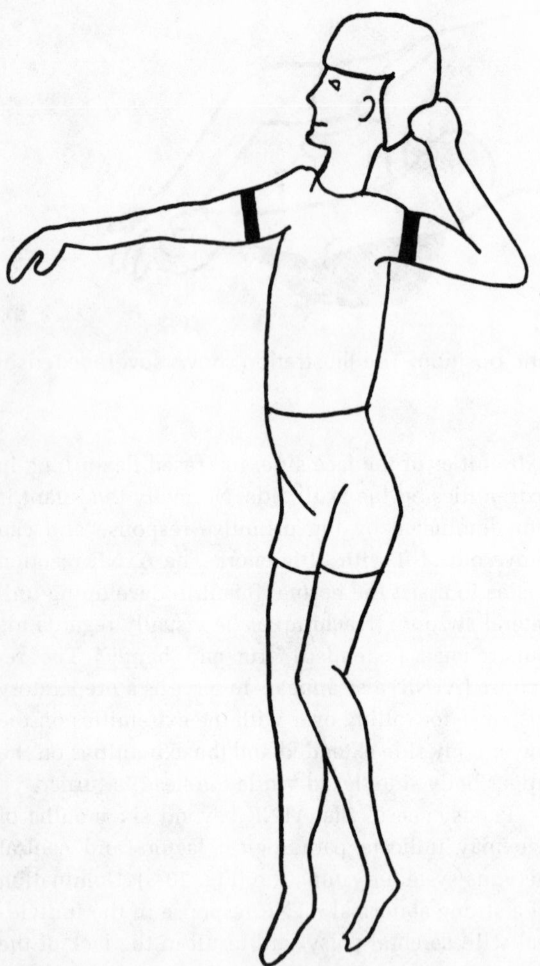

FIGURE 20-3. Pathological tonic neck reflex.

spine with either concavity of the curve on the side with increased extensor tone or convexity of the curve on the side with increased flexor tone. The lower jaw may laterally deviate to the side of increased extensor tone. This is another characteristic of the pathological influence of the ATNR and its abnormal effect on body symmetry.

If the lower jaw deviates to the side, the upper and lower teeth will not be positioned properly for chewing. Feeding problems will result. Difficulty in visual horizontal tracking across the midline can also be observed. In conclusion it is noted that an abnormal increased postural tone will prevent the development of righting, equilibrium, and protective extension reactions, so necessary for normal growth and development.

CLASSIFICATION

There are three main types of cerebral palsy: spasticity, athetosis and ataxia. Most cases, however, are mixed and do not fit into a clear-cut classification. The presence of abnormal postural tone is common to all types. A fourth type of cerebral palsy is flaccidity. This is seen in either an infant or toddler (from one to three years); initially the child is flaccid but later, with maturation, the child will become classified as one of the three main types.

Spasticity

Spasticity refers to increased muscle tone. Spastic individuals usually have quadriplegic, diplegic, hemiplegic, and sometimes paraplegic involvement.

The severe spastic person has strong hypertonus with little change in the degree of tone. There is increased tone or constant co-contraction of the agonist and antagonist muscles which inhibits any type of relaxation while awake or asleep. Because of the maintenance of a few abnormal postures, these individuals are more vulnerable to developing deformities. The deformities may be scoliosis; kyphosis; flexion deformities of the hips, knees, and fingers; forearm pronation contracture; subluxation of the hip; and shortening of the heel cords with inward or outward turning of the foot (equinovarus and equinovalgus respectively). There is little movement except when strongly stimulated. This movement is small and labored within a limited range of motion. Primitive spinal patterns are often completely inhibited by tonic reactions. Startle reactions are common to many cases. Tonic patterns are seen in the tonic neck and tonic labyrinthine reflexes and also a positive supporting reaction. Associated reactions can be felt but little movement is observed. Righting reactions, protective extension, and equilibrium reactions are often absent. Neck righting, however, may be present.

The individual with moderate spasticity may have normal to hypertonic muscle tone. The degree of hypertonicity is influenced by the stimulation of effort, emotion, speech, and sudden stretch. More spasticity is seen in the agonist than in the antagonist muscles and more so distally than proximally. Deformities may develop from the maintenance of abnormal postures, the use of stereotyped abnormal patterns, and the associated reactions in lesser involved parts. These deformities may be in the form of kyphosis; lordosis; hip subluxations or dislocations; flexion contractures of hips and knees; or tight hip inward rotators, adductors, and heel cord shortening with foot rotation.

Although the range of motion is greater in the moderate spastic, it is usually not complete throughout every range. Learned skills are performed in primitive and abnormal patterns without the selectivity of movement. Total movements may be in synergies. There may be voluntary use of spinal and tonic reflex patterns for purposive movements. Primitive spinal patterns of total flexion or extension are common. A strong startle response is usually present. Tonic patterns of the tonic neck and tonic labyrinthine reflexes and positive supporting reactions are often present. Associated reactions in the form of associated movements are strong. Some righting reactions may be present. Equilibrium reactions in sitting and kneeling are often developed but not in standing and walking.

Athetosis

Athetosis which refers to fluctuating muscle tone may be divided into four types: athetosis with spasticity, athetosis with tonic spasms, choreoathetosis, and pure athetosis. Usually there is quadriplegic involvement but sometimes there is hemiplegic involvement.

ATHETOSIS WITH SPASTICITY. The athetoid with spasticity seems to have moderate spasticity in the proximal parts and athetosis in the distal parts. Muscle tone fluctuates between normal and hypertonus. Deformities are less frequent than in the spastic type but may occur as flexor deformities at the hips, elbows, and knees. There may be some co-contraction at the proximal joints. Such individuals often lack selective movement and the grading of muscle action. There is some control throughout the midranges. Postural patterns are similiar to those with moderate spasticity. Primitive spinal patterns are present but modified by involuntary movements. There are strong influences of the tonic neck reflexes (symmetrical and asymmetrical) and the tonic labyrinthine reflexes. Although usually present, righting reactions are unreliable because of the intermittent influence of tonic reflexes.

ATHETOSIS WITH TONIC SPASMS. The athetoid individual with tonic spasms changes from hypotonic to hypertonic muscle tone. Lack of co-contraction causes excessive extension or flexion. Strong postural asymmetry influenced by tonic neck reflexes which are more exaggerated to one side may cause deformities to develop. These may be scoliosis, kyphoscoliosis, dislocation of the hip on the skull side, and flexor contractures of the hips and knees if the individual has been sitting for long periods. Occasionally the hips, fingers, or lower jaw sublux. There is hardly any voluntary control of movements because of strong, intermittent tonic spasms. Extreme postures of flexion or extension are assumed. There seems to be involuntary movement more distally located than proximally located. Because the individual either is in tonic spasm or is hypotonic and unable to move, primitive spinal patterns are usually not present. Strong tonic patterns are seen in the asymmetrical and symmetrical tonic neck reflexes and the tonic labyrinthine reflexes. Righting, equilibrium, and protective reactions are absent.

CHOREOATHETOSIS. The individual with choreoathetosis has muscle tone which fluctuates from hypotonic to normal and from hypotonic to hypertonic. There is no co-contraction. Deformities are rare but there is a tendency for subluxation of the shoulder and finger joints. There are extreme ranges of motion with no grading of midranges. The large jerky involuntary movements seem to be more proximal than distal. Hands and fingers are weak but often coordination is good in free movement. There is a lack of selective movement and fixation of movement. Primitive spinal patterns are present but modified by the athetosis. There are intermittent tonic reflex patterns. Righting and equilibrium reactions are present to some extent, but coordination is abnormal. Protective extension of the arms is abnormal and often absent.

PURE ATHETOSIS. The individual with pure athetosis is rare. His muscle tone fluctuates between being too low to normal. Rarely are there any deformities. There may be some transient subluxations of the shoulder and finger joints, and there is lack of co-contraction. Twitches and jerks of individual muscles or even muscle fibers are seen. Slow, writhing involuntary movements which are more distal than proximal and lack of fixation are characteristic. Primitive spinal patterns are present but modified by athetosis. These patterns are less primitive and more selective than in choreoathetosis. There is rarely any tonic reflex influence. Righting, equilibrium, and protective extension reactions are present but involuntary movements interfere with them.

Ataxia

Ataxic cerebral palsy is characterized by moderate to severe muscular hypotonia with generalized weakness, truncal and head ataxia, incoordinated movement, and intention tremor.[25] Ataxia may be associated with spasticity, athetosis, or a combination of both. Muscle tone is usually hypotonic but fluctuates between hypotonus and normal. There is a lack of fixation and sustained postural control. Coordination is fairly normal although usually primitive. Righting reflexes and equilibrium reactions are highly developed but movements are incoordinated. Intension tremor and nystagmus are common.

Flaccidity

Flaccid cerebral palsy may be seen from birth to about three years of age. With maturation it usually becomes one of the three main types. Involvement generally is quadriplegic. Muscle tone may be so low that tonic neck reflexes are not elicited. Typically the legs go into the frog position, i.e., hip abduction and external rotation and knee flexion. This position may cause hip dislocation. The trunk and chest seem flat, arms are flexed, hands are fisted, and there may be intermittent extensor spasticity. Respiration is usually very shallow. The infant/child has full range of motion which he or she does not use. There may be hypermobility of the joints. There is no ability to co-contract muscles.

ASSOCIATED NEUROLOGICAL ABNORMALITIES AND PROBLEMS

The occupational therapist must be aware not only of the motor implications of cerebral palsy but also of the possible associated problems or neurological abnormalities. Studies have shown that most children with cerebral palsy have anywhere from two to seven additional disorders.[26]

It is estimated that 50 percent of the children with cerebral palsy have *disturbances of vision*. This may be from incoordination of the eyes as seen especially in quadriplegic involvement. There may be internal or external squints or strabismus which may be alternating or fixed and cause lack of accommodation. The lack of conjugate movement may cause an impairment of stereoscopic vision. The child may not be able to move his or her eyes and thus must move the head. Strong neck retraction may limit the athetoid child's ability to look down. A strong asymmetrical tonic neck reflex may fix the eyes to the face side of the head or may prevent the eyes from moving over the midline. Total blindness may be caused by the increasingly rare retrolental fibroplasia and by optic atrophy. It is likely that the cerebral palsied child who may also be hemiplegic will have visual field deficits from optic radiation.[27]

An estimated 25 percent of the children with cerebral palsy have some type of *auditory disturbance*. The most common auditory problem is high frequency deafness. This is most likely to be seen following neonatal jaundice of the athetoid child but is also common in the spastic child. There may be auditory imperception or agnosia.[28]

Speech disturbances are seen in approximately 25 percent of the cerebral palsy cases.[29] The most common problem is dysarthria which is a pseudobulbar palsy seen in the spastic, athetoid, and mixed types. Aphasia is rare. Apraxia of the mouth, throat, and larynx may cause an inability to speak.[30]

The impairment of *stereognosis* is common in the individual with hemiplegic involvement. There may be a more subtle global problem with the spastic quadriplegic child.

Sensory integrative disorders are seen in approximately 14 percent of individuals with cerebral palsy.[31] An apparent higher incidence is seen in the spastic child. This may be from the brain lesion, the child's inability to explore the environment, or learning disorders. (See Chapter 7, Section 3.)

An estimated 50 to 75 percent of the children with cerebral palsy have *below average intelligence*.[32,33] Seizure disorders are seen in approximately 25 percent of the cases.[34] Any type of seizure may occur but the seizure usually is generalized. It is more common with hemipleiga of postnatal origin. It is rare in the athetoid child.[35]

Emotional problems are common among children with cerebral palsy. This is often compounded by emotional immaturity since the child tends to be more dependent upon the family. This may result from physical dependency or because of exclusion from a group of normal children. The degree of acceptance and adjustment to disability is primarily the result of both the birth injury and the reactions of the child with the immediate environment of parents and family.[36]

Some individuals with cerebral palsy exhibit a *weak self-image;* their ability to feel a sense of self-worth and/or responsibility may be minimal. They may demonstrate difficulties in group situations and in interpersonal relationships. In essence, there seems to be a general tendency to withdraw from social interactions.

Limited studies have been done on *personality traits.* It seems that athetoid children tend to have more emotional instability and to be explosive. The spastic child seems to have more of an obsessive compulsive personality and may find it more difficult to adapt to new situations.

It is probable that in some cases the associated problems are more limiting than the motor abnormalities.

ASSESSMENT

Accurate assessment of the individual with cerebral palsy is essential for appropriate functional treatment planning. The person should be evaluated thoroughly in order to find his or her correct developmental levels. Areas that should be considered are physical, sensory, perceptual, emotional, cognitive, cultural, and social.

The occupational therapist should be aware that there is no single evaluative tool that defines the many abnormalities seen in the cerebral palsied child. Instead there are many tools used in conjunction with each other, and the selected combination results in a more accurate evaluation. The following are a variety of evaluative tools with which the occupational therapist should be acquainted and knowledgeable to utilize in the assessment process.

Physical Evaluation

Physical evaluation may include assessment of reflex, motor development, oral motor reflexes, activities of daily living, and the Denver Developmental Test.

1. *Reflex test:* (see Chapter 10 and Figure 20-4). This includes the development and integration of gross reflex maturation from the spinal level to standing equilibrium.

2. *Motor development:* (see Chapter 10 and Figure 20-5). This includes gross developmental activities from raising the head to independent walking and fine developmental activities of reflexive grasp to supination and opposition.

3. *Oral motor assessment:* (see Figure 20-6). This includes pertinent reflexes influencing control to the coordination of fine oral movements.

4. *Activities of daily living:* (see Chapter 10). This test is given to individuals with a mental age of over 6 years.

5. *Denver Developmental Test:* (see Chapter 10 and Figure 20-7). This screening test, developed by Frankenburg and Dodds at the University of Colorado Medical Center, Denver, covers gross motor, language, fine motor adaptive, and personal social development from 0 months to 6 years.

Sensory Evaluation

(See Chapter 10.) Sensory refers to tactile, proprioception, kinesthesia, temperature, pain, sharpness-dullness, and stereognosis.

Perceptual Evaluation

(See Chapter 7, Section 3, and Chapter 10.) Perceptual evaluation is a necessary part of the evaluation process because there are many neurological abnormalities observed in the child with sensory integrative dysfunction, and it is important to be able to pinpoint each one.

Emotional Evaluation

(See Chapter 10.) The emotional evaluation correlates with the developmental level and the individual's stage of adjustment and acceptance.

Cognitive Evaluation

(See Chapter 10.) The Slosson Test of Verbal Intelligence[37] seems to be an adequate evaluative tool of cognition. Bayley,[38] Gessell, and Denver screening also test this area.

Cultural and Social Evaluation

Although formal standardized tests do not seem to be available, the therapist should be aware of the

(*Text continues on p. 512.*)

REFLEX TESTING CHART

Name: Reflex Level:

B.D.: Therapist:

Date:

Reflexes	+	−	*Comments:*
1. Level One—Spinal:			
a. Flexor Withdrawal			
b. Extensor Thrust			
c. Crossed Extension			
2. Level Two—Brain Stem:			
a. Asymmetrical Tonic Neck			
b. Symmetrical Tonic Neck			
c. Tonic Labyrinthine—supine			
prone			
d. Associated Reactions			
e. Positive Supporting Reaction			
f. Negative Supporting Reaction			
3. Level Three—Midbrain: Righting Reactions:			
a. Neck Righting			
b. Body Righting acting on the Body			
c. Labyrinthine Righting acting on the head			
d. Optical Righting			
e. Amphibian			
4. Automatic Movement Reactions:			
a. Moro Reflex			
b. Landau Reflex			
c. Protective Extensor Thrust			
5. Level Four—Cortical: Equilibrium Reactions:			
a. Prone-lying			
b. Supine-lying			
c. Four-foot kneeling			
d. Sitting			
e. Kneel-standing			
f. Standing—hopping			
dorsiflexion			
see-saw			
g. Simian posture			

FIGURE 20-4. Originally from Newington Hospital for Crippled Children, Newington CN, Occupational Therapy Department. In Fiorentino, M. R.: Reflex Testing Methods for Evaluating CNS Development. Springfield IL: Charles C Thomas, 1972, p. 50. Reprinted with permission.

MOTOR DEVELOPMENT CHART

Name: Date:

B.D.: Dominance:

Reflex Level: Therapist:

Motor Development *Comments:*

I. Head Raising:
1. Prone (1–2 mo.): ______
2. Supine (4–6 mo.): ______
3. Sidelying (7 mo.): ______

II. Turning:
1. Supine-sidelying (1–4 wk.): ______
2. Supine-prone (6 mo.): ______
3. Prone-supine (8 mo.): ______

III. Crawling (7–8 mo.):
1. Puppy dog: ______
2. Static—makes amphibian movements: ______
3. Creeps—makes amphibian movements; moves body forward: ______
4. Bunnyhops—assumes 3 point crawling using complete rotation: ______
5. Crawling—assumes 4 point crawling using complete rotation: ______
6. Crawling—uses partial rotation up to sitting then assumes 4-foot kneeling and crawls: ______

IV. Sitting:
1. Maintains (7 mo.): ______
2. Assumes using complete rotation (10—12 mo.): ______
3. Assumes using partial rotation (2–5 yr.): ______
4. Assumes symmetrically (5 yr.): ______

V. Standing:
1. Kneel-stands: ______
2. Kneel-walks: ______
3. Pulls up to standing (10½ mo.): ______
4. Stands unassisted (14 mo.): ______
5. Walks (15–18 mo.): ______

(Continued)

FIGURE 20-5. Originally from Newington Hospital for Crippled Children, Newington CN, Occupational Therapy Department. In Fiorentino, M. R.: Reflex Testing Methods for Evaluating CNS Development. Springfield IL: Charles C Thomas, 1972, p. 51. Reprinted with permission.

MOTOR DEVELOPMENT CHART (*Continued*)

Arm—Hand

	Development	*Comments:*
0–4 mo.	Reflexive grasp—no eye-hand coordination:	
4–8 mo.	Conscious grasp—pronation: a. crude: b. between palmar and fingers—ulnar: c. thumb adducted, not utilized:	
6 mo.	Eye-hand coordination begins: Arms used asymmetrically—control from shoulder and shoulder girdle: Corralling reach;	
7 mo.	Radial palmar grasp:	
8 mo.	Scissor grasp: Thumb envelopes object: Elbow flexible:	
9 mo.	Crude pinch—pincer grasp: Advertent release of grasp: Wrist flexibility: Use of forearm between mid-position and pronation:	
11 mo.	Pincer release: Supination more frequently:	
12 mo.:	Opposition: Supination—cortically controlled:	

many ethnic backgrounds and their cultural influences on the individual's personal environment. These are important cues for the therapist since they assist him or her in understanding that mental thread which gives meaning to the child's life. Thus the therapist is better equipped to plan a treatment program that is compatible with the lifestyle of the child.

The therapist will also gain much information from informal observation of the individual with peers and family. Not only is social interaction seen but also many facets of the entire developmental spectrum. The family is encouraged to assist in the evaluation process. The therapist should be sensitive to the family's understanding and adjustment to their child. This may influence the reliability of their reported observation.

Each member of the therapeutic team evaluates and presents findings to those involved with the individual. An interrelated functional and individualized treatment program may then be planned and executed.

INTERVENTION

The treatment of the individual with cerebral palsy is a twenty-four-hour-a-day process. The entire family should become an integral active part of the treatment team. The treatment team may consist of the occupational, physical, and speech therapists,

(*Text continues on p. 518.*)

CHECK LIST FOR ORAL-MOTOR INVOLVEMENT AND COMMUNICATION

Name ______________________ Sex __________ Birth Date ____________ Examiner ______________

Diagnosis____

	Date:	*Date:*	*Comments*
MOTOR FUNCTIONS *Position for Testing* (1) Passive (2) Active I. *Head and shoulder movements* 1. Shrug one shoulder at a time 2. Turn head w/o associated movement of shoulders			
Neck righting (positive or negative)			
Asymmetrical tonic neck reflex			
3. Flex shoulder forward; does head fall back?			
4. Bring head forward; does shoulder fall back?			
5. Can child lift head—prone? Inf. of L.R.R. (2 mo.)			
Can child lift head—supine? (6 mo.)			
Laughing, crying, and coughing 1. Associated reactions			
2. Phlegm—when crying?			
3. Spontaneous			
4. Voluntary			
II. *Infantile reflexes* (1) Absent (2) Weak (3) Strong 1. Eventual inhibition of: a. Rooting reflex			
b. Suckle pattern			
c. Biting reflex			
d. Hyperactive gag			
e. Mandibular facet slip			

(*Continued*)

FIGURE 20-6. Oral motor assessment.

CHECK LIST FOR ORAL-MOTOR INVOLVEMENT AND COMMUNICATION (*Continued*)

	Date:	*Date:*	Comments
2. Oral movements for facilitation (1) Normal (2) Moderate (3) Poor a. Lip closure 1. While sucking			
2. While chewing			
3. While swallowing			
4. Bilabials in individual words			
5. Bilabials during spontaneous speech			
6. Lips at rest			
b. Sucking Infant feeding—age when solid food was introduced			
1. Grooving of tongue while sucking			
2. Straw placement—on sides			
3. Straw placement—in middle			
3. Chewing (1) Dev. to side (2) Rotary (3) Up and down			
4. Swallowing a. One swallow at a time			
b. Repetitive pattern			
5. Synchronous breathing a. At rest			
b. Upon phonation			
III. *Involuntary movements* (1) None/very little (2) Moderate (3) Much a. Lips			
b. Tongue			
c. Diaphragm			
1. At rest			
2. Upon phonation			
d. Larynx (vocal cords)			
1. Abductor spasms (hoarse, tense speech)			
2. Abductor spasms (breathy, leakage of air)			

CHECK LIST FOR ORAL-MOTOR INVOLVEMENT AND COMMUNICATION (*Continued*)

	Date:	*Date:*	*Comments*
IV. *Dysarthria* Child performs act: (1) Normal (2) With difficulty (3) Not at all a. Lips			
1. Close on command			
2. Pucker			
3. Retract			
b. Tongue 1. Lateralize left			
2. Lateralize right			
3. Dissociate from jaw			
4. Elevate			
5. Protrude			
6. Point			
c. Movement of soft palate			
1. Is speech nasal?			
2. Is speech denasal?			
Breathing 1. Reverse breathing			
2. Hyperventilation			
3. Nasal breathing			
4. Abdominal			
V. *Other observations and comments* a. Drooling 1. Why a. Posture			
b. Motor involvement			
c. Sensory deficit			
d. Lack of motivation			
e. Other			

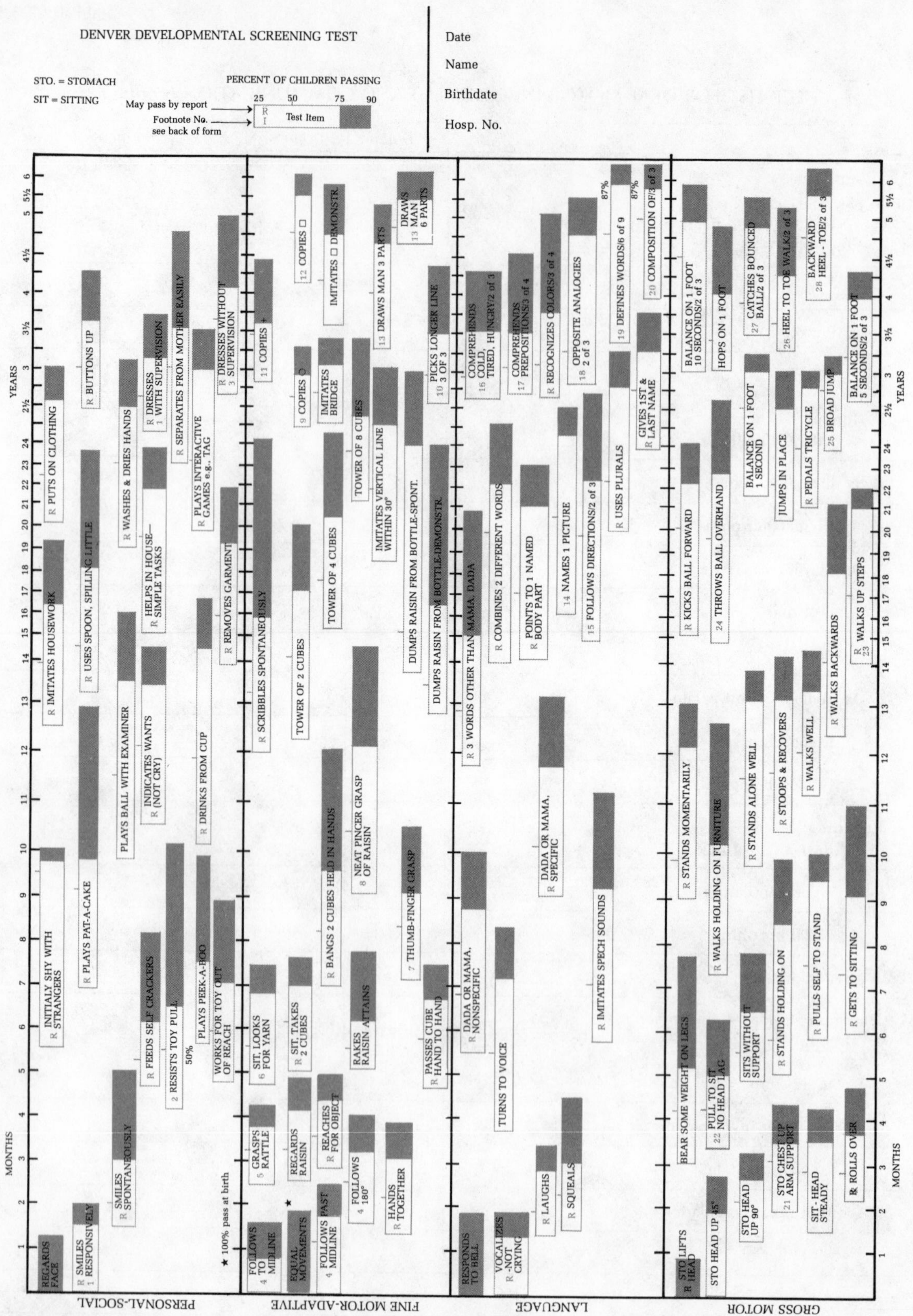

FIGURE 20-7. Distributed as a service by Mead Johnson Laboratories. © 1969 by W. K. Frankenburg, M.D., and J. B. Dodds, Ph.D., University of Colorado Medical Center, Denver. Printed with permission.

DATE
NAME
BIRTHDATE
HOSP. NO.

DIRECTIONS

1. Try to get child to smile by smiling, talking or waving to him. Do not touch him.
2. When child is playing with toy, pull it away from him. Pass if he resists.
3. Child does not have to be able to tie shoes or button in the back.
4. Move yarn slowly in an arc from one side to the other, about 6″ above child's face. Pass if eyes follow 90° to midline. (Past midline; 180°)
5. Pass if child grasps rattle when it is touched to the backs or tips of fingers.
6. Pass if child continues to look where yarn disappeared or tries to see where it went. Yarn should be dropped quickly from sight from tester's hand without arm movement.
7. Pass if child picks up raisin with any part of thumb and a finger.
8. Pass if child picks up raisin with the ends of thumb and index finger using an overhand approach.

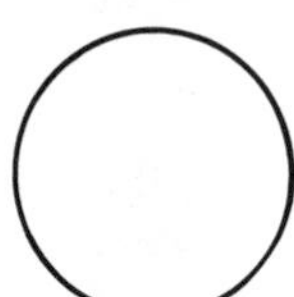

9. Pass any enclosed form. Fail continuous round motions.

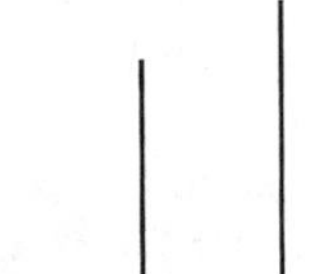

10. Which line is longer? (Not bigger.) Turn paper upside down and repeat. (3/3 or 5/6)

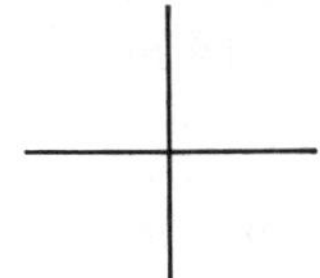

11. Pass any crossing lines.

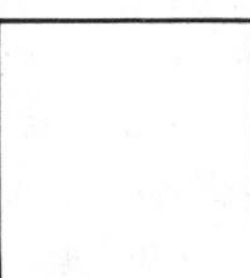

12. Have child copy first. If failed, demonstrate.

When giving items 9, 11 and 12, do not name the forms. Do not demonstrate 9 and 11.

13. When scoring, each pair (2 arms, 2 legs, etc.) counts as one part.
14. Point to picture and have child name it. (No credit is given for sounds only.)

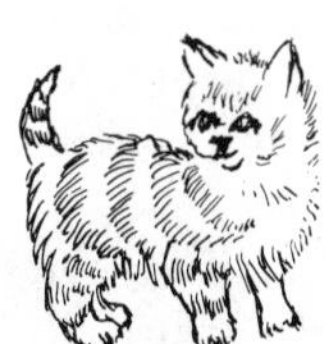 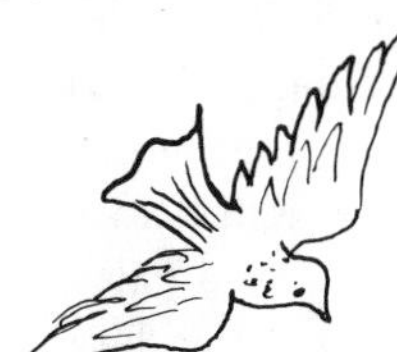 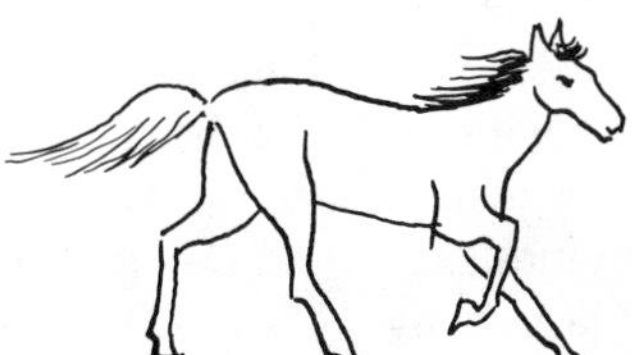 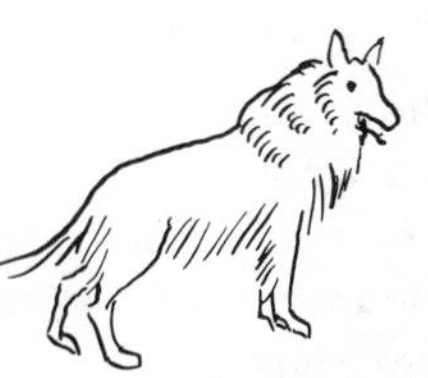 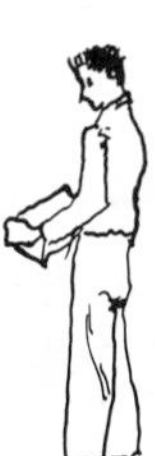

15. Tell child to: Give block to Mommie; put block on table; put block on floor. Pass 2 of 3. (Do not help child by pointing, moving head or eyes.)
16. Ask child: What do you do when you are cold? . .hungry? . .tired? Pass 2 of 3.
17. Tell child to: Put block *on* table; *under* table; *in front* of chair, *behind* chair. Pass 3 of 4. (Do not help child by pointing, moving head or eyes.)
18. Ask child: If fire is hot, ice is ?; Mother is a woman, Dad is a ?; a horse is big, a mouse is ?. Pass 2 of 3.
19. Ask chilkd: What is a ball? . .lake? . .desk? . .house? . .banana? . .curtain? . .ceiling? . .hedge? . .pavement? Pass if defined in terms of use, shape, what it is made of or general category (such as banana is fruit, not just yellow). Pass 6 of 9.
20. Ask child: What is a spoon made of? . .a shoe made of? . .a door made of? (No other objects may be substituted.) Pass 3 of 3.
21. When placed on stomach, child lifts chest off table with support of forearms and/or hands.
22. When child is on back, grasp his hands and pull him to sitting. Pass if head does not hang back.
23. Child may use wall or rail only, not person. May not crawl.
24. Child must throw ball overhad 3 feet to within arm's reach of tester.
25. Child must perform standing broad jump over width of test sheet. (8½ inches)
26. Tell child to walk forward, ⊂⊃ ⊂⊃ ⊂⊃ ⊂⊃ → heel within 1 inch of toe. Tester may demonstrate. Child must walk 4 consecutive steps, 2 out of 3 trials.
27. Bounce ball to child who should stand 3 feet away from tester. Child must catch ball with hands, not arms, 2 out of 3 trials.
28. Tell child to walk backward, ← ⊂⊃ ⊂⊃ ⊂⊃ ⊂⊃ toe within 1 inch of heel. Tester may demonstrate. Child must walk 4 consecutive steps, 2 out of 3 trials.

DATE AND BEHAVIORAL OBSERVATIONS (how child feels at time of test, relation to tester, attention span, verbal behavior, self-confidence, etc.):

the physician, psychologist, and nurse. In addition, the child often sees a pediatrician, neurologist, orthopedist, physiatrist, and psychiatrist. To this team the occupational therapist brings his or her skills in developmental assessment and individual problem solving. The child is viewed as a total being.

Before any evaluation or treatment can be effective there must be a mutual respect and acceptance between the individual and the therapist. The child must realize that there is a genuine caring for him or her because he or she is important and because he or she is himself or herself.

The occupational therapist should identify the physical needs, emotional or maturational level, intellectual level, and specific interests of each person. The therapist then plans a highly individualized program and presents a choice of several appropriate activities to meet the person's specific needs. In choosing activities the therapist should also consider the cultural background, age level, physical ability, interests, and the functional level of the person.

Many remediation techniques may be combined with age-appropriate activities. Besides toys, games, books, and crafts, everyday practical activities may be suggested. These activities may include helping to mix cookies, knead bread, fold laundry, hang up clothes, dry unbreakable dishes, or dust. It may simply be playing near and/or in a cabinet of pots and pans. All of these are normal developmental experiences that the individual with cerebral palsy may miss. The occupational therapist, in his or her unique professional role, provides a therapeutic environment which includes these activities in conjunction with treatment.

GENERAL OCCUPATIONAL THERAPY TREATMENT PRINCIPLES AND REMEDIATION TECHNIQUES

Treatment of the individual with cerebral palsy involves consistent symmetrical handling. This treatment should (1) influence the amount of postural tone by reducing, increasing, or steadying the tonus; (2) inhibit abnormal patterns; and (3) facilitate normal responses. A child should not spend more than twenty minutes in any one position.

Spasticity

There are three basic principles of handling that the occupational therapist should follow when treating the spastic child. They are noted here.

FLEXED POSITION FOR CARRYING. *The spastic child with increased extensor tone should always be picked up and carried in a flexed position.* Before being picked up, the child should be fully positioned in hip and knee flexion with legs abducted. The shoulders should be protracted and the arms slightly abducted. The head should be in the midline and slightly flexed. The child should not be picked up under the arms with legs fully extended. This increases extensor tone.

The child may be carried facing outward with his or her back to the therapist's chest. This allows the therapist to maintain normalized tone and the child to move easily and visually explore his environment.

The child may be carried with hips abducted and flexed while straddling the therapist's hip. The arms should be symmetrically controlled to prevent retraction of the shoulder girdle. This method of carrying distributes the weight more evenly and is easier to use with the older and heavier child.

The adult with cerebral palsy may be lifted from his or her wheelchair using the same symmetrically flexed position. This may require one person on either side.

DECREASING HYPERTONUS AND INHIBITING ABNORMAL PATTERNS. *All movements of the spastic individual should be slow and rhythmical.* Motion should be facilitated proximally, i.e., trunk, shoulders, and hips. This should automatically reduce tone distally. Slow passive rotation of the trunk between the shoulder and hips is a key to postural relaxation.

The individual may be placed prone on a large therapy ball. With arms outstretched over the head and legs abducted and externally rotated, gently rock him or her back and forth or side to side until relaxation occurs. The therapist has more control of the child if held above the knees.

With the child prone over a roll, elbows supported on floor, arms pronated and hands open (Fig. 20-8), the therapist kneels between the child's legs which are in external rotation and abduction. The therapist positions his or her hands on the

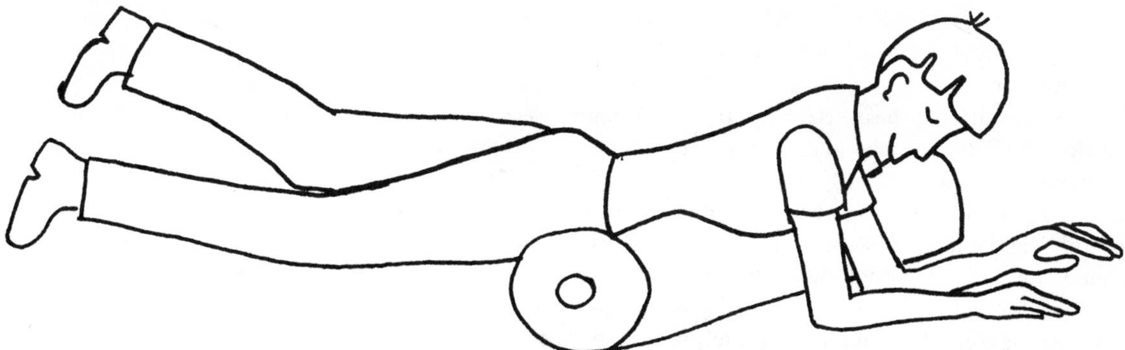

FIGURE 20-8. The child's prone position over a roll or bolster. Used to reduce excessive tone.

child's hips and gently rotates the child from side to side until excessive tone has been reduced.

The spastic person should be prepositioned before being moved and/or placed in the required situation. For example, before putting the child prone over the roll, the therapist positions the child in prone over his or her arms. The child's arms are outstretched over the therapist's arm and legs are abducted and supported over the therapist's other arm.

Side lying on a wedge or firm pillow with the head flexed forward, the hips and knees flexed, and the shoulders protracted (Fig. 20-9) is an excellent position to neutralize tone. The extremities on the upper side should be more flexed than those on the lower side.

A firm pillow should be placed under the head and upper shoulders to inhibit extensor tone. Arms should be positioned across the chest to stimulate midline and finger play and to inhibit external rotation of the arms and retraction of the shoulders. Sand bags, small pillows, or rolled up towels may be placed along the lateral border of the upper arm. The legs should be slightly flexed and abducted with a rolled up blanket or pillow.

Neutral warmth has been used successfully to decrease hypertonicity. The child may be flexed into the correct position, wrapped in a soft blanket, and held in this manner until he or she relaxes. The child may also be positioned in a large box of styrofoam packing chips. The chips support the child as well as act as an insulator for body heat.

FACILITATING NORMAL RESPONSES. After tone has been normalized, the normal postural reflex mechanism is facilitated.

To facilitate the combined action of the labyrinthine and optical righting responses in prone position, the individual may be placed prone over a wedge with arms fully extended over the head. The therapist kneels by his or her side. The therapist places his or her arms under the child's axilla and extends the child's spine by raising the chest off the wedge. This should facilitate head extension

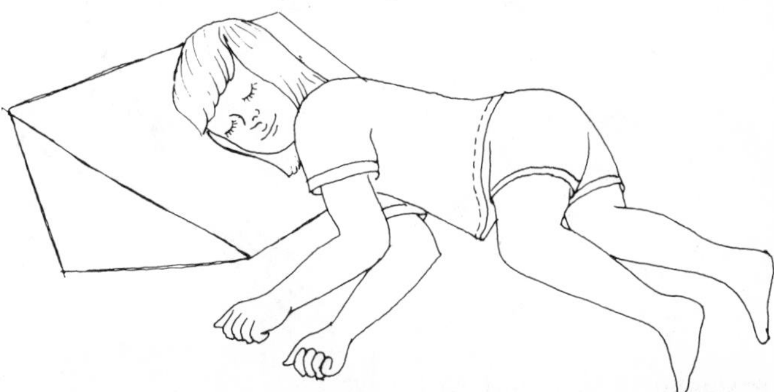

FIGURE 20-9. Side lying on a wedge.

against gravity. Downward pressure on the top of the head through the spine will increase co-contraction of the neck muscles.

After facilitating head righting in the prone position, the child may be placed on a prone board to play at a table (Fig. 20-10). This increases extension of the child's neck for better head and trunk control. The child may be positioned with legs extended and with feet weight bearing in the foot rest box or may kneel in the foot box. Positioning on the prone board is used to inhibit abnormal flexor tone and to facilitate extension.

To facilitate head righting in the supine position, the therapist places the child in a fully flexed position with head on a wedge or firm pillow. The child's knees are flexed to the abdomen, hips adducted and arms folded across the chest. The therapist places his or her arms at the child's shoulders, bringing them forward. Using the shoulders as a key point of control, the therapist diagonally rotates the trunk and slowly assists the child to the semi-upright position within his or her range of neck control. The head must flex forward. Downward pressure on the head may facilitate co-contraction.

To encourage body on body righting reactions which facilitate segmental rolling, the shoulder girdle can be used as a key point of control. The child is placed supine with one arm extended over the head and the contralateral leg flexed at the hip and knee. The therapist places his or her hand on the protracted shoulder and rotates the trunk to assist the child's rolling toward the extended side into the prone position.

To facilitate protective extension in a forward suspended position, the child is placed prone over a roll or small ball. The therapist controls the child by externally rotating and abducting the legs. The therapist gently lowers the child to the floor. The child's arms should automatically extend and his or her hands open with fingers abducted to prepare for weight bearing. To increase co-contraction of the upper extremities, alternate tapping may be provided at the elbows.

To facilitate static equilibrium reactions in the prone position, place the child prone on the floor and on fully extended arms. The therapist gently countertaps the shoulders from side to side while the child maintains his or her balance.

For dynamic equilibrium reactions in the prone position, the child is placed prone on the therapy ball or vestibular board. The child is gently rocked to one side to displace the center of gravity. This should facilitate the head and trunk righting toward the high side causing these extremities to abduct and extend. The extremities on the low or other side will abduct and extend to protect and break the fall.

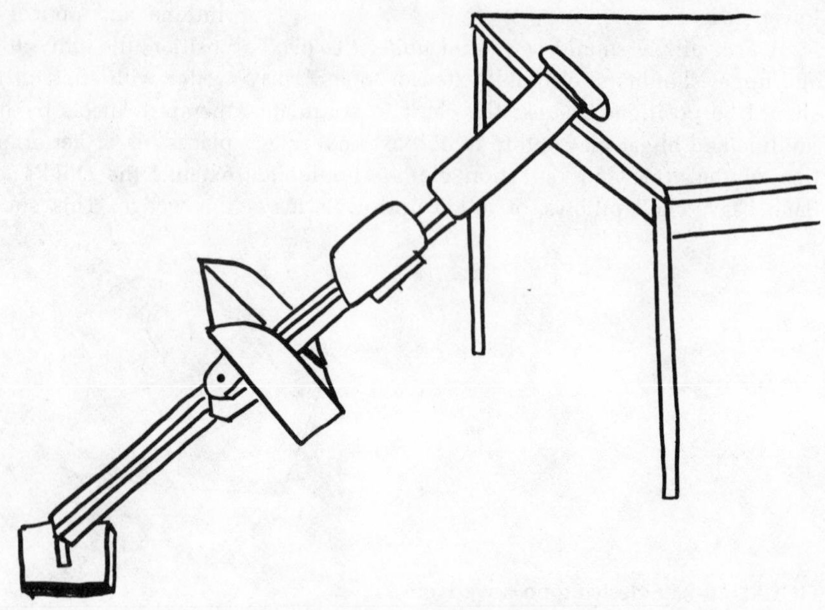

FIGURE 20-10. A prone board.

Treatment should begin in the prone position and should be facilitated according to the normal developmental sequence (see Chapter 3, Section 1).

Athetosis

The individual with athetoid cerebral palsy exhibits fluctuating postural tone between hypertonicity and hypotonicity. Movements are uncontrolled and wide in range. Midline orientation of head and extremities frequently is absent.

In order to control the involuntary movements and obtain body symmetry, proper positioning is essential. The position for carrying the athetoid person involves bringing the individual's arms forward with the carrier's forearms in front of the individual's arms. The child's hands are then placed and held by the carrier's hands over the lower part of the child's knees. The hips should be adducted with the knees flexed higher than the hips. The back should be positioned in front of the carrier's chest[39] (Fig. 20-11).

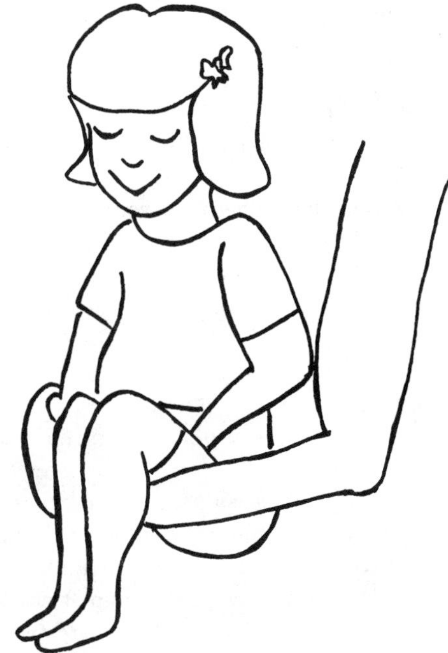

FIGURE 20-11. Position for carrying an athetoid child.

Postural tone should be normalized. If the tone is too low, weight bearing with pressure and resistance can be used to facilitate sustained tone for postural control. The athetoid individual who, in prone, is able to right his or her head against gravity, assume, and maintain prone prop position should advance to the prone on extended elbow position. When the child can maintain this position, he or she should rock slowly from side to side, front to back, and diagonally. This should be followed by assuming a position from extended elbows, going back to prone prop and then advancing again to extended elbows. If this is performed slowly and repetitively, it will help to facilitate co-contraction of the shoulder muscles and control of the arm movements in midrange.[40] The head should be oriented in midline. If the head deviates to the side, the influence of the pathological assymetrical tonic neck reflex (ATNR) can interfere with performance. Likewise, if the head hyperextends or flexes, the influence of the pathological, symmetrical tonic neck reflex (STNR) can result in poor performance as well. Sometimes the athetoid child uses the STNR to maintain weight bearing on extended elbows by increasing head extension. This increases extensor tone in the arms but also causes increased flexor tonus in the legs. Using abnormal reflexes hinders progress and thus should be avoided.

If co-contraction at the elbow is poor, indicating low tone, tone can also be increased by tapping the muscles about the elbow. Tapping should facilitate co-contraction and should enable the individual to bear weight on extended elbows in the prone position.[41]

When tone is too high in the athetoid child, the techniques used to normalize tone in the individual with spasticity should be applied. Positioning in a side lying wedge (see Fig. 20-9) may be an excellent way to normalize tone and inhibit involuntary movements. In fact, this is usually a good position for the individual when participating in play activities that involve hand usage.

Once the individual has gained midrange control of movement in weight-bearing positions, he or she should advance to control midrange movements without weight bearing and without involuntary movement. The individual should also try to maintain body symmetry. Side sitting could be a good position for this intervention. Side sitting to the right involves bearing weight on the fully extended right arm. The trunk should remain straight. The legs are flexed with both knees facing toward the right and equal weight is distributed on the buttocks. Placing and holding techniques are introduced with the free left arm. This involves having the left arm passively moved with minimal support and placed in various positions within the range of movement. The individual with athetosis should control the arm while being moved. When the arm is placed in position, he or she should control or maintain the exact range of position.[42]

The next objective is to facilitate (if absent) or organize (if present) the normal postural reflex mechanism (righting, equilibrium, and protective extension reactions).

Head righting to the side can be facilitated in side sitting position, if present in prone and supine. With the individual side sitting to the right without bearing weight on right arm, the therapist holds the left arm and lowers the individual toward the floor on his or her right side. The individual should right the head laterally to the left. If head control is lost, joint compression should be applied downward on the top of the head. The individual should be lowered only as far to the floor as he or she can maintain head control.[43]

Protective extension reactions may be facilitated while sitting if present in prone position. In side sitting, the therapist sits at the side where protective extension reactions should result. The therapist holds the arm at the elbow with one hand. With the other hand the therapist provides joint compression using the base of the palm of the hand. This helps to facilitate co-contraction and tone in the arm. The individual's arm is then lowered sideways to the floor for weight bearing on the fully extended arm. This technique will be particularly helpful when postural tone is too low as seen in some athetoid persons.[44]

Another method of facilitating protective extension in sitting is to hold the individual's right arm in extension, abduction, and external rotation. Then the individual is gently pushed toward the opposite or left side. The left arm should extend in protection. This procedure can be repeated on the opposite side and the direction can be altered to the front, back, or opposite side.[45]

In the quadruped position, protective extension can be facilitated by the therapist. Using the shoulder girdle as the key point of control, the therapist pulls the shoulders backward and upward, lifting the individual's arms and hands up and down on the supporting surface. This technique also facilitates co-contraction and extension in arms required for weight bearing.[46]

Protective extension can be elicited in kneelstanding and standing as well. It should only be facilitated in the positions in which the individual is able to maintain tone for control.

Equilibrium reactions may be facilitated in sitting if tone is normalized and the individual can maintain the sitting position. With the individual sitting lengthwise on a carpet-lined barrel and legs fully extended, the therapist gently rocks the barrel from side to side. This should facilitate head and trunk righting plus appropriate reactions of extremities.

If the individual sits perpendicular to the length of the barrel and the therapist rocks the barrel forward and backward, equilibrium reactions should result. If tilted backward, the head and trunk should right forward and the arms should come forward as well. When tilted forward the opposite reactions should occur. The vestibular board or therapy ball may be used as a substitute for the barrel.

Another method which may be used to facilitate equilibrium reactions in sitting is to have the individual sit on a bench. The therapist places his or her hands on the lateral aspect of the upper trunk. Using this as the key point of control, the trunk is rotated to each side. The individual should right his head and abduct and extend his arm and leg in the direction which is opposite to the trunk rotation.[47]

On all fours or in the quadruped position, the individual is gently pushed to each side. At the point of the individual's losing his or her balance, the therapist applies a counter push at the shoulder.

Dynamic equilibrium reactions may be facilitated in kneeling, half kneeling, and standing positions. Again these reactions should only be facilitated when the individual is able to maintain the position.

In summary, intervention for the individual with athetosis is usually more static than for the spastic individual, particularly during the process of establishing sustained tone for postural control. When this has been obtained, facilitation of the normal postural reflex mechanism follows. Athetoid persons can move but movement is uncontrolled and/or involuntary and needs to be organized. In the presence of spasticity, these individuals cannot move because of increased tone. They require the sensory input and feedback of normalized tone and movement patterns.

Ataxia

There are three basic principles of handling that the occupational therapist should follow when treating the ataxic individual. They are similar to the principles presented for the spastic child.

FIXED POSITION FOR CARRYING. Since the ataxic individual usually has spasticity and/or athetosis, the same principles of handling apply. The ataxic child should always be picked up and carried as one would the spastic and athetoid child.

DECREASING HYPERTONUS AND INHIBITING ABNORMAL PATTERNS. The basic ideas presented under the treatment of the spastic and athetoid person may be applied to the ataxic individual. Reflex inhibiting postures may be used to reduce hypertonus.

FACILITATING NORMAL RESPONSES: The ataxic individual usually has normal reactions but cannot use them appropriately because of incoordination or tremors. It is necessary to work for sustained co-contraction of agonists and antagonists. This may be done by firmly holding the child in various developmental positions. Sensory feedback in the form of heavy tapping of muscles, joint compression, and weighting of the trunk and/or extremities will provide proprioceptive and kinesthetic feedback in which to steady and increase the muscle tone.

Flaccidity

There are three basic principles of handling which the occupational therapist should follow when treating the infant or child with flaccidity.

FIXED POSITION FOR CARRYING. Since the flaccid infant or child lacks muscle tone, he or she should be well supported. The child should be carried in flexed position with head slightly flexed forward. Added trunk control may be needed.

INCREASING POSTURAL TONE. The flaccid infant or child needs as much controlled sensory input as possible. The therapist can provide this input by bouncing, rubbing, and tapping the infant or child in order to increase the muscle tone. This child needs to be moved often as he or she tends to be content in any position.

FACILITATING NORMAL RESPONSES. To stimulate deeper breathing, the infant or child should be encouraged to both laugh and cry. The developmental scale is followed beginning at prone and head control and continues to supine and then to sitting. It is necessary to work slowly and steadily and to wait for reactions.

SPECIFIC REMEDIATION TECHNIQUES

It is perhaps in the areas of *oral-motor, feeding, dressing* and *communication skills* that the occupational therapist has a unique role. These daily activities are automatic for the normal individual. However, for the individual with cerebral palsy, these are functional activities which are essential for building independence and developing a strong, positive self-image.

Pre-Speech and Feeding (Oral-Motor)

Normal Reflexes

According to the Rood approach,[48] one of the major sequences in normal motor development is the vital function sequence. This sequence includes the coordination of functions of food ingestion, respiration, and speech articulation. (See Chapter 7, Section 2, The Neurodevelopmental Approaches.)

Normal oral-motor behavior begins in prenatal development approximately at seven-and-a-half weeks of menstrual age. (Menstrual age or weeks refers to age of the fetus as measured by the time from the onset of the mother's last normal menstrual cycle.)[49] Tactile stimulation applied to the perioral area facilitates the first oral fetal reflex activity.[50]

Table 20-1 indicates the local fetal reflex activity of the face as a result of tactile stimulation applied to the area innervated by the trigeminal nerve, the fifth cranial nerve. During normal postnatal development, primitive oral reflexes can be observed in the newborn.

Table 20-1. Fetal reflex activity of the face.

Response	*Area stimulated*	*Menstrual age*
Mouth opening	Lower lip	9½ weeks
Swallowing	Lips	10½ weeks
Momentary lip closure and, with repeated stimulation, swallowing	Lips (and/or tongue)	12½ weeks
Maintained lip closure	Lips	13 weeks
Protrusion of upper lip	Upper lip	17 weeks
Protrusion of lower lip	Lower lip	20 weeks
Protrusion and pursing of both lips simultaneously	Lips	22 weeks
Audible sucking	Lips	29 weeks

Based on data from papers of Hooker.[51]

ROOTING REFLEX. This reflexive response can be seen from birth to three to four months of age and up to seven months in the sleeping infant.[52] Characteristic of the reaction is turning of the head toward the direction of tactile stimulation which is applied in a light stroking manner at the corner of the infant's mouth. Touching of the upper lip elicits lip and tongue elevation accompanied by mouth opening and head extension. The opposite reaction occurs when the lower lip is stimulated. The lip and tongue depress, mouth opens, and head flexes.[53] These reactions are thought to be associated with the infant's search for the food source such as the nipple of the mother's breast.[54] Diminishing of the reflexive response can occur immediately after feeding; therefore it is observed best when elicited in a hungry infant.[55] In the newborn most responses to direct tactile input are of an avoidance or protective withdrawal reaction (i.e., the infant moves as far away from the input as possible). However, the rooting response is one of the first reactions of the neonate that enables him to pursue the tactile input, thus allowing him to make contact with his external environment.

SUCK SWALLOW REFLEX. The normal duration of this primitive response is within the first or second day of life to two to five months of age.[56] Tactile stimulation applied to the infant's lips by the nipple of the mother's breast or bottle results in lip closure followed by a rhythmical movement of the tongue and jaw enabling the infant to obtain food. Usually three repetitive sucks followed by swallowing make up the rhythmical pattern.[57] Sucking action is performed by the elevation and applied pressure of the anterior aspect of the tongue against the nipple, and this movement elicits the release of the liquid. The swallowing action and the transferring of the liquid to the back of the oral cavity is the function of the posterior aspect of the tongue.[58] Non-nutritive sucking can be observed in the neonate also. This is referred to as sucking action in the absence of food.

PROTECTIVE GAG REFLEX. An oral reflex normally present from birth gradually becomes weaker when chewing occurs but does persist throughout life. Tactile input to the posterior aspect of tongue or soft palate will normally elicit a gag response. The gag response is thought to be hyperactive if it is facilitated in any other area of the oral cavity.[59]

BITE REFLEX. This reaction can normally be seen from birth and it gradually diminishes around five to six months when rotary chewing develops. Facilitation of the response is by direct application of tactile input to gums, teeth, or tongue resulting in a rhythmical opening and closing of the mouth.[60] Normally the infant's response to tactile stimulation in the oral area is very sensitive. From birth the infant engages in hand-to-mouth activity.[61] By six months of age the total patterns of either complete flexion or extension are modified by combined patterns of flexion and extension enabling the infant to bring his feet to his mouth. Oral exploration of body parts is not only important for the development of body image but also helps to desensitize the low threshold to tactile input. Another important developmental milestone is the object to mouth exploration particularly dominant at six to seven months of age.[62] This not only teaches the child about his external environment but also assists in the decreasing of oral sensitivity. When finger feeding begins and various consistencies of food are introduced, the infant will be able to accept the food and spoon without facilitating the primitive oral reflexes, particularly gagging.[63]

BABKIN REFLEX. This reflex is a normal neonatal response characterized by opening of the infant's mouth when pressure is applied to the palm of the hand.[64]

MENTAL PALMAR REFLEX. This reflex is characterized by light touching of the infant's palm, which facilitates observable movement of the chin and is considered a normal reflexive response.[65]

Abnormal Responses to Normal Reflexes

These oral reflexes can be totally absent or persistent beyond the normal time of inhibition in the child with cerebral palsy. In either case the response is considered pathological, making feeding extremely difficult and an unpleasant experience for the therapist, family, caretaker, and the individual with cerebral palsy.

Pathologically the rooting response can be absent. It can remain persistent but may be obscured by the influence of the tonic reflex activity such as the tonic labyrinthine reflex (TLR) or the asymmetrical tonic neck reflex (ATNR).[66] Domination of the ATNR prevents self-directed hand-to-mouth activity. This activity is a normal and important process for inhibiting the rooting response which is impossible for the atypical infant.[67] Abnormal persistence of the suck swallow reflex beyond five months of age is usually accompanied by an open mouth pattern with protruding or thrusting of the tongue forward during the swallowing process. The tongue pushes the liquid or food from the mouth. Swallowing accomplished in this manner is referred to as a reversed swallowing pattern. Normally, during swallowing, the lips assume closure and the tongue retracts into the oral cavity.[68] Continuation of the suck swallow reflex also prevents the development of nonreflexive sucking as well as disassociation of tongue and jaw movements (necessary for independent tongue movements required for speech).[69]

Absence of the suck swallow reflex makes feeding time very frustrating. Consequently the inexperienced person might think he or she is solving the problem by enlarging the hole in the nipple so that the fluid will flow more rapidly. Also the person may tilt the individual's head backward so that gravity will assist the fluid in being transported down the throat.[70] This is an undesirable feeding technique referred to as "bird feeding." It should not be used because it does not facilitate any normal functioning of the oral motor mechanism.

Developmental Feeding Sequence

During the first few months of life the normal infant uses the suck swallow reflex to remove liquid from breast or bottle and food from a spoon.[71] This activity is accomplished by the rhythmical movements of the tongue and jaw with little active participation of the lips. The elevation of the anterior aspect of the tongue during sucking will later be used to produce sounds such as "d" and "t." Likewise the retraction of the tongue during swallowing will be incorporated into producing deep throaty sounds such as "g" and "k."[72]

At six or seven months of age, when the child has gained sufficient head and trunk control, feeding takes place in a highchair.[73] When fed, the child uses his lips in a closing manner to remove the food from the spoon.[74] The action of lip closure will eventually be used for bilabial sounds such as "m," "b," and "p."[75] Finger feeding is also developing and facilitates biting (vertical jaw movements) and chewing (rotary jaw movements). Simultaneously the tongue and jaw movements become disassociated and tongue mobility increases. The child is able to elevate, depress, protract, retract, and lateralize the tongue to either side. These independent tongue movements enable the child to shift the food within the oral cavity.

Drinking from a held cup starts around seven or eight months of age. The lips close on the cup rim and the liquid is transferred to the back of the mouth for swallowing.[76]

Through continued practice the child becomes independent in spoon feeding at two to three years of age, cup drinking at one-and-a-half years, and straw drinking at three to four years.[77]

The individual with cerebral palsy can have difficulty at any level within the developmental feeding sequence. Some of the most common problems which interfere with feeding include:[78]

1. Release of tonic reflex activity which creates abnormal postural tone throughout the total body including the oral motor mechanism. Abnormal tone prevents the development of central control essential for adequate feeding positioning.
2. Persistence or absence of oral reflexes such as biting or hyperactive gag.
3. Jaw thrusting or retraction interfering with obtaining and/or maintaining jaw closure.
4. Lack of lip closure.
5. Tongue thrusting or retraction and lack of independent tongue movements.
6. Abnormal breathing patterns.
7. Poor sucking, swallowing, chewing patterns or complete absence of those skills.
8. Drooling.
9. Gagging, choking, and coughing.

To better understand the abnormal oral patterns encountered by individuals with cerebral palsy it might be helpful to understand and perform for yourself a few activities stated below.

1. Try swallowing with your head forward in flexion and then with your head hyperextended. Which was more difficult? Hyperextension of the head is part of an abnormal total pattern of increased extensor tone and suggests the importance of maintaining the head in midline with slight flexion.

2. Analyze your pattern of swallowing. In what position is your tongue when you initiate and conclude the swallowing process? Normally the lips are closed and the anterior aspect of the tongue is elevated against the front of the hard palate when beginning the swallowing process. The tongue ripples to transfer liquid to the back of the mouth and the posterior aspect of tongue humps upon swallowing. Try swallowing with your lips and mouth open wide and your tongue protruding beyond the lips. Did you find this difficult and unpleasant? Swallowing accomplished in this abnormal manner is known as a reversed swallowing pattern and is commonly observed in individuals with cerebral palsy.

3. When analyzing your chewing pattern you will note that your lips remain closed, the jaws rotate during chewing, and the independent tongue movements are necessary to transfer the food in the oral cavity for both chewing and swallowing. Now try chewing with your mouth open and your lower jaw laterally deviated to the right side. If the jaw is deviated far enough the teeth do not come together for chewing. Strong pathological influence of the ATNR causes lateral deviation of the jaw in individuals with cerebral palsy rendering the process of chewing impossible.

Respiration

The normal newborn infant is symmetrically flexed in all positions and lacks the ability to extend or right his head and body against gravity. The chest is barrel shaped and respiration is accomplished by a rapid abdominal breathing pattern with minimal involvement of the thoracic area.[79]

At six months babbling increases and a more mature breathing pattern develops which involves greater thoracic participation (due to the action of the diaphragm and intercostals). The chest is elongated and breathing decreases in rate but increases in excursion.[80] Maturation of the respiratory movements is related to motor development. In prone lying the labyrinthine righting reaction enables the infant to gain antigravity control. Extension of the infant's head against gravity increases the extensor tone throughout his or her body, enhancing greater trunk stability and mobility necessary for thoracic breathing. In supine and upright positions such as sitting, the effects of gravity pushing downward on the body assists in elongation of the thoracic cavity. Body righting on body reaction facilitates rotation within the body axis and also enhances a more mature breathing pattern.[81]

Inspiration goes with extension in normal respiration and exhalation goes with flexion. Phonation occurs on exhalation. Respiratory function in the individual with cerebral palsy is frequently impaired by the influence of abnormal tonic reflex activity. This ultimately effects phonation. The presence of strong extensor spasticity results in tightly retracted abdominal muscles causing the rib cage to become flared and flattened. Breathing is shallow with reduced vital capacity making it extremely difficult for the individual to sustain or vary vocal intonations.

A reversed breathing pattern is not uncommonly demonstrated and is defined as an abnormal process in which the individual speaks on inhalation instead of exhalation. Strong flexor spasticity also influences respiration and phonation. The arms are usually pulled very tightly against the thoracic area preventing the development of a deep regular respiratory pattern.

Evaluation Process

Early evaluation of oral motor mechanisms should be done as soon as possible. Functioning of these oral motor mechanisms must be observed in relation to the movement of the whole body since the individual with cerebral palsy most often reacts in more or less total pathological reflex patterns. Mueller has defined ten steps in the oral assessment process which are as follows:[82]

1. *Observation of Facial Expression.* The facial expression accompanied with strong spasticity may be represented as an abnormal spastic grin due to the tightly retracted lips. This can suggest that the individual is happy and content; however, this is not necessarily a true representation of emotional affect. The facial expression of the individual with hypotonicity can be characterized as a droopy, sad expression displaying little interaction with the environment. Due to the abnormal low tone, this expression does not necessarily indicate the individual's inner feelings or level of comprehension.

2. *Oral Reflexes.* Absence or persistence beyond time of usual habituation of the oral reflexes (rooting, suck swallow, bite, gag) can suggest pathology.

3. *Feeding.* Observation of a feeding session can prove to be most revealing. One should note how the individual eats from a spoon, drinks from a bottle and/or cup, and how he swallows, bites and chews as well. His responses to different consistencies of food should also be recorded.

4. *Oral Sensitivity.* The next step would include assessment of the individual's response to digital stimulation around and in the mouth. Individuals with hypertonicity might display a hyperreactive, defensive response whereas those with hypotonicity might exhibit a hyporeactive response. In either case, the reactions can interfere with the feeding process.

5. *Teeth-Palate Development.* Observation of the presence or absence of teeth, the condition of the teeth and placement of teeth during jaw closure should be noted. Is the hard palate highly arched? Any other abnormalities should be recorded.

6. *Jaws.* Observe the position of the jaws at rest (open or closed) and the coordination of jaws during movement (vertical and rotary). Is the lower jaw abnormally protracted, retracted or laterally deviated? Subluxation of the lower jaw is not uncommon.

7. *Lips.* Note the position of the lips at rest and during movement. Are fine coordinated movements such as pursing of the lips possible?

8. *Tongue.* Observe the position of the tongue at rest. Is it retracted or protracted; elevated or depressed? Are involuntary movements of tongue noted? Are fine coordinated movements such as elevation or lateralization of the tongue demonstrated? Are the movements of tongue disassociated and independent from jaw movements?

9. *Respiration.* Evaluate breathing pattern at rest and under stimulation. Is breathing abdominal or thoracic? Many times the pattern is shallow and irregular. Reversed breathing pattern is not uncommon. In the presence of spasticity the chest is commonly flared and flattened; in the presence of hypotonicity the rib cage might be barrel shaped.

10. *Voice.* Does the individual phonate on inhalation or exhalation? Can he sustain and vary vocal intonations?

For additional information, refer to the oral-motor assessment form, Figure 20-6.

Remediation Techniques

THERAPEUTIC FEEDING TECHNIQUES. 1. *Positioning:* Proper positioning which decreases spasticity and involuntary movements and increases normal postural tone is critical during feeding. Central control and body symmetry are imperative. Positioning is a very individualized aspect. Each child will need to be thoroughly and individually evaluated so that the best position for him or her can be determined.

There are certain factors in feeding positioning that are applicable to most individuals. The head should be slightly flexed forward and the trunk as fully extended and straight as possible without any lateral deviation to either side. Hyperextension of the head and trunk should be avoided. The shoulder girdle should be protracted with the arms brought forward and slightly externally rotated and supinated. Hands are open. Retraction of the shoulder girdle should be prevented. Hips should be flexed to 90 degrees and legs should be slightly abducted. Knees should be flexed higher than the hips and the feet supported. With athetoid children the shoulders also should be protracted but with internal rotation and pronation of the arms for better stability.

Suggested positionings are presented here. The semi-upright face-to-face position can be helpful for the individual who lacks head and trunk control (Fig. 20-12). To obtain this position, the therapist sits on a chair close to the table and places a wedge so that the thicker end is supported by the edge of the table and the thinner end positioned in the therapist's lap. The angle of the wedge can be varied by how close the therapist sits to the table. It is most desirable to have the child as close to an upright position as the child can tolerate. The child is placed supine on the ramp as upright as possible. The child's head may require increased flexion and this is accomplished by placing a rolled towel or U-shaped piece of foam at the base of the skull. Direct pressure to the occipital region of the skull should be avoided as this can increase abnormal extensor spasticity. The child's arms are brought forward and the therapist uses his or her body to keep the legs positioned in abduction. Do not feed *anyone* in the supine position. This may result in aspiration of food to the lungs causing pneumonia and/or death by obstruction of the air passageway.

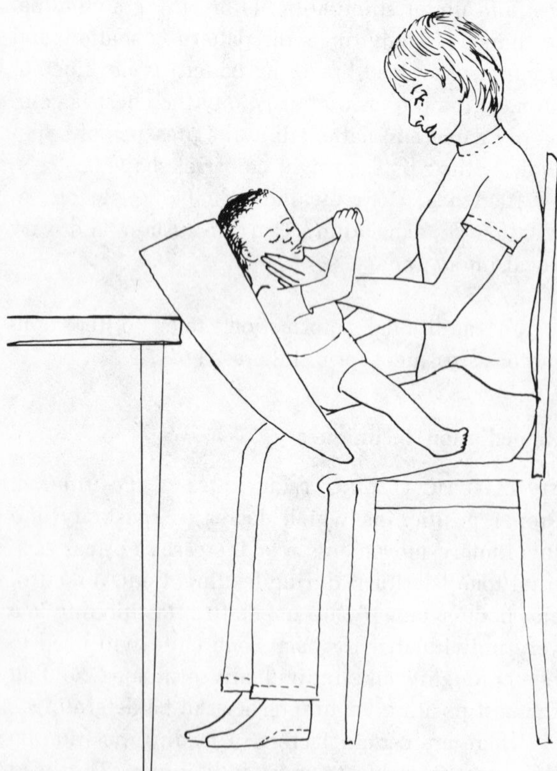

FIGURE 20-12. Semi-upright position used in face-to-face feeding.

An adaptation of this feeding technique involves the therapist's sitting on the floor with hips and knees flexed and the wedge supported on the therapist's thighs. The child is positioned in the same manner, obtaining as close an upright position as can be tolerated. These face-to-face positions are excellent for facilitating eye-to-eye contact and good communication.

Another feeding position involves the therapist's placing the child on his or her lap and cradling the child in the arms. The therapist uses arms and legs for control. One arm is placed around the child and used to provide head and trunk control; the other arm is used to introduce the food. The therapist's leg which is positioned on a small block, elevates the child's knees to provide a functional position.

Prone lying over a wedge or in the therapist's lap with the child lying at a 45 degree angle can be helpful for the individual with severe sucking and swallowing problems.[83]

Side lying on a side lying wedge (Fig. 20-9) can be particularly helpful when severe extensor spasticity is demonstrated.

On some occasions positioning on a prone board (Fig. 20-10) can be useful. With the athetoid child, this position can help to improve stability through weight bearing. The child that is dominated by severe flexor tone can be placed on the prone board to facilitate extension. If the prone board is used for a feeding position, care should be taken to prevent hyperextension of the head when introducing food or liquid.

When the child has gained sufficient head and trunk control, feeding in the upright seated position is most desirable. Triangle chairs with trays can be constructed (Fig. 20-13) and/or high chairs can be adapted to meet the individual's needs.

Some therapists find that an adapted high chair is preferred because of its desirable position and because of its appropriate height. (See Chair Adaptations later in this chapter.)

2. *Jaw Control*: Many abnormal feeding behaviors may necessitate jaw control. Two specific abnormal behaviors are essential for the therapist to note: (1) If the child's jaw is open, thrust forward, and/or laterally deviated and (2) if the lips are open and the tongue thrusts forward pushing liquid or food from the mouth.

The therapist can inhibit these abnormal behaviors by using a three-finger jaw control technique applied directly from the front or from the side. Jaw control from the front (Fig. 20-14) is provided by placing the distal phalanx of the thumb on the center of the chin between the tip of the chin and the center of the lower lip. Direct inward pressure is applied by the thumb. The thumb controls the opening and closing of the jaw and facilitates slight head flexion as the neck extensors are stretched. The thumb should not pull downward as this elicits opening of the mouth. The index finger is placed on the jaw line to prevent lateral deviation of head and jaw. The middle finger is placed under the chin and direct upward pressure is applied at the base of the tongue to inhibit the tongue from thrusting forward and to

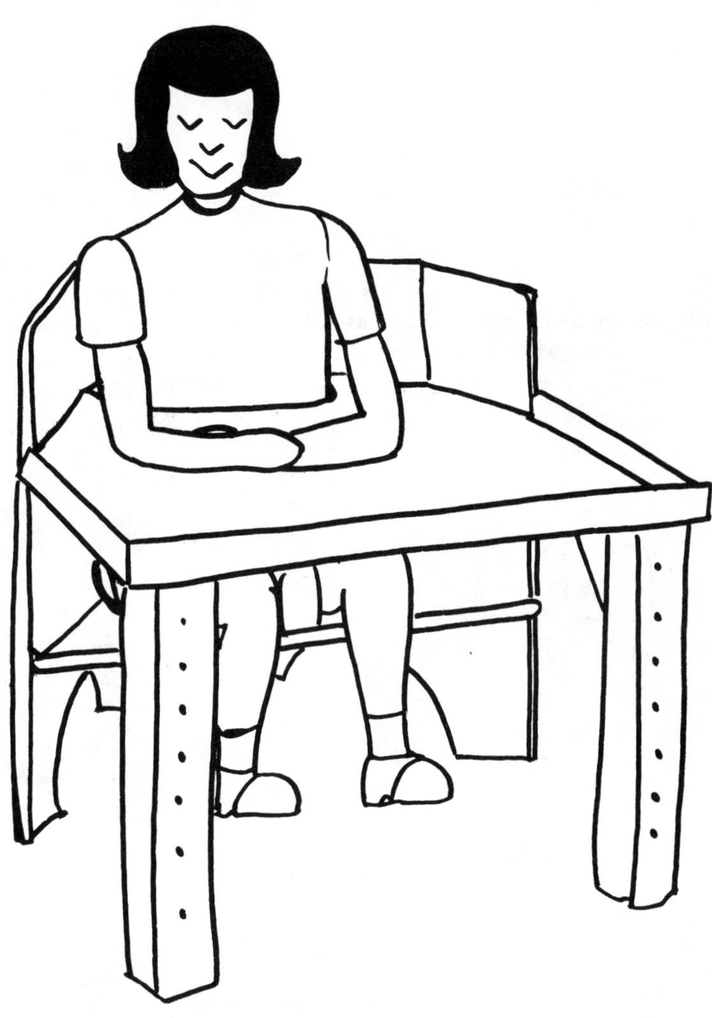

FIGURE 20-13. Triangle chair with tray.

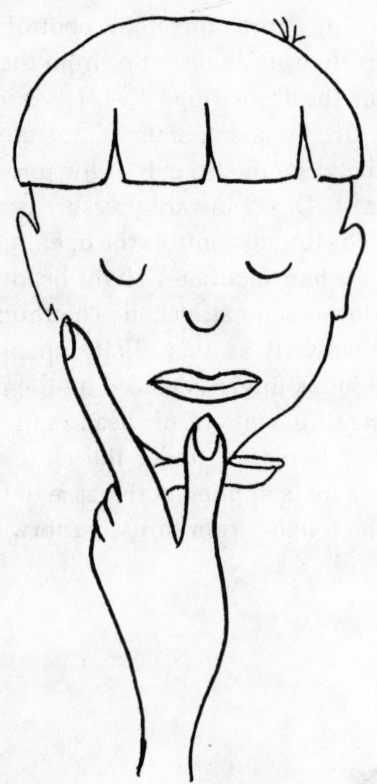

FIGURE 20-14. Three-tinger jaw control applied from the front.

control the jaw from opening. The forearm can apply pressure on the sternum to stimulate additional head flexion and forward positioning of the shoulders.

Jaw control from the side (Fig. 20-15) involves placing the thumb on the jaw line. Using this technique the thumb will inhibit lateral jaw movements. The index finger is positioned on the chin. Direct inward pressure is applied to elicit slight head flexion and to control the opening and closing of the jaw. Direct upward pressure applied at the base of the tongue by the middle finger placed under the chin helps to control tongue thrust and jaw opening. Using this technique, the fifth finger is available for applying pressure on the sternum to assist in bringing head and shoulders forward.[84]

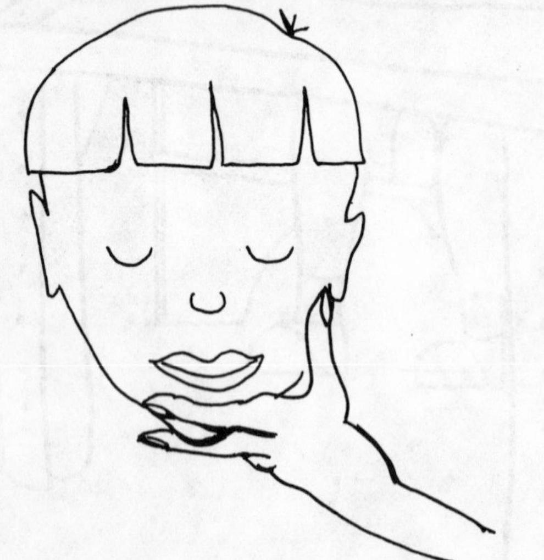

FIGURE 20-15. Three-finger jaw control applied from the side.

3. *Desensitizing Oral Tactile Defensiveness:* Another step in the therapeutic feeding process is desensitizing oral tactile defensiveness. This is a very important process and should be done prior to each feeding session. It should be kept in mind that, when increased oral sensitivity is present, aversive reactions to tactile stimulation applied to other body parts are usually present. Controlled and adequate positioning is essential because the negative response to tactile input can elicit abnormal postural patterns.

Before direct digital stimulation is applied to the gums, firm pressure applied to the upper extremities working distal to proximal will enable the therapist to successfully approach the mouth. An activity that reinforces this movement is playing with dress-up hats. The putting on and taking off of hats either by the child or the therapist will provide firm pressure to the head and this will help to decrease sensitivity to that area. Playing games using puppets and applying firm pressure to the face with the puppets may also be accepted by the child and even found to be fun.

When the child begins to accept tactile input activities as described, direct digital stimulation to the gums may be introduced. Jaw control should be provided during digital stimulation as the gum stimulation increases saliva and swallowing can be facilitated through the control.[85] The index finger is used to provide firm fast pressure beginning at the midline of the gums of the top jaw, which is the most sensitive area of the gums. Proceed with rubbing to the back of the gums and then return to the front of the mouth past the midline. Remove finger from the oral cavity and maintain closure of the jaw with control until swallowing has occurred. Reintroduce finger only after swallowing. Repeat this process approximately three times and then provide the same procedure to the gums on the other side of the upper jaw followed by a repetition of the procedure to the gums on the lower jaw. Always remember to withdraw the finger, maintain jaw closure, and facilitate swallowing. Swallowing can be facilitated by placing index finger horizontally between upper lip and nose and exerting pressure. If a bite reflex is present do not provide digital stimulation inside the teeth, because this will stimulate the reflex and cause the therapist's finger to be bitten. If the bite reflex is absent proceed with the technique applied to the upper gums inside the teeth. Next, the hard palate should be stimulated from front to back and from midline to sides. The tongue can be desensitized last by firm strokes from front to back.[86] However, remember to remove finger, apply jaw control for closure, and facilitate swallowing after each area is desensitized. The *order of sequence* as presented above should be followed *very carefully*. It is unlikely that the entire sequence will be able to be completed when the technique is first introduced. This is a gradual process and the individual will need sufficient time to adjust to the many movements which occur when oral areas are stimulated.

Digital stimulation to the gums is important not only because it decreases tactile sensitivity but also because it improves circulation of the gums. This technique is particularly helpful in the presence of hyperplasia, an abnormal swelling of the gums, possibly due to medication given for seizure control.

In the case of a hyporeactive response to direct oral stimulation (commonly observed in the individual with hypotonia) the same procedure should be introduced; however the tactile stimulation should be given lightly and slowly to facilitate a response.

4. *Drinking:* The individual with cerebral palsy frequently has difficulty achieving adequate jaw and lip closure while drinking and usually liquid flows readily from the corners of the mouth. Abnormal tongue protrusion or retraction also interferes with the tongue's mobility which is necessary for swallowing. These abnormal oral behaviors can be observed during sucking from a bottle or drinking from a cup. According to Mueller, the individual who demonstrates severe deficits of tongue and swallowing patterns or who presents an absent suck reflex should not be given liquids in a bottle. Instead the individual should drink from a cup.[87]

In order to facilitate normal drinking patterns, proper positioning and jaw control are extremely important.

Adapting a plastic cup by cutting out a U shape on one side usually is effective. It enables the therapist to accurately observe the tongue and lip action. Tilting the cup clears the nose and prevents hyperextension of the head (which could facilitate abnormal postural tone throughout the body).

With the jaw and lips controlled in closure, the U shape of the cup is opposite to the rim. The rim side is gently placed on the individual's lower lip. The cup is tilted so that the liquid just touches the lower lip and flows smoothly into the oral cavity through movement from the upper lip. Jaw control for closure is maintained and the cup remains on the lower lip during swallowing.

It is important that the head does not hyperextend during swallowing as swallowing is very difficult in this position. Increased head extension is also likely to facilitate abnormal extensor tone throughout the body. Placing the cup between the teeth should be avoided as this can facilitate a pathological bite reflex or other abnormal oral patterns.[88]

If a child is able to suck from a bottle and demonstrates mild oral deficits, jaw control may still be required in order to facilitate adequate jaw and lip closure and tongue control.

Drinking through a straw should not be introduced until the individual has accomplished coordinated drinking. At that point, straw drinking may facilitate better lip mobility.

5. *Spoon Feeding:* Proper positioning and jaw control should be provided when necessary and in most cases will be essential in spoon feeding. The spoon is always introduced from the front of the mouth at the midline of the lips. The bowl of the spoon should be small (to prevent additional tactile input) and shallow (to facilitate easy removal of food). A small amount of food is placed on the spoon. The spoon is introduced without touching the tip of the tongue or the teeth. It is placed at least one-third back on the tongue with firm pressure. This will inhibit the tongue thrust and reversed swallowing pattern and will facilitate lip closure. Once the lips have closed, the spoon is removed in a straight outward direction from the mouth without touching the teeth. Jaw control for closure is maintained until swallowing occurs. The index finger can be placed between the upper lip and nose, applying

pressure to facilitate swallowing. Remember to avoid touching the tip of tongue and teeth. Stimulation to the tongue tip can result in thrusting of the tongue. With the teeth it can elicit a bite reflex.[89] Do not remove excess food on chin with spoon. The stimulation may elicit abnormal oral reflexes. Instead use a terry cloth towel and a pressure blot (such as patting) to remove the food.

The feeding technique changes as soon as better oral control has been acquired and maximum jaw control is no longer needed. Now the spoon is held slightly below the center of the mouth and the child is required to flex his head forward to obtain the food. He uses only his lips to remove the food from the spoon. Again, the spoon should not touch his teeth. If he has difficulty initiating the swallow, pressure applied under the chin or between the upper lip and nose may be the only assistance required.

Proper positioning is still important in self-feeding. The child may also require some assistance. Observe which hand the child uses for holding a spoon and sit close to that side. Help the child hold the spoon in a palmar grasp with the thumb under the handle.[90] Place your index finger on the dorsal aspect of the child's hand and your thumb at the base of his or her thumb. After the spoon is filled, apply pressure with your thumb to elicit an outward turning of the individual's hand. This technique will help to supinate the child's hand and inhibit overturning of the spoon en route to the mouth.

Some control of the opposite shoulder may be helpful for inhibiting increased extension. Place your arm behind the child's back and your hand on his or her shoulder in order to facilitate protraction.[91] Suggested utensils during spoon feeding include scoop dishes with rubber bottoms to prevent slipping and small-bowled spoons with built-up handles.

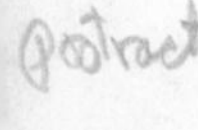

6. *Chewing:* Chewing is defined as rotary jaw movements; biting consists of vertical jaw movements. Place food at the side of the child's mouth between the molars to stimulate the biting action. Do not introduce food for chewing at front center of mouth. After the biting action occurs, apply jaw control and the child should begin to chew. Do not passively move the jaws in a chewing motion for the child because this will reinforce a pathological action.

7. *Drooling:* Drooling can be caused by three major factors: (1) poor head control, (2) impaired swallowing, and (3) lack of jaw and lip closure. Proper positioning of the child throughout the day, improving head control, and using jaw control decreases drooling. In addition, frequent patting of the lips will elicit lip closure. While patting the lips, do not push the lips together since this will only increase further opening. Using a neurophysiological principle which states that a stretched muscle contracts, quick stretch pressure can be applied to the lip area (Fig. 20-16). Stretch pressure applied with the index and middle finger above the upper lip in an upward and outward manner will enhance closure of the upper lip. Likewise, quick stretch pressure applied below the lower lip in a downward and outward direction will elicit closure of the lower lip. Stretching the corners of the mouth outward after each stretch will also facilitate contraction of the lip muscles. After the muscles contract, the therapist may repeat the procedure. Another technique to facilitate lip closure is to lightly stroke across the midline of the lower lip several times.[92]

Cautionary Measures for the Therapist: A continuous verbal reminder to the child to swallow is of little therapeutic value since it is a cortical level command. Remediation is most effective at the subcortical level.

The type of food presented to the individual is very important. In addition to nutritional value, food influences oral motor mechanisms. Therefore the following foods should be *avoided:*

—sweet foods, since they increase saliva and thus increase drooling.

—milk in the presence of congestion, since this increases and thickens the mucus. Powdered milk or oily fluids such as beef or chicken broth help to thin the mucus.

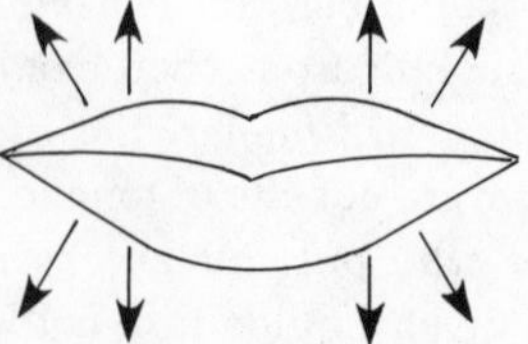

FIGURE 20-16. Quick stretch pressure of lips for lip closure.

—tough meats, since this makes chewing more difficult and can increase abnormal postural tone. Skinless hot dogs, lunch meats, chicken, and cheese are softer and make chewing easier.
—thin liquids, runny food, and foods combining solids and liquids such as soups with vegetables or noodles. Thicker foods are more desirable and easier to manage, e.g., ground hamburger, french fried potatoes, cooked carrots, or green beans. Baby foods may be thickened with wheat germ or dry formula. Milk and fruit juices have thicker consistencies than water.

Note that tepid temperature foods may help to inhibit oral pathology.[93]

NEUROMUSCULAR TREATMENT TECHNIQUES FOR ORAL MOTOR DEFICIT. It is not uncommon for the individual with cerebral palsy who exhibits an absent suck swallow reflex to be fed via a nasogastric tube. This feeding technique ensures adequate nutritional intake but does not facilitate improved functioning of the oral motor mechanisms. Tube feeding may result in a hyporeactive gag reflex.

A neuromuscular technique used to facilitate a gag reflex in the presence of a hyporesponsive reaction involves stretching of the arches of the soft palate (palatopharyngeal and palatoglossal arches) as well as the uvula with the ball end of a metal swizzle stick.[94]

The hyperactive gag reflex can possibly be inhibited by "walking back" on the midline of the tongue and applying pressure with the ball end of the swizzle stick. Pressure should be stopped immediately prior to eliciting a gag response and swallowing should follow. The procedure may be repeated five to seven times.[95] Caution should be taken to avoid touching the tip of the tongue since this might facilitate a tongue thrust if tongue protrusion is present.

Using the ball end of a swizzle stick and gently vibrating on either side of the frenulum under the tongue is a technique used to inhibit the tongue thrust; also vibrating with fingers under the chin may be helpful in facilitating tongue retraction.[96] Another successful technique for the therapist to use is pulling the tip of the tongue out of the mouth with his or her fingers (wrap fingers in a small piece of terry cloth toweling). The underlying principle of this technique is that the stretch of muscles facilitates contraction. Do not push the tongue back into the mouth as this will only increase tongue protrusion.

Hyperretraction of the tongue is noted less often but can be a characteristic of severely increased extensor tone with head hyperextension and shoulder retraction as well. In this case, pushing the tongue farther back in the mouth can help to elicit a more normal position of the tongue.[97]

A technique involving sequential steps to facilitate sucking and swallowing would be to (1) vibrate around the orbicular muscle, (2) vibrate downward on either side of the throat, (3) apply stretch pressure to the lips as previously described, and (4) apply stretch pressure to the laryngopharyngeal musculature.[98]

Dressing

Acquisition of dressing and undressing skills for the child with cerebral palsy should follow the same sequence as for the normal child (Table 20-2).

Initially it is necessary to help the child develop an interest in the dressing and undressing process. As abilities increase and the child is developmentally ready, cooperation should increase.

The most common position for dressing a normal child is in the supine position. With the cerebral palsied child, this may make him more rigid and will unnecessarily complicate the process. By laying

Table 20-2. Acquisition of dressing and undressing skills.

Age	*Skill*
12 mo.	cooperates with dressing, i.e., extends arms to put in sleeve
18 mo.	purposefully removes socks
2 yr.	removes unlaced shoes
	removes pants with assistance over hips
3 yr.	removes clothes completely except for small buttons and back fastenings
	unfastens medium-sized buttons
	puts on underpants, socks, and shoes
4 yr.	fastens large buttons
	laces shoes
5 yr.	fastens medium-sized buttons
	dresses self except for bows and small buttons
6 yr.	ties bows

Adapted from Finnie.[99]

the small child prone with arms and legs extended across the therapist's knees or lap (Fig. 20-17), the child can be cared for with more ease. The child's extremities can easily be manipulated into clothing and the whole child is in a therapeutically functional position.

The position of choice for dressing is to set the child between the therapist's legs with the child leaning forward at the hips, legs abducted and knees flexed; this decreases extensor tone. One should describe and name each article of clothing and body part as it is used or moved. Perhaps, initially, it would help to work in front of a mirror in order that the child can see what is happening. When the child begins to assist the therapist, the mirror should be discontinued as the reversed image may be confusing.[100]

For the child, adolescent, and adult dominated by flexor or extensor tone, the side lying position seems to neutralize the excess tone and facilitates

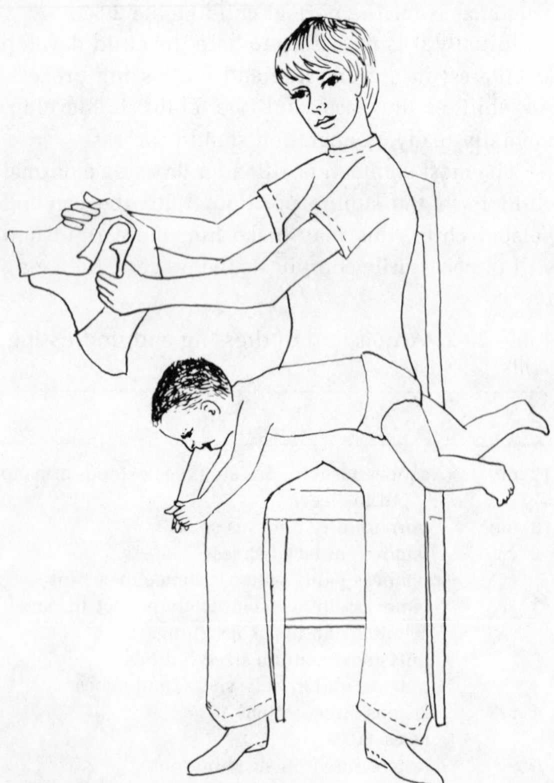

FIGURE 20-17. Dressing may be facilitated by laying the small child on the therapist's lap.

the dressing process. When rolling the individual from side to side, the knees and hips should remain flexed to inhibit extensor tone.

If the person must be supine, he or she should have a hard pillow under the head and shoulders to break up the extensor tonus. Knees and hips should be flexed and abducted.

No matter which position is used for dressing the child, a symmetrical position should be maintained. Note the following suggestions:

1. Put the more affected limb in clothing first.
2. Straighten the arm before putting it in a sleeve.
3. Hold the arm at the elbow or above to move it. If resistance is felt, do not attempt to pull the arm through a sleeve by pulling on the hand. This causes the whole arm to flex and the shoulder to retract.
4. Before putting on shoes or socks, the leg should be flexed.

If the child wears braces, remove them by unfastening at the most proximal point and work distally to the feet. When putting braces on, be sure that the heel is firmly placed down into the shoe before lacing and securely tying the bow. Continue to work from distal to proximal. Two adult fingers should fit under each closure for a comfortable fit.

According to Finnie,[101] a child should be ready to undress himself when he or she (1) knows body parts, (2) is aware of self in space, and (3) can name or recognize clothes.

Some children will dress while sitting in a sturdy low chair. If the child does not have enough balance to sit while leaning forward, several alternatives may be used. The child may sit between the therapist's legs for support. A triangular chair may be used either on the floor (Fig. 20-18) or raised on a platform. A corner or wall may provide additional support (Fig. 20-19).

The older and more severely involved child may not be able to sit. If head control has been attained, he or she may be able to dress and undress either side lying, prone, or supine. A simple pants pusher or pants puller is often needed (Fig. 20-20).

While sitting with hips and knees bent, the child may remove socks by pulling on the toe or by sliding the thumb down the back of the leg and over the heel. The sock may also be rubbed off the toes either using the other foot or the floor. For these purposes, nonstretch and nonelastic socks are helpful. Tube socks are also easier to put on than those with a heel.

In order to put on socks the child should have knees and hips bent. The sock is opened with two hands and the child is encouraged to make a "big mouth with the opening" in order to put all toes in at one time. Some children will try to put the sock on the big toe first and will try to stretch it across to the little toe. This often leaves the little toes out of the sock or pops the sock off the foot. In this case it helps to start with the little toe and stretch to the big toe.

Removing underpants or trousers may be done while sitting or lying down. The child shifts his or her weight to push them over the hips and down the legs.

To put underpants or trousers on, the child is flexed at knees and hips. After feet are in the correct holes, the child may stand up, kneel stand, or roll from side to side to pull them up.

Unlaced shoes may be kicked or rubbed off. Two colored laces may be used to encourage unlacing.

When first putting shoes on the feet, the laces should be very loose. A flexed and abducted leg is necessary. High top shoes are easier to put on if loops are sewn on at the heels. These keep the back of the shoe from being crushed.

Bow tying can be a difficult process. When the child is ready for tying, the same words of instruction should be employed with each treatment ses-

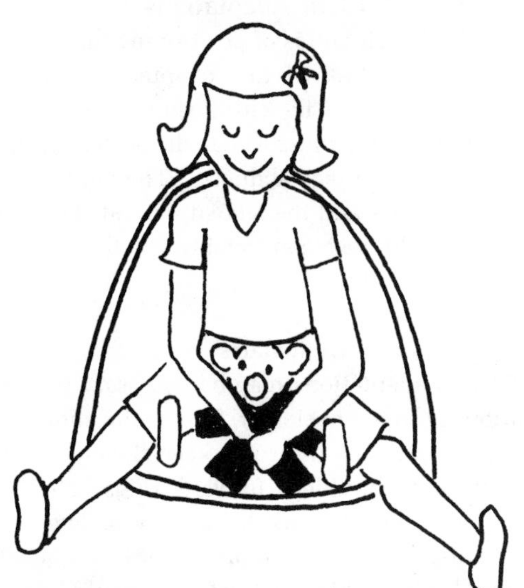

FIGURE 20-18. A triangular chair for use on the floor.

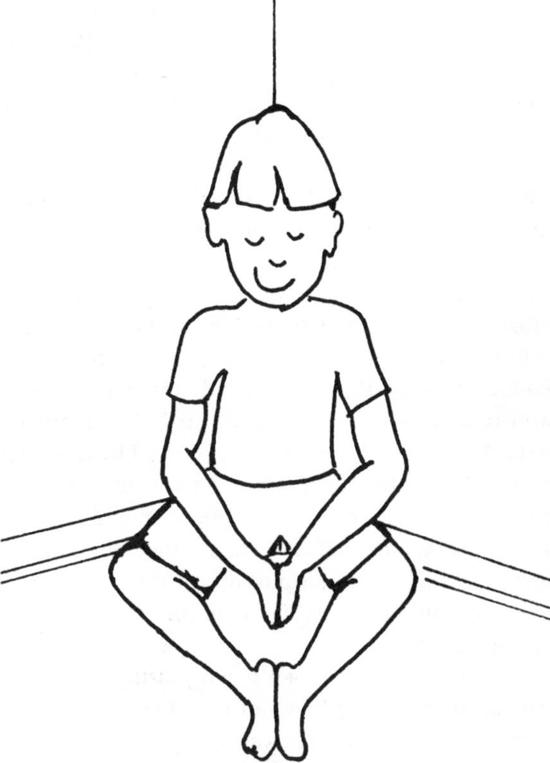

FIGURE 20-19. A corner may provide additional sitting support.

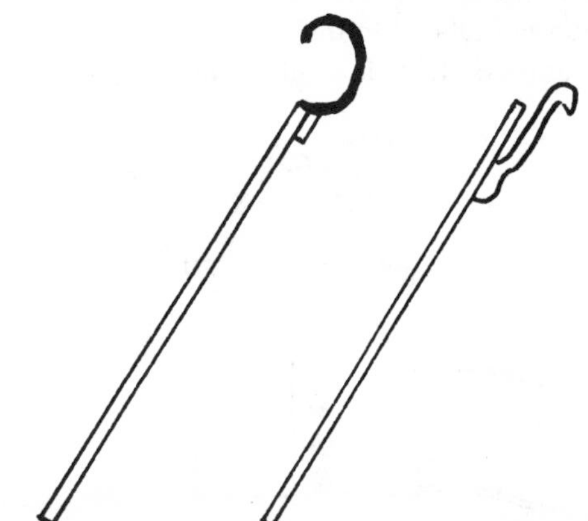

FIGURE 20-20. Pants puller and pants pusher.

sion. Many children seem to benefit from the "backward chaining" method of instruction. Using this method the therapist ties the bow up to the very last step and then asks the child to complete the final step in the process. As one step is mastered, the child continues working backwards until the entire process has been completed. This same process is important to follow with each article of clothing.

The removal of overhead and front opening shirts can be done in several ways. The usual way is to cross one's arms, grasp either side of the bottom, and pull it up and over the head. One or both hands can be used to grasp the neck. Usually the nondominant arm is pulled out of the sleeve first. The dominant side sleeve is either shaken or pulled off by the other hand. Some children prefer to remove both arms from the sleeves, then pull the shirt off and over the head. Another method is to remove the nondominant arm from the sleeve and pull it over the head and off the opposite arm. Most methods can be done while supine or prone.

The process is reversed when putting a shirt on. The arms are put in first and then over the head or vice versa. The more involved side goes in first, over the head, and the dominant arm in last.

To put a front opening shirt or coat on, the "duck the head" method is good to use. The garment is positioned with the collar near the child, label side up. Each arm is placed in the sleeves and the whole shirt placed over the head.

The buttoning and unbuttoning process should be learned on the child's own clothing or on a button vest (Fig. 20-21). (It is our opinion that buttonboards are nonfunctional since they put the buttons in a position not related to the child's body.)

It appears that few clothing adaptations are necessary for the individual with cerebral palsy. Clothing should be loose fitting to facilitate putting on and removing. Velcro closures can be used if coordination is too poor for buttons, zippers, or snaps. Sometimes a buttonhook is helpful and the addition of a large loop to a zipper may prove advantageous. The adolescent may need a pants pusher or puller. Trousers with elastic tops alleviate closure problems.

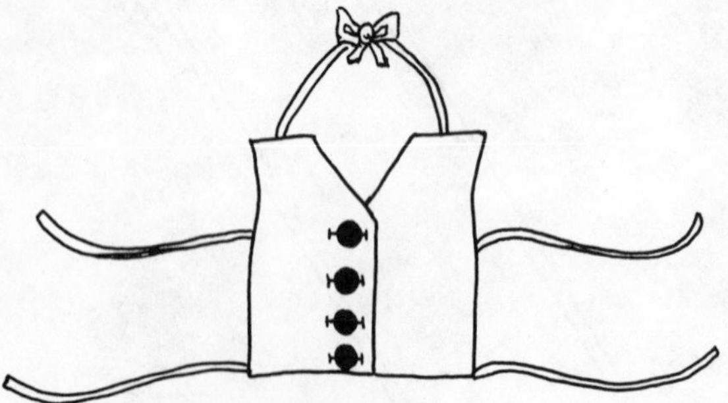

FIGURE 20-21. A button vest.

When an older child is referred to occupational therapy for treatment, the area of dressing is often a prime need. Many times it seems easier for a parent to dress a child than to take the time to teach and allow the child to do it. This may be related to the fact that parents have not been included in the treatment program of their child and have not been given counsel in how to help. This exemplifies how essential it is for the occupational therapist to work with the parents early in the stages of treatment and to continue to do so during the entire treatment process. The occupational therapist may also find that he or she has "itchy" hands and wishes to assist the slow child, so the therapist must also remember the pride children have with mastery of a task and how proud the severely involved adolescent is who says for the first time, "I don't have to wait for someone to dress me. I can do it myself."

Chair Adaptations

The basic principles of positioning mentioned in the feeding portion of this chapter also apply to chair positioning. The child should sit with the trunk straight, hips and knees flexed to beyond 90 degrees, with the legs abducted. The ankles should be at 90 degrees and the feet supported. The child's elbows should rest comfortably on the chair arm rests or lapboard.

Wheelchairs and Highchairs

Certain adaptations may be necessary for proper positioning in a wheelchair. The chairs should have solid seat and back inserts to keep the child's trunk straight and shoulders forward (Figs. 20-22 and 20-23). To prevent trunk asymmetry or lateral flexion, foam-padded wooden projections may be added to the solid back (Fig. 20-22); these should be placed laterally and should extend from several inches under the arm to the waist. Care should be taken

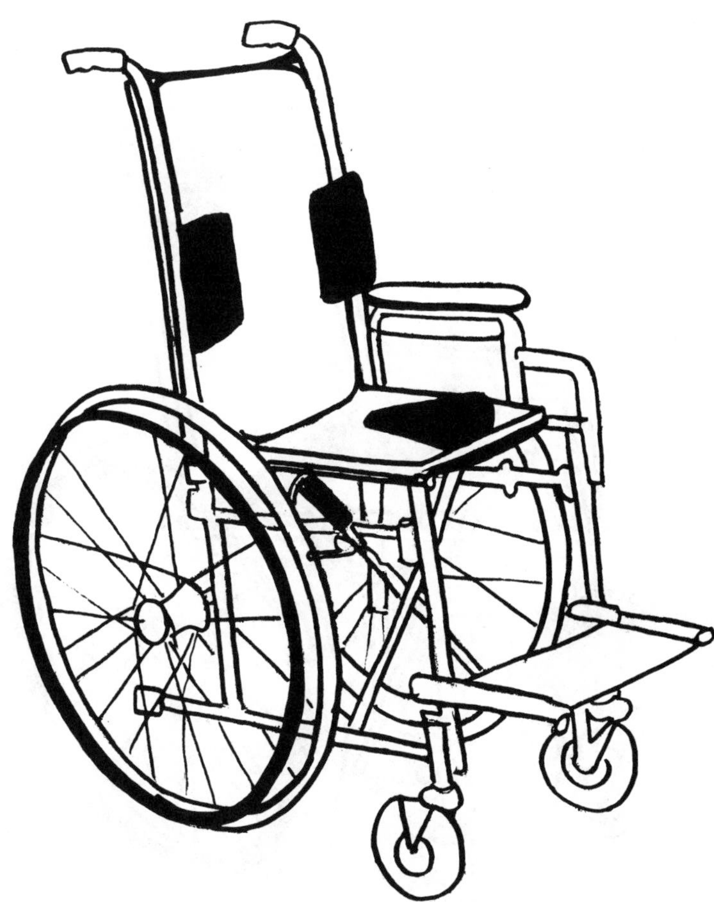

FIGURE 20-22. Wheelchair adapted with solid seat and back inserts, abductor wedge, and lateral support projections.

that the child does not "hang" on the projections causing axilla damage. They should fit close to the child's body. The sensory feedback of leaning to the side assists the child in actively correcting his or her posture.

The depth of the seat should come to an inch or two behind the child's knees to provide normal flexion. A pillow may be placed behind the child to push him forward for proper positioning. For the very small child, the seat upholstery may be removed and a specially made insert put in its place. This should be made to the child's dimensions and should allow the proper depth for the knees. A firm wedge-shaped seat with the highest aspect in the front and lowest part in the back may be used to increase hip flexion (Fig. 20-23).

To inhibit scissoring or adduction of the legs, a padded wooden triangular abduction wedge can be attached to the seat (Fig. 20-22). The widest base of the triangle is towards the front of the chair. If the wedge is two thirds the length of the thigh, it will inhibit adductor spasticity. The footrest must be positioned so that the knees are slightly higher than the hips to decrease extensor tone. It can be made higher and wider by attaching a piece of wood to the footrest (Fig. 20-23). The entire sole of the foot should be supported to inhibit the positive supporting reaction.

If the child has too much abduction of the lower extremities as seen with the atypical flaccid child, padded wooden insets may be attached to the seat parallel to the lateral border of the thighs. This prevents excessive abduction and maintains proper alignment of the thighs with the hip joint.

It is important that children see the world from the upright or sitting position. For the child who

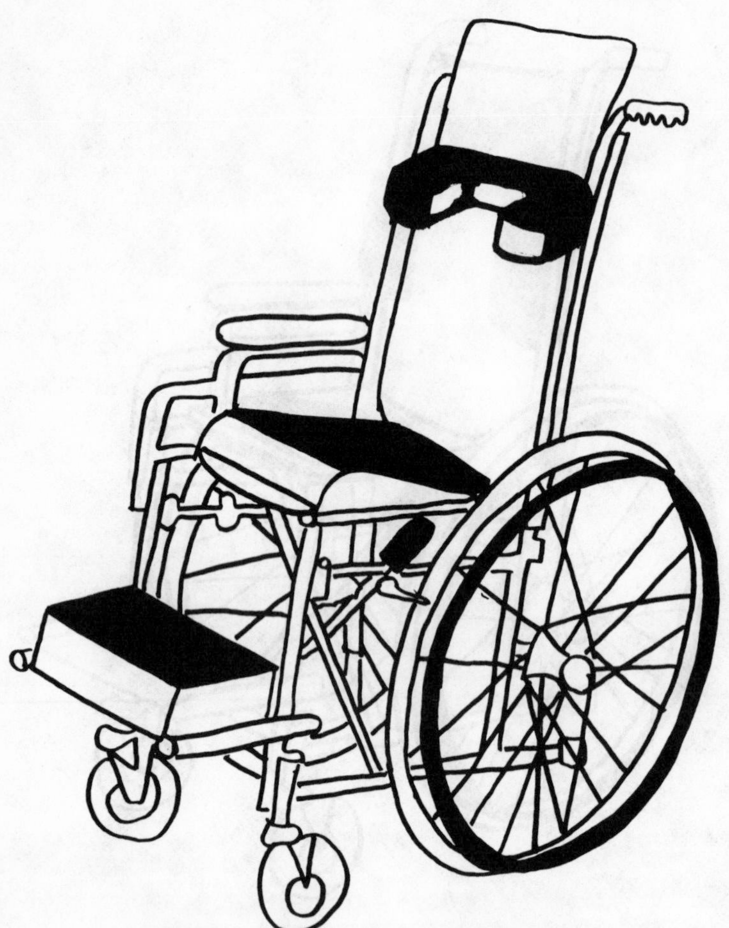

FIGURE 20-23. Wheelchair adapted with inclined solid seat insert, extended solid back insert with U-shaped neck support, and raised footrest platform.

lacks neck righting responses and is unable to hold his head up independently, a U-shaped wedge (Fig. 20-23) may be attached to the solid chair back and positioned at the base of the neck to support the head. Care should be taken to avoid the occipital area.

The same principles and ideas presented for wheelchair adaptations can be applied to highchairs, strollers, potty chairs, and other positioning devices.

Triangular Chairs

A triangular chair provides good support for the individual with cerebral palsy. It may rest on the floor giving the child sitting support while allowing him or her the normal developmental activity of playing on the floor (Fig. 20-18). The back of the chair comes to the shoulder level to provide lateral and back support. The child's knees should come to the edge of the seat to allow slight flexion while "long" sitting. The child is also able to "circle" sit. Abductor posts or wedges may be placed on the seat to inhibit adduction (see Fig. 20-18).

A triangular chair may also be raised on a platform and fitted with a small table (see Fig. 20-13). This gives the individual back, side, and front support. The elbows should rest comfortably on the table. An abductor wedge may be attached to the seat. The individual is able to sit in the chair, eat, play, or even complete schoolwork.

The whole process of chair adaptations is a highly individualized one. The occupational therapist should be aware of the many aspects of the individual's needs in order to problem solve with the child and family the chair adaptations that are most suitable.

Communication

The basic need to communicate one's joys, sorrows, needs, ideas, frustrations, anxieties, and sense of belonging may be thwarted in the cerebral palsied individual because he or she is unable to express himself or herself through the normal channel of the spoken word. The individual may be intelligent but too severely involved physically to talk or to control the head, trunk, and upper extremity. Oral control may be insufficient for speech. The occupational therapist together with the speech therapist can provide a means of nonverbal communication.

In the early stages of treating and handling the young infant, communication between mother and infant should be stressed just as it is with the normal child. Because of the added special needs of the infant, early communication skills often are overlooked. These skills usually begin with the face-to-face confrontation between mother and infant. In order to receive the infant's attention, good external control of the child's head and shoulders is necessary. Initially, with the severely involved child, communication may be started in the side lying position and later it may progress to other positions.

The occupational therapist should be sensitive to the subtle nonverbal messages of a child. Increased muscle tone may mean the child is upset, excited, hurt, needs the bathroom, or wants attention. Darkness under the eyes may mean the child has a headache. Excessive drooling may mean the child is under emotional stress. Closing the eyes may mean he or she is retreating from the environment.

As the child grows older and still has not developed speech, alternate means of language expression should be utilized. The simplest form of communication is indicating "yes" or "no" or by moving a body part. This may be blinking the eyes, looking up, moving an arm or leg, or turning the head. Some intelligent children have learned to blink the Morse code in order to communicate.

The next level for the nonverbal child may be the language board or book. This may be a lapboard secured to the wheelchair or a book or card which is carried. A language board is often about 28 by 18 inches. It is covered with either plexiglass or a clear plastic material to protect it from drooling and everyday wear and tear.[102] The child points to the board using fist, finger, elbow, eyes, paper straw, or headstick. A headstick may be fastened to a headband and protrude from the midforehead level.

Several types of boards are possible. A ring board has plexiglass rings five-eighth to one-half inch thick which are glued to the top of a plexiglass board. Used to reduce involuntary movements, the rings can be large in diameter and spaced far apart or be small in diameter and spaced close together. The written insert is attached under the board with the writing showing through the rings.[103]

An adapted ring board for a headstick has smaller rings about three-quarter inch in diameter. These may be arranged the same as a typewriter keyboard or in a list form with phrases. The child points to the message with a headstick.[104]

Flat boards may list many important words and phrases. The child points to the words or phrases in the appropriate column to convey the message.

A more sophisticated form of language board utilizes number and color coding of the words (Fig. 20-24). Colors and numbers are spaced along the edges of the board. In the center, a color- and number-coded grid has many words or phrases on it. The nonverbal child uses his eyes to point to an appropriate color first and then to a number. This locates a word on the grid to relay a message. Either whole sentences, phrases, or individual words may be placed on the grid.

It is important that the material is positioned within the child's functional area of movement. Correct positioning maintains body symmetry and will not facilitate abnormal postural reflexes.

The language board may grow as the child develops abilities. The first board may have objects on it such as a toy toilet and small cup. The next level may have pictures on it. These may come from magazines, familiar photographs, or simple drawings. Pictures may depict needs such as toilet, drink, food, bed, television, Mother, Father, places to go.[105] As reading skills develop, words replace pictures. Eventually, words may be arranged by parts of speech and increase in complexity. For some nonverbal individuals, an alphabet card and pointer may be sufficient to meet the individual's needs. The letters may be arranged alphabetically or as on a typewriter keyboard.

Electronic aids are now available for the non-

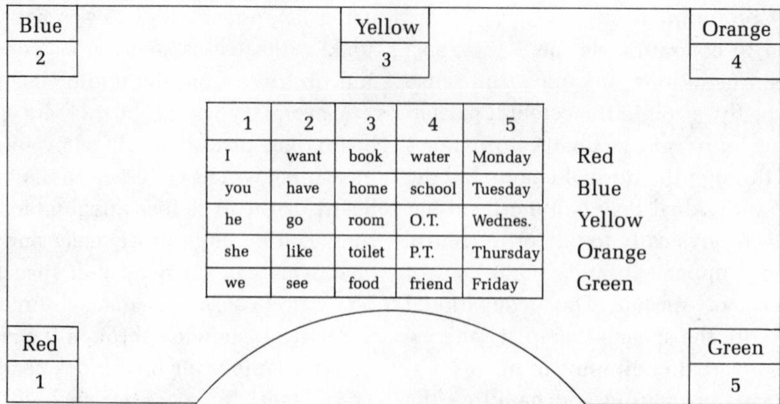

FIGURE 20-24. The language board utilizing number and color coding of words.

verbal individual. Three basic approaches with these aids are scanning, encoding, and direct selection. Scanning generally refers to the placing of appropriate phrases, letters, or symbols in a line or a grid configuration. The individual then controls a system which goes through each step until the desired message is completed. Encoding refers to a more complex system of controls in which a particular pattern of numbers or letters is used to relay a message. Usually there is a series of activating switches. Direct selection refers to communication by direct input. An example would be a small calculator type device in which the individual spells a word or message on the keyboard. This is then displayed on the device.

Communication aids can be controlled using many different switches.* A rocking lever may be activated by gross hand or arm movement or by a mouth- or headstick. A tongue switch may be activated by the tongue or lips. A pneumatic switch is activated by either blowing or sucking. A rocking level may be adapted to a chin switch. An arm slot control holds the arm on a desired switch without activating other ones.

Psychological/Sociocultural Communication

The occupational therapist is appreciative of the many electrical and technical devices that aid the cerebral palsied person in communication. However, these devices are mechanical by nature and do not assist in the development of survival skills from an emotional/sociocultural point of view. Individuals, whether handicapped or not, respond well to a humanistic approach. The occupational therapist, by virtue of skill in interpersonal communication and knowledge of medicine, can be particularly perceptive and sensitive to the cerebral palsied person's needs. The therapist can provide the caring, human warmth, and professional expertise which are so essential for strengthening the cerebral palsied person's adjustment to disability.

The occupational therapist has multiple roles to play in the total treatment program of the physically handicapped. However, the psychological/sociocultural aspects of the treatment have an impact on whether the treatment is successful or not.

According to Versluys,[106] the areas of communication in which the occupational therapist plays a significant role are (1) the use of therapeutic relationships, (2) the elements of a therapeutic environment, (3) the use of interpersonal relationships, (4) the provision of group and individual experiences, (5) the use of activities designed to assist the patient in adjustment to physical dysfunction, and (6) the restructuring of a lifestyle toward independence and productive living.

The occupational therapist can provide the cerebral palsied person with a psychological climate and/or environment that encourages healthy, independent living. He or she can provide individual and group situations that allow the child or adult to express feelings about the disability. Nonthreatening informal discussions can prepare the child or adult for rehabilitation, enhance knowledge about

* Many electronic devices are available from Prentle Romich Company, R.D. 2, Box 191, Shreve, Ohio, 44676.

the disability, provide a release for tense or depressed feelings, and provide practical sessions for problem solving in community situations with which he or she will come in contact. All of these factors will assist the cerebral palsied person in psychological adjustment to life.

FAMILY. The occupational therapist should encourage the family or those closest to the cerebral palsied person to participate as fully as possible in the treatment program. Whatever support a family and/or friends can lend to the person will ease the adjustment and help the person focus on assets which, in turn, will bring satisfaction. It is also to be noted, however, as Versluys suggests,[107] that the family or closest of kin need to air their feelings and thoughts about the disability because they too need emotional support and assistance in the adjustment process.

CULTURE. Underlying the structure of the cerebral palsied person and his family is their cultural system. This includes their values, customs, beliefs, traditions, and attitudes about life which should be keenly recognized by the therapist. They may differ from the therapist's and, if so, it is the responsibility of the therapist to research (as part of the evaluative process) their cultural system. If this is done, the therapist, the individual, and the family will feel infinitely more successful about the rehabilitation. In addition, the therapist will have gained valuable interesting knowledge and will have broadened his or her scope of human understanding.

REFERENCES

1. Samilson, R. L. (ed.): Orthopaedic Aspects of Cerebral Palsy. Clin. Develop. Med., Nos. 52/53. London: Heineman, 1975, p. 1.
2. Ibid., p. 3.
3. Ibid.
4. Bobath, K.: The Motor Deficit in Patients with Cerebral Palsy. Clin. Develop. Med., No. 23. London: Heineman, 1975, preface.
5. Ibid.
6. Ibid.
7. Bobath, K., and Bobath, B.: Cerebral palsy. In Pearson, P. H. (ed.): Physical Therapy Services in the Developmental Disabilities. Springfield IL: Charles C Thomas, Publishers, 1972, p. 31.
8. Gordon, N.: Pediatric Neurology for the Clinician. Clin. Develop. Med. Nos. 59/60. London: Heineman, 1976, p. 134.
9. Bobath and Bobath: Cerebral palsy, p. 33.
10. Berzins, G. F.: Causes of Cerebral Palsy. Mimeographed handout, 1972.
11. Ibid.
12. Ibid.
13. Gordon: Pediatric Neurology.
14. Bobath, K., and Bobath, B.: The facilitation of normal postural reactions and movements in the treatment of cerebral palsy. Physiotherapy 50:246, 1964, p. 4.
15. Ibid.
16. Fiorentino, M. R.: Normal and Abnormal Development: The Influence of Primitive Reflexes on Motor Development, ed. 2. Springfield IL: Charles C Thomas, Publishers, 1976, pp. 26, 28, 31, 32.
17. Fiorentino, M. R.: Reflex Testing Methods for Evaluating CNS Development. Springfield IL: Charles C Thomas, Publishers, 1972, pp. 22-32.
18. Ibid, pp. 38-47.
19. Fiorentino: Normal and Abnormal Development, p. 37.
20. Bobath and Bobath: Facilitation of normal postural reactions, p. 4.
21. Fiorentino: Reflex Testing Methods, p. 37.
22. Bobath, B.: Important Stages of Motor Development. Mimeographed handout, 1970.
23. Ibid.
24. Connor, F., Williamson, G., and Siepp, J. (eds.): A Program Guide for Infants and Toddlers with Neuromotor and Other Developmental Disabilities. New York: Teachers' College Press, 1976, p. 130.
25. Gordon: Pediatric Neurology, p. 130.
26. Samilson: Orthopaedic Aspects, p. 7.
27. Bobath and Bobath: Cerebral palsy, p. 35.
28. Bobath and Bobath: Cerebral palsy, p. 36.
29. Samilson: Orthopaedic Aspects, p. 8.
30. Bobath and Bobath: Cerebral palsy, p. 37.
31. Samilson: Orthopaedic Aspects, p. 8.
32. Ibid.
33. Gordon: Pediatric Neurology, p. 145.
34. Ibid., p. 8.
35. Gordon: Pediatric Neurology, p. 145.
36. Bobath and Bobath: Cerebral palsy, p. 36.
37. Slosson, R. L.: Slosson Intelligence Test for Children & Adults. Slosson Educational Publications, East Aurora NY, 1971.
38. Bayley, N.: Scales of Infant Development. New York Psychological Corporation, New York, 1969.
39. Finnie, N. R.: Handling the Young Cerebral Palsied Child at Home, ed. 2. New York: E. P. Dutton, 1975, p. 50.
40. Connor, Williamson, and Siepp: A Program Guide for Infants and Toddlers, p. 205.
41. Bobath and Bobath: Cerebral palsy, p. 172.
42. Ibid.
43. Ibid, p. 149.
44. Ibid, p. 167.
45. Ibid.
46. Ibid.

47. Ibid, pp. 155-156.
48. Stockmeyer, S.: An interpretation of the approach of Rood to treatment of neuromuscular dysfunction. Am. J. Phys. Med. 46:903, 1967.
49. Shepard, T., and Smith, D.: Prenatal life. In Smith, D., and Marshall, R. (eds.): Introduction to Clinical Pediatrics. Philadelphia: W. B. Saunders Co., 1972.
50. Jacobs, M. J.: Development of normal motor behavior. Am. J. Phys. Med. 46:41-42, 1967.
51. Ibid.
52. Fiorentino: Normal and Abnormal Development, p. 10.
53. Jacobs: Development of normal motor behavior, p. 47.
54. Colangelo, C., Bergen, A., and Gottlieb, L.: A Normal Baby: The Sensory-Motor Processes of the First Year. Blythedale Children's Hospital, Valhalla NY, 1976, p. 5.
55. Ibid.
56. Mueller, H.: Facilitating feeding and pre-speech. In Pearson, P. H. (ed.): Springfield IL: Charles C Thomas, Publishers, 1972, p. 287.
57. Davis, L.: Pre-speech development. In Connor, F. Williamson, G., and Siepp, J. (eds.): A Program Guide for Infants and Toddlers with Neuromotor and Other Developmental Disabilities. New York: Teachers' College Press, 1976, p. 211.
58. Colangelo, Bergen, and Gottlieb: A Normal Baby, p. 5.
59. Mueller: Facilitating feeding and pre-speech, p. 287.
60. Davis: Pre-speech development, pp. 211-212.
61. Brazelton, T. B.: Neonatal Behavior Assessment Scale. Clin. Develop. Med., No. 50. Philadelphia: J. B. Lippincott Co., 1976, p. 41.
62. Gesell, A., et al.: The First Five Years of Life. New York: Harper & Row Publishers, 1940, p. 23.
63. Davis: Pre-speech development, pp. 211-212.
64. Jacobs: Development of normal motor behavior, p. 47.
65. Colangelo, Bergen, and Gottlieb: A Normal Baby, p. 7.
66. Mueller: Facilitating feeding and pre-speech, pp. 286-287.
67. Davis: Pre-speech development, p. 216.
68. Davis: Pre-speech development, p. 216.
69. Ibid., p. 216.
70. Finnie: Handling the Young Cerebral Palsied Child at Home, p. 113.
71. Ibid.
72. Davis: Pre-speech development, p. 212.
73. Finnie: Handling the Young Cerebral Palsied Child at Home, p. 113.
74. Davis: Pre-speech development, p. 212.
75. Ibid.
76. Ibid., p. 213.
77. Gesell: The First Five Years of Life, p. 242.
78. Keen, R. A., and Sullivan, S.: Normal Development: Normal and Abnormal Handouts. Pennsylvania Training Model, 1974.
79. Salek, B.: Normal Motor Development as a Base for Normal Respiration and Pre-Speech Function. Department of Physical Therapy, University of Maryland, Baltimore MD, 1975, p. 3.
80. Ibid., p. 5.
81. Ibid., pp. 5, 6.
82. Mueller, A. H.: Pre-Speech Evaluation and Therapy. Course offered in Zurich, Switzerland, 1973.
83. Mueller: Facilitating feeding and pre-speech, p. 297.
84. Finnie: Handling the Young Cerebral Palsied Child at Home, p. 119.
85. Mueller: Facilitating feeding and pre-speech, p. 299.
86. Ibid.
87. Ibid., p. 300.
88. Ibid.
89. Ibid.
90. Finnie: Handling the Young Cerebral Palsied Child at Home, p. 127.
91. Ibid.
92. Mueller: Facilitating feeding and pre-speech, p. 300.
93. Sullivan: Normal Development: Normal and Abnormal, p. 17.
94. Farber: Sensorimotor Evaluation and Treatment Procedures, p. 59.
95. Ibid.
96. Ibid., p. 60.
97. Ibid., p. 61.
98. Ibid., p. 62.
99. Finnie: Handling the Young Cerebral Palsied Child at Home.
100. Ibid., p. 94.
101. Ibid., p. 96.
102. Schultz, A. R.: Language Boards. Handout from Home of the Merciful Savior, Philadelphia PA, 1970.
103. Ibid.
104. Ibid.
105. Schultz: Language Boards.
106. Versluys, H.: Psychological adjustment to physical disability. In Scott, A. D., and Trombly, K.: Occupational Therapy for Physical Dysfunction. Baltimore: Williams & Wilkins, 1977, p. 21.
107. Ibid.

BIBLIOGRAPHY

Ackerman, N.: Early Identification and Intervention Programs for Infants with Developmental Delay and Their Families: A Summary and Directory. National Easter Seal Society for Crippled Children and Adults, Chicago, 1973.

Ainsworth, M. D. S.: The development of infant-mother interaction among the Ganda. In Foss, B. M. (ed.): Determinants of Infant Behavior, Vol. 2. New York: John Wiley & Sons, 1963.

Ainsworth, M. D. S., and Bell, S. M.: Some contemporary patterns of mother-infant interaction in the feeding situation. In Ambrose, A. (ed.): Stimulation in Early Infancy. London: Academic Press, 1969.

Ambrose, J. A. (ed.): Stimulation in Early Infancy. London: Academic Press, 1969.

An Instructional Guide for Parents. Pennsylvania Consortium for the Preparation of Professional Personnel for the Severely and Profoundly Mentally Retarded/Multihandicapped. School of Education, Duquesne University, Pittsburgh PA, 1974.

Andrews, B., et al.: Cerebral palsy: My baby is slow. Patient Care 21 (1972).

Ardran, G. M., and Kemp, F. H.: Some important factors in the assessment of oral pharyngeal function. Develop. Med. Child Neurol. 12 (1970).

Ayres, A. J.: Sensory Integration and Learning Disorders. Los Angeles: Western Psychological Services, 1972.

Bangs, T. E.: Language and Learning Disorders of the Pre-Academic Child. New York: Appleton-Century-Crofts, 1968.

Banus, B.: The Developmental Therapist. Thorofare, NJ: Charles B. Slack, 1971.

Barnard, K. E., and Powell, M.: Teaching the Mentally Retarded Child: A Family Care Approach. St. Louis: C. V. Mosby Co., 1972.

Barness, A., and Pitkin, R. M.: Symposium on nutrition. Clin. Perinatology 2, no. 2 (1975).

Battle, C. U.: Disruptions in the socialization of the handicapped child. Rehabil. Lit. 35 (1974).

Beintema, D. J.: A Neurological Study of Newborn Infants. Clin. Develop. Med., No. 28. London: Heinemann, 1968.

Bell, R. Q.: Contributions of human infants to caregiving and social interaction. In Lewis, M., and Rosenblum, L. (ed.): The Effect of the Infant on Its Caregiver. New York: John Wiley & Sons, 1974.

Bergen, A.: Selected Equipment for Pediatric Rehabilitation. Blythedale Children's Hospital, Valhalla, New York, 1974.

Berlyne, D. C.: Laughter, humor and play. In Lindzey, G., and Aronson, E. (eds.): Handbook of Social Psychology. Reading MA: Addison-Wesley Publishing Co., 1970.

Berry, M.: Language Disorders of Children. New York: Appleton-Century-Crofts, 1969.

Birch, H. G., and Gussow, J. D.: Disadvantaged Children: Health, Nutrition, and School Failure. New York: Harcourt, Brace and World: Grune and Stratton, 1970.

Black, F., et al.: Congenital Deafness: A New Approach to Early Detection of Deafness Through a High Risk Register. Boulder: Colorado Associated University Press, 1971.

Bly, L.: Normal Motor Development; A New Way of Looking. Presentation at the Pediatric Section Meeting of the American Physical Therapy Association, Washington DC, February 1976.

Bobath, B.: Abnormal Postural Reflex Activity Caused by Brain Lesions, ed. 2. Clin. Develop. Med. London: Heinemann, 1971.

Bobath, B.: The very early treatment of cerebral palsy. Develop. Med. Child Neurol. 9:373-390, 1967.

Bobath, B., and Bobath, K.: Motor Development in the Different Types of Cerebral Palsy. London: Heinemann, 1975.

Bobath, K., and Bobath, B.: An analysis of the development of standing and walking patterns in patients with cerebral palsy. Physiotherapy 48:144, 1962.

Bosley, E.: Development of sucking and swallowing. Cerebral Palsy J., 26, no. 6 (1965).

Bosma, J.: Fourth Symposium on Oral Sensation and Perception. National Isntitutes of Health, Bethesda MD, 1973.

Bosma, J. (ed.): Symposium on Oral Sensation and Perception. Springfield IL: Charles C Thomas, Publishers, 1967.

Bower, T. G. R.: Development in Infancy. San Francisco: W. H. Freeman, 1974.

Bower, T. G. R.: Perceptual functioning in early infancy. In Stone, L. J., Smith, H., and Murphy, L. B. (eds.): The Competent Infant: Research and Commentary. New York: Basic Books, 1975.

Bower, T. G. R.: Stimulus variables determining space perception in infants. In Stone, L. J., Smith, H., and Murphy, L. B. (eds.): The Competent Infant: Research and Commentary, New York: Basic Books, 1975.

Brazelton, T. B.: Infants and Mothers. New York: Delacorte Press, 1969.

Brazelton, T. B.: Psychophysiologic Reactions in the Neonate. J. Pediatr., 58, no. 4 (1961).

Brazelton, T. B., Koslowski, B., and Main, M.: The origins of reciprocity: The early mother-infant interaction. In Lewis, N., Rosenblum, L. (eds.): The Effect of the Infant on Its Caregiver. New York: John Wiley & Sons, 1974.

Breckenridge, M., and Murphy, M.: Growth and Development of the Young Child. Philadelphia: W. B. Saunders Co., 1969.

Broussard, E. R., and Hortner, M. S.: Further considerations regarding maternal perception of the first born. In Hellmuth, J. (ed.): Exceptional Infant. Studies in Abnormalities, Vol. 2, New York: Brunner-Mazel, 1971.

Bruner, J. S.: Volition, skill and tools. In Stone, L. J., Smith, H., and Murphy, L. B. (eds.): The Competent Infant: Research and Commentary. New York: Basic Books, 1975.

Caplan, F. (ed.): The First Twelve Months of Life: Your Baby's Growth Month by Month. Princeton NJ: Edcom Systems, 1973.

Carlsen, P.: Comparison of two occupational therapy approaches for treating the young cerebral palsied child. Am. J. Occup. Ther., 29: 267, 1975.

Cliff, G., and Nymann, C.: Mothers Can Help. A Therapist's Guide for Formulating a Developmental Text for Parents of Special Children. The El Paso Rehabilitation Center, El Paso TX, 1974.

Crickmay, M. C.: Speech Therapy and the Bobath Approach

to Cerebral Palsy. Springfield IL: Charles C Thomas, Publishers, 1970.

Crothers, B., and Paine, R. S.: The Natural History of Cerebral Palsy. London: Oxford University Press, 1959.

Danella, E.: A study of tactile preference in the multiply handicapped child. Am. J. Occup. Ther., 27: 457, 1973.

Dargassies, S.: Neurological maturation of the premature infant of 28-44 weeks gestational age. In Falkner, F. (ed.): Human Development. Philadelphia: W. B. Saunders Co., 1966.

DiLeo, J.: Developmental evaluation of very young infants. In Hellmuth, J. (ed.): The Exceptional Infant: The Normal Infant, Vol. 1. New York: Brunner-Mazel, 1967.

Dreyfus, B. C.: Organization of sleep in prematures: Implications for caregiving. In Lewis, M., and Rosenblum, L. (eds.): The Effect of the Infant on Its Caregiver. New York: John Wiley & Sons, 1974.

Drillien, C.: The Growth and Development of the Prematurely Born Infant. Baltimore: Williams & Wilkins, 1964.

Dubowitz, V.: The Floppy Infant. Clin. Develop. Med. No. 31. London: Heinemann, 1969.

Egan, D. F., Illingsworth, R. S., and MacKeith, R. C.: Developmental Screening 0-5 Years. Clin. Develop. Med. No. 30. London: Heinemann, 1969.

Eimas, P. D., et al.: Speech perception in infants. In Stone, L., Smith, H., and Murphy, L. B. (eds.): The Competent Infant: Research and Commentary. New York: Basic Books, 1975.

Eisenberg, R. B.: The organization of auditory behavior. In Stone, L., Smith, H., and Murphy, L. B. (eds.): The Competent Infant: Research and Commentary. New York: Basic Books, 1975.

Escalona, S. K.: The Roots of Individuality: Normal Patterns of Development in Infancy. Chicago: Aldine Publishing Co., 1968.

Fantz, R.: Visual perception from birth as shown by pattern selectivity. In Stone, L. J., Smith, H., and Murphy, L. B. (eds.): The Competent Infant: Research and Commentary. New York: Basic Books, 1975.

Farber, S.: Sensorimotor Evaluation and Treatment Procedures for Allied Health Personnel, ed. 2. Purdue University at Indianapolis Medical Center, 1974.

Flavell, J. H.: The Developmental Psychology of Jean Piaget. Princeton: Van Nostrand, 1963.

Frailberg, S.: Blind infants and their mothers: An examination of the sign system. In Lewis, M., and Rosenblum, L. (ed.): The Effect of the Infant on Its Caregiver. New York: John Wiley & Sons, 1974.

Frailberg, S.: Parallel and divergent pattern in blind and sighted infants. Psychoanalytic Study Child 22:264-300, 1968.

Frailberg, S.: The Magic Years. New York: Scribners, 1959.

Frailberg, S., Siegel, B. L., and Gibson, R.: The role of sound in the search behavior of a blind infant. Psychoanalytic Study Child 21:327-357, 1966.

Freedman, A. M., Kaplan, H. I., and Sadock, B. J.: Modern Synopsis of Comprehensive Textbook of Psychiatry. Baltimore: Williams & Wilkins, 1972.

Furth, H. G.: Thinking without Langauge. New York: Free Press, 1966.

Gardiner, P., et al (eds.): Aspects of Pediatric Ophthalmology. London: Spastics International Medical Publications, Lavenham Press, 1969.

Gardner, D. B.: Development in Early Childhood: The Preschool Years. New York: Harper & Row, Publishers, 1964.

Gardner, E. Fundamentals of Neurology, ed. 6. Philadelphia: W. B. Saunders Co., 1975.

Gelber, S., Richardson, S., and Leventhal, M.: The Developmental program: Infants and toddlers; normal development of communication. In The Ripple Project: A Nationally Organized Collaborative Project to Provide Comprehensive Services to Atypical Infants and their Families. National Office of United Cerebral Palsy, New York, 1974.

Gesell, A.: The ontogenesis of infant behavior. In Mussen, P. H. (ed.): Carmichael's Manual of Child Psychology, ed. 3. New York: John Wiley & Sons, 1970.

Gibson, J. J.: The mouth as an organ for laying hold on the environment. In Bosma, J. F. (ed.): Symposium on Oral Sensation and Perception. Springfield IL: Charles C Thomas, Publishers, 1967.

Gilfoyle, E., and Grady, A.: A developmental theory of somatosensory perception. In Coryll, J., and Henderson, A. (ed.): The Body Senses and Perceptual Deficit. Boston University Symposium, March 1972.

Ginsberg, H., and Opper, S.: Piaget's Theory of Intellectual Development: An Introduction. Englewood Cliffs NJ: Prentice-Hall, 1969.

Goodenough, F. L.: Anger in Young Children. Minneapolis: University of Minnesota Press, 1931.

Goodenough, F. L.: Expression of the emotions in a blind-deaf child. J. Abnormal Social Psychol. 27 (1932).

Gralewicz, A.: Play deprivation in multihandicapped children. Am. J. Occup. Ther. 27:70, 1973.

Haith, M.: Visual scanning in infants. In Stone, L. J., Smith, H., and Murphy, L. B. (eds.): The Competent Infant: Research and Commentary. New York: Basic Books, 1975.

Hemiplegic Cerebral Palsy in Childhood and Adults. Report of an International Study Group. Clin. in Develop. Med., No. 4. London: Heinemann, 1961.

Herron, R. E., and Sutton-Smith, B. (eds.): Child's Play. New York: John Wiley & Sons, 1971.

Hess, R. D., and Shipman, V. C.: Cognitive Elements in maternal behavior. In Hill, J. P. (ed.): Minnesota Symposia on Child Psychology, Vol. 1. Minneapolis: University of Minnesota Press, 1967.

Hess, R. D., and Shipman, V. C.: Maternal influences upon early learning: The cognitive environments of urban preschool children. In Hess, R.D., and Bear,

R. M. (eds.): Early Education. Chicago: Aldine Publishing Co., 1968.

Hixon, T., and Hardy, J.: Restricted motility of the speech articulators in cerebral palsy. J. Speech and Hearing Disorders 29 (1964).

Holser-Buehler, P.: Correction of infantile feeding habits. Am. J. Occup. Ther. 27:6, 1973.

Holser-Buehler, P.: The Blanchard method of feeding the cerebral palsied. Am. J. Occup. Ther. 20:1, 1966.

Holt, K. S.: Facts and fallacies about neuromuscular function in cerebral palsy as revealed by electromyography. Develop. Med. Child Neurol. 3:255-268, 1966.

Humphrey, T.: The prenatal development of mouth opening and mouth closure reflexes. Pediatric Digest, 11:12, 1969.

Hutt, C.: Exploration and play in children. In Herron, R. E., and Sutton-Smith, B. (eds.): Child's Play. New York: John Wiley & Sons, 1971.

Ilg, F., and Ames, L. B.: Child Behavior. New York: Harper & Row, Publishers, 1955.

Illingsworth, R. S.: An Introduction to Developmental Assessment in the First Year. London: National Spastics Society. Heinemann, 1962.

Illingsworth, R. S.: The Development of the Infant and Young Child: Normal and Abnormal, ed. 4. Baltimore: Williams & Wilkins, 1970.

Ingram, T. T. S.: Clinical significance of the infantile feeding reflexes. Develop. Med. Child Neurol. 4:159-169, 1962.

Initial COMPET (Commonwealth plan for education and training of mentally retarded children). Pennsylvania Department of Education, Harrisburg PA, 1972.

Kagan, J.: Change and Continuity in Infancy. New York: John Wiley & Sons, 1971.

Kagan, J.: Continuity in cognitive development during the first year. In Stone, L., Smith, H., and Murphy, L. B. (eds.): The Competent Infant: Research and Commentary. New York: Basic Books, 1975.

Kagan, J.: The determination of attention in the infant. In Stone, L., Smith, H., and Murphy, L. B. (eds.): The Competent Infant: Research and Commentary. New York: Basic Books, 1975.

Klapper, Z., and Birch, H. G.: A Fourteen-Year Follow-Up Study of Cerebral Palsy: Intellectual Change and Stability. Paper presented at the annual meeting of the American Orthopsychiatric Association, San Francisco, 1966.

Komich, P., and Tearney, A.: The sequential development of infants of low birth weight. Am. J. Occup. Ther., 27: 396, 1973.

Kong, E.: Very early treatment of cerebral palsy. Develop. Med. Child Neurol. 8:198-202, 1966.

Kron, R. E.: Studies of sucking behavior in the human newborn: The predictive value of measures of oral behavior. In Bosma, J. F. (ed.): Second Symposium on Oral Sensation and Perception. Springfield IL: Charles C Thomas, Publishers, 1970.

Kubler-Ross, E.: On Death and Dying. New York: Macmillan Publishing Co., 1969.

Langlois, A.: Respiratory Patterns in Infants Aged Six to Thirteen Months. Unpublished Doctoral Dissertation, Teachers' College, Columbia University, New York, 1975.

Lewis, M., and Rosenblum, L. (eds.): The Effect of the Infant on the Caregiver. New York: John Wiley & Sons, 1974.

McGraw, M. B.: The Neuro-Muscular Maturation of the Human Infant. New York: Hafner Press, 1963.

McNeill, D.: The Acquisition of Language. New York: Harper and Row Publishers, 1970.

Menyuk, P.: The Acquisition and Development of Language. Englewood Cliffs NJ: Prentice-Hall, 1971.

Milani-Comparetti, A., and Gidoni, E. A.: Pattern analysis of motor development and its disorders. Develop. Med. Child Neurol. 9:625-630, 1967.

Miller, A. J.: Neurophysiological Properties of the Swallowing Reflex. Ph.D. Thesis, UCLA Dept. of Physiology, 1970 (unpublished).

Morris, S.: Program Guidelines for Children with Feeding Problems, 1974. Illinois State Pediatric Institute (1640 W. Roosevelt Road, Chicago IL 60608).

Mueller, H.: Feeding. In Finnie, N. R. (ed.): Handling the Young Cerebral Palsied Child at Home, ed. 2. New York: E. P. Dutton, 1975.

Mundy, Castle, A. C., and Anglin, J. Looking strategies in infants. In Stone, L., Smith, H., and Murphy, L. B. (eds.): The Competent Infant: Research and Commentary. New York: Basic Books, 1975.

Murphy, K.: Development of Normal Vocalization and Speech in the Child Who Does Not Talk. Clin. Develop. Med. No. 13. Heinemann, 1964.

Murphy, L. B.: Infant's play and cognitive development. In Piers, M. (ed.): Play and Development. New York: W. W. Norton & Co., 1972.

Mysak, E.: Neuroevolutional Approach to Cerebral Palsy and Speech. New York: Teachers' College Press, 1968.

Northern, J., and Downs, M.: Hearing in Children. Baltimore: Williams & Wilkins, 1974.

Norton, Y.: Neurodevelopment and sensory integration for the profoundly retarded multiply handicapped child. Am. J. Occup. Ther. 29:93, 1975.

O'Donnell, P. A.: Motor and Haptic Learning. Belmont CA: Dimensions Publishing Co. in association with Fearon Publishing Co., 1969.

Ogg, L.: Oral-pharyngeal development and evaluation. J. Am. Phys. Ther. Assoc. 55:3, 1975.

Paine, R. S., et al.: Evolution of postural reflexes in normal infants and in the presence of chronic brain disorders. Neurology 14:1036, 1964.

Paine, R. S., and Oppé, T.: Neurological Examination of Children. Philadelphia: J. B. Lippincott Co., 1966.

Peiper, A.: Cerebral Function in Infancy and Childhood. New York: Consultants Bureau, 1963.

Phelps, W., Hopkins, T., and Cousins, R.: The Cerebral-Palsied Child. New York: Simon and Schuster, 1958.

Piaget, J.: Development and learning. In Lavatelli, C. S., and Stendler, F. (eds.): Readings in Child Behavior and Development, ed. 3. New York: Harcourt, Brace, Janovich, 1972.

Piaget, J.: Play, Dreams and Imitation in Childhood. New York: W. W. Norton & Co., 1963.

Piaget, J., and Inhelder, B.: The Psychology of the Child. New York: Basic Books, 1969.

Prechtl, H., and Beintema, D.: The Neurological Examination of the Full Term Infant. Clin. Develop. Med., No. 12. London: Heinemann, 1964.

Provence, S., and Lipton, R. C.: Infants in Institutions: A Comparison of Their Development with Family Reared Infants During the First Year of Life. New York: International Universities Press, 1962.

Rosenbloom, L.: The consequences of impaired movement: A hypothesis and review. In Holt, K. (ed.): Movement and Child Development. London: Heinemann, 1975.

Rugel, R., et al.: The use of operant conditioning in a physically disabled child. Am. J. Occup. Ther. 25:247, 1971.

Saint-Anne Daregassies, S.: Neurodevelopmental symptoms during the first year of life. *Develop. Med. Child Neurol.* 14, 1972.

Scarr-Salapatek, S., and Williams, M.: The effects of early stimulation on low-birth-weight infants. Child Devel. 44 (1973).

Schaffer, H. R., and Callender, W. M.: Psychologic effects of hospitalization in infancy. Pediatrics 24 (1959).

Smith, D.: Recognizable patterns of human malformation: Genetic, embryologic and clinical aspects. Major Problems Clin. Pediatr., Vol. 7. Philadelphia: W. B. Saunders Co., 1970.

Spock, B.: Baby and Child Care. New York: Pocket Books, 1957.

Stockmeyer, S. A.: A sensorimotor approach to treatment. In Pearson, P. H., and Williams, C. E. (eds.): Physical Therapy Services in the Developmental Disabilities. Springfield IL: Charles C Thomas, Publishers, 1972.

Taft, L., and Cohen, H.: Neonatal and Infant Reflexology. Hellmuth, J. (ed.): In The Exceptional Infant: The Normal Infant, Vol. I. New York: Brunner-Mazel, 1967.

Thompson, J.: Development of facial expression of emotion in blind and seeing children. Arch. Pscyhol. 37, no. 264, 1941.

Twitchell, T. E.: Normal motor development (1965). In Growth and Development: An Anthology. American Physical Therapy Association, Washington DC, 1975.

Tyler, W., et al.: Interpersonal components of therapy with young cerebral palsied. Am. J. Occup. Ther. 28:395, 1974.

Van den Berg, B. J., and Yerushalmy, J.: Studies on convulsive disorders in young children. Pediatrics 3:177, 1969.

Van Riper, C., and Irwin, J.: Voice and Articulation. Englewood Cliffs NJ: Prentice-Hall, 1958.

Vanderheiden, G. C. (ed.): Non-Vocal Communication Techniques and Aids for the Severely Physically Handicapped. Baltimore: University Park Press, 1976.

Walsh, G.: Cerebellum, Posture and Cerebral Palsy. Clin. Develop. Med. No. 8. London: Heinemann, 1963.

Walsh, G.: Measuring ocular motor performance of cerebral palsied children. Am. J. Occup. Ther. 28:265, 1974.

Wilder, C. N.: Respiratory Patterns in Infants: Birth to Eight Months of Age. Doctoral Dissertation, Columbia University, 1972. Dissertation Abstracts International, 1973, vol. 33, 5052B-5053B. (University Microfilms No. 73-93056).

Willard, H. S., and Spackman, C. S. (eds.): Occupational Therapy, ed. 4. Philadelphia: J. B. Lippincott Co., 1963.

Wolff, P. H.: The development of attention in young infants. In Stone, L., Smith, H., and Murphy, L. B. (eds.): The Competent Infant: Research and Commentary. New York: Basic Books, 1975.

Wolff, P. H.: The natural history of crying and other vocalization in early infancy. In Foss, B. M. (ed.): Determinants of Infant Behavior, Vol. 4. London: Methuen, 1969.

Wolff, P. H.: The serial organization of sucking in the young infant. Pediatrics 42:943-956, 1968.

Wyke, B.: The neurological basis of movement: A developmental review. In Holt, K. (ed.): Movement and Child Development. London: Heinemann, 1975.

Yarrow, L. J.: The crucial nature of early experience. In Glass, D. (ed.): Environmental Influences: Biology and Behavior Series. New York: Rockefeller University Press, Russell Sage Foundation, 1968.

Yarrow, L. J.: The development of focused relationships in infancy. In Hellmuth, J. (ed.): Exceptional Infant. New York: Brunner-Mazel, 1967.

ACKNOWLEDGMENTS

To Elizabethtown College, Elizabethtown, Pennsylvania, with special appreciation to Barbara Thome Bagri, who typed and retyped the entire chapter; to Elizabethtown Hospital for Children and Youth; and to Reading Easter Seal Agency, Reading, Pennsylvania.

21
Burns

Maude H. Malick

The United States has one of the highest fire death rates of the five major industrialized nations in the world.* Over 15,000 persons die each year in fires or as a result of thermal injuries. Over one million adults and children are burned annually, requiring admission to a hospital or limiting their activity for more than a day. One hundred thousand of these burned individuals require hospitalization either in burn care centers or in community hospital facilities. However, only 10 percent of these burn patients are cared for in specialized burn care units. Of the approximately six thousand children burned, 50 percent stay in a hospital facility for one month or less, 25 percent for two months, and the remainder for three or more months. Yet, at the same time, youth promotes a higher survival rate. Studies have shown that approximately 50 percent of all burns occur to individuals under twenty years of age, making this a crucial problem for the young. Eighty percent of the burns occur in the home.

* Facts on pages 547–550 are from MacMillan, B. G.: Burns in children. Clin. Plastic Surg. 1:633–643, 1974.

KINDS OF BURNS AND INITIAL TREATMENT

The most common cause of flame burns is clothing ignited from uncontrolled fires, while hot liquids, primarily coffee or boiling water, cause the majority of scald burns in the home. The mortality rate associated with flame burns in children is approximately 25 percent as opposed to 5 percent from liquid burns. Twenty-five percent of all burns among children result from heating units, hot liquids or vapors, stoves, electrical appliances, and matches. The inappropriate use of matches or lighters remains the leading cause of clothing ignition in children with 86 percent of these accidents involving children under ten years of age.

Statistics from the National Burn Information Exchange† indicate that the mortality rate is four times higher in the groups of patients in which burns are associated with clothing. Twenty-four percent of

† The National Burn Information Exchange is a service of the American Burn Association. Its current address is given at the end of this chapter.

the patients sustaining clothing-related burns die in the hospital as compared with only 6 percent of those patients whose clothing had not burned. The National Consumers Bureau has now made it mandatory for children's clothing to be made of nonflammable fibers.

The electrical burn is seen more in males than in females, and the extent of injury is dependent upon the number of volts that the body has been subjected to. In over 75 percent of electrical burns, the upper extremity has been injured or involved. The number of amputations from electrical burn is extremely high with accompanying increased morbidity. The mortality is highest in those suffering severe electrical injury and is caused primarily by respiratory and cardiac arrest rather than by the burn.

The primary objective for all thermal burns is to extinguish all flames, remove smoldering clothing, and position the patient horizontally. Standing often results in smoke inhalation. In chemical burns immerse or wash the area with large amounts of water to dilute the chemical agent.

The initial application of cold to minor burns of limited extent is extremely helpful in reducing pain and edema, provided it is applied soon after the injury. Care should be taken not to use large cold compresses when transporting patients for prolonged periods of time, since severe hyperthermia may result, interfering with capillary profusion and viability of the injured areas.

The burned areas should be covered with a clean material. Ointment or any other remedies should not be applied so that an accurate assessment of the injury can be made at the initial medical facility. The extensively burned patient should not be given water since the dangers of aspiration and water intoxication may jeopardize the future course of the patient.

ANATOMY AND PHYSIOLOGY OF THE SKIN

The skin is the largest organ of the body. It is made up of three layers. The outer layer, which is called the epidermis, is approximately 60 to 120 microns thick, except on the palms and soles of the feet which are from 0.5 to 0.8 millimeters. There are no blood vessels, capillaries, nerve endings, or lymphatics in the epidermis. Directly beneath the epidermis is the dermis, which is five to ten times thicker than the epidermis. This layer contains lymphatics, blood capillaries, nerve endings, hair follicles, sweat glands, and sebaceous glands. These are embedded in a ground substance which also contains collagen fibers, fibroblasts, reticulin, and elastin fibers lying in smooth parallel formations. The subcutaneous tissue lies directly beneath the dermis and epidermis.

In addition to providing a covering for the bony framework of the body and the life-sustaining organs, the skin serves the following purposes:

1. It *protects against infection*. It maintains a physical barrier that keeps out organisms and other bacteria. It has a bacteriostatic and bactericidal capability which can destroy small numbers of bacteria that penetrate the skin.
2. It *prevents loss of body fluids*. Its structure is such that it can assist in maintaining the delicate fluid balance which is required by the body and functions to avoid dehydration.
3. It *controls body temperature*. The increase and decrease of evaporation of water from the sweat glands acts as a temperature control. The sweat glands excrete excess water in small amounts of sodium chloride, cholesterin, and traces of albumin and urea.
4. It is an *organ of sensation*. The nerve endings within the dermis distinguish light or excessive pressure, pain, and low or high temperatures, thus allowing the individual to modify what he or she is doing in order to avoid damage or pain. The sebaceous glands protect the skin by the secretion of oils which soften and lubricate the skin. Vitamin B is made when the sunlight reacts with the cholesterol compounds within the skin.
5. It is *cosmetic*. The skin varies in pigment, texture, and whirls and patterns. This variation from one race to another and from one individual to another serves in identifying individuals.

All of these things are taken into consideration in determining the extent of the burn and its trauma to the patient both in its physical management and in its psychological considerations.

CLASSIFICATION OF BURNS

The extent of the total body burn should serve as the basis for the selection of the treatment facility. Burns of up to 15 percent of the total body surface can be adequately handled in community hospitals and those up to 25 percent in general hospitals. If more than 30 percent of the body area is burned, the patient should be taken to a burn center. Minor burns include partial thickness burns of less than 20 percent of the total body surface and full thickness burns of less than 10 percent. If a decision is made to transfer the patient to a more advanced facility, the evacuation should be carried out as early in the immediate postburn course as possible. All burns of the hands, perineum, and face should be admitted to the hospital.

The severity of the burn is determined by the size and depth of the burn, the age of the patient, past medical history, and the part of the body burned. Only after these factors are determined can the proper decisions be made about disposition, treatment, and prognosis of the patient.

The area of the body burned can be determined in several ways. In adults of 16 years or more the Rule of Nines applies and is adequate for most clinical purposes (Fig. 21-1). For infants and children the burn estimate diagram and table has been modified. A detailed diagram should be completed only after the blisters and dirt have been removed, since dirt and debris of normal skin often have the appearance of burn skin.

The Rule of Nines aids in estimating the percentage of burn for it divides the body surface into areas of approximately 9 percent or multiples of 9 percent. The head, the neck and the upper extremity each represent 9 percent; the lower extremity and the front and the back of the torso each represents 18 percent; and the perineum represents 1 percent. The

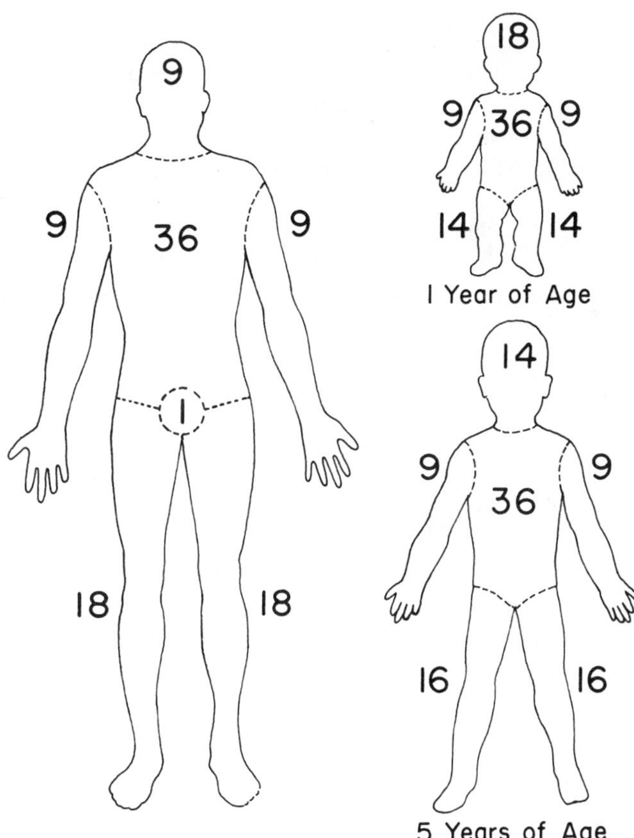

FIGURE 21-1. Rule of Nines.

rule is modified for children from birth to one year of age, allowing from 18 to 19 percent for the head and neck and 13 percent for the lower extremities. One percent is subtracted from the head and neck and added to the lower extremity for each year in ages one to ten. At the time of definitive care more accurate estimate of the extent of burn is made by using a table that more precisely relates to the changes of body proportion to maturation.

Burn injuries are arbitrarily classified as minor, moderate, and severe (Table 21-1). Minor burns rarely require hospitalization. Patients with full thickness burns of less than 2 percent, not involving critical areas, may be treated on an outpatient basis until they require hospitalization for skin grafting. Noting that a patient's hand is about 1 percent of the total body surface, this information can be useful in estimating the area of the burn on admission. The following criteria can be used to determine the degree of the burn.

Superficial first degree burns (Fig. 21-2) are confined to the epidermis and are characterized by erythema which blanches under pressure. There can be slight pain and edema but no blistering. The superficial burn can heal in a week since enough epithelial cells remain in the skin to provide new dermis.

Partial thickness second degree burns involve the dermis and are characteristically more painful and sensitive to pinprick, with blisters and considerable subcutaneous edema. The treatment of partial thickness burns is entirely directed toward the prevention of infection. Bacterial infection can seriously interfere with healing and change a partial thickness burn into a full thickness burn.

Deep partial thickness burns are burns in which the epidermis and part of the dermis are dead. The deep dermis is injured but alive and will provide tissue for spontaneous healing. The hair follicles and sebaceous glands are destroyed. Only the deepest parts of the sweat glands in the epithelium will survive.

Small bits of epithelium will suffice for re-epithelianization on the surface although it occurs more slowly than in the superficial partial thickness burn. This type of burn is sometimes referred to as *deep thermal burn*.

Full thickness third degree burns involve the destruction of the full thickness of the skin with possible muscle, tendon, and bone damage. Spontaneous healing is not possible. Grafting is usually necessary after the necrotic eschar has been removed. The area of third degree burn is usually dry and unblistered, is depressed below the surface of the surrounding burns, and is transparent with thrombosed vessels in its depth. The burn is painfree and insensitive to pinprick. Deep flame burns and some electrical burns may appear charred or black.

Doubtful depth areas are leathery, waxy-white or red, and nonblanching with subcutaneous edema. Occasionally blisters occur. Pinprick sensation can be absent. These burns usually destroy the full thickness of skin in children and areas of thin skin such as ears, eyelids, and inner forearm in adults. The swelling and pain associated with burns of the

Table 21-1. Means of classifying severity of burns.

	Minor	*Moderate*	*Severe*
Percent partial thickness	Less than 15%	15 to 30%	More than 30%
Percent full thickness	Less than 2%	2 to 10%	More than 10%
Hand, face, feet, and perineum	Not involved	Not involved	Involved
Age	Of little significance	Of little significance	Less than 18 months, more than 65 years
Etiology	Of little significance	Minor chemical and electrical burns	Major chemical and electrical burns
Complicating illnesses	Of little significance	Of little significance	Cardiac, renal, and metabolic involvement

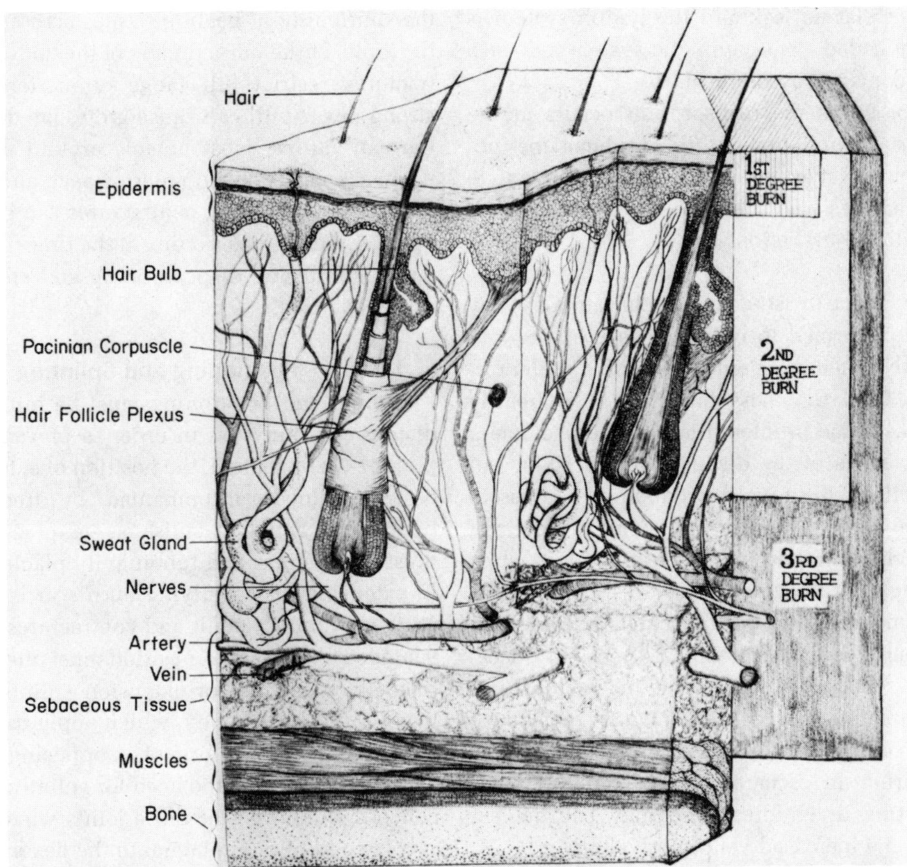

FIGURE 21-2. Cross section of the skin showing the depth of burn in relation to skin damage.

preorbital area, perineum, and both hands and feet frequently make outpatient nursing difficult.

OTHER MAJOR BURN DAMAGE

Respiratory Tract

Respiratory tract injuries are one of the major causes of mortality in burn patients. In considering causes of respiratory distress in the acute burn, it is important to realize that only a few patients with facial burns require an artificial airway or ventilatory assistance and then only rarely during the first twenty-four hours. The oral airway is necessary if the patient is comatose and close observation is necessary for signs of airway obstruction. If the patient has evidence of facial burns with singed nasal hairs and soot about the nose and mouth, careful monitoring is required. A tracheostomy should be performed only if absolutely necessary.

Body Fluid

When the burn occurs there are changes in the distribution of the body fluid. Depending on the temperature and the duration of heat causing the burn wound, a certain depth of injury or tissue death occurs. In minor burns where a thin layer of epidermis and dermis are exposed to heat for a short time, the changes will be minimal and may include redness with a separation of the outer layer of dermis, caused by blistering or slight edema. With prolonged exposure to heat, the capillary bed and the deeper tissues are traumatized and destroyed.

This trauma takes the form of increased capillary permeability or a thrombosis in severe wounds. As capillary permeability increases, the capillaries leak fluid into the interstitial spaces and interspatial fluid is increased. This is called edema. The lymphatic system would normally carry away the increased tissue fluid, but when the burn is large there is a great deal of plasma leak and the lymph system is rapidly overloaded. The lymphatic system may also have been damaged by the heat.

In minor burns the reabsorption occurs at the same rate as accumulation of fluid so edema does not occur. When massive edema does occur, immediate surgical measures may need to be undertaken to avoid vascular constriction.

PREVENTION OF LIMB ISCHEMIA. Escharotomies may need to be performed to both relieve pressure and prevent limb ischemia. Edema developing under circumferential full thickness burns in an extremity may produce a rise in interstitial pressure sufficient to cause cyanosis of the distal unburned skin, impairing capillary filling and producing progressive neurological deficits. Medial and lateral incisions of only the eschar to relieve pressure is painless when made through third degree burns and should be performed promptly if the signs of ischemia develop. In electrical burns, even fasciotomy is necessary occasionally to relieve pressure. With increasing burn edema a circumferential full thickness chest burn may significantly restrict the motion of the thoracic cage, requiring an escharotomy for relief. This is especially true in children who may become exhausted by the increased ventilatory effort.

ROLE OF THE OCCUPATIONAL THERAPIST

The first seventy-two hours after a severe burn injury the patient is in burn shock. During this period the burn team's duty is to stabilize the many internal and external changes caused by the thermal insult. As a result of the burn and loss of skin, the body has lost its ability to protect itself against infection, to maintain a balance in body fluids, and to prevent heat loss. Although most burn units maintain approximately 80 degrees room temperature, heat shields are also often used to maintain body heat.

The occupational therapist plays an important role in the initial phase of burn management by preventing soft tissue contractures, which is the major cause of loss in joint function and distorted skeletal positioning. Because of burn trauma and heat loss the patient quickly assumes the flexed, adducted fetal position for comfort and warmth. This position directly causes contracture deformities resulting from the shortening of healing tissues across and around the joints of the burned parts of the body. These contractures restrict full range of motion, and their strong flexor pull can cause grotesque distortions of the extremities, most notably around the face and neck, especially when anterior neck and face burns exist. The impending contractures can be prevented by careful early positioning at the time of admission, daily monitoring of positioning and splinting, and active exercise.

Positioning and Splinting

Proper bed positioning must be initiated immediately on admission in order to prevent deformity (Fig. 21-3). In general, the position of extension must be maintained, accompanied by frequent short periods of active exercise as is practical during dressing changes and tubbing. By placing the joints in extension, the overlying burn scar is maintained at its maximum length and contractures can be prevented. This extended position must often be accomplished by the use of extension splints across the major joints of the body, which apply traction to the healing tissue in the form of an opposing force (Table 21-2). In evaluating the need for splinting, the major concern should be for those joints where the burns involve a joint or are lateral to the flexor surface of a joint. Uninvolved joints should be free so that tendon shortening and stiffness will not occur.

Exercising

All of the joints should be exercised daily, preferably using active motion rather than passive motion to prevent joint stiffness. Active motion contributes to the maintenance of muscle mass and strength, while passive motion prevents tendon adherence as well as the tightening and shortening of the joint capsules. Passive motion should be gently executed and never pressed beyond tissue resistance.

All wounds should be carefully cleaned, debrided, and dressed at least twice daily. Splints must be thoroughly washed and dried before reapplying. Low-temperature splints such as those made of orthoplast and polyform can be gas autoclaved. Exercise, self-care activities, and night splint regimen must be followed until spontaneous healing of the burned areas occurs and, in the case of third degree

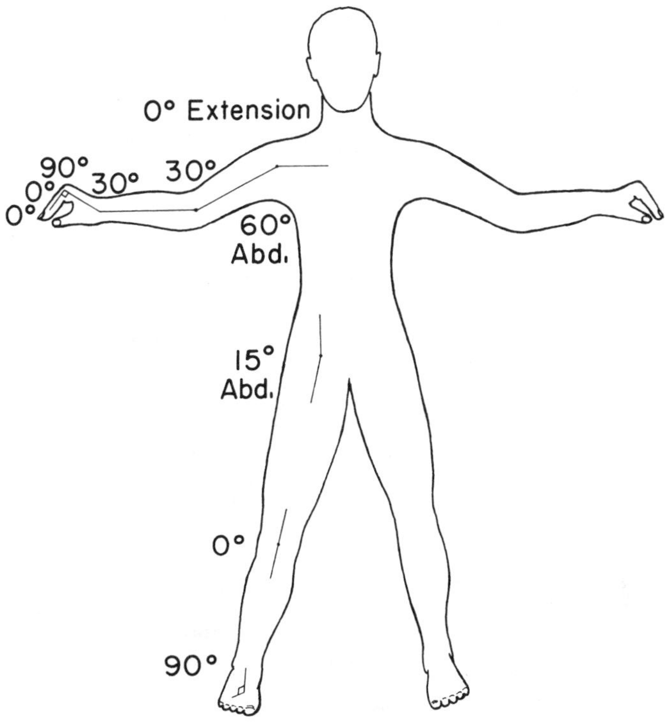

FIGURE 21-3. Initial burn position. In order to maintain maximum joint excursion and prevent contractures, this position may be altered depending on the location and extent of the burn.

burns, until the grafted areas have set, which usually is seven to ten days post-graft.

Pressure Stretch Techniques

A research study conducted at the Shriners' Burns Institute in Galveston, Texas, has indicated that more than 80 percent of patients who have suffered second and third degree burns will develop hypertrophic scarring throughout the burned areas after new skin and grafts have healed (Fig. 21-8). If no attempt is made to control the development of scar hypertrophy, crippling disfigurement is likely to occur as a result of severe contractures and the unchecked formation of thickened, knobby red scar tissue. In normal burn wound healing there is a great increase in vascularity to form the granulation tissue that the body uses to restore the damaged skin site. Studies conducted by Doctor Hugo Linares at the Shriners' Burns Institute indicate that the granulation tissue shows an increase of *fibroblasts.* Fibroblasts are the cells that synthesize mucopolysaccharides and collagen fibers necessary for the development of new connective tissue.

In the development of normal skin dermis, fibroblasts appear to be irregular in shape and flat with a lumpy surface. But the fibroblasts that develop within the reticular layer of a hypertrophic scar are spider-shaped with rounded nodular bodies. These fibroblasts produce an excessive amount of collagen fibers which adhere to each other in an irregular pattern. The nodules of compact collagen permit little or no interstitial spacing as they fill the middle and lower reticular layers of the dermis. The collagen filaments entwine with each other to produce a ropelike appearance (Fig. 21-9). In addition to the irregular shape of the nodules, a hypertrophic scar will synthesize collagen at more than four times the rate of normal skin. It is this pile-up of collagen-filled nodules that gives rise to the rigid, thickened hypertrophic scar which later can cause contractures.

It has been known for some years that the application of controlled, consistent pressure to the surface of an immature hypertrophic scar will, in time, reduce the scar and leave a smooth, pliable skin surface. But the persistent problem remained regarding how pressure could be applied and maintained throughout the maturation of the scar. Pressure

Table 21-2. Directions for positioning and splinting.

Body part	*Positioning*	*Splinting*
Neck	Slight extension No pillows should be used Mouth of patient should be able to be closed	Soft cervical collar (Fig. 21-4) Rigid (low-temperature thermoplastic) neck conformer (Fig. 21-5)
Shoulders	Arms abducted 60 to 90° with slight internal rotation	Traction or axillary splints may be used Small pillow between scapulae will encourage external rotation
Elbow	Full extension when anterior surface of arm is involved Elbow should be ranged with exercise and/or activity during the day and positioned at night in full extension	Three-point extension splint can be worn over dressings (Fig. 21-6)
Hips	Whether prone or supine—neutral extended position	Abduction position can be accomplished by positioning drop foot splints approximately 12 in. apart
	Legs should be abducted 15° from the midline	A bar placed between the knees attached to the three-point extension splints will maintain abduction
Knee	Full extension	Three-point extension splints for night use (Fig. 21-6)
Ankle	90° (which is normal standing position) prevents the shortening of the Achilles tendon	Foot board—drop foot splints When using a posterior splint, the heel must be suspended to prevent pressure sores. When prone, position patient so that foot hangs over edge of the mattress. Extension splints can be attached to tennis shoes to aid in positioning.
Spine	A straight-line position to prevent scoliosis, especially with lateral body burns.	
Hands	*Wrist* 30° extension or dorsiflexion *Metacarpophalangeal joint* 70 to 90° flexion *Proximal and distal interphalangeal joints* full extension Thumb abducted and extended to maintain web space (Fig. 21-7)	Functional pan splint placing interphalangeal joints in full extension maintaining "burn" position

dressings and elastic Ace wraps were tried but all of these materials slipped, bunched up, constricted, or fell off.

The Jobst Institute in Toledo, Ohio, developed a special Dacron Spandex elastic fabric to be used in the construction of carefully fitted pressure gradient garments. Garments constructed from this new fabric, when accurately measured, fitted, and consistently worn by burn patients, provide and maintain adequate pressure to prevent hypertrophic scar formation. In addition, the multidirectional stretch of the fabric allows any normal movement of the body. The garments are custom engineered and constructed for each patient to provide a consistent gradient pressure over the burn scar areas.

The garment can be engineered to apply pressure directly over the burned areas, including the entire body (Fig. 21-10). Often one body area will be grafted or will heal several weeks before the rest of the body is ready for measuring. These areas should be measured and garments ordered as early as possible (Fig. 21-11), leaving large unhealed areas for measurement later.

Healed burns which are ready for measurement can vary greatly in color from a deep purple to a pink. The measurement and fitting of pressure gradient garments may begin as soon as these open areas of newly healed scar tissue are reduced to the size of a dime. In other words, any graft site, whether it is a patch or mesh type, should be almost

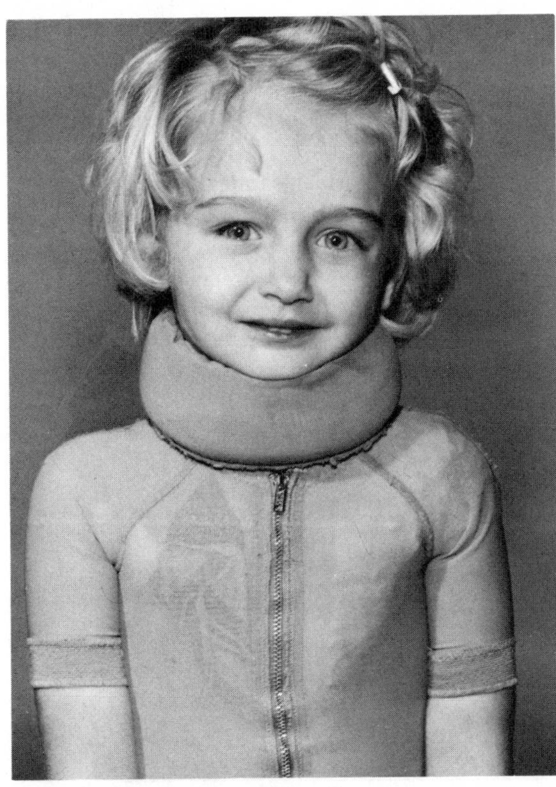

FIGURE 21-4. Soft cervical collar.

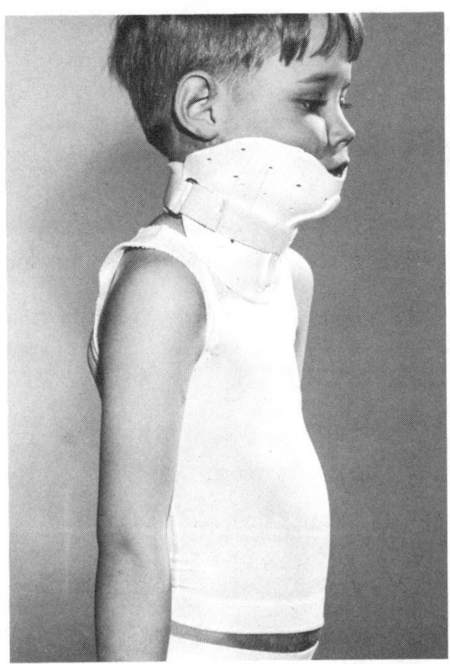

FIGURE 21-5. A rigid low-temperature thermoplastic cervical collar.

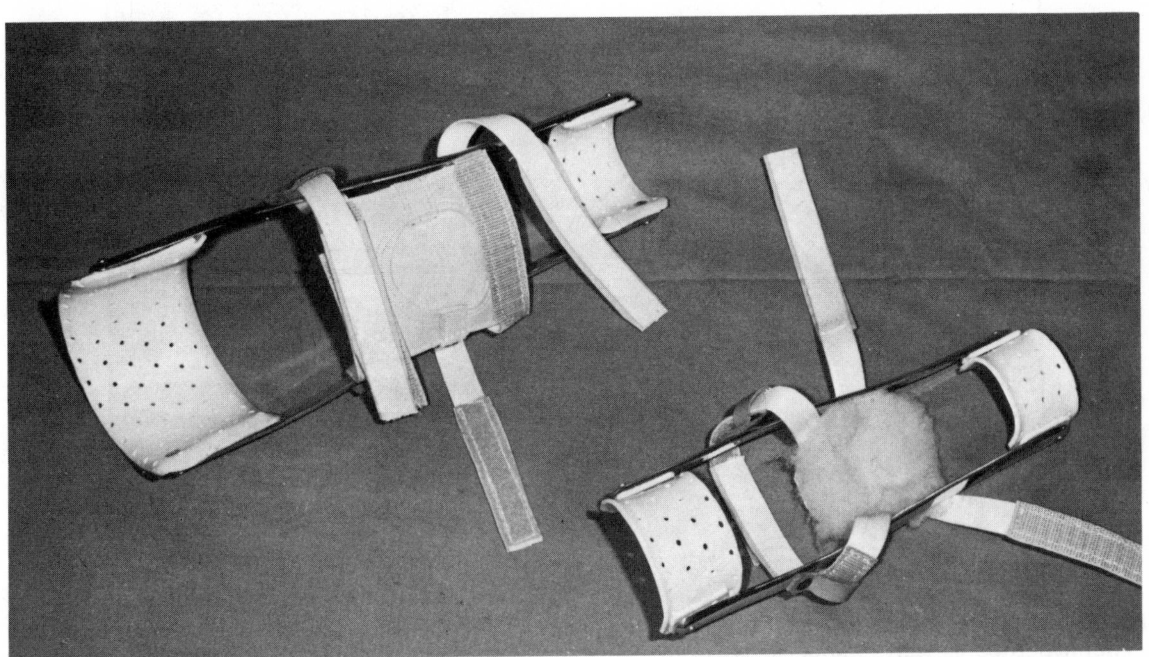

FIGURE 21-6. Three-point extension splints can be used for elbow and knee extension.

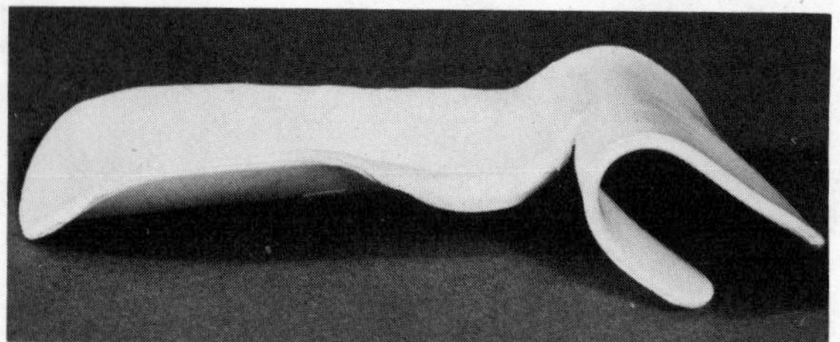

FIGURE 21-7. Functional position splint for the thumb.

completely healed before measurement. In fact, a minimum of seven days post-graft should be allowed before measurement is considered. Donor sites should also be dry and well healed before garments are fitted.

The pressure garments must be very carefully measured and designed in order to provide adequate pressure over the burned areas and still allow normal body mobility. Full length zippers should be desig-

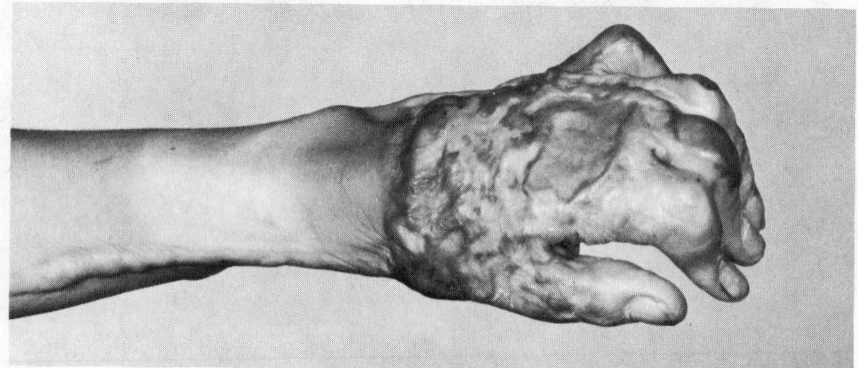

FIGURE 21-8. Scar hypertrophy on a burned hand.

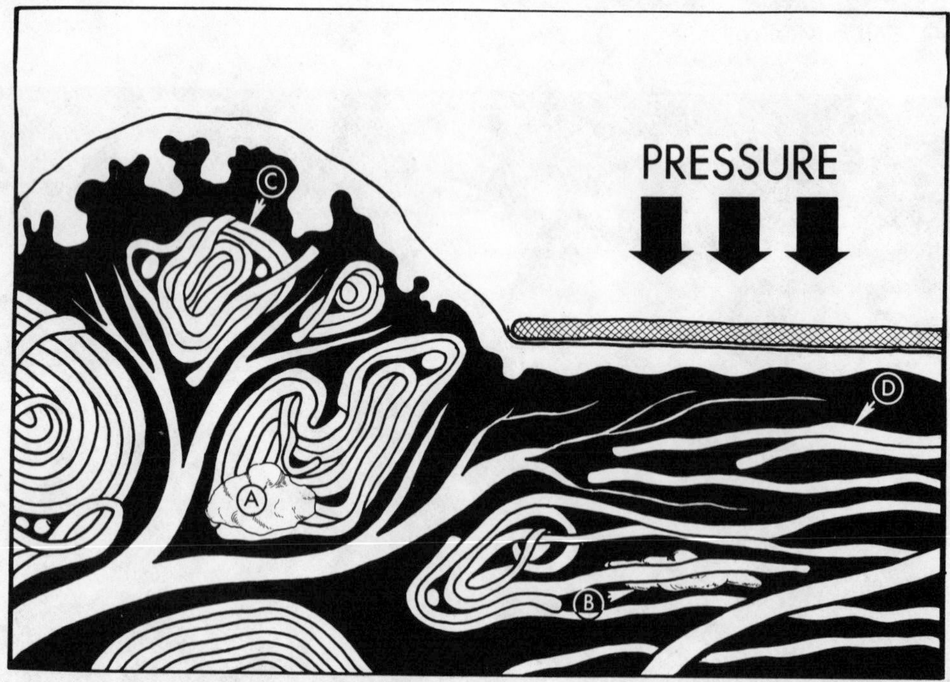

FIGURE 21-9. Effect of pressure on healing scar tissue: *A,* Fibroblast in hypertrophic scar; *B,* Fibroblast in nonhypertrophic scar; *C,* Ropelike collagen filament in hypertrophic scar; *D,* Linear parallel arrangement of collagen filament in nonhypertrophic scar.

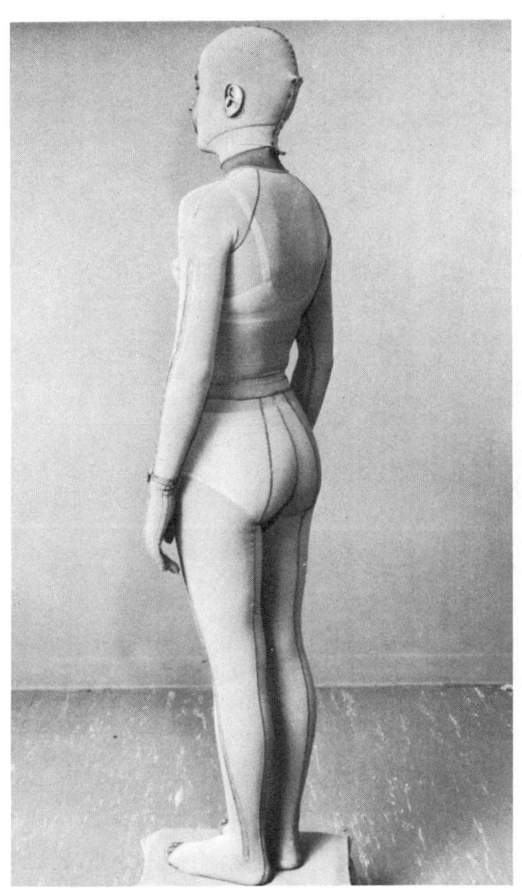

FIGURE 21-10. Jobst pressure gradient burn garment.

nated whenever a burned extremity is involved. In this way all shearing effects can be eliminated when the garments are donned. In order to be wholly effective, the pressure garments must be worn consistently twenty-four hours a day for nine to twelve months or until full scar maturation. The patient and his or her garments and splinting should be followed on a regular outpatient basis (every two weeks and later monthly) in order to monitor the pressure and position management.

The pressure stretch techniques are essential to soften, smooth, and maintain elastic skin during the maturation process and to prevent hypertrophic scarring and subsequent contractures.

The Burned Hand

The burned hand is of major concern to the occupational therapist and is the burn that occurs most frequently; this is because the hand is in an exposed position and is used to extinguish the fire. Dorsal hand burns are the most frequent and the most disabling of hand burns. Dorsal burns of the hand tend to produce a deformity consisting of hyperextension of the metacarpophalangeal joints, flexion of the interphalangeal joints, adduction and extension of the thumb, radial deviation to the wrist, and wrist flexion. The resulting flattening of the transverse and longitudinal palmar arches render the hand nonfunctional. All of these deforming positions will develop into contractures unless the hand is appropriately exercised, splinted, and treated.

The basic burn splint should be designed individually to prevent hand deformities from developing. In addition to preventing wrist flexion, it prevents metacarpophalangeal joint extension deformity and proximal interphalangeal joint flexion contracture commonly called the "claw" deformity (Fig. 21-12). Because the extensor tendons lying on the dorsum of the hand are so poorly protected they are extremely vulnerable to injury as they cross the proximal interphalangeal joint. The classic boutonniere deformity is seen all too frequently. When the wrist is held properly in extension the metacarpophalangeal joints tend to flex because of the effects of gravity and the tension on the intrinsic muscles. This position allows the intrinsic muscles to act on the interphalangeal extension. However, the most vulnerable joint in the hand is the proximal interphalangeal joint.

If, as a result of direct burn damage to the extensor mechanism or through proximal interphalangeal joint flexion, the middle extensor slip is caught between the unyielding eschar and the underlying heads of the proximal and middle phalanges, partial destruction of the extensor mechanism will result. The lateral bands of the joint can be shredded or slip volarly, thus causing the hand to assume the typical burn hand deformity. For this reason careful positioning of these two sets of joints is mandatory, and no fist clenching is permitted until the stability of the extensor mechanism is assured. Internal splints with Kirshner wires can be used to prevent the development of metacarpophalangeal, interphalangeal, and thumb deformities as well.

The main indication for internal splinting is

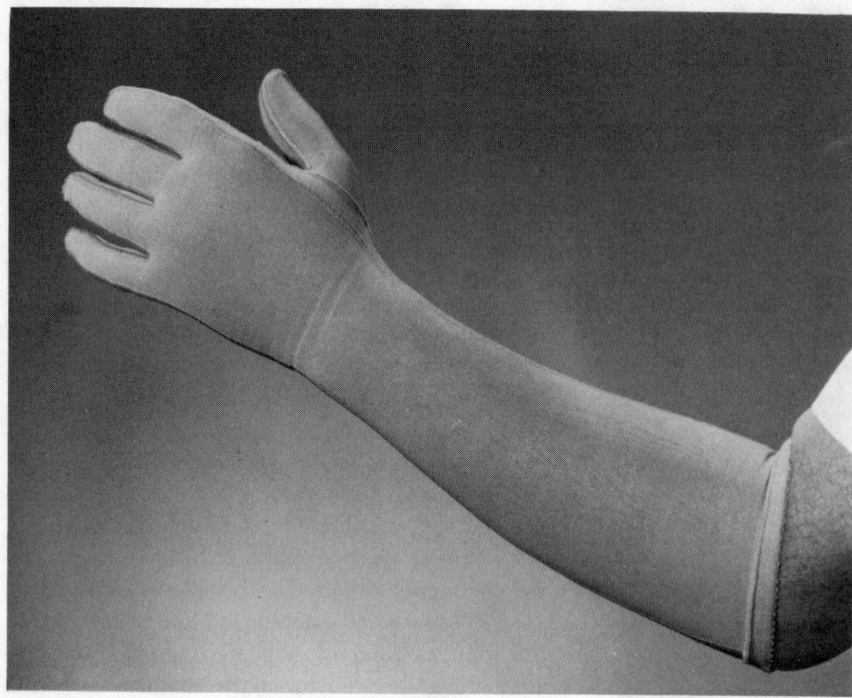

FIGURE 21-11. Pressure gradient gloves.

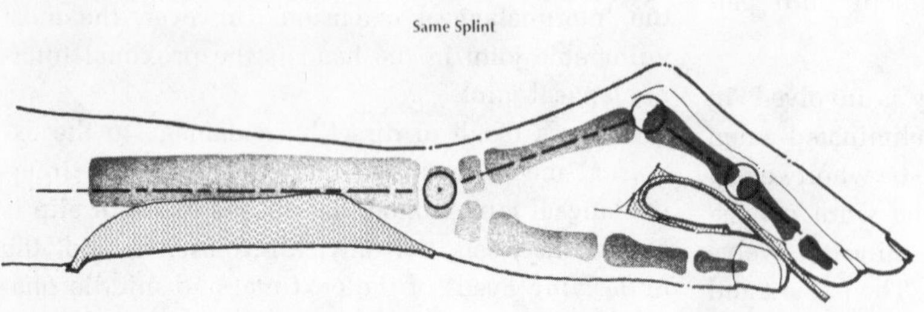

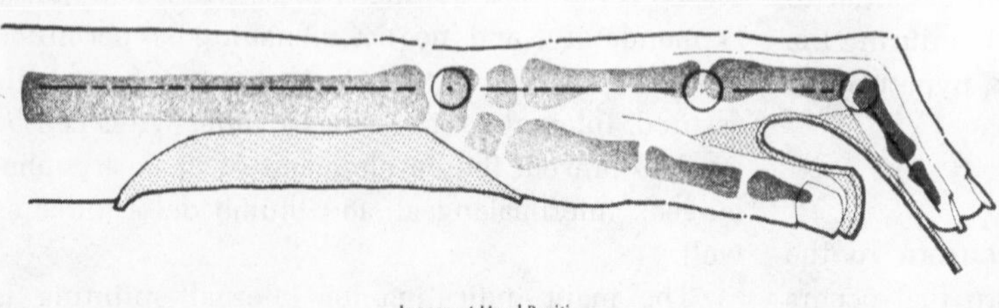

FIGURE 21-12. Burn functional hand splint. If the splint is allowed to slip forward a claw deformity can result.

destruction of a tendon from the burn or bacterial invasion. This most frequently occurs to the extensor mechanism over or just proximal to the proximal interphalangeal joint. Careful external splinting judiciously monitored can prevent the flexion deformity. If the flexion deformity is not corrected, the pull of the flexors, mainly the strong sublimis, will cause the proximal interphalangeal joint to flex often beyond the 90 degrees of flexion. Thumb adduction will also occur unless the thenar web space is maintained and the thumb placed in the position of abduction and opposition. Often direct pressure contour pan splinting is required to soften, stretch out, and oppose existing contractures (Fig. 21-13). Progressive contour pan splinting can stretch out an immature (pink) scar in order to reach maximum extension and motion in a joint.

Treatment Plan

When planning occupational therapy treatment the following factors must be considered: the depth of burn, location of burns, associated injuries, extent of total body injury, extent of injury to the hands, the age of the patient, and patient cooperation. Age is of particular importance. Most children are unable to understand or cooperate in a program of active motion but can understand carefully planned play and self-care activities. The hands of children can be splinted for prolonged periods without producing undue stiffness. Within a few days the full active range of motion can be reached even after numerous days of static splinting. Elderly patients often lack the strength or comprehension to carry out exercises for active motion, so careful splinting and monitoring must be instituted. Early self-care activities can provide the motivation for movement. The members of the burn team or hospital staff should encourage cooperation and repeatedly emphasize correct positioning and active motion. Staff and patient education must be an ongoing effort to aid in the prevention of deformity and to encourage early functional return.

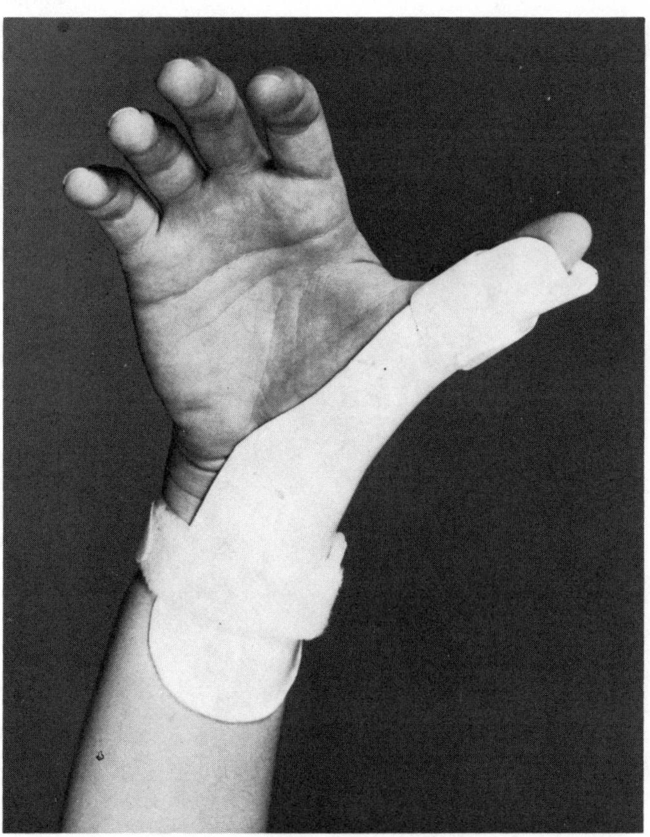

FIGURE 21-13. A pressure contour splint can correct deformity.

Palmar burns to the hand produce contractures and deformity pulling toward the location of the injury. Dorsal splinting or contoured palmar pan splints (Fig. 21-14) holding the hand in full extension should be considered. Wrist flexion contractures and deformities can easily arise with accompanying adduction and flexion contractures of the thumb.

Early self-care activities such as feeding and personal hygiene should be started as soon as the patient is medically stable. Sometimes adaptive devices may be needed but should not be used unless absolutely necessary. Many problems related to functional loss of joint motion and anatomical deformities can be alleviated through normal use of the extremities and activity. Strength will return in weakened and atrophic muscles, especially with early ambulation and normal daily movements of the body. Adhesions of tendons and surrounding structures will also be freed through continuing activities of daily living. Time is an important factor. Capsular structures, shortened by poor positioning or inactivity, can be stretched when appropriate activities are planned.

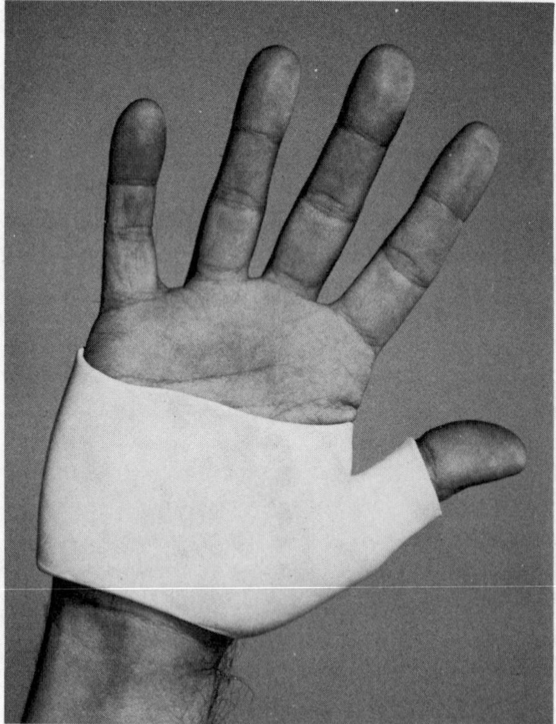

FIGURE 21-14. A palmar extension pan splint can be used to soften scar tissue and correct web space contractures.

The occupational therapist should work towards full self-care independence and increase in extremity function, physical endurance, and muscle strength. A homemaker checkout should be required to see if any additional training is required such as work simplification and energy conservation techniques. Bilateral activities should be stressed and easy-flow work patterns established. Self-care activities can be used as a form for therapeutic exercise.

Early ambulation with good posture should be encouraged. If extensive leg burns exist, wrapping with Ace bandages using the figure-eight technique may be indicated to alleviate pain caused by blood rushing to the lower extremities. If the patient has had skin grafts to the legs, bedrest must be maintained for ten days post-graft. Even though venous circulation has returned to the graft site and the graft appears stable, adequate arterial blood flow will take longer to become established. The patient may be allowed to stand and move about with Ace wraps after ten days to encourage ambulation and proper foot positioning to eliminate heel cord contractures. Pressure leg garments should be considered. Active motion in the form of exercise, self-care activities, planned activities, and ambulation will improve muscle strength, free adhesions, and stretch skin and joint structures.

Dynamic splinting may be required to do corrective positioning, to counterbalance flexion contractures, and to apply a slow traction pull. Splints are indicated when a metacarpophalangeal flexion deformity exists. Early adduction contracture of the thumb can be an indication for dynamic splinting. If the thumb contracture persists, resulting in the adduction deformity, early surgical intervention is often employed.

Contact axillary splinting in the form of an airplane splint is frequently indicated when anterior chest and shoulder burns exist. The airplane splint can be constructed out of reinforced Plastazote or low-temperature plastics with reinforcements. The shoulder should be maintained in 90 to 100 degrees abduction. Strapping will be required to maintain this position.

A variety of graded work and recreational activities can be programmed including leatherwork, weaving, and woodwork projects to increase range of motion, develop work tolerance, and increase personal independence.

Psychological Considerations

The emotional aspects of burn care deserve careful consideration because the patient suffers not only devastating physical trauma but also overwhelming psychological stress. The occupational therapist, as an active member of the burn team, will need to aid in the identification and management of these psychological problems. Age, personality, family support, and social and economic factors influence the manner in which the patient can handle his or her problems.

The fear of death is real for the burn patient when immobility, prolonged and intense pain, separation and isolation, loss of control over one's fate, and association with other dying patients exist. The fear of mutilation and disfigurement can be a traumatic experience, especially as body changes occur throughout the treatment process. Especially threatening are fears of disfigurement experienced by patients with facial burns. Genuine grief must be recognized as the patient faces discharge with the loss of an acceptable body image and fear of nonacceptance by the outside world.

The patient's self-perception has impact on the individual's personality, and feelings of hostility and grief can develop. The patient must also be able to cope with emotional stress not only in relation to feelings towards self but also in relation to feelings towards individuals and circumstances concerned with the accident.

Disruption of a life cycle and separation from the family circle can cause complex problems, especially if hospitalization is for any length of time. The patient may develop, as a substitute for familial emotional support, new methods for gaining gratification and reward.

The severely burned patient frequently is in conflict regarding dependency versus independency. Some patients find it difficult to accept forced dependency and to develop necessary trust relationships with others.

Prolonged hospitalization and convalescence put a strain on not only the patient but also the attending medical team. Each surgical procedure must be interpreted carefully. Strong anxiety in the patient must be recognized, especially in relation to the patient's perception and interpretation of the injuries as they relate to plans and future goals.

When massive burns exist the patient often has a hospital stay of more than ninety days and faces a longer term of continuing medical procedures. Many times these procedures are carried out in a rehabilitation unit or center. The rehabilitation facility is appropriate for aggressive rehabilitation. Transfer to a rehabilitation area also gives the patient a feeling of progress. A physical medicine evaluation should be made early in the acute care stage; management by a physiatrist in a rehabilitation center then can be recommended and planned.

Initially the therapist is involved as part of the burn team in the identification of physical and psychological problems and in planning management of those problems. Development of rapport and an interpersonal relationship between the therapist and the patient is of vital importance in the management of the patient. A kind but realistic approach will be most helpful to the patient in coping with numerous problems as they become apparent. The therapist can be effective by interpreting the problem realistically and reducing the patient's stress by providing sound emotional support. Much of the ongoing anxiety can be alleviated by giving the patient a sense of worth and by maintaining interpersonal relationships.

At the first encounter the therapist should introduce himself or herself to the patient, orient the patient to his or her environment, and interpret the therapist's role. During treatment the therapist aids the patient by explaining what procedures and treatments are necessary and by defining medical terms in lay terminology. In this way a sound rapport and respect can be developed between the patient and the therapist. Thus the patient can more easily express feelings and will be more amenable to reestablishing personal independence and cooperation throughout the longer phase of rehabilitation and scar maturation.

Counseling should be directed towards a return to normal activity as quickly as possible, with the importance of follow-up visits stressed. Often the family and friends must be counseled to aid them in interpreting and understanding the patient's reactions and feelings. This is especially true when there are feelings of grief or hostility.

Group therapy sessions are important for the psychological rehabilitation of the patient. In these sessions the patient should be allowed to openly express fears and anxieties. Here he or she can discuss possible solutions with others in the same situation. The social worker and psychologist should be members of group therapy sessions. The family should be included in discussions with the patient in order to discern ways of handling situations that it will encounter after the patient returns to the home, community, job, or school.

Nutrition

Nutrition must be carefully monitored and modified so that the catabolic phase of metabolism is corrected. The patient should be in positive nitrogen balance or anabolism, which promotes healing. This positive nitrogen balance is necessary and must be maintained through a high-caloric, high-protein diet. The patient must recognize that good nutrition with a well-balanced diet is necessary for tissue repair and maintenance of strength during the rehabilitation period.

Follow-Up Program

A schedule for close outpatient follow-up is necessary to check and maintain a good outpatient protocol. In this way scar maturation, joint problems, pressure garments, and need for reconstructive procedures can be monitored (Fig. 21-15). The social worker should be active in the outpatient program to monitor the home situation, provide home care services as needed, give emotional support, and provide for equipment and transportation needs. Should reconstructive surgery be indicated, whether it be functional or cosmetic, the patient must understand the need for the procedures and the need for time to pass before many of these procedures can be accomplished. The surgeon and the physiatrist work together to correct deformities in order that the patient may gain maximum function.

The most frequent areas of reconstruction are the webbing of the hands, thumb adduction, wrist flexion, axillary contractures, dorsal toe contracture, and posterior knee contractures. Children require the most reconstruction considerations because their scar tissue may not grow as rapidly as developing bone.

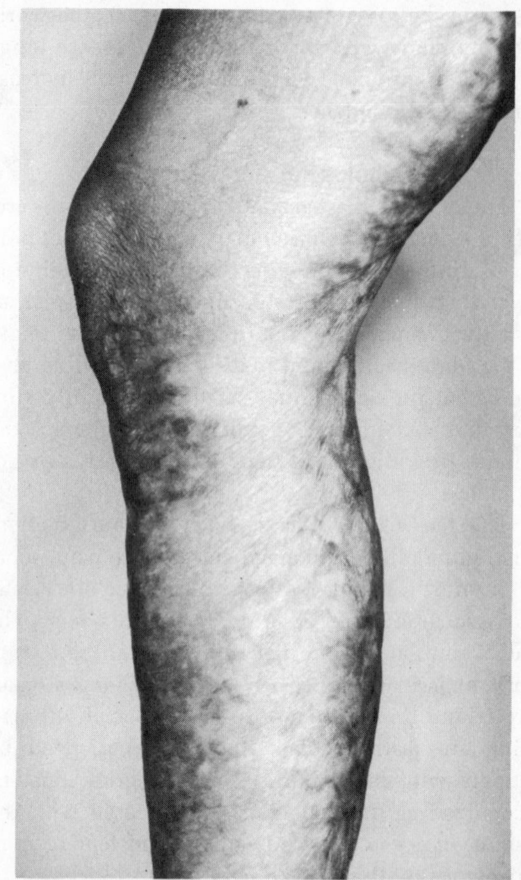

FIGURE 21-15. A blanched mature burn scar can be attained with proper pressure techniques on the burn scar areas. Close outpatient follow-up is necessary to maintain the schedule.

The American Society for Burns Recovered, Inc., is a national organization formed to aid burned individuals and their families to cope with ongoing problems. The national office is in Orange, New Jersey. Local chapters have been formed in most major cities where active burn units exist.

BIBLIOGRAPHY

Baebel, S., Bulkley, A. L., and Shuck, J. M.: Physical therapy for burned patients. J. Phys. Ther. 53:1289–1293, 1973.

Boswick, J. A., Jr.: The management of fresh burns of the hand and deformities resulting from burn injuries. Clin. Plastic Surg. 1:621–631, 1974.

Evans, E. B.: Orthopedic measures in the treatment of severe burns. J. Bone Joint Surg. 48:643–669, 1968.

Evans, E. B.: Preservation and restoration of joint function in patients with severe burns. J.A.M.A. 204:843–848, 1968.

Evans, E. B.: Prevention and correction of deformity after severe burns. Surg. Clin. N. Am. 50:1361, 1970.

Evans, E. B., et al.: Prevention and correction of deformity after severe burns. Surg. Clin. N. Am. 50:1361–1375, 1970.

Feller, I. T., Archambeault, C., Jones, C.: Procedures for Nursing the Burned Patient. Dexter MI: Press of Thomson-Shore Inc., 1975.

Goldberg, R. T.: Rehabilitation of the burned patient. Rehab. Lit. 35:73–77, 1974.

Jaeger, D. L.: Maintenance and function of the burned patient. J. Phys. Ther. 52:627–633, 1972.

Kischer, C. W., Shetlar, M. R., and Shetlar, C. L.: Alteration of hypertrophic scars induced by mechanical pressure. Arch. Dermatology 111:60–64, 1975.

Larson, D. L.: Repair of the boutonniere deformity of the burned hand. J. Trauma 10:6, 1970.

Larson, D. L.: The Prevention and Correction of Burn Scar Contracture and Hypertrophy. Pamphlet, Shriners Burns Institute, Galveston Unit, Texas, 1973.

Larson, D. L., et al.: Development and correction of burn scar contracture. In Matter, P. (ed.): Transactions of the Third International Congress on Research in Burns. Prague, 1970.

Larson, D. L., et al.: Skeletal suspension and traction in the treatment of burns. Ann. Surgery 168:981–985, 1968.

Larson, D. L., et al.: Techniques for decreasing scar formation and contractures in the burned patient. J. Trauma 11:807–823, 1971.

Lavore, J. S., and Marshalls, J. H.: Expedient splint of the burn patient. J. Phys. Ther. 52:1036–1042, 1972.

Linares, H. A.: Granulation tissue and hypertrophic scars. In International Symposium and Workshop on the Relation of Ultrastruction of Collagen to the Healing of Wounds and the Surgical Management of Hypertrophic Scars. Cincinnati OH, 1973.

Linares, H. A., et al.: On the origin of the hypertrophic scar. J. Trauma 13:70–75, 1973.

Linares, H. A., et al.: The histiocytic organization of hypertrophic scar in humans. J. Investigative Derm. 59:323–331, 1972.

MacMillan, B. G.: Burns in children. Clin. Plastic Surg. 1:633–643, 1974.

Malick, M.: Manual on Dynamic Hand Splinting. Harmarville Rehabilitation Center, Pittsburgh PA, 1974.

Malick, M., and Carr, J.: Monograph on Burn Management. American Occupational Therapy Association, Rockville MD. In press.

Shetlar, M. E., et al.: The hypertrophic scar, hexosamine containing components of burn scars. Proc. Soc. Exp. Biol. Med. 139:544–547, 1972.

Shetlar, M. E., et al.: The hypertrophic scar, glycoprotein, and collagen components of burn scars. Proc. Soc. Exp. Biol. Med. 138:298–300, 1971.

Tanigawa, M. P. C., O'Donnell, O. K., and Graham, P. L.: The burned hand—a physical therapy protocol. J. Phys. Ther. 54:953–958, 1974.

Von Prince, K. M. P., Currerri, P. W., and Pruitt, B. A.: The application of finger nail hooks in splinting of burned hands. Am. J. Occup. Ther. 24:156–159, 1970.

Von Prince, K. M. P., and Yeakel, M. H.: The Splinting of Burn Patients. Springfield IL: Charles C Thomas, Publishers, 1974.

Willis, B.: Burn Scar Therapy—A Treatment Method. Pamphlet from Jobst Institute Inc., Toledo OH, 1973.

Willis, B.: Custom splinting the burn patient. In Lynch, J. P., and Lewis, S. R. (ed.): Symposium on the Treatment of Burns. St. Louis: C. V. Mosby Co., 1973, pp. 93–97.

Willis, B.: Splinting the Burned Patient. Galveston: Shriners Burns Institute. Pamphlet distributed by Johnson & Johnson, New Brunswick, NJ, 1971.

Willis, B.: The use of orthoplast isoprene splints in the treatment of the acutely burned child: A follow-up. Am. J. Occup. Ther. 24:3, 1970.

RESOURCES

American Burn Association
(William W. Monafo, M.D.
St. John's Mercy Hospital
615 South New Ballas Road
St. Louis MO 63141)
(maintains an active office providing a full range of educational, medical, research, and patient referral services)

American Society for Burns Recovered, Inc.
439 Main Street
Orange, New Jersey 07050

Jobst Institute
653 Miami Street
Toledo, Ohio 43694

(visual aids and educational material)

22
Hand Rehabilitation

L. Irene Hollis

Rehabilitation of the hand is not only a specialty area in its own right, but it is also touched upon in all aspects of occupational therapy. Patients with physical disabilities of the upper extremities are treated through the use of manual tasks, as are patients with psychosocial problems. The often quoted statement from Reilly's Eleanor Clark Slagle lecture: "Man, through the use of his hands, can influence the state of his health,"[1] is borne out in clinical practice. The blind become dependent upon the use of their hands and latent skills must be fully developed. The deaf communicate with sign language which requires finger agility. From pediatrics to geriatrics hand activities are utilized in treatment because the patient becomes involved in "doing" rather than "having things done to."

ANATOMY OF THE HAND

Basic to the therapist's utilization of hand activities is the understanding of the anatomy of the hand and arm. The usual course in anatomy at school is geared to cover general information, so special effort must be made to learn the details of hand anatomy. This can be done in several ways. There is no better way to do this than to dissect a fresh specimen, but this is not always available. Another avenue for learning is observation of surgical procedures of the hand, which is quite beneficial. There are also well done audiovisual aids. The 16 millimeter movie *Functional Anatomy of the Hand*,[2] made by a plastic surgeon, is a classic in this field. Another classic is the December 1951 issue of the Ciba Clinical Symposia *Surgical Anatomy of the Hand*.[3] This small booklet has a fine text and the drawings by Frank Netter are of special benefit. This issue has been reprinted several times.

Not only should the therapist be knowledgeable concerning specifics of hand antomy, but he or she can also inform patients of their condition. The Ciba booklet provides schematic drawings which can be shown to the patient to illustrate involved structures. The more the patient knows and understands about the injury or condition, the more cooperative the patient may be in carrying out the treatment program. It has been said that patients have to rehabilitate themselves. The therapist can lay out a course but it is the patient who must direct efforts so that maximal improvement will ensue.

The patient's comprehension of the extent of injury to the structures and the value of the diverse therapy routines is fundamental to the treatment. The hand surgeon usually explains details to the patient, but it is not until the therapy program gets underway that the average patient starts asking questions and really understands the scope of the problem. The time spent in informing the patient of pertinent details is well invested. Various models of hand anatomy can be used, but demonstrations of surface anatomy (directions of muscle pull and bulk of contracting muscles) on yourself or another patient are especially valuable.

A clinic in which a number of patients are undergoing hand rehabilitation serves as an excellent laboratory. Usually there is more than one patient with a similar injury. The therapist needs to be available to clarify points at times, but the value of having patients with similar problems at different stages of their recovery being exposed to one another is inestimable. Colored photographs need to be taken from time to time since these can be used to show to a patient in the event no similar case is available.

REFERRAL CRITERIA

When setting up a hand rehabilitation program, just what categories of patients the program will accept should be spelled out. As a general rule any person may be referred to occupational therapy for hand rehabilitation who exhibits one or more of the following conditions of the hand or arm as a result of congenital, traumatic, pathological, or psychological causes:

1. Limited joint range of motion
2. Limited strength or endurance
3. Incoordination and limited dexterity
4. Sensory impairment
5. Physiological amputation of the entire hand or any part thereof
6. Edema
7. Impairment resulting from disfigurement
8. Definite potential for developing any of the above conditions

EVALUATION PROCEDURES

The moment a patient appears in the occupational therapy clinic the therapist can start evaluating by *observing* the patient's use of his or her hands. To understand the disabled hand one must know the normal one. There are individual variations but the position of function is one that calls for wrist dorsiflexion or extension so that (1) the opposed thumb is in line with the radius and (2) the second and third metacarpals, under control of the extensor carpi radialis longus and brevis muscles, are extended about 45 degrees. The two ulnar metacarpals are not extended as much, and this is one reason there is a transverse arch of the hand (Fig. 22-1).

The injured hand is frequently held with the thumb and the two ulnar metacarpals in as much extension as the stable second and third ones. The common digital extensor tendons are called into action to lift the two ulnar metacarpals. These tendons also extend the fourth and fifth metacarpophalangeal (MP) joints, and, as a result, the palmar arch is flattened and a clawhand results. This position (Fig. 22-2) is nonfunctional and should be brought to the attention of the patient so that he or she can relax the thumb and the ulnar extensors and let the fingers fall into the amount of flexion that occurs when the viscoelastic quality of the flexor profundus tendons is unopposed by active extensor pull.

The patient may hold the injured hand motionless. This is unnatural and suggests that the patient may experience pain on motion or has "psychologically amputated" the hand. Hands are connected intimately with our mental processes. Normally a constant stream of sensory impulses pass from the hand to the brain and coordinated motor impulses are

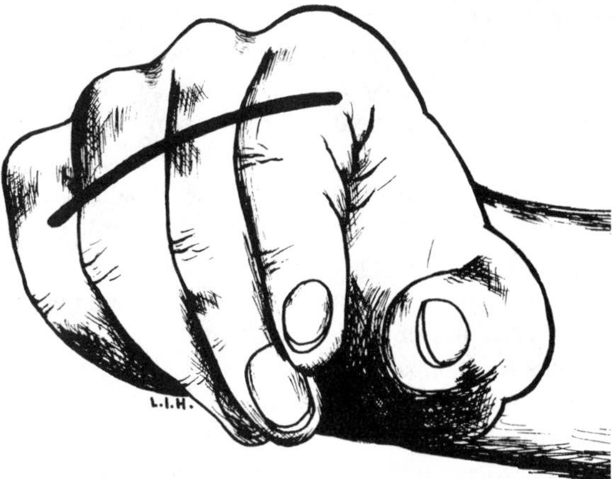

FIGURE 22-1. The functional position of a hand. Note the transverse metacarpal or palmar arch.

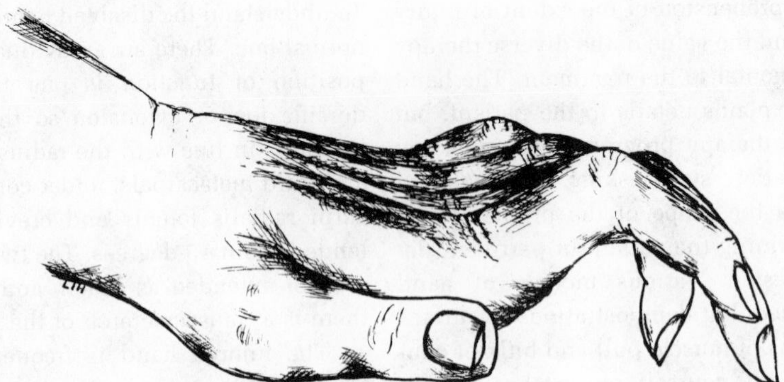

FIGURE 22-2. A nonfunctional position of the hand. The transverse metacarpal arch is flattened.

transmitted from the brain to the hand in response. At times a particular injury or disease process interrupts this pathway so that no impulses are transmitted. This is a physiological state. However, in numerous cases, there is no obvious pathology to account for the lack of transmission of impulses. Instead it may be due to inhibition, usually at a subconscious level, on the part of the patient who has disassociated the injured hand from control by the brain. Such a disassociation can be overcome through purposeful activities in occupational therapy, and the sooner a program is initiated the easier it is to reverse this unhealthy state.

If the protective position is a result of pain the therapy program should be directed toward decreasing the pain. Application of a supportive splint is sometimes effective or the use of heat or cold might help. Both thermal modalities are effective in many cases. The therapist must find the process most beneficial to the patient and instruct in the application of it or, better, suggest daily activities that will incorporate use of one or the other. A patient with arthritis may work in more comfort if hot air from a hair dryer is directed toward the hands. How often washing dishes in warm soapy water is therapeutic!

The therapist may also have to institute a program of sensory bombardment to alter the threshold at which one is able to tolerate stimuli. Very often a patient who has had a crushing injury may have hypersensitivity throughout the hand. Small sensory nerves are involved and, when the bandage is first removed, the initial response to touch or contact is one of pain. As long as the injured hand is wrapped in a bulky bandage there is little or no sensory input and this period of sensory deprivation may lower the patient's pain threshold to the extent that he or she is unable to tolerate having a therapist evaluate joint range of motion. The therapist should start the bombardment by having the patient rub gently over the entire surface of the hand with a soft material, then rub more vigorously and introduce rougher textures. A tool that vibrates is another way of producing sensory bombardment. The patient can respond very rapidly to such stimuli and even during the first treatment session there may be enough improvement to tolerate the therapist conducting the initial evaluation.

The hour invested in a thorough evaluation is time well spent.[4] A formal study should be done initially and this can serve as a baseline. The sample Hand Evaluation is used at the Hand Rehabilitation Center, Chapel Hill, N.C. All or portions of the evaluation should be repeated at intervals to document losses, gains, or areas in which no changes are measurable. Such evaluations are time consuming but they provide the opportunity to become better acquainted with the patient and to learn as much as possible about the type of condition and the resultant decreases in active as well as passive ranges of motion and strength of pinch and grasp. An assessment should be made concerning the areas on the skin of the hand where there is total absence of sensibility and areas that are near normal or hypersensitive to touch. These areas are recorded on the outlines of the hands on the Hand Evaluation Chart.

HAND EVALUATION*

NCMH Unit Number: ______________________ Patient Name ______________________

y=yes; n=no I. Functional Activity	Date: Eval. by:				Date: Eval. by:				Date: Eval. by:				Date: Eval. by:				Date: Eval. by:			
	I	L	R	F	I	L	R	F	I	L	R	F	I	L	R	F	I	L	R	F
A. Key pinch by digit																				
B. Pulp to pulp pinch by digit																				
C. Gross grip FN–PPC (cm)																				
D. Gross grip (mm Hg)																				
E. Pinch grip (lb)																				
F. Pick up a pencil																				
G. Write with a pencil																				
H. Button the button																				
I. Open, close safety pin																				
J. Comb hair																				
K. Use a drinking glass																				
II. Volume Measurement	Norm = Invol. =				Norm = Invol. =				Norm = Invol. =				Norm = Invol. =				Norm = Invol. =			
III. Pain: Ask the patient to describe his pain and record area, resting or in motion, severity (none, mild, moderate, severe)																				

IV. Sensory Evaluation

A. Using light touch. Record yes or no in each of the areas.

B. Coin identification.

C. If sensory deficit is evident, do ninhydrin test and attach record.

R L R L

Date:__________

R L R L.

Date:__________

R L R L

Date:__________

R L R L

Date:__________

R L R L

Date:__________

* Printed with permission of Hand Rehabilitation Center, Chapel Hill, N.C.

HAND EVALUATION *(Continued)*

V. Joint range of motion

		Date:												
			Act.	Pass.	Act.	Pass.	Act.	Pass.	Act.	Pass.	Act.	Pass.	Act.	Pass.
Index:	MP	Ext.												
		Flex.												
	PIP	Ext.												
		Flex.												
	DIP	Ext.												
		Flex.												
Long	MP	Ext.												
		Flex.												
	PIP	Ext.												
		Flex.												
	DIP	Ext.												
		Flex.												
Ring	MP	Ext.												
		Flex.												
	PIP	Ext.												
		Flex.												
	DIP	Ext.												
		Flex.												
Fifth:	MP	Ext.												
		Flex.												
	PIP	Ext.												
		Flex.												
	DIP	Ext.												
		Flex.												

HAND EVALUATION *(Continued)*

		Date:												
			Act.	Pass.	Act.	Pass.	Act.	Pass.	Act.	Pass.	Act.	Pass.	Act.	Pass.
Thumb:	MP	Ext.												
		Flex.												
	IP	Ext.												
		Flex.												
	MC	Abd.												
Wrist:		Ext.												
		Flex.												
Forearm:		Sup.												
		Pro.												
Elbow:		Ext.												
		Flex.												

During the evaluation period the occupational therapist keeps in mind the splinting requirements that will need to be met. The therapist should check for extrinsic, intrinsic, and Landsmeer's ligament tightness. Bunnel[5] introduced these tests many years ago and they help to determine some of the reasons for poor hand function. Considering what motion the muscle group being evaluated performs, the evaluator, in administering these tests, starts with the proximal joint affected and moves that joint in the opposite direction. The evaluator then attempts to move the next more distal joint into the position opposite that which muscle action would be expected to produce.

In testing for extrinsic tightness (Fig. 22-3) the evaluator desires to find out whether the patient's inability to flex the metacarpophalangeal (MP) and interphalangeal (IP) joints simultaneously is due to adhesions along the finger extensor tendons on the dorsum of the hand or whether it is due to limitations within the joints. As the test is administered the MP joint is passively flexed and attempt is made to move the proximal interphalangeal (PIP) joint into flexion. If the PIP joint will not passively flex, the pressure on the MP joint is relaxed and the evaluator again attempts to flex the PIP joint. If this can be done easily the extensor tendon must be adherent along its course on the dorsum of the hand and it is only when slack is allowed in the tendon across the MP joint that the PIP joint can flex. If one is unable to flex the PIP joint regardless of the position of the MP joint, then one surmises that the problem is one of PIP joint stiffness resulting from articular pathology rather than extrinsic tightness.

Intrinsic tightness results in an "intrinsic plus" deformity with the MP joints in flexion and the PIP joints in extension. In the early stages of intrinsic tightness the evaluator can detect evidence of it by moving the finger into extension at the MP joint and then attempting to flex the PIP joint (Fig. 22-4).

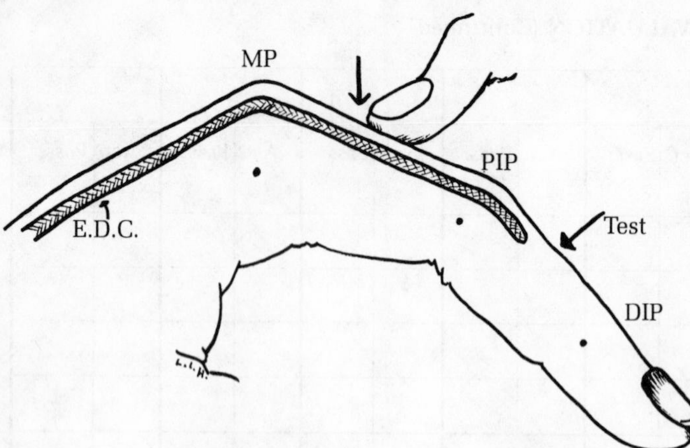

FIGURE 22-3. Test position for extrinsic tightness.

If there is more resistance when the finger is in this test position than when the MP joint is flexed and the PIP joint is also flexed, intrinsic muscle tightness is suspected. This would influence decisions regarding splinting the hand structures.

The third in this series of tests is one called Landsmeer's ligament tightness testing (Fig. 22-5). Milford, in his book on the ligaments of the hand,[6] shows excellent photographs of Landsmeer's ligament (oblique retinacular ligament). This is only a ligament, not a tendon; it is the sole identified structure which crosses *only* the PIP and distal interphalangeal (DIP) joints. It does not cross the MP joint, and so the position of the MP joint has no direct effect upon the test. A finger that has had disruption of the extensor hood and tendon over the PIP joint goes into a boutonniére deformity (Fig. 22-6). The lateral bands slip down volar to the axis of rotation at the PIP joint and when the intrinsic muscles contract to put tension on these lateral bands they pull the joint into more flexion rather than extending it, and the DIP joint goes into more hyperextension. This can be accounted for in two ways since the patient frequently rests his or her fingertips on a flat surface and attempts to pull the finger into an extended position. The patient does not accomplish PIP extension but does force the DIP joint into hyperextension. Once the DIP joint goes beyond zero degrees or into some hyperextension, the lateral band has a more direct pull on its insertion on the distal phalanx and, as a result, the finger goes into even more hyperextension at the DIP joint. Landsmeer's ligament originates on the volar-lateral aspect of the proximal phalanx, runs volar to the axis of rotation at the PIP joint, but joins the lateral bands as they cross the middle phalanx and run dorsal to the axis of rotation of the DIP joint. The ligament joins the lateral bands as they insert on the dorsum of the distal

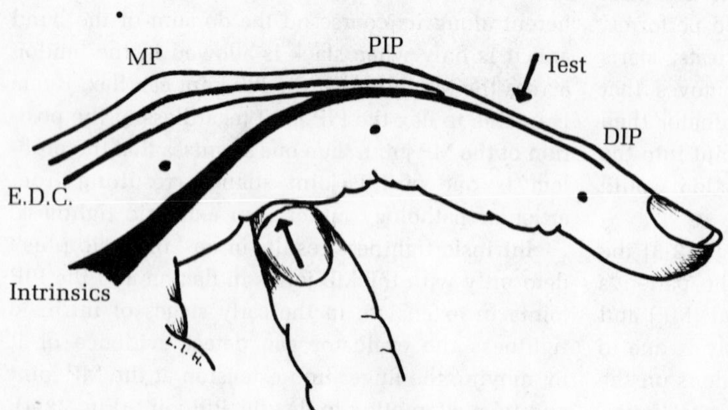

FIGURE 22-4. Test for intrinsic muscle tightness.

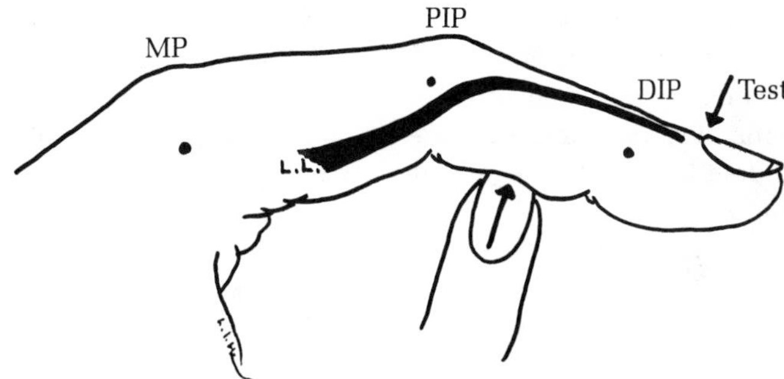

FIGURE 22-5. Test for Landsmeer's ligament tightness.

phalanx. The presence of Landsmeer's ligament tightness complicates a boutonniére deformity since it may become fibrotic in a relaxed, shortened position and there is inability to flex the DIP joint when attempting to extend the PIP joint fully. In fact the patient may be unable to get the DIP joint down to neutral when the PIP joint is in extension. In treating any boutonniére deformity one should check for Landsmeer's ligament tightness and initiate a splinting program if there is any evidence that the DIP joint cannot be flexed when the PIP joint is in extension but can be flexed when the PIP joint is flexed. The position of the MP joint is immaterial since the ligament does not cross that joint. The test position can be compared to the position for intrinsic tightness (see Fig. 22–4) if one moves distal one joint so as to move the PIP joint into extension and attempts are made to place the DIP joint into flexion.

One other important evaluation procedure is measurement of edema. One can compare the normal to the injured hand and either a water displacement method can be applied[7] or a tape can be used to check the circumference of a finger or arm. Edema can be quite pernicious when it accumulates in the hand since the serous fluid, rich in fibrin, can cause the small finger joints to stiffen very rapidly. One has to consider the reduction of edema a high-priority goal.

GOALS IN REHABILITATION

The most practical goal that can be set is that of achieving a functional hand for the patient. The patient must be involved in the setting of goals since he or she knows what vocational and avocational pursuits require, must put forth the most effort to reach the goals, and has to live with the results of rehabilitation efforts. The therapy and medical members of the team must add input to help keep the goals in line with the reality of the situation. Surgery is not indicated in many instances, so the burden of restoration of adequate joint motion falls to the therapists who apply conservative approaches to get improved flexion, extension, abduction, adduction, as the case demands.

One important way in which occupational therapists have contributed to the conservative approach is by designing and fabricating splints. Many of the splints are *supportive* in design since some joints need to be held in a certain position to allow healing to take place in the soft tissues about the joints, or to allow a fracture to be immobilized. In some instances painful hands are made more comfortable with supportive splints.

Corrective splints can be static or dynamic. Usually dynamic splints are more effective since a small amount of force can be exerted by rubberbands or springs over a long period of time similar to the way orthodontic appliances can accomplish so much. Such dynamic splints can be made to get wrists back into an extended position so that finger

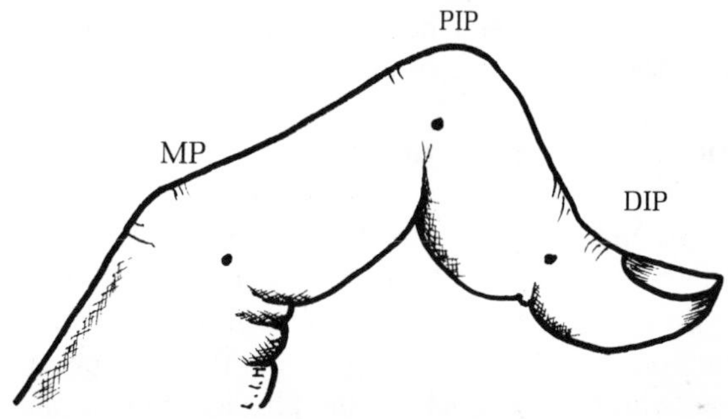

FIGURE 22-6. Boutonniére deformity.

flexors can work more advantageously. Gradual force from a specifically designed splint can gain flexion or extension of an elbow or supination or pronation of a forearm. The amount of force required to move the large joints may be great, but for the small joints of the fingers it is minimal. Caution should be emphasized here since this small force must be applied quite close to the joint axis of rotation to avoid damaging the joint surfaces in the event there are adhesions causing compromise of the gliding motion of the joint.

Some dynamic splints offer resistance to the pull of the tendons. This can be applied when one wishes to strengthen muscles which have the potential for developing a more powerful pull. A small amount of resistance often enables a patient to get a better sense of muscle action. Flexor motion, for instance, may be initiated if a dynamic splint supplies a very gentle extension pull on the fingers. The dynamic force can be used assistively also to aid a patient by augmenting a small amount of active motion. The therapist must closely supervise the patient in the use of dynamic splints since the patient may "fight" the pull of the splint and increase the imbalance between the weak muscle that should be assisted and the stronger muscle that already overpowers the weak one.

The patient may need modifications of the devices used in activities of daily living as well as tools used at work. The occupational therapist can supply these *adaptive* devices. Many of them must be individually designed and can be fabricated in the clinic.

SPECIFIC INVOLVEMENT

Peripheral Nerve Injuries

Many peripheral nerves have two components: sensory and motor components.

Median Nerve Involvement

Of the three major nerves influencing the hand, wrist, and forearm the *median nerve* usually is considered to be the most important one. Its importance is due to the sensory component and its motor function on the intrinsic muscles of the thumb. Specialists who have worked out the physical impairment ratings, which are used in practice to determine what monetary compensation is due a person who was injured on the job, declare that a hand that lacks median sensibility has a 75 percent disability. This is based on sensory loss alone. The hand that lacks tactile sensibility in the thumb and index finger does not function normally. Patients do not know without looking when they hold an article between these numb fingertips, and so they often drop the items held. They lack coordination since they have no position sense. They are unaware of sharp edges and hot surfaces and may inadvertently injure the hand. A burn or cut does not heal easily since the circulation to an insensitive finger is compromised.

One responsibility of the occupational therapist is to instruct the patient in protective measures so the patient will use the eyes to substitute for the absent sense of touch. People who lose their sense of touch gradually due to a disease process such as diabetes or leprosy adjust to this loss and can continue to function quite normally. It is the patient who suffers a total loss instantly from trauma that is unable to adjust. Surgeons repair the severed nerve but seldom does the patient regain perfect cutaneous sensibility. Sensory nerves are so complex in function that with an average repair the patient may get return of protective sensation only. The patient can avoid burning or cutting the hand but lacks the highly discriminatory sensibility that enables him or her to perform finely coordinated activities. A good program of sensory reeducation does improve the ability to function and thus should be instituted as early as possible.[8]

If the motor component of the median nerve is cut at or near the wrist the result is loss of ability to abduct and oppose the thumb. Without these movements the thumb is held close to the palm and when one attempts to circumduct the thumb across the palm so that it can touch the small finger tip-to-tip it slides instead flatly across the palm and the thumb and small fingernails touch. One is unable to position the thumb so as to reach around a glass, for instance. If the nerve is repaired successfully at the wrist level, nerve regrowth will take place at about 1 millimeter a day or an inch each month. Therefore, within three to six months the thenar muscles should be showing some signs of reinnervation.

During this period of waiting for evidence of regeneration of the nerve, the occupational therapist should apply a protective splint to hold the thumb in the functional position described previously. If the thumb is permitted to be pulled into extension by the muscles innervated by the intact radial nerve, the small muscles which make up the thenar group will be on stretch and will not function well even if the median nerve does regenerate. If the hand is splinted so that the thumb is in front of the index finger and some type of C-shaped spacer or dynamic pull is used to hold the first and second metacarpals apart, the patient can make functional use of the index and long fingers to pinch against the thumb. Any number of activities are then possible for the patient and a somewhat normal pattern of hand use can be maintained.

This preservation of purposeful use of the hand during recovery is a significant contribution in itself. Habit pattern pathways account for one's ability to automatically maneuver items between the fingers and perform coordinated tasks. Some of this automaticity is compromised because of the decrease in tactile sensibility but, by supplying the patient with a carefully designed splint which positions the thumb without interfering with the active motion in the index and long finger, one can expect a far better outcome from a median nerve injury. The therapist should be alert to any poor habit patterns or positions of the thumb that will be detrimental.

Ulnar Nerve Involvement

An ulnar nerve injury does not cause quite as great an effect on the sensibility of the hand as a median nerve injury, but the motor loss is far greater. The sensory status of the surface of the ulnar palm plus the volar small finger and half of the ring finger is involved when the volar digital branch of the ulnar nerve is severed. If the dorsal branch of the ulnar nerve, which takes a separate path proximal to the wrist, is severed the entire dorsum of the ulnar half of the hand plus the dorsum of the entire small finger and half of the ring finger are anesthetic. The dorsal branch is injured less often than the volar branch and the presence of adequate sensation on the back and side of the small finger helps to serve as protection against burns and cuts on that side, even though the volar sensory branch may be severed.

The major involvement in the hand from an ulnar nerve injury is the result of the motor loss. Muscles that originate distal to the wrist are called intrinsic muscles. Three fourths of the intrinsic muscles of the hand are innervated by the ulnar nerve. Not only are the intrinsic muscles that make up the hypothenar group on the ulnar side of the palm innervated by the ulnar nerve but also the four dorsal interossei, the three palmar interossei, and the lumbricals to the ring and small fingers. The huge thumb adductor which originates on the third metacarpal and inserts on the proximal phalanx of the thumb has ulnar nerve supply as well as the deep belly of the flexor pollicis brevis muscle. Every digit suffers from loss of the ulnar motor supply. Loss of the adductor power of the thumb is quite disabling to an individual, and the thumb often collapses at the MP joint into what is known as Froment's position (Fig. 22-7). Without the mediating influence of the interossei the fingers are at the mercy of the extrinsic flexors and extensors (those that have their muscle bellies in the forearm with only the tendons running across the wrist and inserting on various phalanges). Without the regulating pull of the interossei, the fingers collapse into a claw position (see Fig. 22-2). Without

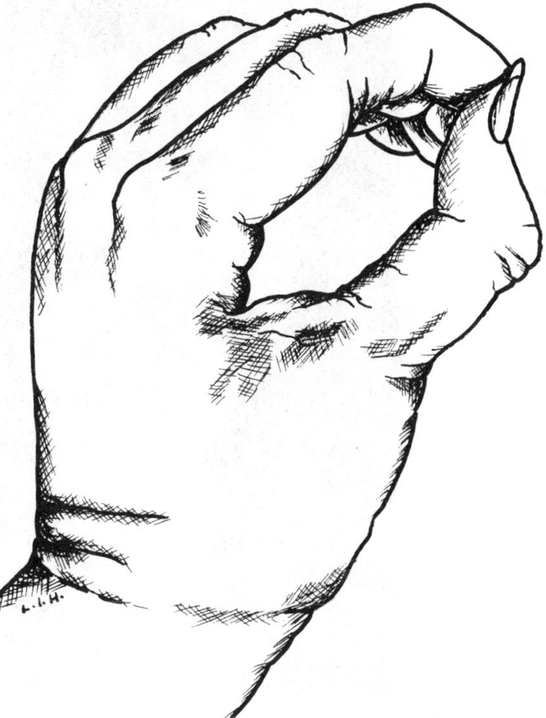

FIGURE 22-7. Froment's sign in the thumb.

early intervention through splinting, this dysfunctional position results in harmful contractures. The hyperextended MP joints allow the collateral ligaments on each side of the joints to become fibrotic in a shortened position so that it becomes impossible, through passive or active motion, to have the proximal phalanx glide around the head of its metacarpal. Early application of a simple MP flexion splint (Fig. 22-8) keeps the collateral ligaments elongated and provides an additional force, even though it is an outside force, that enables the central slips of the common extensor tendons to act on the proximal interphalangeal joints rather than having all of their power exerted to extend or hyperextend the MP joints.

Throughout the waiting period to see whether the repair of the ulnar nerve has been successful and whether the interossei will be reinnervated, the occupational therapist should examine the patient at regular times from two to four weeks apart to check on progress, to repair the splints and modify them if necessary, and to reinforce functional patterns. Sensory reeducation can be applied as well as neuromuscular facilitation techniques. When there is evidence of return of some motor activity the patient should be examined by the therapist more often and provided with meaningful activities which will reinforce use of the minimal motion as it becomes available to the patient. At this time the significance of not over-using and abusing the returning motor functions is just as important as the carefully guided use of these functions. The skills of the therapist are very important in this phase of therapy. For example, there may be a need to devise specific pieces of

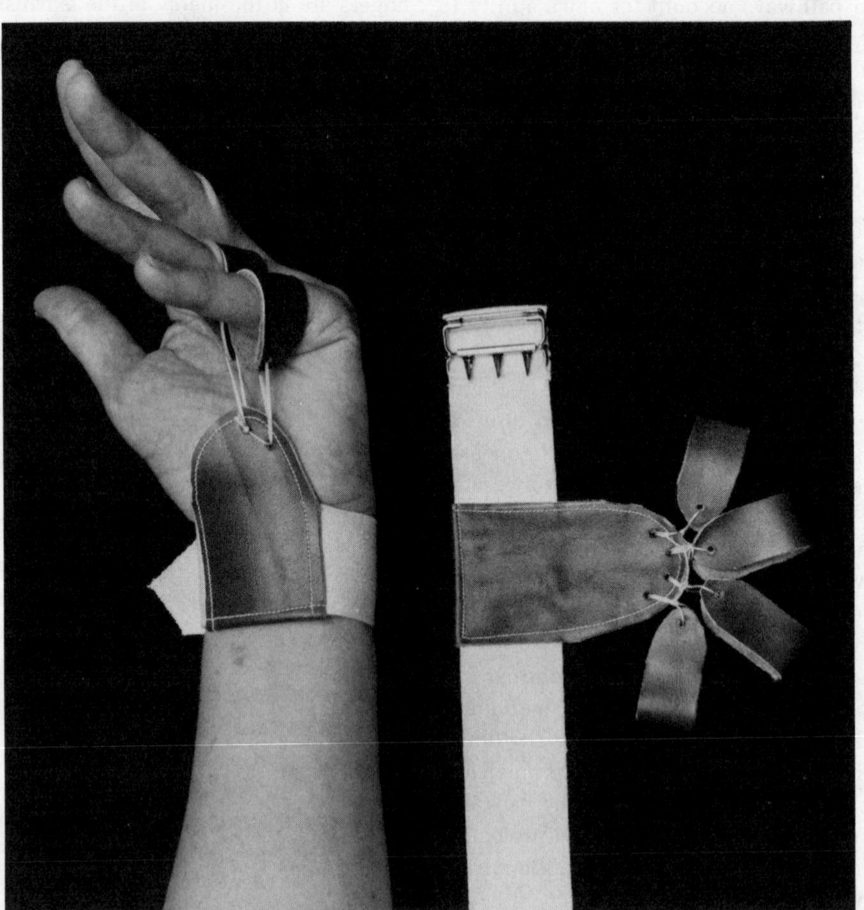

FIGURE 22-8. Simple anti-claw splint. It is used on only two fingers when there is an ulnar nerve injury but on all four when both the median and ulnar nerves are involved.

equipment which the patient can use to strengthen the interossei by flexing the MP joints so the proximal phalanges contact a surface without having the PIP and DIP joints flex. The patient might participate in a leather lacing project and hold the lacing between proximal phalanges and the platform portion of the device worn (Fig. 22-9). Repetitive actions involving simultaneous MP flexion and IP joint extension are beneficial to the patient who is trying to strengthen the intrinsic muscles as they are being reinnervated.

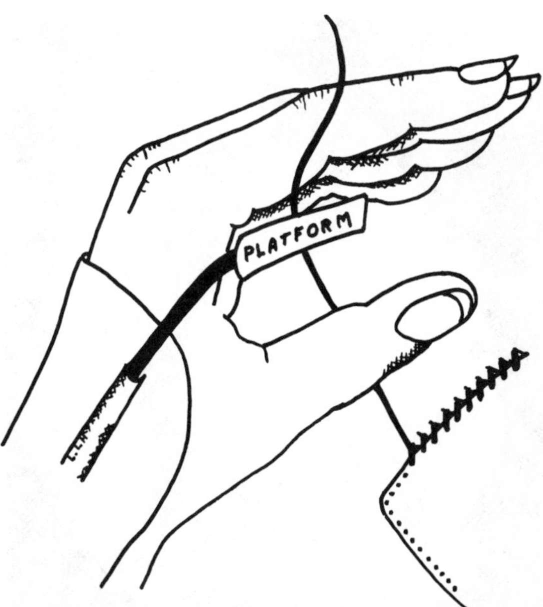

FIGURE 22-9. A splint for use on a patient who is learning to contract the intrinsic muscles to flex the metacarpophalangeal joint and extend the interphalangeal joints. The patient can do leather lacing by having the proximal phalanges contact the platform and hold the lacing.

Combined Median and Ulnar Nerve Involvement

When both median and ulnar nerves are lost the resultant condition is difficult for the patient to tolerate. The total loss of sensibility discourages use of the hand and the motor deficits make it impossible to pinch or grasp. With the thumb and fingers going into hyperextension at the proximal joints and full flexion at the distal joints it is impossible for the thumb to contact the fingertips to pinch. Some lateral pinch or "key pinch" is possible with the thumb contacting the side of the index finger, but this is ineffective except for turning a key in a lock. It can be used for some dressing activities but should be discouraged since it increases the possibility of adduction contracture of the thumb. A splint similar to the one shown in Figure 22-10 holds the thumb in abduction and maintains the MP joints of the fingers in enough flexion to permit the use of the common extensors to extend the IP joints. The position of pinch is reestablished but, since there is no cutaneous sensibility, the patient must be taught to watch closely to avoid damaging the fingertips. Joint mobility can be maintained and the patient will have a more useful hand when the nerve regeneration restores sensibility and muscle function or when tendon transfers are done surgically in the event motor nerve regeneration is insufficient.

Radial Nerve Involvement

The radial nerve must be injured at or above the elbow to have its injury totally affect the hand in the motor realm. There is a branch of the radial sensory nerve which traverses the forearm and is superficial along the distal dorsal border of the radius. This sensory nerve supplies about half of the dorsum of the hand and as far as the PIP joint on the dorsum of the radial digits. Loss of sensation over this area is not disabling; however, an injury to this dorsal sensory branch can cause a pain syndrome that is devastating. Particular attention should be paid to this trigger area and efforts should be made to relieve the discomfort if possible by desensitizing techniques before it reaches a proportion that interferes with functional use of the forearm and hand.

The motor branch of the radial nerve spirals around the lateral, distal third of the humerus and is frequently involved in "Saturday night paralysis" or other compression injuries in this area. As a result of the radially innervated wrist, finger, and thumb extensors' being at least temporarily denervated, the ability to hold the wrist in an extended position is lost so that the grip strength is greatly diminished. There is no way to actively extend the fingers at the MP joint, so patients resort to use of the intrinsic muscles which flex the MP joints even though they do extend the IP joints. A simple splint made from brass welding rod with leather finger cuffs and a wrist and forearm strap (Fig. 22-11) can give support

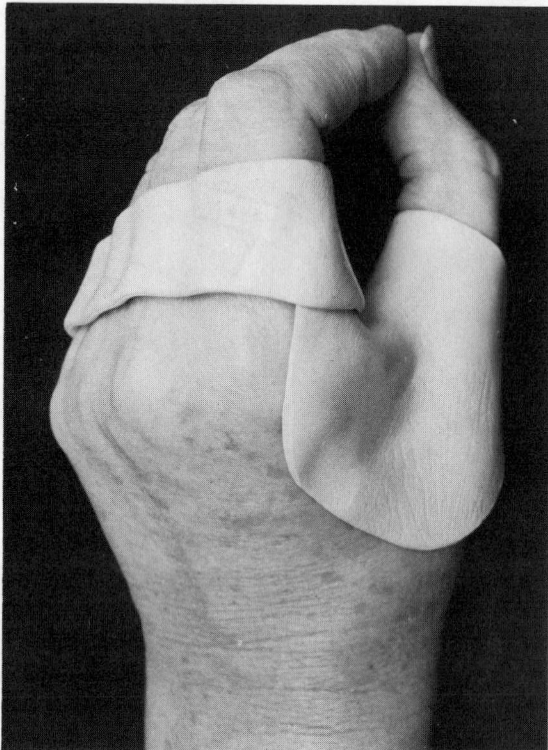

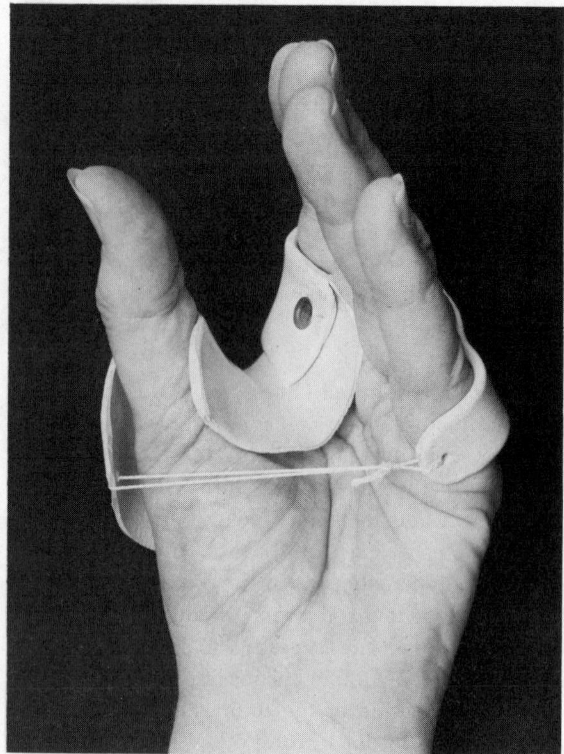

FIGURE 22-10. Two views of a splint for use on a patient who has combined median and ulnar palsy. This splint provides support for the thumb and keeps the fingers from going into a claw position.

to the hand by suspending the fingers from the proximal phalanges. No palmar cuff is necessary so there is nothing to interfere with grasping tool handles. The wrist flexors are actively contracted to get passive extension of the fingers in order to reach around a large article. One joint, either the wrist or the MP joints of the fingers, must give in order for the other one to assume a new position. The splint on the left in Figure 22-11 is the original design and was based upon the use of nylon cords to simulate external finger extensor tendons which were "tenodesed" or secured at the wrist. As long as the patient has mobile joints and active use of wrist and finger flexors he or she can use this type of splint to control wrist drop. The wire is bent to provide built-in wrist extension. The splint may be simplified as seen on the right in Figure 22-11 by eliminating the nylon cord and placing the leather finger cuffs directly on the brass wire which rests above the proximal phalanges. One does need to apply some material at each side of the wire to block the finger cuffs from slipping around the bend. As shown in the illustration, small pieces of Kay splint have been heated and shaped around the wire to serve as stops. A small stop can also be soldered on the wire. This splint is very effective and permits nearly normal use of the hand during the waiting period to see if a compressed radial nerve will have return of function or while awaiting surgical tendon transfers in the event the nerve has been irreparably damaged.

Flexor and Extensor Tendon Injuries

There are controversies among hand surgeons concerning all aspects of reconstructive surgery, but disagreement is perhaps most evident concerning management of flexor and extensor tendon injuries. The therapist must adjust his or her program to be consistent with the philosophy of the surgeon supervising the cases referred for therapy.

One point of agreement among all surgeons is that finger joints must be mobilized as thoroughly as possible prior to surgical intervention. Occupational

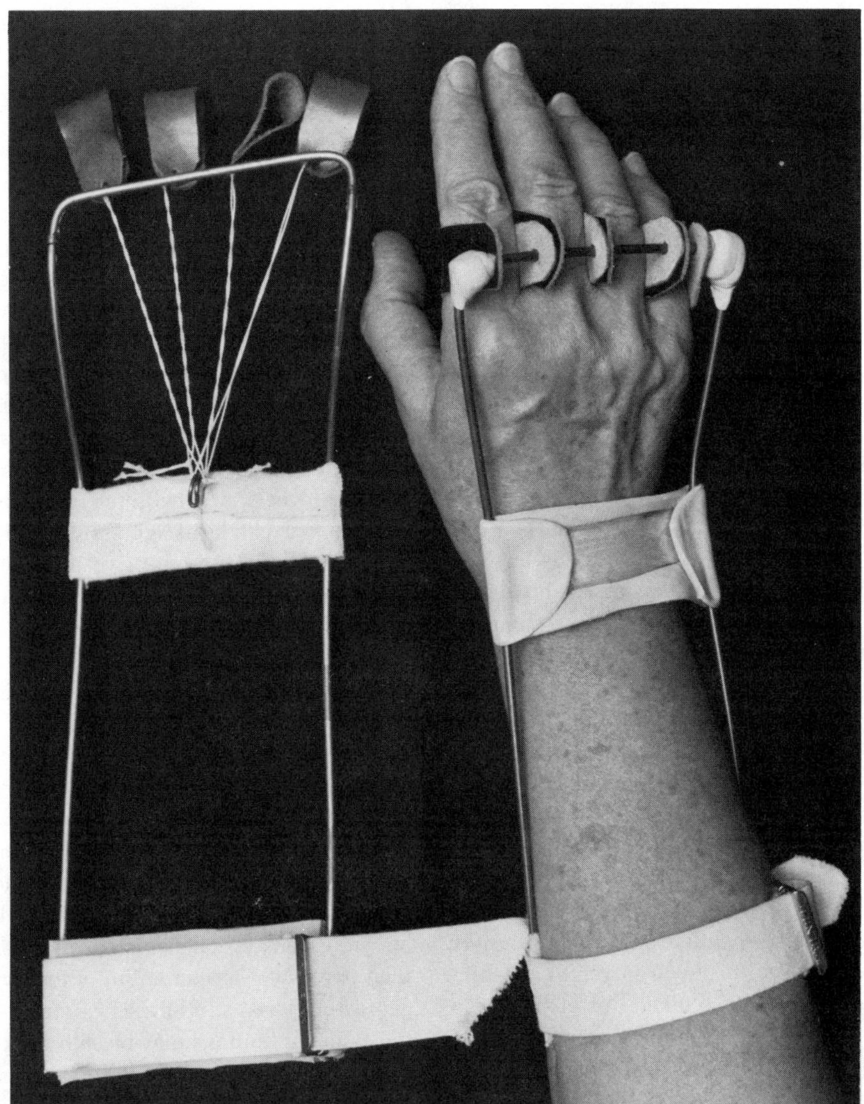

FIGURE 22-11. A radial palsy splint. The splint on the left has nylon cord attached to each leather finger cuff. This cord runs through a small wire loop soldered to the wire frame directly above each finger. The cord is then fastened to a hook on the wrist cuff. The splint on the right has the leather finger cuffs slipped onto the wire frame.

therapists should participate and innovate in the mobilization phase. One can attach a finger in which the flexor tendons have been severed to an adjacent, mobile one by using Velcro to make a fellow traveller (Fig. 22-12). This is preferable to taping two fingers together since the Velcro is double thick between the fingers and keeps them apart, thus avoiding maceration of the skin. If three or four fingers have severed flexor tendons one may resort to using a pair of cotton work gloves and sewing nylon fishing line up each glove finger on the palmar side to serve as external flexor tendons. These lines are tied to rubberbands in the distal palm and the rubberbands are stretched down to hook on a wrist strap. The tension of the rubberbands maintains the fingers in some flexion but the patient can extend actively

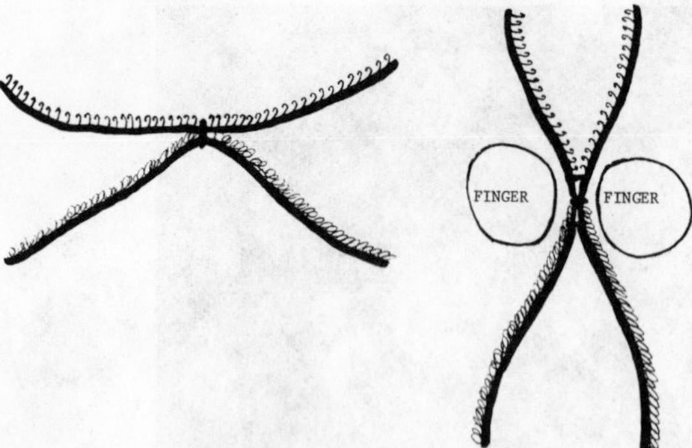

FIGURE 22-12. A fellow traveller made from Velcro. The soft side of the Velcro faces the back of the hook piece when it is sewn together in the middle. Each piece is then turned back upon itself and sewn again.

to open the hand. Both of these methods enable a patient to hold a steering wheel or broom handle without resorting to activating the intrinsic muscles of the injured finger or fingers. Without the aid of the glove or fellow traveller the patient is apt to recruit the intrinsics (which flex the MP joint but extend the IP joints) and the stage is set for development of a very poor habit pattern. This habit pattern is called extensor habitus or paradoxical extension. Never let it develop since it is difficult to eliminate in the presurgical phase. Should a patient overuse the intrinsics following flexor tendon grafting he or she is apt to have an inadequate result from tendon surgery.

On the twenty-first to the twenty-fifth day after surgery when the patient is taken out of the occlusive dressing (which was applied to control edema and position the hand to put slack on the repaired flexor tendon) a protective splint should be used to eliminate the possibility of inadvertently disrupting the tendon repair. This splint should be worn at all times except when the patient is being supervised in an exercise routine. During this period, a padded banding metal splint can be applied on the dorsum of the hand so a distal Velcro strap can be secured around the proximal phalanx without blocking the PIP joint. The MP joint is held in extension and the patient is asked to actively flex the PIP joint. Even though both flexor tendons are cut (the profundus and superficialis), the surgeon frequently prefers to repair only the profundus tendon. When the patient flexes the PIP joint it may seem to be out of line in view of the fact that the patient will use the profundus muscle belly to accomplish this motion. We have found that a better result can be attained early if one concentrates on the PIP joint motion rather than MP or DIP joint motion. One can fabricate a calibrated gauge for the patient to measure active, unresisted PIP motion, but passive flexion and not extension generally are used during the first two weeks out of dressing. In the third week of therapy one may introduce passive extension of only one joint at a time. The MP and DIP joints should be positioned in flexion while gently extending the PIP joint passively. The MP and PIP joints can be flexed while the DIP joint is extended. This method affects the joint tightness, not the tendon anastomosis. By the fifth week of rehabilitation (eight weeks after surgery) one can be as aggressive as one wishes with resistive flexion and passive extension. This time schedule may be altered some according to the philosophy of the surgeon but will be consistent with most programs.

A repaired extensor tendon must be protected at least one week longer than a repaired flexor tendon. The reason for this difference is that flexor tendons and muscles are powerful and can exert too much force if they are permitted to actively pull against the thin weak extensors. The extensors are not designed for power, but for range of motion. If adequate flexor range is not obtained by the tenth week after surgery on an extensor mechanism, the therapist should plan to apply a proper splint of the dynamic type to get further wrist and finger flexion. At this late stage the extensor tendons may be able to extend the wrist and MP joints effectively but, if there are adhesions which limit the patient from achieving an adequate grip, priorities must be altered and flexion range must receive added emphasis.

OCCUPATIONAL THERAPY ACTIVITIES

The therapist should choose wisely when selecting the variety of activities that will be used in a specialty program for hand rehabilitation. If the budget is limited one can concentrate on a few activities rather than investing in equipment and supplies for a wide variety. The main guideline is to select activities that can be adapted readily to provide the motions required in treatment and which permit themselves to be graded as to demands on strength and coordination.

Games provide an endless variety of demands. Many peg games which are available commercially in miniature sizes can be reproduced in larger sizes so that the pegs can be more easily manipulated. The holes in these games can be placed farther apart and early attempts on the part of the patient can lead to success rather than frustration. Some games can be played by one person and several of these should be available, but those that require two or more players are also needed to aid with socialization. A peg game can be used as an early modality for a patient who has had nerve and flexor tendon damage. In the absence of sensation there is no danger of the patient harming the hand, and the fingers can be supported with small splints to channel flexor motion to the joints which must be exercised. For more strengthening the patient can use self-closing, spring-loaded clamps to move the pegs or, for sustained grasp, a pair of pliers can be modified by adding a spring opener made from steel banding metal (Fig. 22-13). The patient has to hold firmly or the pliers will release and the peg will fall.

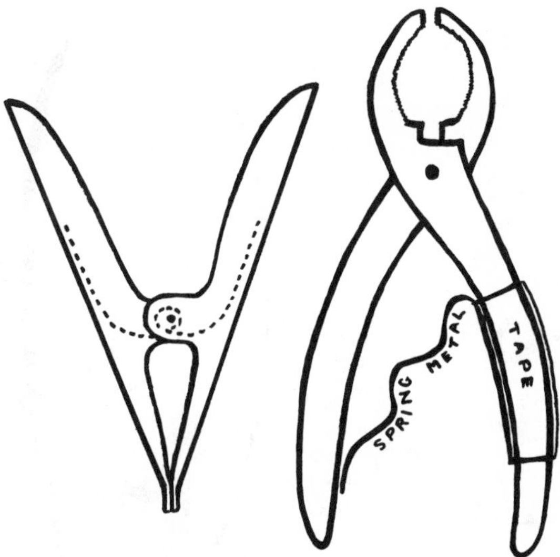

FIGURE 22-13. Self-closing clamps and self-opening pliers for use in playing peg games and doing leather lacing.

Marbles can be used to play the games if one has a reamed out hole for the marble to fit into as well as a drilled hole in the center of each depression deep enough and of the correct size to hold the peg. The marbles provide another challenge to the patient since they are more difficult to handle.

A suspended golf practice ball, a small basket made by cord knotting with a light string around a 4 inch wire loop, and a modified Ping-Pong paddle (Fig. 22-14) can provide a challenging activity to aid a patient in gaining wrist extension. The hand grip is at a right angle to the paddle and encourages balanced wrist extension. An upright post can be attached to a chair back to enable one to strap the forearm in a perpendicular position to ensure use of wrist extension when the patient bats backhand at the ball. A different paddle can be made for use when trying to gain pronation or supination (Fig. 22-15). A file handle or dowel can be provided for the patient to grip. Aluminum clothesline wire can be inserted into the handle and attached to the paddle so that the angle can be changed to fit various needs. For supination or pronation the patient should sit with the forearm resting on a padded shelf

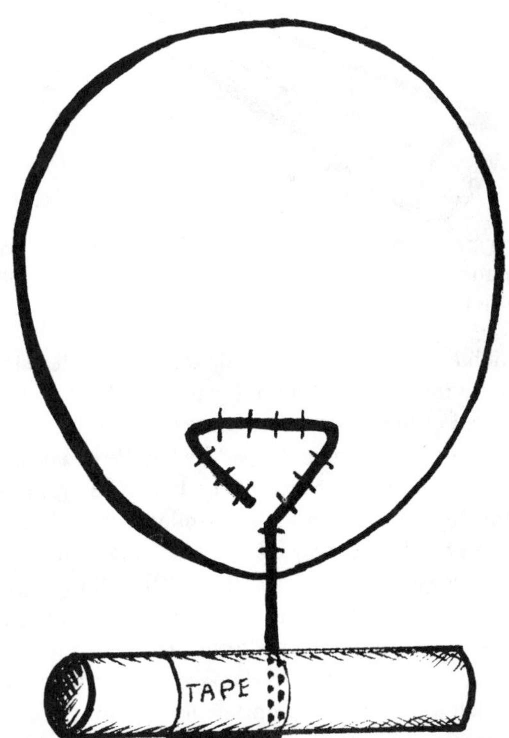

FIGURE 22-14. An adapted Ping-Pong paddle for use in improving balanced wrist extension.

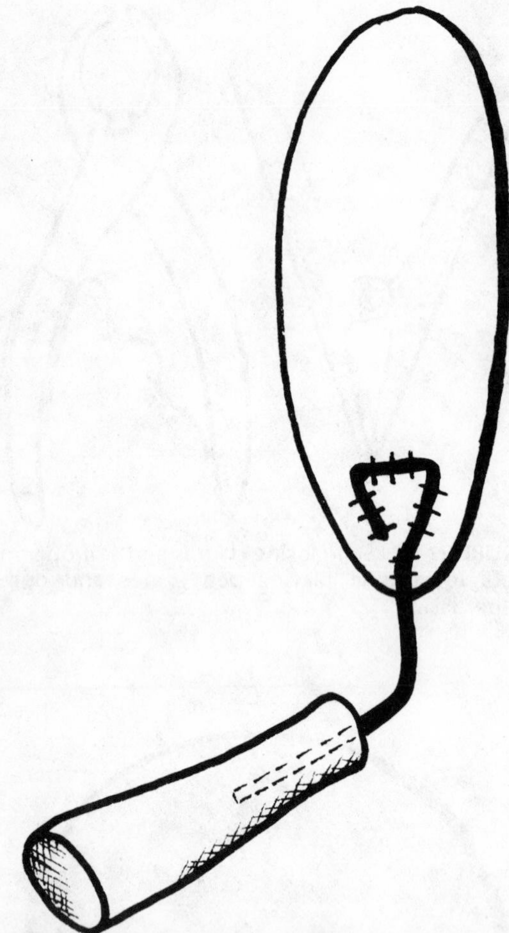

FIGURE 22-15. A Ping-Pong paddle adapted so that a patient can work towards active supination and pronation.

which is horizontal to the chair back and with a strap around the forearm close to the flexed elbow. A strap in this location does not interfere with supination or pronation. The wire in the paddle handle can be bent so that the limited range of motion of the arm can result in contact with the suspended ball.

Leather lacing projects provide opportunities to vary the ways in which a patient will pull the lacing through. A specially designed palmar device provides a patient with a platform placed in the exact position necessary for the damaged finger to contact it. Such a device is appropriate for use for the small finger if one is trying to get a patient to use the flexors of that finger. A lacing platform as shown in Figure 22-9 is designed to encourage MP flexion through use of intrinsic muscle action. A variety of spring-loaded clamps (see Fig. 22-13) can be collected so that the patient can progress from one requiring very weak grip strength to stronger clamps as strength increases. The self-opening pliers depicted in Figure 22-13 require sustained grip or the pliers will open and the lacing will drop out of the jaws.

Stippling of leather belts is a useful therapeutic project. One can take 6 inches of a ¾ inch dowel and drive a small nail into one end. The head of the nail can be clipped off and the end of the nail filed to make a modified point. Sponge rubber can be placed around the dowel handle to build up the size enough to permit the patient to grip the tool firmly and push the nail point into dampened belt leather far enough to make a depression. This is a repetitive task and can result in a rewarding finished product. Stipplers can be modified in design in order to meet the treatment requirements of a variety of patients (Fig. 22-16).

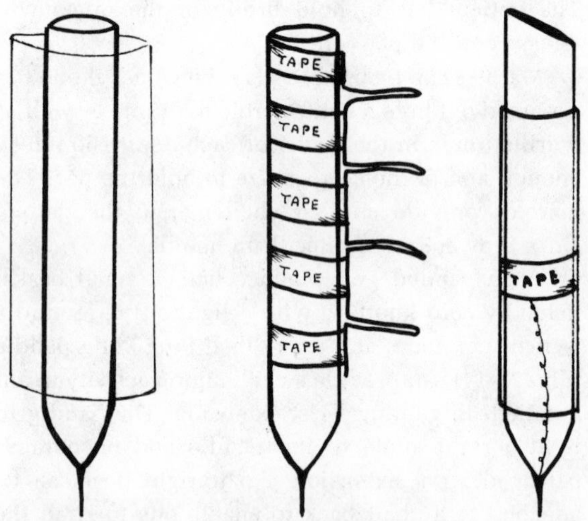

FIGURE 22-16. Leather stippling tools made from wooden dowels with nails driven in the ends. The heads are cut off and the nails are filed to modified points. *Left,* Sponge rubber wrapped to build up the dowel. *Center,* Projections formed from Kay splint and taped to the dowel to make a tool for use by a patient who has ulnar drift of the fingers. *Right,* Inspired by a Volkswagen brake lever. The dowel is slipped through an aluminum tube and a rubberband is taped to the tube and tied to the nail. This stippler is useful when one needs an exerciser for the flexor pollicis longus muscle.

When a patient with rheumatoid arthritis has the common problem of ulnar drift of the fingers, a stippler handle can be adapted to provide projections which fit to the ulnar side of each finger when the dowel is grasped. With each use of the stippler the fingers are forced into radial deviation.

Another useful variation of the stippler depicted is one inspired by the brake lever on a Volkswagen. The aluminum tube is grasped with the fingers; the thumb, through the use of the long flexor, plunges the wooden dowel down so the point contacts the leather. The rubberband offers resistance to the thumb flexion and will return the dowel to its original position. This stippler is good for strengthening grasp in general as well as thumb flexion.

Woodworking projects also offer a variety of adaptations. Many patients work in furniture factories and have introduced therapists to salvage materials that their companies are happy to provide. Table and chair legs that have flaws may often be supplied by some firms. Projects such as foot stools, plant stands, and small tables can be made from the legs in combination with Formica-covered sink cutouts from cabinet makers. In order to sandpaper the round legs a different type of sander has been designed (Fig. 22-17). If the table leg is positioned high on a surface, this strip sander can be used by alternately flexing and extending the arms. The adapted handle encourages use of finger flexors. This activity is also useful for reducing edema since the hand is in an elevated position and all of the hand and arm muscles are actively contracting and relaxing.

Job Simulation

In occupational therapy one frequently needs to find out exactly what strengths and ranges of motion are required of patients on their jobs. These conditions can be simulated as much as possible in the clinic to help in determining whether a patient will be able to return to work. One can use spring scales and attach fabrics or dowels to have patients pull in the manner required to see whether they can pinch firmly enough to hold the material related to their job requirements. Leather, fabric, yarn, sheet metal and variety of tubing sizes have been materials patients may hold or pull. As a therapist works with a patient and realizes what he or she is going to need to hold or maneuver in order to get back on the job the therapy activities can involve materials similar

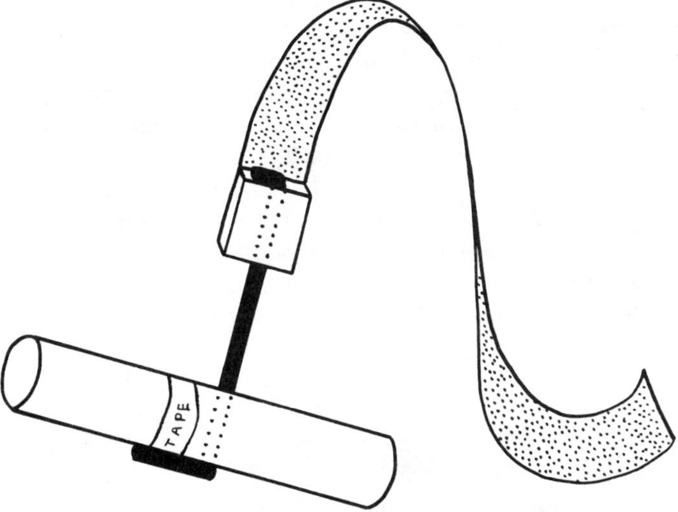

FIGURE 22-17. An adapted strip sander. A hole can be drilled through the center of a wooden dowel and a piece of wire run through and bent at a right angle so it can be taped to the dowel. At the other end the wire runs through a small wooden block to which is tacked and taped a long strip of sandpaper. The strip of sandpaper can be cut from a sanding belt since belts are reinforced with fabric and will not tear easily, or several sheets of sandpaper can be laid edge to edge with a continuous strip of reinforced tape applied across several and then cut into strips.

to those that will be expected to be handled later. Instead of always relying on the routine evaluation forms, the therapist must innovate and add items to fit the evaluation to the individual patient. For a truck driver one might use the round metal frame over which a laundry bag is stretched. The patient sits and places his feet on the braces near the floor and resists the pull of his hands which are using the open circular frame at the top to simulate the steering wheel. A truck steering wheel is usually relatively horizontal rather than vertical, and this simulation can aid the therapist in finding out whether the patient's arm and hand can function adequately to allow returning to employment. Of course, this is only a job simulation, but it does serve to indicate to the patient and therapist how strength is improving.

A torque wrench can provide feedback as to how much force a patient can exert in pulling or pushing levers. Employers will supply information concerning the number of inch-pounds required to shift the levers in a plant so a patient has a realistic goal toward which to aim.

Patients who live in the country may complain that they are unable to carry a bucket of water from the well. As part of such a patient's occupational therapy program, one can make use of a bucket containing sandbags rather than water. The patient carries it with increasing weight and for longer distances as grip strength and upper extremity function improves.

There are limitless possibilities of devising job simulations. An industrial nurse or vocational counsellor, willing to work closely with the occupational therapist, can obtain job descriptions and borrow tools used in patients' occupations. Such coordinated efforts help to make a rehabilitation program more realistic and aid in returning a patient to employment sooner.

OUTCOME CRITERIA

To ensure that patients referred to an occupational therapy program for hand rehabilitation receive optimum benefits, one must examine their records to see the condition of the patient when he or she entered the program and screen the documented evidence to find indications that the treatment processes applied contribute to the patient's overall benefit.

Surgeons frequently refer patients to occupational therapy for assistance in diagnosis. After a massive hand injury it is not always easy to make a decision regarding which structures have been damaged and are in need of repair. The therapist should explore various possibilities and administer specific tests or place the hand in test positions consistent with the nature of the condition to determine patient response. All findings should be recorded carefully so the surgeon has the benefit of all data on which to base clinical and therapeutic decisions.

After a patient has been treated by an occupational therapist the records should reveal the measurable improvement in the range of joint motion, strength, and endurance. Improvement of functional ability, coordination, and dexterity should also be documented. If a patient has been referred because of sensory impairment, the therapist's notes and records should indicate the patient's status at the time of entry into the program. Subsequent notes must indicate the decrease in areas that are totally without response to sensory stimuli with the notes showing improvement delineated carefully. In some cases no improvement is evident but the therapist should indicate how the patient has been helped to cope with insensitive fingers by teaching protective measures.

Since edema has a detrimental effect on the joints of the hand, records should show clearly how successful the efforts toward reducing edema have been. Hand volume measurements can be graphed. This will enable noting when edema is decreased and, if it has been recorded regarding what activity preceded each measurement, conclusions can be drawn regarding which of the activities have been the most beneficial.

The records for amputees who have been referred for treatment should indicate how consistently their full or partial prostheses have been worn and how many activities of daily living they perform using the prostheses. Many amputees and those with severely mangled hands suffer from the trauma imposed upon their self-images. It is difficult to measure the effectiveness of one's input into solution of this problem, but the progress notes should indicate changes in the behavior patterns related to self-image.

As the records are reviewed to determine whether

improvement continues or whether a plateau has been reached, one is made acutely aware of the importance of well-documented progress notes. Patients are referred to occupational therapy for treatment of a variety of conditions and the professional skills of the therapist bring about results that should be documented sufficiently to justify physicians' continued referral of patients to the service.

REFERENCES

1. Reilly, M.: Eleanor Clark Slagle Lecture. Occupational Therapy Can Be One of the Great Ideas of 20th Century Medicine. Am. J. Occup. Ther. 16:1, 1962.
2. *Functional Anatomy of the Hand,* 16 mm movie. Davis and Geck, American Cyanamid Co., Danbury CT 06810.
3. Lampe, E. W.: Surgical Anatomy of the Hand. Ciba Clinical Symposia, Ciba Pharmaceutical Products, Inc., Summit NJ, 1951.
4. Perry, J. F., and Bevin, A. G.: Evaluation procedures for patients with hand injuries. Phys. Ther. 54:6, 1974.
5. Boyes, J. H.: Bunnell's Surgery of the Hand, ed. 5. Philadelphia: J. B. Lippincott Co., 1970.
6. Milford, L.: Retaining Ligaments of the Digits of the Hand. Philadelphia: W. B. Saunders Co., 1968.
7. DeVore, G. L.; and Hamilton, G. F.: Volume measuring of the severely injured hand. Am. J. Occup. Ther. 22:16, 1968.
8. Dellon, A. L., Curtis, R. M., and Edgerton, M. T.: Reeducation of sensation in the hand after nerve injury and repair. Plastic Reconstr. Surg. 53:3, 1974.

BIBLIOGRAPHY

American Academy of Orthopedic Surgeons: Symposium on Tendon Surgery in the Hand. St. Louis MO: C. V. Mosby Co., 1975.

Barr, N. R.: The Hand: Principles and Techniques of Simple Splintmaking in Rehabilitation. London: Butterworths, 1975.

Bunnell, S.: Surgery in World War II, Hand Surgery. Department of the Army, Washington DC, 1955.

Flynn, E. J.: Hand Surgery. Baltimore: Williams & Wilkins, 1966.

Kaplan, E. B.: Functional and Surgical Anatomy of the Hand. Philadelphia: J. B. Lippincott Co., 1965.

Spinner, M.: Injuries to the Major Branches of Peripheral Nerves of the Forearm. Philadelphia: W. B. Saunders Co., 1972.

Weeks, P. M., and Wray, C. R.: Management of Acute Hand Injuries: A Biological Approach. St. Louis MO: C. V. Mosby Co., 1973.

Wynn-Parry, C. B.: Rehabilitation of the Hand. London: Butterworths, 1973.

23

Amputations

Elinor Anne Spencer

To be an amputee is to be without a limb or limbs as a result of injury, disease, or congenital deformity. Bodily functions develop in the presence of anomalies in children with congenital deformities or early post-birth amputations, but post-adolescent amputees suffer the loss of a part of the body which had previously been integrated into the total body image. Function, sensation, and appearance of the involved extremity are affected, and the amputee must rely on a strange mechanical device as a replacement for the natural limb. Since the traumatic amputee has usually matured physically, the circumstances of the amputation, its meaning, and its consequences are different from those of the congenital or very young amputee. This chapter emphasizes the rehabilitation team's work with a person who has suffered traumatic amputation after adolescence.

There are many causes of amputations: trauma, peripheral vascular disease, thrombosis, embolism, malignancy, and trophic changes. The most common cause of upper extremity (UE) amputations is trauma resulting from industrial accidents, which are usually connected with the use of high speed power tools. The most common cause of lower extremity (LE) amputations is peripheral vascular disease.

The physical therapy service is responsible for most of the training of the LE amputee but, since LE amputees are frequently referred to the occupational therapy service for assistance in motivation, physical restoration, self-care independence (ADL), and prevocational assessment, this chapter discusses some appropriate treatment objectives and activities. However, because the occupational therapist participates actively in the prosthetic training program of the UE amputee, this will be the main focus of the chapter.

The patient's reactions to the loss of a limb vary depending on age when the amputation occurred, intelligence, physical development, sex, vocation, avocational interests, social status, and finances. The amputee may also have problems in function because of the presence of phantom sensations, a phenomenon in which the amputee actually feels the presence of part of the limb that has been amputated. This can lead to difficulties in his or her accepting, tolerating, and learning to use the prosthesis (the artificial limb).

The amputee rehabilitation program begins with the decision to amputate and ends with the successful functional and cosmetic integration of the prosthesis into the body schema. Whether the cause of the amputation is trauma or disease, the first step in the total program is the consideration of the type and level of surgery and the psychological and physical preparation of the patient.

SURGICAL CONSIDERATIONS

During the surgical procedure of amputation the physicians try to save as much tissue as possible. The importance of structural length and support of the bone, length and strength of the cut or damaged muscles, and sensation through adequate skin coverage bear out the practicality and necessity of preserving tissue. Regardless of the level of the amputation, the muscles involved directly or indirectly in the function of the amputated part are affected by the loss.

Prior to the operation, the necessity of the amputation, the expected result, the postoperative conditioning program, the possibility of difficulties in adjustment, and the prosthetic training program are explained to the patient. He or she must be prepared both medically and psychologically for the problems which he or she may encounter as he or she prepares to use the prosthesis.

Both during and after surgery, effort is made to form the stump in such a way as to maintain maximum function of the remaining tissue and to provide maximum use of the prosthesis. Blood vessels and nerves are pulled down, cut, and allowed to retract so that they do not interfere with the amputee's use of the prosthesis by causing pain in the stump when the device is used.

Either a *closed* or an *open* amputation may be done by the surgeon. The open amputation allows free drainage of affected material, minimizing the possibility of infection before closure. The immediate closed amputation may reduce the period of hospitalization but it also reduces free drainage and introduces the danger of bacterial growth. When the closed amputation is performed, either immediately or following sufficient drainage, the maximum amount of tissue is saved. However, regardless of the surgical method used, the stump must be strong and resilient and have a snug, comfortable contact with the socket of the prosthesis, for the amputee will exert much pressure on the stump while using the device.

Special Considerations and Problems

There are several problems related to the amputation. Physical problems may affect or hinder the prosthetic training program with either the UE or the LE amputee. Such problems are the length of the stump, its skin coverage, its sensitivity (i.e., presence of hypersensitivity and/or edema), its healing, the condition of the skin, and the presence of infection. For example, an amputee with either a very long stump or a very short one may find the design of the various components of the prosthesis unsatisfactory either cosmetically or functionally. Perspiration, the natural result of physical effort, may result from excessive confinement of the stump in the prosthesis' socket, for the stump lacks ventilation. The occupational therapist must also be aware of the possibility of the amputee's being allergic to plastics and resins from which the socket is made.

The sensation of the stump is important to the rehabilitation of the amputee. If a hand has been amputated and the patient has been fitted with a prosthetic prehension device, he or she no longer experiences functional sensation in the area which has been amputated. Although he or she has sensation in the stump, it is functionally lost when he or she puts on the prosthesis. Therefore, he or she will have to depend on visual cues in order to use the terminal device to handle objects. Sensation can also be a problem if the socket is ill-fitting or if the stump is not well-formed at the distal end. Therefore, the amputee must become adjusted to the pressure of the socket on the stump. He or she also must become used to the pressure of the harness on his or her shoulders and to the weight of the prosthesis.

Levels of Amputations of the Upper Extremity

The higher the level of amputation the more the amputee must depend on the prosthesis for replacement of bodily function and the more extensive the prosthesis must be. Generally accepted levels of amputation are indicated in Figure 23-1.

Amputations at the joints are referred to as *disarticulations* (i.e., finger, wrist, elbow, or shoulder disarticulation). Amputations below the wrist across the metacarpal bones are referred to as *transmetacarpal*. At this level and below, amputations are referred to as *partial hand*. Should the amputation occur between the wrist and the elbow the level is

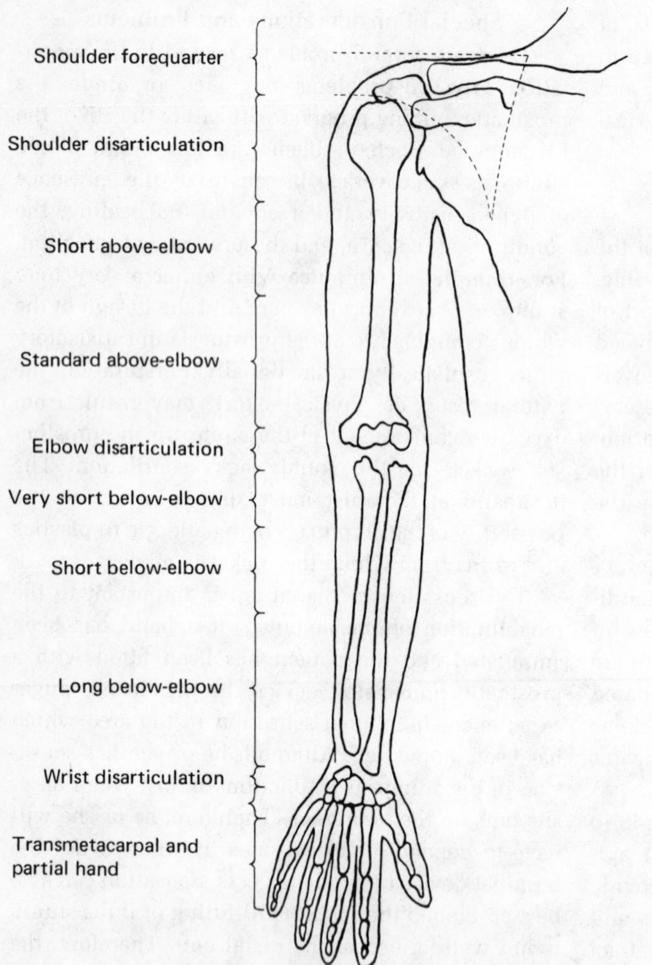

FIGURE 23-1. Amputation levels of the upper extremity.

referred to as *below elbow* (BE), and amputation between the elbow and the shoulder is referred to as *above elbow* (AE). Amputations at the surgical neck of the humerus (distal to the humeral head) to the shoulder articulation are referred to as *shoulder disarticulations*. Amputations above the shoulder joint involving the clavicle and scapula are referred to as *forequarter*.

Although there are general types of prostheses for each level of amputation, each prosthesis is medically prescribed for the person's individual needs and the artificial limb is custom-made and individually fitted.

Phantom Sensations

Phantom sensations are common among amputees. Frequently, crush injuries, with their accompanying sensations of burning or cramping, are the most prevalent causes of phantom sensations. The sensation is that the limb remains a part of the person in spite of the amputation. Although, in most cases, this awareness is painless, at times it can become intolerable to the patient and actual pain may result. In such a case, a revision of the stump through surgical methods may be necessary.

The phantom sensations are usually felt as the distal parts of the extremity (i.e., the amputee senses the existence of a non-existent hand or foot). These phantom sensations seldom involve the total extremity.

Usually the patient describes the feeling of a presence, perhaps a tingling sensation. In addition to supportive counselling, the most effective compensation for the phantom sensation is the early use of the stump combined with either a temporary or a permanent prosthesis. The distal contact of the stump with the socket can have a desensitizing effect on the stump and can thus minimize phantom or painful sensations.

The amputee may also have to accept a new body image; this is difficult for some amputees because major changes in their body images will occur with the loss. Some amputees may be disturbed by this change in body concept and may have subsequent difficulties in prosthetic training. To be functionally useful, the prosthesis must be integrated into the body schema and become a part of the individual.

Cineplasty

Under most circumstances a conventional prosthesis, using shoulder harnessing for suspension and control of prosthetic function which is channeled through a control cable, is provided for the amputee.

However, if the rehabilitation team and the patient wish, a second surgical procedure can be done after the initial procedure is well-healed. The biceps or pectoral cineplasty is done occasionally in order to eliminate the shoulder harnessing and to increase sensory feedback from the terminal device. The more common of the two sites for cineplasty is the biceps muscle. A surgical tunnel is made through the muscle into which a plastic pin is inserted and the control cable is attached to both ends of this pin. The prosthesis is then controlled by the contraction and relaxation of the biceps muscle (Fig. 23-2).

Because the tunnel must be kept clean consistently, there is considerable chance of infection if the amputee does not take sufficient care of his or her hygiene. Additionally, the amputee who has had a cineplasty procedure must be able to accept the cosmetic effect of the tunnel through the biceps muscle.

Limb Replantation

Limb replantation, or the rejoining of the amputated part following direct trauma, has been done with varying success. It is generally accepted that prosthetic replacement is limited as an acceptable substitute for natural appearance and function of the lost part and that it will always remain a substitute. Disadvantages of prosthetic replacement include the necessity of achieving replacement of normal function through mechanical means, loss of functional sensation, periodic breakdown of devices, psychological reactions to loss, and the effects on the concept of self-image. In the effort to provide the amputee with a natural replacement, replantation has been done when immediate medical attention is available and when the amputated part of the limb can be adequately salvaged and replaced safely. Success depends on vascular continuity and nerve and tendon repair. Fibrosis and atrophy can occur, however, and the replanted part may be limited in function and sensation.

Figure 23-3 shows an amputee who has functional amputated digits of her right hand and a hand replantation of her left arm. This was done at the wrist. In this case a 1 inch prehension range was achieved; however, digital sensation is minimal. The

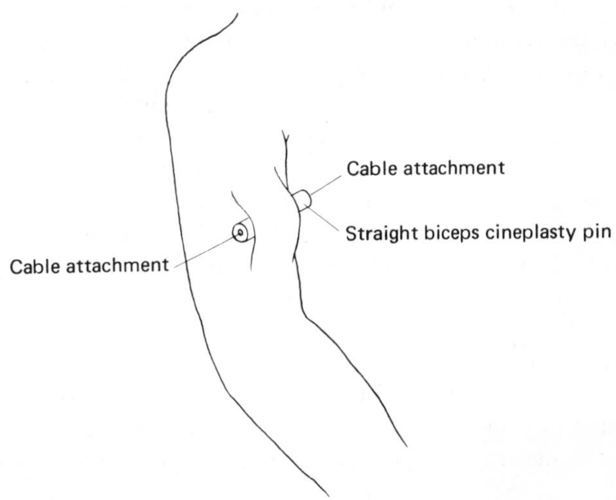

FIGURE 23-2. Biceps cineplasty tunnel with straight cineplasty pin.

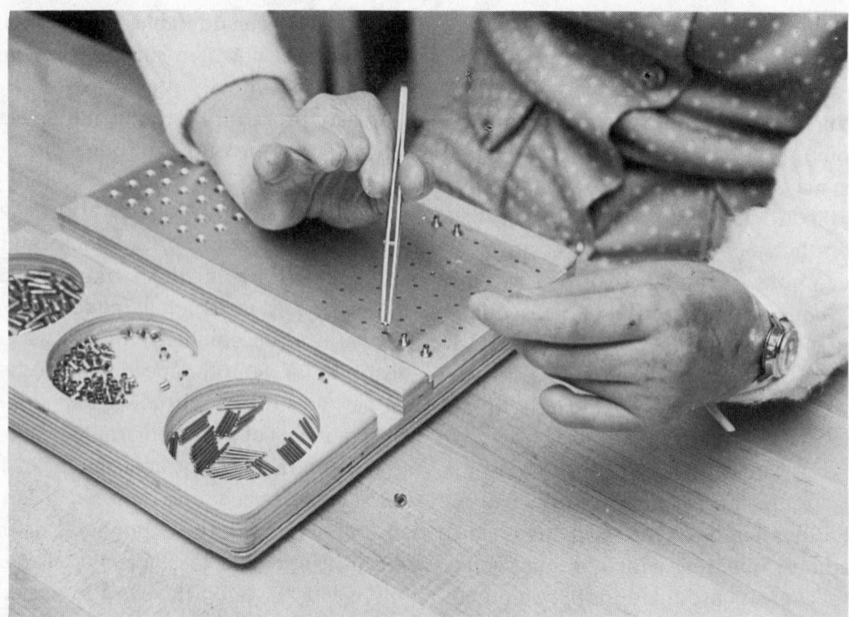

FIGURE 23-3. Bilateral amputee uses right partially amputated fingers to grasp tweezers. The left hand is a replantation and has limited pinch function and acceptable cosmetic value but lacks functional sensation.

amputee shown here uses her hand as a functional assist and enjoys the relatively normal cosmetic look. Since amputees are likely to have different opinions regarding cosmetic value and function it is very important to find out how the amputee feels in regard to the replacement alternatives for both.

PARTS OF THE UPPER EXTREMITY PROSTHESIS

Terminal Devices

The most significant component of the prosthesis is the terminal device (TD), which provides both function and cosmetic worth.

A cosmetic terminal device, used principally for appearance, may be as simple as a flesh-colored glove used to cover a partial hand. Aside from being used to hold light objects or to position objects by pushing or pulling, this cosmetic device may have little functional value for the amputee. However, its psychological value is unquestioned.

A second type of cosmetic terminal device is the functional hand which can be attached to the wrist unit of most UE prostheses (Fig. 23-4) and is operated by cable control. The functional hand consists of a plastic spring-controlled device with fingers which are controlled in flexion and extension at the metacarpophalangeal joints by the control cable of the prosthesis. The thumb of the hand can be placed manually in either of two positions: to grasp small objects or to grasp large ones. A plastic glove fits over the hand, presenting a natural appearance. The gloves are available in a variety of skin tones.

Functional hands have either voluntary opening or voluntary closing mechanisms activated by cable control, and they may either lock in position or be free-wheeling or nonlocking.

The hook is the most functional of the terminal devices. It is made of either steel or aluminum and is canted or lyre-shaped. It is either locking or nonlocking, with either voluntary opening or voluntary closing capacity (Fig. 23-5). The hook is usually lined with neoprene, which protects objects while the amputee is grasping them. The needs of the amputee determine the weight, length, design, and function of the hook device chosen by the rehabilitation team.

Many kinds of hooks are available to provide for the diverse needs of the amputee. Among them are aluminum hooks required for above-elbow and shoulder disarticulation amputees who need mini-

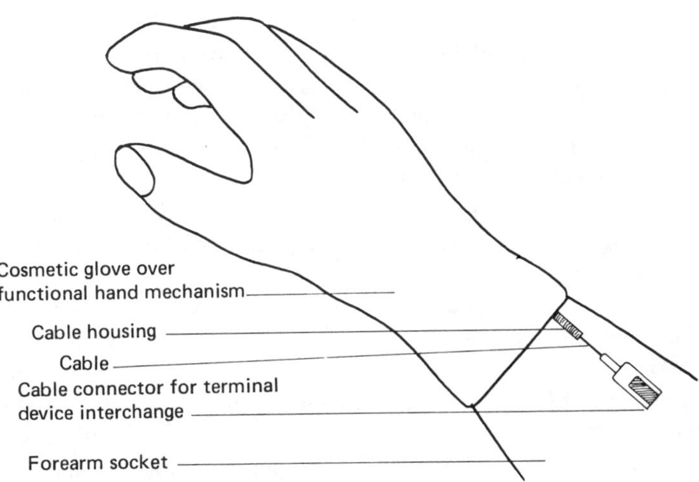

FIGURE 23-4. Functional hand with cosmetic glove and cable attachment.

mum weight of the prosthesis, steel hooks for below-elbow amputees requiring durability, farmers' or carpenters' hooks for ease and safety in tool handling, and narrow opening hooks for use in laboratory or office work. Special hooks are available for bowling and holding a baseball mitt. Hooks and functional or cosmetic hands are generally interchangeable through the common wrist unit attachment which is laminated onto the forearm socket.

Wrist Unit

The terminal device (either cosmetic or functional) is connected to the forearm socket (or shell) by the wrist unit. The three basic wrist units are locking, friction, and oval.

The advantage of the *locking unit* is that it prevents the hook from rotating during heavy industrial work. By pushing a button on it, the amputee manually operates the wrist unit, which allows the posi-

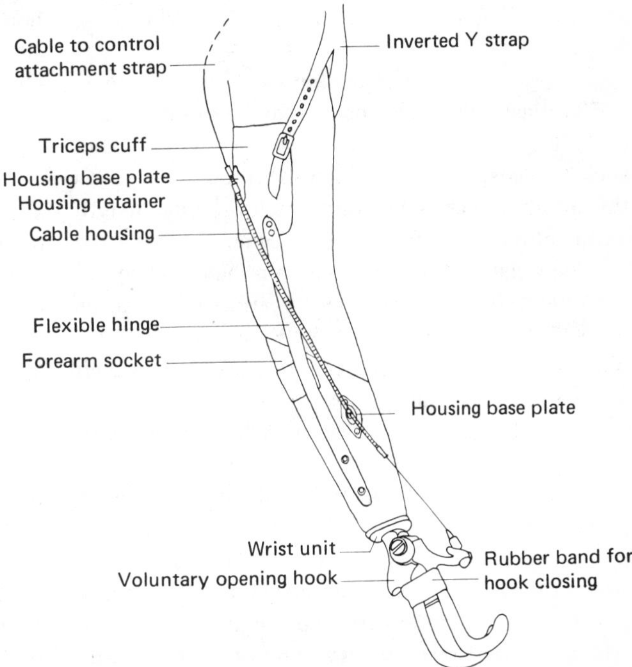

FIGURE 23-5. Right below-elbow prosthesis.

tion of the hook to be changed by rotation. The hook can easily be ejected for interchange of hook and hand.

The *friction unit* has threads and the hook must be screwed into the unit. Although this procedure is more time-consuming than that of the locking unit, the hook can be more easily positioned for specific tasks. Either the locking or the friction unit can be used with both BE and AE prostheses.

The *oval unit* is a special, thin unit for a wrist disarticulation prosthesis; it is used where the length of the components must be minimal in order to make the length of the amputated arm conform to that of the sound extremity.

A wrist flexion unit is available for placement of the hook in three wrist flexion positions for increased function. It is a manually operated device and is usually prescribed for the bilateral amputee for added versatility in terminal device positioning. One activity which is aided by this device is shaving; it helps as well in other activities close to the body.

Terminal devices and wrist units have standard connections. When the desired type of terminal device is chosen, one needs simply to determine the type and size of the wrist unit to accompany it. Usually the wrist unit is chosen according to the way in which the amputee will use the prosthesis in activities of daily living and at work.

The Socket

The plastic laminate socket may be either single- or double-walled. A BE amputee has a double-walled socket consisting of an inner wall which conforms to the stump and an outer wall which provides length and contour to the forearm replacement.

The wrist unit is laminated onto the distal end of the forearm socket. Since the forearm socket can be used by both the AE and the BE amputee to carry objects (i.e., a coat, a handbag, or packages) as well as to push or to pull large or heavy objects, it is made of strong plastic resins which provide lightness and durability.

Since overall weight and bulk must be minimized for the AE and shoulder disarticulation amputees, a single-walled forearm socket, or shell, is best for these prostheses. The socket provides length and contour to the forearm replacement. A double-walled socket is provided for the upper arm stump.

The Munster-type socket was devised mainly for the short stump of the BE amputee to eliminate problems of fit, security, and poor leverage which were prevalent with the conventional split-sockets, difficult to fit on this type of amputee. It consists of a single double-walled forearm socket which extends just proximal to the olecranon process posteriorly and fits around the biceps tendon anteriorly. The figure nine harness of the Munster-type prosthesis is not necessary for the suspension of the prosthesis; thus the figure nine harness can be used with or without a triceps cuff. The socket is preflexed at approximately 35 degrees, thus limiting complete flexion and extension of the elbow. However, even with this disadvantage in range of motion, the fit is adequate for lifting and holding.

Upper-Arm Unit

The upper-arm unit of the AE prosthesis is a double-walled socket with the locking elbow unit laminated onto the socket. Since the AE amputee lacks independent elbow flexion and extension, these are provided mechanically by an elbow unit which is activated, locked, and unlocked by the cable control system. A turntable at the joining of the locking elbow unit and the upper arm socket can be manually moved for internal and external rotation of the forearm, enabling the amputee to work with the hook directly in front of the body or out towards the side. The forearm shell is attached to the locking elbow unit and the upper arm socket (Fig. 23-6).

Shoulder Disarticulation Prosthesis

The shoulder disarticulation prosthesis has a supporting socket portion which sometimes extends to the anterior and posterior aspects of the shoulder, depending on the level of the amputation. Frequently, a passive abduction hinge joint is added at the shoulder for ease in manually positioning the arm and donning clothing.

Hinges

Hinges provide functional alignment and positioning between the forearm and the upper-arm socket or the harness. In addition, the flexible dacron or leather hinges used in the BE prosthesis allow active rotation of the forearm with a minimum of restriction. In the AE prosthesis the steel hinges provide rigidity to the mechanical elbow joint to ensure strength, durability, and dependability.

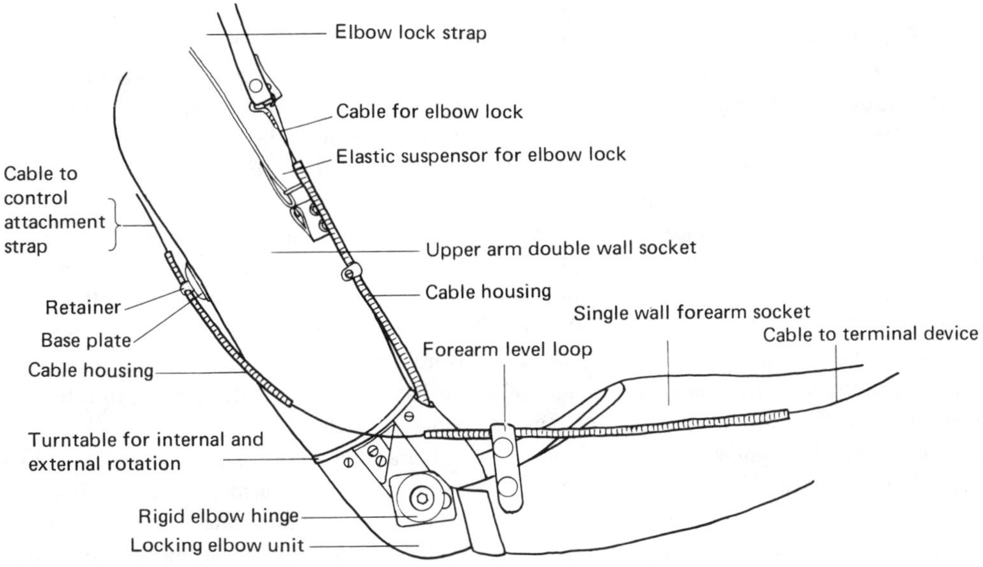

FIGURE 23-6. Right above-elbow prosthesis with locking elbow unit.

Harness

The function of the harness is to provide stable support of the prosthesis to facilitate the amputee's wearing and using of it, to provide attachment for the control cables, and to assist the cables in the operation of the prosthesis. Basically, the Dacron straps are formed in a figure-eight pattern with extra straps added as needed for better support or additional control function. For ease in use, the figure-nine harness is used with the Munster prosthesis. For the wrist disarticulation amputee, a simple cuff socket and a figure-nine harness may suffice.

Stump Sock

A stump sock is worn by the amputee to aid in absorption of perspiration, to provide warmth to the stump, and as padding for comfort and fit of the socket. An AE amputee frequently uses the short sleeve of a T-shirt in place of the stump sock. Use of an under-blouse or T-shirt can alleviate discomfort from the harness straps in beginning training sessions.

Control System

The control system is a very important part of the prosthesis. It determines the functional value of the prosthesis for the amputee. The control cable of the terminal device is attached to the device and to the harness. This cable is guided along the socket and cuff or the upper-arm socket by retainers which hold it in the most advantageous position for ease of function. Terminal device operation is generally accomplished by forward flexion of the shoulder. During the training period the amputee practices this isolated motion and eventually he or she is able to operate the hook or hand with minimal physical strain.

For the AE amputee this basic terminal device control cable also serves in flexion and extension of the mechanical elbow when the elbow unit is unlocked. It is activated by forward shoulder flexion. At times, additional joint motions are used in this cable operation: (1) because of limitation of shoulder control or strength; (2) to provide smooth operation of the prosthesis; (3) to enable the wearer to achieve maximum function of the mechanical arm and hand in reach, grasp, release, and hold. These motions may be shoulder abduction and adduction, scapular abduction and adduction, or shoulder flexion of the unamputated arm.

The second basic cable operates the elbow lock. It is attached internally or externally to the elbow unit and extends to the anterior deltoid-pectoral strap of the harness. A combination of shoulder elevation, depression, external rotation, and extension is used to both lock and unlock the elbow unit.

Control cables for the shoulder disarticulation

and forequarter prostheses are attached to the humeral or scapular part of the upper-arm socket, and their exact design and function are determined by the needs of the individual amputee.

During the training period the amputee is carefully instructed to isolate the patterns of joint and muscle movement which control the operation of the prosthesis. (The instruction process will be discussed in the section on prosthetic training.) The extent to which the prosthesis provides the amputee with increased function depends on the quality of the fabrication of the prosthesis, its fit, the comfort and limitations of the wearer, and the range of mechanical function. The amputee's limitations may be physical, psychological, and/or social. The range of mechanical function of the prosthesis includes grasp, release, hold, push, pull, and reach, which, depending upon the control by the wearer and the types of prescription components, can be extensive for the amputee.

CINEPLASTY PROSTHESIS

As mentioned earlier, the cineplasty prosthesis is a special form of prosthetic device. In this case, the harness functions as additional support and comfort for the wearer but it is not necessary for the actual function of the prosthesis. The same terminal devices, wrist units, and socket design described earlier can be used. However, the control system is different because the surgical procedure consists of forming a tunnel through the biceps muscle (see Fig. 23-2).

This procedure is undertaken following the standard amputation. A plastic pin is inserted through the tunnel. At each end of the pin is a cable attachment from which a cable extends. These cables eventually join in a common adjustment plate and another cable extends from this point to the terminal device (Fig. 23-7).

For added security, a triceps cuff may be strapped around the upper arm (Fig. 23-8). This cuff is attached to the forearm shell with flexible hinges.

In addition to eliminating the necessity of binding harnessing, the cineplasty control system approximates normal isolated muscle function. Rather than joint motion or muscle expansion for control, the cineplasty prosthesis is operated by the biceps muscle. With biceps control there is some simulation in sensation in the terminal device.

A person who has a cineplastic procedure gener-

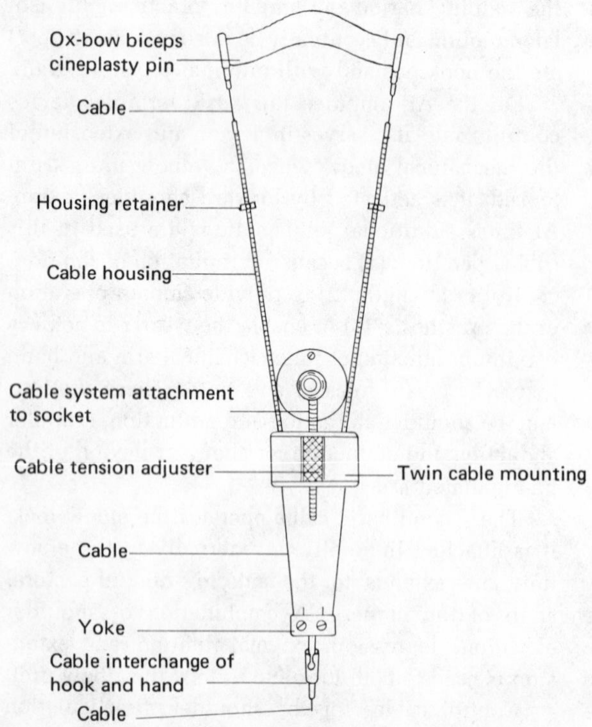

FIGURE 23-7. Biceps cineplasty cable control system.

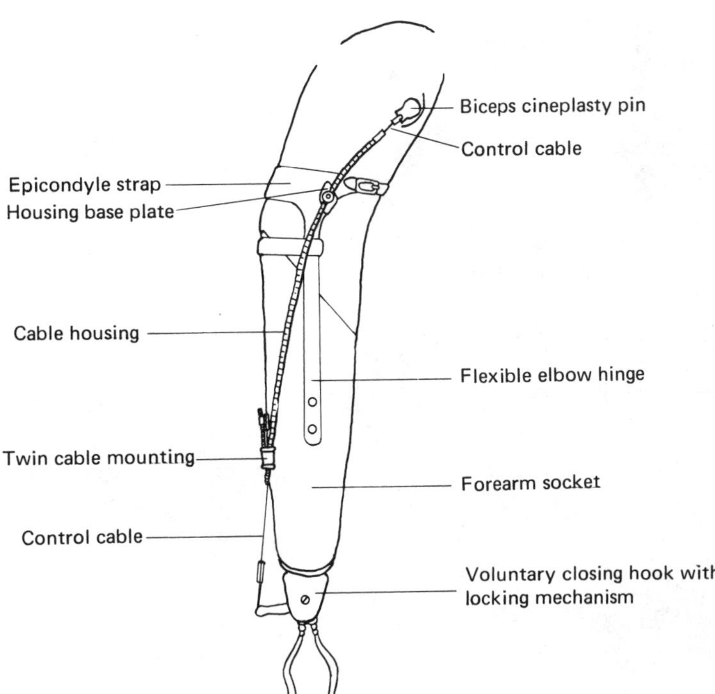

FIGURE 23-8. Right below-elbow cineplasty with voluntary closing hook.

ally has undergone pre-prosthetic training and has learned to use a harness-controlled prosthesis prior to cineplastic surgery and thus, if necessary, can revert to the use of a standard control system.

BILATERAL AMPUTEE

The bilateral amputee faces not only the functional and cosmetic adjustments of the unilateral amputee but also the complete loss of sensory contact with objects while using the prostheses. Prosthetic replacement is prescribed according to the level of amputation. Particular attention is given to minimizing weight and providing ease of bilateral operation of the elbows and terminal devices through the control system. For ease in putting on and removing of the prosthesis by the amputee, as well as for its security and adjustment, the two prostheses are secured to a common harness system. A wrist flexion unit is helpful on one side for added mechanical positioning.

Because sensation is essential to the *blind* bilateral amputee, the Krukenberg surgical procedure may be done if the individual has a long below-elbow amputation of either or both arms. This procedure involves the separating of the radius and ulna and accompanying musculature to enable the amputee to achieve a grasp and release function through supination and pronation of the forearm. Sensation is maintained as grasp is achieved without an external prosthesis. Some amputees can achieve independence with this procedure.

PARTIAL HAND AMPUTATION

The amputee with a partial hand amputation may or may not need or use a prosthesis. In the effort to save as much tissue as possible, the surgeon can often save parts of the hand for motor function and sensation. As shown in Figures 23-9, 23-10, and 23–11 full function can be maintained for the grasping of tools and general coordination and sensation with partial amputation of the fingers. In this case, there is complete function of the metacarpophalangeal joints for adequate positioning of the fingers and strength is preserved in the muscle tendons as is fingertip sensation. Complete amputation of the fingers necessitates prosthetic replacement to provide grasp and prehension. Figures 23-12, 23-13, and 23-14 show the use of a functional replacement to enable the amputee to use tools. The amputee shown here has normal function and sensation in the thumb. Cosmetic replacement can also be provided by a glove with soft or firm fingers which

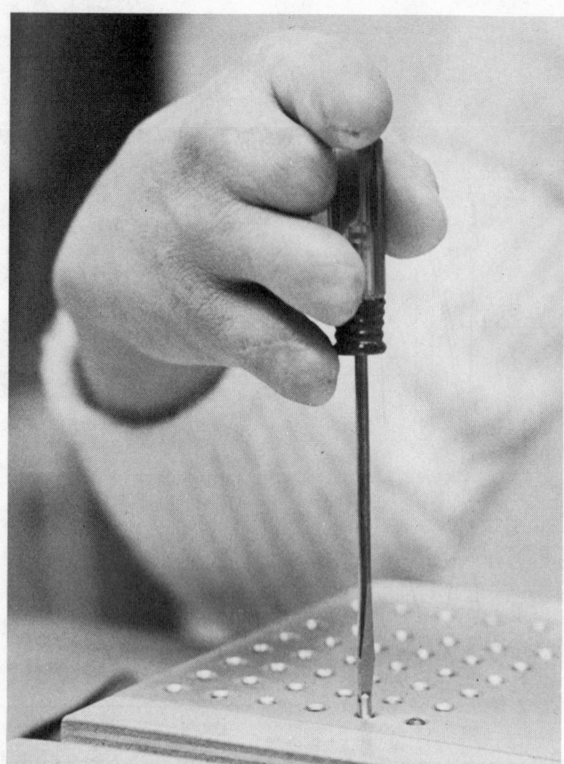

FIGURE 23-9. The amputee grasps a small screwdriver between the partially amputated fingers and the remaining thumb.

can be manually positioned for function and appearance.

OCCUPATIONAL THERAPY AND THE UPPER EXTREMITY AMPUTEE

Physical Considerations

Generally speaking, the longer the stump the more the amputee can do both in the pre-prosthetic program and in the prosthetic training program. With a well-healed, healthy stump, the amputee has a good purchase power on the socket and security in its fit. In the case of a BE amputation, the longer the stump the more active supination and pronation the patient is likely to have. This situation will assist him or her in positioning the hook for grasp and placement of objects. Also, if the stump is long, either AE or BE, it is more useful to the amputee; he or she has a tendency to use it more frequently, thus maintaining normal range of motion and strength.

During the postoperative and pre-prosthetic periods the patient will usually automatically change dominance to the sound extremity. If the dominant extremity has been amputated and the patient is forced to use the non-dominant extremity for grasp and placement of objects, he or she may have some incoordination. In this case, he or she can

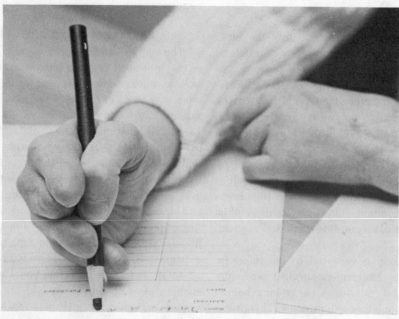

FIGURE 23-10. The amputee with full use of the thumb is able to write normally with adaptive grasp by the partially amputated fingers.

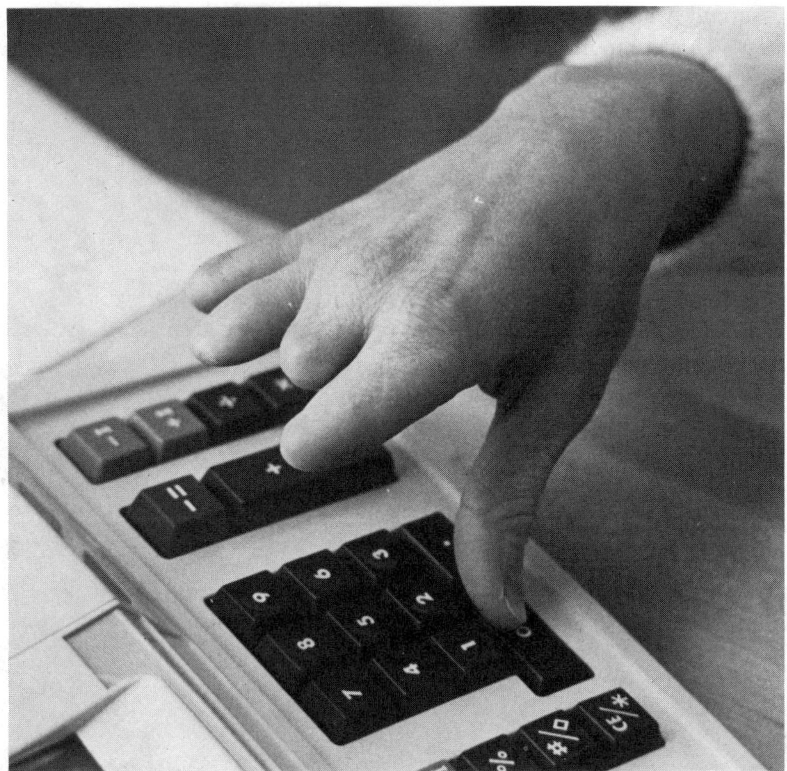

FIGURE 23-11. This individual had partial finger amputation caused by an industrial machine. Full mobility at the metacarpophalangeal joints and complete sensation enable the amputee to use a calculator effectively.

benefit from activities with the sound extremity to improve the fine coordination of the previously non-dominant arm. The amputee who has suffered loss of the non-dominant extremity may be less motivated to use the prosthesis, for he or she will depend on the dominant extremity to compensate for the other arm.

It is important to stress bilateral activities to help the patient adjust to limitations in reaching and in holding large objects as well as to aid the development of bimanual coordination. Involvement in activities aids in the healing of the stump and in learning to use the prosthesis.

The bilateral amputee usually chooses the side with the longer stump to become the dominant side. Sometimes he or she is trained in the use of one prosthesis at a time. However, since the two prostheses have a common harness and the body must adjust to the weight and balance of the mechanical devices, the bilateral amputee may start the training program with both limbs, concentrating on one at a time.

Early Fitting

It is commonly recognized that early fitting of the prosthesis or prostheses aids the training program. Some doctors and therapists think that it is more desirable to fit several temporary prostheses rather than to wait for several months for the arrival of the permanent one. This technique provides early prosthetic training while the permanent limb is being fabricated. There are four approaches to shortening the time between the amputation and the fitting of the permanent prosthesis.

1. In some cases, particularly if the patient has a long stump or stumps, utensils can be fitted into the Ace bandage, which is applied to the stump to facilitate shrinkage.

2. Utensils can be fitted into the pocket of a strap and wrapped around the stump with a Velcro fastening. A temporary prosthetic cuff can be devised from plaster or leather to which either utensils or the terminal device and controls can be attached.

3. Early fitting, several weeks postoperatively, has met with success. This temporary prosthesis consists of a plaster cuff with components and a control system similar to the ones the permanent prosthesis will have.

4. The immediate post-surgical fitting is being done with upper extremity amputees. It has been found that immediate fitting, in addition to shortening the time between amputation and the wearing of the prosthesis, has hastened control of edema, lessened post-surgical pain, encouraged conditioning of the stump, and provided more rapid use of the controls and the prosthesis. The plaster dressing with conventional harness and controls is applied at the time of surgery or during the immediate postoperative period. The plaster casts are changed as the stump shrinks. Provision of this type of immediate prosthesis encourages a positive approach from the patient and early learning of prosthetic use; thus, when the amputee receives the permanent prosthesis, he or she has developed appropriate muscle use and has learned controls.

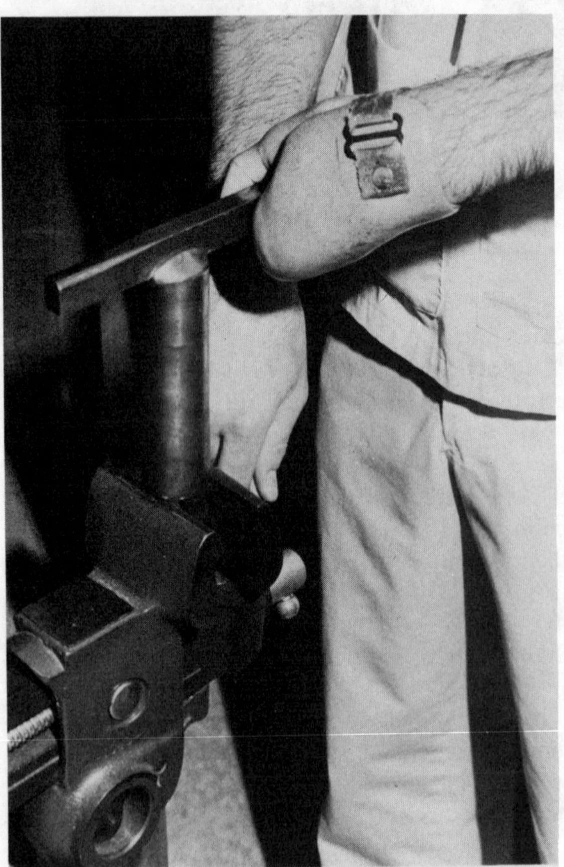

FIGURE 23-12. This partial hand amputee uses a prosthesis to replace the fingers and to provide opposition to the remaining thumb for grasping.

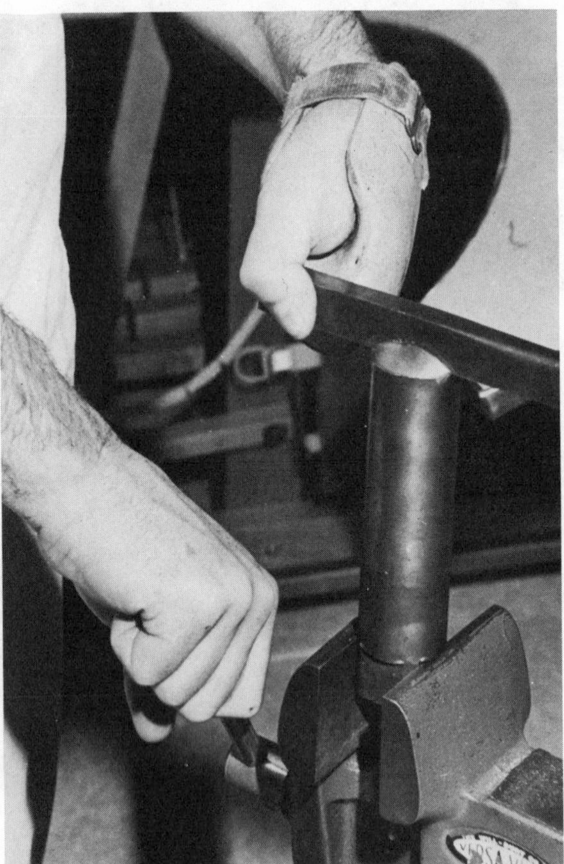

FIGURE 23-13. This finger replacement prosthesis provides opposition to the thumb for grasping.

Psychological Reactions

In assisting the amputee in adjusting to his or her condition and in becoming motivated to learn the function and care of the prosthesis, the occupational therapist must recognize the amputee's psychological reactions to his or her situation. If the patient feels guilt or shame regarding the amputation, his or her relationships with family and friends may be affected, presenting difficulties. He or she may be depressed and may refuse to cooperate with the training program. On the other hand, the amputee may be

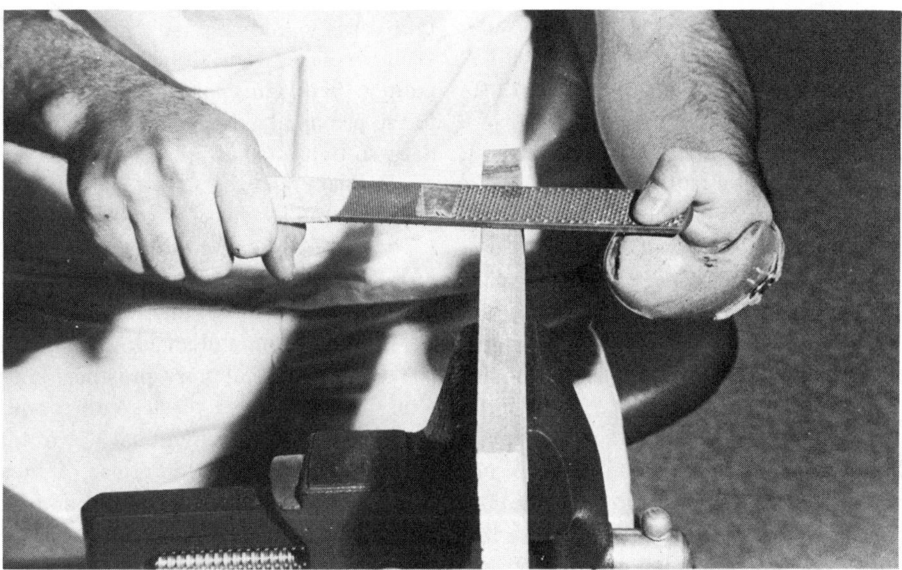

FIGURE 23-14. This patient wears a partial hand prosthesis to hold tool for bimanual wood filing.

interested in compensating for the loss by learning as much as he or she can about the prosthesis, by accepting change and by demonstrating eagerness to learn.

It is very important to consider the patient's feelings and useful attitudes. The prosthesis should be presented in a way that is meaningful to the amputee. For some persons, function is most important; for others, appearance is the greatest concern. For either, prosthetic replacement can help the amputee by providing function and cosmetic value.

Becoming familiar with the prime concerns of the amputee with regard to vocational and social needs as well as self-esteem begins with the initial contact between the patient and the therapist. Careful attention is given to combining the components needed and desired by the individual. Careful initial evaluation, pre-prosthetic preparation, and prosthetic training in all areas of function are necessary for adequate acceptance and use of the prosthesis by the amputee. The therapist's positive attitude toward the amputee, his or her stump, his or her fears, achievement of lost function, and cosmesis through prosthetic replacement reinforce the patient's attitude. Most important is the provision of opportunities for the patient to use the prosthesis in all appropriate activities and to socialize with others in the process. Involvement of family members in the training program may also be helpful.

Pre-Prosthetic Period

The pre-prosthetic period is the time between the amputation and the fitting of the prosthesis. This is the period of "getting ready" for the prosthesis. The patient should be confronted with the importance of the pre-prosthetic program as preparation for prosthetic replacement. A successful pre-prosthetic program hastens physical and psychological adjustment to the prosthesis and minimizes problems in wearing and using the permanent prosthesis. In this period it is important to counsel and guide the amputee regarding both the acceptance of his or her condition and the acceptance of the mechanical device which must substitute for natural motor power, sensation, and physical appearance. Counselling sessions with the amputee should also include his or her family and friends in order to involve them in the training program.

When medically approved, passive and active strengthening activities are started by the physical therapist and the occupational therapist to encourage maximum use of the stump, maximum range of motion (ROM), and maximum use of muscles, especially those of the arm and shoulder. A well-planned pre-prosthetic exercise program contributes to successful adaptation and provides strong muscles for the training in isolated motions for control and use of the prosthesis.

Following the amputation, the loss of the weight of the missing part causes a shift in the amputee's center of gravity. Atrophy of the musculature on the side of the amputation, scoliosis, and compensatory curves may occur if the patient does not have proper exercise. Therefore, the beginning exercise program is geared toward correcting faulty body mechanics and providing the amputee with sufficient ROM and strength to operate the prosthesis.

The first step is to establish good rapport with the patient so that it will be possible to help him or her in working through his or her necessary adjustments and in learning independence in daily living with the aid of an artificial limb. The relationship between the training therapist and the patient is a very important one, for the therapist must understand the patient's attitudes toward the prosthesis in order to help him or her accept and use it. The amputee may have fears of being different, may question the attitudes of others toward him or herself, and may even question him or herself about possible inadequacies.

Before the amputee receives the prosthesis, he or she must develop strength and tolerance in the stump. As soon as possible following the amputation, exercises are begun to maintain and, if necessary, to regain normal passive and active ROM in the joints proximal to the amputation. Since the hospital stay may be short, these exercises are designed so that they can be done in outpatient situations in the clinic. Although this may be painful to the patient, it is important to maintain and encourage maximum movement and use of the extremity during the healing period in order to prepare the amputee for the prosthesis, to prevent weakening of muscles through disuse, and to encourage shrinkage of the stump.

After complete healing, the stump is massaged to encourage circulation, to prevent adhesions from scar tissue, to reduce swelling, to encourage desensitization, and to prevent the patient from fearing to handle the stump. Bandaging with an elastic Ace bandage or "shrinker" is done several times per day to encourage shrinkage and shaping. Wrapping should be done carefully with attention to tightness, unnecessary folds in the bandage, and complete, even coverage of the stump to ensure comfort to the patient. Bandaging should be done from the distal to the proximal end. Care must be taken not to bandage so tightly as to produce muscle atrophy.

To encourage the use of the stump the occupational therapist may strap utensils to it which are used in ADL. Such utensils may include a knife, fork, or toothbrush. The amputee should be encouraged to use the individual implements in ADL.

The shrinking and shaping are also hastened by provision of a temporary prosthesis in the form of either a leather or a plaster cuff to which utensils can be attached for functional use of the extremity.

In this period, maximum use of the arms should be encouraged in both unilateral and bilateral exercise and functional activities. Additionally, since posture can be affected by the loss of a part, balance and posture exercises are necessary to prevent substitution patterns; these exercises help to make the amputee aware of his or her new body image.

Although the pre-prosthetic program can be enhanced by the use of a temporary prosthesis, the amputee's tolerance determines when it may be applied. The temporary prosthesis aids the amputee in overcoming the initial psychological shock of amputation in the following ways—it provides a temporary replacement for the length of the missing arm; it provides him or her with a degree of independence, since a fork or a tool or other utensils may be attached to it to provide functional use of the amputated extremity. Additionally, a temporary prosthesis aids in cosmetic lengthening of the stump and, most significantly, is a device with which the amputee can perform bimanual and bilateral activities. One of the most important parts of the training program lies in the amputee's early involvement in activities which show results.

At this time, the amputee should be encouraged to use the sound arm in one-handed activities, even though he or she may not be naturally motivated to do so. If the amputated arm had been the dominant one, he or she may have temporary difficulties in accepting the loss and in using the non-dominant arm. In this case, he or she may need exercises to develop coordination patterns in the remaining limb. Activities such as eating, dressing, writing, and bathing may be difficult with the non-dominant hand. It is very important at this time to provide a program to encourage successful one-handed use in daily activities.

For the amputee with a cineplasty, the biceps muscle becomes the motor for the prosthesis, thus providing the link between the muscle and the prosthetic mechanism. Because the cineplasty provides increased arm ROM and the amputee is free of a harness, it allows the amputee to hold the prosthesis in any position without affecting the operation of the terminal device. For maximum use of the cineplasty prosthesis, it is necessary to have a 1½- to 2-inch excursion of the surgical tunnel. Routine exercises to maintain this excursion include isolated muscle exercise of the biceps, isometric contractions and holds, and sufficient relaxation for the excursion and the opening of the terminal device. The cineplasty prosthesis is reported to provide improved dexterity and sensitivity to the amputated limb by the physiological use of the stump muscles.

In preparing the patient for prosthetic wear and in providing the prosthesis appropriate to the patient's needs and expectations, the occupational therapist must consider several important questions. First, does the patient need it? This will depend on the patient's limitations as a result of the amputation, his or her vocational and avocational needs and interests, and his or her attitude towards the value of the prosthesis. Another question relevant to the prescription is what does the amputee need it for, and will he or she wear it? This depends largely upon attitude towards the loss of the limb, loss of function, and relationships of the amputee with other people. Does he or she need and want function or cosmetic acceptance or both? What is most important to him or her in homelife, at work, in hobbies, and in social life?

Following the pre-prosthetic program, or near its end, these questions are taken into serious consideration in order to prescribe the appropriate prosthetic components for the maximum benefit to the amputee. At this point the rehabilitation team comes together for consultation.

Prior to the prescription the physiatrist measures the stump and examines the patient. The parts and controls of the prosthesis are determined by many factors: range of motion, strength, length, skin coverage and appearance, incision site, shoulder strength, and job requirements. Ideally, the physiatrist prescribes the prosthesis at the amputee clinic in the presence of the rehabilitation team and the patient and with the consultation of those who will be training the patient to adjust to and to use the prosthesis. At this time, if not before, the occupational therapist can acquaint the new amputee with the various components and harnessing which he or she is likely to have and perhaps can introduce him or her to another amputee who has completed the training program and is using the prosthesis successfully.

The accompanying pre-prosthetic evaluation form can be used by the occupational therapist as a guide to determine what are appropriate components (hook and hand) for the amputee. If the patient has not remained in the hospital during the postoperative, pre-prosthetic period, the evaluation form is helpful in determining his or her limitations and needs in terms of strengthening the extremity and trunk for prosthetic wear and use. Should an amputee return to the hospital's amputee clinic for prescription of a new prosthesis, this form is helpful in evaluating whether he or she should be given the same type of prosthesis or if different components would be more helpful. The occupational therapist can also assess the amputee's needs for further training, especially if he or she has not used the prosthesis extensively in daily activities.

Check-out of the Prosthesis

Before the amputee begins his or her training program, members of the rehabilitation team examine the prosthesis to make sure that it conforms to the prescription and that it is mechanically sound. In performing the check-out of the prosthesis, the occupational therapist evaluates its fit and comfort for the wearer and checks the motion and function of the components. Should adjustments need to be made in any part or parts of the prosthesis the rehabilitation team makes recommendations to the prosthetist in order to ensure that the amputee does not begin the training program with an uncomfortable or mechanically mediocre device. The physician makes the final approval of the prosthesis.

OCCUPATIONAL THERAPY PRE-PROSTHETIC EVALUATION

Name: ______________________ Date: ______________
Address: ______________________ Telephone No. ______________
Age: ______________ Dominance: ______________
Date, cause, and type of amputation: ______________________
____
Level of amputation: ______________ Length of stump: ______________
Prosthesis: #1 ________ #2 ________ #3 ________ #4
Type of present prosthesis: ______________________
Occupation: ______________________
____
Date last worked: ______________________
R.O.M. in shoulder: ____________ elbow: ____________ wrist: ____________
supination-pronation: ______________________
Strength in shoulder: ______________ elbow: ______________
Pain in stump: ______________________
Phantom sensations: ______________________
Current use of limb without prosthesis: ______________________
Use of previous prosthesis: ______________________
Attitude toward new prosthesis: ______________________
a) function: ______________________
b) cosmesis: ______________________
Additional remarks: ______________________
____
____
Prescription at clinic: ______________________
____
Prosthetist: ______________ #Training sessions: ______________
Signed: ______________

At the time of the check-out, which occurs during the first training session, the occupational therapist begins to acquaint the amputee with prosthetic terminology. The amputee learns the names of the parts and their functions, and learns the proper attachment of the harness and the components so that he can keep the prosthesis clean and can interchange the terminal devices efficiently.

In instructing the patient in the care of the prosthesis, the occupational therapist teaches the amputee the proper use of the hook, wrist unit, and cable system. The amputee is instructed to use just enough motion to open or close the hook, to watch for worn rubberbands, to avoid putting unnecessary strain on the cable, and to watch for spreading of the housing and excessive friction between the cable and the housing.

The socket should be kept clean with soap and water; the stump socks should be washed daily; and the harness should be washed at least once per week. Leather parts can be cleaned with saddle soap. If the tips of the Dacron harness straps begin to fray, they can be sealed at the edge by singeing with a match.

The amputee should be instructed to use only cable control to operate the functional hooks and hands. Manual operation may damage the mechanism. The amputee should also be warned never to use the terminal device in such activities as hammering nails or removing screws as this can tear threads and damage hook neoprene.

The cosmetic gloves on the functional hand are very perishable. It is important to guard the glove against tearing, since it functions as a protection of the hand mechanism from dirt and wetness. Also, these gloves soil easily, can be stained or marked if laid on dirty surfaces, and darken with age. Substances such as certain foods, ink, newsprint, and chemicals can damage the glove and lessen its cosmetic effect. The occupational therapist should recommend that the amputee keep the hand in a plastic bag when it is not in use. The amputee should be warned against oiling parts of the prosthesis or removing the glove from the hand, and should be counselled to return to the prosthetist for any assistance needed.

Training Program

A successful training program for an amputee requires the coordinated efforts of a rehabilitation team. This team includes the surgeon, nurse, physiatrist, physical therapist, occupational therapist, social worker, prosthetist, rehabilitation counsellor, and psychiatrist or psychologist. A coordinated effort of these persons is necessary for the provision of appropriate prosthetic replacement and training in the use of the prosthesis.

At the beginning of the training program, the prosthesis should be put on over a light-weight shirt so that the occupational therapist and the amputee can see the prosthesis function and so that it is not hindered by tight clothing. The amputee should become accustomed to using the mirror as a guide to learning the correct positioning of the harness straps in back and in learning the control motions.

Loose clothing is recommended for the amputee to facilitate putting on, wearing, and using the prosthesis. Clothing with front fastenings, Velcro closures, and wide shirt cuffs are helpful. The use of a buttonhook (Fig. 23-15) designed especially for the amputee can assist him or her with the problem of fastening the sleeve button on the sound side. Sewing the buttons on with elastic thread enables the amputee to leave the button fastened when removing the shirt, even if the cuffs are narrow, for the cuff will then stretch enough to allow the hand and arm to be removed from the sleeve. When putting on the shirt, the amputee should remember to put it on the amputated side first. One-handed shoe tying and special closures can simplify dressing procedures.

There are two approaches commonly used in training amputees. In one, the training program is directed toward developing the potential level of the amputee's performance. With this approach a unilateral amputee learns to develop fine coordination with the prosthesis, so that he or she can have maximum use of it even in case of an injury to the remaining extremity. The other approach varies from the potential approach in that the amputee is trained in the use of the prosthesis only as an aid in bimanual activities. Regardless of the approach, activities should be chosen which are suitable to the amputee's needs. The occupational therapist should encourage the amputee to indicate any additional and special training which he or she desires.

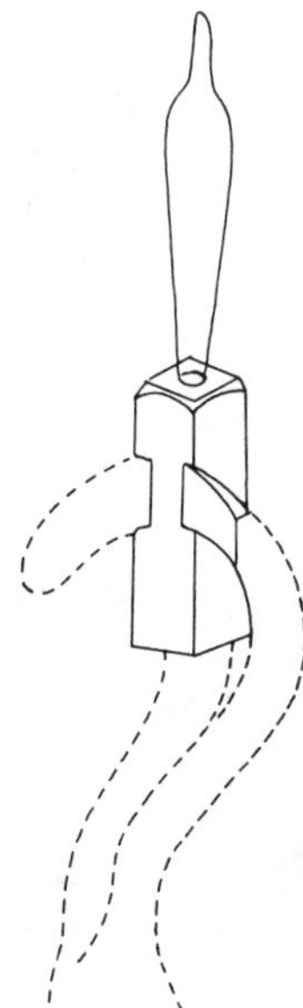

FIGURE 23-15. Amputee buttonhook.

The training period serves as a "try out" period to check the efficiency of the prosthesis and the practicality of the components to suit the amputee's individual needs as well as to make adjustments of malfunctions of the device.

The length of the training sessions should be increased as the amputee's tolerance and adaptation increase. He or she must master its use in training before combining the prosthesis and remaining extremity in bimanual activities and before wearing the prosthesis outside the clinic. Wearing it outside the clinic for an overnight period is advised for the first out-of-clinic experience. This is preferable to having the amputee wear it at home for an entire weekend. Training with the hand should be delayed until use of the hook has been mastered unless the amputee has only a hand provided.

The general goals of training include (1) independence in self-care and ADL, (2) return to former work or to a better job, (3) improved appearance, (4) return to hobbies and recreation, and (5) mastery of new skills.

Certain factors affecting the amputee's capacity to learn may, unfortunately, be detrimental. They include poor habits uncorrected in pre-prosthetic training, lack of motivation, lack of sensory feedback from the nonsensory prosthesis, time needed for training, age, inability to learn, and lack of a sense of accomplishment. The occupational therapist must attempt to minimize an amputee's negative attitude toward any or all of these factors.

The positive attitude of the amputee is very important; he or she must want to learn. The occupational therapist must encourage the amputee to have varying positive attitudes toward the prosthesis, such as considering it as a tool, a device to conceal his or her disability, an improvement of his or her body image, and/or a substitute for loss. Since it is important for the amputee to eventually integrate the prosthesis into his or her bodily function, he or she must become acquainted with it as a potential part of self, both functionally and cosmetically. The amputee should have a feeling of success after each training session.

Early training in successful use of control motions can enable the amputee to feel that he or she will be successful in future training activities. He or she should be cautioned against using the opposite shoulder to control the device and should be taught to operate the prosthesis with the amputated extremity as much as possible. Control motions should be minimal to save strength and thus to extend the time during which the amputee can wear and use the prosthesis.

In the first training session, the amputee should be taught the use and care of the stump sock (mentioned earlier).

Sensation is a natural guide to motor control. We recognize objects by shape, texture, size, and movement. But the amputee must often substitute vision for sensation (e.g., using visual cues in observing the amount of hook opening). He or she combines this with the sensation of cable tension to provide visual-sensory training, using the perception of both position and force. The proprioceptive sensation in the stump and the arm can aid here. He or she also uses auditory cues, such as the clicks in the elbow lock, hand, and hook for efficient operation of the prosthesis.

During the first session it is important to acquaint the amputee with the actual function of the hook by teaching exercises for opening and closing it. Since many voluntary opening hooks are prescribed for amputees, let us use them as an example.

Following the cable pull by shoulder flexion, the cable tension is released by shoulder extension and the hook is pulled closed by its rubberbands, which yield 1 pound of pressure each. The standard number of rubberbands employed is usually three or four, although up to eight and more may be used for the BE amputee for added grip strength. (Fig. 23-16 shows a device for applying rubberbands.) The amputee begins his or her training by learning to isolate the control motions needed to activate the hook. Then, using visual cues and sensing in his or her shoulder the resistance of the rubberbands, the amputee learns how to control the exact opening of the hook. In order to minimize the energy expenditure needed to use the hook, the amputee should be encouraged to open the hook only slightly more than the size of the object he or she wishes to pick up—just enough to grasp the object. The amputee should practice with objects of different sizes and weights in order to achieve control. Additionally, drills requiring the grasp of objects of different forms, textures, and materials are necessary for the amputee to learn the basic motions used in operating the hook. Since

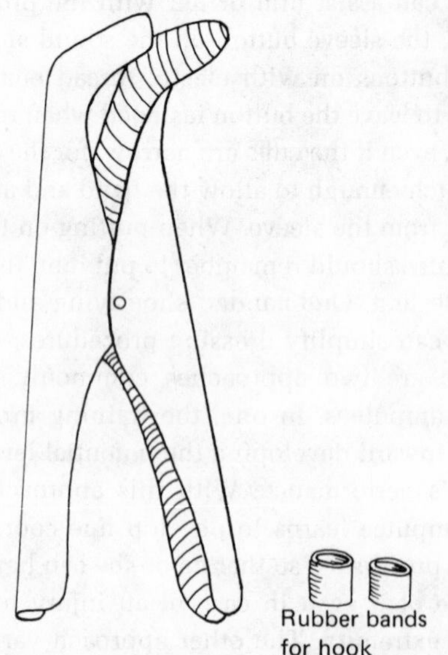

FIGURE 23-16. Band applier for voluntary opening hook.

some materials are light, breakable, or easily crushed (i.e., a paper or plastic cup), it is important to teach the amputee to employ a minimum of pressure by maintaining tension on the cable during grasp. The amputee should also learn to operate the hook in different planes of arm movements, so that he or she will achieve maximum functional use.

These drills for grip control should be extended to other components of the prosthesis. The amputee must learn how to preposition the terminal device at the wrist unit, how to operate the elbow unit, how to use the turntable, how to coordinate the elbow lock and elbow flexion and extension, and how to preposition the shoulder. In these drills the use of the terminal device is combined with a number of gross arm functions. The amputee learns the grasp, placement, and release of objects on shelves, tables, and the floor and learns to depend on the grip of the hook or functional hand.

During this early drill period, use of the sound extremity should be encouraged. During the rest periods the amputee should be encouraged to practice unilateral activities as well as bilateral ones. It is through these more complicated coordination activities that the prosthesis begins to be functionally integrated into the bilateral UE activities of the amputee. Although the unilateral amputee may already have become independent in ADL during the preprosthetic period, there are many things which we are accustomed to doing with two hands. For example, the amputee may find it difficult to cut meat, button a shirt sleeve, tie shoes, or wrap a package with one hand. The prosthesis may help him or her to accomplish these things, or the occupational therapist may discover that additional adaptive devices are needed.

Whatever the problem, the occupational therapist should encourage the amputee to become skillful in the use of the hook and to devise ways to increase independence in function. Participation in woodworking, sewing, weaving, or other avocational activities can be motivating for the amputee, can provide coordination and strength, can show how his or her prosthesis can help in doing things, and can aid in integrating the prosthesis into bodily function.

Using a worksheet checklist of activities accomplished can be helpful in recording the amputee's progress of training in both the clinic and the home. Since there are many activities that the patient will do at home that cannot be simulated in the clinic, the therapist should continue to encourage the amputee to do new things at home following each training session and to report successes or difficulties with new tasks. In this way, the therapist is able to assist the patient not only in controls, training drills, and activities, but also in tasks and responsibilities in the routine of daily living. Thus, the program becomes relevant to each amputee's needs.

Activity categories on the worksheet should include basic prehension activities, dressing and grooming (including putting on and taking off the prosthesis), eating and social skills (using keys and opening an umbrella), homemaking, clerical activities, and activities related to vocational and avocational interests.

Another training aid is a prosthetic training board with common objects (locks, light switches, pencil sharpener) attached to it.

Recreational activities during the pre-prosthetic and prosthetic training periods provide general body conditioning and development of a new image for the amputee.

Prevocational Training

Because industrial accidents are a frequent cause of UE amputations, a prevocational assessment should be included in the training program to assist the amputee in recognizing capabilities in prosthetic function and whether or not he or she, as an amputee, can safely return to a former occupation or whether he or she needs to consider a change of occupation and additional vocational training. Specific tasks related to the individual's type of work should be included in the prosthetic training program to assess his or her safe and efficient handling of tools, power equipment, and heavy and light materials. Work tolerance can be assessed by the use of timed job-simulated tasks.

Prevocational considerations include training in general household activities. Training in the accomplishment of homemaking tasks such as meal preparation, cleaning, and household repairs are included.

Child care is also included in the prevocational program.

External Power

Research is continuing into more effective control systems and sites and for the development of improved components to simulate natural movements and functions. Efforts are being made to lessen weight, to improve locking and grasping mechanisms in the hand and the hook, to improve the glove material, and to increase the overall cosmesis of the prosthesis. Specific considerations are development of a more efficient elbow unit, rerouting of the cables to the inside of the arm instead of the outside, improved cosmetic appearance, higher operating efficiencies, and decreased wear on clothing. There is also research interest in providing active wrist rotation.

The electric arm, a complex experimental mechanism, provides the amputee with an electric elbow and forearm rotation control. This mechanism is controlled by small batteries and a motor which are placed on the arm structure or in the amputee's pocket. The experimentation into electric control is an effort toward providing the mechanical extremity with a total coordination pattern and better integration into the body system. The aim is to provide a link between the person and the mechanical device by using a stimulus from the person's energy to activate the prosthesis.

Another idea is the use of phantom sensations to aid in the control of the BE prosthesis, using the signals from the forearm muscles for prehension and forearm rotation (pronation and supination). This method does not apply to the AE amputee, since the forearm muscles are gone and the power source muscles are removed from the terminal device.

In addition to the prohibitive cost of these experimental devices, another problem with an external power source is the replenishment of power. But efforts to produce designs which will simulate characteristics of normal muscle functions continue, in hope of achieving the goal of successful integration of the device and the person.

With the continuing research into the use and application of external power, the concept of "man-machine," or the integration of the person and the assistive device, is often cited. Since the physician and the prosthetist recognize the need for an engineer who can provide devices operated with external power, the engineer or a specialist in bioengineering has become a new member of the rehabilitation team.

OCCUPATIONAL THERAPY AND THE LOWER EXTREMITY AMPUTEE

Amputations of the lower extremities are generally more common than those of the upper extremities because of the high incidence of peripheral vascular disease and traumatic injuries to the lower limbs. Psychological reactions mentioned earlier concerning the upper extremity amputee pertain also to the lower extremity amputee. Since age, body build, physical and medical condition, vascular supply, and motivation are factors in the rehabilitation of the lower extremity amputee, there are some patients for whom provision of a prosthesis is contraindicated. These persons are encouraged to maintain maximum independence and mobility with the aid of a wheelchair, crutches, and other necessary assistive devices. The amputee for whom a prosthesis is appropriately prescribed can usually look forward to partial restoration of basic functions, independence in self-care, and the opportunity of returning to work of some kind.

Basically, the detailed study of lower extremity (LE) function, pre-prosthetic preparation, prosthetic prescription, check-out and training, and the management of problems encountered by the LE amputee are handled by the physician and the physical therapist. However, there are many ways in which the occupational therapist can also contribute to the functional rehabilitation of the LE amputee. In a general hospital or a rehabilitation center the occupational therapist may actually work with as many or more LE amputees as UE amputees.

Pre-Prosthetic Period

Passive and active exercises of the lower extremities are performed or supervised by the physical therapist during the early postoperative period of healing. The nurse or physical therapist teaches the amputee to bandage the stump to encourage shrinkage and forming of the stump for prosthetic fitting. Proper positioning of the body in the wheelchair is important to prevent contractures in the joints proximal to the amputation, scoliosis of the spinal column, and edema—all of which could hinder successful prosthetic function. In the case of below-knee (BK) amputation, the use of a seat-board adapted for the individual amputee can be used in a regular chair or a wheelchair to maintain the knee in passive extension with knee flexors stretched while the amputee is performing activities in a sitting position.

The LE amputee may be referred to occupational therapy in the pre-prosthetic or the prosthetic phase of training or both. In either case, the occupational therapist should become familiar with the medical aspects of the patient's care and the goals of the rehabilitation program. Pertinent information the occupational therapist should learn from the chart or from the staff members should include:

1. Location, type, level, and cause of amputation.
2. Condition of the stump and amputated extremity.
3. General body condition.
4. Precautions.
5. Previous prosthetic replacement, if any.
6. Recommendations for passive and active positioning of the joints of the amputated extremity.
7. The appropriate amount of standing and walking to encourage and the degree of safe support needed by the amputee.
8. Complicating factors.

Throughout the pre-prosthetic and prosthetic stages of training the amputee may go through changes in attitude and behavior as he or she gradually realizes the extent of the loss and its effect on his or her life. Continual counselling is often necessary to help the amputee to adjust to the amputation, the change in body image, and the wear and use of the mechanical device to substitute for natural function. He or she must also adjust to working with his or her arms, gearing him or herself to abilities rather than disability, finding new interests, and socializing in the new situation.

The seat-board mentioned previously can be made by the amputee as part of an upper extremity exercise program. It can be made of ½ or ¾ inch plywood which conforms to the measurement of the inside of the chair seat; one side extends to the end of the amputee's stump. The extended side should be narrow enough to prevent interference with the comfort of the sound leg in a sitting position, and at the same time should provide passive extension to the knee of the amputated leg. The seat-board should be padded sufficiently for comfort, and particular attention should be paid to such sensitive areas as the end of the stump.

In this pre-prosthetic phase the amputee may come to occupational therapy either in a wheelchair or walking with crutches. A variety of treatment techniques can be used. Since balance and upper extremity and trunk strength will be very important in prosthetic use, maximum function of these areas is encouraged. Insofar as the amputee can tolerate the exercise, his or her sitting tolerance and balance is challenged by the use of upper extremity activities. Although at first an amputee with a high above-knee (AK) amputation or bilateral leg amputations may need to hold onto the chair with one hand to support himself or herself in a sitting position while using the other hand, he or she should be encouraged to depend on the trunk for balance to leave both arms free for UE activities. As upper extremity strength and confidence in balance increase, ROM and resistance required in performing manual activities should be increased to further challenge trunk balance. Activities such as woodworking, weaving, and printing may be adapted to the amputee's individual needs. An activity in which the patient has a vocational or avocational interest may provide motivation in the activity so that he or she can increase tolerance of the given position and redirect energies from anxieties regarding his or her condition toward purposeful activity. Activities at this stage are directed toward the amputee's achieving independent function of arms and trunk while seated in a wheelchair.

Another aspect of independence regards self-care tasks. These include bathing and care of the stump, transfers, and dressing. A unilateral amputee should have little or no difficulty in this area. However, aids such as grab bars for bath and toilet, a transfer board or tub seat for bathing, and a raised toilet seat can be helpful as the amputee adjusts to a new body image and copes with the problems of balance. Phantom limb sensations can be a complicating factor if the amputee suddenly moves to get up and forgets that he or she cannot stand on the amputated limb, even though feeling is there. Continued physical and psychological support in these instances is necessary to minimize fear and to encourage confidence. Dressing is usually easier from a sitting position on the bed. Front fastenings and loose clothing also help to minimize frustrations.

Maximum independent function should be encouraged both with and without the prosthesis. For example, the amputee should be encouraged to stand on the sound leg in front of a table for short periods of time. This will encourage hip extension of the amputated side and will develop balance. However, attention must be paid to the amount of standing time so as not to encourage scoliosis of the spine.

Therapists have found that immediate postoperative fitting of a prosthesis or the use of a temporary pylon and the working prosthesis after the amputee's scar tissue has healed is beneficial to the LE amputee training program. The temporary pylon provides the amputee with early replacement of the amputated limb to encourage functional activity while the stump is being conditioned and the permanent prosthesis is being made.* The pylon consists of a plaster stump socket to which a pylon is attached to provide length and base support to the amputated leg. With the pylon the amputee can stand and ambulate soon after the amputation.

A working prosthesis is permanently attached to the machine that the amputee will use for exercise (i.e., to the foot-powered lathe or the bicycle jigsaw). It also consists of a stump cuff which is laced up the sides for ease in putting on and provides a comfortable fit for different persons. It is open at the distal end to eliminate pressure on the end of the stump.

When the patient has put the cuff on the stump, he or she fits the pylon shafts into the cuff. As the base is attached to the bicycle jigsaw or the lathe, the amputee is then able to operate these machines and thus engage in active LE exercise of the amputated limb. The working prosthesis could be used with a foot-powered floor press, treadle sewing machine, or loom if properly adapted to the needs of the amputee. ROM and resistance can be graded, and the amputee can engage in an activity requiring coordination, balance, and strength of all four extremities and the trunk.

* For specific designs of the pylon, see M. S. Jones: *An Approach to Occupational Therapy*. London: Butterworths, 1964, Chapter 6.

It must be remembered that at first the amputee fatigues more rapidly, even in the activity of maintaining sitting and standing positions, and that until tolerance increases, energy is directed toward these basic functions.

Prosthetic Training Program

The LE amputee depends on the prosthesis for support of the body in standing and walking. It is important that the prosthesis be appropriately prescribed, that it fit comfortably, and that it provide adequate functional assistance. The prescription and mechanical function of the prosthesis are checked thoroughly by the physical therapist. Function of the parts, how the amputee should put on the prosthesis, and how he or she should use it are taught by the physical therapist.

Independent locomotion depends on the fit and comfort of the prosthesis as well as on the general condition and tolerance of the amputee. Some may be able to discard their wheelchairs fairly soon. However, the amputee with poor tolerance of the prosthesis or a poorly fitting one may need the security of the wheelchair for a long time. In either case, the occupational therapy program can benefit the amputee by encouraging work in the treatment room doing activities in a standing position when he or she can tolerate it. Even if the amputee is still dependent on the wheelchair early in prosthetic training, he or she must eventually adjust to the mechanical, insensitive prosthesis by learning to judge where it is relative to the rest of the body, and he or she must learn how to function with it.

When the amputee receives the prosthesis, most of his or her attention will be on the fit and use of it. Since he needs rest periods from ambulation training, he or she continues in an occupational therapy program for upper extremity strengthening and prosthetic tolerance. The activities outlined in the preprosthetic period are continued. At this point, they are done with the prosthesis on unless the amputee is resting the stump or it is irritated by the prosthesis. His or her program is geared toward encouraging acceptance of the prosthesis (to function in activities challenging UE and LE coordination and function), prosthetic tolerance, development of ADL independence, UE and LE activity exercise program, realization of his or her capacities, and vocational and avocational guidance.

Wearing time of the prosthesis is gradually increased according to the comfort and tolerance of the socket in sitting and standing positions. As the amputee will be weightbearing in the standing position, he or she must adjust to the sensation of bilateral weightbearing and the sensitivity of the stump to the hard edges and base of the socket. According to his or her tolerance and balance, the amputee can decrease the support he or she uses while standing. Engagement in UE activities in a standing position, which provides a wide range of motion and resistance, helps to challenge and to increase standing balance. Walking to cabinets to get and replace materials or tools and walking around tables and machines should be encouraged to increase functional independence. Carrying articles from place to place also further challenges balance and independent function. Aids such as a cart with wheels or a tray can minimize the stress of carrying items.

In ADL, the patient now learns to incorporate the prosthesis into bodily activities. He or she learns at what point in dressing activities to put on the prosthesis so that it will aid, rather than interfere with, ease and speed in dressing.

An important part of the prosthetic training program is aiding the amputee to realize his or her capabilities. In the occupational therapy environment tasks both to improve the amputee's tolerance and function with the prosthesis and to relate to the requirements of his or her job may be set up.

Prevocational Exploration

Amputation may prevent a person from returning to a former line of work and it may be a great source of anxiety. When the amputation prevents the individual from returning to a former occupation, the occupational therapist can provide valuable information to the vocational rehabilitation counsellor regarding the functional capabilities of the amputee. Information regarding interests, intelligence, physical abilities and skills, work tolerance, work habits, and general motivation for achieving new skills assists the counsellor in investigating new possibilities for the employable amputee in vocational planning.

BIBLIOGRAPHY

Amputees, Amputations, and Artificial Limbs. An Annotated Bibliography. Committee on Prosthetic-Orthotic Education, Division of Medical Sciences, National Academy of Sciences, National Research Council, Washington DC, 1969.

Anderson, M. H., Bechtol, C. O., and Sollars, R. E.: Clinical Prosthetics for Physicians and Therapists. Springfield IL: Charles C Thomas, 1959.

Bender, L. F.: Prostheses and Rehabilitation after Arm Amputation. Springfield IL: Charles C Thomas, 1974.

Blakeslee, B.: The Limb-Deficient Child. Berkeley and Los Angeles: University of California Press, 1963.

Fishman S., and Kay, H. W.: The Munster-type below-elbow socket, an evaluation. Artif. Limbs 8:4, 1964.

Garrett, J. F., and Levine, E. S. (eds.): Psychological Practice with the Physically Disabled. New York: Columbia University Press, 1961.

Gerhardt, J. J., et al.: Immediate post-surgical prosthetics: Rehabilitation aspects. Am. J. Phys. Med. 49:3, 1970.

Hartman, H. H., et al.: A myoelectrically controlled powered elbow. Artif. Limbs 12:61, 1968.

Jones, M. S.: An Approach to Occupational Therapy. London: Butterworths, 1964.

Kay, H. W., et al.: The Munster-type below-elbow socket, a fabrication technique. Artif. Limbs 9:4, 1965.

Klopsteg, P. E., and Wilson, P. D., et al.: Human Limbs and Their Substitutes. New York: Hafner Press, 1968.

Licht, S. (ed.): Rehabilitation Medicine. Baltimore: Waverly Press, 1968.

Long, C., and Ebskov, B.: Research applications of myoelectric control. Arch. Phys. Med. 47:190, 1966.

Loughlin, E., Stanford, J. W., and Phelps, M.: Immediate post-surgical prosthetics fitting of a bilateral, below-elbow amputee, a report. Artif. Limbs 12:17, 1968.

Mital, M. A., and Pierce, D. S.: Amputees and Their Prostheses. Boston: Little, Brown & Co., 1971.

Mulhern, F. P.: Biceps cineplasty exercise. Am. J. Occup. Ther. 11:322, 1957.

Munroe, B., and Nasca, R. J.: Rehabilitation of the upper extremity amputee. Military Med. 140:6, 1975.

Newman, J. B. (acting ed.): Newsletter . . . Amputee Clinics. Committee on Prosthetic-Orthotic Education, Division of Medical Sciences, National Academy of Sciences, National Research Council, Washington DC.

Reilly, G. V.: Pre-prosthetic exercises for upper extremity amputee with special reference to cineplasty. Phys. Therapy Rev. 31:183, 1951.

Review of Visual Aids for Prosthetics and Orthotics. Committee on Prosthetic-Orthotic Education, Division of Medical Sciences, National Academy of Sciences, National Research Council, Washington DC.

Santschi, W. R.: Manual of Upper Extremity Prosthetic, ed. 2. Los Angeles: Department of Engineering, UCLA, 1965.

Sarmiento, A., et al.: Immediate postsurgical prosthetics

fitting in the management of upper-extremity amputees. Artif. Limbs 12:14, 1968.

Scott, R. N.: Myoelectric control of prosthesis. Arch. Phys. Med. 47:174, 1966.

Shaperman, J. W.: Learning techniques applied to prehension. Am. J. Occup. Ther. 14:70, 1960.

The Control of External Power in Upper-Extremity Rehabilitation. National Academy of Sciences, National Research Council, Publication #1352, Washington DC, 1966.

Tohen, Z., and Alfonso, M. D.: Manual of Mechanical Orthopaedics. Springfield IL: Charles C Thomas, 1973.

Tosberg, W. A.: Upper and Lower Extremity Prostheses. Springfield IL: Charles C Thomas, 1962.

Wellerson, T. L.: A Manual for Occupational Therapists on the Rehabilitation of Upper Extremity Amputees. New York, published under the auspices of the American Occupational Therapy Association, 1958.

Willard, H. S., and Spackman, C. S.: Occupational Therapy, ed. 3, p. 308, Philadelphia, J. B. Lippincott Co., 1963.

The following journals are invaluable to the occupational therapist working with amputees:

Artificial Limbs: A Review of Current Developments. Committee on Prosthetics Research and Development, Division of Engineering and Committee on Prosthetic-Orthotic Education, Division of Medical Sciences of the National Research Council, National Academy of Sciences, Washington DC.

Inter-Clinic Information Bulletin. Available from Prosthetics and Orthotics, New York University Post-Graduate Medical School, 317 E. 34th St., New York NY 10016.

ADDRESSES

Cosmetic restorations:

Realistic Industries
3010 Lyons Road
P.O. Box 6158
Austin, Texas 78702

ACKNOWLEDGMENTS

Thanks to Patricia A. Curran for editorial and typing services, Barry W. Kaufmann for assistance in preparing the illustrations, and Ron Gregory for photography.

24

Occupational Therapy Theory, Assessment, and Treatment in Educational Settings

Nancy Allen Kauffman

The original role of the occupational therapist in educational settings was primarily the treatment of orthopedically handicapped children. Learning impaired children became a new focus of the therapist's attention in the early 1970s. As educators became aware of the role of motor, sensory, and perceptual development in the continuum of learning, therapists were hired to work in school settings. They worked with preschool and young learning disabled children in readiness skills and movement exploration. They treated older children who had deficit level gaps in developmental skills necessary for learning. Perceptual-motor training and, later, sensory integrative therapy were used in treatment. Educators also began to place new emphasis on profoundly retarded and severely multiply handicapped children who had previously been denied public education. Therapists were hired to provide treatment as well as to help educators establish developmental sequencing for perceptual-motor, psychosocial, and self-care goals.

A survey by the American Occupational Therapy Association in 1976 identified 584 registered occupational therapists employed in public schools. One hundred of their positions had been created during the previous two years. This number continued to increase rapidly as the range of services expanded to include not only full time treatment but also itinerant programs, screening, and preventive programs providing evaluation, interpretation, and recommendations. Therapists also provide consulting services or inservice workshops for teachers, parents, and school district administrators.[1]

The occupational therapist in the early 1970s was a new addition to school systems, with a new frame of reference for looking at the educational needs of handicapped children. Lack of uniformity of policy, problems of communication, and blurring of roles between educational and therapeutic personnel resulted. With the passage of new legislation the need for appropriate personnel in every school district was mandated. Pressure on school boards and administrative personnel by parent advocate groups became an effective method of creating positions in many states.

LEGISLATION

President John F. Kennedy's Panel on Mental Retardation in 1962 recommended that education of the handicapped should help every individual make the most of his or her potential. To fill the gaps in services, Congress passed the Developmental Disabilities Services and Facilities Construction Act in 1970. Lawsuits against school systems in two areas (Pennsylvania Association for Retarded Children versus Commonwealth of Pennsylvania, 1971, and Mills versus Board of Education of the District of Columbia, 1972) established that handicapping conditions could no longer be a reason for excluding children from public education.

Many states then passed similar legislation and in 1975 President Gerald Ford signed into law the Education of All Handicapped Children Act (PL 94-142) which requires that handicapped children must receive a free *and appropriate* public education. Education in its broadest sense is the intent, regardless of the child's type or level of disability, and should not be restricted to academic ability. Handicapped children include the learning disabled; speech, language, hearing, or vision impaired; or physically, mentally, or emotionally impaired. In some states, by 1980, the handicapped must be educated from age three to twenty-one. Parents or guardians participate with professionals in developing a diagnostic-prescriptive Individualized Educational Program (I.E.P.) which must be written for each child annually.[2]

The Cascade System (Fig. 24-1) is a theoretical prototype used in many states as a conceptual framework for devising appropriate placements for children. It assumes that the greatest number of handicapped children can be absorbed into the mainstream of education. Children are placed in "the least restrictive alternative," i.e., the class which best fits their needs and is as close as possible to the everyday classroom. This allows financial resources

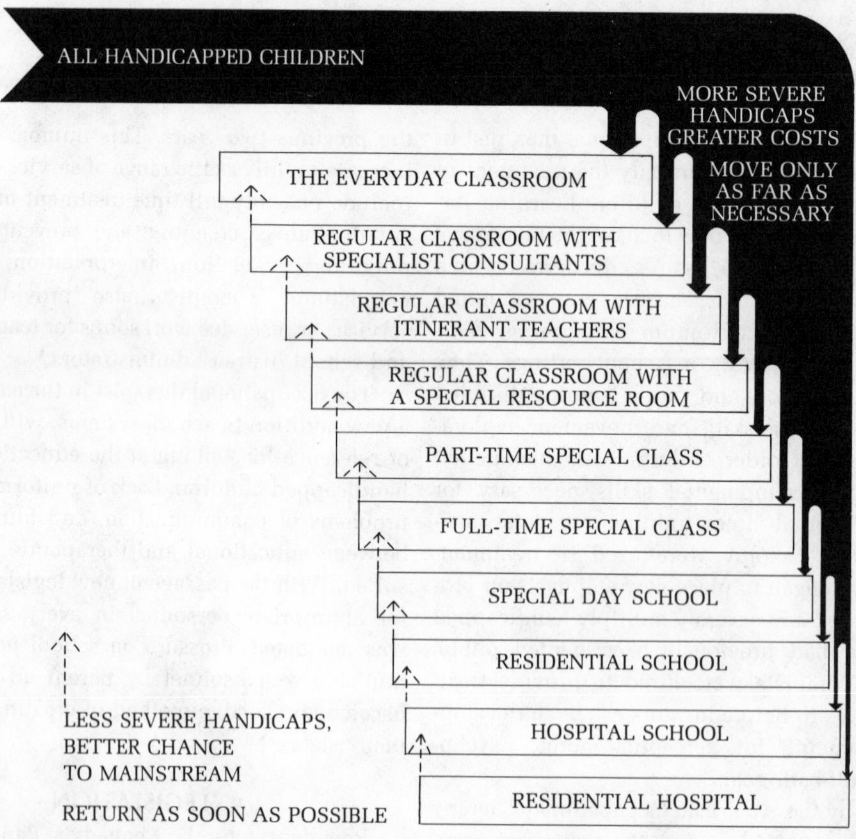

FIGURE 24-1. The Cascade System. From One Out of Ten: School Planning for the Handicapped, 1974, p. 7. Courtesy of Educational Facilities Laboratories, New York.

to be directed to the most handicapped children and is in agreement with the normalization principle which recommends conditions as close as feasible to the mainstream of society. The educational objectives for each student include movement toward the least restrictive alternative as soon as possible. Ideally, support from counseling, educational, and therapeutic services is provided as needed to facilitate the transition at each step.[3]

Parents have the legal right to examine all school records and to disagree with placement decisions. They may bring legal counsel and other professionals of their choice before an impartial hearing officer and question school personnel involved with program development or appropriate placement decisions for their child. Advocacy groups, often comprised of parents, use legal recourse to bring about educational changes on behalf of children.

TEAM APPROACH

Local school systems have interdisciplinary committees which make decisions about placement of children in programs at various levels of the Cascade. These decisions are based on such things as developmental level, academic performance, social maturity, and behavior and never simply on age or Intelligence Quotient (IQ). The committee recommends placement based on the primary cause of the child's learning problem. If a secondary problem, such as emotional overlay, has developed, appropriate education emphasizing treatment of the primary problem often eliminates it.

Team members who serve on the interdisciplinary committee within school systems may be occupational therapists, psychologists, speech and language clinicians, educational diagnosticians, teachers, school counselors, principals or program directors. The role of these team members is described later. Others who may serve as interdisciplinary committee members or may provide consultation are medical, neurological, psychiatric, optometric, and physical therapy personnel. Important team members who do not serve on interdisciplinary committees are teachers of art, music, and physical education. These teachers may have been specially trained to work with handicapped children. The parent, child, classroom aide, and volunteer also play important roles in the team effort of teaching the handicapped child.

Interdisciplinary Team Members

All members of the interdisciplinary committee assist in formulating decisions on appropriate placement of children.

OCCUPATIONAL THERAPIST. The unique function of the occupational therapist is to report results of sensory integrative, visual perceptual, self-help, and motor testing. The therapist may also write programs or make suggestions to be carried out by teachers, aides, parents, or volunteers.

PSYCHOLOGIST. Psychologists in many states report mental age or I.Q. scores. They may have responsibility for labelling the primary cause of the child's learning impairment, in which case other committee members simply determine the appropriate placement level on the Cascade. Test results which form the basis for the psychologist's recommendations may include, among others, the Wechsler Intelligence Scale for Children—Revised (WISC-R) or the McCarthy Scales of Children's Abilities. Experience has shown that consideration of subscores of tests given by the psychologist have given diagnostic information which has reduced the amount of time spent in evaluation by the therapist. Figure 24-2 and Figure 24-3 suggest interpretations of subtest scores. A breakdown of subtest scores may have to be specifically requested.

SPEECH AND LANGUAGE CLINICIAN. This member of the interdisciplinary committee reports test results of the child's receptive language (comprehension or decoding of what is heard) and expressive language (encoding through the use of linguistic symbols). For both expressive and receptive language, consideration is given to the child's use of sounds (phonology), meaning (semantics or vocabulary and concepts), and grammar (syntax and morphology). Integration (inner associative language processing such as categorization and understanding of analogies) is also considered as well as retention (memory) and such perceptual problems as auditory discrimination and speed of verbal response.

THE TESTS	Spatial	Quantitative	Sequencing	Perceptual organization	Conceptualization and verbal comprehension	Ability to concentrate: Distractibility	Visual motor integration: Fine motor	Verbal expression
• VERBAL SCALE								
Information					✓			✓
Similarities					✓			✓
Arithmetic		✓			✓	✓		
Vocabulary					✓			✓
Comprehension					✓			✓
Digit Span		✓	✓			✓		
• PERFORMANCE SCALE								
Picture Completion	✓					✓		
Picture Arrangement			✓		✓			
Block Design	✓			✓				
Object Assembly	✓			✓			✓	
Coding	✓		✓				✓	
Mazes	✓						✓	

FIGURE 24-2. Content of test items of the Wechsler Intelligence Scale for Children (WISC-R). Modified from Waugh, K. W., and Bush, W. J.: Diagnosing Learning Disorders. Columbus: Charles Merrill, 1971.

EDUCATIONAL DIAGNOSTICIAN. This specially trained teacher reports results of standardized tests of academic and readiness achievement levels in number concepts and in the developmental sequence of listening, speaking, reading, and then writing. The diagnostician also makes observations about the child's learning style which may differ widely from the child's strengths and weaknesses in tactile, kinesthetic, visual, or auditory modalities. For example the child may score low in tests of auditory processing but may learn to read better through listening than looking tasks.[4] The diagnostician may report on perceptual, language, and motor performance if they are not tested by other services.

SPECIAL EDUCATION TEACHER. Teachers sometimes have responsibility for making reports to the interdisciplinary committee as well as actually teaching children. The classroom teacher is the most significant person in the educational program because of having the most consistent contact with the handicapped child. This teacher makes recommendations about the everyday social maturity and behavior as well as academic, perceptual, and language performance of children in the classroom. The resource room teacher sees mildly handicapped children for a portion of each day to work on specific deficit areas. The itinerant special education teacher travels to schools or homes for the purpose of either

THE TASKS	Verbal	Perceptual-Performance	Quantitative	General Cognitive	Memory	Motor
1. Block Building		P		GC		
2. Puzzle Solving		P		GC		
3. Pictorial Memory	V			GC	Mem	
4. Word Knowledge	V			GC		
5. Number Questions			Q	GC		
6. Tapping Sequence		P		GC	Mem	
7. Verbal Memory	V			GC	Mem	
8. Right-Left Orientation		P		GC		
9. Leg Coordination						Mot
10. Arm Coordination						Mot
11. Initiative Action						Mot
12. Draw-A-Design		P		GC		Mot
13. Draw-A-Child		P		GC		Mot
14. Numerical Memory			Q	GC	Mem	
15. Verbal Fluency	V			GC		
16. Counting and Sorting			Q	GC		
17. Opposite Analogies	V			GC		
18. Conceptual Grouping		P		GC		

Chart showing the contribution of the eighteen tasks to the six scales

FIGURE 24-3. Plan of the McCarthy Scales. From McCarthy, D.: McCarthy Scales of Children's Abilities, 1972. Courtesy of the Psychological Corporation, New York.

screening and teaching children or suggesting to regular teachers academic intervention methods for mildly impaired children.

COUNSELOR. The counselor brings to the interdisciplinary committee awareness of both the child's family milieu and a variety of placement services within the community and the school system.

SCHOOL PRINCIPAL AND PROGRAM DIRECTOR. These committee members interpret local administrative policies in special education.

Testing

Occupational therapists should become familiar with tests frequently used by each of these disciplines in order to better interpret results. A task analysis, after observing pertinent tests being administered, is one effective means of doing this.

Testing by the therapist as well as other team members is only important if it results in program planning to benefit children. Along with educators and language specialists, occupational therapists play a key role in district-wide and local school policies for identifying handicapped children who may need special services. Procedures that have proven effective in various school districts will be described.

SCREENING

Children with severe handicaps are placed in appropriate programs at an early age. For some children the need for special education is not readily apparent. Screening procedures for identifying these children before the end of kindergarten or first grade allow early detection of children with learning disabilities, minimal brain dysfunction, mild mental retardation, or mild emotional disturbances. Proper school placement or special help within the everyday classroom at an early age helps prevent development of secondary emotional overlay resulting from learning failure in later grades. It also provides intervention procedures at a time in the child's life when they will be most helpful. Keeping the child in the everyday classroom or returning the child there at the earliest opportunity is currently considered most desirable. The goal of screening is to identify children who need help without interfering in the lives of children who have only a mild and temporary developmental delay. Various screening methods have been used for investigating children's motor, language, perceptual, cognitive, and behavioral deficits. The following are several examples of screening procedures that have been used in kindergarten and first grades.

Color coded name tags were used in one school district to call attention to children whom classroom teachers knew were having difficulty. Occupational therapists observed the whole class performing a battery of informal screening tasks, then made recommendations for training of problem children based on the results. A small percentage of children was recommended for further standardized testing.

Another school district sent a team of medical and educational personnel to individually observe and screen a few problem children identified by each teacher. Recommendations were made to the teacher and parents for managing the specific educational and behavioral problems. Later the team returned and used additional test measures for the one or two children who, in spite of several months of maturation and special teaching techniques, still had the greatest problems.

Volunteers were used in Fort Worth Public Schools to assist professionals in testing children using a locally developed screening instrument.[5]

The School District of Philadelphia developed a learning disabilities checklist to be marked by classroom teachers for each of their students.[6] It eliminated the need for screening by specialists. Although the attempt was made to write items observable during normal classroom activities, many teachers resisted the extra burden of evaluation. Such a checklist could be used for parent observation or for school use where teachers have been trained and motivated. The checklist, typical of many developed around the country, did serve one of its purposes: to familiarize teachers with behavioral and performance characteristics of young children with subtle learning problems. Easily understood phrases were checked as occurring frequently or seldom and cover the topics listed below:

1. *Behavior.* Items in this section cover hyperactivity; distractibility and impulsiveness; overreaction to change, excitement, unexpected touch, sounds, or smells; hypoactivity; focusing on irrelevant details; difficulty completing tasks; perseveration; inconsistent academic performance; difficulty with peer relations.

2. *Motor Coordination.* These items test for placing two feet per tread when climbing or descending stairs; clumsiness or awkwardness in moving or catching a ball; inability to hop three times or skip; difficulty copying pantomimed body positions especially when crossing the midline; difficulty touching the tip of the nose with the little finger with eyes closed; inability or awkwardness in bead stringing, coloring, pasting, buttoning, cutting, or holding a pencil.

3. *Orientation.* Items tested are body image; drawing a person; under- or over-reaching for objects or colliding with people or things; environmental disorientation; confusion of directional words such as up and before; inappropriate placement or size of drawings or writing on paper; difficulty understanding schedules and elementary time concepts.

4. *Visual Motor Integration.* These test items include difficulty matching symbols or pictures and recognizing a figure when only fragments are presented; difficulty with puzzles or connecting dot patterns; switching of hand use while cutting, throwing, drawing, or eating; inability to copy correctly a circle, cross, square, or X.

5. *Language.* These items test for poor auditory figure-ground and discrimination; inability to categorize or classify objects ("mistakenly groups large with small, round with flat, toys with clothing, etc."); inability to reproduce simple sound rhythms; poor auditory sequencing of three spoken simple directions; inability to repeat the sequence of three words or numbers and to easily and rapidly recall words or names of familiar items (note: a combination of poor rote auditory memory plus difficulty with word calling often means the child will need long-term special education services); avoidance of spoken language; inability to rhyme; difficulty communicating events sequentially or in complete sentences.

A fifth screening procedure that some school districts have instituted is the use of published rating scales. Some are criterion referenced tests which have instructional activities suggested for each test item or section in which the child needs additional help. Criterion referenced tests, now widely used by educators for establishing goals and objectives, evaluate performance on specific skills or knowledge without comparisons between individuals as in standardized testing. An attempt is made to list skills in the order in which they are normally acquired, and the criterion of the test is 100 per cent mastery.[7] Examples of this type of testing procedure are the Learning Accomplishment Profile,[8] which gives developmental age expectations from age one month to six years for all areas tested, and the very thorough Behavioral Characteristics Progression[9] chart and program. The Santa Clara Inventory of Developmental Tasks[10] and Diagnostic and Prescriptive Technique: Handbook I[11] offer many instructional activity suggestions for children who do not meet certain perceptual, language, and other behavioral criteria.

Using the developmental chart in Table 24-1, a therapist can quickly determine the normal age at which children acquire commonly tested abilities. The chart reads developmentally down from the top to the bottom. It also reads across from left to right, as some developmental sequences on the right side of the chart may be interrupted because of deficits in developmental sequences on the left side. This type of chart can be helpful in talking with parents, recommending developmental activities, or making judgments about children's performance levels.

Screening procedures in this section may be conducted by therapists or may be recommended by them for others to do. Such procedures help to identify the mildly handicapped child whose physical, emotional, or learning problems have been difficult to pin down specifically or have gone completely undetected. Further testing and remediation of physical and emotional problems and mental retardation have been covered in earlier sections of this book.

STANDARDIZED TESTING

Standardized testing which compares a child's performance with that of many other children may be helpful if it results in appropriate program planning. The test procedures described here, as well as the treatment suggestions in the next section, will emphasize learning disability symptoms sometimes associated with minimal brain dysfunction (see Chapter 14). Application to school settings for five- to ten-year-old children with normal intelligence will be stressed. Because learning disability type deficits often complicate the problems found in mental retardation, cerebral palsy, emotional disorders, and sensory deficits, methods described here may be a useful adjunct to testing and treatment practices for those handicapping conditions.

Southern California Sensory Integration Tests

This battery is the most comprehensive instrument for the occupational therapist to use for testing children with subtle learning problems and has been described previously in this book (Chapter 10). However, some therapists may not be qualified to give the complex battery or may be in a school situation where it is not available. Therefore alternative tests will be suggested.

Standardized Screening

The Meeting Street School Screening Test[12] and Slingerland Screening Tests[13] have subscores which indicate proficiency in language, perception, and visual-motor skills.

Visual Perception

The easy to administer Motor-Free Visual Perception Test (MVPT)[14] results in a perceptual quotient which tells how successfully the child pointed to the figure which matched each stimulus. The correct answers require perception of visual space, form, figure-ground (picking out figures from a distracting background), closure (visually completing figures that are only partially represented), and memory. No subscores are given. In a second test choice, Marianne Frostig's Developmental Test of Visual Perception, the perceptual quotient has been found to predict academic success, but the five subscores are no longer considered valid indicators of specific deficit areas.

Visual Motor Integration

Form copying ability often correlates highly with neurological impairment. Beery and Buktenica's form copying test[15] is recommended because it is easy to score and may be administered in a group. The manual has suggestions for developmentally sequencing remediation. Care must be taken in the scoring and it is important to resist the tendency to score too hard. Other good tests of visual motor integration are the Bender Motor Gestalt test used by psychologists, Slosson Drawing Coordination Test and Benton Visual Retention Test.[16]

Gross Motor Ability

Testing for mild motor deficits is often accomplished using the Purdue Perceptual-Motor Survey or reflex testing mentioned in Chapter 10. A second choice would be the Devereux Test of Extremity Coordination,[17] which requires an assistant to time speed of responses in four separately scored subsections: sequential motor activity, fine motor ability, static balance, and perceptual motor activity.

Language

Nonstandardized assessment of the child's language processing should be included in the therapist's test battery if formal language testing has not been done by a speech and language clinician. Use of the language section of the screening checklist

(Text continues on page 624.)

Table 24-1. Child Development Chart

Items closer to top of each column suggest remedial sequences for problems observed closer to bottom of column. Items in left hand columns suggest possible causes of problems in certain columns further to the right.

	General reflex development	*Sensory development*	*Body scheme*	*Equilibrium*
0–3 mo.	• 0–2 mo. Phasic/movement spinal cord reflexes predominate. Limbs coordinated in total flexion or extension. • 0–6 mo. Static, brainstem mediated reflexes are present. Stimulation of labyrinths or neck muscle feedback changes distribution of muscle tone throughout body.	• 1–4 wk. Infant differentiates: Tactile (touch, pressure) Temp. (hot, cold) Taste (sweet, sour, salty, bitter) Vision (see vis. percept. column) • Infant also experiences vestibular input, internal chemical changes, audition.	• 1 mo. Mass motor activity reaction to stimuli. • 3 mo. Plays regarding hands.	
3 mo. to 1 yr.	• 4–15 mo. Midbrain mediated reactions in all-fours position help child right self, turn over, assume crawl & sit positions. Maximum concerted effort 10–12 mo. • 6 mo. Equilibrium reactions under cortical control begin to gradually modify, inhibit & dominate righting reactions if muscle tone is normal. Results in standing, walking, well-coordinated person.	• 3 mo. Tickle reaction.	• 4–6 mo. Plays with hands and feet in supine. Hands come together in play.	• 7–9 mo. Sits. 4-point kneel; rocks back & forth.
1–2 yr.			• 12–18 mo. Points to 2 of own body parts.	• 12–13 mo. Kneel/ stands. • 14 mo. Stands. • 14–18 mo. Walks; feet wide apart, arms in primary balance role

Developed from Ayres. Banus, Beery, Berry, Bobath, Cattell, Colarusso, Cratty, Dale, Denhoff, Erhardt, Fantz, Fiorentino, Frostig, Gesell, Gilfoyle, Grady, Hammill, Hull and Hull, Kephart, Llorens, Moore, Norton, Oseretsky, Pearlson and Piaget.

Age norms are approximate. Authors vary. Children vary. Development does not really occur in separate rows and columns. All parts of the nervous system influence each other.

Bilateral integration	*Visual perception*	*Eye-hand coordination*	*Language*
• 1–4 wk. Assymetrical postures predominate.	• 3–4 wk. At 10″ discriminates ⅛″ stripes from plain surface. • 1–2 mo. Discriminates stylized face from oval pattern. Also color. • 2 mo. Visual size & near distance constancy developing. Unable to apply them simultaneously.	• 0–4 wk. Reflexive grasp. No eye-hand coordination. Touch tells when to grasp. • 1–4½ mo. Fixates on light monocularly. • 2 mo. Prone, head and chest up for forward vision. • 3 mo. Eye follows past 90°. • 3 mo. Plays regarding hands.	• 1 mo. Responds to sound. Undifferentiated crying. • 3 mo. Vocalizes pleasure in response to social stimuli. Vocal noises resemble speech.
• 4–6 mo. Hands together in play. • 6 mo. Symmetrical arm use & postures predominate. • 7 mo. Transfers toy 1 hand to the other. Hands cross midline. • 7–8 mo. Creeps amphibian; tactile stim. to stomach. • 7–8 mo. Bunny hops. • 7–9 mo. 4-point crawl; homo then hetero-lateral.	• 6–7 mo. Discriminates + ○ □ △. 3-dimensional discrim. easier than 2-dimensional. • 8–24 mo. Convergence to 2″ from nose. Divergence to 20″. Primitive depth perception.	• 4 mo. Rotates head to inspect surroundings. • 4–6 mo. Visually pursues lost toy. • 6 mo. Eye-hand coord. begins. • 6 mo. Palmar grasp. • 6–12 mo. Imitates scribble. • 10 mo. Crude release. Pokes finger in holes.	• 4 mo. Turns to noise & voice. • 6 mo. Distinguishes angry-friendly voice. • 6 mo. Intonational jargon. • 9 mo. Comprehends a few gestures, intonations, "no-no," "hot." Echolalia. • 10 mo. Word-like syllables: ma-ma-ma, da-da-da. Comprehends & waves bye-bye.
• 11–12 mo. Cruises sideways, holding furniture.		• 12 mo. Neat pincer grasp. Supinated grasp developing. • 13 mo. Good release. • 15 mo. Places objects into & out of containers.	• 12 mo. First word, usually noun. • Action response to commands. • 1–5 word vocabulary.

Table 24-1. Child Development Chart. *(Continued)*

	General reflex development	*Sensory development*	*Body scheme*	*Equilibrium*
1–2 yr. (Cont.)				usually at or above shoulder height. • 17 mo. Stoops to pick up toy without losing balance.
2-yr. old			• Identifies 2 body parts from picture. • Touches tummy, cheek, arm, leg, mouth, hair.	• Up & down stairs independently, 2 steps per tread holding on. • 2½ yr. Jumps, 2-foot take off. Tiptoes briefly. • Runs. Walks sideways & backwards.
3-yr. old		• Vision occluded, matches grossly different textures, e.g., sandpaper & satin.	• Knows front, back, side of self. Also chin, neck, forearm.	• Jumps from 12″ height, feet together or 1 ft. lead. • Up stairs 1 foot per tread, no support. Down 2 steps per tread, no support. • Hops 1 foot 2, 3 times. • Climbs 3 rungs. • Squats. • 3½ yr. Tandem walks 10 ft.

Bilateral integration	*Visual perception*	*Eye-hand coordination*	*Language*
		• 18 mo. Turns pages, 2 or 3 at a time. • 21 mo. Puts large pegs in pegboard.	• 1-word sentences. • Can mentally perform behavior before physically perform. • Object permanence. • Produces all vowel sounds. • 1½ yr. Extension of word meanings; over-generalizations. • 50-word vocabulary, mostly nouns.
• Rhythmical bounce, sway, nod, swings arms.	• Enjoys watching moving objects. • Simultaneous visual size & distance constancy developing. • 20/70 visual acuity. • 2½ yr. Adds chimney to 3-cube train	• Hand preference beginning. • Tower of 6–7 cubes. • Strings large beads. • Throws. • Imitates / • 2½ yr. Imitates —, ○ • Copies /	• 2-word sentences that are functionally complete. • Imitates absent models; pretends; reconstructs memories. • Knows "in" and "under." • 2½ yr. Telegraphic speech. • 3-word sentences.
• Walks swinging arm with opposite leg, arms free of shoulder ht. balance position. • Pedals tricycle. • Weight shift in throwing. No step into.	• Tends to react to entire stimulus rather than label separate parts, especially if unfamiliar. • Picks longer line 3 of 3 times. • 3½ yr. Imitates cube bridge	• 10 pellets into bottle in 30 sec. • Tower of 9–10 cubes. • Copies —, ○ • Grasps with extended wrist, & good thumb opposition. • Turns doorknob, forearm rotation. • Unbuttons accessible buttons. • May shift handedness. • Catches large ball, arms extended. • 3½ yr. Imitates X.	• Has adult grammatical structure. Complete simple-active sentences. • Uses sentences to tell understandable stories. • 3½ yr. Speech disfluency. • "Why" questions. • Names 1 color.

Table 24-1. Child Development Chart. *(Continued)*

	General reflex development	*Sensory development*	*Body scheme*	*Equilibrium*
4-yr. old		• Names heavier of 2 weights. • Discriminates different scents. • Compares different textures, e.g., soft, smooth.	• Draws man with head and legs.	• Stands 1 foot 4 sec. Broad jumps . . . • standing—8–10″ • running—23–33″
5-yr. old	• Primitive reflexes inhibited or dominated. In supine & all-fours child can turn head side-to-side, up, down without elbows, shoulders, or knees changing angle. • Can flex in supine & extend in prone positions for 10 sec. • Sits and stands symmetrically from supine with only slight body rotation.	Vision occluded . . . • discriminates ○□ ☆ blocks (stereognosis). • points to touched finger 1/2 times. • points to within 3″ of stimulus spot on arm. • points to hand &/or cheek touched singly or simultaneously.	• Copies Simon Says postures. • Draws 6-part unmistakable man with body. • Points front, back, near, up, down, with eyes closed. • Can clench and bare teeth. • Aware of, but confuses left and right. • In pictures identifies object that is beside, between, in middle, in front of.	• Down stairs, alternating feet, no support. • Stands 1 foot 6–8 sec. • Balances on tiptoe, 1/3 trials. • Running broad jump 28–35.″ • Jumps 10″ high hurdle. • Begins balance beam backwards. • Tries roller skates, jump rope, stilts.
6-yr. old				• Jumps over rope 20 cm. high. • Standing broad jump 3 ft.

Bilateral integration	*Visual perception*	*Eye-hand coordination*	*Language*
• Runs with good arm-leg coordination. • Gallops. • 4½ yr. Skips, 1 foot only (lame duck skip).	• With increasing age child tends to differentiate stimuli in environment, esp. when specific language labels applied to them. • Slow down of rapid visual acuity development since birth. • Matches shapes (same color and size). • Can find simple familiar overlapping outline figures. • Builds 6-block pyramid. • 4½ yr. Copies gate	• Follows moving object smoothly with eyes ↔ ↕ ⤡ ⤢ • Copies + • 10 pellets into bottle in 25 sec. • Bounces ball awkwardly.	• Transforms kernel sentences. • 4-word sentences, some complex or compound. • Intuitive thought begins, less concreteness. • Little word analysis; deals with whole sentences. • Names primary colors. • Counts 3 objects, though imperfectly. • Uses slang. • Understands syntax, grammatical contrasts beyond production ability. • Repeats 3 digits • 4½ yr. Perceives differences in concrete events.
• Mimics pointing to ipsi- or contralateral ear or eye. 2/3 trials. • Can reproduce simple rhythmic clapping. • Marches in time to music.	• 20/30 visual acuity. • Difficulty with orientation. Can detect ↕ reversals easier than ↔ reversals after instruction. • Difficulty performing closure necessary to distinguish ○ □ ▭ • Simultaneous size constancy & form discrim. developing. • Imitates 10-block pyramid. • 5½ yr. Begins to mentally rotate simple shapes for solving puzzles.	• Copies / □ \ X • Imitates △ • Sequential finger opposition (1, 2, 3, 4) with visual regard and minor associative movements. Slow. • Throws 16″ playground ball 10–11 feet. Catches bounced large playground ball.	• Embeds phrases, clauses in sentences. • Develops percepts of number, speed, time, space. • Inner logic & imaginative thinking. • Categorizes by likeness & difference. • Marked increase in vocab. comprehension (not use). • Repeats 4 digits • 5½ yr. Mean length of response = 4.9 words.
• Skips alternately. • Throws stepping with foot opposite throwing arm.	• Begins to identify imbedded familiar outline figures. • Recalls 3½ of the 9 Bender Gestalt figures.	• Copies △ ✳ • 6½ yr. Hand dominance established.	• Command of every form of sentence structure. • Mean sentence length rapidly increasing. Now 6.5 words.

Table 24-1. Child Development Chart. *(Continued)*

	General reflex development	*Sensory development*	*Body scheme*	*Equilibrium*
6-yr. old (Cont.)				
7-yr. old	• Arises from supine to standing in 1–1.5 sec.	• Vision occluded, can reproduce - X O drawn on back of hand 1/2 trials.	• Good jumping jacks. • Can knit eyebrows. • 7½ yr. Stabilizes arms and trunk against much resistance. • Knows left and right on self.	• Stands on 1 foot, eyes closed, 3 seconds. • Can hop and jump accurately into small squares. • Walks 2″ wide balance beam.
8-yr. old			• Eyes closed, points right & left. • Can wrinkle forehead.	• Crouches on tiptoes without falling 1/3 trials.
9-yr. old			• 9½ yr. Discriminates left & right on facing person.	• Runs 16–17 ft./sec. • Jumps over rope 15″ high 2/3 trials. • Jump, clapping hands 3 times, 1/3 trials.
10–12 yr.				• 10 yr. Hops 50 ft. on 1 foot in 5–6 sec. • 11 yr. Standing broad jump 4½–5 ft. • 12 yr. Standing high jump 3 ft.

Bilateral integration	*Visual perception*	*Eye-hand coordination*	*Language*
	• May still reverse some letters or numbers.		• Asks for and attempts to verbalize explanations, causal relationships.
• Can tap floor alternately with feet.	• 20/20 visual acuity. • b-d, p-q confusions resolved. • Builds 6-block pyramid from memory.	• Grips pencil tightly, often close to tip. Pressure may be heavy. • Good sequential finger opposition (1, 2, 3, 4). • Drops 20 coins, one at a time, into open box in 16 sec. • Accurately taps swinging suspended ball 2/5 tries. • 7½ yr. Copies	• Good speech melody & facial/hand gestures. • Good inner language. • True communication; shares ideas. • Mean length of response 7.2 words.
• Good 2-2, 2-1, 1-2 hop. • Can run into moving jump rope but cannot alter step.	• Identifies heavily embedded familiar figures. • Notices and labels component parts of stimulus more than does younger child. • Capable of attending to both whole and part.	• Laces 8 beads in 20 sec. • Places 10 pairs of matchsticks in box in 16 sec.	• Skilled use of grammatical rules. • Acceptable articulation.
	• Closure figure recognized and seen as incomplete. • Notices wholes & parts simultaneously in figures composed of familiar objects.		
	• 11 yr. & above. Recalls 5½–6 of the 9 Bender Gestalt figures.	• 1p yr. Draws 3-dimensional geometric figures. • 10 yr. Judges & intercepts pathways of small balls thrown from a distance. • 12 yr. Linear perspective seen in drawings. • Anticipates locomotor & manual responses to rapidly moving objects, e.g., where to catch ball whose complete trajectory is not observable.	

developed by the School District of Philadelphia is recommended.[18] Some other informal screening instruments also include language items.[19,20,21] Language capability is an important consideration as it sometimes gives information about cerebral hemisphere functioning. In addition it is an essential component of understanding test and treatment instructions.

Complete lists of tests for screening and evaluating learning impaired children are available from federally funded Area Learning Resource Centers and local centers, sometimes called Special Educational Instructional Materials Centers (SEIMC). These centers, in many locations around the country, also have samples and lists of educational curriculum materials. *The Mental Measurements Yearbook*, edited by Oscar K. Buros[22] and published every several years, is an important reference book which groups tests by topic and includes several critiques of each one by authorities in the field.

TREATMENT

The only two treatment methods that have consistently produced academic gains in learning disabled children, according to numerous research studies, are special education classes and medication.[23] The correlation between improved academic performance and therapeutic intervention in visual perception and motor performance is still the subject of great controversy in the field of education. Language training has recently been heralded as the new area of emphasis for the learning impaired child and its correlation with reading skills is more direct. It is, however, important to avoid the tendency to apply one treatment method exclusively or to follow a bandwagon approach in solving children's problems. School therapists should be alert to relevant scientific reporting in their own and other professional literature and should continually investigate and scientifically evaluate their own testing and treatment data.

After initial testing the therapist may write either a specific prescription or general recommendations for the teacher, parent, or volunteer to carry out. Volunteers are trained and supervised by therapists. The itinerant therapist travels to several different schools or homes. Sometimes children leave the classroom to come to therapy several times a week. They may be seen individually or in small groups. In some cases therapists see whole classes of eight to twelve students in order to demonstrate to the teacher appropriate classroom activities or children's performance deficits.

Table 24–2 shows one method of organizing treatment goals on an evaluation record showing performance levels for groups of young children. It is a modification of a sensory integrative profile by Llorens and Seig.[24] It shows deficit areas often found in learning disabled children and test items that can be used to identify them. The therapist administers only those tests most suitable to the age and capability levels of the child.

While one inadequate score within a particular heading is usually insignificant, clusters of low scores indicate treatment goals. The long term objective of occupational therapy for the five- to ten-year-old learning disabled child would be good psychosocial adjustment and age-appropriate performance within each heading. This should result in a well integrated youngster at a readiness level for learning academics if there were no complicating behavior or language problems. It would not result in increased academic performance unless accompanied by an appropriate educational program. Academic proficiency is of paramount importance and the therapist should avoid removing a child from the classroom unless therapy is clearly warranted and ongoing assessment indicates progress is being made. Individual subtests cannot be considered as separate entities and caution should be used in determining the importance of any one subtest score. Drilling in splinter skills should be avoided and a broad developmental program should be emphasized.

Columns in the chart are listed more or less in the sequence that a normally developing child would acquire them, which would suggest the developmental sequence for therapy. However, the learning disabled child's abilities are characterized by inconsistencies, with peaks of performance in some areas and valleys of inadequacy in others. The treatment goal is to fill in the gaps so the child can achieve a consistently high level of performance.

Test results of five-and-one-half-year-old Richard are recorded on the chart as an example of the use of this evaluation record. A diagnostic-prescriptive program for improving motor and perceptual function-

TABLE 24–2. Evaluation Record For the Mildly Neurologically Impaired.

	Head-ings					*Reflex development*											*Bilateral integration*								*Body scheme and tactile discrim.*													
CLASS DAYS: ______ TIME: ______ TO ______	*Column items*	Classroom #	Age	I.Q.	Behavior	ATNR	Prone Ext. (Kep)	Supine Flex.	Cocontract'n	Postrot. Nystag. (SC)	Sitt'g Blance	Forw'd Bal. Beam (Kep)	Sideway Bl. Bm. (Kep)	Backw'd Bl. Bm. (Kep)	Stand'g Bal. (SC)	Static Bal. (Dev)	STNR creep (Bndr)	Midline Xing (SC)	Bilat. Mot. Cord. (SC)	Dbl. Circles (Kep)	Skip (Kep)	2-2, 2-1 hop (Kep)	Dominance Hand	Eye / Foot	Imitate Post. (SC)	Imitate Post. (Kep)	Perc. Mot. (Dev)	Sequ. Mot. (Dev)	Point Body Parts	Angls in Snow (Kep)	Kinesthesia (SC)	Man. Form. (SC)	Fing. Identif. (SC)	Graphesthesia (SC)	Loclzt'n Tac. Stim. (SC)	Dbl. Tact. Stim. (SC)	Tactile Dfsivenes (SC)
Richard	*Test scores*		5½	93	α	α	↓	↓	↓	+1.2	α	α	α		+.1 / -.2	α	α	↓					R	R / R	-20				↓		+.7	+ 1.2	-.9		-1.9	-.5 / -.7	α

Evaluation Record for the Mildly Neurologically Impaired—(*Continued*)

	Fine motor											*Spatial orientatn*						*Vis. discrim. & fig. grnd.*				*Memory*						*Language*						
																						Vis'l				Aud								
	Mot. Acc. (domin.) (SC)	(non-domin.) (SC)	Vis. Mot. Integr. (Beery)	Design Copy (SC)	Pencil Grip	Handwriting	Sequent. Fing. Tip Touch	Fine Motor (Dev)	Ocular Fixation	Ocular Pursuit (Kep)	Ocular Converg. (Kep)	Envirnmtl Disorientation	Posit. in Space (SC)	Space Visualiz. (SC)	Reversals: letter—word	Reading L. to R. direct.	R-L Discrim. (SC)	Percptual Quotnt (MVPT)	Figure Ground (SC)	Letter Recogntn	Recogntn of error (Beery)	Sequence of 4 color beads	Sequ. of 3 vis. instrctns	Memory test items (MVPT)	Posit. in Space mem. (SC)	Repeat 3 wrds or #'s	Sequ. of 3 audit. directns	Receptive	Expressive	Integrative (Associative)	Auditory Discrim.	Word finding (naming)	Sound-symbol assoc.	Speed of Auditry Process'g
Richard	-24				↓	↓	↓		α	↓	↓	OK	-9	-7	—			↓	-1.9	↓	↓	α	α		α	↓	↓	α	α	↓	α	↓		↓

Code for standardized tests indicated in parenthesis:

- Kep —Kephart's Purdue Perceptual Motor Survey
- SC —Southern Calif. Sensory Integration Tests
- Dev —Devereux Test of Extremity Coordination
- Beery —Beery-Buktenica Test of Visual Motor Integration
- MVPT—Motor Free Test of Visual Perception

Blank score indicates item not tested because (a) it was not age appropriate, or (b) new insight into deficit areas would not result.

After testing use soft pencil to fill in scores on pages 1 and 2 for only those items tested. Then with soft red pencil make hachures in boxes of pertinent low scores indicating current treatment objectives. Use the Evaluation Record to see goals common to the whole group, to zero in on particular children's deficits when part of the group is suddenly absent, and for ready reference when talking with parents and teachers. Erase and change scores often as children show progress.

ing might be correlated as follows: through sensory integrative techniques the therapist would use both vestibular and tactile stimulation to enhance reflex development, ocular control, visual perception, and body scheme. Several auditory sequential directions using the scooter board, could frequently be included in the activities. The physical education teacher could emphasize prone extension and supine flexion along with games involving moving specific body parts. The classroom aide, volunteer or resource room teacher could supervise Richard's copying of specifically selected inch cube and pegboard designs to help fine motor and prereading perceptual skills. Independent desk work could include worksheets emphasizing imbedded geometric shapes and alphabet letters for visual figure-ground discrimination. Parents should provide daily tacticle stimulation at home. Such a complete program could be organized by the therapist or may be planned and agreed upon by all the professionals at a team meeting. The language therapist would be emphasizing Richard's associative language processing and the speed with which he makes oral responses. Awareness of the language problems helps all members of the team understand his learning style better.

The columns listed in the chart are only examples of test results or developmental activities that could be listed. Other standardized or observational score columns could be substituted, for example, pertinent subtests of the WISC-R or McCarthy tests.

Interpreting Performance

Testing and treatment of the youngster in the special education setting may be complicated by mild undetected deficits in visual, auditory, or tactile acuity. On the other hand a child may hear well and express him or herself well verbally but have a severe impairment in auditory reception. In that case, automatic or learned reliance on visual cues may cause misinterpretation of such instructions as "I'm drawing a line on top of the black line. If I go off the black line by accident [like this] I come back on the black line again [like this]"[25] One bright language impaired child with excellent auditory acuity proceeded half way around the Southern California Motor Accuracy Test with regularly spaced pencilled projections off the tracing line in spite of many verbal efforts by the examiner to halt the practice. On the other hand, "Do this, this, and this after you roll to the ladder," may be an impossible activity for the child who cannot remember the sequence of three visual stimuli or does not understand the temporal concept "after." It is important to know a child's sensory, language processing, and cognitive deficits as well as to analyze the testing and treatment requirements in order to understand the full impact of a child's performance.

Management of Behavior

Hyperactivity often causes behavior management problems and inaccurate interpretation of performance capability, particularly in a large group of developmentally impaired children. Helping a child learn to manage his or her own behavior may be one goal of therapy. In addition, it is important for children to leave therapy quietly controlled and ready to resume desk work without disrupting the academic classroom.

Medicine prescribed by the child's doctor is likely to be helpful if the cause of the hyperactivity is organic, particularly if the child consistently demonstrates hyperactivity, poor impulse control, and short attention span. The central nervous system stimulant Ritalin is most often effective, while the amphetamine Dexedrine is a good second choice. It is thought that possibly the stimulants may act on the reticular activating system, a part of the brainstem that receives and sorts out stimuli. In a few cases the tranquilizers Thorazine and Mellaril may help reduce anxiety.[26,27] The use of medication should be accompanied by special education, environmental control, and, sometimes, counselling.

Hyperactivity may also be psychogenic. It may be caused by emotional overlay secondary to a learning problem or it may reflect an inconsistent childrearing approach. In this case the child is physically able to control his or her own behavior but is preconditioned not to do so.[28]

Management of hyperactive behavior, particularly if it is of psychogenic origin, requires firmness, structure, and environmental controls. Such controls might include reducing distractions, defining performance expectations clearly, and giving clear warnings of impending minor changes. Keeping accurate daily records of types and forerunners of inappropriate behavior in the classroom helps determine the cause of hyperactivity and effectiveness of intervention procedures.[29]

Behavior modification, currently widely used in the field of education, is a particularly useful method of managing hyperactive behavior of psychogenic origin and of bringing about improvement in specific performance goals. Performance is first assessed and terminal goals or behavioral objectives are established. Positive rewards or reinforcements which are important to the child are determined so that they may be used upon successful completion of each small step approaching the goal. Negative or incorrect behavior or performance are usually ignored and are not given negative reinforcement by scolding or criticism. Primitive rewards are often edible. Interim rewards, such as paper tokens which can be traded in for treats or privileges, are more therapeutically desirable, and social rewards such as a handshake or smile are the highest level. Frequency of rewarding is decreased as the child's performance improves.[30,31]

Learning disabled children, even the very hyperactive, learn to sit quietly on their special spots waiting for treatment to begin when they know the star they will receive can later be exchanged for free play time. They understand when newly performed activities are listed on an "I can do" sheet to take home. On individually written self-paced activity sheets, each step leading to appropriate and correct behavior can be checked off as it is mastered.

Consistency of expectations and rewards is important, especially when working with a group. Motivating and allowing a child to make the decision to cooperate has more positive results than trying to force conforming behavior. Having a child help establish his or her own goals often fosters cooperative behavior.

If a whole class is difficult to control, activities for the whole class to do simultaneously may be required. In that case formal structure or very calming activities at least at the beginning and end of the session may be necessary to establish control.

A finely delineated sequence of steps might be helpful when working with more than one or two students simultaneously: (1) have equipment ready and highly motivating activities planned (some will have been selected by the students); (2) position children with enough space between them to perform the task; (3) gain undivided attention of the group; (4) introduce equipment and wait until reaction subsides; (5) briefly and clearly explain the task using three or fewer sequential directions; (6) demonstrate; (7) gain undivided attention; (8) have one or all children demonstrate verbally or through performance to be sure that directions are understood; (9) gain undivided attention; (10) signal start of task; (11) continually reward appropriate performance verbally or with a pat, handshake, star, privilege, or other reward; and (12) conclude task specifically by change in positioning of children or equipment or by some other specific means. Avoid the temptation of rushing into a new activity before the children have had time to "change gears."

The experienced therapist may wish to make efficient use of time with a well controlled group of mildly impaired children by using learning stations or circuit training. At several positions around the room equipment or activities are placed for use by one or two children. It is important for each unsupervised activity to provide its own feedback so the child knows whether he or she performed correctly. (Did the beanbags go in the can? Did you catch the ball?) Children change stations at their own volition or as "the gong sounds" or as the therapist directs. With this method all children are therapeutically engaged with activities or equipment which can be used by only one child at a time. The therapist stays with the station that is least safe or needs to have feedback provided. Each child could be directed only to those particular stations within his or her own treatment program. Classroom and physical education teachers are often experts in using this method and would be helpful models.

Gross Motor Therapy

Many educators are skeptical of claims that improvement in reflex development, balance, bilateral integration, and body scheme have any positive correlation with reading and academic performance. Research on perceptual motor training has been inconclusive. While a positive correlation cannot be documented between academics and improvement in individual motor tasks such as skipping, evidence is mounting that the central nervous system basis of motor deficits frequently seen in learning disabled children may also be the cause of poor academic achievement.[32,33,34] Treatment which improves central nervous system functioning pertinent to both problems would be warranted. Research has begun to show favorable results of such therapy in improving both academic performance[35] and motor performance[36] in spite of the absence of any form of skill training.

Adequate balance and coordination allow cognitive skills to be directed towards the task at hand rather than towards the execution of postural and manipulative movements. Here are some additional considerations which may be enlightening for the skeptic: (1) motor training is known to improve motor performance; (2) this results in increased self-help skills and peer-related playground and neighborhood activities; (3) this, in turn, results in improved self-image; (4) improvement in self-image by itself may result in improved academic performance; and (5), in addition, the increasing amount of central nervous system research mentioned above is becoming more convincing.

Sensory Integrative Therapy developed by Ayres[37] is an important remedial technique and is one of the primary foundations for occupational therapy's uniqueness in treating learning disabled children. Bender[38] offers a specific training program for tonic neck reflex problems. Helpful perceptual-motor activities and group games have been developed by several authors.[39,40,41,42] Training in specific skill development is sometimes self-integrating (such as the bilaterally integrating activity of skipping casually around the playground once the correct movement has been learned). Skill development in peer-related activities such as ball skills also has a place in treatment or may be recommended to the physical education teacher or volunteer.

Tactile Discrimination

The role of the tactile system in establishing body scheme and spatial orientation is well defined in sensory integrative theory. One research study investigated the use of tactile input to teach letter and word recognition. Results suggest a method of teaching children who have good visual and spatial imagery and good visual motor integration (primarily right hemisphere functions) and major deficits in reading or sound-symbol correspondence: these children may benefit from tracing on their skin, letter or word shapes with which to make visual and possibly speech associations.[43,44] Children's asymmetrical response to tactile learning in later experiments by that researcher may have implications for cerebral hemisphere dominance and integration.[45]

Fine Motor Training

While the pursuit and convergence functions of the extraocular muscles have sometimes been noted to improve following vestibular stimulation and tonic neck reflex inhibition, at other times it is necessary to refer children for examination by an optometrist or ophthalmologist or specifically to train ocular pursuit.

Therapists are often asked about fine motor classroom problems. In addition to general gross and fine motor planning activities, direct teaching in sequential progression is usually necessary. Hammill[46] and Robinson[47] recommend handwriting techniques and the Beery-Buktenica test manual[48] recommends form copying sequences. Pencil grippers manufactured by Developmental Learning Materials are invaluable. Use of geometric-shaped template cut-outs, chalkboard size graded up to large then small desk size, should precede letter formations. For most learning disabled children cursive writing is recommended even though manuscript printing may not have been mastered. Before recommending methods for teaching handwriting, rule out problems of eye-hand coordination (by determining whether the child reproduces letters better with the eyes closed), kinesthetic feedback, finger dexterity, spatial orientation, and visual memory.

Training in Visual Perception

Research about the development of visual perception has been reported in Scientific American[49] and by Douglas.[50] The efficacy of testing for and training specific subdivisions of visual perception without relating the training to academic skills has been questioned and should be employed cautiously. When appropriate, general training in visual tasks requiring spatial orientation, discrimination, perception of figure-ground relationships, and memory is primarily done by teachers in some schools. In others the therapist assumes the responsibility. More often teachers of four- to six-year-old learning disabled children stress these pre-reading skills while other teachers stress academic skills. In any event the therapist should be prepared to treat and make recommendation for treatment in any of these problem areas and should be aware of the developmental sequences in each. In some cases the child's ability to perceive is improved; in others the child is taught to compensate for the deficit.

Catalogues from Teaching Resources, Boston MA, and Developmental Learning Materials, Niles IL, give ideas for commercially available materials and inspiration for making original activities and supplies. Both have cross-referenced indexes telling perceptual and language goals of each of their programs and supplies, and Teaching Resources has a glossary of perceptual terms.

Worksheets printed from ditto masters,[51,52] although in disfavor in some schools because of their overuse in normal classrooms, do offer a wide variety of sequenced tasks which can be individually selected to train specific deficits of learning impaired children. Their use under plastic overlays with erasable crayons extends their lifespan. Because they are only two dimensional, their use should be interspersed with such things as beads, geometric-shaped blocks, building cubes, and manipulative toys.

Bush and Giles[53] suggest activities for visual memory training. When a deficit exists in this skill it is important to determine that the child can discriminate well visually and has age-appropriate visual spatial skills before attempting to train visual memory per se. Children can sometimes learn to compensate for poor visual memory by using subvocal language, kinesthetic and tactile tracing, frequent rehearsal, and specific attention to patterns and details.

Training in Language Processing

As in the case of visual perception subdivisions, caution should be used in training language processing subdivisions. They are all interrelated, not separate, subskills. Children with observed deficits should be referred to a speech and language clinician who is the best source of information about problems in this area. Auditory discrimination, word finding, memory, and speed of processing might be included in occupational therapy programming if appropriate. The classroom teacher may also be emphasizing these, as well as comprehension, expression, and categorization.

Program Development

Motor, tactile, perceptual, and language remedial suggestions have been given for use by the therapist in treatment or for recommending to educators, parents, or volunteers. Appendix C provides further examples of program suggestions that can be made for improving gross and fine motor development in young learning disabled children. The activities recommended are for behavioral characteristics which have been developmentally sequenced and are also suitable for children with many other handicaps. A therapist might wish to prepare such a program guide in the areas of visual perception, memory, or self-help skills. The Appendix C Program guide for motor development is based on developmental and sensory integrative theories as well as current educational practices.

Other sources of remedial or training ideas in motor, tactile, perceptual or language areas are the published rating scales[54,55,56,57] and the writing of Miner[58] and Hayes and Komick.[59]

Record Keeping

Therapists keep daily records of treatment programs and of recommendations made to teachers, administrators, or volunteers. At least twice a year therapists who treat children send descriptive report cards home and write progress notes which are added to the child's school records. In accordance with PL-142 schools may require from the therapist written annual long-term goals and short-term behavioral objectives as part of the child's Individualized Educational Program. An example of a short-term objective is the following: By November 13 Johnny will be able to choose through tactile cues triangle-, rectangle-, and diamond-shaped objects on request from a group of five objects with 90 percent accuracy.[60] Specific documentation is now required by law, and professionals in education are held accountable for children's progress.

Central storage of reports and objectives by all services encourages interdisciplinary communication and a unified approach to treatment.

FUTURE ROLE OF OCCUPATIONAL THERAPY

As occupational therapists establish the uniqueness of their contribution to the total education program, current requirements for educational certification may be relaxed in many of the school districts which now require them. On the other hand, some school district therapists are choosing to broaden their professional expertise by taking graduate courses in special education or early childhood development. Consultancy and supervisory positions may become more prevalent, particularly for those therapists who also choose to take special education training.

Early identification, infant stimulation, and special preschool programs in some school districts are beginning to employ occupational therapists. At the secondary level, education for the handicapped was formerly little more than academic maintenance, and often the handicapped were not admitted to vocational high schools. New secondary education programs are being established for mildly impaired children. The new programs emphasize compensation for perceptual and language deficits as well as counseling and vocational adjustment in preparation for setting realistic and challenging life goals.

The unique contribution occupational therapy could make in such programs is apparent. Parents should be encouraged to demand appropriately trained personnel at all levels of public schooling, and therapists should make their qualifications known to local school boards. Increasing professional contributions and involvement by therapists in local chapters and national conventions of organizations for the handicapped will offer opportunities for reciprocal sharing between educators, parents, and therapists. Listed in the Glossary are three such organizations for those who have educational problems: The Association for Children with Learning Disabilities, The Council of Exceptional Children, and The Association of Retarded Citizens.

Future expectations include a larger percentage of school age children receiving direct occupational therapy services and contributions by therapists to each child's annually written Individualized Educational Program. In addition a larger number of therapists would be expected to serve in advisory or supervisory capacities in school districts to help develop procedures for early identification and curriculum adjustment in motor and pre-academic areas as well as counseling and vocational programs for adolescents. Because this is a newly developing field, original research should be undertaken by therapists when possible to verify clinical observations. It is also imperative to keep abreast of other pertinent research in occupational therapy, education, psychology, and neurology.

REFERENCES

1. Occupational Therapy in the Public School System. American Occupational Therapy Association, Rockville MD, 1976.
2. Public Law 94-142 Education for All Handicapped Children Act, As reviewed in Legislative Alert. American Occupational Therapy Association, Rockville MD, 1976.
3. One Out of Ten: School Planning for the Handicapped. Educational Facilities Laboratories, 850 Third Avenue, New York, 1974.
4. Newcomer, P., and Hammill, D.: ITPA and Academic Achievement: A Survey. The Reading Teacher, May, 739, 1975.
5. Kurko, V., Crane, L. L., and Willemin, H.: Preschool Screening Instrument. Fort Worth: Fort Worth Public Schools, 1973.
6. The Cornman Diagnostic Center Learning Disabilities Checklist for Kindergarten and 1st Grade, ed. 2. School District of Philadelphia, Philadelphia, 1975.
7. Gillespie, P. H., and Johnson, L.: Teaching Reading to the Mildly Retarded Child. Columbus OH: Charles Merrill, 1974.
8. Sanford, A. R.: Learning Accomplishment Profile and Manual, 1974. Kaplan School Supply Corporation, 600 Jonestown Road, Winston-Salem NC.
9. Behavioral Characteristics Progression, 1972. Developed by Santa Cruz County Office of Education, P.O. Box 11132, Palo Alto, VORT Corporation.
10. Gainer, W. L. (ed.): Santa Clara Inventory of Developmental Tasks, 1974. Santa Clara Unified School District, California, Richard L. Zweig Associates.
11. Farrold, R. A., and Schamber, R. G.: A Diagnostic and Prescriptive Technique: Handbook I. Sioux Falls SD: ADAPT Press, 1973.
12. Hainsworth, P. K., and Siqueland, M. L.: Meeting Street School Screening Test. Crippled Children and Adults of Rhode Island, Inc., Providence, 1969.
13. Slingerland, B. H.: Slingerland Screening Tests for Identifying Children with Specific Language Disability. Cambridge MA: Educators Publishing Service, Inc., 1969.
14. Colarusso, R., and Hammill, D.: Motor-Free Test of Visual Perception. Academic Therapy, San Rafael CA, 1972.
15. Beery, K. E., and Buktenica, N. A.: Developmental Test of Visual-Motor Integration. Chicago: Follett Publishing Co., 1967.
16. Benton, A. L.: Visual Retention Test, 1963. Psychological Corporation, 304 E. 5th St., New York.
17. Devereux Test of Extremity Coordination in Individual Motor Achievement Guided Education. Devereux Foundation, Devon PA, 1974.
18. Cornman Diagnostic Center Checklist.

19. Behavioral Characteristics Progression.
20. Gainer: Santa Clara Inventory.
21. Farrold and Schamber: Diagnostic and Prescriptive Technique.
22. Buros, O. K. (ed.): Mental Measurements Yearbook (1st to 7th). Highland Park NJ: Gryphon Press.
23. Silver, L. B.: Acceptable and controversial approaches to treating the child with learning disabilities. Pediatrics 55:406, 1975.
24. Llorens, L. A., and Seig, K. W.: A Profile for Managing Sensory Integrative Test Data. Am. J. Occup. Ther. 29:205, 1975.
25. Ayres, A. J.: Southern California Sensory Integration Tests. Western Psychological Services, Los Angeles, 1972, p. 27.
26. Haslam, H. A., and Valletutti, P. J. (eds.): Medical Problems in the Classroom. Baltimore: University Park Press, 1975, p. 294–297.
27. Lecky, P.: Drug Management and Survival Techniques for Parents and Teachers. Lecture during Programming for Learning Disabilities Conference, St. Joseph's College, Philadelphia, 1974.
28. Murray, J. M.: Is There a Role for the Teacher in the Use of Medication for Hyperkinetics? J. Learning Disabil. 9:30, 1976.
29. Ibid.
30. O'Leary, K. D., and O'Leary, S. G.: Classroom Management: The Successful Use of Behavior Modification. Elmsford NY: Pergamon Press, 1972.
31. Stephens, T. M.: Directive Teaching of Children with Learning and Behavioral Handicaps. Columbus OH: Charles Merrill, 1970.
32. Frank, J., and Levinson, H.: Dysmetric dyslexia and dyspraxia. Am. J. Child Psychiatry 12:690, 1967.
33. DeQuiros, J. B.: Diagnosis of vestibular disorders in the learning disabled. J. Learning Disabil. 9:39, 1976.
34. Ayres, A. J.: The Effect of Sensory Integrative Therapy on Learning Disabled Children. Center for the Study of Sensory Integrative Dysfunction, Pasadena CA, 1976.
35. Ayres, A. J.: Improving academic scores through sensory integration. J. Learning Disabil. 5:339, 1972.
36. Kantner, R. M., et al.: Effects of vestibular stimulation on nystagmus response and motor performance in the developmentally delayed infant. Phys. Ther. 56:414, 1976.
37. Ayres, A. J.: Sensory Integration and Learning Disorders. Western Psychological Services, Los Angeles, 1973.
38. Bender, M. L.: The Bender-Purdue Reflex Test and Training Manual. Academic Therapy, San Rafael CA, 1975.
39. Kephart, N. C.: The Slow Learner in the Classroom, ed. 2. Columbus OH: Charles Merrill, 1971.
40. Cochran, N. A., Wilkinson, L. C., and Furlow, J. J.: Learning on the Move. Dubuque IA: Kendall-Hunt Publishing Company, 1975.
41. Cratty, B.: Developmental Sequences of Perceptual Motor Tasks. Educational Activities, Inc., Freeport NY, 1967.
42. Belgau, F. A., and Basden, B. V.: Perceptual-Motor and Visual Perception Handbook of Developmental Activities. Perception Development Research Associates, LaPorte TX, 1971.
43. Scheville, H.: Tactile Discrimination and Learning Disabilities: An Analysis of Four Prototypes. Unpublished paper. Smith Kettlewell Institute of Visual Sciences, San Francisco, 1974.
44. Scheville, H.: Tactile Reception as Sensory Enhancement for Learning Disabled Children. Unpublished paper. Smith Kettlewell Institute of Visual Sciences, San Francisco, 1975.
45. Scheville, H.: An Experimental Tactile Program for Children with Reading Disabilities. Unpublished paper. Smith Kettlewell Institute of Visual Sciences, San Francisco, 1975.
46. Hammill, D. D.: Problems in writing. In Hammill, D. D., and Bartel, N. R. (eds.): Teaching Children with Learning and Behavior Problems. Boston: Allyn & Bacon, 1975.
47. Robinson, J.: Vanguard School Handwriting. Lectrolearn, Inc., Berwyn PA, 1975.
48. Beery and Buktenica: Developmental Test of Visual-Motor Integration.
49. Held, R., and Richards, W.: Perception: Mechanisms and Models. San Francisco: W. H. Freeman and Company, 1971.
50. Douglas, A. G.: A tachistoscopic study of the order of emergence in the process of perception. In Dashiell (ed.): Psychological Monographs 61: 1–133, 1947.
51. Frostig, M., and Horne, D.: The Frostig Program for the Development of Visual Perception. Chicago: Follett Publishing Co., 1964.
52. Visual-Motor Skills, Visual Readiness Skills and Seeing Likenesses and Differences. Elizabethtown NJ. Continental Press, 1974.
53. Bush, W. J., and Giles, M. T.: Aids to Psycholinguistic Teaching. Columbus OH: Charles Merrill, 1969.
54. Sanford: Learning Accomplishment Profile and Manual.
55. Gainer: Santa Clara Inventory.
56. Farrold and Schamber: Diagnostic and Prescriptive Technique.
57. Behavioral Characteristics Progression.
58. Miner, M. B.: A perceptual-motor training program in the public schools. Am. J. Occup. Ther. 25:193, 1971.
59. Hayes, M., and Komick, M. P.: The Development of Visual-Perceptual-Motor Function. In Banus, B. S. (ed.): The Developmental Therapist. Thorofare NJ: Charles B. Slack, 1971.
60. Ibid.

ACKNOWLEDGMENTS

The support and suggestions graciously offered by Joanne Gressang, Ed.M, O.T.R., and Moya Kinnealey, M.S., O.T.R. Thanks also to Dr. Kenneth Bovée for his extensive editorial assistance in preparation of the manuscript.

25

Community Home Health Care

section 1/In the Urban Setting/Ruth Ellen Levine

The first section of this chapter presents a theoretical overview of the health care delivery system, descriptions of home care services and funding sources, and the roles of the home-based team. The second section deals with application and presents a model for the delivery of home care services. Case studies are included in each to illustrate ideas presented.

Practice is the area in which knowledge and skills are put to the test. The essence of home-based occupational therapy is working with people. The therapist is drawn into the family's inner sanctum—its home—to deliver services. Here the family will be taught how to help maximize the client's level of functional performance.

This chapter can never capture the excitement and fun of the home care treatment process. Every home presents unique problems, new relationships and challenges. After working in the field for a while, therapists begin to wonder whether they might be gaining as much as they are giving.

While the information this chapter contains applies directly to urban, home-based occupational therapy, with some modification much of it can also apply to other aspects of community practice.

CONTEXT AND THEORY

The Health Care Delivery System

While the majority of occupational therapy programs have been housed in institutions, care can be offered in a variety of settings. Home care and community programs are emerging as a dynamic and expanding area of occupational therapy practice.

The fundamental reasons for the movement away from institutions include (1) societal changes, such as the decrease in the birthrate and the increase in numbers of older people, (2) environmental factors, such as the scarcity of natural resources and increased dependence on technology, and (3) financial matters, such as the decrease in funds available to health service operations. All of these factors affect the quality of life in general and the structure of the health care delivery system in particular.

Medical care has evolved into a complex industry. From an individual service model like the practice of the fabled country doctor, there has evolved a multiple-entry, technology-based business. The science of healing has vastly improved, but the cost has been enormous: the result of the expansion has been an explosion of knowledge which has served to divide health care into isolated fragments, where few practitioners comprehend the whole.

This approach might be efficient when problems are purely physical. However, there is a growing body of research that indicates that most basic physical problems have some psychological overlay, and psychological problems have physical effects. The art of healing the whole person is as important as medical science and technology.

In the present situation, the patient comes to feel fragmented and alienated. The medical delivery system is viewed as a business rather than a service. The patient becomes a consumer, and the professional a delivery agent.

There is a movement to control the soaring costs, excessive waste, and inefficiency of the medical empire. Consumers are attempting to organize for their own interests. Watch-dog government agencies are proliferating and the interest in accountability for the professional is growing. Nonetheless, to date in the United States, there is no national system to coordinate and organize the delivery of all health services.

The American medical system has made significant advances in many areas, but its sophisticated technology and theory do not serve all of our citizens. In many areas basic health care is not available to needy consumers. As costs soar and technology is increasingly used, access to the system becomes more difficult. Also, the general focus remains on pathology rather than prevention.

During the 1960s, more funds were available and the theme of practice seemed to be expansion at every level. There seemed to be hope of reaching all Americans with vital health services, and practitioners felt less need to set priorities. In contrast, one of today's difficulties is adjusting to a shrinking health dollar. Practice in the 1970s emphasizes accountability and priority setting. In a tight financial situation, goals and objectives determine the use of limited resources. Practitioners are responsible and accountable for their actions. Within these boundaries, home care can prove an important solution to some of the problems neglected during the years of rapid expansion and growth.

Description of Home Care

Home care includes a wide variety of services that are delivered to clients in their own homes or in some home-like setting, such as a boarding house. At home, the client is in familiar surroundings where the family is often central to the care process. Another benefit is that home care services can cost less than institutionalization. Goals for home care services are maintaining and/or restoring health and promoting the maximum level of independence in functional activities. Other goals are to help the individual live in the home setting and to teach family members and friends how to care for the client. Clients who do not need the constant monitoring skills of the institution staff can appropriately use home care services.

Home Care for Patients Who Have Been Hospitalized

There are several ways in which home care can be used. Patients who are hospitalized for an acute problem can receive rehabilitation services while still in the institution. After this training, they can continue to be treated in their homes. All services—the hospital, the rehabilitation center and the home care team—must work toward a common goal. In home care, institutional goals can be translated so as to meet the client's needs. The following case study demonstrates the need for that kind of translation.

CASE STUDY

Before making the first visit, the home-based therapist called Mrs. G.'s therapist at the rehabilitation center. Mrs. G., a 67-year-old hemiparetic patient, had received training in ADL, bilateral hand exercises, and kitchen activities and had completed the two-month stay in the rehabilitation center successfully.

The home-based therapist found Mrs. G. upstairs in her bedroom. The therapist asked why she was there when she could be dressed and seated downstairs. Mrs. G. reported that she did not feel as if she could do anything. When the home-based therapist asked Mrs. G. about her previous training, Mrs. G. looked puzzled. Then a flash of understanding spread over her face. "I made a colonial salt box," she said with a note of pride in her voice. "I also made a cutting board."

The homebound therapist pressed her for additional information: "What about the dressing and kitchen activities?"

Mrs. G. said that she could do those activities in the hospital but had no idea how to proceed in her own home. "Things are all turned around here. Anyway," Mrs. G. added philosophically, "I don't eat jello."

In eight visits the homebound therapist was able to translate the institutional program goals into activities that were available in Mrs. G.'s own home. Mrs. G. was involved in every activity choice. Basic dressing and undressing techniques were reviewed in one visit. The one-handed cutting board was retrieved from the back of the china closet and its use demonstrated in preparing potatoes which were then used to make Mrs. G.'s favorite casserole. Bilateral sanding was replaced with ironing.

Mrs. G. wanted to assume her former household chores. The home-based therapist reviewed the institutional goals and then taught Mrs. G. how to organize her housework. The success that Mrs. G. achieved in gaining independence was based on the work of the hospital team, the rehabilitation team, and the follow-up of the home care practitioner.

Home Care for Patients Never Hospitalized

Another important use of home care involves clients who were never hospitalized for their condition. They are under a doctor's care and are referred to a home care agency. The doctor determines the treatment goals for the client; the home care team carries out the plan and reports any changes to the doctor. Included in this category of home care referrals are clients who may not be covered by any kind of insurance. (Insurance often does not cover treatment for learning disabilities, undiagnosed mental health problems, preventative techniques, maintenance, and/or other supportive services.) If the client has sufficient funds, the occupational therapist can carry out the treatment process under a doctor's orders.

The Home Care Team

Home care teams are made up of the appropriate specialists, the client, and the caretakers (family and/or friends, neighbors, clergy, and nonprofessional help). This diverse group is most effective when it functions as a cohesive unit. Each individual views the client from a different perspective. The client is the focal point of the delivery process; client views must be valued and respected. All of the unique goals and skills of all of the team members must be organized into a unified whole (Fig. 25-1). The client and the caretakers, who are with the client for most of the day, must form the hub of the wheel

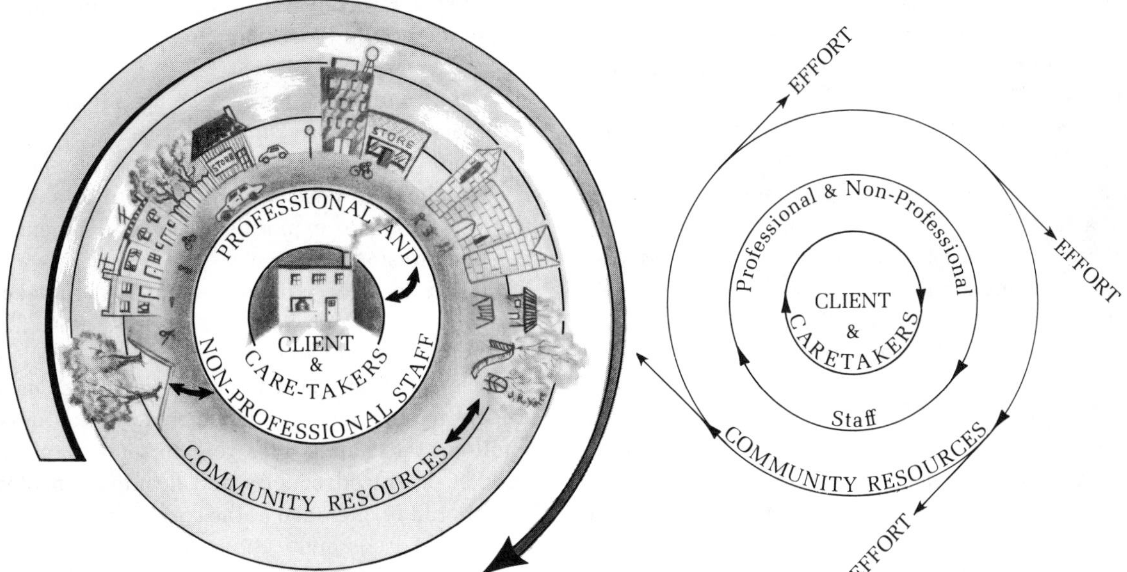

FIGURE 25-1. The wheel of team effort. All of the unique goals and skills of all of the team members must be organized into a unified effort. All members must move in one direction so that the treatment can move forward.

of effort. All members' efforts must move in the same direction. Such a wheel can not roll forward unless all of the forces that are operating around it move in the same direction. Figure 25-1 illustrates this concept.

The team should focus on the client's assets and strengths as well as on disability and liabilities. The client's premorbid life-style should be explored in an effort to understand the present situation. This exploration should also facilitate the therapist's selection of appropriate activities and setting of goals. The assets and liabilities of the individual team members must be assessed. Roles can then be assigned with regard to their best effect on the client's condition.

Roles of Home-based Team Members

Communication is vital to the team effort. All members must be aware of their individual roles and of how the roles influence the achievement of the team's long term goals. Briefly, the roles of the team members are as follows:

The *nurse* carries out skilled duties that include supervising medication, giving injections and nutritional advice, caring for wounds and dressings, monitoring vital signs, and teaching and supervising the client and caretakers regarding daily care. The nurse is usually the coordinator of the client's care; he or she supervises other nursing personnel such as home health aides.

The *home health aide* carries out the nursing care plan. Duties include bathing, dressing, and feeding the client; carrying out and/or reinforcing therapeutic activities and exercise regimes; maintaining the environment; assisting in the preparation of meals; and providing assistance with ambulation and self-administered medications. The home health aide also offers psychological support.

The *physical therapist* employs physical agents such as heat, light, water, electricity, massage, radiation, and exercise to restore clients to their maximum level of physical function.

The *speech therapist* uses knowledge about speech, hearing, and language to plan and implement a realistic program to increase the client's communication skills. The client's emotions affect speech; thus psychological aspects are an important part of speech therapy.

The *occupational therapist* uses specified therapeutic, self-care, homemaker, and creative activities to facilitate and/or maximize the client's level of function. Both the psychosocial and the physical aspects of the client's condition are assessed in terms of the total context for treatment.

The *social worker* uses a problem solving approach to help clients help themselves. Options and resources are presented to the client and caretakers in an attempt to maximize the client's level of adjustment.

Not all of the possible home care professionals were presented in this section. Others may include a podiatrist, optometrist, dentist, homemaker, dietician, and home-visiting physician.

COMMUNICATION. Communication is the essential part of any team effort. Training in group dynamics is helpful in opening channels for communication. In the home setting there are three basic forms of communication—face-to-face interaction and telephone and/or written interaction.

Face-to-face communication takes place in the client's home or in the agency. This type of interaction may be difficult to arrange for a team because each team member has a different schedule and visits the client at a different time. Team goals and roles must be resolved early in the treatment process because they could block communication and progress.

Written communication may be used in lieu of a face-to-face interaction. On an informal level, notes may be left in the client's house for other team members. Telephone discussions may prove to be a more effective method of exploring issues and potential areas of confusion.

Another form of written communication takes place after each client visit—the progress note. The importance of documentation cannot be avoided in the home situation. Many fiscal intermediaries have stringent requirements for documentation that must be followed to qualify for reimbursement. Notes should be organized, concise, and clear to the reader. Goals should be included at the end of the record of each visit. All communication with team members should be noted; contrasting pen colors can be used for easier reference. Additional information on this form of formal communication can be obtained from Chapter 26.

Communication creates a sense of teamwork that

is satisfying to all of the members. The following quote underscores the effort that one must invest to develop a team.

> . . . It is naive to bring together a highly diverse group of people and expect that, by calling them a team, they will in fact behave as a team. It is ironic indeed to realize that a football team spends 40 hours per week practicing teamwork for those two hours on Sunday afternoon when their teamwork really counts. Teams in organizations seldom spend two hours per year practicing when their ability to function as a team counts 40 hours per week.[1]

COORDINATION. It is difficult to create a home care team. However, if several professionals assume the responsibility for coordination, the communication channels can begin to open. The client who is the focus for care should be informed of and included in all communication. No decisions can be made without his or her participation. If the client is unable to take part in decision making, a family member or caretaker should be included in the discussions. In keeping with this spirit of family participation, conferences can be held in the client's house, or the client or caretaker invited to the home care center.

A healthy team should have conflicts and problems. Issues should be identified and aired. Skilled group members are able to separate subjective issues from objective goals. This is why the home care practitioner needs to understand group dynamics. Such knowledge can be gleaned from a balance of practical experience and a theoretical base. (The group reflects life; it is a microsociety that has ups and downs.)

The analogy of the team Wheel of Effort discussed earlier is useful here (see Fig. 25-1). Understanding this diagram helps in understanding the breakdown in services if forces work in opposite directions. The wheel cannot make any progress toward its goals if forces are not pushing in one direction. Even tiny forces, if opposing, can prevent forward movement. The best way to prevent this type of breakdown in progress is to air issues and to express feelings about a given problem. Communication is the key to the client's success.

The Role of the Urban Therapist

The role of the urban home-based or community occupational therapist is unique. The therapist who works in an institution usually specializes in physical or psychosocial dysfunction while the home-based therapist should be a generalist. The nature of home care delivery requires a pragmatic individual who can solve problems using materials and equipment available in the client's own environment. The ability to adjust to different settings and a variety of individuals is also important. Effective communication skills are essential. Treatment must lead to functional activity and be relevant to the client's life-style.

The home care occupational therapist must function in the client's total environment. Thus, both the physical and psychological aspects of the client's problem must be considered. The client, the home environment, the caretakers, the illness, the resulting disability, the family resources, the community and the other team members form a whole unit or gestalt.

The word gestalt is defined as an organized field that has unique properties which cannot be derived merely from the sum of its various component parts. The client is perceived as a complex and dynamic person who has assets and/or liabilities in the areas of cognition, perception, sensation, movement, emotion, social interaction, and cultural background. All of these areas are factors in the client's gestalt. (The concept of a holistic approach to a person is explored in greater depth in the earlier chapter in human development, Chapter 3.) The therapist must be aware of the factors that influence the client's internal and external world. Both aspects affect planning and treatment.

History

The role of the home-based occupational therapist has changed little since the idea's inception. Home-based services emerged around 1920, usually as a part of a Visiting Nurse Association. Referrals were made by a nurse with a doctor's approval. Supplies were donated or purchased. The focus was on activity, usually handcrafts that were to increase self-esteem, channel energy into constructive tasks, keep the mind occupied, and increase functional performance. The patient's interests and attitudes determined activity choices. The concept of activity has since remained the same although activities chosen have been changed in response to differing life-styles and mores. Also, there is an increase in knowledge regarding the use of particular activities to effect specific improvements in function.

Present Practice

Today therapists may work in several different ways. The common practice is for an agency to hire an occupational therapist and pay a salary. A large agency may even pay for supplies and offer the use of an agency car.

PRIVATE PRACTICE. Some therapists are engaged in private practice. They divide their time among several agencies or settings. These practitioners may also receive private referrals. Payment may be a combination of part-time salary and fees-for-service. A fee-for-service is a lump sum of money that is paid to the therapist for each visit. The therapist is not a bona fide member of the agency; no benefits are paid. Note-writing and travel time is included in the fee. At times the agency will pay for attendance at staff meetings and conferences.

One advantage of private practice is the freedom that it affords the therapist. Treatment times and hours and patient-load and demands can be varied. Practice can be carried out in several specialty areas; programs that could not afford occupational therapy can begin to offer the service. This modest beginning does not put the service in a make-it-or-break-it position. Some therapists are combining part-time institutional work with private practice.

GROUP PRACTICE. Another convenient way to deliver part-time occupational therapy is in a group practice with one therapist acting as coordinator. A registry of local therapists who wish to pursue part-time work is compiled. Once the names are organized, the process is not complex. State laws must be researched for local requirements. This is usually a simple matter for a lawyer to handle. When the group is organized, referrals can be received. Contracts can be signed with several agencies or single referrals can be accepted.

Individual therapists are assigned to a location near their home or work. Referrals are assigned by location. At least one member must be available during the day for phone calls, referrals, and attendance at meetings.

The benefits of a group practice are numerous. The agency can deal with one coordinator instead of several part-time workers. A broad geographical area can be serviced without wasting time in travel. The group seeks its own members and is better able to evaluate member skills. Service to clients is not interrupted by vacations, illness, and other obligations —the group and not just one person is responsible for the referrals.

The group members benefit because the work is part-time. More therapists can participate in home care delivery. Agencies with small case loads can still provide occupational therapy services. Therapists can join or leave the group without any major disruption of service. The group name becomes familiar to agencies and community centers even if individual therapists have to drop out of the group.

Social Roles and Home Care

This section reviews research in sociology. This information provides a foundation for differentiating the practical roles of the therapist in an institution and of the home-based therapist. Stated simply, the difference lies in the power they hold. "Power refers to the ability to secure one's ends in life, even against oppression."[2] In the institution, the client has only a minimal amount of power over other team members and within the treatment process. The reverse is true in home-based therapy, where the practitioner becomes a guest in the client's world.

Each person has a role in the social system. This social system is composed of numerous subsocieties which reflect parts of the total society. The social system is stratified; it reflects a hierarchy. The social group or society is arranged ". . . into a hierarchy of positions that are unequal with regard to power, property, social evaluation, and/or psychic gratification."[3] The roles at the top of the social structure have more authority and status than those at the bottom. This ordered hierarchy of roles creates an arrangement of society that facilitates function.

Medical practitioners rarely consider the sociological aspects of the health care delivery system. Whether it is acknowledged or not, the practice of any aspect of medicine is a social act. Each practitioner has a place in the social system. The professional's role is shaped by the social system as well as by individual skills, knowledge, and attitudes. Any role, regardless of the individual who occupies the role, has certain values and functions that transcend individual differences. Professional education, liaisons, job descriptions, and status in the social hierarchy all shape individual behavior. Individuals express their roles in unique fashions while societal pressures determine the outer boundaries.

In general, the larger the social unit, the more numerous, specialized, and rigid are the roles of the participants. Communication among professionals becomes difficult. People organize around different specialty areas; those who are outside of this area do not tend to socialize and/or meet informally on a frequent basis. Territory becomes an important issue. The overall goals of the institution become abstract and less obvious to members of the broader society. Individuals at the bottom of the social system do not interact with those at the top.

In an institution the patient is at the bottom of the social system. An individual patient is not a permanent member of the institution's social system and such a role has little power. The patient role can become depersonalized in a world of experts. Yet the goals of the institution are said to be based on serving the patient. While staff members are sensitive to individual patients, they often neglect the powerless state of this role. The recent popularity of a discussion regarding Patient Rights in the institution merely exaggerates their lack of real power.

This situation is reversed in the home setting. The therapist is a guest in the client's house. The practitioner is a temporary addition to the family social system. The client and the caretakers determine the therapist's role as much as do the therapist's job description and training. If the therapist does not meet the client's needs, suggestions will be ignored or services cancelled. The client has more control over the practitioner; therefore, the client has more control over the treatment.

Funding

Home health agencies are funded by both public and private sources. Public sources include federal, state, and local monies. Private sources include insurance companies, religious groups, charities, endowments, and fees collected for services.

In the United States, most home care programs receive some of their funds from Medicare or Medicaid reimbursement. It therefore seems important to review some aspects of Title XVIII, Title XIX, and Title XX of the Social Security Act. Since Medicare is a national program, guidelines for any national health care program may be based on this legislative package.

Medicare

Title XVIII of the Social Security Act provides legislation for Medicare funding. Medicare provides medical benefits primarily for older Americans, but persons who have been disabled for more than twenty-four months can also qualify for Medicare benefits. Medicare has two types of coverage. Home care can be provided under Part A (hospital insurance) or Part B (medical insurance).

Specific requirements are established for all of the services that Medicare will fund. Not only do these guidelines influence current practice, but they will also affect the future. The importance of Medicare extends beyond funding; it sets national standards for practice. In short, Medicare establishes national priorities regarding the services that will be covered, the quality and nature of those services, and the degree to which the practitioner and the agency will be held accountable for the care they give.

Unfortunately, the current Medicare program does not consider occupational therapy a primary home care service. As a result of this distinction, skilled nursing care, physical therapy, and/or speech therapy must also be required by a client for their occupational therapy to be covered. Thus, occupational therapy is never used independently in the home unless an alternative funding source is available. Another factor is that the primary services evaluate the need for occupational therapy and influence the number of visits that will be covered. The specific boundaries of occupational therapy services covered by Medicare are presented later in this section.

The occupational therapist must also be aware of the criteria which must be met prior to reimbursement. Part A and Part B have different criteria.

Six criteria that must be met to qualify for Medicare under Part A (hospital insurance) are as follows:

1. The client must be admitted to a qualified hospital for at least three consecutive days.

2. Home health care must provide further treatment in the area which required hospital care.

3. Care must include part-time skilled nursing, physical therapy, and/or speech therapy.

4. The client must be homebound.

5. The client's doctor must assess the need for home care and establish a plan for the client within fourteen days following the client's discharge from the institution.

6. The home health agency must be a participant in Medicare.

If all of the above criteria are met, Plan A will pay for not more than one hundred visits for one year following a client's discharge.

If no hospitalization was required, Part B (medical insurance) will pay for one hundred home visits. For a client to be eligible, the following criteria must be met:

1. The client's condition must require the services of one of the primary services listed above.

2. The client's doctor must determine the need for one or more of the primary services and must establish a health care plan.

3. The client must be confined to the home setting.

4. The home health agency must be a participant in Medicare.

After the client pays a deductible fee, Medicare will reimburse the agency for the home services.

Medicaid

Medicaid or Medical Assistance, Title XIX of the Social Security Act, is a program for people who have no other means to pay for medical care. The program is based upon a formula for matching federal and state dollars. For example, the state must contribute a percentage of its per capita income. The ratios for the contributions are set by law. Some states do not contribute large sums of money to this program. Their reimbursement rates for home care may not cover the actual cost of the services. If services are rendered, the agency must deal with the resulting deficit. If no alternative income is generated, the agency assets will be eaten away. Usually monies from other sources are used to reduce the loss. However, this solution creates a complex and, at times, precarious funding situation. This is one of the reasons for establishment of rigid eligibility criteria. States may also develop their own criteria for eligibility.

Home health may or may not be part of a Medicaid treatment package. Coverage varies from state to state. In some cases Medicaid will pay for 180 days of home care after hospitalization. In other states only a fraction of the cost of home care is reimbursed. This situation will strain an agency that wants to serve clients with limited resources.

Social Service Program

Title XX of the Social Security Act may also influence occupational therapy. This program provides funds specifically to support social service programs for older Americans. Services may include hot meals that may be delivered to homebound individuals or served in a nearby community center twice a day. There are other offerings such as legal services, counseling, escort and homemaker or home health aide services, referral and follow-up on individual needs, and social activities. The program was designed to attract individuals to a nearby service unit where services could be organized and delivered efficiently. Even the homebound can be reached. Complex problems, once identified, can be referred to other appropriate agencies. For the occupational therapist, Title XX programs can provide a source of home care referrals and/or utilize occasional occupational therapy services when clients come in to eat their meals.

Other Funding Sources

Other sources of revenue include third party carriers like private insurance companies such as Blue Cross. Coverage varies with the company, the state, and the region of the country. Third party carriers are beginning to recognize the value of home care services. They save expensive hospital inpatient days; services are less costly. Local communities, through public health departments and/or grants to private agencies, may commit tax dollars or federal revenue sharing monies to support home care. Hospitals may develop their own home care departments. These groups, like the agencies that provide nonreimbursable services, may use private funds to ease their deficit. Included in this private category are donations, endowments, and contributions from charities like the United Way.

Some organizations offer specific services to clients. Two examples are the loan of adaptive equipment and the purchase of drugs. Religious groups may also contribute to home care assets. Members may volunteer to help with a problem; this may even include human resources that will relieve strained family members for a specific period of time during the day. Hot meals and the purchase of necessary equipment are other examples. Another source of private funds is the collection of fees for services. This may be based on a sliding scale to accommodate for different family incomes.

Another emerging source of referrals and financial support for home care is the federally approved Health Maintenance Organization (HMO). All federally approved HMOs must offer home care services. The HMO is a prepaid group practice. Each subscriber pays a fee which entitles him or her to receive a wide range of health (not just medical) services. Some services that are covered are routine check-ups, dental care, and prenatal care. All are oriented toward the maintenance of health. When and if a member becomes ill, the HMO provides complete medical care. Therefore, it behooves the HMO to utilize preventative rather than remediation services. If not, all of the practice finances will be absorbed by medical costs.

Another source of money can be used to initiate new programs. This source is grant money, which may be public or private monies. The therapist must identify a particular community need, find possible funding sources, and draft a grant proposal. There are a number of references and guides to assist with this task. If funded, money could be used to initiate new programs or provide services in an innovative area that is not reimbursed in any other way. There are two problems that are inherent in the grant structure. The first is the amount of time and effort that must be devoted to the development of the grant proposal. There is no guarantee that the proposal will be funded. The second concern is the temporary nature of grants. Alternative sources of support must be established for the program to continue.

In summary, there are a number of sources from which home care services can be funded. The agency tries to develop the broadest coverage for the services that it has to offer. Without a solid financial base, the future of the program is limited. No agency can operate at a loss indefinitely.

Medicare and Occupational Therapy

Medicare regulations have established national guidelines for all reimbursable services. Guidelines determine the diagnoses and care that will be covered. These guidelines establish the narrowest definition for occupational therapy services. Therefore it seems reasonable to outline this base, although therapists will hopefully be able to deliver broader services. In general, Medicare coverage dictates that the client must be able to improve significantly in a reasonable and generally predictable period of time. Claims for reimbursement for custodial care and/or maintenance are not accepted by Medicare.

On the first visit of a treatment program to be funded by Medicare, the client must be evaluated and appropriate goals must be established. Some agencies require a projection of the number of visits that will be needed during the next sixty days. Each visit must move the client closer to the long-range goals. Every sixty days the case must also be reviewed with other team members. The client has a limited number of home visits that will be covered (this issue was discussed in the previous section on eligibility criteria); visits must therefore be shared among all of the team members.

At present Medicare defines occupational therapy as a "medically prescribed treatment concerned with improving, or restoring functions which have been impaired by illness or injury or, where function has been permanently lost or reduced by illness or injury, to improve the individual's ability to perform those tasks required for independent functioning."[4] Services may include:

1. the evaluation and reevaluation as required of a patient's level of function by administering diagnostic and prognostic tests;
2. the selection and teaching of task-oriented therapeutic activities designed to restore physical function . . .;
3. the planning, implementing, and supervising of individualized therapeutic activity programs as part of an over-all 'active treat-

ment' program for a patient with a diagnosed psychiatric illness, . . .;
4. the planning and implementing of therapeutic tasks and activities to restore sensory-integrative function, . . .;
5. the teaching of compensatory techniques to improve the level of independence in the activities of daily living, . . .;
6. the designing, fabricating, and fitting of orthotic and self-help devices, . . .; and
7. vocational and prevocational assessment and training.[5]

There are other restrictions: services must be prescribed by a physician and performed by a qualified occupational therapist or certified occupational therapy assistant who works under the therapist's supervision. The most important clause in the criteria for coverage is that services are considered "reasonable and necessary" only where the client's condition indicates that there will be a significant practical improvement in the level of function in a "reasonable" period of time.[6] Occupational therapy must be goal-directed, purposeful activity that can maximize the client's level of function in a predetermined period of time.

Not all programs are governed by Medicare, but the number of older Americans increases daily and this will in itself expand Medicare services. Also, unfortunately for occupational therapy, Medicare standards are national and therefore influence coverage throughout the country. It is hoped that efforts will be rewarded that seek the expansion of Medicare coverage to include occupational therapy as a primary service.

Programs other than those that are totally dependent on Medicare funds may regard occupational therapy in a different light. In some settings the value of custodial and maintenance services are recognized and undiagnosed mental illness may also be treated. The boundaries of Medicare coverage are presented here to establish a base for home care practice. Services should not be narrowed further. The home care therapist should define the role of occupational therapy so that the maximum number of clients can be reached. However, if the role were too broadly defined, other services could be duplicated and the unique focus of occupational therapy may be lost. A balanced, well-defined role should be developed and should function within the boundaries of the home care agency's financial resources.

Future Legislative Influences

Home care and occupational therapy coverage may be affected by several emerging forces. Public Law 93-641, the National Health Planning and Resources Development Act of 1974, has established regional health planning agencies which will attempt to organize and distribute regional health resources. Duplication and unnecessary waste could be avoided so that health care costs could be controlled. Any future national health insurance bill will also have an effect on home care and occupational therapy practice. There are a number of bills that are under consideration. Some offer broader services than others. The exact form that this program will take cannot be determined at this time. Future practice will be influenced by forces in the legislative arena.

APPLICATION

This section describes the treatment process during which occupational therapy services are delivered to a homebound client. At first, in this process, there is a period of gradual building during which relationships and treatment regimes are established. After this a plateau period frequently occurs during which fewer gains take place. During this time learning and therapeutic patterns are reinforced. Finally the client and caretakers return to a daily routine that incorporates both the treatment regime and their former life scheme. This treatment process is presented in Figure 25-2.

Each of the five divisions in the diagram represents a phase in the treatment cycle. The umbrella of prevention pervades the entire cycle; it is a fundamental consideration throughout the delivery process. Each of these phases, as well as some of the issues that arise during that period, will be discussed in detail in this section. Generally, discussions will be pragmatic and oriented to describing and facilitating action taken by an occupational therapist in a home-based treatment program. In brief, the five phases of the treatment process are:

1. *Intervention*. This includes the referral, initial visit, and process of data collection.

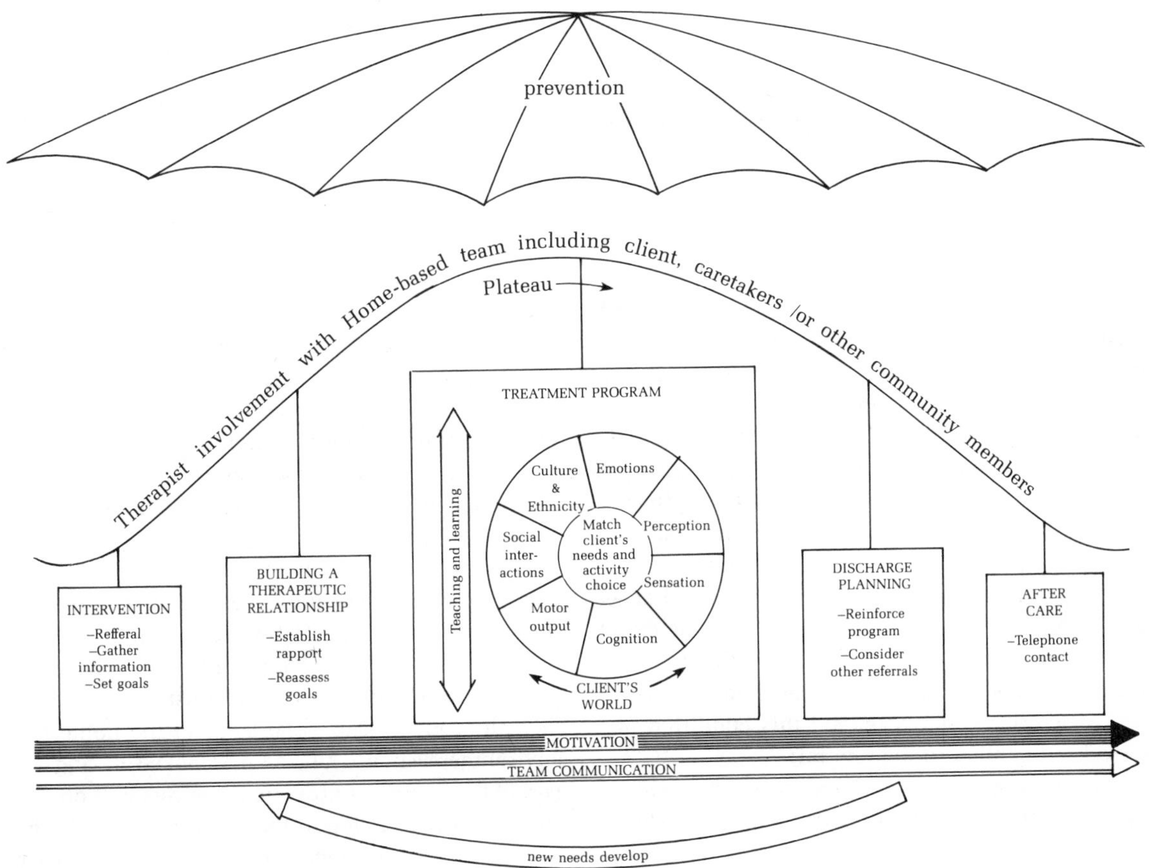

FIGURE 25-2. An urban delivery model: home-based occupational therapy.

2. *Building a Therapeutic Relationship.* In this period, the initial assessment is completed. Long- and short-term goals are established defining the focus of the occupational therapy care plan. The initial foundations for a trusting relationship are being built.

3. *Carrying Out the Treatment Program.* This is a time to teach the client and the caretakers how to maximize the client's level of function. Therapeutic exercises and modalities are introduced. The thrust of the team effort is to integrate the skills that the client gains into the daily life style.

4. *Discharge Planning.* During discharge planning goals are reassessed and new resources are sought out. Preparation is made for the termination of direct services. The full responsibility for care shifts back to the client and the caretakers.

5. *After-Care.* This is a time when contact with the client is maintained by telephone conversations. If new needs arise the process begins again with a referral.

Intervention

Referral

The referral or a call for service initiates the home care delivery process. There are a number of sources for occupational therapy referrals. Common agents outside of the agency include doctors, social workers, and hospital public health coordinators. Sources within the agency include nurses, physical therapists, speech therapists, and nursing supervisors.

The community occupational therapist must be willing to educate referral agents with regard to potential referrals. Most professionals will begin to utilize occupational therapy if they come in contact with proof of client progress. Talking about occupational therapy in a staff conference often is not as effective as demonstrating its value in actual treatment settings. Funding sources should be secure prior to any education campaigns.

The referral contains a brief medical history and present diagnosis of the client. Data such as age, sex, address, phone number, type of insurance, or fee status are given as well as the names of the client's doctor and of a person who is responsible for the client. A telephone call to the referral source may yield additional information.

A sample referral may be organized similar to the example given here. The referral briefly summarizes the client's current problem. Nonetheless, the client's past medical history should be reviewed with the client and his or her family. Occasionally a major medical problem is not listed on the referral sheet. For example, a Cerebral Vascular Accident client, with a recent acute heart problem, may not have mentioned his emphysema at the time he was admitted for emergency care, and this condition may have been omitted in the referral.

Once the general orders are received, each discipline involved in the home care process should receive more detailed instructions. For example, the nurse will require a list of medications and the physical and the occupational therapist will need specific instructions as to the client's tolerance to activity. All professionals should also be aware of the need for skill in observation.

Building a Therapeutic Relationship

Preparation for the Initial Visit

There are two aspects to preparing for the initial visit. First, if treatment was given previously, the client's former occupational therapist should be called and the client's program reviewed. Second, the client should be called or visited by the primary provider and given a brief introduction to occupational therapy service. The occupational therapist can then call the client and establish a mutually agreeable visit time. This time will depend on the visit appointments of other professionals, the family's needs, and the occupational therapist's schedule. A number of visits in one area of the city can be planned for the same day to avoid unnecessary travel time. If the client or caretaker sounded unsure of the appointment time, it is best to call again shortly before the visit.

Initial Visit

The initial visit is crucial to the entire treatment process. Not only must the client be assessed, but the entire environment including architectural barriers, caretakers, and resources must all be considered. Treatment goals must be established and the therapist must decide on the best way to interact within the client's social system. During the initial visit the therapist should act as a participant-observer, taking in information as much as giving it out.

The therapist must determine the best way to facilitate communication. (This topic is explored in Section 2 of this chapter.) The client's nonhuman environment is a rich source of information. How are objects arranged? Do any appear to be treasured? Is the furniture accommodating or uncomfortable? Is there a cherished pet? These and many other questions must be raised in the therapist's mind during the initial visit. (The importance of the nonhuman environment should not be overlooked during any part of the treatment program.) Answers will provide cues on how to relate to the social system. The following case study demonstrates a therapist's effective use of the nonhuman environment.

CASE STUDY

The occupational therapist walked up a flight of freshly scrubbed marble steps and rang the doorbell of a twin house. Peering through the double glass doors of the glass enclosed porch, he noted an orderly, modestly furnished porch and living room. Starched white ruffled curtains stood out from the window sills. Crocheted doilies adorned the dated, overstuffed sofa and arm chairs. Tiny, delicate china objets d'art were displayed on the sofa endtables. The focal point of the living room was a religious statue which was situated on an altar. The front windowsill was lined with large, potted plants. The potting soil in several pots was decorated with china figurines and had large satin bows stuck in it.

A neatly attired, elderly woman hobbled to the door; she seemed hesitant and fearful. The therapist displayed his arm patch and loudly mentioned his name and their earlier telephone call. The woman could see the agency insignia on the therapist's car door. She smiled and opened the door.

The therapist analyzed his observations. Signs indicated that the family might have little contact with young men. If he made enthusiastic gestures,

HOME CARE DEPARTMENT

REFERRAL FORM

HOSP. NO. ______

H.C. CASE NO. ______

H.I. CLAIM NO. 164-53-4173 A

PATIENT Ralph Norton

ADDRESS 51 Highware Ave.

CITY Canton, Pa. ZIP 10001 TEL. NO. 243-6741

DATE OF BIRTH 12/6/11 AGE 66 SEX M

MARITAL STATUS S (M) W SEP. DIV. HOSP. ACCOM. P S/P W OPD

RESPONSIBLE PERSON IN HOME Wife Adele

ADDRESS Same ZIP

SOURCE OF REFERRAL City Hospital

HOSP. OR S.N.F.: ADM. DATE 3/4/78 DISCH. DATE 3/20/78

PARTY RESPONSIBLE FOR CHARGES TO PATIENT ______

B.C. OR INS. CERT. NO. ______ GR. NO. ______

IS ILLNESS EMPLOYMENT RELATED? YES ☐ NO ☒

PATIENT'S EMPLOYER Retired

ADDRESS Same ZIP

PLAN OF TREATMENT—TO BE COMPLETED BY PHYSICIAN

DIAGNOSIS (PRIMARY AND SECONDARY—IN ORDER) MI CVA (L) Hemiplegia, Diabetes Mellites, HT

SURGICAL PROCEDURE – DATE ______

PROGNOSIS Fair

PATIENT INFORMED: DIAGNOSIS YES ☑ NO ☐ PROGNOSIS YES ☑ NO ☐

FAMILY INFORMED: DIAGNOSIS YES ☑ NO ☐ PROGNOSIS YES ☑ NO ☐

THERAPEUTIC GOALS Increase Independence in Self-Care + Ambulation

MEDICAL SUPERVISION IN HOME BY Dr. Jay Zaller TEL. NO. 234-5000 (PAGE)

ADDRESS 64 WINGDALE AVE. CITY ______ ZIP ______

HOME HEALTH SERVICES ORDERED: NURSING ☒ PHYSICAL THERAPY ☒ MEDICAL SOC. SER. ☐ SPEECH THERAPY ☐ OCC. THERAPY ☒ HOME HEALTH AID ☒

MEDICATIONS
Digoxin 0.25 mg. O.D.
Lasix 40 mg. O.D.
Aldomet 250 mg. B.I.D.
Diabenese 250 mg. a.m.

LABORATORY TESTS Electrolyte 1X mon Digoxin level / q.o mon.
Blood Sugar 1X mon

DIET Low Salt 1500 Cal A.D.A.

ACTIVITIES ALLOWED No Stairs graded program

TREATMENT AND SPECIAL EQUIPMENT Hospital Bed, commode

SPECIAL INSTRUCTIONS, REACTIONS TO BE REPORTED TO PHYSICIAN ______

PATIENT TO BE SEEN BY PHYSICIAN: DATE 5/4/78 HOME ☒ OFFICE ☐ OPD ☐

HOME HEALTH SERVICES TO BE PROVIDED ARE NEEDED TO TREAT THE CONDITION(S) FOR WHICH THE PATIENT RECEIVED SERVICES DURING THE RELATED STAY IN A HOSPITAL OR SKILLED NURSING FACILITY. YES ☐ NO ☐

I CERTIFY THAT THE PATIENT IS (1) HOMEBOUND, (2) REQUIRES THE HOME HEALTH SERVICES INDICATED ABOVE ON AN INTERMITTENT BASIS, (3) THE PATIENT IS UNDER THE CARE OF A PHYSICIAN WHO WILL REVIEW THIS PLAN OF TREATMENT PERIODICALLY.

3/20/78
DATE

Jay Zaller MD.
PHYSICIAN'S SIGNATURE REG. NO.

JAY ZALLER
PHYSICIAN'S NAME — PLEASE PRINT

(371–HC–1)

HOSPITAL COPY
HOME CARE DEPARTMENT
REFERRAL FORM

PATIENT Norton HOME CARE CASE NO. 3143 A

TO BE COMPLETED BY HOME CARE NURSE

REVIEW OF PATIENT'S ILLNESS (INCL. PREVIOUS HOSPITALIZATION, LAB. FINDINGS AND SOCIAL DATA SIGNIFICANT TO PATIENT'S CARE)

Pt. had c° severe pain in chest to wife. Taken to Emergency Room. Treated for M.I. While in hospital suffered CVA 3/7. Treated + placed in ICU 2 days. Condition stabilized. Hx ↑ B/p + HT last 16 years. Started PT + OT in hospital. Discharged to home for continued treatment. Presently oriented, no acute distress. S.O.B upon exertion. Unable to ambulate w/out asst. Unable to grasp w/ Ⓡ UE. Diabetes controlled w/ medication + diet

BP 150/90 T. 98° R. 70 weak + irreg.

SERVICES ORDERED:	NURSING	P.T.	S.T.	O.T.	M.S.S.	H.H.A.
DATE OF FIRST VISIT:	3/21					
FREQUENCY OF VISITS:	2-3	2X		1X		5X WK

PERTINENT INFORMATION REGARDING CARE TO BE GIVEN 3X WK

Monitor B/p + Meds.
max level Ⓘ A.D.L.
MAX strength Ⓑ UE + Ⓑ LE-S
↑ Balance + Co-ordination

NOTE:
MAX. LEVEL OF FUNCTION W/IN BOUNDARIES OF CARDIAC STATUS

MEDICAL SUPPLIES AND EQUIPMENT PROVIDED Hospital Bed, Commode

DATE 3/20/78 SIGNATURE Dee Jackson TITLE M.S.W.

(371–HC–2)

Printed with the permission of Helen L. Rawlinson, Director, Home Care Department, Blue Cross of Greater Philadelphia. The form is used by all hospitals participating in the Blue Cross of Greater Philadelphia Home Care Program and Demonstration Study. (The patient on pages 645 and 646 is fictitious.)

for example, they might be unfamiliar and arouse suspicion. The orderly rooms implied a formal, respectful demeanor; a boisterous person might not be well received in this home. One might also speculate that changes should be introduced gradually; abrupt decisions should be avoided. The therapist used these cues from the nonhuman environment to enhance the effect of his communication.

A home-based therapist needs to develop the ability to establish a rapport with people in various social systems. Developing this kind of skill depends on making good observations and at evaluating what is observed. The therapist must also be aware of his or her own value systems and how they affect the perception of others.

Setting Goals

Part of the initial visit must be devoted to goal setting. The client, caretaker(s), and therapist must establish the long term goal(s). This is actually the desired end of treatment. The client's life-style, assets and liabilities, environment, motivation, resources, and support network are all instrumental in making this decision. Using the long-term goal as a base, the therapist will develop an occupational therapy care plan. Since the long-term goal will take 2 to 6 months to accomplish, short-term goals must be established to maximize the client's mastery. The therapist uses a graded plan to achieve success. The long-term goal will also guide all visit and modality decisions.

An example for a bedridden arthritic client is to "increase independence in A.D.L." To accomplish this task the following short-term goals must be completed: increased functional use of affected extremities, increased independence in A.M. care, increased independence in dressing skills, work simplification techniques (dressing), and use of an adapted stocking donning device.

Not only must the client understand the short-term goals, but the caretaker(s) must be part of the teaching process also. The caretaker(s) will reinforce the occupational therapy program in the therapist's absence.

A short-term goal takes from 2 to 4 weeks to accomplish. From this experience the client can gain confidence and increase his or her self-esteem. Therapeutic activities are used to accomplish the short-term goals. They reinforce learning and exercise appropriate body parts. An example of a therapeutic activity is "brushing teeth and combing hair using built-up holder." This activity will increase the client's performance in A.M. care, one of the short-term goals listed earlier.

Goals can be useful to facilitate communication. Each discipline has a plan and all professionals are coordinating their efforts. The client outcome can be assessed periodically without much effort merely by reading the list of long- and short-term goals and activities.

Physical and Psychosocial Assessment

The assessment of the client's liabilities is organized and the findings are presented on an evaluation form. This must be brief and goal-oriented. The focus of the agency and the requirements of the funding source will determine some of the criteria included in the assessment. Although most medical professions acknowledge the value of prevention, most funding is based on acute short-term problems.

The clinical forms presented in other sections of this text can be adapted for home use. An example of a form that is aimed at a population of clients who all have Medicare benefits is given here. No matter what form is used both the physical and psychosocial aspects of the client must be evaluated and discussed.

Treatment Process

The most important aspect of this treatment phase is the client's progress. One major difference between clinic-based and home-based occupational therapy is that, in home-based services, the therapist frequently will not see the client for several days. Carry-over must therefore last longer. Also, in the home situation, it is helpful to make use of the resources and objects around the house rather than to rely upon more specialized therapeutic tools. Architectural barriers, liabilities, and assets must be taken into account and can be used to the advantage of the therapy program.

Teaching and Learning

A common method of maximizing the client's exposure to occupational therapy is to teach family

OCCUPATIONAL THERAPY EVALUATION AND CARE PLAN

Name ____________________ H.I.C. No. ____________________
Date of Evaluation ____________ Age ______ Medical Record No. ______________
____________________ Date of Onset ____________________
Diagnosis ____

Communication Ability ______________________________________

HOME SITUATION

Architectural Consideration ______________________________________
Family Members ______________________________________
Daily Routine ______________________________________

PHYSICAL CAPACITY

	Right	Left	COMMENTS
RANGE OF MOTION/UE			
Active	___	___	
Passive	___	___	
MUSCLE TONE	___	___	
STRENGTH	___	___	
HAND CAPACITY			
Appearance	___	___	
Hook Grasp	___	___	
Lateral Pinch	___	___	
Palmer Grasp	___	___	
3-Jaw Pinch	___	___	
Opposition	___	___	
COORDINATION			
Gross	___	___	
Fine	___	___	
Bilateral	___	___	
PRONATION/SUPINATION	___	___	
SENSORY			
Sharp/Dull	___	___	
Stereognosis	___	___	
Proprioception	___	___	

Physical Endurance ____________________
Visual Deficits/Aids ____________________
Present Use of Same ____________________
Hearing Deficits/Aids ____________________
Visual Motor Perception ____________________
Hand Dominance __________ Change Required? __________
Comments from Perceptual Evaluation: __________

This plan was developed by Ruth E. Levine, Lynn Marcus, Jane Roda, and Carmella Strano, Community Occupational Therapy Consultants Group, and is printed with permission.

Name ______________________ Medical Record No. ______________________

ACTIVITIES OF DAILY LIVING

I - Independent
A - Minimal Assistance
M - Maximum Assistance
D - Dependent

Feeding:

Eat with Fork ______
Cut Meat ______
Butter Bread ______
Drink from Glass ______

Hygiene:

Comb Hair ______
Brush Teeth ______
Cosmetics/shave ______
Wash Upper Body ______
Wash Lower Body ______
Shower/Tub ______
Nails ______
Urinal/Toilet ______

Transfers:

Chair ______
Bed ______
Toilet ______
Tub/Shower ______
Car ______

Dressing:

UE Dressing ______
UE Undressing ______
LE Dressing ______
LE Undressing ______
Buttons ______
Fasteners ______
Shoes/Braces ______
Ties/Laces ______
Sling ______

General Abilities:

Phone ______
Turn Pages of Book ______
Wristwatch ______
Doorknob/Key ______
Writing ______
Open/Close Drawers ______
Operate TV ______
Lights ______
Faucets ______
Flush Toilet ______
Pick Up Articles From Floor ______

Ambulation Ability ______________________
Patient's Homemaker Skills (Meals prepared by) ______________________

Medical Equipment Available ______________________
Additional Equipment Needed ______________________
Comments ______________________

Short Term Goals ______________________

Long Term Plans ______________________
Treatment Frequency
and Duration ______________________

____
OCCUPATIONAL THERAPIST

members and/or home health aides the client's program. The client can carry out the program daily if caretakers are willing to help.

A difficulty in this process is that modalities and activities must be taught to nonprofessional team members. Therefore, techniques should be simplified. For example, if it is possible, exercise should be presented in the form of an activity. (The need for daily, concentrated therapeutic exercise might be better served in a rehabilitation center.) It is helpful to outline instructions briefly on paper. This will serve as a reference for all team members.

Simplifying techniques and sharing skills with caretakers is helpful even if funding sources allow daily exercise to be done by the occupational therapist as there will be a time when the actions that the client learns must be translated into some activity that can be continued after the home-based occupational therapy service ends.

Some Common Home Care Programs

The home care therapist must understand activity analysis and be able to translate activity choices into the client's gestalt. The theoretical base previously presented should be consulted (see Chapter 5).

Many factors influence treatment outcomes. Physical aspects of the environment as well as the ethnic background, culture, social interaction patterns, resources, educational background, social class, and emotions must be considered. Other important issues are the value systems, availability of medical services, religion, and family/neighbor support networks. These factors provide information and cues regarding the client's life-style. The therapist has a rich source of data which may facilitate the selection of treatment modalities in the home setting.

The home care therapist must adapt successful clinical practice modalities for home use. Several examples are the use of a towel under the affected arm and a smooth table top to duplicate the internal and external shoulder motion obtained when using a ball-bearing skate board; a bowl and household objects for grasp-place-release exercises; old kitchen chairs for bathtub transfers (one inside and one outside of the tub) instead of a costly shower seat; canned goods placed in an old pocketbook or sock for strengthening exercises replace the need for sandbag weights: paper towels or a wash cloth wound around handles and secured with a rubberband for building-up utensils; a soup bowl instead of a plate guard; and a damp rag used under kitchen equipment to stabilize them.

Transfers

All home care personnel must be skilled in transferring clients in less than ideal circumstances. Family members are unfamiliar with the process; they may fear that they will injure the client or themselves. The occupational therapist must frequently position the client for activities. This is commonly done without assistance. Since caretakers and neighbors frequently observe therapy, good technique and an air of competence are essential.

Architectural Barriers

A factor that affects the outcome of a home care program may be physical in nature. Architectural barriers can impede client progress. Economic factors limit large-scale changes in many homes. Few people have access to the resources that would be needed to renovate basic necessities such as the bathroom and kitchen fixtures. The therapist must assess the type of changes that would be helpful and possible. Little can be gained from an exploration of changes that can never come about.

Another less obvious factor is cultural in nature. While some people enjoy change that will facilitate their daily performance, others regard adjustment with new discomfort. The total expenditure of energy needed for change is not considered possible. The daily, but smaller, energy expenditure attached to the current inconvenience seems more acceptable. Sometimes the only stable part of the client's world is the unchanging nonhuman environment. The illness may have upset and altered everything else including roles and relationships. Investment in the secure and unchanging environment may be more reasonable to some people.

The therapist who blindly suggests extensive change in this type of situation may find a brittle and resistant audience. It seems logical to suggest minor changes like moving a bookcase one foot to the left to free a passage for wheelchair accessibility. However, the client may not wish to crowd the picture that hangs next to the bookcase. The therapist can gently offer suggestions which may be remembered at some later date. The nonhuman world may be the last place that remains unscathed by the client's illness.

The best approach for the therapist to use cannot be precisely outlined. Clients must be assessed in the context of their nonhuman environment and social interaction patterns. There is no need for the therapist to invest energy in attempting to foster change when the client does not think that any benefit can be gained from the alterations.

Change was precluded in the next case study because of cultural and economic factors. This family was limited in income and parochial in outlook. It would not be acceptable to readily accept suggestions from an "outsider." The therapist could raise questions but could never expect to see immediate results. The therapist's role regarding changes to the environment was, at best, one of a catalyst. The only change that she considered was the addition of a snack table to the right side of the refrigerator. Any other considerations would have been too costly. The family seemed to accept the idea, but the item was never purchased. Possibly after the case was discharged, the family was able to develop its own solution to the problem.

CASE STUDY

The Hagers have resided in their small row house for thirty years. The brick house is over 150 years old; it is situated in a blue-collar residential district in a large metropolitan area.

Mrs. Hager is fifty-four years old. She has a residual left hemiparesis. Her recovery is complete except for a decrease in shoulder function. A Winter-Haven perceptual test revealed a possible deficit in visual memory and spatial relations. She can dress independently although her performance is slow. The occupational therapist has been actively involved with Mrs. Hager's training for two months. The long-term goal is to "maximize independent functioning." The short-term goal is to help Mrs. Hager be independent in the kitchen.

The therapist found that Mrs. Hager used her disability. She could now garner the sympathy and support of her two teenaged children. She agreed to try to work in the kitchen only because her children could not cook very well. The biggest problem that hindered progress was the layout of the kitchen and the breakfast room. (See floor plan in Fig. 25-3.)

Whenever Mrs. Hager wished to take things out of the refrigerator, she had to walk back several feet to place the objects on the table. The food then had to be transferred into the pantry. Mrs. Hager refused to consider carry-all baskets. She felt that they "looked funny." The therapist suggested that a snack table be placed next to the refrigerator. The client agreed but never was able to procure the item. The stove was also a problem; it did not have an automatic pilot light. After a few unsuccessful attempts

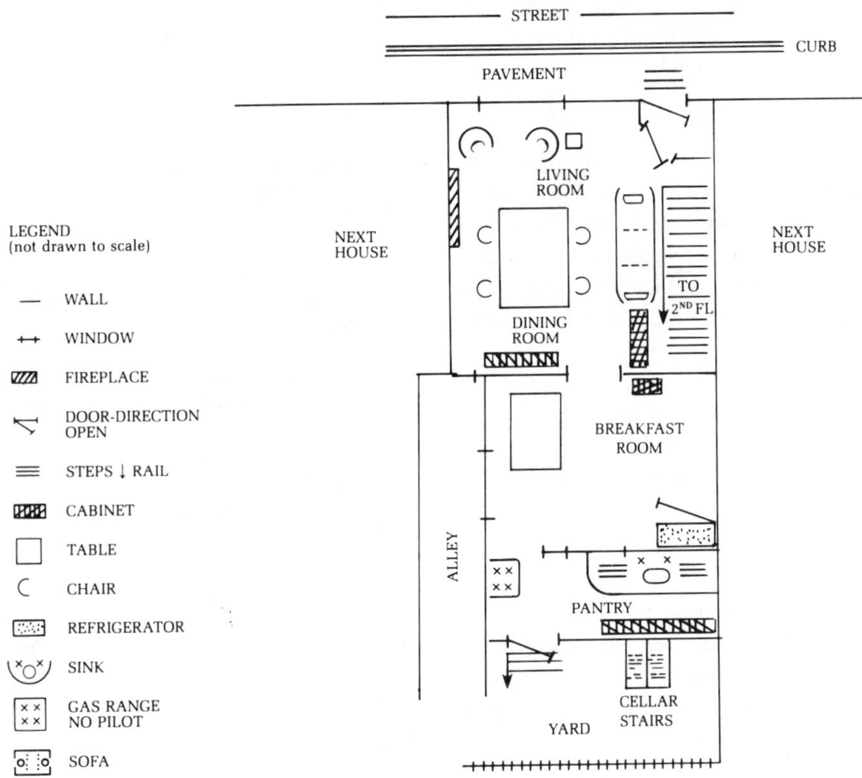

FIGURE 25-3. Floor plan of the first floor of the Hager house. The floor plan depicted here is common in a blue-collar neighborhood near the industrial center of a large city. The houses are over 150 years old. Streets are narrow and barren. Small yards extend for 15 to 20 feet from the back doors. The average income is $10,000 a year for a family of four. This particular neighborhood is close-knit and insular. Relatives live "two doors" away or "around the corner."

at cooking, Mrs. Hager was willing to turn this responsibility over to her oldest daughter. "I guess that she is old enough after all," she said.

The Hagers could not afford any extensive changes. Their culture did not support do-it-yourself innovations. The nonhuman environment was one of the only stable things in their lives. There was little energy left to invest in change.

Plateau

After a period of time that usually varies between one and six months, the client's performance may reach a plateau. No other gains—physical or psychosocial—may be made in this phase although this does not preclude further improvement at a later date. Once the client has not advanced in approximately four to six visits, the therapist should begin to plan for a reduction in visit frequency. If the agency has resources for chronic care, the client can be carried indefinitely. In this case the therapist visits periodically to check on the program and readjust the goals. A common problem is that funds for chronic care are limited. Instead of periodic visits the case must be discharged. This is true for Medicare clients.

If discharge is necessary, discuss the discharge plan with other professionals. The client's assets and liabilities should be considered and additional suggestions and actions should be shared during a discharge conference. Another agency's help may be needed in which case a referral must be forwarded to the new agency.

Discharge should be preceded by a gradual reduction of visits during a two-month period. The family should be weaned from the daily support it has received so far. All professionals should share their plans with the client and the caretakers. Abrupt changes should be avoided.

After-Care

The client may develop a need for service at a later date. Brief phone calls can be made every few months to evaluate any concerns. Newly developed capacities, relapses, or changes in the support network may necessitate additional treatment. If so, the case is referred to the agency again and the cycle begins all over. This is not uncommon.

REFERENCES

1. Fry, R. E., Lech, B. A., and Rubin, I.: Working with the primary care team: The first intervention. In Wise, H., et al. (eds.): Making Health Teams Work. Cambridge MA: Ballinger Publishing Co., 1974, p. 56.
2. Tumin, M. M.: Social Stratification. Englewood Cliffs NJ: Prentice-Hall, 1967, p. 12.
3. Ibid.
4. Home Health Agency Manual for Medicare, 205.2, A. Social Security Administration, Health Information Manual No. 11. Department of Health, Education and Welfare. U.S. Government Printing Office, Washington DC, 1975-210-829:430.
5. Ibid.
6. Ibid., 205.2,B.

BIBLIOGRAPHY

Brill, N. I.: Teamwork: Working Together in the Human Services. Philadelphia: J. B. Lippincott Co., 1976.

Brill, N. I.: Working with People: The Helping Process. Philadelphia: J. B. Lippincott Co., 1973.

Goffman, E.: The Presentation of Self in Everyday Life. Garden City NY: Anchor Books, 1959.

Hall, E.: The Hidden Dimension. Garden City NY: Anchor Books, 1969.

Jaco, E. G. (ed.): Patients, Physicians and Illness: A Sourcebook in Behavioral Science & Health, ed. 2. New York: Free Press, 1972.

Leininger, M.: Some anthropological issues related to community mental health programs in the United States. Community Mental Health J. 7:50–61, 1971.

Mechanic, D.: The concept of illness behavior. J. Chronic Disease 15:189–194, 1962.

Mills, T. M.: The Sociology of Small Groups. Englewood Cliffs NJ: Prentice-Hall, 1967.

Olmstead, M. S.: The Small Group. New York: Random House, 1959.

Rogers, C.: Freedom to Learn. Columbus OH: Charles E. Merrill Publishing Co., 1969.

Sanchez, V.: Relevance of cultural values. Am. J. Occup. Ther. 18:1–5, 1964.

Scott, C. S.: Health and healing practices among five ethnic groups in Miami, Fla. Public Health Reports 89:524–532, 1974.

Suchman, E. A.: Social patterns of illness and medical care. J. Health Human Behav. 6:2–16, 1965.

Suttles, G. D.: The Social Order of the Slum. Chicago: University of Chicago Press, 1973.

Zborowski, M.: People in Pain. San Francisco: Jossey-Bass, 1969.

section 2/In the Rural Setting/Elizabeth B. Devereaux

Just as each individual patient, each urban setting, and each ghetto has unique characteristics, so does each rural community. To be even minimally effective, the occupational therapist functioning in a rural community must understand the people: their culture, values, and attitudes. Even the therapist who has grown up in a rural community and returns there to practice may find that he or she is considered an "outsider" by virtue of his having been away, and even more, having obtained an education while he was away.

It is natural to assume that, while there are cultural and subcultural differences in this country, we all want pretty much the same things, generally in the form of a "better life"—and a better life demands a better job and a higher income to get there. But these assumptions and the next action—that of the therapist's imposition of his or her own values onto treatment direction—will only lead to frustration in dealing with many of the clients in a rural culture. Actually the characteristics discussed here do not belong exclusively to the rural culture. The distinction should not be made between rural and urban; the distinction should be made between the middle class and a "folk class," which is a working class that seems to fit somewhere between the lower class and lower middle class.[1,2] The folk class appears to exist *wherever* people have been limited or defeated by their environment[3] whether this happens in the urban ghettos, the Western plains, or Appalachia.

Most rural areas also have a professional class and a middle class which are influenced by the culture of the folk class but usually can be dealt with more nearly as one would deal with such groups anywhere. These two classes generally are seeking the better life, will serve on committees and work for the common good, and want good health care including preventive health care. There is also the lower class, and they would be approached in the rural area as in any other area of the country. They are characterized as a group dealing inadequately with life's problems, with families often having multiple problems that are perpetuated from one generation to another. These people may have aspirations for a better life but are lacking in basic resources such as education, problem-solving ability, work skills, and just plain know-how to even work toward the fulfillment of their dreams.

It is not intended that this chapter give an in-depth view of the folk class or the folk culture. Rather, the overview given is aimed toward raising the therapist's level of awareness of the attitudes, mores, and values of the culture; the gradations of its influence throughout the various strata of the populations encountered; the lack of results when a therapist works counter to the culture; and some types of approaches and interventions that might work. Much of the material in this chapter is drawn from my own experiences while living and working in West Virginia and Ohio and visiting rural areas in many other parts of the country. This is mentioned to confirm the suspicions of those readers who may detect a strong flavor of Appalachia in these writings. It is true—I have been influenced by the culture.

A SOCIOCULTURAL OVERVIEW

There is men's work and there is women's work in this culture and seldom the I'll-wash-and-you-dry cooperative sharing often seen between husband and wife in the middle class. It's up to the husband to make a living and the wife to take care of the house and children. The wife often does the painting and wall papering, the yardwork and the gardening, although the husband may work in the garden too. Even small children are expected to do their share of helping with the chores.

Frequently the men in this society have fewer years of schooling than the women do. The men have worked outdoors doing physical labor, farming, ranching, lumbering, hunting, fishing, mining where formal education wasn't needed and where social skills weren't particularly needed and there was little opportunity to learn them. Women, though, have learned from each other the skills of cooking and canning, sewing and quilting, and housekeeping and raising children and have learned a higher level of social skills than the men. Parents, children, aunts, uncles, cousins, and all the other possible relations in an extended family usually live close by. This is particularly true in mining and lumber camps, where houses are often built side by side in a string up the valley until they run into a mountain. This factor makes it easier for women to have social interaction than the men.

Husbands and wives don't seem particularly close to each other and, when groups of people get together, the men congregate in one group and the women in another and there is little interaction between them. Individuals often seem to lack a feeling of self-worth, gain most of their acceptance and approval from their group, and so tend to avoid taking sides in controversial issues, not wanting to offend members of their group and risk becoming alienated from the security the group represents.

Rural Poverty

The rural poor is composed of the unemployed of any category, including miners, sharecroppers, ranch hands, farm workers, lumbermen, and so forth. The rural poor also includes those whose income falls below the poverty income: migrant farm workers, hired hands, tenant farmers, those who live on the land they own, American Indians, Mexican-Americans, Puerto Ricans, blacks, and whites.[4]

Some who have studied the problems of poverty maintain that the use of a specific subsistence income level to define what is "poor" is less meaningful than a definition that is relative to the society in which the person lives. John Kenneth Galbraith is one who contended that even if people have a subsistence income, if that income is a great deal less than that of the rest of the community, they are poverty-stricken since they do not have a level of existence that is considered decent or acceptable to their community.[5]

Whatever the accustomed level of existence, even that is often in jeopardy. The farmer who is poor generally farms with hand tools on land with poor soil, often on a hillside, and is at the mercy of the weather as well. Miners sometimes lose their jobs with no warning, being told at the end of a shift that the mine is closing. They have been surviving and providing for their families, even though they may live in a company house or a shack on their own land. Every room is usually used for sleeping and there's a television set, but the miners and migrant workers often owe their "whole pay to the company store." When there is no work and no other jobs available there is no pay and, after trying to exist for awhile with no income, even a welfare check (if they are eligible) raises their subsistence level.

With no other marketable skills there's no use moving to the city. The emotional shock that comes with the realization that he can't get a job sometimes causes a man to stop the risk of trying. Feeling controlled by other people and other things and unable to provide for their families, many men just give up. To some outsiders this looks like a loss of interest in work. Eventually it leads to his becoming physically unemployable after a few years. All this results in a fatalistic attitude, with an "It ain't no use tryin', nothin's gonna make any difference anyhow. Things is meant to be this way, an' you can't do nothin' to change 'em. It's the Lord's will."

Dependence and Independence

Every culture has its own survival system and one aspect of particular importance in the folk class is the relationship of individuals to their peer groups: men to men, women to women, and each to his or her family. Each is dependent on a peer group and a family for acceptance and security. The family does not seem to know how to nurture its members so they can develop the security to become independent. Being so emotionally dependent only leads to deeper feelings of insecurity.

Some have been able to leave their rural homes and find jobs in the city. These have usually been the younger people with more education and ambition than those left behind who, in turn, have been least capable of changing things for the better.[6] The largest migration at any one time in the United States occurred during World War II. Those who migrated went either to war or to the city to work. They tended to stick together, in living quarters and neighborhoods, and tried to recreate and preserve their culture, returning home frequently to visit "the folks." Many said they would return to their rural area immediately if they could find a job.

With the younger people leaving and birth control methods being used more, the birth rate has been declining and the percentage of elderly increasing in rural communities. This, therefore, means an increase in the group most steeped in tradition with little or no desire or energy to change.

The pioneers and early settlers, ancestors of many of today's folk classes, were noted for their independence, which conveyed a sense of identity, autonomy, self-direction, but did not exclude working cooperatively with neighbors and projects of benefit to all. Weller[7] says that independence has changed to individualism, which has a self-centered focus, so that things are done independently but always with the "what's in it for me?" attitude. Each person's affairs are an individual matter and people are basically against joining anything except one of the political parties. A man may attend a Parent-Teachers Association meeting or go to church occasionally (while many of his wife's activities center around church and school) but, if there's no immediate gratification of his self-interest, he probably won't go back to the next meeting. Living and becoming accustomed to unpredictable rapid changes out of their control, these people see no benefit in planning for the future. There's no concept of committee work or long-term goals or of planning and working for community improvement.

The Children's Place

Family planning is a recent development, and large families have been common in this culture. A high rate of illegitimacy seems accepted. Illegitimate children are seldom given up for adoption, and may be raised by the mother and/or her parents.

Babies are to be cuddled and played with, but as they begin to assert their individual personalities and become more difficult to control parents play with them less and less, and the children form their own peer groups. The adage that "children are to be seen, not heard" operates in this culture, as opposed to the middle class culture where the children are the center of attention. Children are to behave as "little adults," may play if it does not disrupt adult activities, and boys have a lot of freedom where girls are expected to stay close to home.

As contradictory as it seems, child-rearing is permissive, impulsive, and indulgent, yet physical punishment is nearly always used rather than taking away a privilege or scolding. A mother may repeatedly tell a child to "do this" or "don't do that," yet the child keeps right on until the mother spanks, switches, or in some physical way gets the child's attention. But when father speaks or gives a stern look, the child generally obeys immediately. With these kinds of inconsistencies and double messages, children learn to ignore the words and hear the tone and the feeling behind them and they tend to continue to respond that way as adults.

Sometimes a father's physical discipline is very harsh and a mother will try to stop it or connive with the child so that the father doesn't find out about the child's misbehaving. This makes the child even more dependent on the mother. And just like all children, they can often talk mom into a less severe punishment or none at all. The child develops a fear of punishment because it's aimed at control of the child, and so the child develops resentment toward authority and fears it. This carries over into adult attitudes. These children are threatened with the law, the doctor, with being given away to strangers, all in an effort to keep them in line. Is it any wonder that these children are often sober and sad looking? They lose their spontaneity and playful qualities at an early age.

The "Flying Feds" Syndrome

In planning and developing a program in a rural community, the therapist will be involved with those from the professional class and the middle class. Although they are generally committed to a better life for their community and for themselves, it is well to remember that they have been influenced by the folk culture around them. Often they are not at all conscious of how their behavior has been affected, but a sensitive observer frequently can spot the patterns.

The occupational therapist works with people who are of the folk culture but have moved out of it somewhat. However, under stress, all people tend to revert to old patterns of behavior. Therefore if programs being developed run counter to cultural influences in the rural communities they simply will never get off the ground. Program planning must accommodate to the cultures involved if it's going to succeed.

All these cultural influences were seemingly ignored by the Flying Feds after the Buffalo Creek, West Virginia, flood in 1972. When mobile homes were assigned, the lowest paid laborer in the mine might find his home situated next to that of the superintendent of the mine. How much easier and quicker would have been the adjustment to the loss if the worker had been surrounded by the familiar cluster of family and friends from his old neighborhood. These people have all too often had things done to them and for them and seldom *with* them.

The flying feds syndrome affects many people in rural communities and occurs in reaction to outsiders' promises to develop programs to meet community needs that (1) never materialize, (2) are superimposed on the community, (3) have criteria so restrictive that, even in the same family, some members may be provided service but others with the same needs may not be, (4) are so general in scope that the particular needs unique to each community are not being served, (5) infringe so much on the rights, freedoms, and dignity of the community and individuals that the community refuses it because the "cost" is too high, (6) duplicate or compete with existing services, or (7) any combination of the above. The flying feds syndrome also makes the people who are affected by it suspicious of anybody who says, "Let's write a federal grant for this program" and of any outsider who comes into the community talking about developing a new program.

The folk culture is suspicious of outsiders and their ideas. It was the outsiders who cheated some of them out of the mineral rights of their land, sometimes because they couldn't read the contract they were signing; who bought their timber for badly needed cash but at a fraction of its worth; who ran railroads and highways over their lands, perhaps paying for them but taking the land whether or not the owners wanted to sell it. The person isolated geographically and culturally, outside of the mainstream of commercial trade, seldom realized the real or potential value of the coal, oil, gas, or timber on the land. Much needed cash and goods were received when the deal was made, but years later he found out that he had also sold land that he wanted to keep in the family. He was lied to and tricked by land agents who told him that they had a prior deed to his land; to avoid going to court he would sign a quit claim which gave the land company mineral and timber rights and, in return, allowed him to continue living on the land. He did not understand the law and courts. He was afraid to speak out in a meeting let alone a courtroom and was afraid that a person like he would not get a fair deal—he would be the victim again. He didn't have money for a lawyer anyway. The people of this culture, even the children, carry a constant level of fear, uncertainty, and anxiety because much of the control of their lives comes from outside of them—an environment that has defeated them and authority that comes in the form of employer, the law, welfare workers. They do not trust strangers, "experts" in particular.

These are independent people, with a lot of pride and dignity, who are used to taking care of themselves and their neighbors. They really don't like "somebody out there"—some expert—telling them what to do and how to do it. Every so often the leaders of a rural community will refuse to accept federal money rather than accept all the restrictions and the superimposition of control from outside of their community.

Those from the folk class may attend an initial meeting to hear a discussion of a project but probably will not become involved or attend future meetings. However, they will use the service if it is of benefit to them and is suited to them.

There are two reasons, primarily, to include people in planning. First, it is a way to get their support for the program during both its development and its implementation. Secondly, and this is probably more important, by involving the people for whom the plan is intended, chances are you'll come up with a better plan. They know their real and felt needs better than anyone else. A program specifically tailored to these needs has a better chance of receiving the support of the community and of being used.

Attitude Towards Health Care

People in the folk class are used to taking care of things themselves as much as possible, using folk medicine remedies passed down from generation to generation: herbs; cough medicine made from brown sugar or honey and turpentine, kerosene or whiskey; berries; teas from tree roots; special tonics, brews, and poultices. As a last resort they'll go to a doctor. As a further last resort, they'll go to the hospital, maybe. Hospitals are frightening, impersonal, outside the scope of comprehension; they are where you go to die.

Sickness is feared and health care is mostly sought in crisis situations. Interestingly, Kent and

Smith describe similar behavior among ghetto poor (". . . the resistance to involvement and the crisis orientation of the poor . . ."[8]) as needing to be considered in developing health programs in the ghettos.

The concept of preventive health care is not understood, and if Johnny cries because the brace hurts his leg he will not have to wear it even if the purpose is to prevent further deformity. Prenatal care is generally nonexistent. Some babies are born in the hospital but many are born at home.

If an older person has to hire a neighbor to take him to the doctor where he waits all day to get heart medicine, and the expense of the trip to the doctor and the medicine means the difference between that and money for food for several days, he's likely to choose the latter. His fatalistic attitude may be that "I'll live 'til my time comes and no medicine will make the difference. It don't matter nohow."

Folk language includes many terms to describe disease and illness which will not be found in a medical dictionary and it is essential to learn the language in order to communicate. A "bealed toe," "low blood," "bad nerves," "running off," and "the bloody flux" are but a few.

The concept of mental health has no meaning in this culture. Mental illness is little understood and is blamed on "bad nerves" or "poor nerves." If the person becomes violent or causes too much of a disruption he may be sent to a state hospital, but many are kept at home, particularly in isolated areas.

I once went on a home visit to a 79-year-old woman who lived with her two brothers, one 81 and the other 83. It was a hot summer day and after driving on a dirt road as far as it went, I walked to the creek, took off my shoes and stockings, waded the stream, put shoes and stockings back on, followed the path around the cornfield and up a hollow. There was an old log cabin, very clean and neatly kept, and stepping inside was like stepping into the 1800s. There was no carpeting on the floors, but the cabin was filled with antiques, including a harpsichord against one wall. Sister had "worn-out nerves," played the harpsichord and did beautiful needlework, but was too disoriented and distracted by her voices to do much more. So the "boys" cooked, farmed, did the housework, and took care of her. As the gentlemanly 83-year-old brother escorted me back to the car to show me where to cross the creek on the stepping stones, he confided that his sister's nerves had started "wearing out" about 30 years before but that the three of them got along just fine. His attitude was one of a completely unquestioned acceptance of responsibility for taking care of his sister, and her "peculiarities" were just something to accommodate to. Their system was in balance and, as a therapist, the best thing I could do was to leave it alone.

THE OCCUPATIONAL THERAPIST IN A RURAL SETTING

Acceptance as a Person, Therapist, and Outsider

Men and women of the folk culture do hard physical work, often for long hours. To endure this, day after day, they have to pace themselves. One of the ways they pace themselves and break into the monotony of their lives is the "come set a spell" approach to business transactions and interaction with neighbors and friends. They have none of the rush-rush-state-your-business-and-leave impersonal encounter of the middle and professional classes. A trip to the store, to buy or sell, includes a "visit," talk about the weather, the family's health, politics, the cow that's about to come fresh.

A visiting therapist needs to build time into the schedule to "visit" with the client and his family, that is, to build a personal relationship along with giving treatment. The therapist may be accustomed to a more structured schedule and a set routine, but he or she can't expect the client to be comfortable or cooperative if the therapist sticks to business only. The therapist plans a schedule, makes it flexible, and keeps it to himself or herself. If the therapist is in the area, he or she should stop and chat even if the purpose is not therapy, because the therapist needs first to be accepted as a person before being effective as a therapist. The therapist is reminded that it took several hundred years for things to get where they are today and no doubt it will take a few years to have things heading in the direction we want them to be. Changes usually occur slowly; perhaps there will be three steps forward and five back and then six forward and only two back. If you know where you're going, you'll eventually get there.

Folk people cannot be hurried or pushed. They

will balk just like a two-year old in the negative stage. Passive-aggressiveness is one power of the powerless.

The therapist must talk the language of the people. The folk class person does not understand logic and concepts and the nuances of speech, and he or she generally has a short attention span. If the therapist speaks the language without being condescending toward the client's space- and experience-limited world, communication will begin. This may involve telling a story or using an anecdote to make a point—use the imagery that's within the folk culture's world to get a concept across.

The Therapists's Attitude

It is often difficult for the therapist to separate personal values from those of the client's and to not superimpose expectations onto the client. Using a story (not of the folk class but of the professional class) to illustrate the point, an occupational therapist was working with a handicapped homemaker, and the client was progressing very well with personal grooming skills but very little with cooking and other homemaking skills. This was very frustrating and the therapist couldn't understand it until one day a neighbor of the client's dropped in while the therapist was in the home. After a few minutes chatting about what the client and therapist were doing, the neighbor said, "Huh, why *should* she learn all those things now when it will be twice as hard? Before she got sick she spent all her time playing bridge and her husband did all those things. I wouldn't want to learn either if I was her!" The therapist made an assumption based on her own values and attitudes and her past experiences working with handicapped homemakers: that one of the purposes of therapy and using adaptive equipment should include enabling the handicapped homemaker to achieve maximum functioning ability with homemaking skills. In this particular case this was not applicable; the client had a life-style that differed from that which the therapist expected.

While the rural community may be resistant to the influence of outsiders, these same outsiders are needed as models to expose the community members to different methods of doing things. There is opportunity for the stranger to the community to perceive problems from a vantage point that the inhabitants do not have, the latter having been saturated by the cultural traditions and attitude "we've always done it this way." By the same token, because it is a tradition does not mean it is inappropriate and should be discontinued. Many traditions serve a useful purpose and need to be continued, but each tradition should be assessed for its present usefulness. Traditional ways of doing things generally give the individual a sense of place in the world and help to anchor him or her in a world that sometimes changes too quickly. In other words, "Don't throw the baby out with the bath water," an expression not infrequently heard in rural communities.

Professional Isolation As a Therapist

Being the only occupational therapist in any community can be a lonely existence professionally. During field work experiences there were occupational therapy supervisors and other occupational therapy students with whom the student could discuss difficult treatment decisions or the relative merits of one splinting material as opposed to another. They could use each other as sounding boards without a lot of explanation because they spoke the same language. They didn't have to redefine the scope of Activities of Daily Living (ADL) first before discussing what was happening with a particular client. Some occupational therapists have had work experience in a clinic setting well-staffed with other occupational therapists prior to moving to a rural setting and, therefore, have a greater depth of practical experience to bring to their new setting. But many occupational therapists in a rural area are newly graduated and are there because of personal reasons. They feel a keen need for professional interaction with other occupational therapists.

DEVELOPING YOUR OWN CONTINUING EDUCATION PROGRAM. Geographical isolation from occupational therapists does not need to include isolation from their ideas. To keep knowledgeable about the people, issues, and concepts involved in the current practice of occupational therapy, read each issue of *The American Journal of Occupational Therapy*, and the AOTA Newspaper. If an article in the Journal is of particular interest, select additional reading from the references listed. There may not be a library nearby, but many rural areas are served by a bookmobile and the state's interlibrary loan service can provide many books and journals that would not be found on the average community library's shelves. Letters to the editor and to the special information exchange sections of the American Occupational Therapy Association publications can result in much up-to-date information from other therapists. Monographs, thesis copies, and other publications which may be ordered from the American Occupational Therapy Association national office are another source of materials.

One of the fringe benefits of working with those trained in disciplines related to occupational therapy is the exchange of reading material. Although they may not relate directly to the practice of occupational therapy the concerns and theories expressed in such literature are often transferable to the occupational therapy framework and can enrich existing knowledge.

When possible, the therapist should attend state, regional, and national conferences and workshops for the professional stimulation and idea exchange so necessary for continued growth.

STATE AND NATIONAL OCCUPATIONAL THERAPY ASSOCIATIONS AS RESOURCES. Each of the fifty states has a state occupational therapy association related to the national organization, the American Occupational Therapy Association (AOTA). Both state and national associations are invaluable resources for the isolated therapist. In my experience, a letter or phone call to various members of the state association has resulted in help in presenting a workshop, written material to assist with the treatment of a client, assistance with legislative matters, and newfound friends. Occupational therapists living in the same state generally have specific information about resources and political structures and influences within the state and knowledge of the total health and social systems.

The AOTA may be used in similar ways, although it should not be expected that it would have breadth and depth of information about each state and its organization membership. A list of printed publications and films and other audiovisual material is available from the national office upon request. The AOTA offers a variety of other services.

Demands for Time and When to Say No

As the therapist becomes accepted as both a person and a therapist and as his or her skills and knowledge become apparent, the therapist will be asked to do many things in the community, to speak to various groups, to help plan and lead workshops, and to serve on committees, advisory groups, and boards, to name a few. This is an excellent opportunity to contribute to the community and influence the direction and integration of services. It also provides opportunities to get to know more people in the community and representatives from various agencies with which the therapist will be working. It is the beginning of the development of a lateral network, which will be discussed in greater detail later in this chapter.

When the therapist is the only occupational therapist in a fifty-mile or more radius, such demands for time increase to such an extent that the therapist has to become selective. Some therapists make this determination by accepting only those appointments within which they feel they can make a unique contribution. When others can perform a service, the therapist should not do the job.

One therapist was asked to accept the position of Research Chairman on a community board, with the specific assignment to research the literature pertaining to mental retardation. Innovative programming and research being done were of particular interest to this board and, since the therapist had access to this type of information and recognized that reviewing the material would benefit her own continuing education, she accepted the appointment. At the first board meeting she was informed by another board member, "Oh, by the way, you are also in charge of distributing and collecting coin containers." The therapist acknowledged that she *could* do that and do it very well but that she *would* not. She explained that the demands on her time were great, that she had accepted the appointment because she felt she could make a unique contribution here, but that there were any number of people in the community who could perform very well the tasks involved with the coin containers. If the board wished to select someone else to do both tasks, she would be happy to resign so that they could do that. The chairman asked that the therapist remain as Research Chairman and assured the board that someone else would be found to assume the coin collection tasks.

PROGRAM DEVELOPMENT

Program development is an art. A variety of skills are required to plan and implement a community program, but it also requires a certain finesse, a flair, to make a plan work.

Some occupational therapists who move into a rural area fill positions in an agency that has an existing occupational therapy program. Others are hired to develop an occupational therapy program. Some are hired by an existing community program that is adding an occupational therapist to the treatment team. Some deal with combinations of the above. But many occupational therapists moving into a rural area are in the position of creating their own jobs. Especially for the latter group, the first step is to work out a definition of occupational therapy that will have meaning in the culture and experience of those with whom the therapist will deal, because he or she will be asked many times "What is it?" and "What does an occupational therapist do?"

Assessment of Needs

Program development should start with an analytical assessment of the needs of the community to be served. What needs are currently filled by existing programs? What are the gaps in service and who is not being served? Can any of the gaps be filled by expanding the scope of an existing program or does a new program need to be started?

In assessing needs it is helpful to gather comparative statistics for the geographic area the program is to serve. Compared to the rest of the state and nation, is the suicide rate higher or lower here? rate of unemployment? illegitimate birth rates? what percentage of population is over 55? are there many admissions to state psychiatric institutions? what is the number of school drop-outs, their average age, and sex? Problems areas and developing trends can be detected through comparative analysis. Further analysis often suggests when, where, what, and how intervention should occur.

Many states have regional planning agencies whose staff keeps current statistics of this type. Other sources include United States Census Reports, Health Systems Agencies, the State Health Planning and Development Agencies, departments of state government, and local county offices.

Assessment of the data may reveal needs not being met in the community and yet the local population may deny that this is a problem. On the other hand, these same people may express felt needs which are not supported by the data analysis at all. If this situation exists, chances are that the latter will receive community support no matter how logical the former is. If possible, the therapist should integrate the two needs and emphasize, when selling it to the community, that the "felt" needs are being met.

In assessing needs and developing a program it is important to be aware of the "communities within the community." These may be a particular ethnic or religious group clustered in the same neighborhood, all children under the age of six, all people over the age of 55, or other peer groups. In some communities the folk class might be the "community within." What differences does each subgroup have to which the program could respond, making it more accessible and more used by them? One county with which I am familiar has two rather small towns less than 15 miles apart. During the Civil War the residents of one town sympathized with the Union and the other with the Confederacy. Today, over 100 years later, if a meeting for county residents is held in one of the towns, the people from the other town will not attend.

Programs the Community Will Support

Find out what programs have been started in the community within the past few years. To what extent are they fulfilling their original purpose? Has the program been modified? Why? What financial supports does each have? Who are the people serving on their boards?

Often it is more important to determine which projects were proposed but never developed. What were the blocks that prevented it from happening? What individuals or groups of people kept it from getting started, and why? In other words, who comprises the informal power structure in this community? Once the blocks are identified that might prevent your program from developing, a plan can be formulated to remove or circumvent them.

It may be necessary to define the steps needed to activate the program, although not trying to accomplish them in sequence. For example, sometimes step 6 might be done easily, then step 3, step 11, and so forth, until the entire plan is operational, with minimal resistance having been raised to each step individually, whereas much resistance might be raised to the project in its entirety.

IDENTIFYING PERSONAL INTERESTS. Everyone wants something and, whether it is in treating a patient or developing a program, it is in the occupational therapist's self-interest to discover the payoff for each person, (group or agency) with which he or she is dealing. A home health care program may be in the personal interest of the state Commission on Aging because many persons receiving the services will be senior citizens; it may be in the president of the local bank's self-interest because his mother had a stroke, is now home from the hospital, and needs rehabilitative services; it may be in the physician's self-interest because he knows his patients need more help than he has the time and energy to provide.

Integration of Services

Every health care professional has an obligation to work toward the integration of services, to make them as visible and as accessible as possible, with continuity of care having one of the highest priorities. In any community there are a number of the same people receiving services from several different health and social welfare agencies, partly because of the fact that they are multiproblem families. It may be because they have problems for which there are no satisfactory solutions but they are still looking. Realistically, it may be because no one agency provides services which deal with every one of their problems. One wonders, how much is due to the fragmentation of services or the widely different approaches to problem resolution from agency to agency with the same family? This pattern of service delivery divides the client into many pieces and results in no one agency being able to use the "whole person" or "whole family" approach. How confusing and frustrating it must be for the client to be dealt with in so many different ways! And how costly in terms of the inefficient use of available resources.

One community's approach toward integration of services and the development of a coordinated plan for clients served by several agencies has been for people offering services to meet every other Saturday morning over coffee and doughnuts for case reviews. Representatives from community agencies, physicians, ministers, teachers, and other community caregivers discuss the clients they have in common and a consistent approach for helping an individual client or a family is developed. This informal evaluation facilitates the delivery of higher quality of service at a lower total cost to the community.

Another approach toward the integration of services is especially practical in a rural community, where duplication of programs for comparatively few clients probably would not occur because of the limits on resources available. Many needs within the community could be met and the health/social services/mental health/education dollar could be stretched by sharing facilities, equipment, staff, transportation, and supplies with day care for the mentally retarded, with partial hospitalization facilties for the emotionally disturbed and the physically handicapped, with the senior citizens program, and with facilities open to community groups, especially youth groups. Separate programs would be required for the groups identified, but activities such as meals, outings, and so forth could often be held jointly. The community will often provide the facilities in the form of church classrooms, empty stores, or areas in city or county buildings for such joint endeavors, and funding can be broad-based by virtue of the funding sources of the groups involved.

The use of health service facilities by community groups would do much to create the image, not of "this is a place for the aged and handicapped," but "this is a place for people." . . . Eventually this supports the awareness that the aged and handicapped are people, first, and people who may have problems, second. Resulting from this interaction should be a synergistic effect having impact on community understanding, education, prevention; a focus on health rather than illness; an emphasis on people's strengths and what they can do rather than what they cannot do; and a concern for their well-being expressed in the strengthening of supports within the community.

Transportation

Transportation is a critical problem in most rural areas, particularly for the disadvantaged. Some places have small buses run by Community Action and a few states now permit the use of school buses for transporting senior citizens and special population groups, but public transportation is often virtually nonexistent. Many people live "up a hollow" or in isolated geographic areas and may have no private means of transportation, except walking, if they are able.

The county seat is the center for schools, shopping, doctors, and courthouse services and is usually the location of any clinics and at least the hub for countywide services. It is frustrating and defeating to have facilities, staff, and program in a central area and to know that those in the outlying areas who need the service are unable to get there.

Some programs have been able to include transportation costs in their budgets and have found it works well to hire a driver living at the edge of the geographic area to be served. The driver can pick up people on the way to the center and take them home when going back in the evening.

Another answer is to take the services to the people via a mobile unit. The optimal benefit of some kinds of services is not gained with this method of delivery, but other kinds can be provided very effectively. Taking services to the people of the folk culture by this method may be the only way to get them to accept the services, at least in the beginning.

Varying levels of success have been achieved by using volunteers to provide transportation. Volunteers often are reluctant, however, to use their own cars to transport clients because of the possible liabilities. For many years the National Therapeutic Recreation Society* has had a service for member agencies through which liability coverage for volunteers can be obtained for a nominal fee.

Providing transportation can be a costly budget item, but service integration in a central area would at least promote maximum benefit for the dollars expended. The bus driver could pick up a senior citizen at one house and the child with cerebral palsy next door, and then stop up the hollow for a mentally retarded teenager.

Community Money Sources

In addition to the usual money sources in any community, such as stores, car dealers, banks, industries, and private citizens, in rural areas there are granges, 4-H Clubs, Future Farmers of America, and Homemaker Clubs. Most of these groups cannot afford to make large contributions, but some may give $25.00 to purchase supplies or buy a piece of equipment, or a church may donate a special lenten offering to help support the work of the therapy program. Unions and union auxiliaries and fraternal organizations are another source. Most of the people living in rural communities are generous in giving what they can and they are accustomed to helping each other.

If there is a college in the area that the program serves, its various clubs may support the program. National college fraternities and sororities support national and local philanthropic endeavors. Local chapters will often organize and carry out fund-raising projects and bring good publicity to your efforts. They are also a good source of volunteers.

Community Linkages—Lateral Networks

There may be formal cooperative agreements between the boards or directors of community agencies, but work between agencies is most often accomplished through an informal lateral network, the linking of one staff member to another. Relationships in an informal lateral network are worth care and nurturing. Red tape can be eliminated much more quickly by staff within an agency than by someone from without. Processes usually can be set in motion by a phone call. The result is better service performed more rapidly on behalf of the occupational therapist's client and is a vital link in the advocacy role taken by the therapist on the client's behalf. The therapist can then reciprocate when network members request assistance from within the therapist's agency.

Those of us involved in the health care and social service delivery business can be pretty grim at times when we get together to discuss what we are and are not getting done and the lack of resources to meet all the needs. This suggestion is not meant to minimize the seriousness of the job but to suggest a way of freeing the energy to keep going: have fun!

Get together with the caretakers in your informal network for lunch, at a party, or at social affairs. Just as a short-cut language is developed between occupational therapists, the same thing can happen

* National Therapeutic Recreation Society, 1601 North Kent Street, Arlington, Virginia 22209.

between those who work together in community systems, especially when they take the time to get to know each other as people.

The same type of approach can be used very profitably in joint programming. I was involved for several years in camping programs for residents of state mental hospitals. One part of the program focused on linking the senior citizens of a geographic unit with the area's senior citizens' center, community mental health center, welfare department, county extension agents, and employment security and social security offices in an effort to secure community placement for those from the state hospital who could function in the community with varying levels of assistance. Staff members for the camping program were drawn from all the agencies involved and, in addition to many other positive spin-offs, they had such a good time many were involved year after year. As one staff member said, "I've never worked so hard in my life, nor enjoyed it more!" And there was a definite carry over during the time between the yearly camping programs in the interaction between the community caretakers involved. They had their own informal lateral network.

Volunteers

The strengths of a volunteer program lie in selection, training, and placement and in helping each to know that time is being spent in a useful, meaningful way rather than in doing busywork. Volunteers should be placed in jobs for which they have the education, training, and demonstrated competence while receiving adequate ongoing supervision. They should be hired and fired just as any paid employee. Volunteers should not perform staff functions but be utilized to enhance existing programs.

Volunteers often have skills that are useful in activity programs, advisory and governing boards, interviewing, and community "buddy" services. While clients are aware of and appreciate the many extras paid staff give, they have a special feeling for volunteers: they are here because they really care and not because they are being paid.

A valuable fringe benefit is that the involvement of volunteers in community programs enables them to tell others about the goals, objectives, and services of your program. Their understanding helps to dispel the prejudice and discrimination which still, unfortunately, often surround mentally and physically handicapped individuals.

The content and extent of training programs the occupational therapist develops for volunteers should be determined by such things as the job they are expected to do, the size of the program, and the number of volunteers. Whatever determinants are factors in training program design, it is essential that training be given. A well-trained volunteer is more confident, becomes involved more quickly at a deeper level, and feels more rewarded. Commitment follows, and involved and committed volunteers who are appreciated for their contribution tend to stay with the program longer.

My approach is to teach empathic listening/responding skills[9] and crisis intervention techniques, using roleplaying to integrate the two, as basic training for all volunteers. Specialized training in the specific task areas assigned to them and information concerning ethics and confidentiality are then given. There is always a psychological component involved when a person is ill or disabled, whether physically or mentally. The combination of empathy/crisis intervention and task-related skills provides each volunteer with tools for interaction with clients in nearly any situation and is useful for building initial and ongoing relationships. Having these skills gives confidence to volunteers and enhances the contributions they can make.

Referrals

The hospital or clinic-based occupational therapy program generally receives many of its treatment referrals from sources in the medical system. Whether in an urban or rural setting, the community-based occupational therapist receives some referrals from medical sources, but frequently receives many more through community contacts, such as those community agencies represented in the therapist's lateral network, the local storekeeper, or law enforcement personnel, to name just a few. The county health nurse and the county extension agent are two particularly good sources, as they visit many homes in the rural area. With referrals originating from so many nonphysician sources the occupational therapist needs to decide which clients' conditions warrant also securing a physician's referral for occupational therapy.

The referral may state only "referred for occupational therapy," but that is acceptable as it gives the therapist an opportunity to discuss the client's condition with the physician and to begin the process of physician-education regarding occupational therapy through discussion and reports sent to the physician regarding the occupational therapy treatment plan and the client's progress.

The community-based therapist often spends more time working with groups such as those that focus on the development of work habits or those for the parents of handicapped children than in doing individual treatment. Such groups seldom need a physician referral. However, this decision requires the therapist's determination in relation to each individual situation.

THE OCCUPATIONAL THERAPIST AS A CONSULTANT IN A RURAL COMMUNITY

The occupational therapist may not feel skilled enough yet to function as a consultant, but the chances are that in a rural community the therapist knows more than anybody else about such things as ordering a wheelchair, the kinds of fastenings that make it easier for handicapped children to dress themselves, and many other aspects of helping people to function at their optimal level. The thought of being a consultant can be scary to the therapist who has not realized that he or she has often functioned in such a role in relation to the parents and families of clients and to other members of the health care team as part of his or her daily work as a therapist. Furthermore, most occupational therapists can be a consultant to the architect designing housing for senior citizens and to the teacher of the homebound, as well as other community caregivers and can contribute much to the health and quality of life of people in the community.

If a therapist desires to be a consultant to a particular group or system, i.e., schools, welfare, ministerial alliance, one way to get their attention is to ask them for consultation concerning a problem. Such a tactic introduces you to personnel within the system, starts a dialogue that shares attitudes, thinking, and skills, and eases the way for their asking for assistance; it may even provide an opportunity for you to offer it.

Extrapolation

The occupational therapist knows the dynamics and process involved in treating the individual client. This same basic model can be extrapolated and built upon in working with groups and in working with the entire community. In other words, assess needs, define goals, specify what needs to be done and the methods to be used, implement the process, and evaluate the results. The following case study is presented as a further illustration of this.

The occupational therapist is functioning as a team member in an interdisciplinary approach to a problem. The role-blurring evident in this situation is a realistic expectation for the occupational therapist working in a rural community. Professionals are few and far between and "one does what one can" to get the job done. As an occupational therapist, one may be uncomfortable losing this much identity and feel that one has lost his or her place. However, it is essential to have a firm sense of identity in order to role-blur. However, human resources must be utilized in the most effective and efficient way possible; there is an overlap between many disciplines (occupational therapy, social work, recreation therapy, etc.) and there is a common base shared by these disciplines. We each see the same things when we examine a particular situation but we see these things from the unique perspective of our own disciplines.

HOTLINE EXPANSION PLAN FOR REGION X

Hotline, Inc., is a 24-hour crisis-intervention telephone service staffed by volunteers and based in A County. It accepts collect calls from the eight county catchment area (Region X—A, B, C, D, E, F, G, and H counties) served by the Region X Community Mental Health Center, Inc. (CMHC). A cooperative agreement exists between Hotline and the CMHC. The occupational therapist who developed the plan is being interviewed and questioned as to the purpose of some of the steps detailed in the plan.

What are you trying to accomplish by developing this plan?

"The overall goal for this community organization project is to expand Hotline services throughout these eight counties, with each county's operation having a satellite relationship to the A County unit. The maximum objective is for each county to have its own phone service, trouble teams, and information and referral services with the necessary organizational structure including funding, training, community support, and inter-agency linkages to maintain this. The minimum objective is for each county to have its own trouble teams, information and referral material which will be used by the A County based phone service to respond to callers' needs, with persons from some of the other counties committed to taking the training and working on the phones in A County and the necessary organizational structure including funding, training, community support, and interagency linkages to support this. Since the 178,000 population of this catchment area breaks down with A County—98,000 and G County—32,000, the other six counties ranging from 15,000 down to 2,000, with eight-party phone lines being prevalent in the smaller counties, the assumption is that no county other than A can reach the maximum objective, but that some of the larger ones may choose to operate somewhere in between the maximum and minimum objectives."

You mentioned maximum and minimum objectives several times and then made the assumption that only County A could reach the maximum. What's the purpose of going through all that?

"Well, this project will be asking an existing organization and a number of volunteers to commit valuable resources—time, energy, and money—and it is important that all involved know not only the *total* of what they want to happen but also what they're willing to settle for. The assumption helps us to be realistic in our expectations. If we did not go through this process of 'thinking through,' we would probably have some people pushing for the maximum objective, wasting energy, and getting frustrated, going right by what realistically could be accomplished, and ending up not accomplishing anything! The minimum objective says that 'this is the bottom line'—if we can't accomplish even that much, then we are better off not using our resources here. It gives us a place to stop without feeling we have failed because we have known all along what the cut-off point was going to be, and why."

There must be a real need for this kind of service for so many people to be so committed to the expansion of it.

"Yes, at the time this plan was developed, Hotline in County A was receiving over 1100 calls each month, and the number climbs steadily. This type of service is based on the theory that crisis intervention at this level by trained volunteers has definite value in the total mental health effort. Our needs assessment included the number of calls being received in County A, including the number received from the outlying counties in Region X, requests for the service from community leaders in each county, requirements of Federal Regulations for National Institute of Mental Health (NIMH) construction and staffing grants for community mental health services, and requirements of the state's Department of Mental Health licensing regulations for psychiatric programs and facilities.

"The primary target population in each county will be a cross-section of community leaders, including representatives from government, law enforcement, education, health, and social service agencies, industry, news media, churches, ministerial alliance, and so forth, those people who have the power to develop the linkages needed to support this kind of program, whether through funding, direct service, cooperation, or whatever. The individuals in this group may, or may not, wish to be involved in Hotline direct services as a phone worker or trouble team worker and so forth. The secondary target will be those persons from the community who wish to be involved in this latter capacity.

"We will be dealing with geographical communities but also the functional communities within the geographical areas. Since the governing board of the CMHC is composed of representatives (community leaders) appointed by the County Court of each of the eight counties, the initial strategy would be to meet with these board members in their county (G County, being the next largest after County A, would be the first county; also the CMHC now has a satellite office there to provide professional back-up services) and discuss the expansion plans with them. The board members are already familiar with the County A Hotline operation and, as a board, have given sanction to the existing Hotline and to expansion of these services. They will be asked to identify and *personally contact* the community leaders in preparation for the first meeting. Past experience has indicated that personal contact by board members is very successful for this type of thing in these smaller counties. Announcement of the meeting to the general community would be by prepared news releases, church bulletins, local radio (if any), and word of mouth. Since none of the counties except A have televison stations, it would be necessary to identify the stations watched most in each county for coverage via talk shows, community service announcements, and so forth, and the same process would be used for radio coverage. Periodic checking with the board members prior to the meeting date will provide an indication of any changes needed in this strategy to get key people to attend the meeting.

"A strategy will be to have three or four knowledgeable and experienced A County Hotline members, including the current chairperson and myself, at the organizational meeting to present the concept and purpose and to answer questions. The tactics used will be education, and persuasion through the Hotline representatives' presentations and hand-outs of printed material discussing the organization of, and factors to be considered in developing, a crisis intervention telephone service in rural and semi-rural areas. Strategy at this meeting will be the selection of a local steering committee with positions paralleling those of the A County Hotline so that A County staff members can work with their G County counterparts (training chairpersons, finances, public relations including a speakers' bureau, scheduling, etc.). I think it is very important for the *local* people to develop the interagency linkages to support this program, but we would be there to facilitate their assessing the various community power structures and help them look at the differences in organizational structures of agencies and therefore differences needed in approach.

"Such a service as Hotline provides does not presently exist in these counties, but what we will be taking away from the existing agencies will be any exclusivity of turf, or autonomy, they presently have in dealing with clients in crisis. This may, or may not be, a threat to an individual agency and will need to be dealt with on an individual agency basis, with those needing such to be determined through ongoing analysis and evaluation of progress of the plan toward the stated goal. Tactics for dealing with an agency would probably emphasize education and informing, persuasion, and using existing laws and probably not include conflict and coercion, though coercion could be used subtly by those in the community power structure if the agency is resistant."

From what you've just said, I'm getting the impression that established agencies might really feel threatened by a new program being organized in the community!

"Yes, this does happen sometimes. You know, agencies, just like individuals, tend to act in their own vital self-interest. In this respect, they are not altruistic! By the same token, agencies are seldom willfully self-destructive, so we need to make cooperation as profitable for them as we possibly can, or make noncooperation so painful or costly that they can't afford not to cooperate!

"Anyway, back to the description of the plan. At this point the staff has made the commitment for County G that the A county Hotline will pay expenses and conduct the first training and will also pay travel expenses for A County members to work with them during the initial organizational phase. The same type of commitment to the other counties in the catchment area has been discussed, but since we are not ready to expand into those counties now, staff has not yet voted on this. The County G people will be involved in every step of setting up and conducting the training, even though they will also be trainees so that they can learn the process. They may choose phone worker training, trouble team training, or both. We are also giving them the opportunity to tie into an existing program, and sharing knowledge we have gained in developing it. The community is getting a coordinated service to fill some of the present gaps, plus education on the worth of another level of mental health service. The counties will each have members on the staff of the A County Hotline, because it is the parent organization. This type of representation was provided for in the original articles of incorporation and bylaws.

"In developing any plan, it is important to identify negative consequences and the risks involved. We constantly ask the question, 'If we do this, what is going to happen? What are possible negative results from our action?' Once the negative results are identified we can plan what we will do to counter them *if* they happen.

"Some of the negative consequences and risks which are possible consequences of the strategy and tactics planned have been discussed already, but there are others that also need to be considered. If key agency representatives do not attend the initial meeting in spite of our efforts, then we will assess who in the community has the clout, power, or control to bring pressure to bear on them. For instance, the County Court partially funds many community agencies and the CMHC board members could remind agencies of this; it would be in the agencies' self-interest to cooperate. This is an example of the type of assessment and counter-strategy tactics which will be employed throughout the process.

"It is essential to be flexible and do your homework. Then, if the catastrophes occur, you are prepared. In this type of community organization much resistance to being 'overwhelmed' by an outside group (in this case, A County Hotline) can be minimized by the basic view that there are two reasons to involve people in planning: one is to get their support and the other is that, by involving those for whom the plan is intended, chances are you will come up with a better plan because they know their needs, strengths, and weaknesses better than do you as an outsider. People also tend to defend that which they help to create. Flexibility helps in this type of effort. It becomes counterproductive to react defensively to small deviations from the goal and objectives. It is much more productive to give most things time to settle and to know what is *important* to act on immediately.

"A definite time table is difficult to establish for all eight counties. This type of volunteer program needs professional back-up services, and there are few professionals of any discipline with mental health training in the counties other than A, G, and F. Back-up help via the telephone could answer some of the needs, except that the demand for services on all levels already far exceeds the capacity of the small CMHC staff to provide it. So, part of the time table is affected by the amount of funding for additional staff provided by the state legislature and Department of Mental Health. An educated guess is that this will continue to be a problem to community mental health programs for a long while yet. This is an external variable. An internal variable would be the level of service each county selected and training time required to teach necessary skills.

"The time table projected allows that the minimum objective could be accomplished in each county in six to nine months. There is no set deadline, so it is not necessary to set up a calendar chart, working backwards from the deadline date, filling in tasks to be accomplished by specific dates, as I do with projects having a fixed target date. After G County is going, then *they* could organize adjacent F County with consultative assistance and support from A County, while the A County team started with adjacent C County. Then C and F could organize E and B, two counties adjacent to them, with A and G again providing consultative assistance and support, and so on until each county in the catchment area was organized. Which groups would organize D and H would depend on who had the time and other resources at that point, and that should be determined later. Total time required would probably be two to three years, and a positive spin-off of this type of approach would be the involvement of a number of different leaders, increased commitment, and the reinforcement and up-grading of skills for those involved which will in turn strengthen their local organizations." (See Fig. 25-4.)

How will you measure the success of this project?

"Actually, evaluation of the progress of the project will begin along with implementation of the plan and will be ongoing. Success or failure will be evident in the extent of accomplishment of the minimum objectives, any levels above them, and the stated goals. This continuous monitoring of what is happening is crucial in each aspect of the plan so that critical revisions can be made when and where needed to keep things moving, not after the programs are obviously bogged down.

"In this type of service the number of calls tends to increase in direct proportion to the publicizing of service. Therefore, evaluation as to effectiveness of publicity and adequacy of service rendered can be monitored by keeping statistics relative to number and type (i.e., depression, sexual, dating problems, etc.) of calls received each month in each of the local counties and/or increases in calls received by the A County Hotline from the local counties. The completeness of this type of evaluation is further augmented by feedback from community agencies regarding comments of clients who have utilized the Hotline service."

THE FUTURE IN THE RURAL COMMUNITY

As interstate highways have cut through the rural areas and access and secondary roads have been improved, the geographical isolation has become less acute for many. Improved roads have also resulted in less economic isolation and have opened areas to cultural influences from outside the rural communities. In recent years any number of college educated young adults and their older counterpart, the industrial age dropouts, have bought or rented land in rural areas, showing an appreciation for the slower pace and less complicated, less stressful lifestyle found in the rural culture. Television in nearly every house and shack has undoubtedly created an awareness of different cultures, different ways of doing things, and different ways of thinking. Resistance to change is particularly apparent in the men of the folk culture, but the awareness created by television has rather insidiously removed one of the barriers to change: they can now at least "picture" how some of the other folks live.

There is relatively little in the rural areas in the way of community health services. Sieg[10] has indicated that there are more hospitals in rural areas than in urban areas, that rural people are hospitalized more than their city neighbors, and that they tend to stay longer because of the inaccessibility to alternative health care. For years, county health nurses and private physicians have provided the only other health care services in many rural areas.

There are wide gaps in health services available in rural areas. The occupational therapist has more to offer than most other disciplines to the process of filling these gaps because of his or her diversification of skills and knowledge, the whole person treat-

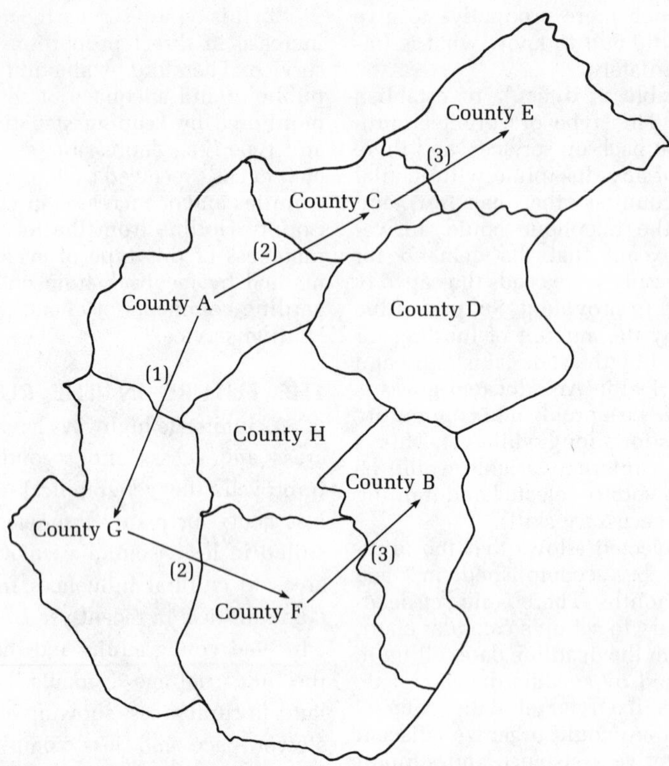

FIGURE 25-4. Flow chart for Hotline expansion.
County A—original Hotline organization.
County G—first satellite Hotline.
Counties F and C—second and third satellites, organized concurrently by G and A respectively.
Counties E and B—fourth and fifth satellites, organized concurrently by C and F respectively.
Counties H and D—satellites to be organized last with organizing satellites to be determined later.

ment approach, and the goal of optimal functioning. The education of an occupational therapist produces a generalist, one who has studied, and usually had direct experience with, the mentally retarded, the physically handicapped, the visually and hearing impaired, the psychiatrically handicapped, the socially and culturally disadvantaged; taken a wide range of courses from anatomy to weaving, group dynamics to individual evaluation; and studied aspects of development from conception to senescence, in illness and in health. The generalist occupational therapist can give direct treatment to many as well as screen and refer others to the proper specialists, disciplines, or services. A positive result expected from this type of functioning would be decreased overall health care costs with a higher quality of care provided as more people would receive the type of care needed.

Occupational therapists function within all the levels of prevention in the community defined by Caplan,[11] originally in relation to mental health, but used here to pertain to the very broad area of prevention. Intervention with populations at risk, those who as yet have no symptoms of maladjustment or disease, is defined as primary prevention[12]; intervention in the form of early diagnosis and effective treatment, aimed at shortening the duration of illness of those who are showing symptoms, sometimes in the acute stage, is defined as secondary prevention[13]; and intervention with those who are past the acute stage, needing rehabilitation to reach their optimal level of functioning and/or to prevent further deterioration, is defined as tertiary prevention.[14]

The teaching/training offered by an occupational therapist working in the rural community can have tremendous impact on the quality of care given and create an ever-widening area of influence for the fundamental beliefs and practices of occupational therapy. Teaching families of clients, Home Health Aides, Homemaker Aides, nursing home staff and personnel, or adult family care home proprietors when to call the occupational therapist, what to do until the therapist gets there, and what to do between visits enhances the effectiveness of the total treatment process. It will also probably facilitate the referral of many more people in need of the occupational therapist's services.

Several occupational therapists[15,16] have recently written of the necessity for the revision of professional curricula to include special skills needed to work in the community, particularly in settings that are not traditional for the occupational therapist. This would indeed contribute much to the preparation of the therapists needed to make a difference in the delivery and quality of health care in the rural community.

The Folk Class

The occupational therapist working with the folk class will first have to know these people better than they know themselves. Their patterns of behavior should become more apparent to the therapist than they are to themselves since the therapist is an objective observer. One of the occupational therapist's strengths is the ability to adapt and, when working with people of the folk class, it is crucial to adapt to them—their culture, their world, their way of doing things—if assistance is to be given them towards resolution of some of their problems.

Long-range planning has little meaning to these people. Therefore, it is up to the occupational therapist, perhaps with the involvement of those in the lateral network, to develop the long-range plan and, starting *where they are* in their life and culture, involve the folk class people initially in quick success projects that are steps in the plan and later in those that take longer to complete and are a little more complex, just as in developing an individual treatment plan working toward delay of gratification. The folk class is beginning to be more accessible and *will* tend to get involved in projects that they think will be successful and that will enhance their own self-esteem.

The impetus to change and the solutions to the problems of the folk class must come from within their group, but their resistance to involvement and lack of a concept of the planning process make the former nearly impossible. If the therapist focuses on a situation which needs to be changed and which would *have their support,* whether a real or felt need, and structures their participation to their need for *action,* the therapist will have achieved the first step toward their involvement. Since the people in this class function most of the time from their feelings, structuring the first project around a "felt need" would no doubt enhance the project's chance of success.

The occupational therapist working in the rural community will, of necessity, devote much time and effort to taking an advocacy role on behalf of clients. Taking the "whole person" or "whole family" approach to treatment means that all those factors impinging on the client's ability to function at his optimal level need attention. Mrs. Jones, aged 79 and living alone, may have held things in tenuous balance on a limited income before she broke her hip and was hospitalized; now she is back home, receiving Home Health Care, but really cannot get out to the grocery, nor is she sufficiently mobile to take care of the house, laundry, and cooking. She is afraid that she will have to go to a nursing home and leave her home, afraid she will fall again and no one will be there to help her, worrying in so many ways about her future. Mrs. Jones is in a "situational crisis." The situation that precipitated her present crisis was the fracturing of her hip. As an occupational therapist concerned with restoring physical functioning, it will quickly become apparent that intervention in the situational crisis is needed to prevent Mrs. Jones' moving into a severe depression and the intervention must occur before she can regain enough energy to focus on improving her physical condition. As an advocate, the occupational therapist will facilitate Mrs. Jones' securing the temporary services of a homemaker from the county Welfare Department, or a neighbor who will help Mrs. Jones an hour a day, or whatever resources are available to be tapped through the informal lateral network. This, along with the physical restoration, is both secondary and tertiary prevention.

Many of the members of the folk class are quite skilled in the various arts and crafts that have a significant place in their culture. These can usually be adapted to improve or restore functioning, and it is important to utilize them this way to assist clients to keep their "place" in their culture. As clients learn to trust the therapist, the introduction of new experiences and activities may be indicated and possible. In other words, focus is on the use of activities that can be translated into *their* community in both work and play situations. The home visits that are necessary to personalize the therapist's relationship with members of the folk class will also provide the opportunity for observing and finding out what the client needs to function in his or her setting. This enables the therapist to gather the information needed to design an overall treatment/activity plan focusing on total needs. People are judged in their community by what they can do that has meaning in that community. Occupational therapy has a vital role to play in making that doing possible.

With the men in one group, the women in another group, the youth in their group, and the children in yet another group, family activities, except perhaps work projects such as the garden, are practically nonexistent. The occupational therapist who can help a family learn to do something creative together will be breaking into an alienating culture pattern and replacing the alienation with an integrating, constructive activity that moves the members toward the closeness they crave.

To be a change agent in the rural community does not always mean that the therapist is the best person to make the personal contacts. Particularly with the folk class, at least initially, the therapist will be looked upon as an expert. Kent and Smith[17] are among those who have found the use of indigenous (a member of the same subculture) workers, as "bridge" persons or links between the persons being served and those providing the services, particularly effective. This is another approach which probably will be used more in the future, because these workers know the culture and how to work with those within it.

THE RURAL COMMUNITY AS A WHOLE

Much of this chapter has dealt with the characteristics of the folk class as a whole. But it is of the utmost importance to be aware that while a total class may have certain characteristics, each member of that class is an individual and one should not attempt to deal with the member in terms of the class, and/or the class in terms of its members.[18] For instance, within the folk class there are those who want a better life and will respond readily to efforts to help them move closer to middle class values and characteristics as well as those who want to stay with the status quo. Different approaches will be needed with each of these two groups, as well as with the individuals within each group.

The middle class and professional class in the rural areas, and the individuals within them, will require still different approaches. And as the rural areas grow and turn into more commercialized communities and towns, this will lead to less personalization, and will eventually force those in the folk class to change even more.

As the sparsely settled areas reach a greater density of population, the more people available to work for community betterment the greater proportion of the population will get involved.[19] This is another trend that will affect approaches used by occupational therapists working in rural areas of the country. This concept was a definite factor in defining maximum and minimum objectives in the case study of the Hotline expansion. The smaller counties simply could not support the maximum objective.

REFERENCES

1. Weller, J.: Yesterday's People. Lexington KY: University of Kentucky Press (with the collaboration of the Council of the Southern Mountains, Inc.), 1966, p. 3.
2. Gans, H.: The Urban Villagers. New York: Free Press, 1962, p. 25.
3. Weller: Yesterday's People, p. 5.
4. James, D.: Poverty, Politics and Change. Englewood Cliffs NJ: Prentice-Hall, 1972, pp.11–12.
5. Galbraith, J.: The Affluent Society, New York: New American Library, 1958, p. 251.
6. James: Poverty, Politics and Change, pp. 11–12.
7. Weller: Yesterday's People, pp. 30–31.
8. Kent, J., and Smith, H.: Involving the Urban Poor in Health Services Through Accommodation—The Employment of Neighborhood Rrepresentatives. Foundation for Urban and Neighborhood Development. Denver CO, p. 2. Paper presented before the Maternal and Child Health Section of the American Public Health Association at the Ninety-Fourth Annual Meeting in San Francisco, November 1966. Requests for copies ($2.50) should be addressed to:

FUND, Inc. (Foundation for Urban and Neighborhood Development, Inc.), 830 Kipling Street, Suite 304, Denver, Colorado 80215.
9. Carkhuff, R.: Helping and Human Relations, Vols. 1 and 2. New York: Holt, Rinehart and Winston, 1969.
10. Sieg, K.: Rural health and the role of occupational therapy. Am. J. Occup. Ther. 29:76, 1975.
11. Caplan, G.: Principles of Preventive Psychiatry, Vol. 1. New York: Basic Books, 1964.
12. Ibid., p. 26.
13. Ibid., p. 89.
14. Ibid., p. 113.
15. Ethridge, D.: The management view of the future of occupational therapy in mental health. Am. J. Occup. Ther. 30:627, 1976.
16. Cromwell, F., and Kielhofner, G.: An educational strategy for occupational therapy community services. Am. J. Occup. Ther. 30:629–630, 1976.
17. Kent and Smith: Involving the Urban Poor, pp. 1–5.
18. Watzlawick, P., Weakland, J., and Fisch, R.: Change Principles of Problem Formation and Problem Resolution. New York: W. W. Norton & Co., 1974, p. 6.
19. McNeil, H.: Increasing Membership Participation in Voluntary Organization—Some Considerations. Appalachian Center Information Report 4, West Virginia University, Morgantown WV, 1972, p. 6.

Part Eight

Organization and Administration

26

Management and Documentation of Occupational Therapy Services

section 1/Management/M. Carolyn Baum

The occupational therapist has the skills to implement the management process. It is a matter of transferring the occupational therapy treatment process to administrative situations that allow the occupational therapist to achieve program objectives. In planning the care of the individual client the occupational therapist collects data, identifies problems, identifies assets, plans long-term goals, plans short-term goals, and identifies the service or treatment to be used to reach the goals. In this chapter management tools are presented which allow the occupational therapist to collect data and plan appropriate strategies for meeting goals and management techniques are presented that provide the therapist with a process for implementing change.

The changes in the health delivery system requiring accountability by demonstration of appropriateness of service has had a major impact on the occupational therapy delivery system. Occupational therapists are entering a profession which is highly regulated by federal laws and accrediting agencies. It is the responsibility of the professional to realize standards that effect them in their daily activities. At one time there was an expectation for therapists to be involved in direct service for the entire work day. This is no longer a reality and would be impractical in light of the regulations placed on health professionals. The occupational therapy supervisor as well as the facility administrator must recognize these regulations and assure that staff members have adequate time to complete their required professional responsibilities. In Table 26-1 some of these responsibilities are explored.

The scope of occupational therapy service ranges from early detection and prevention, acute medical management and rehabilitation, to long-term management. Occupational therapy practitioners work in many settings to deliver services but all have one thing in common: the requirement to work within a system that utilizes people to accomplish its objectives. People require a management process that identifies for them expectations and structure in order to function individually within a system. The management structure of settings will vary from extremely informal to the most structured sophisticated system. As professional occupational ther-

Table 26-1. Professional responsibilities of occupational therapy staff members.

Professional responsibilities	*Source of regulation or activity*
Establishment of plan of care for each client	Joint Commission on Accreditation of Hospitals and American Occupational Therapy Association
Regular progress reports	Joint Commission on Accreditation of Hospitals and American Occupational Therapy Association
Patient conferences	Medicare, Joint Commission on Accreditation of Hospitals and American Occupational Therapy Association
Developing audit criteria and medical audit activities	Joint Commission on Accreditation of Hospitals, Professional Standards Review Organization and American Occupational Therapy Association
Family conferences	Joint Commission on Accreditation of Hospitals and American Occupational Therapy Association
Coordination for patient management	American Occupational Therapy Association and Joint Commission on Accreditation of Hospitals
Planning for discharge	Joint Commission on Accreditation of Hospitals and American Occupational Therapy Association
Developing home programs	Joint Commission on Accreditation of Hospitals and American Occupational Therapy Association
Medical record review	Legal consideration, Joint Commission on Accreditation of Hospitals and Professional Standard Review Organization
Supervision of assistants	Medicare and American Occupational Therapy Association
Communication with support staff (transport personnel, aides)	Legal consideration (can delegate to person only within their level of competency)
Patient scheduling	To coordinate patients' care within tolerance for activity
Student supervision	Requirement in a clinical education setting
Medical rounds	Professional communication
Program planning	To update and expand services
Interpretation of test results	Standardized tests require careful interpretation before reports are submitted to the referring physician

apists we are required by our Principles of Occupational Therapy Ethics to understand these systems as well as uphold the standards that direct their operation. Two Ethics that speak of our responsibilities are:

RELATED TO EMPLOYERS AND PAYERS: *The occupational therapist shall render service with discretion and integrity and shall protect the property rights of the employers and payers.*

RELATED TO LAW AND REGULATIONS: *The occupational therapist shall seek to acquire information about applicable local, state, federal and institutional rules and shall function accordingly thereto.*[1]

The traditional science of management is not discussed in this chapter. A study of basic management principles should be made by students and practitioners. A vocabulary of management science is included in the glossary at the end of this chapter. Since I am not presenting these materials as an integration of management and occupational therapy theory, no direct references are given. References that support the theories are acknowledged in the bibliography.

THE OCCUPATIONAL THERAPY MANAGEMENT PROCESS

Data Collection

The management assessment presented in this chapter provides the occupational therapist with a tool to use in determining the effectiveness of current operations. The questions have no absolute answer but a yes answer in most questions relates the current level of operation to basic management principles. The therapist must determine the degree of the problem based upon understanding of the system in which the problem exists. I developed this assessment while in the position of Director of Physical Medicine and Rehabilitation at Research Medical Center, Kansas City, Missouri. For an additional data collection see the section on Medical Care Evaluation Studies near the end of the chapter.

MANAGEMENT ASSESSMENT

I. *Department Organization*	Yes	No
Does the department have written objectives?	___	___
Does the structural design of the department allow for the implementation and the achievement of objectives?	___	___
Are the objectives designed to compliment and support other departments that have similar objectives?	___	___
Is the administrative staff aware of and do they support the departmental objectives?	___	___
The objectives are: (write them out)		
Do all staff participate in the establishment of objectives?	___	___
Are staff held accountable for writing and meeting objectives?	___	___
Are all positions described in current job description?	___	___
Are the job responsibilities for all staff clearly defined and formally documented?	___	___
Is there a table of organization?	___	___
Are the lines of communication clearly defined?	___	___
Are all staff kept informed of the organizational changes that effect their functions?	___	___
Are facility policies available for staff to review and do the staff know responsibilities in carrying out policy?	___	___
Are departmental procedures written and approved by administration?	___	___
Is there a systematic plan for development, review and approval of departmental procedures?	___	___
Are the procedure manuals current?	___	___
Does the administrative staff have an appropriate understanding of the department's functions?	___	___

II. *Departmental Management*	Yes	No
Are all staff required to write yearly goals?	___	___
Is scheduling coordinated with other services?	___	___
Are regular staff planning sessions held?	___	___
Are interdisciplinary conferences held?	___	___
Does staff participate in medical rounds?	___	___
Are *all* physicians aware of the department's services?	___	___
Is the nursing staff aware of the department's services?	___	___
Have units of measure been established to determine staffing needs?	___	___
Is the staffing pattern correct for current programming?	___	___
Are patient records designed and maintained to meet AOTA, JCAH, and Medicare standards?	___	___
Are all staff members aware of their importance in the department?	___	___
Are regular performance appraisals done on all staff?	___	___
Is the morale of the department good?	___	___
Has the turnover been minimal?	___	___
Does the department receive professional medical guidance?	___	___

III. *Physical Facilities*	Yes	No
Is there adequate space for treatment?	___	___
Is there adequate storage space?	___	___
Is equipment properly maintained?	___	___
Is there a preventative maintenance program?	___	___
Does this department have an outside entrance with sufficient parking for outpatients?	___	___
Is the department easily accessible to non-ambulatory as well as ambulatory patients?	___	___
Are all doorways wide enough to get a wheeled stretcher or wheelchair through?	___	___
Are sufficient waiting room facilities provided that will handle peak loads?	___	___
Is there adequate secretarial space?	___	___

IV. *Personnel*	Yes	No
Does the personnel department provide hospital orientation to new employees?	___	___
Are employee benefits equal to or higher than other local facilities?	___	___

Are salaries equal to or higher than other local facilities? ___ ___
Is the personnel file kept current with all the employees' outstanding as well as poor performances? ___ ___

V. *Purchasing of Supplies*

Is there a written procedure concerning supply purchases? ___ ___
Is there an inventory control on supplies? ___ ___
Does the department head utilize the purchasing department in reviewing new equipment and materials? ___ ___

VI. *Departmental Budget*

Is the budget set up on a control system? ___ ___
Does the department head receive monthly reports on budget expenditures and income? ___ ___
Is the department able to generate enough income to maintain itself? ___ ___
Does the department head participate in budget planning? ___ ___
Is the budget adequate to handle all necessary supplies? ___ ___
Are charges established in relation to both direct and indirect costs for each type of treatment procedure? ___ ___
Are rates approved by the Executive Director? ___ ___
Are departmental charges comparable to other area hospitals? ___ ___

Identification of Problems

The degree of the problems identified in the assessment must be determined. This should be done in consultation with others in the health care delivery system, which may include the administrator, other department chairmen, the medical staff, the community, and the staff members. Most important in this problem-identification phase is relating the problems to program objectives. Priorities should be established so that short-term goals can be written in sequence.

Identification of Assets

The program strengths (assets) must be identified. It is with these assets that the problems which have been identified are solved.

Long-Term Goals

The long-term goals reflect the end-result or the status that will be achieved when the problems are solved. The long-term goals should be identified and supported by the administrative structure if the activities that will be performed affect an established procedure or require an expenditure of funds. A completion date should be identified which will assist in allocating the time needed to solve the problem as well as carry on the normal functions of management.

Short-Term Goals

Short-term goals identify the step by step process a manager uses in meeting long-term goals that support the program objectives. Each of these goals requires a "how to" component. The short-term goals must have a process or a well-thought-out procedure with it as well as a projected completion date. In establishing the procedures to implement short-term goals one should investigate all resources to assist in the process. These may include management engineers, internal auditors, fiscal advisors, medical records personnel, personnel consultants, and many community resources. Developing these working relationships provides visibility not only for the manager but also for the occupational therapy service.

Process for Implementing Change

Budget

The budget is a management tool. Through the budgetary process the manager has the ability to change program objectives by getting financial support for the program. In planning a projected budget (1) develop the objectives of the service and (2) justify the expenses that will be required for implementation. Approval of the budget would then allow the manager to carry out objectives independently.

A series of questions must be asked prior to the establishment of a budget:

1. What is the net income of the occupational therapy service per year and does it support the current operation?
2. What is the facility's percentage of reimbursement for occupational therapy from private, federal, and self-pay clients?
3. What costs are considered direct costs?
4. What costs are considered indirect costs?

5. What percentage of income is required of the department to contribute to the indirect costs of the facility?

6. What is the bad debt percentage?

These questions will be answered differently in each setting and are critical to understanding of the management function.

The information required for the budgetary process itself may include the following:

Direct Costs	*Explanation*
Salaries	actual including merit raises
Payroll taxes	Social Security taxes (currently 5.85%)
Overtime	usually 2% of total hours
Vacation relief	self-explanatory
Supplies	consumable department and clerical services
Student programs	stipends or meals
Educational expenses	tuition and travel to workshops
Inservice	money to pay speakers
Reimbursable supplies	adaptive equipment—articles to be sold to clients

Indirect Costs	*Explanation*
Administrative	administrative support for necessary department personnel, accounting, purchasing, etc.
Housekeeping	cleaning and maintenance of facility
Laundry	linens
Plant operation	maintenance, utilities

For the purpose of demonstration an example of the budgetary process is given.

Step I. Identifying direct costs

Direct Costs

Salaries	68,000
Payroll taxes (5.85%)	3,978
Overtime	1,360
Supplies	3,000
Student programs	2,000
Education	1,500
In-service	350
Reimbursable supplies	2,400
Total	82,588

Step II. Determining indirect costs

Indirect costs are usually delegated by square footage and in the author's experience have approximated 40% of the total budget. These indirect costs can be determined by the following formula once the direct costs are established.

$$\frac{\text{Direct costs}}{X} = \frac{60\%}{40\%}$$

$$60X = 40\,(\text{direct costs})$$

$$X = \frac{40\,(\text{direct costs})}{60}$$

$$X = \text{Indirect costs}$$

In the example we would find the indirect costs to be:

$$\frac{\$82{,}588.00}{X} = \frac{60\%}{40\%}$$

$$60X = 40\ (\$82{,}588.00)$$

$$X = 40 \times \frac{\$82{,}588.00}{60}$$

$$X = \$55{,}059.00$$

Indirect costs—$55,059.00

Step III. Determining bad debt allowance (8% is used for the example)

Direct costs	$ 82,588.00
Indirect cost	$ 55,059.00
Total cost	$137,647.00
	X 8%
	$ 11,011.76
Bad debt allowance	$ 11,012.00

Step IV. Determining total budget requirements

Direct costs	$ 82,588
Indirect cost	55,059
Bad debt allowance	11,012
	$148,659

Step V. Determining the fee for service

Divide the total budget by the number of procedures projected for the budget periods.

Number of procedures for budget period = 20,000

$$\text{(procedures) } 20{,}000 \overline{)\ \$148{,}659}\ \text{(total budget)} = \$7.43$$

Cost for each procedure —$7.43
Charge for each procedure —$7.50*

Step VI. Planning a control budget

Divide the total budgeted procedures by 12 to determine the number of planned procedures per month. Divide the total budget by 12 to determine the planned income per month.† Record these figures and compute each month the

* Determine this in consultation with the financial administrator.

† Once data is collected it is important to vary the monthly proposals according to the variations in caseloads per month. (Example: December may be a light month because of the holidays.) The number of work days in the month can be a guide.

actual with the planned (Table 26-2). Explain any significant differences (.05) either positive or negative to the administrator in charge of the occupational therapy service.

Table 26-2. Planning a control budget.

Month	*Procedures*		*Income*	
	Planned	*Actual*	*Planned*	*Actual*
Jan	1666		12388	
Feb	1666		12388	
Mar	1666		12388	
Apr	1666		12388	
May	1666		12388	
Jun	1666		12388	
Jul	1666		12388	
Aug	1666		12388	
Sep	1666		12388	
Oct	1666		12388	
Nov	1666		12388	
Dec	1666		12388	
Total	20000		148659	

Report Writing

One of the most important skills a therapist must develop is management report writing. This skill is necessary to submit reports that are ready for executive action or to report actions to subordinates. It is through written communication that the manager maintains a historical file of actions and data that support change. A report is defined as an official statement of facts, their sources, an analysis of their importance, and recommendations for how they may be used.

A report must be understood at many levels and must be written in the style acceptable within the facility's system. Basic to a successful report are the following characteristics:

1. *Directness.* Get to the point at once, avoid suspense.
2. *Summarize.* Begin each section with a summary before you go into details.
3. *Conciseness.* Include only pertinent details.
4. *Readability.* Use correct grammar.
5. *Objectivity.* Because a report is a statement of facts, recommendations must be based on facts and not on personal prejudice.
6. *Appearance.* The appearance contributes greatly to the attention the report is given.

A report justifying additional staff or the expansion of services or requesting program changes may be written in the following sequence:

1. *Summary.* State the objectives of the report.
2. *Introduction.* State the problem.
3. *Study.* Present the data.
4. *Conclusions.* What you expect to occur with the proposed change.
5. *Recommendations.* Changes requested, including alternatives.
6. *Physical facilities.* The effect of change on physical plant.
7. *Equipment.* Equipment needs.
8. *Personnel.* Changes in personnel.
9. *Costs.* The cost of the change.
10. *Appendix.* Support data.

The outline format to be used is:

I.
    A.
        1.
            a.
                1)
                    a)

References are available and should be used in developing a style of management report writing.

Methods Improvement

Methods improvement can be described as management work simplification. The occupational therapist's preparation in this area can easily be transferred. In looking at a job to be accomplished use an orderly approach to develop a solution. This process includes (1) select the task to be improved; (2) question if the task can be eliminated; (3) describe the components of the task; (4) question each component of the task; (5) develop the new method of implementing the task; and (6) implement the new method.

Step 1. Select the task to be improved. These might be tasks that take too long, cost too much, tasks where materials are wasted, or tasks that people do not like to do.

Step 2. Question if the task can be eliminated. Question whether the objectives of the program can be met without the task being performed.

Step 3. Describe the components of the task. Describe every detail and challenge it for its contribution to the total process.

Step 4. Question each component of the task. To each component ask the following questions. *What* is done? *Where* is it done? *When* is it done? *Who* does it? and *How* is it done?

Step 5. Develop the new method of implementing the task. The method should specifically relate to the program's objectives and may be presented to staff in procedural form so that all persons involved know what their responsibilities are in the implementation.

Step 6. Implement the method. Implement the method but review it periodically to see that it is necessary and meets specific objectives.

Personnel Management

The management process requires people to carry out objectives. It is unfair to assume that people know what is to be done and can do it without direction. Individuals work effectively if they know what is expected of them and can define the structure in which they can work without supervision. It is the manager's responsibility to assist and support employees in their professional development. It is sometimes necessary to make decisions which will not be supported by all your staff members. The manager has the responsibility of bringing the staff into line with established objectives.

A personnel problem with a staff member requires the management process that is outlined in this chapter. First, identify the problem; second, establish goals; and third, develop a plan for improvement. This process will accomplish the following objectives: identify to the employee the performance level that is acceptable and provide the manager with the data to terminate the relationship if necessary, after having fully implemented a plan to encourage satisfactory performance.

This area of management should be studied further by persons in supervisory positions because it relates so much to the professional developmental process of the occupational therapist.

Collective Bargaining

Collective bargaining is an area where managers must have current knowledge. Resources are available from the American Occupational Therapy Association as well as from personnel departments of individual facilities.

Change

All managers have experienced staff members who are resistant to change; therefore, it is important to involve persons who will be affected by the change in the planning and implementation phases. Important to remember is that the change must be understood by the employees as it relates to the program objectives. The employees' understanding of the need for change should alleviate much of the anxiety so often exhibited. Any occupational therapy department must maintain enough stability to function yet not allow itself to become static or unconscious of the health system and its needs to adapt to changing conditions. A balance of stability and change are necessary for survival and growth. The occupational therapist must learn to recognize how to maintain this balance. This is possible through the writing of objectives and the accepting of responsibility for meeting them.

Resources for Managers

The American Occupational Therapy Association can provide the manager with copies of current standards, model job descriptions, examples of procedures, current laws that affect the manager's performance, and many potential resource contacts to assist in problem solving. The manager can contact the federal government for guidance either through the regional offices or at the federal level for help in interpreting any federal regulation. These contacts and addresses can be obtained from the American Occupational Therapy Association, Government Affairs Division.

In addition to library resources perhaps the manager's greatest ally is the administrator who can provide assistance and support for developing effective management skills. The manager of occupational therapy is an important link in the administrator's management system because it is through just such managers that the objectives of the facility are accomplished.

section 2/Documentation

The documentation of plans and accomplishments with clients reflects the therapist's pride in the profession and indicates the individual's degree of confidence in his or her skills. Documentation is a professional responsibility. The Principles of Occupational Therapy Ethics identifies this responsibility as one of its ten principles:

RELATED TO RECORDS, REPORTS, GRADES, AND RECOMMENDATIONS: The occupational therapist shall conform to local state and federal laws and regulations applicable to records and reports. The occupational therapist abides by the employing institution's rules. Objective data shall govern over subjective data in evaluation, grades, recommendations, records and reports.[2]

The medical record is the communication network that links a team of specialists together so that a patient/client can receive care that is designed and implemented to solve his or her problems.

Legal Liability

The record can be used in legal transactions; however, this should not alter the purpose of documenting the course of the patient's illness and medical care. There are legal considerations that affect the use of the medical record both in and out of court. The facility must provide procedures to the therapist for directions in use of the record because laws vary considerably from state to state.

In some states patients now have the right to see their records. Facility policies should reflect state laws.

The Recording Process

Traditionally the medical record has been the communication tool for professionals. Every facility has its own procedure for documenting the care being delivered. It is the responsibility of the occupational therapist to follow the procedure adopted by the facility and to follow the procedures relating to disclosure of information.

In 1970 Lawrence L. Weed, M. D., published a book entitled *Medical Records, Medical Education and Patient Care.*[3] His concept of medical records is now being taught in health professional programs throughout this country. Many medical centers have fully implemented this process. It has significant application for occupational therapy as the problems the patient is experiencing are recorded and the entire progress section of the record relates to the problems. Dr. Weed recently has supported that the patient should maintain a record so that he or she takes the responsibility for his or her own health status and controls the information. The record traditionally has been the property of the facility but we may see this change in time.

Occupational Therapy Records

Occupational therapy records are currently mandated by standards; two examples of these are Standard III of the Rehabilitation Section of the Joint Commission on Accreditation of Hospitals Standards and standards established by the Representative Assembly of the American Occupational Therapy Association. Each medical record must include a current, written plan of care. The plan must include the problems, goals, and treatment.

Problem Oriented Record—Its Application to Occupational Therapy

In its totally implemented status the physician identifies the patient's problems from a data base. The therapist contributes to this data base through the initial assessment and plan of care.

Many facilities have not implemented the problem oriented record. Nevertheless it is possible and very practical for the occupational therapist to record in this format. The advantages of using the problem oriented record are:

1. A note is not written unless there is data to record.
2. The format provides the opportunity for self-evaluation as well as peer evaluation.
3. It allows for collection of data to support the need for occupational therapy services.
4. It provides a clear description of the status of the patient's condition and rehabilitation potential.
5. It is possible to state specifically what service was delivered and the result of the service.

The process for recording the problem oriented record is called SOAP.

S stands for *Subjective*, what the patient tells the therapist. To avoid confusion in recording this information S can be introduced by the phrase, "The patient states . . ."

O stands for *Objective*. This is where evaluation results and observations are recorded. Progress is recorded here.

A stands for *Assessment*. This is where the occupational therapist can give a professional opinion. Example: "Patient will require post-hospital care as family states they cannot manage the patient in the home until he is at a minimal assist level of self-care." It is also the place to assess the effectiveness of the plan and recommend change in the treatment plan. Example: "Patient will not be able to ambulate to accomplish homemaking tasks. Recommend he be fitted with a wheelchair."

P stands for *Plan*. This part must reflect what services will be provided. As the patient progresses the therapist states program goals for other professionals to see. Examples: Announce a planning conference, state the follow-up that will be provided, or identify the objectives of the home program.

A traditional occupational therapy note might be written as follows:

1/26/77—Occupational Therapy

Patient was instructed in and shows understanding of work simplification techniques. Patient's endurance for sitting is two hours but fatigues after ten minutes of standing. Patient should be able to independently prepare meals but will need assistance in cleaning and home maintenance tasks. Patient states she is ready to go home and try to maintain household. Patient's family will be informed of patient's abilities and their need to provide support. Recommend a home visit in one week to see how patient is implementing techniques and as needed if patient requires support or additional learning experiences.

Carolyn Baum, OTR 1-26-77

The problem oriented record would appear as follows:

Problem: Decreased Endurance

S: Patient states she is ready to go home and try to implement learned techniques in managing her home responsibilities.

O: Patient shows understanding of work simplification techniques. Sitting tolerance is two hours, fatigues after ten minutes of standing.

A: Patient should be able to prepare meals independently but will need assistance in cleaning and home maintenance.

P: Patient to demonstrate to family her abilities and limitations to gain support of her desire to be as independent as possible. Home visit by occupational therapist at one week after discharge and as needed until patient has made appropriate adjustment.

Carolyn Baum, OTR 1-26-77

Medical Care Evaluation Studies

Occupational therapists must learn the technique of medical care evaluation. This technique provides the therapist with data with which to evaluate services. The technique provides the manager with a process to collect data which may support necessary administrative changes. Medical Care Evaluations are required by the Professional Standards Review Organization (PSRO) and the Joint Commission on Accreditation of Hospitals. The American Occupational Therapy Association provides educational programs and materials to assist members in understanding the process and its implications. Medical care evaluation studies are developed from the basic audit process (Fig. 26-1). These steps are outlined here.

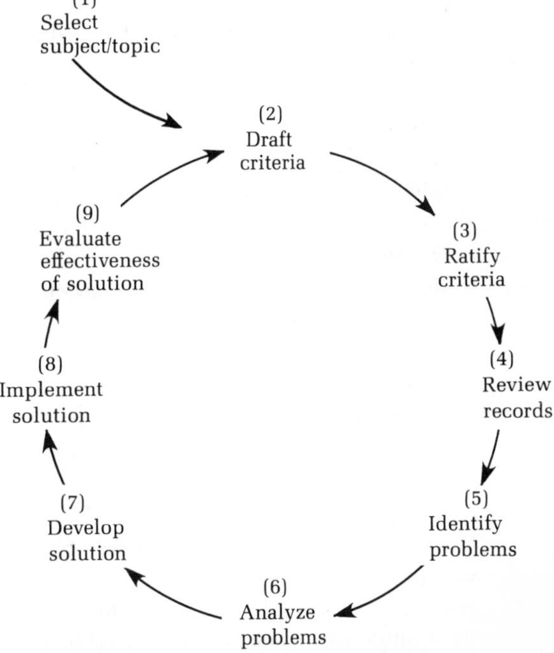

FIGURE 26-1. Basic procedure for audit. (See text for explanation.)

1. *Select Subject*
   a. The subject for the audit can be:
      —a diagnosis (admission or discharge)
      —a problem (i.e., spasticity, dependency in self-care, student failing a course)
      —an abnormal evaluation result
      —a therapeutic measure (use of specific facilitation technique, use of gross motor activities)
      —a procedure, to measure persons conformance to it
      —the effectiveness of course content
      —the students' response to a course
      —the effectiveness of service relative to costs
      —the appropriateness of occupational therapy utilization in a facility
   b. Some facets of occupational therapy service that can be looked at using the audit process:
      —justification of occupational therapy service
      —accuracy of test results
      —effectiveness of a procedure
      —effectiveness of a course
      —appropriateness of treatment
      —the extent of follow-up in patient management
2. *Draft Criteria*
   Limit yourself to five criteria. The criteria *must be* designed to be:
      —reasonable
      —understandable
      —measurable
      —behavioral
      —attainable
3. *Ratify Criteria*
   All those affected by the criteria must accept it (clinicians, curriculum, staff, etc.)
4. *Review Records*
   a. Records may be the patient's chart, the student's comments regarding a course, the student's records, incident reports, administrative reports, expenses of the department. It may be the medical records report if you are looking at how many patients receive occupational therapy, or it may be that you will have to design an assessment tool to have students or staff fill out to critique a certain situation.
   b. It is not necessary to review many records to find out if objectives or outcomes have been met; as few as three or as many as fifty may do. Ten to twenty would be ideal.
5. *Identify problems*
   Compare the actual with the expected.
6. *Analyze problems*
7. *Develop Solution*
   a. Were there adequate records kept?
   b. Is education needed?
   c. Do you need more personnel?
   d. Does the policy or procedure need changing?
8. *Implement Solutions*
9. *Evaluate the Effectiveness of the Solution*
   a. Wait six to nine months—re-audit with the same criteria.
   b. If necessary revise your criteria and have it ratified again.

GLOSSARY

Administration. the total activity of a manager

Audit. study of performance usually through a review of objective data. Results of audit may indicate a need for change

Authority. the sum of the powers and rights assigned to a position

Controlling function. making sure the results conform to the plan

Coordinate. to time, unify, and integrate work as it takes place

Decentralization. the systematic and consistent delegation of authority to the levels where the work is performed

Leadership, management. the work of planning, organizing, leading, and controlling performed by a person in a leadership position to enable people to work most effectively together to attain identified ends

Management by exception. a process whereby the manager is given the authority to carry independently all functions that are within the context of established procedures and/or approved budget

Management by objectives. a process whereby superior and subordinate managers agree on common goals. Through this agreement each individual's major areas of responsibilities are defined in terms of the results expected.

Manager. one who enables people to work most effectively together by performing the work of planning, organizing, leading, directing, and controlling

Organizing function. the work a manager performs to arrange and relate the work to be done so it can be performed most effectively by people

Performance standards. the criteria by which methods and results will be evaluated

Planning function. the work a manager performs to predetermine a course of action. The following questions are asked: what am I going to do? and what is the best way to do it?

Procedure. a standardized method of performing specified work

Relationship, line. the relationship of those persons and organization components that are accountable for objectives and who have delegated authority to make decisions with respect to those objectives

Relationship, staff. the relationship of those persons and organization components that provide advice and service in the accomplishment of objectives

REFERENCES

1. Principles of Occupational Therapy Ethics, American Occupational Therapy Association, 1977.
2. Ibid.
3. Weed, L. L.: Medical Records, Medical Education and Patient Care. Chicago: Year Book Medical Publications, 1970.

BIBLIOGRAPHY

Gallagher, W. J.: Report Writing for Management. Reading, MA: Addison-Wesley Publishing Co., 1969.

Hospital Medical Records, American Hospital Association, Chicago, 1972.

Hurst, J. W., and Walker, H. K.: The Problem Oriented System. New York: Medcom, 1972.

Kast, F. E., and Rosenziverg, J. E.: Organization and Management: A System Approach. New York: McGraw-Hill Book Co., 1974.

Organizing For Health Care, A Tool for Change. Boston: Beacon Press, 1974.

Ratcliff, J.: The Physical Therapy Problem Oriented SOAP Note. Self-Instructional Material Project, Chapel Hill NC, 1974.

Supervisory Management Course For Hospital Supervisors, Part I. Management Principles, 1969, and Part II, 1969. Supervisory Management Association, founded by the American Management Association, Chicago.

Weed, L. L.: Your Health and How To Manage It. Essex Junction VT: Essex Publishing Co., 1975.

ACKNOWLEDGMENT

A very fortunate experience for me occurred during the period from 1967 to 1976. When at Research Medical Center in Kansas City, Missouri, I worked directly with two of the best possible teachers because they demanded learning. I would like to credit them for the input they have had on the profession of Occupational Therapy: Wayne E. Conery, Assistant Director for Professional Services, and A. Alan Transue, Assistant Director for Fiscal Services.

Part Nine

Consultancy and Research

measurement of change constitutes a significant barrier to occupational therapy research productivity.

Ayres serves as an example of an occupational therapist researcher who was motivated by wanting to improve the lives of children who were handicapped by the inability to process and use sensorimotor information. Her long and sometimes arduous path toward developing theory began with simple clinical observation. Her interest in determining relationships between the clinical facts she discovered so they could be organized into a coherent whole was based upon wanting to do a better job as an occupational therapist. The clinical researcher in occupational therapy obtains the reward of serving patients or clients in numbers far beyond those she could reach in a one-to-one clinical therapy program. She also enjoys the excitement that comes from the discovery of new knowledge and the pride that emanates from contributing to the future development of the profession.

The clinical researcher in occupational therapy needs free access to a clinical facility. He or she possesses specialty expertise in a particular area of occupational therapy, knowledge and skills in research design and methods, the ability to identify needs for consultation in the area of statistical analysis or other means of data analysis, time and other resources to carry out the research, writing skills to enable the research to be published for the scrutiny of all, and a high degree of motivation to enable him or her to persist in spite of the obstacles he or she will encounter in the real world of people and capriciousness. Whitehead once called research "a welcoming attitude toward change." A most important quality for a researcher is openness to change, openness to the data that do not fit, especially the data which tend to refute the theory in question.

The clinical researcher must maintain a high level of consciousness of the ethics involved in protecting the rights of human subjects. All human beings who take part in occupational therapy research have the right to give or withhold their informed consent to participation in the project. The subject needs to know what, if any, risks could accrue to him or her as well as any benefits to be obtained for him or herself or humanity for participating in the research. He or she must be informed that he or she can withdraw from a project at any time without fear of reprisal. He or she needs to be assured that privacy and anonymity will be preserved by the researcher.[11] Signed informed consents must be retained by the researcher as evidence of the subject's willingness to participate in the research project. Informed consent for minors creates a difficult ethical question: who should provide the consent? Researchers considering the participation of children as subjects should refer to the entirety of the published Department of Health, Education and Welfare Research Guidelines.[11]

Research in occupational therapy is beginning to formulate and test unique theory. Occupational therapy needs to encourage more researchers to enter the profession by emphasizing the excitement and challenge of research in the publicity which attracts students to the field. The profession itself needs to establish more in-depth doctoral level occupational therapy educational programs to provide the skills, knowledge, and attitudes necessary to produce quality research.

For those who seek a career which requires a deep personal commitment and provides substantial rewards in the excitement of discovery, the generation of new knowledge and fields of practice for occupational therapy, the role of occupational therapy researcher or consultant offers a career of unlimited growth along with the opportunity to become self-directed, pioneering, and a leader in determining the future direction of the profession.

REFERENCES

1. Pavalko, R.: Sociology of Occupations and Professions. Itasca IL: F. T. Peacock Publications, 1971, pp. 33–36.
2. Livingston, F. M., and O'Sullivan, N. (eds.): Occupational Therapist Consultant Manual. Southern California Occupational Therapist Consultants Group, Los Angeles, 1977. (For a discussion of the occupational therapist consultant's role in skilled nursing facilities.)
3. Frostig, M.: Developmental Test of Visual Perception. Consulting Psychologists Press, Palo Alto CA, 1966.
4. Kephart, N.: The Slow Learner in the Classroom. Columbus OH: Charles E. Merrill Publishing Co., 1960.
5. von Bertalanffy, L.: General System Theory. New York: George Braziller, 1968.
6. Yerxa, E., and Gilfoyle, E.: AOTF Research Seminar. Am. J. Occup. Ther. 30:509–514, 1976.

27

The Occupational Therapist as Consultant and Researcher

Elizabeth J. Yerxa

A significant characteristic of professional persons is that they are able to work with a considerable degree of autonomy.[1] An example of such professional autonomy is the characteristic of being selected directly by clients and deciding what needs to be done for them. Doctors and lawyers determine, independently, what needs to be done to benefit their clients. Occupational therapy as an emerging profession is beginning to demonstrate such autonomy, although to a lesser degree than the older, more established professions.

In contrast to the hospital or clinic-based occupational therapist who usually evaluates and plans therapy for patients only upon physician referral, some occupational therapists are working as consultants, many in private practices owned and operated by themselves. Other occupational therapists serve as the principal investigators of research projects which they conceive, implement, evaluate, and report in the profession's literature. These new roles require a high degree of autonomy along with the need to collaborate with other professional persons on a peer level. The researcher and consultant are exciting new roles for occupational therapists to play because their self-directed contribution to the quality of life for persons, the health of institutions, and the development of new knowledge contributes substantially to society and the evolution of the profession.

THE OCCUPATIONAL THERAPIST AS CONSULTANT

A consultant occupational therapist is one who offers his or her unique occupational therapy knowledge and skill to create change in a system. The occupational therapist's services may be sought by an individual or more commonly by an organization such as a school, skilled nursing facility, community agency, or hospital.[2] The consultant provides occupational therapy expertise to the individual or institution which contracts for it. The service may be sought on a one-time-only basis to solve a particular problem or on an ongoing basis to provide for a continuing need. Consultants are often at the leading edge of the profession, creating new programs and innovative roles for occupational therapists.

CASE EXAMPLE

Maureen Hayes, registered occupational therapist, was employed as a consultant for a school district within a large metropolitan area. She was sought by the school district to help teachers identify children with possible learning disorders and to initiate programs of early intervention so that these children could develop the basic academic skills necessary for successful performance in school. Several teachers had reported their frustrations with children who had to flunk kindergarten or who were so disruptive that they required inordinate amounts of attention. The teachers' efforts had thus far been ineffective in solving the problem. The older the children became the more they fell behind in their schooling. Ms. Hayes provided the teachers with new knowledge and skills so that they could perform their jobs more effectively in assuring that their students learned.

The consultancy process with institutions requires a similar thought process to the therapeutic process with individuals. However, the consultant looks at the problem as one component of a complete system. The problem must be determined as one appropriate for occupational therapy intervention. Data are gathered, then analyzed to produce hypotheses as to appropriate forms of intervention. Hypotheses are selected, implemented, and evaluated as to their effectiveness in solving the problem.

Ms. Hayes identified the problem as "probable learning disorders," which presented an appropriate area for occupational therapy consultation. She had worked with children with learning disorders for three years. She prepared herself for entry into the system by meeting with kindergarten teachers informally to identify their perception of the learning problems they were confronting.

Ms. Hayes began the process of data gathering by instituting screening devices such as the Frostig Tests[3] and the Kephart Motor Evaluations[4] with children in kindergarten classes. A strong correlation was discovered between the children who were having problems identified by the teachers and those who showed sensorimotor and perceptual deficits on the screening tests. Ms. Hayes developed programs of classroom intervention which were carried out by the teachers and teachers' aides. She conducted one-hour classes daily for some of the more severely disabled children on an intensive basis. Families were advised as to appropriate play activities which could be carried out at home. At six-month intervals the children were retested for changes. These data along with data on their performance in the classroom were used to assess the effectiveness of the intervention programs. The evaluations showed that the childrens' performance improved substantially.

Several unique qualities of the consultancy process emerge from this discussion of Ms. Hayes' role and function. First, she viewed the problem from a perspective of the entire school district, recognizing each school and classroom as a subsystem of the district. She knew how the components of the system related to one another, i.e., superintendent to school principal to teacher to parent to pupil. She needed to intervene in the school system in such a way as to recognize its integrity and preserve its functioning. In this case, she had to obtain the understanding and support of every component of the system without posing a threat to anyone, especially to the teachers who were accustomed to being considered the experts on learning.

A consultant usually has no *authority* within the system. He or she only creates change as the system allows change to take place. The consultant offers advice but the components of the system determine whether the advice will become input to create change. The openness or closedness of the system to advice is greatly influenced by the professional competency, systems knowledge, and interpersonal skills of the consultant. A failure in demonstrating any of these characteristics may result in a closed system. A consultant prepares others to carry out the advice provided rather than intervening personally. In addition to giving advice the consultant must prepare the persons who are going to implement the advice with the skills to do so. The successful consultant obtains the reward of seeing problems solved, clients served, and new programs developed as a result of his or her skill. He or she often enhances the understanding and increases the utilization of occupational therapy services.

The special qualifications of the occupational therapy consultant are (1) highly developed expertise in an area of occupational therapy; (2) knowledge of systems theory[5] and how to relate it to organizations (the "big picture"); (3) good interpersonal skills; and (4) the capacity to teach others how to carry out intervention programs.

Consultants face unique dilemmas in addition to the usual ethical constraints of professionalism. If others are to carry out intervention programs ethically, how much should be expected of persons who are not educated in the skills, knowledge, and values of occupational therapy? For example, when should the consultant teach teachers to carry out programs for the learning disabled and when should he or she advise that occupational therapists be employed to do so? Could clients be harmed by the inappropriate application of occupational therapy knowledge? In the case of Ms. Hayes, the registered occupational therapist maintained control of the screening and program development phase of the consultancy while the teachers carried out the classroom intervention program under her supervision.

As more occupational therapists become consultants, the autonomy of the profession will increase as will the importance of preparing occupational therapists to develop the prerequisite skills to be effective consultants applying the ethical tenets of consultancy.

THE OCCUPATIONAL THERAPIST AS RESEARCHER

Research in occupational therapy is in its infancy. Many leaders in the profession emphasize that research should have the highest priority in order to develop the knowledge base of the profession.[6] Much of the research which has been done in occupational therapy thus far is descriptive of client characteristics or occupational therapist characteristics or is concerned with the outcome of occupational therapy education.[7] Occupational therapy clinical research is needed now as never before to assure the profession's accountability to the public. The rise of the consumer movement in the late 1960s identified the need for accountability by the providers of health care as well as the providers of other products in the United States.[8] Increasing pressure has been exerted on occupational therapy to prove the efficacy of its services and to produce tangible results. AOTA task forces have decried the lack of a research base for professional practice. States which have moved toward licensure have experienced great difficulty in defining occupational therapy legally so that it is differentiated from other professions such as physical therapy, psychology, and speech therapy. Occupational therapy educators who have sought conceptual models for occupational therapy curriculums which were based upon unique occupational therapy knowledge found multiple theories but little theory which had been put to the test of research.

The current state of research in occupational therapy represents a stage in the normal evolution of professions which proceeds from the intuitive practice of untested art to the logically rigorous practice of science. Most professions, including medicine, are still a mixture of the two, although more rigorously tested than occupational therapy. As Kuhn points out, the presence of competing theories in a field often leads to a scientific crisis which can result in a new paradigm.[9] Some authors view occupational therapy at the stage of a crisis, in the Kuhnian or positive sense. However occupational therapy is viewed, most professional and outside observers agree that research to develop and test the occupational therapy knowledge base is crucial to its future development, especially in the area of clinical research related to occupational therapy outcomes.

Ayres provides a current model of an occupational therapy clinical researcher. In 1963 she published her first papers describing the discovery of a heretofore unidentified group of perceptual motor syndromes.[10] These syndromes had been identified through a painstaking period of clinical observation, followed by hypothesis formation, testing of the hypothetical observations in a controlled fashion, careful analysis of the data gathered, and finally the drawing of tentative conclusions about hypotheses. Note the similarity of this thought process to the process outlined before as the consultation thought process. As one occupational therapist plans a treatment program for an individual client, Ayres extended the thought process to apply to whole groups of individuals in a scientifically rigorous way. She presented her data for the scrutiny of the disinterested scientific community so her observations could be tested and evaluated by others. Occupational therapy theory is developed and tested through this process. Isolated and meaningless facts must be interrelated and rendered meaningful in the fabric of a theory just as isolated threads must be woven into the fabric of a garment to create a design. Each new experiment tests the strength of a theory and either supports its validity or fails to support it. Ayres developed and validated a battery of objective tests in order to evaluate her theory. At present, occupational therapy possesses few such standardized tests for theory testing. This lack of objective instrumentation for the

7. Yerxa, E.: Occupational Therapy Research in 1974: Models of Enlightenment. Proceeding World Federation of Occupational Therapists, pp. 674–680, 1974.
8. Somers, A.: Health Care in Transition. Hospital Research and Education Trust, Chicago, 1971.
9. Kuhn, T.: The Structure of Scientific Revolutions, Chicago: University of Chicago Press, 1962.
10. Ayres, A. J.: The Development of Perceptual-Motor Abilities: A Theoretical Basis for Treatment of Dysfunction. The Eleanor Clarke Slagle Lectures, American Occupational Therapy Association, Rockville MD, 1973.
11. The Institutional Guide to DHEW Policy in Protection of Human Subjects, Part 46, Title 45. U.S. Department of Health, Education and Welfare, Washington DC, October 1973.

Part Ten

Projections for the Profession

28

The Profession of Occupational Therapy: Today and Tomorrow

Elizabeth J. Yerxa

This chapter explores the following questions regarding the profession of occupational therapy: What are the criteria of professionalism? How well does occupational therapy meet these criteria? How do individual occupational therapists provide competent services to patients or clients? What are some of the pitfalls of professionalism? What are the unique contributions of occupational therapy to health care? And, finally, what does the future hold for the profession of occupational therapy?

Occupational therapy is viewed by its members as a profession. However, from the outside, Pavalko[1] views occupational therapy as a marginal profession in the company of such other groups as nurses, social workers, and even the police. In his view, occupational therapy is "on its way" as a profession but hasn't quite made it. On what basis does he make his assessment?

Many definitions exist for the term "profession." For Pavalko, the characteristics of a true profession include having a systematic body of theory and knowledge, relevance to basic social values, a long period of specialized training, motivation to serve humanity, autonomy, a sense of commitment to a "calling," a sense of community, and a code of ethics. Moore[2] adds that a profession is a full-time, paid occupation. These characteristics are widely accepted as criteria of professionalism.

In applying the criteria of professionalism to occupational therapy, the first limitation which appears is the lack of a *systematic body of theory and knowledge*. Unique theories and models of occupational therapy are only now emerging and are far from being tested to generate new knowledge. Much of occupational therapy's knowledge is still empirical and unsystematized. However, hopeful signs exist in the very formulation of new models and theories which can be used to organize and interpret observations in the future. Examples exist in the theories and models of Ayres, Reilly, Mosey, Llorens, and Fidler.

Occupational therapy is relevant to the *social values* of humanism, independence, productivity, self-directedness, and freedom of choice which are inherent to a democratic society. The application of such values in the patient-occupational therapist relationship is discussed later in this chapter.

The *period of specialized training* or education

for an occupational therapist now requires four to five years leading to a bachelor's or master's degree. The length of such training is shorter than that required for medicine or law but similar to that required for nursing and social work. The degree to which occupational therapy training can be specialized at present is limited by the lack of a systematic theory and knowledge base. However, initial training to the level of the master's degree is becoming more common. The AOTA Mental Health Task Force recommended in 1976 that the entry level of education for all occupational therapists be at the master's level.[3] That recommendation is still being discussed and has not yet been implemented. The length and content of the education of occupational therapists is still highly variable. Future decisions as to the length and specialization of occupational therapy education will have a profound effect on the knowledge base and status of occupational therapy as a true profession.

A *motivation to serve humanity* has been demonstrated consistently in the literature of the profession since its origin. This motivation is conveyed, for example, in all of the Eleanor Clark Slagle lectures presented by occupational therapists who have received the highest academic award of the profession. The service motive is also conveyed in the literature that is used to recruit new members into the profession, thus assuring that those who enter the profession ascribe to the service motive.

The characteristic of *autonomy* is described by Pavalko as "self-regulation and self-control." Mathewson[4] and Pavalko[5] agree that the major limitation to occupational therapy's status as a true profession is its lack of autonomy since most occupational therapists rely upon receiving a physician's prescription or referral prior to initiating occupational therapy. Mathewson relates this dependence upon the physician to occupational therapy's status as a "feminine" profession since approximately ninety-five percent of its members are women. Currently most occupational therapists do not possess a high degree of autonomy.

A *sense of commitment to a calling* can be demonstrated by the numbers of those entering the profession with a life-long commitment to continue working within it. Except for the interruptions posed by marriage and child raising, the majority of occupational therapists do demonstrate such a commitment. They perceive their work as an end in service and satisfaction rather than a means to the end of remuneration.

A *sense of community* in a profession is demonstrated by a bond of common identity and a distinctive culture shared by the members of the profession. In considering the unique language of occupational therapy and the organization called the American Occupational Therapy Association, which exerts control over its members, occupational therapy does demonstrate a sense of community. Mathewson,[6] however, feels that the sense of community is weak since women often give first priority to that community represented by their husband's profession.

The final characteristic, a *code of ethics*, is evolving for occupational therapy. Standards of ethical practice are developed by the members of the AOTA Commission on Standards. These are published in the AOTA Bylaws[7] and the AOTA Principles of Occupational Therapy Ethics[8] for public scrutiny. Professional ethics in occupational therapy assure such protections as the patient's right to competent practice of occupational therapy, confidentiality of the patient-therapist relationship including records, and professional responsibilities such as seeking information regarding the major health problems of society and educating the public.

Occupational therapy is on the threshold of becoming a true profession according to the accepted criteria of professionalism. The two characteristics which appear to need the greatest strengthening are (1) the development of a systematic body of theory and knowledge and (2) the attainment of a greater degree of autonomy.

With the advent of the consumer movement in the 1960s and its influence upon the health care system, society no longer accepted a profession's implicit assurance of competency but rather demanded that professional persons be held accountable for demonstrating their competence to peers and consumers.

A crucial dimension of professional competence is the quality of the therapist-patient or therapist-client relationship. Often the student in his or her first contact with the patient is anxious and confused about how to relate in his or her new role as a professional. He or she doesn't yet possess the knowledge and skills of a full-fledged professional. However, the patient expects him or her to provide professional occupational therapy services. At this point the student may say to him or herself or the supervisor, "Why can't I just be the patient's friend?" Being able to move from the role of the "lay" friend to the role of professional "therapist" is one of the most challenging and significant components of professional development.

In 1976 occupational therapy students at the University of Southern California who were at the end of their six-month field work experience identified the characteristics in Table 28-1 to differentiate a friendship from a professional therapeutic relationship. This comparison is by no means exhaustive nor is it agreed upon universally. It is presented to stimulate thought and discussion. The person who needs help needs *both* kinds of relationships. But the professional person brings unique knowledge and skills to the therapeutic relationship.

Table 28-1. Comparison of helping relationships.

Friendship relationship	*Professional relationship*
Subjectivity	Objectivity
Seek immediate comfort	Seek long-range good
Reciprocal sharing of feelings	More one-way communication of feelings
Give and take	Give
Peer relationship (no special knowledge)	Non-equalitarian relationship (specialized knowledge)
Lifelong or long-term commitment	Short-term commitment of therapist
Mutual choice in relationship	Patient/client choice limited by service goals
Expectation of friendship	Expectation of professional benefits

Results of an Occupational Therapy Student Seminar discussion, University of Southern California, Los Angeles, Fall 1976.

Occupational therapy's emphasis upon the patient acting independently creates a unique demand upon the therapist-client relationship. Occupational therapy cannot be done *to* a person in the sense that surgery or massage are done to a patient. The *patient* must do what is therapeutic. The therapist is an enabler. Meyeroff states that, "Caring involves trusting the other to grow in his own time and in his own way."[9] Such trust is basic to the concept of the patient as an active participant. Also, Meyeroff identifies therapist empathy when he states: "In being with the other, I do not lose myself. I retain my own identity and am aware of my own reactions to him and his world. Seeing his world as it appears to him does not mean having his reactions to it; and thus I am able to help him in his world."[10]

Professional objectivity about the patient-therapist relationship enables the therapist to escape being personally wounded by the client's coping mechanisms including the anger which might mark such coping. It also requires the capacity to recognize therapist behavior which is dependency-producing and counterproductive to the goal of occupational therapy, self-directedness. The provision of choices for the patient is a significant component of occupational therapy which affirms the dignity and competence of the client.[11] Developing the capacity to relate therapeutically is a lifelong process requiring the thoughtful examination of the quality of each relationship based upon the criterion of how well it enabled the client to move toward greater self-direction and competence.

In addition to the nature of the professional relationship, occupational therapists have responsibilities which assure their professional contribution to society. These include providing evidence of the maintenance of competency, active participation in the professional organization, development and maintenance of standards of professional education, and ethical conduct.

Maintenance of competency in occupational therapy is presently based upon voluntary activity such as attendance at continuing education programs and workshops. Such continuing education is designed to enable occupational therapists to keep their knowledge and skill current with new developments in the profession and to attain more specialized knowledge which can be applied in practice. However, as more states adopt occupational therapy licensure laws, demonstration of competency regularly through proof of participation in continuing education programs or passing examinations is becoming more of a necessity. The American Occupational Therapy Association is currently developing a continuing certification plan which is designed to assure the maintenance of competency on a national basis by establishing criteria for recertification every three to five years. Such criteria have not as yet been adopted.

In order to develop a sense of professional community and to serve the public an occupational therapist needs to participate in the American Occupational Association and the local Occupational Therapy Association. These organizations are increasingly serving as advocates for the consumers of health care as well as for the profession itself. Legislation for the provision of occupational therapy services to clients who need such services is often initiated and/or supported by the professional association. Standards of practice to assure quality services are developed and ratified by the members of the association. Each American Occupational Therapy Association member has the right to influence the future direction of the profession by making his or her concerns known to his or her representative who sits in the American Occupational Therapy Association Representative Assembly, the policy-making body.

The quality of professional education in occupational therapy is protected through standards of education which are developed by the American Occupational Therapy Association Commission on Education in collaboration with the American Medical Association and ratified by the American Occupational Therapy Association Representative Assembly. Such standards are published for public scrutiny in the Essentials of an Accredited Educational Program for the Occupational Therapist. They protect the public interest by establishing minimum standards for entry into the profession. The successful passage of the American Occupational Therapy Association certification examination is also required for entry into the profession. The designation of O.T.R. after one's name assures the public that an individual has demonstrated entry level competency for the practice of the profession. Ethical standards of practice have already been discussed in the first portion of this chapter.

Social scientists have identified some of the pitfalls of professionalism which can interfere with the public interest.[12] Among these are professional territoriality, self-interest, status concern, imposition of foreign value systems upon the client, and establishment of professional status hierarchies or "pecking orders" within the health care system. These pitfalls need to be kept in mind by occupational therapists to assess to what extent the profession's activities interfere with its ability to improve the life opportunities for clients.

Professional territoriality disputes often occur as a result of the division of labor in the health care delivery system caused by the knowledge explosion. Who does what is not necessarily clear cut. Ambiguities of practice may lead to conflicts in such areas as who treats what part of the person or who uses such modalities as exercise or sensory integrative therapy. Such disputes become counterproductive when they drain off time and energy which should be available to the patient. Interdisciplinary clinically-based educational experiences for occupational therapy students and other health care disciplines help prevent such disputes later on by developing communication and respect early in professional practice.

Professional self-interest may become confused with the public interest. For example a profession might expend a great deal of its resources protecting "standards of practice" which actually might be devoted to protecting its practitioners from competition by other groups who could perform the service just as well but at a reduced cost to the consumer. In occupational therapy the advent of the Certified Occupational Therapy Assistant was sometimes resisted on the basis that it would lower the standards of occupational therapy practice. In fact, the profession has devoted considerable effort to establishing and maintaining the standards of practice and education for Certified Occupational Therapy Assistants in order to assure the provision of quality occupational therapy services. The dental profession has adopted a similar course with the introduction of the dental hygienist.

Overconcern for status is another pitfall of professionalism. Status concern may be determined by the arguments which are used in support of higher standards of education and practice. If such standards are justified on the basis of higher salaries and higher status among professional peers rather than increased quality and breadth of services, overconcern for status might be suspected. Such overconcern for status is contrary to the humanitarian and non-self-serving concept of professionalism.

A professional pitfall which can be counterproductive to occupational therapy is the imposition of contrary value systems upon the client. Since most occupational therapists are white, female, and from the middle socioeconomic level of society, occupational therapists also represent the value systems of their culture. They have expectations about appropriate attitudes toward work and leisure time, family structure, and sex roles. It is difficult to eliminate these often unconscious values from the professional relationship so that occupational therapists do not impose foreign values upon the patient. Such imposition might interfere with the patient's ability to regain an appropriate role in his or her particular community. Some self-help groups such as Synanon and the Center for Independent Living in Berkeley, California, express antiprofessional attitudes. Such attitudes seem to reflect a reaction against imposition of foreign values. Self-help groups may arise when the attitudes of professionals are perceived by clients as condescending and authoritarian.

Within the traditional medical model, a status hierarchy or hospital pecking order can often be identified. Considerable striving can be observed by those professions who wish to move up within the hierarchy. The hierarchy is often constructed with the physician on top, the other professions below in varying order, and the patient on the bottom.[13] The end-result of status hierarchies is harmful to patients since energy is lost in striving and the patient's low status interferes with participation in the decisions which affect him or her profoundly.

The unique contribution of occupational therapy to society might be viewed at three different levels: (1) the occupational therapy services level, (2) the health care delivery level, and (3) the health care system level.

Occupational therapy services are provided by three categories of personnel, the occupational therapist, the certified occupational therapy assistant, and the occupational therapy aide. The functions of each vary according to the needs of the setting. However, the registered occupational therapist is usually responsible for determining the particular theory of treatment to be practiced, selecting and administering the evaluation instruments and formulating the specific treatment plan for clients. The certified occupational therapy assistant is most active in administering the therapeutic program, observing the client's reactions and reporting these to the registered occupational therapist who then may initiate changes in the program. Some certified occupational therapist assistants work as activity directors in skilled nursing facilities under the supervision of registered occupational therapists who consult with the facility. The occupational therapy aide has received on-the-job training for filling this role in the delivery of services. He or she assists both registered occupational therapists and certified occupational therapy assistants in carrying out treatment, and maintaining the physical facilities, schedules, and transportation of clients. The effectiveness of the performance of these three persons is highly dependent upon their ability to work as a team. Some characteristics of good occupational therapist teams are open communication, active participation in decision making, respect for the contribution of each member, sharing of rewards such as praise for a job well-done, and patient-centeredness. The most effective OTR-COTA-OT Aide teams include the patient as an active participant.

At the health care delivery level, the occupational therapist often interacts with other members of the health care team such as administrators, dieticians, nurses, physicians, physical therapists, psychologists, social workers, speech pathologists, teachers, and vocational counselors. The occupational therapist's successful functioning on the health team is influenced by a confidence in his or her unique contribution to patient care, an ability to articulate that contribution in clear statements (free of jargon), the capacity to relate well to others, and skills in the area of consensual decision making, conflict resolution, authentic self-exposure and feedback.[14]

At the health care system level the profession of occupational therapy has an opportunity to influence public policy. Since more and more health care services are being financed by the government and private insurance companies, occupational therapy is increasingly making its services known to third party payers for services. Such insurance coverage often makes the difference as to whether occupational therapy services are provided by hospitals, clinics, home care services, and so forth. Because congress and the state legislatures play a vital role in establishing health care policy, occupational therapists need to stay informed and politically active. Since numbers influence legislators, occupational therapy has strengthened its political voice by joining together with other professions with whom it shares goals to form coalitions such as the "Coalition of Independent Health Professions." In this way occupational therapy has contributed to the writing of legislation which is better able to serve the needs of consumers. Occupational therapists also serve the health care system by acting as advocates for client groups whose needs require social change. Occupational therapists have been instrumental in activities which improved the lives of the handicapped, such as the removal of architectural barriers and of the physical restrictions for obtaining driver's licenses, and the obtaining of transportation for the handicapped. Occupational therapists have led the way in demonstrating new uses of purposeful and meaningful activity for the prevention of disability in infants and children and in the improvement of life satisfaction for the chronically disabled in their communities.[15] Occupational therapy is beginning to make its voice heard in the land but must expend even greater efforts to inform the public of its services.

Quo vadis occupational therapy? Even a crystal ball does not provide a perfect prediction of the future. The signs of the present may point in the right direction but the future always remains inscrutable. With the limitations of prediction in mind, the following trends are apparent.

The profession of occupational therapy will enter an era of developing its unique knowledge base through accelerated theory building and clinical research which tests theory. Such research will be facilitated through the development of several new doctoral level educational programs in occupational therapy departments. These programs will prepare students with greater skill and motivation to perform clinical research.

Occupational therapy is entering a decade in which federal and state governments will exert greater control over the development and delivery of health care services. Occupational therapy will influence government legislation so that persons with chronic disability receive adequate resources to attain a better quality of life. The move toward national health insurance carries with it the danger that most of the country's resources will be spent on acute care leaving millions of chronically ill with the prospect of living their lives as subhuman fixtures rather than as self-directed persons. Occupational therapy will increasingly serve as a visible advocate for the chronically ill and handicapped.

Occupational therapy will develop new roles and functions particularly as consultants in the development of new occupational therapy programs in schools, community mental health centers, prisons, juvenile halls, primary health care clinics, and labor unions. Occupational therapy will remain within the medical milieu, broadening it to include more emphasis on the social and behavioral aspects of patient reintegration with the community. However, occupational therapy will also take a more active role within the educational and social systems of the "well" community. Increased emphasis will be placed upon screening clients for potential problems and intervening early to prevent disability. For example, occupational therapists will work with labor unions in the development of pre-retirement programs so that workers will learn healthy and satisfying ways of using their new leisure time.

The profession will apply more and more of its resources to communicate with the public about the services it has to offer. Such efforts will lead to the development of a definition of occupational therapy for the lay public which will make the services of occupational therapy understandable to more persons who need them. More potential consumers will then actively seek occupational therapy services. The profession will also be more clearly defined for other professions in the health care delivery system. The number of referrals for occupational therapy services will be increased as knowledge of what occupational therapy offers is increased. Finally, those within the profession will define occupational therapy for occupational therapists in a new way which encompasses a biopsychosocial view of persons and emphasizes the significance of purposeful and meaningful activity in all stages of human development. This will enable the profession to unify its efforts for more effective public education, clinical research, service, and a more definitive curriculum for tomorrow's occupational therapy student.

REFERENCES

1. Pavalko, R.: Sociology of Occupations and Professions. Itasca IL: F. T. Peacock Publications, pp. 33–36, 1971.
2. Schein, E.: What is a profession? In Professional Education. New York: McGraw-Hill Book Co., 1972, pp. 7–14.
3. Allen, C.: Report of the American Occupational Therapy Association (AOTA) Mental Health Task Force. AOTA Newspaper, September 1976.
4. Mathewson, M.: Female and married: Damaging to the therapy profession. Am. J. Occup. Ther. 29:601–605, 1975.
5. Pavalko: Sociology of Occupations and Professions, pp. 33–36.
6. Mathewson: Female and married.
7. American Occupational Therapy Association Bylaws, Section XIII.
8. Principles of Occupational Therapy Ethics. AOTA Newspaper, November 1976. (See Appendix B.)
9. Meyeroff, M.: On Caring. New York: Harper and Row, Publishers, 1971, p. 20.
10. Ibid., p. 42.
11. Yerxa, E.: Authentic occupational therapy. Am. J. Occup. Ther. 21:1–9, 1967.
12. Zimmerman, T. F.: Is professionalism the answer to improve health care? Am. J. Occup. Ther. 28:465, 1974.
13. Gellman, W.: Attitudes toward rehabilitation of the disabled. Am. J. Occup. Ther. 14:189–190, 1960.
14. Rubin, I., et al.: Improving the Coordination of Health Care. Cambridge MA: Ballinger, 1975.
15. Weimer, R.: Some concepts of prevention as an aspect of community health. Am. J. Occup. Ther. 26:1–9, 1972.

Appendices

Appendix A
Occupational Therapy Definition for Purposes of Licensure

Occupational Therapy is the application of occupation, any activity in which one engages, for evaluation, diagnosis and treatment of problems interfering with functional performance in persons impaired by physical illness or injury, emotional disorders, congenital or developmental disability, or the aging process in order to achieve optimum functioning and for prevention and health maintenance. Specific occupational therapy services include, but are not limited to, activities of daily living (ADL); the design, fabrication and application of splints; sensorimotor activities; the use of specifically designed crafts; guidance in the selection and use of adaptive equipment; therapeutic activities to enhance functional performance; prevocational evaluation and training; and consultation concerning the adaptation of physical environments for the handicapped. These services are provided to individuals or groups through medical, health, educational and social systems.

Adopted by the Representative Assembly, American Occupational Therapy Association, April 18, 1977. Published in 1977 Representative Assembly Minutes. Am. J. Occup. Ther. 31:594, 1977. Reprinted with permission of the American Occupational Therapy Association; Jerry A. Johnson, President.

Appendix B
Principles of Occupational Therapy Ethics*

Preamble

This association and its component members are committed to furthering man's ability to function fully within his total environment. To this end the Occupational Therapist renders service to clients in all stages of health and illness, to institutions, other professionals, colleagues, students and to the general public.

In furthering this commitment the American Occupational Therapy Association has established the Principles of Occupational Therapy Ethics. It is intended that they be used by all occupational therapy personnel, including practitioners in all settings, administrators, educators, and students. These principles should be reflected in and supported by licensing laws, regulations, consultation, planning and teaching. They are intended to be action oriented, guiding and preventive rather than negative or merely disciplinary. Professional maturity will be demonstrated in applying these basic principles while exercising the large measure of freedom which they provide and which is essential to responsible and creative occupational therapy service. For the purpose of continuity the following definitions will support information in this document: Occupational therapist includes registered occupational therapists, certified occupational therapy assistants, occupational therapy students. Clients include patients and those to whom occupational therapy services are delivered.

* Adopted by the Representative Assembly, American Occupational Association, April 1977. Published in Am. J. Occup. Ther. Newspaper, November 1977. Reprinted with the permission of the American Occupational Therapy Association; Jerry A. Johnson, President.

I. RELATED TO THE RECIPIENT OF SERVICE

The occupational therapist demonstrates a beneficent concern for the recipient of services, maintains a goal directed relationship with the recipient which furthers the objectives for which it is established. Services are evaluated against objectives and accountability is maintained therefore. Respect shall be shown for the recipients' rights and the occupational therapist will preserve the confidence of the patient relationship.

II. RELATED TO COMPETENCE

The occupational therapist shall actively maintain and improve one's professional competence, represent it accurately and function within its perimeters.

III. RELATED TO RECORDS, REPORTS, GRADES, AND RECOMMENDATIONS

The occupational therapist shall conform to local, state and federal laws and regulations, and regulations applicable to records and reports. The occupational therapist abides by the employing institution's rules. Objective data shall govern subjective data in evaluations, grades, recommendations, records and reports.

IV. RELATED TO INTRA-PROFESSIONAL COLLEAGUES

The occupational therapist shall function with discretion and integrity in relations with other members of the profession and shall be concerned with the quality of their services. Upon becoming aware of objective evidence of a breach of ethics or substandard service the occupational therapist shall take action according to established procedure.

V. RELATED TO OTHER PERSONNEL

The occupational therapist shall function with discretion and integrity in relations with personnel and cooperates with them as may be appropriate. Similarly, the occupational therapist expects others to demonstrate a high level of competence. Upon becoming aware of objective evidence of a breach of ethics or substandard service the occupational therapist shall take action according to established procedure.

VI. RELATED TO EMPLOYERS AND PAYERS

The occupational therapist shall render service with discretion and integrity and shall protect the property and property rights of the employers and payers.

VII. RELATED TO EDUCATION

The occupational therapist implements a commitment to the education of society and the consumer of health services as well as to the education of health personnel on matters of health which are within the purview of occupational therapy.

VIII. RELATED TO EVALUATION AND RESEARCH

The occupational therapist shall accept responsibility for evaluating, developing and refining service and the body of knowledge and skills which underlie the education and practice of occupational therapy, at all times protects the rights of subjects, clients, institutions and collaborators. The work of others shall be acknowledged.

IX. RELATED TO THE PROFESSION

The occupational therapist shall be responsible for gaining information and understanding of the principles, policies and standards of the profession. The occupational therapist functions as a representative of the profession.

X. RELATED TO LAW AND REGULATIONS

The occupational therapist shall seek to acquire information about applicable local, state, federal and institutional rules and shall function accordingly thereto.

XI. RELATED TO MISCONDUCT

The occupational therapist shall not appear to act with impropriety nor engage in illegal conduct involving moral turpitude and will not circumvent the principles of occupational therapy ethics through actions of another.

XII. RELATED TO BIOETHICAL ISSUES AND PROBLEMS OF SOCIETY

The occupational therapist seeks information about the major health problems and issues to learn their implications for occupational therapy and for one's own services.

Appendix C

Program Guide for Gross and Fine Motor Development of the Learning Disabled Child

Nancy Kauffman

This appendix to Chapter 24 is a motor development guide for use in creating non-academic program ideas to share with teachers, physical educators, parents, and aides and thus is written in nontechnical language. It is intended for use with four- to eight-year-old learning disabled children but may be adapted for other mildly impaired youngsters. It is based on developmental sequences in the Child Development Chart in Chapter 24. The program guide is divided into four sections; (1) Body Scheme (which includes sequenced items listed under Sensory Development on the Child Development Chart); (2) a combined section of Reflex Development and Balance Skills (the latter from the Equilibrium section); (3) Coordination of the Two Body Sides (from Bilateral Integration section of the chart); and (4) Eye-Hand Coordination (which includes some developmentally sequenced items under Visual Perception).

Behaviors in the left column of each of the four sections are arranged approximately developmentally, and some include approximate age norms. Therefore they can be used by educational personnel for informal evaluation/data gathering to determine *general* areas which need remedial help, for developmental program planning, and for reevaluation. This would not, of course, replace the standardized and developmental testing to be done by the therapist. The behaviors in the left column may also be stated in positive terms by therapists or educators for writing behavioral objectives as a part of diagnostic-prescriptive Individualized Educational Programs (I.E.P.s).

BODY SCHEME

Body scheme is the unconscious awareness of the physical and sensory components of the self. It includes awareness of the physical structure, movement/functions, and positions of the body and its parts in relation to each other and to objects in the environment. As used here it also includes the ability to recognize and interpret touch and pressure to the skin. Children with good body scheme accurately imitate new body postures or movements; have smoothly coordinated movements on the playground, particularly when trying new actions; adequately point to or name body parts (assuming that language comprehension and memory are adequate); draw human figures age appropriately; and interpret touch/pressure to the skin comfortably and accurately.

If these behaviors are observed	*Try these activities, strategies, or materials*
Cannot comfortably accept ordinary new or unexpected touch/pressure to skin. Has aversion to haircuts, new clothes, sand play, mudpies, love-pat on shoulder, injections, bare feet in grass, wind through hair.	• Apply firm, well-modulated pressure in rapid rhythm. Teacher rubs back/arms during rest time. • "Time out" four times daily for child's *self*-rubbing of arms, tummy, legs, neck, and face. With rapid back and forth motions use *child's* choice of soft or rough fabric, carpet piece, baby oil, hairbrush, or paint brush. • Present a variety of textures/sensations in calm, well-structured atmosphere: ice cubes, warm water, textured fingerpaints, sand play, rotary electric shoe polish brush, vibrator, tug of war on tummy in grass, electric hair dryer, inchworm race on back on grass or thick carpet. • Avoid unexpected touch by teacher/students. Encourage "thinking space" between children in line; position desk to avoid accidental touch; praise verbally rather than with love-pats unless child sees the pat approaching. • Slowly encourage physical contact within child's toleration level—lapsitting, arm around shoulders, hand pat on hair.
Is unable to imitate simple body postures/movements accurately.	• Give visual, verbal, *and* tactile clues. Manually move child to appropriate position so movement/position can be felt and learned through experiencing it. • Encourage movement/contact of all body parts with different textures and surfaces: mat, shredded paper, blankets, floor, grass, brick wall, and smooth wall. • Mimetics, pantomime, obstacle courses, animal walks, Simon Says "do this," "See a Lassie." • Trampoline, cheerleader yells, signal flags, mat stunts. • Child wiggles through rungs of leaning, suspended, or sidelying ladder with predetermined movements or climbs in and out of holes in refrigerator shipping cartons. • Action songs: I'm a Little Teapot, Inky Dinky Spider, Two Little Ducks, Little Cottage in the Woods, My Hat It Has Three Corners.

If these behaviors are observed	*Try these activities, strategies, or materials*
	• Child performs familiar movements in slow motion: walking, walking backwards, crawling, skipping, especially against resistance. • Child reproduces silhouette of partner's body positions (use film projector light), then verifies by measuring/feeling silhouette against wall.
Inaccurately uses and points to own body parts as directed.	• Beginning with easiest to learn (facial features, arm, side, etc.), teach body part awareness, being alert to child whose problem is not poor body image but poor language comprehension or poor auditory-motor match (can understand words but can't carry out appropriate movement response without visual clue). • Then work on behavior required for identification "... front, back, side, in ..." Later work on identification of more difficult body parts (wrist, knee, shoulder, etc.) • One sequence of teaching body parts (achieved over a long period of time) is to have child: touch and move part while repeating his/her name touch and move part, eyes shut touch part to object (from standing, sitting, lying down positions) while repeating its name touch part to object, eyes shut touch part to part ("put your ankle on your knee") touch part to part, eyes shut name part independently "place ankle higher than shoulder," or "back higher than head," or "ear lower than knee" • Refer to body image instructional sequences recommended in *Developmental Sequences of Perceptual Motor Tasks.*[1] • Child rapidly and firmly rubs body parts while naming: "paint" with wet or dry brush rub off "mud" or "ice cream" with hand-sized towel/carpet wrap body part with yarn or bandage at goal line rub powder off "hurt" ankle or wrist held in air during lame puppy race. • Point out body parts and movements during doll play or on pop-singer posters.

If these behaviors are observed	*Try these activities, strategies or materials*
	• Sing Dem Bones, Head and Shoulders—Knees and Toes, Looby Loo, Hokey Pokey. • Play Busy Bee (partners touch back-to-back, ankle-to-ankle, etc.) • Be alert to the idea that pointing to or naming body parts is only one step in "knowing" body image.
With eyes closed, cannot point to location of one or two touches on body parts (approximately age 5).	• Emphasize identification of and tactile stimulation to body parts. • Emphasize activities suggested for imitation of simple body postures/movements.
Does not know meaning of front, back, side, in, up, above, out (approximately age 5). Has difficulty negotiating obstacles and judging distances, especially if blindfolded.	• Eyes closed, child points to objects in familiar room, then verifies by looking, approaching, and *touching* with specified body parts. • Place three to five 8-inch numbers around room. Eyes closed, children point to numerical answer to simple verbal math problem, then verify. • Eyes closed, child touches one body part to another; touches body part to object in environment; goes through obstacle course; follows thick-rope path; touches environmental objects to front, side, top of body planes. • Child applies verbal directional labels to gross body movements and fine manipulative placement of small objects. • Child uses beanbags or plastic or playground balls for target or goal throws or dodge ball. Increase spatial awareness through eye-body, eye-hand, and foot-eye coordination activities.
Is unable to draw six-part recognizable person with body (approximately age 5).	• Look for other indications of delayed eye-hand coordination. • Emphasize awareness of body parts and imitation of postures (above).
Cannot discriminate simple shapes traced on skin with eyes closed.	• Help child identify large simple shapes traced on back, hand, or tummy using "point to the answer" method instead of "draw the answer" (eye-hand coordination may be poor) or naming answer (language deficits may be present). Advance to more complex shapes and to naming shapes. • Seat teams facing forward. Trace shape or letter on back of last child on each team. Each child traces

If these behaviors are observed	*Try these activities, strategies or materials*
	on back of person in front. Child in front of each team traces that team's shape on chalkboard. • Identify hand-sized objects felt in bag but not seen. • Child identifies finger touched by partner when eyes closed or points to spot(s) touched by partner or by "it" in circle game.
Cannot name heavier of two weights (approximately age 4); with eyes closed cannot tell whether one finger has been moved to up or down position by partner/teacher; cannot stabilize arms and trunk against much resistance (approximately age 7½).	• Children do tug of war while standing, sitting, and lying down. • Encourage pressure on joints through resistance: walrus, crab, seal walk, wheelbarrow race, crawling with partner facing child and pushing against shoulders, stretching inner tubes, partners trying to force wrists together or apart. • Compression of joints through jumping, leaping, trampoline, and bouncing board.
Has poorly developed sense of rhythm. Awkwardly performs rapid alternating motions using opposite muscle groups.	• Rhythm band, marching, dancing, musical activities, and Lummi sticks. • Provide definite, clear auditory rhythm signal (drum or triangle beat) with each separate motion response. This may need to be accompanied by touch/pressure clue. Example: angels in snow movements slowly to beat of metal triangle, with touch to appropriate limb for those children who need this extra clue. • Child performs rapid opposing motions on signal or to beat of music: palms down, palms up index finger touch tip of nose, tip of finger held at arm's length tongue protrudes straight forward, retracts into mouth protruding tongue touches one side of open mouth, then opposite side child repeatedly says sound "puh, puh, puh" or "buh, buh, buh" or "tuh, tuh, tuh" heel-toe, heel-toe tap while sitting, standing.
Does not know right/left on self with eyes closed (approximately age 8); right/left on facing person (approximately age 9½).	• Point out freckle or tiny scar on child's right or left hand to help in discrimination. • Child identifies randomly distributed right and left hand/foot cutouts. • Footsie Game. Advance player on game board number of spaces written on correctly identified foot "playing card" drawn from pack.

If these behaviors are observed	*Try these activities, strategies or materials*
	• Zip Zap. (Circle Game. Zip means name right neighbor, Zap means name left neighbor. Encourage speed.) • Blindfold one child. Others give verbal directions to lead child to target, e.g., three steps to right, two steps backwards, two steps to left. • Use facing pairs of objects such as trucks, TV sets, chairs, to demonstrate and quiz diagonal aspect of right and left before applying labels to right or left of facing object. *Later* teach right and left on facing persons.

REFLEX DEVELOPMENT AND BALANCE SKILLS

As early primitive postural reflexes decrease in importance, the normally developing child acquires more advanced balance skills which allow automatic equilibrium responses. These responses first develop with the infant in a lying down position, then in sitting and kneeling on hands and knees, and finally in standing and walking positions. Training for delayed balance skills should proceed in the same developmental sequence. Early behaviors are generally, although not absolutely, prerequisite to later behaviors and should be mastered first. Grade school children with good balance skills have good head and trunk stability while sitting and/or standing, walk with feet close together and with hands swinging reciprocally at sides, and hop, jump, leap, and walk a balance beam easily.

If these behaviors are observed	*Try these activities, strategies, or materials*
Has very inadequate sitting balance and difficulty "leading with the head" when rolling.	• Log and egg rolls, somersaults on mats or down inclines. (Make more difficult up incline, against resistance, or holding beanbag between knees.) • Move head separate from body in backlying position to look in various directions on cue, including looking at toes without lifting back.
Is unable to lie on stomach on small pillow and hold head, shoulders, arms, knees and toes off floor (for 10 seconds, approximately age 5½).	• Back raises with feet held; leg raises with trunk held. Kraus Weber position. Push ups. • Scooter board activities on stomach.
Is unable to curl up in a ball while lying on back and hold head, arms, feet off floor (for 10 seconds, approximately age 5½).	• With chin on chest and arms folded, child kicks ball across floor with sole of foot, kicks balloon over short "net," rides bicycle motion with legs while hips off floor, blows tissue off chest. • Child rides gym scooter on back, with head and feet up, using hands to pull forward on suspended rope or ladder rungs.

If these behaviors are observed	*Try these activities, strategies, or materials*
	• On monkey bars and jungle gyms, child attains and then holds upside down, curled up position while looking forward.
Cannot stand from back-lying position almost symmetrically (approximately age 5½ or 6). Must turn nearly onto stomach or hands-knees position before reaching standing.	• From back-lying child quickly jumps up and runs or moves to goal or target with minimal trunk rotation. • From standing position child stoops, reaches for object across midline, picks it up from floor, and returns to standing position.
Squirms or readjusts posture often in sitting position. Has difficulty sitting on unsteady or tipsy equipment, especially if not holding on.	• Child seat walks on buttocks—race or stunt. • Play musical chairs on tipsy seats, no hands. • Partners sit back to back, lock elbows, then try to stand. Partners face each other, hold hands and touch soles of feet while rocking far forward and backward. • Child sits on and rides swing, seesaw, sliding board, barrel lying on its side, board with hubcap screwed under it so curve touches floor, scooterboard, one rope swing.
Has difficulty balancing in hands and knees position on unsteady surface or in three-point position (one hand or foot raised), especially if head is turned toward one side.	• In hands and knees position child rocks forward and backward, head facing forward. With forehead, taps suspended ball so it hits target on wall or knocks over bowling pins on chair. • Vary head position during hands and knees balance activities so eyes look at targets forward and at either side. • In hands and knees position child rocks side to side or uses one hand or knee to push ball or beanbag to goal. • Place color card (or vocabulary word, letter or number) under each hand and knee. Instruct child to "lift yellow (or #7) hand (knee) and hold for 5 seconds." Advance to lifting two limbs, later three.
Is unable to jump in place, climb stairs one foot per tread without holding on, squat or briefly tiptoe (approximately age 4).	• Child jumps off of short, then taller objects, then jumps over flat, then taller obstacles. • Child runs up incline and jumps off in various directions and postures. • All teachers and parents cooperate to remind child about one foot per stair tread.

If these behaviors are observed	*Try these activities, strategies, or materials*
	• Stunts or musical games encourage squatting (ducklike), walking on tiptoes (fairies and tall people), and jumping (over imaginary brooks, obstacles).
Cannot heel-toe walk, broad jump, hop on one foot briefly, descend stairs one foot per tread without holding on (approximately age 5).	• Play potato-on-a-spoon race, dodgeball with plastic beach ball, hopscotch with two feet and later one foot, potato sack race, hopping tag, and trampoline. • Child heel-toe walks on tape, fat rope, balance beam, and side of ladder.
Does not try roller skates, stilts, jump rope (approximately age 6). Cannot high jump 8 inches, broad jump 3 feet.	• Introduce skates, coffee can stilts, wooden pole stilts, jump rope (first teacher turns, later self-turning occurs).
Is unable to crouch on tiptoes (approximately age 8), jump clapping hands three times (approximately age 9), hop 50 feet in 5 seconds (approximately age 12).	• Advanced balance beam activities. • Simple track and field events.

COORDINATION OF THE TWO BODY SIDES

This skill indicates the body's motoric ability to function as a whole. Developing children first initiate purposeful movement with both arms/legs similarly, and later reciprocally (i.e., with one limb after another in steady rhythm). Children also first perform movements without crossing the body's midline (a theoretical plane or line drawn from the center of the forehead straight down to a point between the feet), and later with midline crossing. It is recommended that training of motorically-delayed children proceed in the same sequence. Children having good coordination of the two body sides have adequately established hand dominance with adequate assist by the nondominant hand; spontaneous crossing of the midline when appropriate; and smooth, coordinated patterns of walking, running, and skipping.

If these behaviors are observed	*Try these activities, strategies, or materials*
Is unable to creep, tummy off floor, with opposing hand and knee moving almost simultaneously (approximately age of 12 months).	• Bunny hopping with two knees moving ahead simultaneously is an immature pattern which should be discouraged in the school-aged youngster. • Child creeps facing target at eye level, hands and tops of feet flat on floor, and pointing straight (not away from or toward midline of body). See *The Bender-Purdue Reflex Test & Training Manual.*[2]

If these behaviors are observed	*Try these activities, strategies, or materials*
	• As correct reciprocal pattern of arm/leg movement develops, add resistance to forward movement at the shoulders and ankles. Resist backward creeping at the buttocks. • Introduce puppy, kitty, and wild animal walks and races, and obstacle courses.
Walks and runs without opposing, reciprocal arm and leg movements (approximately age 4).	• If hands are held at shoulder level during walking/running, train balance skills. • Invert tricycle. Child rotates wheel with reciprocal hand motion on pedals. • Child pulls rope, hand-over-hand, to move gym scooter seat toward goal, to lift weighted pulley rope. Pedal gym scooter with hands moving reciprocally. • Introduce tricycles, pedal cars, Big Wheels, Sit 'n' Spin, Irishmail cart.
Cannot gallop, sashay, slide-step well, or skip with one foot only (lame duck skip) (approximately age 5).	• Encourage reciprocal hand and foot rhythms: xylophone, bongo drums, Ali Babba and the Forty Thieves, wheelbarrow walk, step-together-step sideways to music. • New skills may have to be taught and learned with two hands moving together first, later hands moving reciprocally. • Teach component skill parts of gallop, sashay, slide-step, lame duck skip, and crab walk.
Inaccurately imitates pantomimed midline crossing postures (approximately age 5). Avoids spontaneous midline crossing.	• Play Simon Says with midline crossing, Lummi sticks, crepe paper humming lasso motions, target throws across midline (also during scooter rides), partner hand-clap games (Peas porridge, Miss Mary Mack, Oh Little Playmate, Pretty Little Dutch Girl), folk dancing steps (Heel-toe cross over; grapevine). • Hurry-Hurry Relay (team game: pass each of many items, two hands together, sideways to team mates until all items reach winning bucket). • Child taps suspended ball sideways with palms. Advance to backs of hands, then palms when arms crossed. • Child creeps along rope or line with knees straddling, hands crossed to opposite side. If necessary, give touch clue to indicate next hand movement.

If these behaviors are observed	*Try these activities, strategies, or materials*
Cannot skip alternately and exhibits much difficulty learning to throw a ball with proper weight shift onto foot opposite the throwing arm (approximately age 6½).	• Skipping: teach slow step-hop pattern on each foot. Place straight rope between feet, or place one foot on board, one foot on floor. Thus child can see and feel difference between the two feet and can begin to predict the feel of the slow step-hop rhythm. (If the board on which one foot practices step-hop is unsteady and clatters on the floor with each step-hop, it gives an additional auditory clue.) Teach reciprocal arm rhythm simultaneous to step-hop by moving arms correctly for the child. • Introduce component skills of throwing, pitching, and catching.
Has not established good hand dominance (approximately age 6½ or 7).	• Check for assymmetry of discrimination in identifying small objects by touch; in recognizing shapes drawn on hand; in recognizing which finger is touched. Train accordingly. (Hand that doesn't feel things adequately may "refuse" to accept dominant role.) • Check again for midline crossing. If each hand works independently only on its own side of the body, neither accepts dominant role.
Cannot perform good jumping jacks or tap floor alternately with feet (approximately age 7). Cannot hop alternately 2 right—2 left or 3 right—1 left foot patterns (approximately age 8). Cannot throw small ball 40 to 60 feet (approximately age 9).	• Child performs angels in snow, jumping jacks and commando crawl (tummy touching floor) with variety of specified arm/leg movements. • Introduce advanced reciprocal hand/foot rhythms, slowly advancing up to need for balance while performing. Sample sequence: 2 right, 2 left rhythm on xylophone 2-2 stamp of feet while sitting 2-2 stamp of feet while standing 2-2 hop *once* while holding teacher's two hands 2-2 hop *once* without holding hands 2-2 hop several times, holding hands 2-2 hop several times, not holding hands • Child bounces ball in pattern or 2 right-2 left or 3 right-1 left.

EYE-HAND COORDINATION

Good eye-hand coordination is seen in the child who cuts, writes, works puzzles, manipulates small materials, and performs motor self-care activities age appropriately and with a good dominant/assistive hand use pattern. Behaviors are listed approximately by degree of difficulty (i.e., in the sequence in which they are normally acquired). Success in more difficult classroom behaviors can be expected only if earlier levels have been mastered.

If these behaviors are observed	*Try these activities, strategies, or materials*
Is unable to focus on object with both eyes as it moves nearer to and farther from face (convergence).	• Teacher or other child slowly moves straw as child tries to put toothpick inside. • Child tries Forward Pass ball-on-rope toy by Developmental Learning Materials.
Is unable to follow moving object (with eyes only, head not moving) thru 160° arc vertically, horizontally, diagonally, and in a circle. Eyes do not move smoothly and together. (Be sure visual acuity has been examined. Persistent or exceptional ocular problems should be referred to a vision specialist.)	• Child tries ball activities using first balloons, large plastic beach balls, whiffle balls, and later large playground balls, then firmer balls, then smaller balls. • Coat-hanger bats for balloons can be made by stretching nylon stockings over hanger pulled to square shape.
Does not poke finger into small hole. Is clumsy in picking up small items between thumb and index finger.	• Child places small objects into and fishes them out of small necked container. This can be timed. • Child tears—tissue (easiest), paper, manila folder, rag (hardest)—while holding between thumb and index finger. • Pinch and squeeze seeds or small discs (toward target), clothespins, and metal clips.
Has difficulty using wrist in side-to-side movements and palms-up/palms-down rotation. Grasps without wrist slightly extended.	• Child rings handbells, turns doorknobs, and unlocks with keys. • Child unscrews nuts and bolts, bicycle spokes from their end-casings or lids from small photo-film can containers.
Balances poorly on floor and chair so hands and forearms are not free to develop manipulative skills.	• Train sitting balance.
Has difficulty rolling clay into snake shape, later ball shape. Is clumsy when pasting, gluing, using even large paint brush, throwing ball with voluntary release. Displays generally inadequate eye-hand coordination in spite of adequacy in previously mentioned eye-hand behaviors.	• Child practices spreading fingers apart and squeezing them together while they are *straight.* * squeeze tiny sponges, eye droppers between fingers squeeze cardboard between straight fingers or finger and thumb so it cannot easily be pulled away spread rubberband wide with straight fingers suddenly spread apart straight fingers without moving wrist, and knock beads or blocks off desk. • Finger plays: Inky Dinky Spider; church and steeple.*

* Fine motor dexterity activities.

If these behaviors are observed	*Try these activities, strategies, or materials*
	• Child walks balloon up and down wall with fingertips. Advance to small plastic ball, Ping-Pong, golf, and playground balls.* • Look for body scheme difficulty and train accordingly.* • Introduce coloring accurately, dot-to-dot, tracing, mazes, lacing cards, pipe cleaners, beads, jacks, chalkboard road (trace on, wet fingers on, wet paintbrush on).† • Child glues outline of letters, then sprinkles on glitter.† • Squirts out lit candle with water pistol.† • Pastes tiny things accurately (e.g., holes punched) using toothpicks.† • Try commercial games such as Perfection, Numbers Up, Drop in the Bucket, Pick Up Sticks, Operation, Etch a Sketch, Cross Fire.† • Child traces on graph paper through empty squares as directed (right, left, up, down); guesses letter reproduced.†
Has not established use of one dominant hand at a time with other hand helping, e.g., in stringing large beads, later small beads; folding paper with definite crease (although inaccurately).	• All of the above activities plus Origami paper folding. • Look for and train problems in coordination of two body sides.
Does not reach across midline of body spontaneously to pick up and put down objects.	• Look for and train problems in coordination of two body sides.
Has difficulty making tower of 9- or 10-inch-cubes, or 3-cube bridge (approximately age 4) or placing small pegs in pegboard holes.	• Child practices block building, pegboards, and copying simple models. • Look for and train visual perception problems.
Cannot copy | — or ○ holding crayon/pencil with appropriate grip and using good assistance of nondrawing hand (approximately age 4).	• Use plastic, three-sided pencil grippers for correct and comfortable pencil position (from Developmental Learning Materials). • Encourage correct grip in all pencil, crayon, and painting activities. • Move arm, later hand, through correct motion on chalkboard, paper, and fingerpaint.
Cannot unbutton accessible buttons (approximately age 4).	• Emphasize self-help skills, breaking each into component parts.

* Fine motor dexterity activities.

† Eye-hand coordination activities. (Can be adapted to all later age activities.)

If these behaviors are observed	*Try these activities, strategies, or materials*
Does not use hands reciprocally.	• Look for and train coordination of two body sides difficulty. • Child winds thread on spool evenly, sharpens pencil, uses manual egg beater.
Is unable to cut paper fringe (approximately age 4). (All cutting activities are listed developmentally here. Actually more advanced cutting skills develop in conjunction with more advanced eye-hand coordination skills.)	• Use four-holed scissors which can be held by both child and teacher. • Introduce cutting tasks in sequence listed under Behaviors. • Encourage: elbow near waist, not away from body wrist slightly extended, not slightly flexed palm facing midline or face, not floor all fingers flexed while cutting, not extended and wide apart scissors held comfortably and consistently in thumb-finger position, preferably near knuckle of thumb but near middle of middle finger assisting hand adjusting paper position to scissors, not cutting hand adjusting position to paper.
Is unable to cut across paper, generally following straight, later curved line.	• Prevents jagged edges by placing paper against center of X.
Is unable to cut out simple shapes having very wide outlines and no sharp angles.	• Child cuts slowly, rotating paper slowly.
Is unable to cut out small ○, △, ▭, □.	• Encourage accuracy.
Is unable to cut cloth.	• Grade up from thin to heavier cloth.
Is unable to cut out complex pictures following outlines.	• Look for and train visual figure-ground problems.
Has great difficulty bouncing and catching large playground ball (approximately age 5); accurately tapping swinging suspended ball two out of five tries (approximately age 7).	• Teach handball skills in sequence of throw, catch, bounce and catch, toss and catch, and strike. • Teach foot-eye skills in sequence of kick, run and kick, and catch with feet.
Cannot put 10 pellets into bottle in 25 seconds (approximately age 5); 20 coins into open box, one at a time, in 16 seconds (approximately age 7).	• Encourage speed of fine motor response.
Is unable to copy +, /, \, □, × (approximately age 5).	• Walk outlined shapes on floor. Then use templates of straight line plus simple geometric forms.

If these behaviors are observed	*Try these activities, strategies, or materials*
	Begin with chalkboard size; advance to desk size.
Cannot draw unmistakable 6-part man including body (approximately age 5).	• Look for and train other indications of body image difficulties.
Cannot oppose thumb and each finger tip sequentially while looking at fingers, even slowly and with similar but incomplete movements of opposite hand (approximately age 5); is unable to do this competently (approximately age 7).	• Encourage competency, later speed in this skill.
With inch cubes, is unable to reproduce 6-block pyramid and gate (approximately age 4½); copy △, ✳ (approximately age 6).	• Look for and train other indications of visual perception problems.
Hand dominance has not been established (approximately age 6½ or 7).	• Look for and train problems in coordination of two body sides.
Is unable to copy many letters and numbers (approximately age 6).	• Encourage correct position of pencil and child's body. Paper position may vary with child's preference, but should be consistent. • For most learning disabled children, cursive handwriting is easier to master than manuscript. • If child forms letters consistently better with eyes closed, allow child initially to learn feel of making each letter without the need for placing it on lines or tracing letter shapes. Later child can learn to visually direct hand. • Use salt tray, heavy crayon tracing, VAKT (Visual Auditory, Kinesthetic Tactile System developed by Fernald[3]). • Use Dubnoff School Programs 1, 2 and 3 by Teaching Resources Company. • Read pages 107–122 in *Teaching Children with Learning and Behavior Problems.*[4]
Is unable to reproduce letters and numbers from memory.	• Encourage visual memory and imagery as well as adequate visual perception. • Read pages 191–247 in *Aids to Psycholinguistic Teaching.*[5]
Has not resolved letter and number inversions (approximately age 6) or b-d, p-q reversals (approximately age 7). Tries to write or read in right to left direction.	• Mark frequently confused letters for easier discrimination, e.g., put a "stinger" (b) on all b's to represent buzzing bee. • Use nondominant index finger to point out direction of pencil movement, e.g., left index finger

If these behaviors are observed	*Try these activities, strategies, or materials*
	points toward round movement for right hander's b ( ), 6 ( ), 3 ( ). • Put arrow pointing to right in upper left hand page corner indicating left-right progression. • Encourage right-left body part discrimination.

REFERENCES

1. Cratty, B.: Developmental Sequences of Perceptual-Motor Tasks. Educational Activities, Freeport NY, 1967.
2. Bender, M.: The Bender-Purdue Reflex Test and Training Manual. San Rafael CA: Academic Therapy Publications, 1975.
3. Fernald, G.: Remedial Techniques in Basic School Subjects. New York: McGraw-Hill Book Co., 1943.
4. Hammill, D., and Bartel, N.: Teaching Children with Learning and Behavior Problems. Boston: Allyn & Bacon, 1975.
5. Bush, W. I., and Giles, M.: Aids to Psycholinguistic Teaching. Columbus OH: Charles E. Merrill Co., 1969.

ADDRESSES

Developmental Learning Materials
7440 Natchez Avenue
Niles, Illinois 60648

Dubnoff School Programs (1 and 2*)
Teaching Resources Corporation
100 Boylston Street
Boston, Massachusetts 02116

The Bender-Purdue Reflex Test and Training Manual
Academic Therapy Publications
P.O. Box 899
San Rafael, California 94901

* 1 (for writing skills) and 2 (for pattern board perceptual exercises).

ACKNOWLEDGMENTS

Thanks to Thomas DiRenzo, physical education teacher, for his contribution to the game and activity suggestions.

Glossary

A.A.M.D. American Association on Mental Deficiency

Accommodation. the response or the motor process of adjusting the body to react to the incoming stimulation

Achievement motivation. the will to perform or to achieve, using some standard

Low achievement motivation: minimal will to try

High achievement motivation: high level of performance

A.C.L.D. Association of children with Learning Disabilities: a non-profit organization, whose purpose is to advance the education and general welfare of children with normal or potentially normal intelligence who have learning disabilities of a perceptual, conceptual, or coordinative nature

Acquisitional. referring to behaviors, attitudes, and ideas which have been learned through experience

Acting out. action rather than verbal response to unconscious drives or impulses; brings temporary relief of tension-situation; may be a substitute for the impulse that originally gave rise to the action.

Active listening. in conversation or interview, attending carefully to what is said by the other—awareness of both verbal and nonverbal communication

Adaptation. any change in structure, form, or habits of an organism to suit a new environment—in reflex action, decline in the frequency of impulses when the sensory nerve is stimulated repeatedly; in psychiatry, those changes experienced by an individual which lead to adjustment

Adaptive behavior. manner with which the individual deals with the cultural, social, physical, and mental demands of the environment

Adaptive skills. learned patterns of behavior which enable the individual to fulfill his/her own needs and the needs of others

Addiction. habit of drug (or alcohol) use, in which the addicted individual has symptoms of distress when deprived of the drug and the irresistible impulse to take the drug

Adolescence. stage of the life cycle lasting from onset of puberty until psychological and biological maturity is reached

Adulthood. stage of the life cycle that begins when the individual attains biological and psychological maturity and ends with the gradual onset of old age

AE. above elbow

Affect. emotional feeling tone-inner feelings and external manifestation-mood

Aggression. forceful, goal-directed behavior
Agitation. motor restlessness with anxiety
Agnosia. loss of comprehension of auditory, visual, or other sensations although the sensory sphere is intact; inability to recognize an object
Agonist. the muscle directly engaged in contraction as distinguished from muscles that have to relax at the same time
AJOT. American Journal of Occupational Therapy
AK. above knee
Akinesia. absence or diminution of voluntary motion
Alienation. feelings of detachment from self, others, or society in general; avoidance of emotional experiences
Alimentation. giving nourishment
Alloplastic. changing or moving things other than self; the external environment
Amaurosis. partial or total blindness from any cause
Amblyopia. lazy eye; dimness of vision, especially that not caused by refractive errors or organic disease of the eye; may be congenital or acquired
Amnesia, anterograde. loss of memory of events after an injury
Amnesia, retrograde. loss of memory of events immediately preceding injury
Amniocentesis. removal of fluid containing fetal cells from the amniotic sac. The fluid is analyzed relative to metabolic disorders and chromosomal content.
Amphetamine. a central nervous system stimulant
Amputation. cutting off of a limb or part of a limb, the breast, or other projecting part
Amyotrophic lateral sclerosis (ALS). a degenerative disease of the pyramidal tracts and lower motor neurons, characterized by motor weakness and a spastic condition of the limbs associated with muscular atrophy, fibrillary twitching, and final involvement of nuclei in the medulla
Anal phase. second stage of psychosexual development (ages 1-3); interests, activities, and pleasure centered in anal zone
Anastomosis. a natural communication, direct or indirect, between two blood vessels or other tubular structures; an operative union of two hollow or tubular structures, as divided ends of intestine or blood vessels
Anergia. lack of energy, passivity
Aneurysm. circumscribed dilation of an artery or a blood-containing tumor connecting directly with the lumen of an artery
Animism. belief that inanimate objects are alive
Ankylosis. natural fixation of a joint; abnormal immobilization of a joint caused by destruction of articular cartilage enabling bony surfaces to fuse
Anoxia. oxygen deficiency
ANSI. American National Standards Institute
Antagonist. certain muscles opposing or resisting the action of others
Antecedent. refers to that which goes before; preceding circumstance, event, or condition
Anxiety. unpleasurable affect, with physiological and psychological changes; real external danger or threat does not exist; feelings of impending danger, powerlessness, tension, and readiness for expected danger
Apgar test. objective test of newborn's health
Aphasia. impairment or loss in ability to receive or to express verbal symbols or ideas; speech and hearing mechanism may be intact
Appendicular. relating to the limbs, as opposed to axial which refers to the trunk and head
Apraxia. inability to perform purposeful voluntary movements, the nature and mechanism of which are understood in the absence of motor or sensory impairment
A.R.A. The Association of Retarded Citizens: a parent-founded non-profit association which promotes the general welfare of retarded citizens by encouraging research, advising parents, developing better understanding of retardation by the public, distributing information, and raising funds
Arteriosclerosis. hardening of the arteries
Arthrodesis. fusion of a joint by removing the articular surfaces and securing bony union; operative ankylosis; the surgical fixation of a joint
Arthroplasty. surgical formation of a joint
Artificialism. belief that an action was a result of an outside agent
Art therapy. treatment technique using spontaneous creative work of patients to explore and analyze and express underlying emotional problems
Assimilation. sensory process of "taking in" or receiving information that is external to and/or within the self system
Association. the organized process of relating the sensory information with the motor act and or relating present and past experiences with each other
Astereognosis. loss of the power of judging the form of an object by touch
Asymmetrical. denoting a lack of symmetry between two or more parts
Ataxia. incoordination of voluntary muscle movements, particularly those used in reaching and walking
Atresia. congenital absence or pathological closure of a normal opening, passage, or cavity
Atrophic, atrophy. pertaining to a wasting of tissues, organs, or the entire body
Audiometrist. one who evaluates a person's hearing

qualitatively and quantitatively by use of an audiometer

Audit. an official examination and verification of accounts and records

Autition. acoustic ability; hearing

Autogenic. autogenetic; self-producing

Autonomic nervous system (A.N.S.). part of nervous system functioning outside of consciousness—directs, for example, breathing, heart rate, and digestion

Autonomy. quality of being self-governing and self-determining (striving toward independence)

Autoplastic. changing or moving one's self

Aversive. causing strong feelings of repugnance, distaste, dislike, or displeasure

Axial. relating to or situated in the central part of the body, in the head or trunk as distinguished from the extremities

Axon. the essential conducting portion of a nerve fiber continuous with the cytoplasm of a nerve cell

Barbiturate. highly addictive CNS depressant (ex. phenobarbitol, pentothal)

Basal ganglia. the basal nuclei of the endbrain (telencephalon)

BE. below elbow

Biofeedback. technique in which patient is made aware of unconscious or involuntary physiological processes and learns to control them

BK. below knee

Body image. conscious or unconscious image of one's body (including function); sum of all feelings concerning the body

Body language. system by which a person expresses feelings and thoughts through posture, gesture, and/or movement

Body scheme. refers to the automatic adjustment of skeletal parts and to the tensing and relaxing of muscles necessary to maintain a position

Boutonniere deformity. PIP flexion with DIP hyperextension

Breech delivery. presentation of the buttocks instead of the head in childbirth

Carpal tunnel syndrome. compression of the median nerve in the carpal tunnel at the wrist causing thenar atrophy and paralysis as well as trophic changes of the finger tips and sensory disturbance of the first three fingers

Catabolic phase. breaking down in the body of complex chemical compounds into simpler ones, often accompanied by the liberation of energy

Cataracts. partial or complete opacity of the crystalline lens or its capsule

Catchment area. a defined geographical area, representing a specified number of people to be served by a mental health center

Catharsis. release of ideas, thoughts, repressed materials from the unconscious, with emotional responses and release of tension (psychoanalytical term)

Causalgia. a neuralgia distinguished by a burning pain along certain nerves

C.E.C. Council of Exceptional Children: an associated organization of the National Education Association, for the advancement of education of exceptional children and youth, both gifted and handicapped

Centering. ability to focus on only one aspect of situation at a time

Cerebellum. the posterior brain mass; it consists of two lateral hemispheres united by a narrow middle portion

Cerebral contusion. bruising to brain causing diffuse disturbance with edema and hemorrhage and destruction of brain tissue

Cervical. pertaining to the neck and the eight cervical vertebrae

Cesarean section. removal of the fetus by means of an incision into the uterus, usually by way of the abdominal wall

Chaining. in behavior therapy, the process by which behavioral patterns are learned by reinforcements given for behaviors which are associated or related to an established behavior

Childhood. stage of the life cycle lasting from the end of infancy until the onset of puberty

Chromosomes. the bodies in the cell nucleus which carry the genes

Circ-o-lectric bed. a circular frame containing a bed on which a patient can lie and be passively positioned from supine to prone on an 180 degree axis, by an electric mechanism. The patient can be tilted at any angle on the axis.

CMHC. community mental health center

C.N.S. central nervous system

Cocontraction. contraction of the agonist and antagonist muscles to provide stability

Cognition. the conscious process of awareness and knowledge of objects through perception, memory, and reasoning; mental process of knowing and understanding; an ego function—thinking, judgment

Cognitive development. the development of a logical method of looking at the world; knowing and understanding

Collagen fibers. protein of the white fibers of connective tissue, cartilage, and bone

Compensation. a process in which a tendency for change in a given direction is counteracted by another change so that the original change is not evident; an unconscious mechanism by which an individual tries to make up for fancied or real deficiencies

Competence. quality of adequacy or possession of required skill, knowledge, or capacity

Conceptual. referring to the formation or construct of ideas and thoughts

Conceptual model. an organization of theoretical constructs or of knowledge upon which a frame of reference for action can be based

Concrete operations. the third stage in Piagetian theory during which the seven- to eleven-year old begins to think logically although thinking is still limited to what is seen

Conditioning. procedure used to alter behavior
classical: through pairing of stimuli to evoke response
operant: through presentation of reinforcements

Confidentiality. medical ethics, holding secret information which a patient has divulged

Conflict. clash of two opposing emotional forces

Conjugate deviation. forced and persistent turning of the eyes and head toward one side; observed with some lesions of the cerebrum

Conscious. (as a noun) that part of the mind which is experienced in awareness (psychoanalytical)

Consensual validation. comparison of thoughts, feelings, and perceptions with others—results in effective reality testing (Harry Stack Sullivan term)

Conservation. a cognitive ability as described by Piaget as occurring with concrete operations; the time when a child begins to understand physical properties of matter equivalence

Constancy. property of remaining the same, as in perceptual constancy, in which things are perceived as unchanged in form even if position or distance may change

Contract. explicit agreement to a well-defined course of action, as in therapy or in supervision

Contracture. a permanent muscular contraction resulting from tonic spasm or loss of muscular equilibrium, the antagonists being paralyzed

Contralateral. originating in or affecting the opposite side of the body

Coordination. the harmonious working together of several muscles or muscle groups in the execution of complicated movements; the working together of different systems of the body in a given process as the coordination between the system of glands and involuntary muscles in digestion

Cortex. the layer of gray matter which invests the surface of the cerebral hemispheres and the cerebellum

Countertransference. conscious or unconscious responses of therapist to the patient, determined by therapist's need; transferred feelings, not necessarily relevant to the real situation (psychoanalytical)

Crisis intervention. brief therapeutic encounter in time, with limited structure, aimed at amelioration of symptoms

Crossed diagonal. a highly integrated pattern with flexion of the upper extremities and extension of the lower extremities on the face side with extension of the upper limbs with flexion of the lower limbs on the opposite side (reciprocal)

Cutaneous. relating to the skin

C.V.A. cerebrovascular accident, a lesion in the brain resulting in paralysis of contralateral side of the body

Cyanosis. a dark-bluish or purplish discoloration of the skin and mucous membrane resulting from deficient oxygenation of the blood

Cytomegalic inclusion disease. caused by the cytomegalovirus, transmitted transplacentally to the fetus from a mother with a latent infection

Dance therapy. technique of using movement and nonverbal communication to aid in rehabilitation; may be group or individual

Debride. to remove (surgically) foreign or devitalized tissue

DB-decibel. a tenth of a bel, a unit frequently used to measure the intensity of sound

Decerebrate rigidity. forceful extension of all joints of the lower extremities, and extension and internal rotation of the upper extremities; caused by brain stem contusion

Decubitus ulcer. a defect of the surface of an organ or tissue caused by prolonged pressure (also known as a bedsore or a pressure sore)

Defense mechanism. unconscious intrapsychic process (ego defenses) to relieve anxiety and conflict from unconscious drives which are not acceptable; includes conversion, denial, displacement, dissociation, idealization, identification, incorporation, intellectualization, introjection, projection, rationalization, reaction formation, regression, repression, sublimation, substitution, symbolization, transference, and undoing

Deformity. congenital or acquired unnatural distortion or malformation of a part of the body

Degenerative disease. progressive deterioration of tissue, particularly true of diseases of the central nervous system

Degenerative joint disease. a degenerative, noninflammatory, localized form of arthritis which causes breakdown of cartilage and results in limitation of motion and formation of bony outgrowths at the joints affected (osteoarthritis)

Denial. unconscious defense mechanism in which an aspect of external reality is blocked from awareness

Dependency. the state of needing someone or something for support

Depersonalization. sense of unreality about self, others, and environment

Deprivation. a negative reinforcement used to weaken or eliminate an undesired action

Desensitization. reciprocal inhibition (Wolpe); person is conditioned to associate comfortable, supportive surroundings with anxiety-producing stimuli and gradually learns to reduce the adverse effects.

Development. changes in the structure, thought, or behavior of a person which occur as a function of both biological and environmental influences (which may be quantitative or qualitative)

Developmental disability. the result of any condition, trauma, deprivation, or disease which interrupts or delays the sequence and rate of normal growth, development, and maturation

Developmental sequence. an established progression pattern of growth and development

Differentiation. the process of discriminating those essential elements of a specific behavior which are pertinent to a given situation, distinguishing those that are not, and thereby modifying or altering the behavior in some manner

DIP. joint. distal interphalangeal joint

Diplegia. paralysis of similar parts on both sides of the body

Diplopia. perception of two images of a single object (double or binocular vision)

Disability rating. classification of loss of function

Disequilibrium. lack or destruction of equilibrium

Disintegration. psychic disorganization

Dislocation. displacement of a bone from its normal position in the joint

Disorientation. inability to judge time, space, and personal relationships

Displacement. unconscious defense mechanism in which the feeling-laden part of an unacceptable idea or object is transferred to an acceptable one

Dissociation. unconscious defense mechanism in which an idea is separated from its accompanying feeling tone

D.O.T. Dictionary of Occupational Titles

D.S.M. Diagnostic and Statistical Manual of Mental Disorders of the American Psychiatric Association

Dyadic. refers to relationship, as between two people—one-to-one

Dynamic splint. splint which allows for or provides motion. Motion is provided by transfer of motion from other body parts or by use of outside forces such as springs, rubberbands, carbon dioxide, or electricity

Dysarthria. motor speech deficit

Dysfunction. inability to perform and interact effectively with the environment; impairment of normal function of a body part or organ

Dyskinesia. impairment of voluntary movement

Dyspnea. shortness of breath

Eclectic. choosing from various sources; not following any single system or frame of reference; selecting and using the best elements of several systems

Edema. a condition in which the body tissues contain an excessive amount of tissue fluid. It may be local or general.

Efferent. conducting (fluid or a nerve impulse) outward or centrifugally

Ego. one of three components of psychic structure (with id and superego); mediates between instinctual drives and external reality demands (Freud)

Egocentric. preoccupied with one's own needs; self-centered; lacking interest in others

Ego functions. ego's management of defense mechanisms to meet person's needs—defense mechanisms mediating between id, superego, and reality; reality testing

Ego strength. effectiveness of ego functions. Strong ego can mediate between id, superego, and reality with enough flexibility to retain energy for creativity and other needs

Embolus. clot brought from a larger vessel to a smaller one causing obstruction

Empirical. founded on practical experience but not proved scientifically; based on observable fact or objective experience

Encephalitis. inflammation of the brain

Encopresis. incontinence of feces

Encounter group. a form of sensitivity training, experiencing individual relationships within a group; focuses on present (J. L. Moreno)

Endocept. intrapsychic primitive organization of perceptions, memory traces, and images; preverbal; cannot be shared, experienced vaguely (Arieti)

Engrams. mnemic hypothesis—the theory that stimuli or irritants leave definite traces on neruons

ENT. ears, nose, and throat

Enuresis. bedwetting

Environment. a composite of all external forces and influences affecting the development and maintenance of an individual

Epicritic function. denoting a set or system of sensory nerve fibers, supplying the skin and oral mucosa, enabling one to appreciate the finer degrees of the sensation of touch, pain, and temperature and to localize same; distinguished from protopathic

Epithelium. tissue composed of contiguous cells with a minimum of intercellular substance

Equilibration. process of finding a balance between accommodation and assimilation

Equilibrium. a state of balance or equality between opposing forces; bodily stability or balance
Equilibrium reactions. bodily reactions to retain state of balance in relation to gravity
Erythema. a redness of the skin occurring in patches of variable size and shape
Erythemia. a condition characterized by an increased number of red blood cells; polycythemia
Eschar. a thick coagulated crust or slough which develops following a thermal burn or cauterization of the skin
Escharatomy. an incision in a burn eschar to lessen constriction of a distal part
Etiology. study of causes of a disease
Euphoria. a sense of well-being; the absence of pain or stress which might be exaggerated
Exacerbation. an aggravation of symptoms of a disease
Excitatory. stimulating, increasing the rapidity of the physical or mental processes
Existential psychotherapy. treatment which puts emphasis on here-and-now—confrontation and feeling experiences; based on philosophy that one has responsibility for one's own existence
Exocepts. images (intrapsychic) of actions, movement; kinesthetic-proprioceptive images (Arieti)
Expressive aphasia. impairment of the ability to use speech and to write communicatively
External powered flexor-hinge splint. use of an outside source to provide power for prehension
Exteroceptive. outside the organism, e.g., sense organ of the skin located on the surface of the body
Extrapyramidal. referring to central nervous system control of involuntary motor behavior
Extrinsic motivation. will to act based on external standards or incentives
Extrinsic muscles. muscles which have their origin in some part of the trunk outside of the pelvic or shoulder girdle
Facilitator. a person who helps to make a process easier, assists progress toward a goal
Family therapy. treatment of family in conflict; focus is on interactions among all members, not on pathology of one
Fasciotomy. incision through a fascia, used in the treatment of certain vascular disorders when marked swelling is anticipated which could compromise blood flow
Fatigability. susceptibility to fatigue
Fear. unpleasurable feeling with psychological and physical changes in response to realistic threat or danger
Febrile. pertaining to or characterized by fever
Feedback. response to behavior
Festination gait. small-stepped shuffling gait seen in Parkinson's Disease; involuntary increase in momentum to compensate for displaced sense of center of gravity
Fibrillation. a small local involuntary contraction of muscle fibers
Fibroblasts. cells which synthesize mucopolysaccharides and collagen fibers necessary for the development of new connective tissue
Fibrotic. pertaining to or characterized by formation of fibrous tissue, usually as a reparative or reactive process
Field dependent. highly motivated to conform to standards or pressures which are external
Flaccid. relaxed, flabby, having defective or absent muscular tone
Flexor hinge. splint or surgery which is used to provide grasp function of the hand through stabilization of the interphalangeal joints of the first two fingers in slight flexion, the thumb in position of opposition, and providing movement at the metacarpophalangeal joint to effect prehension
Forearm orthosis. ballbearing feeder
Formal operations. the fourth and final stage of Piagetian theory beginning at twelve to fifteen years and characterized by logical thinking and a grasp of abstract concepts
Formative evaluation. along the way
Frame of reference. belief system based on conceptual models—in therapy, organized basis of theory, delineation of function and dysfunction, evaluation and treatment approaches, postulates regarding change
Froment's sign. flexion of the distal phalanx of the thumb when a sheet of paper is held between the thumb and index finger in ulnar nerve palsy
Functional treatment. relates to a specific function which has been lost and is being relearned or to a function which is being learned for the first time
Gastroschisis. a congenital defect in the abdominal wall, usually with protrusion of the viscera
Gavage feeding. feeding by a stomach tube
Gene. any portion of the chromosome which transmits hereditary characteristics
Genital phase. final stage of psychosexual development, during puberty; pleasure centered on genital to genital contact (Freud)
Geriatrics. physiology and pathology of old age
Gerontology. the study of later maturity and old age in its biological, psychological, and sociological aspects
Geropsychiatry. branch of psychiatry dealing with problems of the aged
Gestalt. an organized field that has unique properties which cannot be devised merely from the sum of its various component parts; the whole or total quality of the image

Gestalt therapy. psychotherapeutic technique focusing on treatment of person as a whole, focuses on here-and-now experience; use of role playing to promote individual or group growth (Frederick S. Perls)

Glaucoma. disease of the eye marked by heightened intraocular tension; may lead to blindness

Gliosis. proliferation of neurological tissue in the central nervous system

Grand mal. a complete epileptic seizure

Graphesthesia. recognition of the form of a number or letter drawn on the skin

Gray matter. substantia grisea; the ganglionic or cellular portion of the brain and spinal cord

Growth. biological/structural changes of the body; increase in size, function, or complexity up to some optimal point

GTO. Golgi tendon organ

Guillain-Barré syndrome. a spreading paralysis, sometimes reversible, with involvement of nerves, nerve roots, cord, brain and meninges, separately or combined

Gustatory. pertaining to the sense of taste

Habilitate. to educate or train (the mentally or physically handicapped, the disadvantaged) to function better in society

Habituation. the ability to become used to certain stimuli and no longer respond to them

Hallucination. false sensory perception without concrete external stimulus; may be visual, auditory, olfactory, gustatory, or tactile

Haptic. pertaining to touch; tactile

Hematoma. accumulation of blood within a tissue

Hemianopsia. blindness in one half of the visual field; may be bilateral or unilateral; also called hemiopia, hemianopia

Hemiparesis. muscular weakness of one side of the body

Hemiplegia. paralysis of one side of the body

Hemorrhage. bleeding, escape of blood from the vessels

Heuristic. quality that encourages further discovery or investigation

Histologically. dealing with the science of the minute structure of cells, tissues, and organs in relation to their function; microscopic anatomy

HMO. Health Maintenance Organization

Homeostasis. the maintenance of steady states in the organism by coordinated physiologic processes

Homolateral. ipsilateral pattern, with the head, thorax, and pelvis turned toward the flexing upper and lower extremities with extension of the contralateral extremities (camel walk)

Hyaline membrane disease. airlessness of the lungs, seen especially in premature neonates with respiratory distress; pulmonary collapse

Hydrocephalus. a condition marked by an excessive accumulation of fluid dilating the cerebral ventricles, thinning the brain, and causing a separation of cranial bones

Hydroureter nephrosis. distention of the ureter with urine because of blockage from any cause

Hyperactivity. excessive or increased activity

Hyperalimentation (HA). overfeeding, superalimentation, forcing of food upon a patient in excess of the demands of the appetite or of the nutritional needs of a person in health

Hyperesthesia. increased sensitivity to touch

Hyperplasia. rapid growth; abnormal increase of cells without formation of a tumor but with increase in size of an organ or part

Hypertension. tension or tonus above normal; a condition in which patient has a higher blood pressure than normal for his age

Hyperthermia. abnormally high fever; also hyperexia

Hypertonicity. hypertonia; an increased effective osmotic pressure of body fluids

Hypertrophic scarring. enlargement of the scar; excessive growth of the scar

Hypertrophy. the enlargement or growth of an organ or other part of the body; the growth is independent of natural growth and is caused by unnatural increase in the size of cells

Hypoesthesia. dulled sensitivity to touch

Hypotension. decrease of systolic and diastolic blood pressure below normal; deficiency in tonus or tension

Id. one of three components of psychic structure (with ego and superego); unconscious, unorganized, the seat of basic instinctual drives and energy (Freud)

Idealization. unconscious or conscious defense mechanism; person overestimates an attribute or aspect of another person

Ideational apraxia. inability to correlate purpose and accomplishment of tasks

Identification. unconscious defense mechanism in which a person patterns himself/herself after another (distinguished from imitation which is a conscious process)

Ideomotor apraxia. inability to imitate gestures or perform purposeful activities on command while retaining ability to perform automatic routine activities

Imitation. conscious process of patterning oneself after another

Impotence. inability to perform sexual intercourse; may be erective (inability to achieve erection); ejaculatory (inability to expel seminal fluid); or orgastic (inability to attain full orgasm)

Imprinting. the process by which animals develop a social attachment for a particular object

Incontinence. inability to retain urine or feces through the loss of sphincter control
Indwelling catheter. a catheter left in place in the bladder
Infancy. stage in the life cycle lasting from birth until approximately eighteen to 24 months
Inhibitory. restraining; tending to inhibit
Integration. the organization and incorporation into the personality and functioning of the individual of data and experience gained
Integrative. helping toward wholeness, organization of thoughts, feelings, and actions
Intelligence quotient. a number assigned to express intellectual capacity obtained by multiplying mental age by 100 and dividing by chronological age
Intension tremor. tremor precipitated or increased on attempt to perform a voluntary coordinated movement
Interoceptive. within viscera; inside the organism
Interstitial. situated between important parts; occupying the interspaces or interstices of a part
Intrinsic motivation. will to act based on personal internal standards, incentives, desires, and needs
Intrinsic muscles. muscles of the extremities whose origin and insertion are both in the same part of the limb (e.g., hand)
Intuitive thought. part of the preoperational period (approximately five to seven years of age) when a child is able to separate mental from physical reality and understand multiple points of view
Ipsilateral. on the same side; denoting especially paralytic or other symptoms occurring on the same side as the brain lesion causing them
Ischemia. local anemia or diminution in the blood supply resulting from obstruction of inflow of arterial blood or to vasoconstriction
IV. intravenous
Jacksonian. spasmodic contractions in certain groups of muscles or paroxysmal paresthesias in certain skin areas as a result of local disease of the cortex
Jaundice. a condition marked by yellow skin and eye whites, caused by changes in the liver cells or obstructions, which cause the bile pigment, bilirubin, to be diffused into the blood
Job tryout. placement of client on actual job in industry
Kinesthesia. the conscious perception of movement, weight, resistance, and position of a body part; also kinesthesis
Kirshner wire. an apparatus for skeletal traction in long bone fracture
Kyphosis. a convex backward curvature of the spine; humpback
Lability. state of being unstable, changeable, or having lack of emotional control
Laminectomy. surgical removal of the lamina or posterior arch of the vertebrae
Latency. a state of inactivity, where potential is hidden or dormant
Latency phase. stage of psychosexual development (age five to puberty) apparent cessation of sexual preoccupation (Freud)
L.E. lower extremity
Learning. relatively permanent change in behavior or in the capacity for behavior resulting from either experience or practice
Lesion. structural or functional alteration of a part caused by injury or disease
Libido. basic psychological energy inherent in every person; the energy supplies the sexual drive whose goal is to obtain pleasure (Freud)
Locus of control. the source or origin of direction of events (Rotter)
External locus of control: control of life events from outside oneself
Internal locus of control: control of life events by one's own thoughts, abilities, and actions
Lordosis. hollow back; anteroposterior curvature of the spine
Lower motor neuron lesion (LMN). lesion occurring in the anterior horn cells, nerve roots, or the peripheral nerve system resulting in flaccid paralysis
Lumbar. pertaining to the lower back and the five lumbar vertebrae
Malignancy. condition of being resistant to treatment occurring in severe form and frequently fatal
Mastery. command or grasp of a subject
Maturation. emergence of an organism's genetic potential; includes a series of preprogrammed changes which comprise changes in the organism's structure and form as well as in its complexity, integration, organization, and function
M.B.D. Minimal brain dysfunction; diagnostic and descriptive category of neurodevelopmental lags
Microthorax. abnormally small chest
Micturition. urination
Milieu. surroundings; social and physical environment
Milieu therapy. treatment using the manipulation of the socioenvironmental setting to benefit the patient
Modeling. setting an example for imitation
Monoplegia. paralysis of one limb
Morality. a sense of what is right and wrong
MP joint. metacarpophalangeal joint
Multiple sclerosis (disseminated) (MS). patches of demyelination in the white matter of the nervous

system, sometimes in the gray matter; progressive disease of the nervous system

Muscular dystrophy (MD). a progressive, familial hereditary disorder, marked by atrophy and stiffness of the muscles and observed when voluntary action is first attempted

Music therapy. use of music as treatment modality

Myasthenia gravis. a disease characterized by an abnormal exhaustibility of the voluntary muscles, manifesting itself in a rapid diminution of contractility, both when the muscle is activated by the will and when stimulated by electric current

Myelination. myelinization; the process of supplying or accumulating myelin during the development or repair of nerves

Myelin sheath. sheath formation of myelin substance which covers axons and nerve fibers

Myelomeningocele (MM). spina bifida with protrusion of both the cord and its membranes

Myoneural junction. the point at which a motor nerve joins with the muscle it innervates

NARC. National Association for Retarded Citizens

NASA. National Aeronautic Space Administration

Necrotic eschar. dead scar tissue

Neonate. a newly born individual, especially an infant during its first month of life

Neoplasm. a new formation of tissue, abnormally, as a tumor or growth

Nephrostomy. the establishment of an opening between the pelvis of the kidney and the external surface of the body

Neuritis. inflammation of a nerve or nerves, usually associated with degenerative processes

Neurodevelopmental treatment approach. movement as primary modality of treatment (Bobaths)

Neuromuscular spindle. muscle proprioceptor

Neuron. unit of the nervous system, consisting of the nerve cell body and its various processes, the dendrites, axon, and ending

Neurophysiological treatment approach. the activation, facilitation and inhibition of voluntary and involuntary muscle action through the reflex arc (Rood)

Neurotendinous organ. a proprioceptive sensory nerve ending in which branching nerve fibers are spread over a bundle of encapsulated fibers near their attachment to muscle; Golgi's organ

NIMH. National Institute of Mental Health

NMS. the coordinated actions of the nervous, muscular, and skeletal systems

Nociceptive response. response to stimuli that could cause harm, injury, or pain

Normal development. determined by wide range of data collected for a particular population within a given time and culture, referring to a specific area or segment of development

Nystagmus. involuntary rapid movement of the eyeball which may be congenital or acquired

Object permanence. the assumption that objects continue to exist when they are out of sight, touch, or some other perceptual contact

Object relations. emotional attachment for another person or object (that which is other than self)

Occiput. occipital area of the skull; the back of the head

Occlusion. act of closing or the state of being closed

Occupational behavior. organization and action based on skills, knowledge, and attitudes to make functioning possible in life roles (Reilly)

Occupational performance skills. those skills required for successful performance of the roles which are assumed by individuals in their lives. Most human roles fall into the categories of play, self-care, and work.

Oedipal conflict. conflict that appears during the phallic stage. It consists of sexual attraction to the parent of the opposite sex and hostility toward the parent of the same sex

Olfaction. sense of smell; the act of smelling

Ontogeny, ontogenetic. relating to the biological development of the individual (distinguished from phylogeny)

Operant conditioning. procedure through which subject is conditioned by use of reinforcement techniques to learn a desired behavior (B. F. Skinner)

Opisthotonic. relating to a tetanic spasm in which the spine and the extremities are bent with convexity forward, the body resting on the head and heels

Optometrist. one who measures the degree of visual powers; a refractionist

Oral phase. earliest stage of psychosexual development (to 18 months); oral zone is pleasure center (Freud)

Orthotics. science that deals with the making and fitting of orthopedic appliances

Osteoarthritis. a degenerative, non-inflammatory, localized form of arthritis which causes breakdown of cartilage and results in limitation of motion and formation of bony outgrowths at the joints affected

Osteosclerosis. osteopetrosis; a rare developmental error of unknown cause but of familial tendency, characterized by excessive radiographic density of most or all of the bones

Otologist. one versed in the science of the ear, its anatomy, functions, and diseases

Paleo-. prefix meaning older, e.g., paleocortex, the older portion of the cerebral cortex

Paralinguistics. communication through intonation, gestures, and other nonverbal aspects of speech
Paralysis. loss or impairment of motor and/or sensory function of a part caused by injury to nerves or neurons
Paranoid. psychiatric syndrome characterized by delusions
Paraparesis. partial paralysis or weakness in lower extremities
Paraplegia. paralysis of muscles in lower extremities
PARC. Pennsylvania Association for Retarded Citizens
Parkinson's disease. (synonymous with parkinsonism, Parkinson's syndrome) neurological symptom-complex characterized by four major symptoms: rigidity, tremor, akinesia, and loss of spontaneous and automatic movement
Peer. another person of one's own age or status
Perception. mental process by which intellectual, sensory, and emotional data are organized meaningfully; the process of conscious recognition and interpretation of sensory stimuli
Peripatologist. one who teaches a blind person to travel
Peripheral. located or pertaining to an outer portion of the body away from the center, such as the extremities
Petit mal. brief lapse in consciousness
Phallic phase. third stage of psychosexual development (ages two to six); interest, curiosity, and pleasure centered on penis or clitoris. The oedipal conflict is present during this phase (Freud)
Phasic reflexes. observable movements in response to a touch, pressure, or movement of the body or to sight or sound received
Phenomenology. study of consciously-reported experiences
Phenylketonuria (PKU). the presence of a phenylketone in the urine
Phylogeny, phylogenetic. evolutionary development of any plant or animal species; ancestral history of the individual distinguished from ontogeny, the development of the individual
Physical impairment. weakening, damage, or deterioration, e.g., as a result of injury or disease
PIP joint. proximal interphalangeal joint
Plateau. a period or state of relative stability following or preceding fluctuating change
Pleasure principle. the notion that a person tries to gain pleasure and avoid pain (psychoanalytical)
PNS. peripheral nervous system
Poliomyelitis. a common virus disease of man which may progress to involve the central nervous system and result in a nonparalytic or paralytic form of the disease, the latter being the classical form of acute anterior poliomyelitis
Polyneuritis. simultaneous inflammation of many nerves which is usually in a symmetrical pattern
POMR. Problem oriented medical record
Postulate. a theoretical proposition assumed without proof
Postural adaptation. righting; midline; stability; equilibrium
Pragmatic. practical; concerned with actual practice
Praxis. the performance of a purposeful movement or group of movements; ability to motor plan
Pre-conceptual. the first part of the preoperational period lasting from age two to four in which there is new use of symbols and symbolic play
Prefrontal lobotomy. neurosurgical procedure in which one or more nerve tracts in the prefrontal area of the brain are severed (also called leukotomy)
Prevocational evaluation. evaluation of activities of daily living (ADL), educational abilities, and physical capabilities and deficits as required for participation in vocational activity
Primary circular reaction. involves an action on the part of the infant that fortuitously leads to an event that has value for him and is centered about his body. The infant learns to repeat the behavior in order to reinstate the event. The culmination of the process is an organized scheme.
Prism glasses. for use by the patient lying supine to prevent eye strain by enabling the patient to see in front of him by looking up to the ceiling
PRN. abbreviation of Latin pro re nata according to needs, sometimes used in prescriptions or written orders
Prodromal. referring to early or premonitory symptoms of disease
Prognosis. predicted course of an illness over a given period of time
Projection. unconscious defense mechanism. Person attributes ideas and feelings to another, the ideas, feelings, and impulses which are his/her own but which are unacceptable to him/her
Projective techniques. loosely structured procedures in which the patient reveals feelings, personality, and unconscious material
Prophylactic. preventing disease; an agent (e.g., vaccine) that acts as a preventive against any disease
Proprioception. appreciation of position, balance, and changes in equilibrium of a body part during movement by receiving stimulus within body tissue such as muscles, tendons, and joints
Protopathic function. denoting a set or system of peripheral sensory nerve fibers furnishing a low order of sensibility, enabling one to appreciate pain and temperature but not to a very delicate extent and definitely not localized; distinguished from epicritic

Pseudobulbar paralysis. paralysis resembling bulbar paralysis but caused by lesion of cortical centers

Pseudohypertrophy. increase in size of an organ without increased size of one or more of its components

PSNS. parasympathetic nervous system: the craniosacral division of the autonomic nervous system

PSRO. Professional Standards Review Organization

Psychomotor. referring to combination of physical and emotional activity

Psychopharmacology. study of drugs, medications, and their effects on psychological and behavioral processes

Psychotherapy. treatment of mental disorder in which trained person interacts with patient on the basis of a therapeutic contract. Treatment is based on communication processes

Ptosis. drooping of the upper eyelid, abnormal prolapse or falling down of an organ or part

Puberty. the period of life when an individual's sexual organs become functional and secondary sex characteristics appear

Pubescence. period of about two years prior to puberty. It is a period of physiological change which triggers the emergence of primary and secondary sexual characteristics.

Pulmonary stenosis. narrowing of the opening into the pulmonary artery from the right ventricle

Purposeful activity. treatment when directed to a response that enhances neural integration

Quadriparesis. partial paralysis or weakness in all four extremities

Quadriplegia. paralysis of muscles in all four extremities

Qualitative changes. subjective elements; no scale to measure

Quantitative changes. measurable and thus easily understood

Rapport. conscious, harmonious accord or relationship between people

RAS. reticular activating system

Rationalization. unconscious defense mechanism. Person uses a feasible, acceptable reason to explain irrational behavior, motives, or feelings

Reactions. complex and inconstant responses developing from integration of simultaneous sensory stimulation such as tactile, vestibular, visual, and auditory

Reality testing. fundamental ego function; objective evaluation of world outside self; testing of real world—human, nonhuman, concrete, ideational

Reality therapy. treatment method in which milieu and therapeutic relationships are based on real and present situations and cause and effect relationships (Glasser)

Recapitulation of ontogenesis. repetition of passage through stages of human development

Receptive aphasia. impairment in interpretation of the meaning of spoken and written words

Reciprocal innervation. contraction in a muscle is accompanied by a loss of tone or by relaxation in the antagonistic muscle

Reenactment. acting out of a past experience as if it were happening in the present—person can feel, perceive, and act as he/she did the first time

Reflex. fetal or neonatal responses that are simple, predictable, resulting from tactile and vestibular stimulation

Reflex action. an immediate unconscious involuntary response of a limb or organ to stimulation of the sensory branch of a reflex arc

Reflex arc. the pathway from the receptor in the skin to the effector organ through which an impulse travels

Reflexes. when a specific event in the environment occurs, the organism automatically responds (Piaget)

Regression. unconscious defense mechanism; person returns to earlier patterns of adaptation

Rehabilitation. the restoration to a disabled individual of maximum independence commensurate with his limitations by developing his residual capacities

Reinforcement. in behavior therapy, strengthening a response by using a stimulus immediately after the response (may be positive or negative)

Reliability. degree to which a test produces the same results on repeated administrations

Remission. an abatement or lessening of symptoms of a disease

Repression. unconscious defense mechanism; removal from consciousness, usually of ideas, impulses, and feelings which are not acceptable (Freud)

Reticular formation. a fine network formed by cells or formed of certain structures within cells or of connective tissue fibers between cells

Retinitis pigmentosa. slowly progressing connective tissue and pigment cell proliferation of the entire membrane with wasting of its nerve elements

Retrolental fibroplasia. a blinding disease of the eye affecting premature infants

Reward. a positive reinforcement used to strengthen a desired action

RH factor. a potent antigen and its presence or absence in the blood is referred to as RH positive and RH negative

Rheumatoid arthritis. a chronic progressive inflammatory systemic disease which causes pain, swelling, limitation, and deformity in the joints, with accompanying involvement of tendons and sheaths, nerves, and muscles

Righting reactions. reflexes which through various

receptors in labyrinth, eyes, muscles, or skin tend to bring an organism's body into its normal position in space and which resists any force acting to put it into a false position, e.g., on its back

Rigidity. inflexible and tonic contraction of muscles giving consistent resistance to passive movement through total range of movement

Rorschach test. projective test in which subject reveals attitudes and emotions through response to inkblot pictures

Rote. habit performance, without meaning; in a mechanical way

Rubella. german measles; an acute, contagious eruptive disease; also called epidemic roseola, French measles

Rural. counties with populations up to 10,000 (additional population begins to be semi-rural) accompanied by geographic isolation, likely cultural and economic isolation as well

Schedule of reinforcement. pattern set up for presentation of reinforcers in behavior therapy

Schemata. Piagetian term which refers to the structure or framework into which one's experiences are integrated

Schwann cell. one of the cells of the neurolemma; a cell that enfolds myelinated and unmyelinated nerve fibers

Sclerosis. hardening of a part with growth of fibrous tissue resulting from atrophy or degeneration of nerve elements

Scoliosis. lateral curvature of the spine

Scotoma. abnormal blind spots

Sealing over. covering up unconscious material

Sebaceous glands. composed of fat, keratohyalin, granules, keratin, and cellular debris

Secondary circular reaction. actions involving events or objects in the external environment. It is the ability to develop schemes that reproduce interesting events which were initially discovered by chance in the external environment.

Sedative. drug which produces calming, relaxing effect—CNS depressant

SEIMC. special education instructional materials centers

Selective inattention. blocking out stimuli which generate anxiety; failing to notice, see, or hear things which the individual may not wish to deal with

Sensibility. the ability to perceive, appreciate, and transmit nerve impulses

Sensorimotor stage. the first stage of Piaget's cognitive theory in which the child from birth to two years of age seeks to integrate perceptions and bodily motions

Seriation. arranging or organizing in orderly series

Sex typing. process of acquiring the behavior and attitudes regarded by the culture as masculine or feminine

Shaping. in behavior therapy, system of establishing desired behavior patterns through reinforcement given for each successive approximation—moving closer to goal

Shearing. distortion of a body by two oppositely directed parallel forces

Shock treatment. psychiatric treatment through use of chemicals or electric current (insulin-ECT or EST)

Situational or simulated job tryout. placement of client in actual work situation in a sheltered workshop or other such institution

SMS. sensory-motor-sensory; sensory feedback integration with the initial sensory input and motor accommodation

SNS. sympathetic nervous system

SOAP. subjective, objective, assessment, plan; used in problem oriented medical record

Social bond. underlying quality of attachment between two persons

Social interaction. active affectionate reciprocal relationship between two persons

Somatosensory. concerning sensation of the body as distinguished from the viscera or mind

Spasm. a sudden involuntary contraction of muscle or group of muscles

Spastic. characterized by spasms and resulting in hypertonia and awkward movements from stiff muscles

Spasticity. state of hypertonicity, involuntary resistance of weak muscle caused by passive range of motion, followed by sudden relaxation of muscle, associated with exaggeration of reflexes and loss of voluntary muscle control; increased muscle tone

Spatial relations. the relationship of the skeletal parts of the body to each other and to objects in the environment

Spatiotemporal adaptation. continuous, ongoing state or act of adjusting those bodily processes required to function within a given space at a given time

Standardized. having established and tested norms

Static splint. splint with no moving parts, maintains a joint in desired position

Stereognosis. the perception and identification of the form and nature of an object through the sense of touch

Stereoscopic. vision in which things have the appearance of solidity and relief as seen in three dimensions

Strabismus. deviation of the eye which the individual cannot overcome

Stress. physical, emotional, or intellectual strain or tension disturbing normal equilibrium

Stroke. a sudden and severe seizure or fit of disease; a popular term for cerebral vascular accident (CVA)

Stryker frame. a bed-turning frame which enables a patient to be rotated from front to back but does not allow tilting

Sublimation. unconscious defense mechanism; replacement of unacceptable wishes, drives, feelings, or goals with those which are acceptable

Subluxation. incomplete or partial dislocation of a joint

Superego. one of three components of psychic structure (with id and ego); (Freud) incorporation of standards, moral attitudes, and conscience

Support system. people, agencies, or institutions which serve to help sustain a person in stress or problems

Supportive. reinforcing the patient's defenses and reassuring him/her (as opposed to probing into conflicts)

Supportive treatment. relates to the psychological and emotional needs and problems

Suppression. conscious act of controlling unacceptable impulses, feelings, or behavior (different from repression which is unconscious)

Suprapubic catheter. a catheter positioned above the pubic arch

Surrogate mother. someone or something that takes the place of a mother in an organism's life

Symbol. something used for or representing an object, idea, image, or feeling

Symbolization. unconscious defense mechanism; idea or object comes to stand for another, based on similarity or association

Synapse. the point at which an impulse passes from one neuron to another

Synergies. combined or correlated actions of different organs of the body, as of muscles working together

Synoptic. affording or taking a general view of the whole or of the principal parts of a subject

Synovectomy. surgical excision of the synovial membrane

Synovial membrane. connective tissue which lines a synovial joint

Synthesize. to form by combining parts into a single whole

Tactile. pertaining to touch

Tactile defensiveness. the quality of being unable to tolerate touch; resistive and uncomfortable at certain kinds of touch (believed to be a form of sensory integrative dysfunction)

Tactile localization. the ability to determine the location of a cutaneous stimulus

Task-oriented group. group whose focus is on reaching a goal, finding a solution to a problem, or making a product

Tay-Sachs disease. amaurosis; a familial disease occurring almost exclusively in Jewish children characterized by flaccid muscles, convulsions, decerebrate rigidity, and blindness

TD. terminal device in upper extremity prosthetics

Tenodesis splint. functional handsplint which operates on the tenodesis principle of wrist extension and finger flexion

Tertiary circular reaction. the interest in novelty and curiosity about an object; the child no longer relies on previous schemes.

Thematic apperception test. projective psychological test. Subject looks at series of ambiguous pictures and interprets what he/she sees. Interpretation will be based on subject's own feelings and attitudes

Theory. a set of logically interrelated statements used to explain observed events; a proposed explanation whose status is still conjectural, in contrast to well-established propositions that are regarded as reporting matters of actual fact

Therapeutic recreation. the utilization of recreational experiences for the prevention and/or amelioration of handicapping conditions

Thoracic. pertaining to the chest and ribs and the twelve thoracic vertebrae

Thrombus. a collection of blood or a clot causing vascular obstruction

TIA. transient ischemic attack

TLC. tender loving care

Toxoplasmosis. a disease caused by infection with the protozoa, Toxoplasma gondii; in the congenital form it causes destructive lesions of the central nervous system, jaundice, and anemia

Tracheostomy. surgical formation of an opening into the trachea and suturing of the edges to the skin in the neck for an airway or passage of a tube

Tranquilizer. psychotropic drug inducing calming, soothing effect without clouding consciousness —major tranquilizers, antipsychotic drugs; minor tranquilizers, anti-anxiety drugs

Transaction. interaction between two or more people

Transactional analysis. system centering on study of interactions between people in treatment—four parts: (1) structural analysis of intrapsychic processes; (2) determination of dominant ego state (parent, child, adult); (3) game analysis; and (4) script analysis (finding causes of problems); used in both group and individual psychotherapy (Eric Berne)

Transductive reasoning. refers to the preoperational child's tendency to use associative reasoning rather than inductive or deductive thought (Piaget)

Transference. projection of feelings, thoughts, or wishes on to another who has come to represent someone from the past; inappropriate applied in present context; used in therapeutic process (psychoanalytical)

Trapeze bar. triangular bar attached to a traction frame on the bed so that the patient lying in bed can reach the bar to assist in rolling over, coming to a sitting position, or transferring from the bed to a chair

Trauma. injury as a result of physical or emotional means or insult

Tremor. alternate contraction and relaxation of opposing groups of muscles resulting in involuntary rhythmic and oscillating movements such as quivering or trembling

Trophic changes. changes in function concerned with nourishment of tissues caused by vascular, neurological, nutritional, or endocrine problems or inactivity (disuse)

Trouble team. team composed of two or three people specially trained in crisis intervention, face-to-face counseling skills; usually sent out to meet with the caller when the situation (runaways, attempted suicides, etc.) seems to require more intervention than can be accomplished on the phone

UE. upper extremity

Unconditional positive regard. the quality of accepting another person and communicating that acceptance regardless of what that person says or does (Rogers)

Unconscious. part of the mind in which psychic material—primitive drives, repressed desires, and memories—is not directly accessible to awareness (psychoanalytical)

Underactive. lacking or slow in taking the initiative to act

Underreactive. responding minimally or slowly to stimuli

Upper motor neuron lesion (UMN). lesion occurring in corticospinal or pyramidal tract located in brain or spinal cord resulting in paralysis, increased muscle tone, and pathological reflexes

Validity. statistical term; the degree to which a given measure indicates quality or attribute it attempts to measure

Values. ideals, feelings, and beliefs which are acted upon

Vascularity. containing blood vessels

Ventricular septal defect. flaw or defect between ventricles of the heart

Viscera. organs of the digestive, respiratory, urogenital, and endocrine systems as well as the spleen, heart, and great vessels

Vocalization. the utterance of sounds

Vocational evaluation. assessment of all factors (medical, psychological, educational, social, environmental, cultural, and vocational) that affect successful employment

Volition. will or purpose

WHO. World Health Organization

Work evaluation. evaluation of vocational strengths and weaknesses through utilization of work (real or simulated)

Work sample evaluation. sample of actual job tasks or a mock-up of actual tasks to determine client's job skills and abilities

Wrist driven flexor hinge splint. use of wrist extension to provide prehension

INDEX